Cardiovascular
and Pulmonary
PHYSICAL THERAPY

Cardiovascular and Pulmonary
PHYSICAL THERAPY

Evidence and Practice

FOURTH EDITION

Donna Frownfelter, PT, DPT, MA, CCS, RRT, FCCP
Assistant Professor and Program Director
Post Professional Doctor of Physical Therapy
College of Health Professions
Rosalind Franklin University of Medicine and Science
North Chicago, Illinois

Elizabeth Dean, PhD, PT
Professor
School of Rehabilitation Sciences
Vancouver, British Columbia, Canada

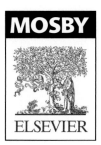

MOSBY

ELSEVIER

11830 Westline Industrial Drive
St. Louis, Missouri 63146

ISBN-13 978-0-323-02775-5
ISBN 0-323-02775-X

Cardiovascular and Pulmonary Physical Therapy Evidence and Practice
Fourth Edition
Copyright © 2006, Mosby Inc.

Previous editions copyrighted 1978, 1987, 1996

ISBN-13 978-0-323-02775-5
ISBN 0-323-02775-X

Acquisitions Editor: Marjory Fraser
Developmental Editor: Donna Morrissey
Publishing Services Manager: Patricia Tannian
Project Manager: Ryan Hastings
Cover Designer: Paula Ruckenbrod
Text Designer: Paula Ruckenbrod

Printed in the United States of America

Last digit is the print number: 9 8 7 6 5 4 3

Contributors

Michael Wade Baskin, PT, RRT
GT Physical Therapy
Louisville, Mississippi

Gary Brooks, PT, DrPH, CCS
Associate Professor
Department of Physical Therapy Education
Upstate Medical University
Syracuse, New York

Meryl I. Cohen, DPT, MS, CCS
Instructor, Department of Physical Therapy
Miller School of Medicine
Therapist, Sylvester Cancer Center
University of Miami Medical Group
Coral Gables, Florida
Adjunct Instructor, Department of Physical Therapy
Massachusetts General Hospital Institute of Health
Professions
Boston, Massachusetts

Simone Dal Corso, PT, PhD
Physiotherapist of Respiratory Division
Federal University of São Paulo
Respiratory Division
Rua Prof. Francisco de Castro n 54
Bairro Vila Clementino
São Paulo, Brazil

Linda D. Crane, MMSc, PT, CCS
Instructor, Division of Physical Therapy
University of Miami School of Medicine
Miami, Florida

Carol M. Davis
Professor & Assistant Chair for Curriculum
Department of Physical Therapy
University of Miami Miller School of Medicine
Coral Gables, Florida

Elizabeth Dean, PhD, PT
Professor
School of Rehabilitation Sciences
Vancouver, British Columbia, Canada

Anne Mejia Downs, MPH, PT, CCS
Adjunct Clinical Assistant Professor
Department of Physical Therapy
Indiana University
School of Health and Rehabilitation Sciences
Indianapolis, Indiana

Christian Evans, PhD, PT
Associate Professor
Physical Therapy Program
College of Health Sciences
Midwestern University
Downers Grove, Illinois

Donna Frownfelter, PT, DPT, MA, CCS, RRT, FCCP
Assistant Professor and Program Director
Post Professional Doctor of Physical Therapy
College of Health Professions
Rosalind Franklin University of Medicine and Science
North Chicago, Illinois

Rik Gosselink, PT, PhD
Professor Rehabilitation Sciences
Respiratory Rehabilitation
University Hospitals Leuven
Faculty of Kinesiology and Rehabilitation Sciences
Katholieke Universiteit Leuven
Leuven, Belgium

Willy E. Hammon III, BSc, PT
Chief of Rehabilitative Services
Oklahoma University Medical Center
Oklahoma City, Oklahoma

Ryan Hartley, DPT
Praxis Physical Therapy and Human Performance
Vernon Hills, Illinois

Gail M. Huber, PT, PhD
Assistant Professor
Department of Physical Therapy & Human Movement Sciences
Northwestern University, Feinberg School of Medicine
Chicago, Illinois

Patrick Knott, PhD, PA-C
Associate Dean, College of Health Professions
Associate Professor and Chair, Physician Assistant Program
Rosalind Franklin University of Medicine and Science
North Chicago, Illinois

Stacy J. Laack, MS, PA-C
Physical Assistant Program
College of Health Professions
Rosalind Franklin University of Medicine and Science
North Chicago, Illinois

Mary Massery, PT, DPT
Massery Physical Therapy
Glenview, Illinois

Susan M. Butler McNamara, PT, MMSc, CCS
Team Leader, Division of Rehabilitation Medicine
Maine Medical Center
Portland, Maine

Lisa Sigg Mendelson, MS, RN, CPAN
Rush University Medical Center
Olympic Fields, Illinois

Victoria A. Moerchen, PT, PhD
Assistant Professor
Department of Physical Therapy and Rehabilitation Science
University of Maryland School of Medicine
Baltimore, Maryland

Claire Peel, PT, PhD
Associate Dean and Professor
School of Health Related Professions
University of Alabama at Birmingham
Birmingham, Alabama

Christiane Perme, PT, CCS
Senior Physical Therapist
The Methodist Hospital
Houston, Texas

Arthur V. Prancan
Associate Chair
Department of Pharmacology
Rush University Medical Center
Chicago, Illinois

Elizabeth J. Protas, PT, PhD, FACSM
Professor and Chair
Department of Physical Therapy
University of Texas Medical Branch
Galveston, Texas

Susan A. Scherer, PhD
Associate Professor
Department of Physical Therapy
Regis University
Denver, Colorado

Alexandra J. Sciaky, PT, MS, CCS
Cardiopulmonary Clinical Specialist
Center Coordinator of Clinical Education
Physical Therapy Department
Veterans Administration Healthcare System
Ann Arbor, Michigan

Linda Crane has been honored by the Cardiovascular and Pulmonary Section for being a dedicated member who was passionate about the practice of physical therapy and exhibited excellence in teaching as well as clinical practice. Linda prepared a survey of practice in Cardiovascular and Pulmonary Physical Therapy that resulted in Entry Level Clinical Practice Guidelines. She was one of the first three APTA Board Certified Specialists in Cardoiovascular and Pulmonary Physical Therapy in 1985. Linda served as Program Chairman and Chairman of the Section (1982-1986), as well as Delegate to the House of Delegates. She received the Lucy Blair Service Award for distinguished service to the profession.

Her focus in clinical practice in neonatal and pediatric cardiovascular and pulmonary therapy was groundbreaking and has endured the test of time. She made a huge difference in the care and direction of practice in this field. Linda wrote our pediatric chapter in the second edition, and in the third edition she worked with Victoria Moerchen on the revision. Vickie commented that this fourth edition was much more

difficult without Linda's guidance and input and she missed her collaboration, as we all do.

Linda found great meaning in her life through her work. She loved clinical practice and teaching, but also loved connecting with her students and colleagues. She was honored by students from two different universities for excellence as teacher of the year and was known as an expert in curriculum development. However, some of the most memorable times for friends and students were when she hosted parties and celebrations. She loved to have fun, her laugh was memorable, and she cared deeply about people. She was a good friend and colleague.

As Meryl Cohen stated in the first Linda Crane Memorial Lecture (February 5, 2000): "We are all better for having known Linda Crane. Our patients receive better care because of Linda Crane. Our students receive better training because of Linda Crane. We are a better profession because Linda Crane worked with us."

Thank you, Linda. Peace be to your memory.

Foreword

It is for me a privilege to be invited to write a foreword to this fourth edition of a highly rated textbook dealing with principles and many aspects of physical therapy management. It has been a very stimulating and instructive reading. The title of the book, *Cardiovascular and Pulmonary Physical Therapy: Evidence and Practice,* concentrates on the cardiopulmonary diseases, but throughout the text it is emphasized that the heart and lungs are interdependent and function as a single unit. Therefore, lung or heart disease must be considered in conjunction with the other organs and in the context of overall oxygen transport. The text points out that oxygen transport is a basis for physical therapy. The links in this transport, from inspired air to the mitochondria, are well described in healthy individuals as well as in patients with various diseases. Mobilization and exercise! Exercise testing and training are described in detail. It is stated that the absence of gravitational stress and exercise are two primary factors contributing to bed-rest deconditioning. Therefore, mobilization and exercise are the two most important physiological interventions available for the physical therapist to remedy cardiopulmonary dysfunction. The authors of many chapters knowledgeably present information about the physiological responses and adaptations to physical activity and this link's application in the rehabilitation not only of patients with cardiopulmonary diseases, but with other diseases as well. One strength of this book is its holistic approach, which includes medical, physiological, psychological, psychosocial, therapeutic, practical, and methodological aspects for taking care of the patient who not only has a very specific and dominating medical diagnosis, but other complicating problems as well. That is apparently too often ignored by physiotherapists and also by physicians. A narrow focus on one clinical problem can lead to neglect of underlying problems, such as arthritis, obesity, high blood pressure, stroke, back pain, and kidney problems in an individual with ischemic heart disease. It is pointed out that one must realize that patient groups can include secondary cardiovascular and pulmonary conditions in addition to the primary presentations of these conditions. The introduction is a good start and includes a review of epidemiological studies discussing lifestyle and diseases of civilization affecting not only adults but also children and adolescents. An "urgent request" is written: "Physical therapists need to consider the underlying risk factors for 'diseases of civilization' irrespective of their specialty or area of practice and primary reason or diagnosis for the consultation… Physical therapists have the potential to be primary health care professionals who are uniquely positioned to develop, support, and promote innovative health programs. Thus, they strengthen the health of communities 'en masse' as well as doing so one person-at-a-time in the clinic." That is one important, at times repeated, message.

The text is very well updated with impressive reference lists. An advantage is that the references are included in the text and not, as in many textbooks, presented more "anonymously" at the end of each chapter. In many sections and critical discussions it is stressed that more research is warranted, providing good ideas and motivation for students to do research! The contributors have generously provided well designed tables, boxes, and figures. Chapters end with review questions.

According to the Oxford Advanced Learner's Dictionary, holistic medicine is treating the whole person rather than just symptoms of a disease (and, I will add, not only the primary disease). That is a common feature of this textbook. I do agree with the statement that "physical therapists have a primary role as noninvasive practitioners in a health team with invasive practitioners, nurses, nutritionists, pharmacists, social workers, psychologists, respiratory therapists, spiritual leaders, and others as each case requires." I do recommend this textbook to everyone included in this team!

Per-Olof Åstrand
Stockholm, Sweden

Preface

Since the publication of the third edition, the Cardiopulmonary Section of the American Physical Therapy Association (APTA) changed its name to the Cardiovascular and Pulmonary Section to reflect changes in medicine and the way that we look at diseases and impairments.

This fourth edition has incorporated that change in focus with a change in title to *Cardiovascular and Pulmonary Physical Therapy: Evidence and Practice*. As the new title also indicates, greater emphasis has been placed on evidence-based rationales, and we have built upon the foundations laid by the original book first published in 1978. Each subsequent edition has included more evidence, and the contents have increasingly reflected the wealth of evidence-based practice in the context of health care and epidemiologic trends.

For this edition, content covers the spectrum from acute- to long-term conditions with a table of contents that unfolds in a logical sequence for the student; evolving from the management of the stable patient with a chronic condition to the more unstable patient with complex and often multiple disorders.

Renowned for its user-friendly approach, *Cardiovascular and Pulmonary Physical Therapy: Evidence and Practice, 4th edition*, continues to be a core textbook in its field. Uniquely balanced in its coverage of cardiac and pulmonary systems in health and dysfunction, the content is based on the latest scientific literature and research, making it highly applicable in the clinical setting. Each chapter has key terms and review questions for discussion to help the reader focus on the important concepts discussed in the chapter. The fourth edition also has additional content on health care trends related to evidence-based management to promote cost-effective management.

Responding to feedback from those using the text, the fourth edition incorporates updates and revisions that make the book unique in its content, including an integrated pulmonary/cardiac approach, coverage of secondary cardiovascular/cardiopulmonary conditions as well as primary conditions, and emphasis on understanding that "every patient is a cardiovascular/cardiopulmonary patient."

The accompanying *Clinical Case Study Guide* has been reformatted into a web-based product that gives readers an opportunity to interactively review the physiological principles presented in the text through the real-life case studies that physical therapists deal with every day in their practice. Our hope is that this will be used widely in teaching physical therapy students and will facilitate their understanding of how to effectively integrate cardiopulmonary concepts in each of their patients, not just in patients with a primary cardiopulmonary diagnosis.

Acknowledgments

There are so many people to thank for coming alongside me and helping in the journey to the fourth edition of this book. One of the common themes for all of us is that our lives are busier than ever and health care delivery is changing daily. As an educator and clinician it is hard to keep up. We know that what is important is to have the foundational concepts and critical thinking skills that allow the clinician to make decisions about the examination and identification of impairments and select appropriate interventions and treatment plans. We are seeing the necessity of emphasizing to people with chronic illness the need to be self managers of their own care, not just a "patient." We need to be educators, coaches, and resources, and occasionally we must provide hands on care and support.

To Elizabeth Dean, how can I thank you for your friendship, insight into cardiovascular and pulmonary physical therapy, and vision for new directions this book can take in the future? You have taken on the wonderful challenge of seeing things in a new way, addressing the direction our profession is taking, and being concerned not just locally but globally. The first chapter that you prepared, which looks at the "diseases of civilization" and the need for physical therapists to be involved in prevention of disease rather than just treatment, is imperative. You have been a "prophet" to the world, performing several sabbatical trips and international consultations and seeing people's needs globally. What a role model you are for our profession. How grateful I am that we have collaborated in this book to see the oxygen transport system as it applies to all patients and how it gives a framework to our examination and treatment of all patients. You have highlighted cardiovascular and pulmonary issues around the world and how they can be prevented with healthy diets, lifestyles, and exercise. How I value our friendship and collaboration over many years and how I look forward to what we will do together in the future.

I want to especially thank my family, who has been so supportive and encouraging to me, especially during the last few months of stressful deadlines and never enough time! Your love and ability to take me away from the pressures of work and writing have made all the difference in keeping me focused and having some time to play with you! When I look back on pictures in the first edition, in which my daughter Lauren, at about six months old, was the baby for the postural drainage positions, I smile and think of the journey of raising three wonderful kids and four editions of our book! Daniel and Kristin joined the pediatric chapter in subsequent editions. It was truly a family project, especially when they would bring "their book" to school for show and tell! I love you all and am so grateful for your presence in my life and the joy you bring. My husband, Dave, has been a solid support and source of encouragement since physical therapy school. He has accommodated my busy schedule and shared family responsibilities and for that I am most grateful.

My deepest thanks to the chapter authors who have taken the time and effort to make this book a success. It is because of you we have been able to remain on the cutting edge of cardiovascular and pulmonary physical therapy. We have new chapters and are grateful to Carol Davis and Meryl Cohen for a wonderful review and application of complementary therapies. We welcome Rik Gosselink and Simone Dal Corso who share their research and knowledge of respiratory muscle training. I enjoyed working with a graduating DPT student, Ryan Hartley, who is my co-author for the patient in the community chapter. Thanks to my colleagues from Rosalind Franklin University Patrick Knott and Stacy Laack for revisions of two previous chapters. You all put this project on the front burner with all your other responsibilities, and we are so grateful to you!

To Mary Massery, most special colleague, former student, mentee, mentor, consultant, confidant, master clinician, but most importantly my dear friend, how I value our relationship personally and professionally. How I love to giggle with you. I wish every clinician could have at least one person they could always go to to discuss issues, patients, families, and concerns with confidence and a sense of collaboration. You are a gift to me!

To our students past and present, thank you for your questions, comments, and challenges. You help keep us in the moment and having fun. We are counting on you to direct the future of our profession, especially relating to people with cardiovascular and pulmonary issues.

Many thanks to our editors, Marjorie Fraser and Marion Waldman, for your support and expertise. You have gone above and beyond the call of duty and we appreciate your work.

To the College of Health Professions at Rosalind Franklin University, especially the Physical Therapy Department, thank you for your support and encouragement and understanding that this is more than my "scholarly activity," but a passion. Thanks for letting me share my passionate belief that "every patient is a cardiovascular and pulmonary patient."

I thank God for the inner strength and comfort, especially during the stress of final preparations. Finding peace in the midst of chaos is an incredible blessing. I feel this book has come together in a special way and I am grateful.

Donna Frownfelter,
PT, DPT, MA, CCS, RRT, FCCP

As is so often said, a written work is never the work of a single individual. Translating one's ideas into a unique package—in this case the fourth edition of our text, which sports the new title *Cardiovascular and Pulmonary Physical Therapy: Evidence and Practice*—reflects the input of many people, directly and indirectly. It is a daunting task indeed to convey one's sincere gratitude to each and every one.

Donna Frownfelter's original 1978 book laid the foundation for what this text is today. Each edition reinvents itself to include more evidence and contents that increasingly reflect the wealth of evidence-based practice in the context of health care and epidemiologic trends. This evolution attests to Donna's insight and adaptability. I continue to marvel at her energy and enthusiasm for the profession and her specialty and adaptability as our world and its health care challenges change. These trends have clearly charted physical therapy's course for the next 100 years. This is an exciting time to be in the profession and an exciting time for me to continue to work with Donna in enabling physical therapists to serve our global society to the maximum. The diseases of civilization are clearly best prevented and managed, and cured in some cases, noninvasively. Our power is awesome. Thank you, Donna, for sharing this remarkable journey.

On the home front, Doug, I cannot thank you enough for your quiet support as the hours wiled away on the computer.

How many times did you hear the "team" shout first thing in the morning? How many times did you hear "almost done?" You have been a treasure.

To other members of my family and friends, there are no words to express my appreciation for your unending support, inquiries, and quality time.

Marjory Fraser and Marion Waldman of Elsevier have been marvelous at keeping things on track and outstanding people to work with. I would like to convey my sincere thanks to you both and to your production team, which has given a face to the fourth edition.

I see that by the fifth edition, physical therapists around the world will have increasingly made their mark as primary health care professionals and leaders in the assault on the diseases of civilization by being effective agents of change. I thank my international colleagues for the pleasure of having them as both colleagues and friends and for working toward a shared vision of "health and participation for all." Together, by translating our substantial knowledge base to address the world's leading health care problems, we shall make a difference.

Elizabeth Dean, PT, PhD

Contents

PART I CARDIOVASCULAR AND PULMONARY FUNCTION IN HEALTH AND DISEASE, 1

Chapter 1 Epidemiology as a Basis for Contemporary Physical Therapy Practice, 3
Elizabeth Dean

Chapter 2 Oxygen Transport: The Basis of Cardiopulmonary Physical Therapy, 37
Elizabeth Dean

Chapter 3 Cardiopulmonary Anatomy, 53
Elizabeth Dean

Chapter 4 Cardiopulmonary Physiology, 73
Elizabeth Dean

Chapter 5 Cardiopulmonary Pathophysiology, 85
Willy E. Hammon III
Elizabeth Dean

Chapter 6 Cardiopulmonary Manifestations of Systemic Conditions, 115
Elizabeth Dean

PART II CARDIOPULMONARY ASSESSMENT, 127

Chapter 7 Measurement and Documentation, 129
Claire Peel

Chapter 8 History, 137
Willy E. Hammon III

Chapter 9 Pulmonary Function Tests, 151
Donna Frownfelter

Chapter 10 Arterial Blood Gases, 157
Donna Frownfelter

Chapter 11 Imaging of the Chest, 163
Patrick Knott

Chapter 12 Electrocardiogram Identification, 169
Christian Evans
Gary Brooks

Chapter 13 Multisystem Assessment and Laboratory Investigations, 187
Elizabeth Dean

Chapter 14 Special Tests, 193
Gail M. Huber

Chapter 15 Clinical Assessment of the Cardiopulmonary System, 211
Susan M. Butler McNamara

Chapter 16 Monitoring Systems in the Intensive Care Unit, 229
Elizabeth Dean
Christiane Perme

PART III CARDIOVASCULAR AND PULMONARY PHYSICAL THERAPY INTERVENTIONS, 245

Chapter 17 Optimizing Outcomes: Relating Interventions to an Individual's Needs, 247
Elizabeth Dean

Chapter 18 Mobilization and Exercise, 263
Elizabeth Dean

Chapter 19 Body Positioning, 307
Elizabeth Dean

Chapter 20 Physiological Basis for Airway Clearance Techniques, 325
Anne Mejia Downs

Chapter 21 Clinical Application of Airway Clearance Techniques, 341
Anne Mejia Downs

Chapter 22 Facilitating Airway Clearance with Coughing Techniques, 363
Donna Frownfelter
Mary Massery

Chapter 23 Facilitating Ventilation Patterns and Breathing Strategies, 377
Donna Frownfelter
Mary Massery

Chapter 24 Exercise Testing and Training: Primary Cardiopulmonary Dysfunction, 405
Elizabeth Dean
Donna Frownfelter

Chapter 25 Exercise Testing and Training: Secondary Cardiopulmonary Dysfunction, 441
Elizabeth Dean
Donna Frownfelter

Chapter 26 Respiratory Muscle Training, 453
Rik Gosselink
Simone Dal Corso

Chapter 27 Complementary Therapies as Cardiopulmonary Physical Therapy Interventions, 465
Meryl I. Cohen
Carol M. Davis

Chapter 28 Patient Education, 495
Alexandra J. Sciaky

PART IV GUIDELINES FOR THE DELIVERY OF CARDIOVASCULAR AND PULMONARY PHYSICAL THERAPY ACUTE CONDITIONS, 505

Chapter 29 Individuals with Acute Medical Conditions, 507
Elizabeth Dean

Chapter 30 Individuals with Acute Surgical Conditions, 529
Elizabeth Dean

PART V GUIDELINES FOR THE DELIVERY OF CARDIOVASCULAR AND PULMONARY PHYSICAL THERAPY CHRONIC CONDITIONS, 543

Chapter 31 Individuals with Chronic Primary
Cardiopulmonary Dysfunction, 545
Elizabeth Dean
Donna Frownfelter

Chapter 32 Individuals with Chronic Secondary
Cardiopulmonary Dysfunction, 569
Elizabeth Dean
Donna Frownfelter

PART VI GUIDELINES FOR THE DELIVERY OF CARDIOVASCULAR AND PULMONARY PHYSICAL THERAPY CRITICAL CARE, 595

Chapter 33 Comprehensive Management of Individuals in the
Intensive Care Unit, 597
Elizabeth Dean
Christiane Perme

Chapter 34 Intensive Care Unit Management of Individuals
with Primary Cardiopulmonary Dysfunction, 611
Elizabeth Dean
Christiane Perme

Chapter 35 Intensive Care Unit Management of Individuals
with Secondary Cardiopulmonary Dysfunction, 625
Elizabeth Dean
Christiane Perme

Chapter 36 Complications, Adult Respiratory Distress
Syndrome, Shock, Sepsis, and Multiorgan System Failure, 639
Elizabeth Dean
Christiane Perme

PART VII GUIDELINES FOR THE DELIVERY OF CARDIOVASCULAR AND PULMONARY PHYSICAL THERAPY SPECIAL CASES, 655

Chapter 37 The Neonatal and Pediatric Patient, 657
Victoria A. Moerchen
Linda D. Crane

Chapter 38 The Aging Patient, 685
Elizabeth J. Protas

Chapter 39 Multisystem Consequences of Impaired Breathing
Mechanics and/or Postural Control, 695
Mary Massery

Chapter 40 The Transplant Patient, 719
Susan A. Scherer

Chapter 41 The Patient in the Community, 735
Donna Frownfelter
Ryan Hartley

PART VIII RELATED ASPECTS OF CARDIOVASCULAR AND PULMONARY PHYSICAL THERAPY, 747

Chapter 42 Body Mechanics—The Art of Positioning and
Moving Patients, 749
Donna Frownfelter
Mary Massery

Chapter 43 Respiratory Care Practice Review, 759
Donna Frownfelter
Michael Wade Baskin

Chapter 44 Care of the Patient with an Artificial Airway, 773
Donna Frownfelter
Lisa Sigg Mendelson

Chapter 45 Respiratory and Cardiovascular Drug Actions, 785
Stacy J. Laack
Arthur V. Prancan

GLOSSARY, 797

INDEX, 809

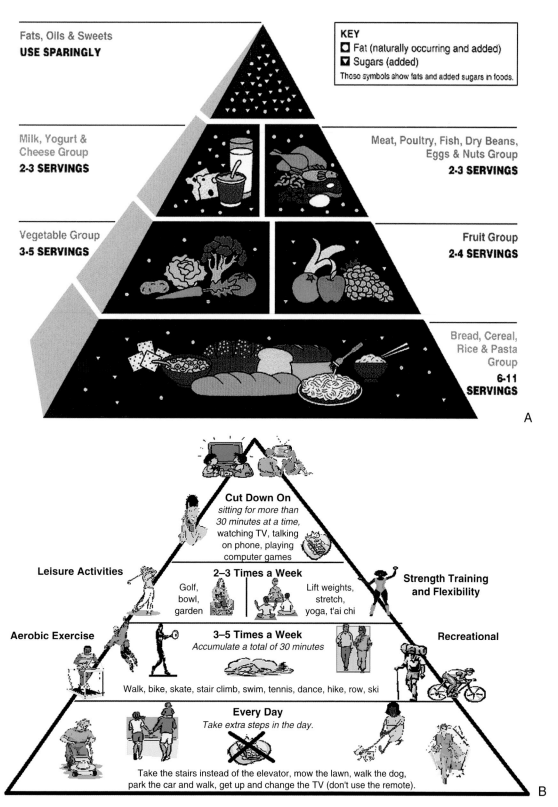

FIGURE 1-1 A, Nutrition pyramid. Limit highly glycemic foods (e.g., sugar and added sugar), pastries, sweets, refined carbohydrates, trans fats, highly preserved and highly processed foods. Include 5 to 8 glasses of water daily. **B,** Physical activity and exercise pyramid. Rest is an important component. Daily physical activity should include 10,000 steps a day*; a minimum accumulated 30 minutes of aerobic exercise three times a week; two to three sessions per week of 20 to 30 minutes of strength training; management of daily stress; breathing of clean air (no active or passive smoking); and several hours of restful sleep daily.
(**A** *Adapted from the U.S Department of Agriculture and the U.S. Department of Health and Human Services*).
*Tudor-Locke, 2004.

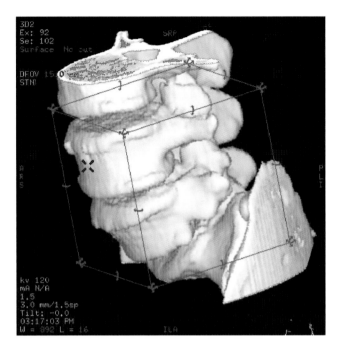

FIGURE 11-10 Three-dimensional reconstruction generated by a CT scanner.
(*From GE Healthcare.*)

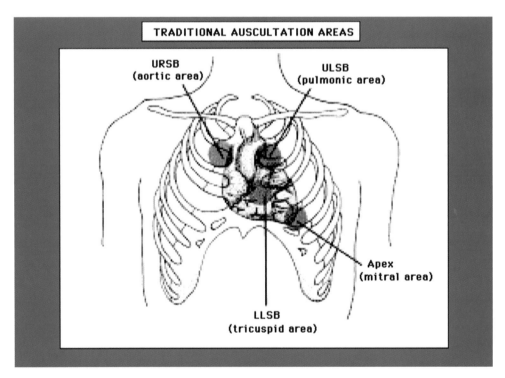

FIGURE 15-10 Cardiac auscultation. (*From http://www.kumc.edu/kumcpeds/cardiology/tofmsllecture/auscultaitonareas.gif; retrieved.*)

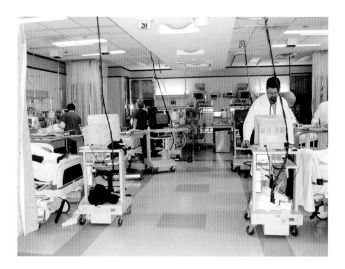

FIGURE 16-1 General view of an intensive care unit.

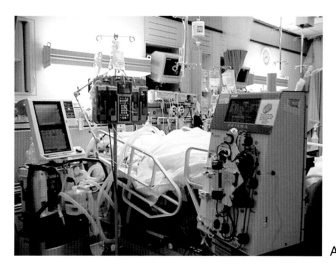

A

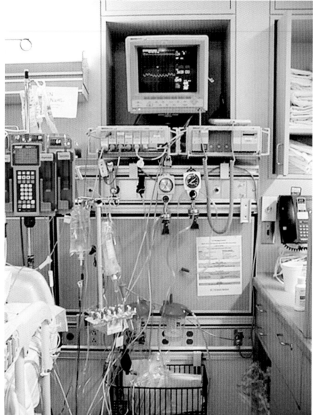

B

FIGURE 16-2 A, Closer bedside view of a patient in the intensive care unit. Note that with all the equipment, the patient is almost lost. **B**, Bedside monitoring equipment.

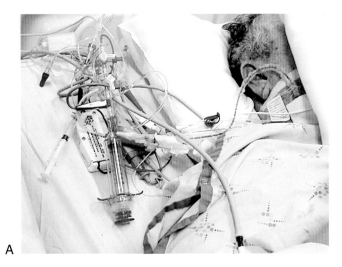

A

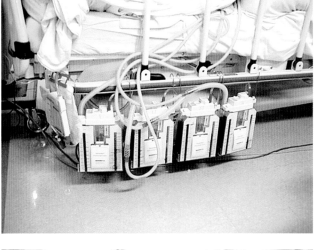

A

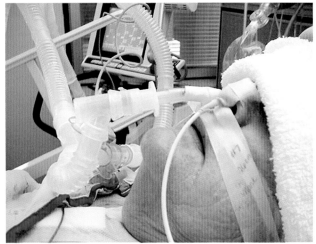

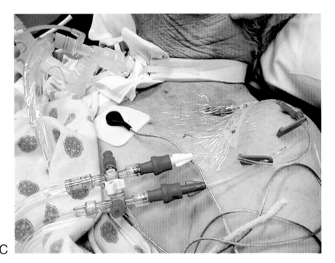

B

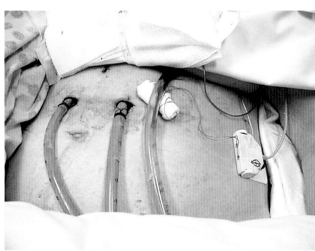

B

FIGURE 16-4 **A**, Chest tube drainage. **B**, Anterior view; mediastinal drains.

C

FIGURE 16-3 **A**, Note the Swan-Ganz catheter on the right jugular vein. **B,** The patient is on a ventilator with a nasoendotracheal tube in place. **C**, Tracheostomy and left subclavian central venous catheter.

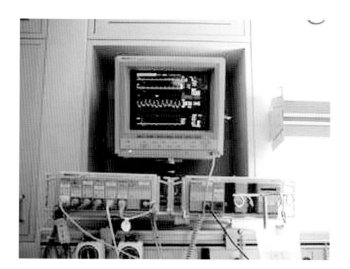

FIGURE 16-5 ECG monitor.

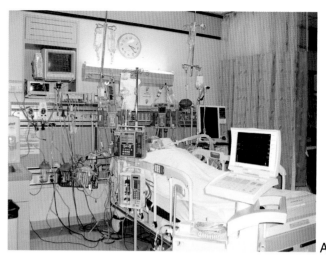

A

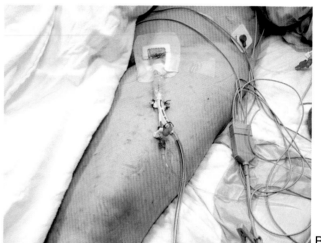

B

FIGURE 16-8 **A**, Patient on an intraaortic balloon pump (IABP) support. **B**, Closeup of the IABP insertion on the femoral artery.

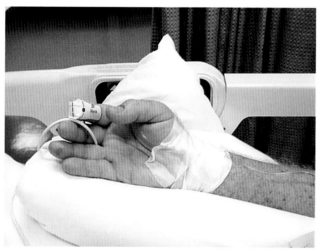

A

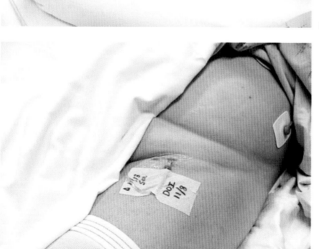

B

FIGURE 16-6 **A**, Radial arterial line. Also note the pulse oxymeter sensor on the finger. **B**, Femoral arterial line.

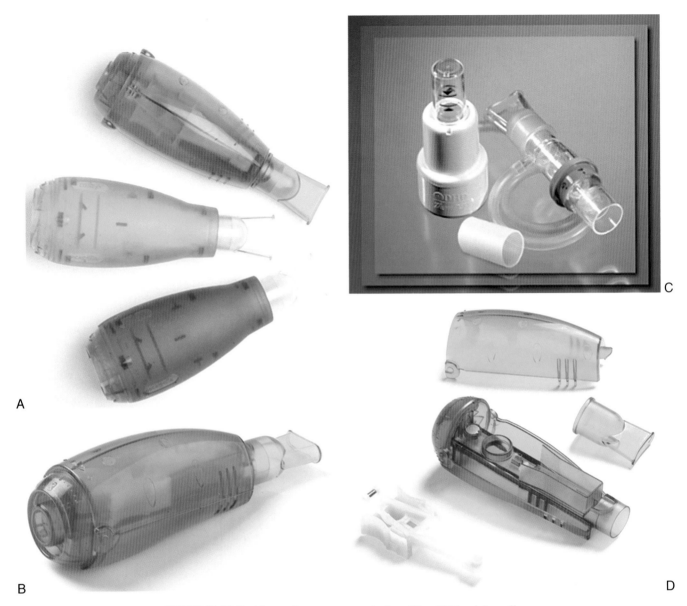

A

B

C

D

FIGURE 21-14 Positive expiratory pressure devices: TheraPEP and Acapella.

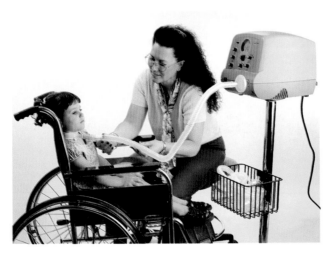

FIGURE 22-16 Cough Assist Machine.

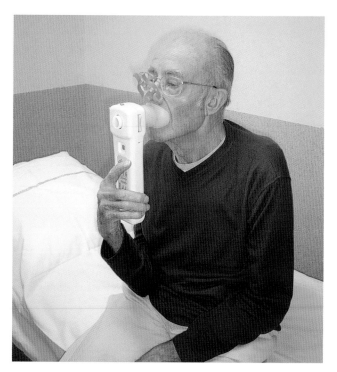

FIGURE 26-2 Assessment of respiratory muscle strength with measurement of mouth pressure.

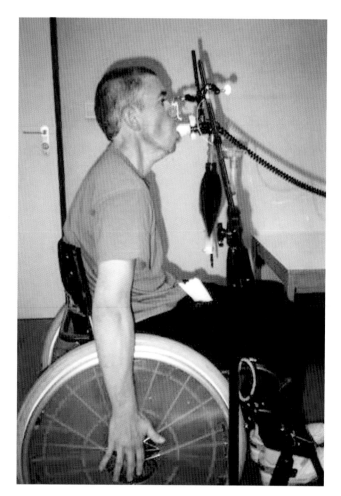

FIGURE 26-5 Normocapnic hyperpnea equipment.

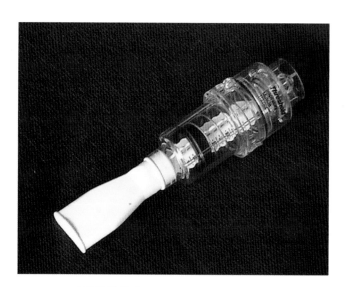

FIGURE 26-4 Threshold loading device.

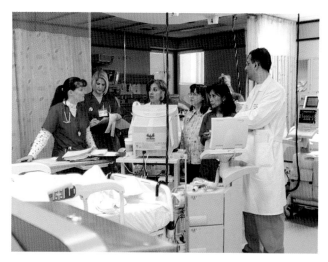

FIGURE 33-2 Multidisciplinary rounds in the ICU. Team work in the ICU is essential to facilitate communication and patient outcome. Note the presence of the nurse, respiratory therapist, pharmacist, social worker, physical therapist, and physician.

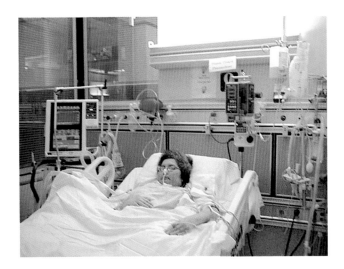

FIGURE 34-1 Patient receiving mechanical ventilation.

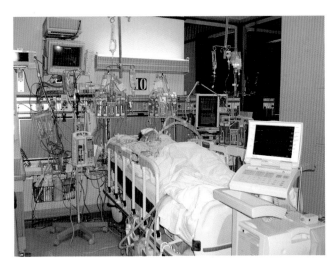

FIGURE 34-4 Patient after open heart surgery. Note mechanical ventilator, mediastinal drains and chest tubes, intraaortic balloon pump, and multiple intravenous drips.

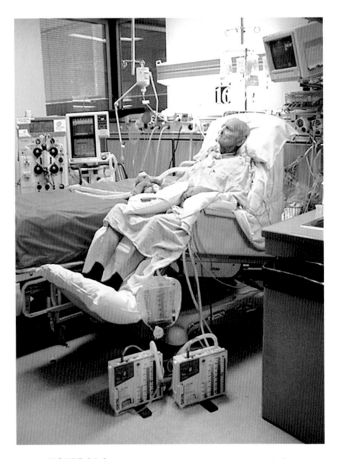

FIGURE 34-2 ICU patient sitting in a stretcher chair.

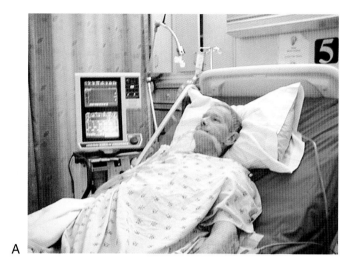

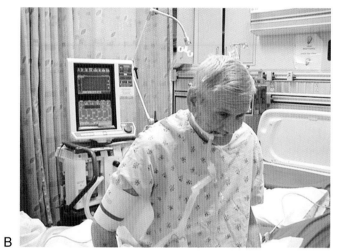

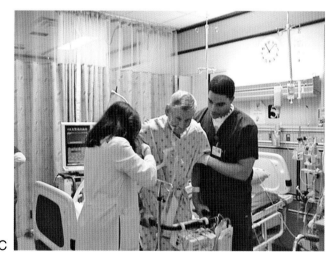

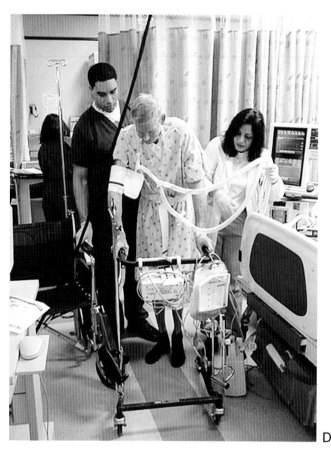

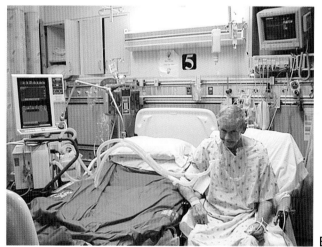

FIGURE 34-3 ICU patient receiving physical therapy treatment. **A,** Patient is on mechanical ventilation with an oral endotracheal tube. **B,** Patient sitting on the edge of the bed. **C,** Standing at the edge of bed with walker and assistance of two people. **D,** Walking around the bed. **E,** Patient sitting on a bedside chair after physical therapy treatment. Specific safety precautions must be followed at all times to safely mobilize the patient and to prevent accidental extubation.

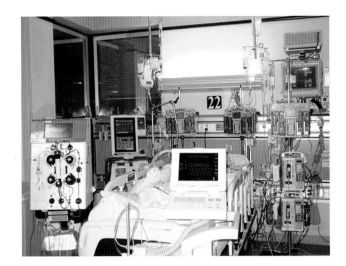

FIGURE 36-2 Patient in the ICU with multiorgan system failure. Note the ventilator, continuous dialysis, intra-aortic balloon pump and multiple intravenous drips.

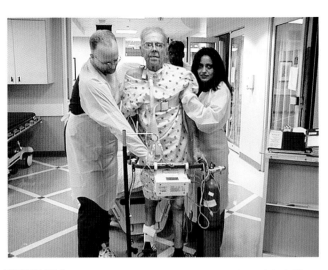

FIGURE 36-3 Mobilizing a patient in the ICU with critical illness polyneuropathty. Note the presence of marked muscle atrophy on both lower extremities.

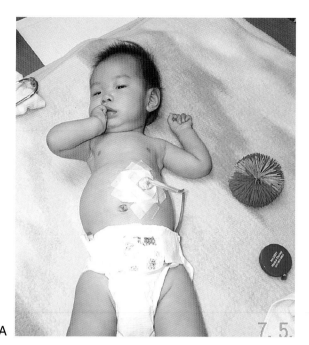

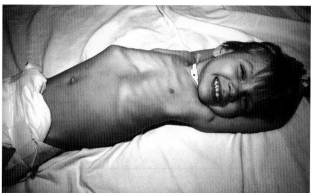

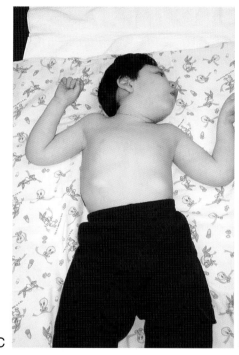

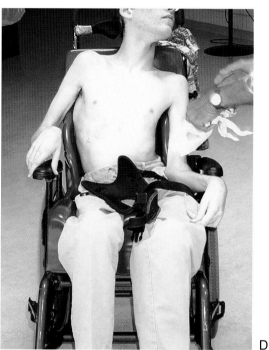

FIGURE 39-2 A, Caitlin, six months of age. Caitlin has spinal muscle atrophy, type I. Note persistent immature triangular shaping of chest wall secondary to pronounced muscle weakness and an inability to counteract gravity effectively. **B,** Melissa, three-and-a-half years of age. Melissa has a C5 complete spinal cord injury due to birth trauma. Melissa's chest wall has become more deformed than Caitlin's chest due to the prolonged exposure to the severe muscle imbalance of the respiratory muscles within gravity's constant influence. Note the marked pectus excavatum and anteriorly flared ribs in supine. **C,** Carlos, 5 years of age and **D,** Kevin, 17 years of age. Both have spastic cerebral palsy. Note the lateral flaring of the lower ribcage, the asymmetry of the trunk, and the flattening of the entire anterior ribcage, all of which are more noticeable in the older child.

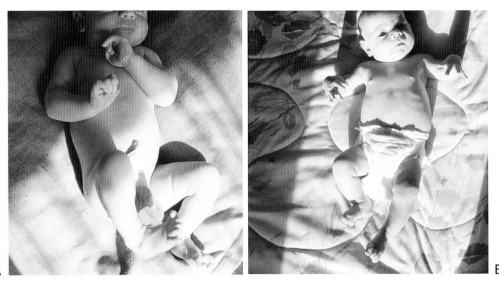

A   B

FIGURE 39-3 **A** and **B,** Newborn chest. Note triangular shape, short neck, narrow and flat upper chest, round barreled lower chest. Muscle tone is primarily flexion and breathing is primarily diaphragmatic and on one plane: inferior.

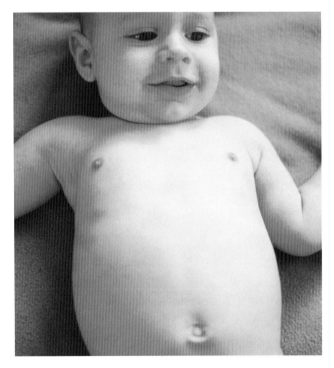

FIGURE 39-4 Infant chest wall at three to six months of age. Increased upper chest width. More convex shaping of entire chest as antigravity movements are becoming possible. Still has a short neck and two functionally separate chambers: thorax and abdomen.

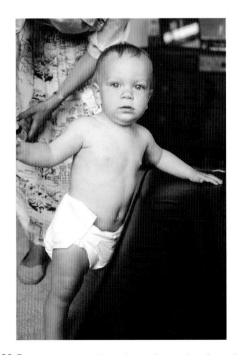

FIGURE 39-5 Infant chest wall at six to 12 months of age. The infant spends more time in upright. The activation of abdominal muscles, gravity's influence, and increased postural demands result in a more elongated chest wall, wider rib spacing, and increased intercostal muscle activation, as well as a functional interface of the ribcage onto the abdomen with the abdominal and intercostal muscles. This improves both the respiratory dynamics by giving more external support to the diaphragm at the mid chest level, and the postural stabilization potential needed for more complex motor tasks. Note that the base of the ribcage is no longer barrel shaped like it is in the newborn.

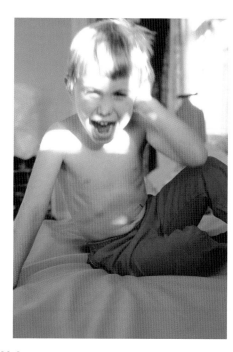

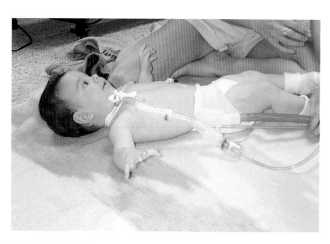

FIGURE 39-11 Nicholas, one year of age. Nicholas was born with both hemi-diaphragms paralyzed and requires full-time mechanical ventilation. When he is off the ventilator for brief periods of time to assess his independent breathing pattern, he demonstrates the second type of paradoxical breathing: a rising upper chest and falling abdomen during inhalation.

FIGURE 39-6 A four-year-old boy. Note the elongated chest, which occupies more than half of the trunk space, the wide intercostal spacing, the effective muscle stabilization of the lower ribcage with the abdominal muscles, the rectangular shaping of the chest from a frontal view, and the elliptical shaping of the chest from a transverse view.

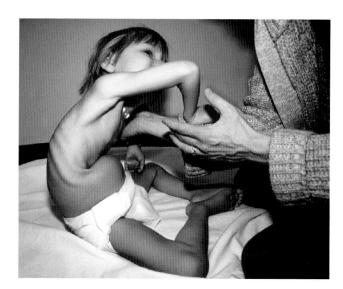

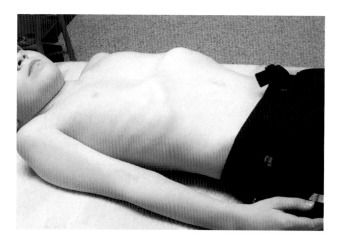

FIGURE 39-8 Melissa, age three-and-a-half years: C5 complete spinal cord injury due to birth trauma. Clinical example of a crushed trunk resulting in severely compromised respiratory mechanics in spite of the fact that her lungs are normal. Melissa was incapable of generating adequate positive pressures to counteract the constant force of gravity and atmospheric pressure upon her developing skeletal frame.

FIGURE 39-12 Justin, nine years of age. Justin has a congenital pectus excavatum. No neurological impairment. His breathing pattern is primarily diaphragm and upper accessory muscles. Note the persistent elevation of the ribcage and the inward collapse of the lower sternum (pectus excavatum). Justin's sternum moved paradoxically with every inspiratory effort, especially during high respiratory and postural demand.

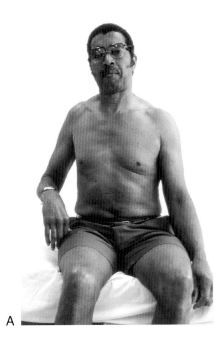

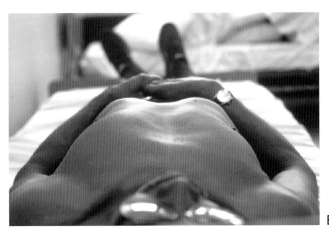

FIGURE 39-13 Charles. Right hemiparesis from a CVA. **A,** Note asymmetry of trunk in sitting during breathing and postural control. **B,** Note the weakness in the right upper chest. Charles' right upper chest moved less during inhalation than the left, which accentuated his asymmetrical trunk alignment and was probably a contributing factor to his impaired posture and upper extremity function in stance and during gait.

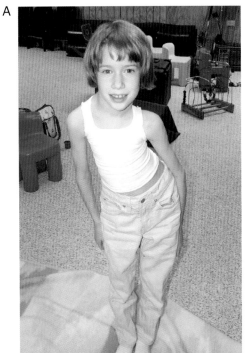

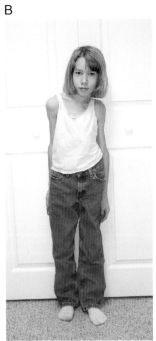

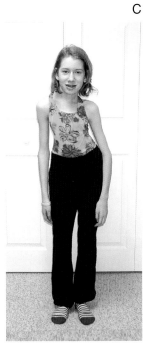

FIGURE 39-14 A, Katie nine years of age; diagnosis of infantile scoliosis. Presurgical workup showed her FVC at 33% of predicted value. **B,** Katie age 10 years, one year later. Her surgeon felt that the improvements in lung volumes and a slight reduction in the scoliosis would allow him to postpone the surgery in order to allow Katie more time to grow before the surgery fixed her adult height. Katie's loose shirt partially occludes the severity of the spinal deformity. **C,** Katie age 13 years, six months after back surgery. Scoliosis reduced as far as possible given her fused ribs (from surgery as a toddler) and other joint limitations.

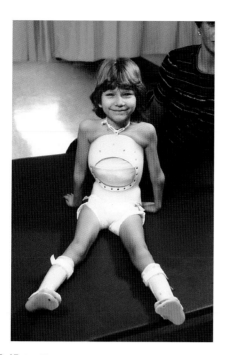

FIGURE 39-15 Melissa, six years of age. Note the use of the TLSO with an abdominal cutout supported by an abdominal binder. This provided support for her developing spine and trunk while still allowing for optimal support for breathing mechanics. Note that the TLSO provided an ideal alignment of the proximal extremity joints (shoulders and hips) as well as the ideal head alignment for normal functions such as talking and eating.

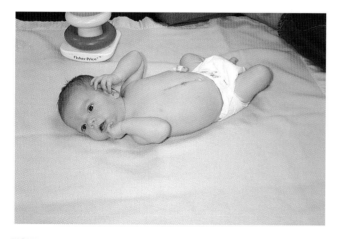

FIGURE 39-17 Jonathan, six months of age. His severe gastro-esophygeal reflux required surgical support (gastrostomy tube and Nissen fundoplication procedures) at five months of age. His mother reports that his favorite posture when in supine is extreme trunk extension and right head rotation. This may have developed as a compensatory strategy against the noxious stimulus from reflux and a possible upper airway obstruction that was yet undiagnosed.

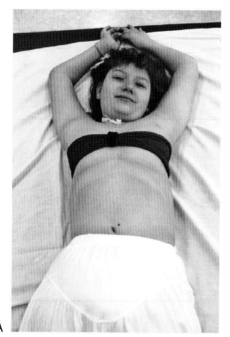

A

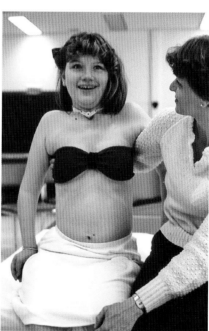

B

FIGURE 39-16 Melissa, 12 years of age, after orthopedic surgery to reduce scoliosis. **A,** Note that the chest wall deformities that were so prevalent at age three are almost completely absent. The only noticeable skeletal restriction is the slight reduction in mid chest expansion noted around ribs six through eight, which looks like a high "waistline" just under her bra strap line in supine. The intercostal muscles, which were paralyzed, are the only support for the ribcage at that level. Melissa used her upper accessory muscles to support breathing and chest wall alignment of the upper chest, and the diaphragm for the lower ribcage. **B,** Melissa continues to wear an abdominal binder in upright postures, but it was removed for this picture.

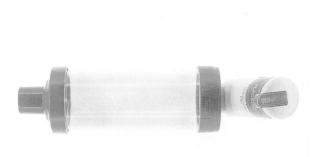

FIGURE 45-1 Metered-dose inhaler (MDI) with spacer.

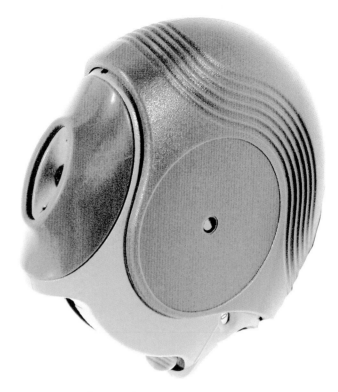

FIGURE 45-2 Multi-dose powder inhaler.

PART I

Cardiovascular and Pulmonary Function in Health and Disease

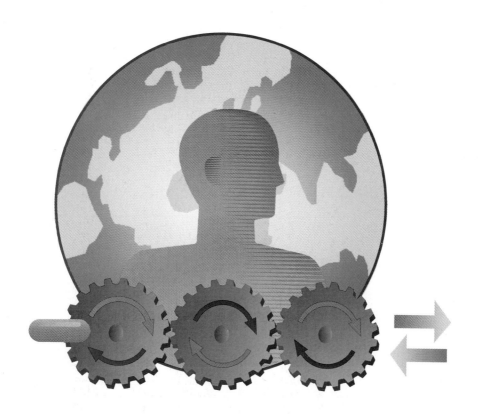

C H A P T E R 1

Epidemiology as a Basis for Contemporary Physical Therapy Practice

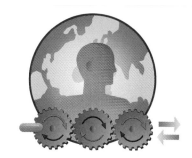

Elizabeth Dean

KEY TERMS

Building healthy communities
Diseases of civilization
Epidemiology
Global health
Healthy people
International classification of function

Magic bullet
Noninvasive practitioner
Our village
Paradigm shift
World Health Organization

This past century, health care priorities have shifted from the prevention and management of acute infectious diseases to the prevention and management of "diseases of civilization," or "diseases of affluence." These include ischemic heart disease, smoking-related conditions, hypertension and stroke, diabetes, and cancer. Not only have the morbidity and death toll resulting from these conditions escalated to their current pandemic proportions, but the probability that an individual (child or adult) might have one or more risk factors is high.

To address the gap between lifestyle practices and the body of knowledge regarding the relationship between lifestyle choices and health (Steptoe et al, 2002), a societal commitment to reducing the number of patients, rather than increasing the focus on drugs and surgery, has never been more urgent than it is now. Physical therapists are uniquely qualified and strategically positioned as health care professionals to be leaders in the translation of this well-established body of knowledge into daily practice (Smith, 1998). Positive attitudes about health and the prevention of illness should be adopted as priorities in health care that supersede the conventional biomedical focus. A consideration of the risks of the diseases of civilization in every individual is consistent with a

comprehensive model of best practice in the context of epidemiological trends—that is, *evidence-based practice in the context of evidence-based planning*. This chapter expands these concepts and outlines principles for applying them proactively and as a priority in the management of every patient. Physical therapists can have a major impact on the leading priorities of health care, one individual at a time.

WHAT IS HEALTH?

The World Health Organization (WHO) defines health as emotional, spiritual, and intellectual, as well as physical well-being, and not merely the absence of disease and impairment (WHO, 2004). Although physical well-being contributes to health in the other dimensions, it does not ensure health. Thus emotional, spiritual, and intellectual well-being should be assessed as systematically as is physical well-being in a model of care based on health. Collectively, these domains of health translate into an individual's capacity to perform activities that enable him or her to participate fully in life (WHO, 2000). The WHO's definition of health has not been amended since 1948. Although having withstood time, this definition of

TABLE 1-1

Concepts of the Health Belief Model

CONCEPT	DEFINITION	APPLICATION
Perceived susceptibility	One's belief of the chances of getting a condition	Define the population(s) at risk and their risk levels Personalize risk based on a person's traits or behaviors Heighten perceived susceptibility if too low
Perceived severity	One's belief of the seriousness of a condition and its consequences	Specify and describe consequences of the risk and the condition
Perceived benefits	One's belief in the efficacy of the advised action to reduce risk or seriousness of impact	Define action to take—how, where, when Clarify the expected positive effects Describe evidence of effectiveness
Perceived barriers	One's belief in the tangible and psychological costs of the advised behavior	Identify and reduce barriers through reassurance, incentives, and assistance
Cues to action	Strategies to activate "readiness"	Provide how-to information Promote awareness Provide reminders
Self-efficacy	Confidence in one's ability to take action	Provide training, guidance, and positive reinforcement

From Stretcher, V.J.R., & Rosenstock, I.M. (1997). The health belief model. In K. Glanz, Lewis, F.M., Rimer, B.K. (Eds). Health behavior and health education: theory, research and practice. San Francisco: Jossey-Bass.

health has failed to be incorporated as the primary goal of contemporary health care.

Over the past century, the primary determinants of improved health have been the provision of clean water, sanitation, basic nutrition, shelter, and security, rather than biomedical advances. In addition, education, and socioeconomic and employment status are important independent determinants of health. Biomedical care has had greatest success in controlling infection, providing symptomatic relief of acute problems, and providing emergency care. Such care, however, has not had the impact on health that the primary determinants of health have had overall, nor has it had major success in preventing and managing the diseases of civilization—the leading killers.

By the time an individual has entered the biomedical system, health care in its truest sense has failed. From this perspective, our state-of-the-art hospitals can be viewed as monuments to our failures rather than to our successes. Without question, there is need for invasive care (drugs and surgery) and well-equipped hospitals. On the other hand, as practitioners committed to noninvasive care, physical therapists have the capacity to promote health and well-being with the global goals of reducing the number of patients and minimizing the need for invasive care.

Because of widespread immigration, the cultural and ethnic profiles of high-income countries such as those in North America and Europe are changing rapidly. Beliefs, attitudes, values, cultures, ethnicity, and traditions significantly affect health, ill health, and their interactions. For example, Asian immigrants to the United States report fewer stress-related and psychological problems than do non-Hispanic Caucasians (Uppaluri et al, 2001). With increasing time in the States, however, reports of stress increase. This might reflect cultural differences in the acceptability of reporting psychological

distress, hence, underreporting; sensitization to the definition of and the awareness of stress with increasing duration of residence; or the compounding effect of increasing stress in the new culture. How best to reduce racial and ethnic disparities through culturally competent health care is a matter of debate and requires such outcomes as client satisfaction, improved health status, and culturally appropriate management and delivery across racial and ethnic groups (Anderson et al, 2003).

Since the psychobiological adaptation model was posited 20 years ago (Dean, 1985), the few models of physical therapy practice that have been reported have included psychosocial and other nonphysiological components. Psychosocial components include health belief, self-efficacy, and perceived control. The Health Belief Model is useful in appreciating the ways in which belief affects health, illness, and the responses and reactions to them (Table 1-1) (Stretcher & Rosenstock, 1997). Assessment of self-efficacy provides an index of an individual's sense of mastery over his or her health and well-being. These concepts can be used in a clinician's practice setting. A few questions will help to assess a patient's perception of susceptibility to risk or a condition. These concepts can provide a basis for health education that includes increasing the patient's awareness of the effects of lifestyle factors on health and of their consequences. The action necessary to avoid the condition or minimize its risk can be selectively targeted for each individual when the individual's context is known.

The International Classification of Function advocated by the WHO interrelates structure and function, activity, and participation in life (WHO, 2000). The biomedical model focuses primarily on impairment (i.e., structure and function), with little attention to health and wellness, sickness impact, life satisfaction, and quality of life (i.e., participation in life and associated activities). One problem that occurs when the primary focus is on the remediation of limitations of structure and function in the management of the leading health care problems of our day is that such limitations do not necessarily affect activity and participation—the essence of life. These relationships should be evaluated in each case, not assumed.

The integration of health belief and motivational models has been a means of incorporating psychosocial dimensions of care, interventions, and outcomes so as to directly address an individual's limitations of activity and participation. As a result of this paradigm shift, an increasing number of measurement tools are available to assess the essential dimensions of health. These tools can be categorized as generic; as having general application across individuals and conditions; or as having specific application to a cohort of individuals, based on age, condition, or some other variable (see examples in Chapter 17). Many of these scales have been validated only on a subset of these cohort groups. Physical therapists must use these tools knowledgeably and specifically to assess outcomes in their practices, just as they use conventional tools to assess and evaluate anatomic structure and physiological function. Health-related quality of life as reflected in the Short Form-36 is an established tool for general use and has been adapted cross-culturally (Mitani et al, 2003; Ware & Sherbourne, 1992). Such tools report the individual's perception of health improvement, which is essential in contemporary health care and is supplemental to conventional objective clinical measures.

The Paradox

People living in high-income countries (e.g., countries in North America and Europe) and, increasingly, in countries whose economies are growing are experiencing a paradox: an increase in the negative impact of lifestyle is combined with an increase in advances in biomedicine, including genome and protonomic research. Technological and economic advances have been proposed as factors contributing to an obesity-conducive environment (Franklin, 2001). The effects of low activity (hypokinesis) and poor nutritional choices on health in Western countries have been reported to be synergistic and partially additive (Vuori, 2001), although a potent interaction may exist. The power of nonpharmacological interventions and solutions to affect global health problems can no longer be considered secondary to pharmacological solutions (Kingsley & Gupta, 1992; Sorrentino, 2000). If pharmacological interventions are indicated in nonemergency situations, those interventions should be viewed only as short-term solutions where possible, until the effects of non-pharmacological interventions and lifestyle changes are apparent.

A nationwide, population-based strategy to improve lifestyle is the only means of improving the country's health en masse and minimizing morbidity and premature mortality with the least risk and cost (Kavanagh, 2001; Wahlqvist, 2002b; Wood, 2001). A modest reduction in cardiac risk factors, for

example, can save approximately three times as many life-years as invasive interventions (Critchley et al, 2003). Preserving and optimizing health in the most cost-effective, low-risk, and ethical manner should be the universal health care priority.

LIFESTYLE AND THE DISEASES OF CIVILIZATION

Poor nutritional choices and sedentary lifestyles coupled with stress, tobacco use, and excessive alcohol consumption underpin the diseases of civilization in high-income countries, and they pose the greatest threats to public health (Bijnen et al, 1994; Musaiger, 2002; WHO, 2003). Eight major risk factors related to lifestyle and their documented impacts on health are shown in Table 1-2. This trend has given rise to dramatic increases in a newly defined condition, metabolic syndrome, which includes insulin resistance, high blood pressure, elevated triglycerides and cholesterol, and obesity. With industrialization and technological advances, the diseases of civilization are on the rise in low- and middle-income countries as well (Cheng, 2001; Ebrahim & Smith, 2001). Despite their prevalence, however, the WHO has proclaimed that the diseases of civilization are largely preventable (WHO, 1999-2003).

Atherosclerosis is the major common denominator and contributor to the leading health problems of our time, including ischemic heart disease (IHD), hypertension and stroke, and diabetes. Factor analysis supports a two-factor solution for heart disease and possibly for other diseases of civilization, which includes family history (factor 1) and lifestyle factors (i.e., smoking, serum cholesterol, blood pressure, nutrition, exercise, and weight control) (factor 2) (Wright et al, 1994). At the population level, choosing health, including optimal nutrition and exercise throughout life, can enhance the quality of life, decrease the prevalence of chronic disease, and reduce the burden of disease on individuals, families, communities, and countries, including suffering and health care costs (Cheng et al, 2002; Ebrahim, 2000; Mann, 2002).

LIFE CYCLE AND THE DISEASES OF CIVILIZATION

The diseases of civilization have their foundation in childhood because their associated underlying health behaviors are rooted during this critical period. IHD secondary to atherosclerosis continues to be the leading cause of mortality and disability in industrialized countries. The prevention and management of risk factors of systemic atherosclerosis should be a primary target of contemporary care for children as well as for adults (McCrindle, 2001; Misra, 2000; Zafari & Wenger, 1998). Ischemic cerebrovascular, coronary, and peripheral vascular diseases are manifestations of the same underlying pathologic process, blood vessel narrowing caused by atherosclerosis and thrombosis. Smoking, a high-fat diet, and inactivity can precipitate damage to the endothelium and cause atherosclerotic deposition on the arterial walls. This common pathway has been associated with increased fibrinogen and C-reactive protein, markers of inflammation (Sakakibara

TABLE 1-2

Major Modifiable Risk Factors for the Diseases of Civilization

	CONDITION					
RISK FACTOR	CARDIOVASCULAR (IHD & HYPERTENSION) AND PERIPHERAL VASCULAR DISEASE	OBSTRUCTIVE LUNG DISEASE	STROKE	DIABETES	CANCER	OSTEOPOROSIS
Smoking	X	X	X	X	X (↑ risk of all-cause cancer*)	X
Physical inactivity	X		X	X	X	X
Obesity	X	X	X	X	X	
Nutrition	X		X	X	X	X
High blood pressure	X		X	X		
Dietary fat†/blood lipids	X		X	X	X	
Elevated glucose levels	X		X	X	X	
Alcohol‡	X		?	X	X	X

*Smoking is not only related to cancer of the nose, mouth, airways, and lungs, but smoking increases the risk of all-cause cancer.
†Partially saturated, saturated, and trans fats are the most injurious to health.
‡Alcohol can be protective in moderate quantities, red wine in particular.
Modified from the Heart and Stroke Foundation of Canada, 2003; Bradberry, J.C. (2004). Peripheral arterial disease: pathophysiology, risk factors, and role of antithrombotic therapy. Journal of the American Pharmacy Association 44(2 Suppl 1):S37-S44; Charkoudian N, & Joyner, M.J. (2004). Physiologic considerations for exercise performance in women. Clinics in Chest Medicine 25:247-255.

et al, 2004). The primary focus of biomedical research has shifted to the role of inflammatory mediators and the contribution of low-density lipoproteins to the cause of atherosclerosis and away from the concept of degenerative vessel disease. Fibrinogen is an inflammation mediator and a clotting factor. People with cardiovascular disease have high fibrinogen levels, which further increase the risk for thrombosis and manifestations of circulatory disease. Inflammation has been implicated in a growing number of chronic conditions, such as IHD, stroke, asthma, gastrointestinal ulcers, cirrhosis of the liver, Alzheimer disease, cancer, and autoimmune conditions (Anonymous, 2003; Brod, 2000). Unhealthy lifestyle choices have been thought to contribute to a proinflammatory state, giving rise to low-grade infection in various organ systems and leading to the signs and symptoms associated with chronic degenerative processes. Although this is an important finding, a proinflammatory milieu and inflammation are not the causes of the chronic conditions with which they have been associated but, rather, are precipitating effects of traumas resulting from lifestyle.

Promotion of healthy lifestyles early in life transfers responsibility to the individual as much as possible and away from some inherent pathophysiological cause. Although conventional invasive biomedical care with medications and surgery may provide symptomatic relief, only fundamental changes in lifestyle can address the root cause in the majority of cases of the diseases of civilization. The physical therapist as a contemporary health care provider must be an excellent health coach and in this role should serve in the management of every patient, both child and adult.

The diseases of civilization are no longer considered adult conditions or age-related conditions. Children are exhibiting signs of cardiovascular disease, including heart failure, hypertension, type 2 diabetes mellitus, and obesity. As a consequence, the children of today will die prematurely and will have prolonged morbidity associated with chronic disease, secondary complications of these conditions, associated adverse responses to other health complaints, increased iatrogenic problems (secondary to health care interventions, including drugs and surgery), and potentially increased end-of-life morbidity and shorter life expectancy than their parents (Katz, 2003). Health-promotion strategies directed toward parents and young children will help to offset the population's health threat by the diseases of civilization.

The post–World War II baby-boom generation characterizes the demographics of many industrialized countries. This cohort has lived in prosperous times, and life expectancy has almost doubled since 1900. Certain behavioral-physiological and psychosocial age-related changes are common among people who live in Western cultures. Although the manifestations of the diseases of civilization are associated with aging, they are not necessary consequences of aging. Evidence for this statement is based on differences among non-Western cultures and differences across cultures. Optimal nutrition, exercise, and stress control, the absence of smoking, and moderate alcohol consumption are central to reducing the probability of disease and disability caused by chronic conditions and to maximizing quality of life as people age (Woo, 2000). In particular, increased quality of life with a higher threshold for chronic disease and less morbidity in the final years of life is the objective.

FIRST DO NO HARM

As primarily a noninvasive health care profession, physical therapy is uniquely positioned at the level of population health to have a primary role in the promotion of health and wellness, and the prevention, cure, and treatment of these pandemic conditions. In the pursuit of the commitment to "first do no harm," health care providers in general have failed to exploit evidence-based, holistic, noninvasive practices as the primary goal in addressing our leading health care priorities; rather, they have continued to favor invasive solutions based on drugs and surgery. Triage of individuals by *both* noninvasive practitioners and invasive practitioners would constitute a bold initiative in health care. Such triage could establish whether a patient's complaint is best managed in the short and long term wholly noninvasively, wholly invasively, or by some combination, with a view to weaning the patient off medications or minimizing the medication. Similarly, every effort should be made to avoid surgical intervention and its risks whenever possible (i.e., surgical intervention as a last resort rather than a first resort) by exploiting noninvasive interventions and strategies to restore health and promote lifelong health. If surgery is indicated, physical therapists should participate at all levels of perioperative care. As a member of the surgical team (see Chapter 30), the physical therapist has much to offer in preparing a patient for elective surgery to improve short- and long-term outcomes and reduce surgical risk. Optimal surgical outcomes extend beyond technically competent surgery. They include empowerment of the individual to manage her or his health, prevention of recurrence of the precipitating problem, reduction of invasive care and support postoperatively, reduced complications, reduced hospital stay, and lifelong health. When an individual enters the health care delivery system her or his receptivity to health information is likely to be high. This is a prime opportunity to evaluate risk factors and prescribe a lifelong health plan.

The efficacy of nonpharmacological treatments in the management of chronic conditions has been well documented, but implementation has been poor (Clini et al, 2003). Physical therapists have a primary role as noninvasive practitioners on a health team that includes invasive practitioners, nurses, nutritionists, pharmacists, social workers, psychologists, respiratory therapists, spiritual leaders, and others, as each case requires. On a broader level, physical therapists can serve in a multisector capacity as consultants and work alongside health care policy makers, corporate business people, urban planners, and architects in developing healthy and safe homes, workplaces, recreational facilities, and communities. The role of the physical therapist has shifed from the acute care hospital and private practice to the community, schools, industry, home, and playing field—wherever people are, physical therapists have appeared.

Biomedical research that evaluates drugs and surgery is often deficient because the research design does not include a potentially superior, noninvasively managed group where feasible. For example, a 12-month exercise program involving selected individuals with stable coronary artery disease has shown superior event-free survival and exercise capacity when compared to individuals who received percutaneous coronary intervention (Hambrecht et al, 2004). In favor of biomedical advances, these types of high-impact advances are rarely profiled as lead articles in the *New England Journal of Medicine*, *Nature*, *Science*, or the popular press, such as *Time* magazine. Yet it is these types of noninvasive advances that show the promise of having a great impact on the population's health, including increased probability of lifelong health and minimal cost, as compared with the results of invasive interventions, which frequently do not address the cause or contributing factors. Such findings must be integrated into contemporary practice to ensure that an individual is not subjected to the undue risk of taking prolonged courses of medication and undergoing unnecessary invasive interventions, with their associated risks and the high probability of repeated invasive procedures. Noninvasive interventions have the distinct advantage over drugs and surgery of empowering individuals to manage their own long-term health by learning skills that will change deleterious lifestyle habits and reduce the risks and costs of rehospitalization and procedures such as revascularization. The number of needless deaths in the U.S. due to drugs is estimated to be approaching 100,000 per year. Loss of life due to other causes, such as infectious disease, would be a focus of national concern.

Epidemiological indicators support the need for a paradigm shift in physical therapy practice based on the capacity to effect lifestyle change. The combination of effective health education (concerning the health benefits of physical activity and exercise, good nutrition, weight control, smoking cessation, and stress management) and exercise prescription can prevent, "cure," and remediate the diseases of civilization (WHO, 1999-2003). These interventions must be a basis for assessment and management in every patient. The conditions may be present as primary diagnoses or as secondary diagnoses in patients who come to a physical therapist. Each individual should be assessed for the risk factors related to these conditions, and prevention strategies should be implemented. Mastering effective health education strategies may be considered the sine qua non for maximizing physical therapy health outcomes in the management of contemporary health care problems. Physical therapists need to adopt this as the primary objective of contemporary practice for each client or patient, as they pursue the primary mission of the WHO— health for all—which may be extended in physical therapy to "health and participation for all," thereby affecting the health of the population.

Consistent with the tenets of Hippocrates to which all health care professions aspire—"first do no harm" and "the function of protecting and developing health must rank even above that of restoring it when it is impaired"—the primary objective is to promote wellness, to prevent illness and disability and, in the event that these occur, to exploit the least invasive interventions (Svendsen, 2003), rather than consider them after invasive interventions have been made (Doyle & Creager, 2003; Scott et al, 2002). Pharmaceutical agents, however, may be needed for immediate symptomatic relief and for reasons of comfort and safety. The goal thereafter is to wean the individual from the medication and promote lifelong health and well-being. The physical therapist's role is to determine how best this can be done in every patient under her or his care. All drugs have potential side effects, including personal disempowerment and psychological dependence. The costs of invasive care and injudicious noninvasive care include the immediate direct and indirect economic cost to the patient and the insurer and the burden of disease on the individual, his or her family, the community, and society. The burden of disease affects the socioeconomic status of the individual (in terms of employability), the state or province, and the country. The mortality rate of individuals with heart disease, for example, has been estimated to be reduced by 20% to 25% with cardiac rehabilitation, which is comparable to the results of established therapies such as beta blockers (Marota Montero & Velasco Rami, 1995). In addition, cardiac rehabilitation is noninvasive; thus it is cheaper and is associated with few side effects. The focus of management is to change negative health behaviors and lifelong health.

Changing one's lifestyle is more challenging than taking a drug or undergoing surgery; in both the latter cases, the patient passively receives treatment. Being an effective agent of change and promoting active participation by their clients in their own health are fundamental to the expertise of the physical therapist who specializes in noninvasive, long-term health and care. In societies with open and free marketplaces such as the United States and Canada, physical therapists need superior skills in educating people regarding their lifestyle choices and promoting healthy lifestyle choices.

EVIDENCE-BASED PLANNING
Addressing the Health Care Needs of the Day

Physical therapists treat individuals with the diseases of civilization as either primary or secondary diagnoses. Smoking is currently the leading cause of death in the United States, with poor diet and sedentary lifestyle anticipated soon to overtake tobacco use (Mokdad et al, 2004). Obesity and sedentary living are second to smoking in terms of negative impact on health. Television viewing, an indicator of sedentary living, is associated with obesity and is a marker of cardiovascular disease independent of total reported physical activity (Jakes et al, 2003). Thus, as noninvasive practitioners, physical therapists have a responsibility to manage these conditions and their risk factors in all patients so as to prevent or control their physical, psychosocial, economic, and societal impact and to promote health.

Our Village

Fundamental to the principle of evidence-based planning is responding to epidemiological indicators and an understanding

of the changing demographics and face of our "village." The diseases of civilization are the leading killers in our village. Men can expect to live 75 years, and women 82 years (National Vital Statistics Report, 2004). Functional capacity, however, is estimated to decrease 10% per decade, and half of this decrement is due to sedentary living. Raising children to be healthy and physically active will promote a generation of healthy middle-aged and older people and will thereby delay their physical dependence by 10 to 20 years.

Health care workers with international health organizations are trained to manage the unique needs of their villages. This entails knowing the health care priorities of the village and making decisions that affect the problems positively and reduce their impact on the community as a whole. A health care worker who focuses on malaria, for example, when intestinal parasites are the priority is a hindrance rather than a help to that village. Similarly, in our current health care climate, physical therapists must make it a priority to meet the leading needs of their own village. Smoking cessation, good nutrition and weight control, exercise, and stress management are evidence-based noninvasive interventions consistent with the needs of contemporary physical therapy practice; the therapeutic potential and impact of those elements on the health of our village is enormous. For example, each kilogram of weight loss has a dose-dependent beneficial effect on health outcomes. Further, as little as 30 minutes of moderately intense activity on most days of the week offsets the deleterious effects of sedentary living (Varo Cenarruzabeitia et al, 2003). With the aging of the people of our village and the signs of the diseases of civilization now evident in children and young adults, the burden of chronic disease will be prolonged in these individuals, particularly toward the end of life. That life expectancy will plateau or decrease as a result has been suggested.

Indigenous peoples in North America and Australasia have unique health challenges and needs. They tend to be less well educated than the dominant culture, have fewer employment opportunities, experience more violent injuries and deaths, and have poorer health and shorter lives. They have significant health risks because of sociocultural factors and genetic predisposition, such as higher rates of diabetes, obesity, hypertension, tobacco use, and alcoholism. Large-scale intervention programs are needed for the indigenous American Indian population based on studies of the health of American Indian children (Story et al, 2003). The past few generations have witnessed a shift from indigenous foods to refined grains and foods high in fat and sugar and from active to inactive lifestyles. These trends have exacted an enormous toll in terms of health.

As individuals age in industrialized countries, their activity levels tend to decline. With relatively long life expectancy in these countries, sedentary lifestyles may prolong end-of-life morbidity. A study of individuals who adhered to exercise programs and those who did not revealed the importance of variables such as self-efficacy, perceived fitness, social support, and enjoyment (Stevens et al, 2003). The results of this study have important implications for urban planning; they can inform the design of healthy communities as well as individual activity and exercise programs.

The study of black Seventh-day Adventists has provided a unique opportunity to isolate the effects of lifestyle on African Americans. Seventh-day Adventists promote spiritual well-being and a healthy diet and lifestyle. As a result, the health of black Seventh-day Adventists is better and the incidence of chronic disease lower than those of black Americans who are not Seventh-day Adventists (Nyenhuis et al, 2003). In addition, based on the results of a study of a large cohort, Mormons tend to be more fit and have fewer risk factors for IHD than other Americans (LaMonte et al, 2000).

The physical activity profiles of African American women have been compared with recommendations for moderate levels of activity (Whitt et al, 2003). The findings showed that only a small proportion of the subjects met the recommended levels of daily physical activity. Exercise was performed on fewer than the recommended number of days per week and for less than the recommended 8 to 10 minutes per session. Attention to frequency and duration may be particularly important when counseling African American women about regular physical activity.

African American women have a higher risk of cardiovascular disease and stroke than Caucasian American women (Wilbur et al, 2003a). Based on a cross-sectional study of 399 urban African American women, correlates of physical activity within this cohort were identified. Programs to promote physical activity must address the safety of the physical environment and psychosocial factors. Inactive women with less than a high school education and those who perceive themselves to be in poor health should be considered special target groups.

Latina women have a higher risk of cardiovascular disease and stroke than do Caucasian American women; this has been attributed to the higher incidence among them of obesity and type 2 diabetes mellitus (Wilbur et al, 2003b). The facilitators and barriers to exercising in this cultural cohort have been examined in a cross-sectional study of 300 Latinas. Physical activity has been reported to be higher in younger women, in married women, and in women who had confidence that they could become more active, saw people exercising in the neighborhood, and attended religious services (Wilbur et al, 2003b). The church was recommended as a suitable community setting for initiating programs that provide women with the knowledge, skills, and motivation to become more active and to transmit this information to others in the community through their families.

The impact of gender is being increasingly appreciated in terms of health affliction, access to health care, and physiological responses and psychological reactions to illness (Charkoudian & Joyner, 2004; Holund et al, 1997). In a Swedish cohort of elderly individuals, obesity-related health indicators and risk factors were reported to differ in men and women and also to differ on the basis of socioeconomic status (Cabrera et al, 2003). In response to cardiac rehabilitation, gender-specific effects on high-density lipoprotein cholesterol

have been documented (Savage et al, 2004). Women demonstrate greater improvement in high-density lipoprotein than do men.

Urbanization, modernization, and immigration are affecting global health. Within industrialized countries, indigenous people are moving from rural to urban areas; this is occurring in the United States, Canada, Australia, New Zealand, and many African countries. Rather than seeing improvements in their health, relocated rural people are succumbing to the diseases of civilization in high numbers. Middle-aged black men who move to urban areas from rural South Africa, for example, increase their risk of IHD and stroke (van Rooyen et al, 2002). One explanation for this response is increased autonomic reactivity to the stress of relocation. Other lifestyle factors, however, may be implicated. These patterns have been reported for other groups, too, such as among Mexicans and Asians who move to more affluent industrialized countries (Suh et al, 2001). The health advantage for people who move from certain Asian countries such as Japan to the West is lost with increasing numbers of years in the new culture (Goel et al, 2004).

Principles of an Evidence-Based Planning Approach

The efficacy of the quick-fix (drugs and surgery) approach to the management of chronic conditions, particularly the diseases of civilization, is being seriously questioned. With respect to long-term outcomes, noninvasive interventions may often be more successful (Simonds, 2003). Mortality rates can be significantly reduced with regular physical activity, optimal nutrition and weight control, and avoidance of smoking (Woo et al, 2002). Hospitalization is inversely related to physical activity, as is the reporting of depressive symptoms. Nonsmokers have lower mortality rates and better self-reported health. These findings are unequivocal and warrant being integrated into a contemporary model of health care. Paradoxically, relative to invasive care, noninvasive physical therapy management is low in cost, yet access to it is commonly more limited than access to invasive care.

The Priorities of Our Village

Health risks and the cause of death in those living today will be found primarily in the diseases of civilization, namely:

- Heart disease
- Smoking-related conditions, including chronic lung disease
- Hypertension and stroke
- Diabetes and metabolic syndrome
- Cancers

These conditions are frequently either the primary or the secondary diagnoses of the patients treated by physical therapists; this positions them favorably to make direct assaults on the risk factors involved in the diseases of civilization in their patients. Physical therapists have the advantage of prolonged patient contact during treatments, and such contact can be exploited in targeting teachable moments and health education opportunities.

The goal is to exploit the benefits of lifestyle modification and supplement those benefits with medication only if necessary (Haskell, 2003), rather than supplementing medication with lifestyle modification. A healthy lifestyle is the treatment of choice for the diseases of civilization as well as the primary intervention for their prevention (Gibbons & Clark, 2001). The translation of these research findings into health care practice is a priority.

Ischemic Heart Disease

The risk factors for IHD are well established (Williams et al, 2002). They contribute to atherosclerotic deposits throughout the systemic vasculature (Bradbury, 2004). Nonmodifiable risk factors include age, gender, family history, and past history. Modifiable risk factors include increased cholesterol, increased homocysteine, smoking, inactivity, high blood pressure, diabetes, weight, and stress (Keller et al, 2003; Shapiro, 2000; Twisk et al, 1997). Less commonly acknowledged risk factors include elevated levels of C-reactive proteins (markers of inflammation; Anonymous, 2003); sharing a lifestyle with someone who has IHD (Macken et al, 2000); and having overweight parents (Paterno, 2003). Further, a shared lifestyle confers increased evidence of IHD in and health risk for children (Gidding, 1999). Other emerging risk factors include passive smoking, level of education, depression, anger coupled with hostility, and social isolation (Graves & Miller, 2003; Panagiotakos et al, 2002).

Based on epidemiological evidence, a 1% reduction in cholesterol reduces the risk of IHD by 3% and a long-term reduction in diastolic blood pressure of 5 to 6 mm Hg reduces the risk by 20% to 25% (Sleight, 1991). Thus even modest changes can have a sizable impact on health. Most risk factors are associated with behavior and can be modified effectively (Sebregts et al, 2000).

Risk factors for IHD are prevalent in the general population. When a cross section of late-middle-aged people was screened, it was found that atherosclerosis involving the femoral artery affected two thirds of them (Leng et al, 2000). Further, a direct relationship was found to exist between the degree of atherosclerosis and cardiovascular and circulatory health. Individuals with peripheral artery disease have a several-fold increased risk of IHD; thus peripheral artery disease can be considered a marker of systemic atherosclerosis. It is estimated that optimal lifestyle could reduce cardiac events related to atherosclerosis by 70% to 80%. Regular walking has a significant effect on reducing the risk for IHD, as has vigorous activity (Bauman, 2004). In men with left ventricular hypertrophy, moderate physical activity reduces the risk of stroke by 49% when compared with sedentary men who do not have left ventricular hypertrophy (Pitsavos et al, 2004). Diabetes has been reported to be a strong risk factor and hypertension a less strong risk factor for IHD in women when compared with men (Burkman, 1991).

Self-reported fitness is independently related to fewer risk factors for IHD and angiographic evidence of IHD in women undergoing coronary angiography for suspected ischemia (Wessel et al, 2004). Measures of obesity are not independently associated with these outcomes. Thus fitness appears to be more important than body weight for cardiovascular risk in women. Physical activity and fitness warrant detailed assessment. They should be an integral part of the cardiovascular risk-factor stratification, and interventions should aim at long-term increases in physical activity and fitness. Assessment of physical activity and exercise programs should be included in the management of all people, particularly those at risk for IHD, and especially women.

Nutrition is a well-established independent risk factor for health or disease. People who consume fish twice a week have a 47% reduced risk of cardiac mortality compared with those who eat fish less often than once a month (Mozaffarian et al, 2004). Cereal fiber (two whole-grain slices of bread daily) is associated with a 14% reduced risk of myocardial infarction or stroke. Cereal fiber consumption even later in life is associated with a reduced incidence of cardiovascular disease (Mozaffarian et al, 2003). One alcoholic drink a day is associated with the least number of cerebrovascular abnormalities. Moderately and highly physically intense leisure-time activities predict 28% and 44% lower mortality rates, respectively, compared with little activity. Low, moderate, and high levels of exercise are associated with 30%, 37%, and 53% more years of healthy life, respectively. Aerobic training can reduce serum lipids even in older individuals. High-density lipoproteins increase in number and low-density lipoproteins decrease (Park et al, 2003). With lifestyle change, atherosclerosis can regress and associated cardiac events can be minimized (Haskell et al, 1994; Niebauer et al, 1997; Ornish et al, 1998; Srinath et al, 1995).

Psychosocial factors have been identified as risk factors for IHD. Difficulty in managing anger and hostility is one such risk factor, irrespective of whether a person has a type I or a type II personality (Anonymous, 2004). Stress is a significant risk factor that can be classified as minor daily stresses or hassles as opposed to negative long-term life events. Lipoprotein levels increase with both; however, coping style and subjective appraisal of stressors are powerful mitigating factors (Twisk et al, 1999). Cumulative daily hassles may be underestimated in terms of their impact on health as compared with major life-event stressors. After an individual's first coronary event, avoidance strategies are negatively associated with healthy lifestyles, whereas positive reappraisal and problem solving are positively associated (Henrichon & Robichaud-Ekstrand, 2002). Positive reappraisal and problem solving, program participation, and the avoidance of distancing and escape strategies predict adaptation to lifestyle changes after a coronary episode. Stress management must consider the type of stressor and help to modify the individual's coping strategies and interpretation of stressors.

The risk of a subsequent cardiac event after the first one is high (Hannan et al, 1990; Weintraub et al, 1997). Thus there is a high prevalence of repeated revascularization procedures and the prescription of more drugs with increased potency to help offset worsening pathophysiological changes. Ornish (1998) reported that 194 individuals with previous revascularization procedures were able to avoid repeat procedures for at least 3 years (the duration of follow-up in the study) with participation in a comprehensive lifestyle-change program. Compared with individuals who also had had a previous revascularization procedure but did not participate in the lifestyle-change program, those who did participate reported less angina to the same extent as that achieved with revascularization. The effects of noninvasive intervention can be considered long term, given their multisystem benefits. Revascularization focuses on the repair of an impairment and does not provide the additional multisystem benefits of the lifestyle-change program.

To date, efforts to effect aggressive modification of risk factors have been marginally successful. Optimal control of modifiable risk factors for coronary atherosclerosis, including cigarette smoking, dyslipidemia, hypertension, and sedentary lifestyle, are well known to reduce the incidence of IHD and, in turn, to reduce the need for revascularization and the utilization of health care resources (Squires, 1996). Our major health crisis can be addressed only by means of an integrated system of care committed to health, wellness, aggressive risk-factor prevention and lifestyle modification. Elucidation of the connections between deleterious behaviors and chronic conditions is urgently needed, especially with respect to health education. We need to clarify what works, what doesn't, for whom, and why.

Smoking-Related Conditions

Smoking is the leading cause of preventable death in the world, including in the United States (Mokdad et al, 2004). Despite the well-documented health hazards, smoking remains prevalent in industrialized and nonindustrialized countries and is estimated to shorten life by 11 minutes for each cigarette smoked (Shaw et al, 2000). Thus smoking cessation is a primary health care goal as well as a professional goal. (In 1996, the American Physical Therapy Association [APTA] adopted guidelines from the Agency for Health Care Policy and Research [AHCPR], which have been revised; see reference AHCPR Supported Clinical Practice Guidelines, 2000). The danger of smoking extends beyond chronic obstructive lung disease (COPD) and cancer. Overall morbidity and all-cause mortality, including cancer of organs other than the respiratory tract, are higher in smokers.

Of the leading causes of mortality worldwide, COPD is typically among the top killers and is associated with the loss of a million years of life each year (Pierson, 2004). In the United States, COPD ranks fourth behind IHD, cancer, and stroke. Long-term smokers have higher incidences of all-cause morbidity and mortality (Box 1-1); thus, smoking leads to life-threatening conditions that are systemic and are related not just to the respiratory tract (Mozaffarian et al, 2004). Former and current smokers have 25% and 44% fewer healthy

years of life, respectively, compared with lifelong nonsmokers. Smoking cessation is a priority for *all* individuals, not only those with lung disease, regardless of disease severity (Yohannes & Hardy, 2003). Smoking by children is highly associated with parental smoking; thus, smoking by adults with young families is a primary focus of public health initiatives (Paterno, 2003).

Pulmonary rehabilitation has demonstrated sustainability of smoking cessation and other health benefits in individuals with COPD (Calverley & Walker, 2003); thus its use is warranted as a preventive measure as well as for the remediation and management of disease (Ockene & Miller, 1997). Rehabilitation programs have proven efficacy independent of pharmacotherapy, so they should be considered primary interventions rather than priorities after conventional expensive medical care has failed (Maltais & Bourbeau, 1995). Only with health coaching and follow-up can these individuals be able to effect life-long health behavior change to reduce exacerbations, reduce doctor and hospital visits, continue working, and reduce overall morbidity. Innovative smoking cessation programs warrant development so that they have maximal impact in the most significant window of opportunity and stage of readiness of a smoker to quit. One such program consisted of 5 weeks of counseling (McDaniel, 1999). The mean time to deliver the intervention was 44 minutes. At 1 month, 70% of participants had continued to abstain. The mean cost of the intervention was approximately $50 a person.

Smoking cessation is the most cost-effective intervention for individuals with heart disease. Treatment of hyperlipidemia and referral to cardiac rehabilitation are highly cost-effective per quality-adjusted life-year and are relatively cost-effective per year of life saved. Smoking is an established risk factor for ischemic stroke, subarachnoid hemorrhage, and intracerebral hemorrhage (Kurth et al, 2003). The risk is directly proportional to the amount smoked. Risk-factor detection and management are the cornerstones of high-impact and high-quality care of cardiovascular disease.

Hypertension and Stroke

Hypertension is pandemic. Atherosclerosis and IHD are commonly associated with high blood pressure (Cucchiara & Kasner, 2002). The manifestations of IHD are increased in people with hypertension, including abnormal lipid profiles, hyperglycemia, increased fibrinogen, obesity, and abnormal electrocardiogram (ECG) readings (Kannel, 1990). These risks can be accentuated by cigarette smoking, elevated cholesterol levels, glucose intolerance, inactivity, and obesity (Shinton, 1997). Other serious consequences of hypertension include stroke and renal disease. Increased sympathetic reactivity has been implicated in the causes of stroke (Everson et al, 2001). Assessment of risk for hypertension is an important component of each patient's assessment. The management strategy should be based on an analysis of the overall risk assessment rather than on blood pressure alone. The prevention of hypertension requires more than normalization of the blood pressure if the deadly manifestations

---

BOX 1-1

Tobacco Facts and Multisystem Consequences of Smoking

Smoking is the single most important preventable cause of illness
  and death
Mortality from smoking:
  Tobacco causes 30% of all deaths of people between 35 and
    69 years of age
  Tobacco reduces a person's life as follows:
    Aged 35 to 59 years: Those killed by tobacco lose about
      27 years of life
    Aged 60 to 69 years: Those killed by tobacco lose about
      16 years of life
Brain:
  Stroke
Mouth:
  Lip and oral cancers
Pharynx and larynx:
  Cancers of the pharynx and larynx are more common in
    smokers
Esophagus:
  Cancer of the esophagus cancer is more common in smokers
Lungs:
  Cancer of the lungs is more common in smokers
Heart:
  Ischemic heart disease, hypertension and circulatory diseases
    are more common in smokers

Chronic lung disease:
  Bronchitis and emphysema; 90% of deaths from chronic lung
    disease attributable to smoking
  Upper respiratory tract infections and days of absenteeism are
    more common in smokers
Gastric and duodenal ulcers:
  Higher risk in smokers
Bladder and kidney cancers:
  Higher risk in smokers
Bone:
  Postmenopausal women who smoke have reduced bone
    density compared with nonsmokers
  Increased risk of bone fractures and delayed healing
Fertility and Pregnancy:
  Infertility
  Smoking increases the risk for spontaneous abortions, still
    births, pre-term deliveries, low-birth-weight babies, and
    sudden infant death syndrome
  Potential developmental and learning delays in children

Data from National Cancer Institute. Cancer Facts, 2005; U.S. Department of Health and Human Services. The Health Consequences of Smoking: A Report of the Surgeon General. U.S. Department of Health and Human Services, Centers for Disease Control and Prevention, National Center for Chronic Disease Prevention and Health Promotion, Office on Smoking and Health, 2004; Peto, R., Lopez, A.D., Boreham, J., Thun, M., & Heath, C. Jr. (1992). Mortality from tobacco in developed countries: indirect estimation based on national vital statistics. Lancet 339:1268-1278; Twardella, D., Kupper-Nybelen, J., Rothenbacher, D., Hahmann, H., Wusten, B., & Brenner, H. (2004). Short-term benefit of smoking cessation in patients with coronary artery disease: estimates based on self-reported smoking data and serum cotinine measurements. European Heart Journal 25:2101-2108.

of high blood pressure, including IHD, are to be avoided. Because of the dire consequences of hypertension the American Heart Association now advocates more stringent blood pressure limits, specifically less than 130/85 mm Hg, irrespective of age (American Heart Association, 2005).

In the adult population in the age range of 60 to 74 years, almost 75% of African Americans have high blood pressure as do 50% of Caucasians (Chobanian et al, 2003). As with heart disease, risk factors for high blood pressure consist of nonmodifiable and modifiable risk factors. Nonmodifiable risk factors include age, gender, race, and other genetic factors. Modifiable risk factors include diets high in sodium and low in potassium, alcohol consumption, reduced physical activity, and being overweight (Slama et al, 2002). Obesity is a strong predictor of hypertension (Shaper, 1996). Although significant reduction of hypertension has been attributed to low-dosage thiazide diuretics and beta blockers, the first line of defense to prevent high blood pressure and normalize blood pressure should be nutritional approaches, weight reduction, and exercise (Hamilton & Hamilton, 1997). In individuals whose hypertension is controlled, the combination of a Mediterranean diet and physical activity can significantly reduce health risk (Pitsavos et al, 2002). Like other diseases of civilization, hypertension is increasingly common in children and should

be included in routine pediatric assessments (National Institutes of Health, 2004).

Although weight reduction is an essential component of hypertension prevention and management, the protective effect of physical activity may be unrelated to the degree of obesity (Hu et al, 2004). A 4% to 8% reduction in body weight can reduce blood pressure by 3 mm Hg, and physical activity can reduce blood pressure by 5/3 mm Hg (Costa, 2002). In normotensive African American men, aerobic exercise can attenuate an exaggerated blood pressure response (Bond et al, 2002). Similarly, normotensive fit African American women have blunted blood pressure responses to experimental stressors (Jackson & Dishman, 2002). One study reported no relationship between physical activity and hypertension, flow-mediated dilation of the brachial artery, or an index of angiogenesis assessed with plasma vascular endothelial growth factor (the latter two being indicators of endothelial dysfunction) (Felmeden et al, 2003). In this study, however, physical activity was based on self-report in a questionnaire rather than on fitness outcomes, so the results of the study are difficult to interpret.

Stroke is a preventable tragedy for nearly 750,000 people a year in the United States; hypertension is the most common risk factor (Kirshner, 2003). Although lowering blood pressure below 130/85 mm Hg is well accepted across age, the success of blood pressure control has been reported to be less than 25% in the hypertensive population (Chalmers & Chapman, 2001). Stroke risk is far from being well controlled despite considerable understanding of its causes, and it remains a major health threat. Risk factors for stroke include previous stroke, hypertension, IHD, atrial fibrillation, hyperlipidemia, diabetes, abnormal ankle-to-brachial pressure index, reduced exercise endurance, retinopathy, albuminuria, autonomic neuropathy, smoking, alcohol consumption, and lack of exercise (Cohen et al, 2003; Hart & Halperin, 1999; Kirshner, 2003; Kurl et al, 2003; Piravej & Wiwatkul, 2003). Walking as short a time as 2 hours a week can reduce the risk of stroke by 50% (Costa, 2002). With respect to nutrition, high sodium and low potassium have been implicated in hypertension and stroke, as have lipids. Low plasma vitamin C is associated with a several-fold increased risk of stroke, particularly in men who are overweight and hypertensive (Kurl et al, 2002). A minimal reduction in diastolic blood pressure (5 to 6 mm Hg) reduces the risk of stroke by 35% to 40% (Sleight, 1991). Thus, weight control; regular exercise; a diet rich in fruits, vegetables, and whole-grain cereals; smoking cessation; and blood pressure control are central to stroke prevention as well as to the comprehensive management of stroke.

To affect the health of the population, stroke prevention depends on the dissemination of these well-established and widely available interventions to a large number of people. Advice given by a health provider to individuals with stroke for the purpose of prevention of a second stroke has a significant impact. In one study, individuals were simply advised to eat fewer high-fat and high-cholesterol foods and to exercise more (Greenland et al, 2002). Compared with a control group that received no advice, those receiving advice reported fewer days with limited activity, fewer days that "were not good physically", and more "healthy" days. The results of this study are compelling in that even simple advice by a health care provider can have a major impact on important health behaviors and on potential health outcomes.

Physical activity and optimal nutrition can reduce the risk of early atherosclerosis in lifelong nonsmokers (Luedemann et al, 2002). Smokers do not show this protective effect. Physical activity seems not only to reduce the risk of stroke but also can provide a potent prophylactic strategy for increasing blood flow and reducing brain injury during cerebral ischemia (Endres et al, 2003). A possible mechanism is augmented endothelium-dependent vasodilation via up-regulation of endothelial nitric oxide synthase in the vasculature. Aerobic exercise three times a week reduces cerebral infarct size and functional deficits in a mouse model and improves endothelium-dependent vasorelaxation (Endres et al, 2003).

Recommendations by the American Heart Association concerning physical activity and exercise guidelines for survivors of stroke concur that physical conditioning is a primary goal in these individuals, who have to contend with both the pathologic effects of stroke and the effects of deconditioning (Gordon et al, 2004). Improved conditioning may help to reduce limitations of activity and participation and hence improve quality of life. The burden of disease and disability and their risk factors may be correspondingly reduced.

Type 2 Diabetes and Metabolic Syndrome

Type 2 diabetes is a serious multisystem condition that has rapidly become pandemic in Western countries and in some other countries where previously its incidence was minimal. In addition to its serious physical and functional consequences, perceived health status and quality of life are compromised (Gregg et al, 2002). By 2010, an estimated 250 million people will be affected worldwide (Turtle, 2000). Formerly known as adult-onset diabetes, type 2 diabetes is now being diagnosed in children, predisposing them to blindness, heart disease, stroke, renal disease, peripheral neuropathies, vascular insufficiency, and amputations (Abraham, 2004; Ten & MacLaren, 2004). Inositol is a poison that forms on the membranes of cells in the presence of high blood sugar, and it has been implicated in the deadly systemic consequences of diabetes. The primary consequences include pathologic changes to the macrovasculature and microvasculature and to the nerve endings. Impaired glucose tolerance is a marker of vascular complications in the large and small blood vessels, independent of an individual's progression to diabetes. Early detection of glucose intolerance allows intensive dietary and exercise modifications, which have been shown to be more effective than drug therapy in normalizing postprandial glucose and inhibiting progression to diabetes (Singleton et al, 2003). Diabetic autonomic neuropathy as an independent risk factor for stroke may reflect increased vascular damage and effect on the regulation of cerebral blood flow in individuals with diabetes (Cohen et al, 2003).

Individuals with type 2 diabetes mellitus have increased risk for cardiovascular disease compared with individuals without diabetes, so strict control is mandatory. Moderate physical activity, including a faster walking pace (Hu et al, 2001), along with weight loss is a powerful combination to reduce the risk of type 2 diabetes, as well as to reverse it. These interventions combined with a balanced diet can reduce the risk of developing diabetes among those who are at high risk by 50% to 60% (Bauman, 2004). Cigarette smoking is an independent risk factor for type 2 diabetes (Wannamethee et al, 2001) and is particularly dangerous for individuals with diabetes (Abraham, 2004).

Metabolic syndrome refers to a virulent and lethal group of atherosclerotic risk factors, including dyslipidemia, obesity, hypertension, and insulin resistance, and it affects some 47 million people in the United States (Scott, 2003). The incidence of the syndrome is increasing and warrants aggressive noninvasive management. Insulin sensitivity is predicted primarily by body mass index, smoking, age, and daily physical activity. Weight reduction counters the effects of metabolic syndrome and may counter the associated hypertension and dyslipidemia as well. Diet and exercise are primary components of the multifactorial approach to prevention and management of this lethal condition.

Obesity

Obesity has doubled over the past decade; 61% of the American population is overweight (Keller & Lemberg, 2003). Obesity is becoming a global pandemic that rivals malnutrition as a health priority in some low-income countries (World Health Organization, 1998), and it contributes to health risks for all diseases of civilization. The complications and risks for which each patient should be assessed include IHD, cardiac myopathy, and chronic heart failure; hypertension and stroke; some cancers; insulin insensitivity and type 2 diabetes mellitus; gall bladder disease; dyslipidemia; osteoarthritis and gout; and pulmonary diseases, including alveolar hypoventilation and sleep apnea (Anonymous, 2000; Grundy, 2002; Hu, 2003; Kannel et al, 2002; Tanaka & Nakanishi, 1996). With each kilogram of weight over normal, the risk for hypertension, heart disease, and diabetes can increase proportionately. Obesity is commonly linked with insulin resistance and high blood pressure, which may reflect reduced activity and exercise. Reduced physical activity is a significant predictor of obesity (Wenche et al, 2004). Insulin resistance associated with lack of exercise in people who are overweight may be further compounded by insulin resistance associated with chronic inflammation observed in fat cells (Xu et al, 2003). Abdominal obesity, lipid metabolism, and insulin resistance are interrelated markers for coronary artery disease (Frayne, 2002). In addition to cardiovascular and general health risk, being overweight affects quality of life (Eckel & Krauss, 1998; Trakas et al, 2001).

Comprehensive care of an individual who is overweight and has abnormal blood sugar levels includes normalization of blood sugar (with recommendations for low-glycemic foods and small, frequent snacks rather than infrequent large meals), weight reduction, trans-fat and saturated-fat restriction, strict blood pressure and lipid control, regular physical activity and exercise, and avoidance of tobacco (Wilson & Kannel, 2002).

Nutritional habits during childhood are associated with diseases in adulthood (Caballero, 2001). Obesity in children is associated with parental obesity (Paterno, 2003). Maintaining weight within a healthy body mass index range throughout life is recommended for optimal health. As a tool, however, the body mass index is limited with respect to assessing adiposity because it fails to discriminate between muscle and fat and identify regional adipose depositions (Liu & Manson, 2001). Physical therapy has a primary role in preventing and managing obesity in every client or patient, irrespective of age, given obesity's serious multisystem consequences, psychosocial sequelae, and threat to life participation and satisfaction (Racette et al, 2003).

Cancer

The risk factors for cancer are well documented and include environmental and behavioral factors, such as nutrition (fats and low fiber), inactivity, poor air quality and smoking, psychological factors, and ingestion of and exposure to chemicals. Cancer, hallmarked by an overgrowth of cells, eventually compromises normal organ function. Cancer prevention and rehabilitation have become a specialty that requires an integrated knowledge of pathophysiology, psychosocial implications, and management interventions (Glassman et al, 2001; Rashbaum et al, 2001). To date, evidence that walking is a strategy to prevent cancer has been best established for colon cancer (Bauman, 2004).

Cancers associated with the highest mortality rates include lung cancer, colorectal cancer, breast cancer, and prostate cancer (Centers for Disease Control and Prevention, 2002). Smoking has been implicated as a risk factor for many cancers, not only those involving the respiratory tract. The role of lifestyle factors in cancer remission has not been studied in detail.

Musculoskeletal Health

Osteoporosis and arthritis may lead to considerable morbidity and secondarily to mortality. Because both have lifestyle components, a risk-factor review to provide a baseline should be included in every initial assessment. Moderate levels of physical activity, including walking, are associated with a substantially lower risk of hip fractures in postmenopausal women (Feskanich et al, 2002). Thus, risk factor assessment of both nonmodifiable and modifiable risks is a major component of the health assessment as a means of minimizing morbidity and potential mortality (APTA, 2001). Osteoporosis and associated morbidity, particularly in older age groups, is a serious health issue that warrants monitoring. Establishing baseline information on bone health in every patient is prudent, given the relationship between lifestyle behaviors (e.g., activity and nutrition—heavy consumption of meat, alcohol, and coffee, and smoking) and bone health. Although older, postmenopausal women have been the focus of bone health studies, other groups are also at risk for osteoporosis and should not be overlooked: older men; inactive children, particularly girls; and individuals with chronic conditions who may be less able to undertake weight-bearing activities and physical activity. In a study of the development of bone mass and strength in girls and young women, only exercise (not daily calcium intake) was associated with bone density and strength (Lloyd et al, 2004). This finding stresses the singular importance of bone building in young people to help offset osteoporosis later in life.

Psychological Health

Mental health problems and depression are prevalent in Western society despite its affluence. Based on one descriptive study, individuals with other mental health conditions such as schizophrenia have poor physical health and die prematurely of cardiovascular disease (McCreadie et al, 2003). Compared with women who have schizophrenia, men with the condition consumed less fruit, vegetables, whole grains, and rice than recommended. Further, the incidence of smoking and obesity in both sexes was higher than in the general population. Cholesterol levels were high and activity levels low. This study suggested cause for concern about both the physical and psychological well-being of individuals with mental health problems and indicated the need for further investigation of the physical health and well-being of persons with mental challenges.

Dementia and Alzheimer disease appear to be increasing. This trend may reflect the aging of the population, lifestyle factors, and improved awareness and detection of these conditions. The factors that have been associated with Alzheimer disease also decrease cerebral blood flow (Krill & Halliday, 2001). Understanding the vascular component of this disease will be an important advance in its prevention and management. In a cohort of older African Caribbean individuals, vascular risk has been associated with cognitive impairment and physical activity is inversely related to impaired cognition (Stewart et al, 2001). Exercise training has been reported to improve physical health and depression in individuals with Alzheimer disease (Teri et al, 2003). Whether this reflects a vascular component of the pathogenesis of the disease that is offset by exercise warrants elucidation.

Dental Health

Periodontitis, characterized by low-grade infection of the gums, is widespread and may be associated with serious systemic health problems. In a study of 39,461 men, periodontitis risk decreased with increased physical activity, independent of such risk factors as age, smoking, diabetes, body mass index, alcohol consumption, and total calories (Merchant et al, 2003). Inactivity and the typical Western diet have been described as proinflammatory. Whether the benefits of a physically active lifestyle and an optimal diet can extend to dental health in general warrants investigation.

Promoting Healthy Living: The Contemporary Physical Therapist's Role

Lifestyle changes have an unequivocal effect on the prevention of the diseases of civilization. They have the potential to reduce the population's health risk and thereby contain the economic cost of these leading killers (Fletcher et al, 1996). Knowledge of healthy patterns can be put into practice in every patient interaction (Giannuzzi et al, 2003). Increased consumption of meat, fat, and sugar has contributed to the increased prevalence of the diseases of civilization in low- and middle-income countries, as well as in high-income countries (Larsen, 2003). An associated increase in the prevalence of insulin-resistance syndromes is further increasing the incidence of cardiovascular disease (Nesto, 2003). Anthropologists have argued that food abundance and inactivity may be altering evolutionary processes and that these factors further contribute to the current pandemic of chronic disease (Chakravarthy & Booth, 2004). Attitudes toward the factors contributing to the diseases of civilization reflect the values and behaviors of society, and optimal control will be achieved only with widespread social action, involving health care providers, and with an increase in individual responsibility.

Why Physical Therapists Need to Understand and Advocate Optimal Nutrition

Physical therapists use exercise as a primary intervention to prevent, remediate, or mitigate the effects of disease and disability. As clinical exercise physiologists, they must have a substantial understanding of healthy nutrition, nutritional assessment, and nutritional regimens that will maximize human performance in patient populations who are not unlike athletes, as well as maximize good health. Without this knowledge, assessment and exercise prescription are suboptimal and, in turn, therapeutic outcomes are suboptimal.

Given that an association has been established between diet and chronic disease, the question of what the optimal nutritional regimen is for humans has been widely debated. The anatomic structure and physiologic (endocrine) function of humans is consistent with an organism designed for a largely plant-based diet, that is, having hands rather than claws, a particular tooth type and skin type, salivary glands, acidity in the saliva, ptyalin in the saliva, a specific level of hydrochloric acid in the stomach, and an intestinal tract of a certain length (Sorenson, 1992).

Cultures that consume a diet based primarily on plants have superior health outcomes. The diets of octogenarians in Asia and of centenarians in general tend to be low in saturated and trans fats and refined sugar and high in fiber as compared with the diets of Western people (Sanders, 2003). Recently, the Mediterranean diet, which includes fruits, vegetables, fish, and vegetable oil, has shown health benefits and has been associated with lower incidence of chronic disability and premature death compared with the typical Western diet (Pitsavos et al, 2002; Pitsavos et al, 2004). Cultures in that area also tend to have higher activity levels, and that influences metabolism and physiological responses to food.

Weight-loss diets are a multibillion dollar industry in Western cultures. Many are unsubstantiated or may theoretically work but are not well balanced in terms of macronutrients and micronutrients that are needed on a daily basis for optimal health. Low-carbohydrate diets have been popular, but weight loss associated with these diets results from calorie restriction and the duration of the diet rather than from a reduction in carbohydrate consumption (Astrup et al, 2004). Weight control is achieved by the balance between optimal caloric and nutrient content consumed and optimal energy expenditure. Given the pandemic of obesity in industrialized countries, physical therapists need to understand the normal physiologic adaptations to poor food choices and sedentary lifestyles— weight distribution, endocrine changes, cardiopulmonary changes, and musculoskeletal changes—in order to prescribe the best lifelong management programs.

Obesity has become a life-threatening pandemic that warrants management before the manifestation of one or more of its deadly consequences, in addition to its associated psychosocial and economic consequences. Along with obesity, glucose intolerance may complicate the picture, or the patient may have subclinical intolerance. Central adiposity, in particular, has been associated with a high incidence of insulin resistance, which may explain the high rates of dyslipidemia, hypertension, and diabetes in these individuals (Ferreira et al, 2002). Thus the physical therapist has a primary role in basic nutrition counseling, commensurate with the promotion of optimal health, and in providing information about nutrition (related to exercise energetics and glucose control) to support a prescribed dosage of regular exercise and physical activity. A nutritionist may have to be consulted to provide nutrition counseling beyond fundamental needs, especially in complicated cases.

Nutrition guidelines have been revised by the U.S. Department of Agriculture (2005) and Health Canada (2005). Compared with previous versions, the revisions are more closely aligned with the literature than with the interests of lobby groups from the food industry, nutrient supplement producers, and organic food producers. Some authorities have argued that the current pandemic of the diseases of civilization reflects adherence to guidelines over which food-industry lobbyists had significant influence, rather than lack of adherence by consumers. Contemporary consumption of fats and refined foods and of vegetables, for example, has failed to meet the recommended revised guidelines. Diets high in refined foods and fat and low in servings of fruit and vegetables have been implicated in the diseases of civilization.

The revised guidelines are more evidence based and are designed to optimize health and reduce the risk of chronic diseases. Earlier guidelines fell short with respect to this objective. Adherence to established dietary guidelines for Americans as assessed by the healthy eating index was only weakly associated with risk for major chronic conditions in men (McCullough et al, 2000a) and was not associated at all with risk for major chronic conditions in women (McCullough et al, 2000b). Thus dietary guidelines and the healthy eating index require further refinement to achieve more favorable outcomes and to allow them to be assessed.

An optimal food pyramid, on which the revised nutrition guidelines are based, is shown in Figure 1-1, *A*. The pyramid illustrates general guidelines for optimizing health in the general public, and these guidelines have been shown to offset the diseases of civilization (Polidori, 2003). Each individual's diet should conform with these guidelines for optimal lifelong health. The nutrition food pyramid emphasizes abundant servings of vegetables at the base; followed by vegetable or lean-meat protein sources and dairy; beans, lentils, and whole grains; and low-glycemia foods. Red meat and eggs, positioned at the top of the pyramid, are to be consumed most sparingly. The typical Western diet is short on vegetables, fruits, and fiber (particularly insoluble fiber) (Liu et al, 2000a; Liu et al, 2000b; Shike, 1999) and includes excessive amounts of highly refined foods and saturated and trans fats (McBurney, 2001). Diets high in grain-based foods are associated with reduced cardiovascular risk, independent of other behaviors (McBurney, 2001; McKeown et al, 2002). Unless a person has an objectively identified deficit, there is no evidence that nutrient supplementation adds benefit to a daily nutritious diet.

Attention to nutrition is important not only in relation to body weight. Cholesterol and tryiglycerides are risk factors for IHD (Giles et al, 1996). To address this major health threat, lipid-lowering drugs have glutted the pharmaceutical market and one-stop coronary cholesterol clinics have been advertised. However, a cardioprotective diet, which has been well described in the literature, should be the goal, in conjunction with lipid-lowering agents in selected cases. Even when these medications are used, weaning individuals off them as lipids and cholesterol are lowered by noninvasive means is an important goal of physical therapy, in conjunction with a lifelong program of exercise, good nutrition, no smoking, moderate alcohol consumption, and stress management.

Why Physical Therapists Need to Understand Exercise in the Context of Population Health

The physical activity and exercise pyramid is shown in Figure 1-1, *B*. This pyramid has a physically active lifestyle at the base, followed by aerobic exercise three to five times a week, followed by strengthening exercise and flexibility, with rest and inactivity at the top. The physical activity pyramid and the food pyramid are good reminders of the priority of each for optimal health (Foss & Keteyian, 1998). Generally, 10,000 steps a day is consistent with an active lifestyle and good health in an adult (Tudor-Locke & Bassett, 2004). Fewer than 5000 steps a day is consistent with a sedentary lifestyle, and 7500 to 99,999 steps a day is consistent with a somewhat active lifestyle. More than 12,500 steps a day is consistent with a highly active lifestyle.

With increased physical activity, the risks for IHD, stroke, and colon cancer are reduced. The precise dosage-response relationships between physical activity and health and between physical fitness and health have yet to be clarified and may differ among people (Blair et al, 2001). Moderate physical activity, which does not have to be strenuous or prolonged, includes leisure activities such as walking and gardening and is associated with marked health benefits (Wannamethee & Shaper, 2001). Even light to moderate physical activity in middle and old age confers significant benefit to cardiovascular health and is protective against all-cause mortality (Katzmarzyk et al, 2000). The U.S. Surgeon General recommends 30 minutes of moderately intense exercise on most days, with an accumulated duration of 180 minutes a week (Gunnarsson & Judge, 1997).

Exercise has a profound effect on the endothelial function of blood, which has been implicated in atherosclerosis, IHD, cerebrovascular disease, and gastrointestinal conditions, and could explain exercise's multisystem benefits. Moderate levels of physical activity reduce the risk of stroke, independent of other factors (Lee & Blair, 2002). In addition to dietary habits, reduced physical activity has been implicated in all the diseases of civilization, including osteoporosis, and exercise is recognized as an essential component in their primary prevention. Even mild physical activity has an important role in the primary prevention of type 2 diabetes mellitus through its direct effect on increased tissue sensitivity to insulin

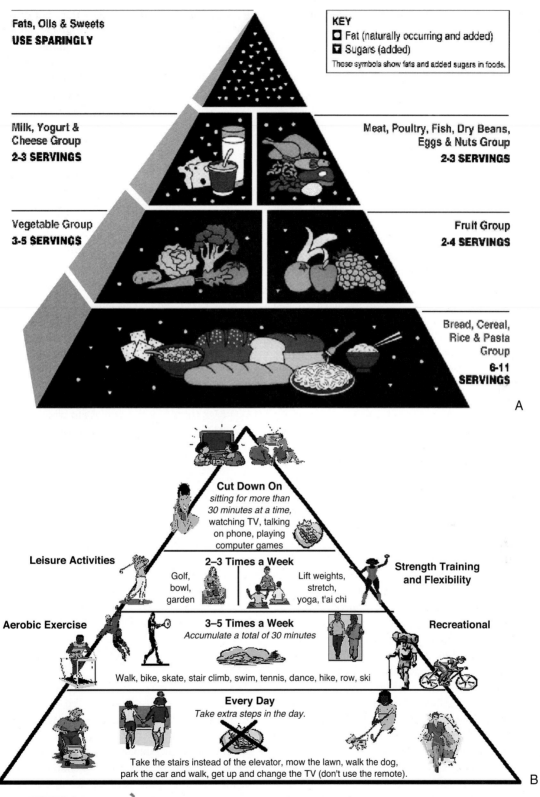

FIGURE 1-1 A, Nutrition pyramid. Limit highly glycemic foods (e.g., sugar and added sugar), pastries, sweets, refined carbohydrates, trans fats, highly preserved and highly processed foods. Include 5 to 8 glasses of water daily. **B,** Physical activity and exercise pyramid. Rest is an important component. Daily physical activity should include 10,000 steps a day*; a minimum accumulated 30 minutes of aerobic exercise three times a week; two to three sessions per week of 20 to 30 minutes of strength training; management of daily stress; breathing of clean air (no active or passive smoking); and several hours of restful sleep daily.

(**A** *Adapted from the U.S Department of Agriculture and the U.S. Department of Health and Human Services*).

*Tudor-Locke, 2004.

(Sato, 2000). Nonpharmacological interventions for the prevention and management of hypertension have been strongly advocated to maximize their therapeutic benefit and to minimize the risks of medications (Orozco-Valero, 2002). Furthermore, in older people, regular physical activity has an important role in preventing chronic disease and prolonged end-of-life suffering (Messinger-Rapport & Sprecher, 2002).

Why Physical Therapists Should Promote Smoking Cessation

Smoking is the leading cause of death. It results in premature death and higher rates of all-cause death (Mokdad et al, 2004). Although Caucasian Americans have a higher rate of smoking than do African Americans, African Americans and women who smoke have significant respiratory problems at a younger age, despite having started smoking later and having a lower overall pack-year smoking history (Chatila et al, 2004). Men with a strong intention to quit have been reported to have a more favorable attitude toward quitting and a stronger sense of perceived control than those with a less strong intention to quit. In addition, men who had a strong intention to quit smoking had greater success (Nguyen et al, 1998). Advocating smoking reduction and cessation is an important responsibility of the physical therapist, regardless of the patient's problems, with a view to promoting lifelong health.

Over time, smoking cessation can reverse many of the lethal effects of smoking (see Boxes 1-1 and 1-2). For smokers unable to quit, advocating "competing" health strategies has been proposed (Naslund et al, 1996a). Improved diets and increased physical activity and exercise, however, do not counter the negative effects of smoking (Luedemann et al, 2002).

Why Physical Therapists Must Understand Ethnic and Cultural Differences

Industrialized countries are becoming increasingly ethnically and culturally diverse as large numbers of people migrate across the globe, particularly to high-income countries where the diseases of civilization are prevalent. With birth rates on the decline in these countries, immigration is being encouraged. Thus the role and impact of ethnicity and culture as important factors influencing health, ill health, use of health care services, the types of health education that are needed, and the ways in which they should be disseminated must be understood (Kromhout et al, 2002).

The prevalence of and the mortality rates associated with COPD increase with age, and the rates are higher in Caucasians than in other ethnic groups in North America (Chatila et al, 2004). Among people with advanced COPD, however, African Americans and women are more prone than other groups to the adverse effects of tobacco smoke. Cardiovascular disease in Mexican Americans and Native American Indians is a particular concern, and it has implications for optimal care and service delivery (Luepker, 2001; North et al, 2003; Storey et al, 2003). Obesity, hypertension, and the metabolic syndrome are also more prevalent in these groups,

---

BOX 1-2

Health Benefits of Quitting Smoking

Immediate Benefits

Family	Quitting smoking removes harmful environmental tobacco smoke that pollutes nonsmokers' breathing space
Individual	Your body starts to heal itself; the levels of carbon monoxide and nicotine in your system decline rapidly; heart rate and blood pressure drop quickly; peripheral circulation improves

Benefits after 1 Year

Increased risk for ischemic heart disease decreases 50%

Benefits after 3 Years

Risk for heart disease declines to levels similar to those of lifelong nonsmokers

Benefits after 5 Years

Risk for cancers of the oral cavity and esophagus reduced by 50%
Risk for bladder cancer reduced by about 50%
Risk for stroke can return to levels similar to those of nonsmokers
Risk for cervical cancer is significantly reduced

Benefits after 10 Years

Risk for lung cancer decreases 50% to 70%

Benefits after 15 Years

Risk for ischemic heart disease is similar to that of lifelong nonsmokers
Risk for death is similar to that of lifelong nonsmokers

Data from the American Cancer Society, 2004; U.S. Department of Health and Human Services. The Health Consequences of Smoking: A Report of the Surgeon General. U.S. Department of Health and Human Services, Centers for Disease Control and Prevention, National Center for Chronic Disease Prevention and Health Promotion, Office on Smoking and Health, 2004; American Lung Association. http://www.lungusa.org/site/pp.asp?c=dv LUK9O0E&b=22938; Manson, J.E., Tosteson, H., Ridker, P.M., Satterfield, S., Hebert, P., O'Connor, G.T., Buring, J.E., & Hennekens, C.H. (1992). The primary prevention of myocardial infarction. New England Journal of Medicine 326:1406-1416.

---

so their special needs should be recognized by physical therapists. Currently, Eastern Europe, the Middle East, and Asia have the highest smoking prevalence in the world.

The health advantages that people of other cultures enjoy in their homelands (Asians, for example) are compromised when they immigrate to Western countries and adopt Western dietary and exercise habits (Egusa et al, 2002; Goel et al, 2004; Wahlqvist et al, 2002a). Although they may benefit from improved health services and access, the diseases of civilization exact more of a toll on new immigrants with each passing year. The physical therapist has a unique role as health educator in promoting optimal lifestyle practices in new immigrants as well as in long-term residents.

People from Utah, 72% of whom are Mormon by faith and follow a strict lifestyle code, have among the best health indexes in the country and some of the lowest rates of chronic disease (LaMonte et al, 2000), but ethnic minorities in Utah are at increased risk of heart disease and stroke, among other conditions. Designing preventive and management strategies requires responding to the needs of different groups. A training program designed specifically for African Americans with stroke and complex comorbidities can be highly effective in improving fitness and reducing risk for further disease and disability (Rimmer et al, 2000). Racial differences have been documented with respect to the interactions of obesity, hypertension, and diabetes between African American and European American women (Dubbert et al, 2002). Greater emphasis must be placed on targeting risk factors in various ethnic and cultural groups. For example, alcohol consumption in Caucasian Americans and weight control in African Americans and Caribbean groups are among the targeted priorities (Dundas et al, 2001). For each individual, the severity of the problem, the risks, and the willingness to change must be assessed to effectively target management strategies. Sensitivity to cultural as well as to individual differences when designing health-education strategies, is essential to the long-term success of the intervention.

Cultural differences in self-reports of body functioning have been described (Owens et al, 2002). These differences, as well as low education status, have explained the overrating of functional status in self-reports when they are compared with objective measures of performance. These observations support the need for greater cultural sensitivity and awareness in the clinic, particularly when the patient belongs to a minority group and the therapist is part of the dominant Caucasian American group. These findings support the need for objective functional assessment in addition to self-reported functional status.

Another important cultural factor in health care is the reporting of discomfort and pain, which affect activity and participation. Studies have looked at the expression of pain and the responses of health care providers to the pain expressed by people from cultures different from those of the health care provider. In addition to cultural differences in pain expression, patients from cultures that are highly expressive in expressing discomfort and pain have been reported to receive less analgesia and fewer pain control interventions than individuals who are less expressive, a characteristic consistent with the dominant culture (Cleeland et al, 1997; Todd et al, 1993).

Physical Therapists as Agents of Change in Health Behaviors

Direct patient access is fast becoming a reality for physical therapists worldwide. With this trend comes the additional responsibility of knowing whom not to treat as well as whom to treat. The physical therapist may be the entry to health care for many, so she or he must consider the patient's overall health and risk factors in addition to focusing on the specific

physical problem that brought the patient to physical therapy. Even if the patient has been referred for physical therapy, the therapist has a responsibility to ensure that the patient's health status is optimal so as to maximize the patient's response to treatment and to address factors contributing to the patient's other complaints, which may be the more serious and important considerations. In a direct-access model of health care delivery, the physical therapist needs to know what is not amenable to noninvasive physical therapy management and, in such cases, should have the patient referred back to or managed concurrently with an invasive medical care practitioner.

Based on the discordance between the extant knowledge of the diseases of civilization and health-promoting lifestyles, health care has failed to significantly reduce the prevalence of these diseases and their risk factors. The issue of why people do not always make appropriate lifestyle choices is of central importance to their health and to the practice of the health care provider. Patients may be more inclined to make follow-up visits to their health care providers than to change their lifestyles (Bergman & Bertero, 2001). One explanation for the failure of conventional models of health education (Baxter et al, 1997; Cupples & McKnight, 1999; Egan, 1999; Joseph et al, 1999; Nisbeth et al, 2000; Rausch & Turkoski, 1999; Sumanen et al, 2004) is that traditionally they have been based on a unidirectional model of information delivery—that is, from the health care provider (a dominant person) to the individual or patient (a subordinate person), in the form of brochures, books, videos, magazine articles, and television and radio announcements. These formats typically are not well targeted to a specific demographic or to the needs of the learner. Smoking cessation programs, for example, have been reported to be more effective when targeted to the specific needs of middle-aged men, including resources that promote a perceived sense of control over health behavior (Nguyen et al, 1996). Changes in behavior are effected most successfully in a personal, bidirectional model, including rapport building, trust, commitment, and follow-up. Other important factors include receptivity, susceptibility, beliefs, timing, message delivery, barriers, reinforcers, and external stimulus-control factors (Guise, 2000). Such a strategy is the so-called AIM approach: Assess the learner, Identify barriers to learning, and Motivate the individual to make change (Kingsbury, 1998).

People may not be receptive to health information because they do not recognize the seriousness of the concern and they find their health behavior is more rewarding to them than is punishing. Cardiovascular disease is the leading cause of death in women, particularly those over 60 years of age. This cohort of women believes they are at low risk for heart attack, yet 82% of coronary events in women are explained by the absence of a low-risk lifestyle (Carlsson & Stein, 2002). Although women may respond favorably to risk-reduction initiatives, their awareness of risk factors and prevention strategies may be poor (McPherson, 2000). When health information (low-fat vegetarian diet, exercise, smoking cessation, and stress management) is delivered in a highly supportive group environment, in innovative multiple formats (e.g., a retreat and group meetings), people make sustainable lifestyle changes that reduce health-risk factors, decrease the need for medication, and improve the quality of life (Billings, 2000; Toobert et al, 2000). Furthermore, health education is more effective when cultural differences that affect health beliefs, attitudes, and behaviors are considered (Khattab et al, 1999; Kok et al, 1982; Nakamura et al, 2003).

Understanding poor adherence to health behavior change is as important as understanding the factors contributing to good adherence. In healthy middle-aged men at increased risk for IHD, for example, poor adherence to the recommendation to increase dietary fiber is related to smoking, high hostility levels, perception of barriers to diet change, and poor knowledge of risk factors (Naslund et al, 1996b). Poor adherence to following a low-fat diet is related to smoking, younger age, and having no family members or friends with heart disease. Poor adherence to an exercise program is associated with younger age and having small children at home. Such information for various target groups is important in planning effective health-education interventions. The results of studies, however, are based on group outcomes. Individual assessments are needed to determine the barriers to and facilitators of learning for each person. The physical therapist must anticipate that these may change for an individual over time.

Education is common to every patient's management, with the possible exception of those who are unconscious, severely mentally challenged, or cognitively incapable of responding to the information. Even in these cases, education of the attending health care providers and care givers can be the priority. The success of health education reflects the individual's expectations (Lau-Walker, 2004). Most physical therapists and other health care providers have little background in assessing expectations. Physical therapists would benefit from formal education in assessing the learners' needs and wants, expectations, and readiness to learn and implement positive changes in their behaviors. Varying expectations may be particularly important when the patient is from a culture different from that of the physical therapist.

Various theories have been proposed to explain people's health choices and to promote improved choices. One such theory is the theory of reasoned action or planned behavior (Azjen, 1983). Based on this theory, an individual's decision to engage in a healthy behavior such as exercise is based on his or her intention. Intention is a function of the person's attitudes, perceived control and self-efficacy, and social factors. The elements of the McEwen model of health motivation are comparable and have been applied to effect positive lifestyle changes in individuals participating in cardiac rehabilitation (Demarais & Robichaud-Ekstrand, 1998). The assessment includes the individual's current knowledge, perceived severity, perceived susceptibility, perceived value of action, background variables, internal and external aids and hindrances, and the catalyst factors. Understanding the factors that affect an individual's lifestyle choices is vital for targeting health education so as to produce sustained outcomes.

BOX 1-3

Prochaska's Stages of Readiness to Change

Precontemplation

- Not currently engaged in the target behavior
- Not seriously thinking of change in the next 6 months
- Unaware of the need to change or denies the need to change

Contemplation

- Not currently engaged in the behavior
- Seriously considering making a change within the next 6 months
- Acknowledges that the behavior is unhealthy
- Seeks out information regarding the pros and cons of changing

Preparation

- Planning to change within the next 30 days
- Has attempted to change in the previous year
- On the verge of taking action to change behavior
- Begins to reevaluate self in light of the new behavior

Action

- Engaged in the desired behavior
- Has implemented the change only in the past 6 months
- Tries the behavior but is at high risk for relapse

Maintenance

- Has maintained the behavior for 6 months

An individual can be at different stages for different health behaviors.

The transtheoretical model of "readiness to change behavior" (Prochaska & DiClementi, 1982) outlines several behavioral-change stages, including precontemplative, contemplative, preparation, action, and maintenance. In designing health-promotion education programs, this model helps to identify the stage of readiness to change, so that interventions can be tailored to and timed with an individual's readiness to interact with the information, thereby enhancing outcomes. The five stages of change are shown in Box 1-3. Key questions can be asked to establish the stage at which an individual may be in terms of readiness to change (Box 1-4).

A study of change in exercise behavior employing the transtheoretical model in sedentary women compared psychological variables and the capacity for a moderate or vigorous exercise program, either at home or at a center, to effect change in their exercise habits over 18 months (Cox et al, 2003). Self-efficacy for exercise competence increased as women moved from the contemplative to the action stage and was particularly marked in the groups involved in vigorous exercise. Almost half of the women shifted from the action stage to the maintenance stage. The intervention was effective regardless of the setting and the intensity of the exercise program.

When patients are in the preparation and action stages, the physical therapist can teach a range of self-monitoring

---

BOX 1-4

Assessing Readiness to Change by Using a Quiz

The *Stage of Readiness to Change* model is designed to help people adopt new health behaviors. Knowing the readiness to change stage helps you to understand the steps you should take to move to subsequent stages to achieve lifelong sustainable health behaviors.

Circle a response to each question using the "Y" or the "N."

Y = Yes, I meet my health objective on this question.
N = For each "N" you circle, circle the readiness to change number.
1 = not thinking about change at this time (precontemplative)
2 = thinking about change (contemplative)
3 = preparing to change (preparation)

Readiness to Change Checklist	Response			Readiness to Change	
Do you exercise moderately intensely at least 3 times a week for 20 to 40 minutes?	Y	N	1	2	3
Are you physically active during your average day (walk, walk briskly, take stairs)?	Y	N	1	2	3
Is your weight within normal range?	Y	N	1	2	3
Do you eat at least 5 servings of fruit and vegetables daily?	Y	N	1	2	3
Do you minimize the trans and saturated fats in your diet?	Y	N	1	2	3
Do you minimize highly refined carbohydrates in your diet (sugar and white flour)?	Y	N	1	2	3
Do you drink alcohol less often than 5 times a week?	Y	N	1	2	3
Are you a nonsmoker?	Y	N	1	2	3
Are you generally relaxed during your day and do you feel in control?	Y	N	1	2	3

---

skills and recording strategies along with information about circulatory and heart disease, risk factors, and disease prevention. Blood pressure self-monitoring can be taught, provided the equipment is calibrated and checked by the physical therapist, standardized procedures are used, and the patient's measurement proficiency is evaluated (Mengden et al, 2000).

Psychological principles, including cognitive and behavior-modification strategies, are central to behavior change; they include stimulus control and events antecedent to the behavior, the reinforcement of the behavior, and consequent events (Wierenga & Oldham, 2002). Shaping, feedback, and reinforcement schedules are powerful strategies. Complex behaviors such as lifestyle behaviors may be shaped by the introduction of small, progressive, easily achievable steps toward a larger goal, a process comparable to the integrated stepwise approach used to improve dietary habits (Srinath et al, 1995). These principles can be incorporated into a model of lifestyle modification that incorporates other factors such as culture (Guise, 2000; Wierenga & Oldham, 2002).

Education and effecting change in health behaviors are perhaps the most important components of the physical therapist's expertise because such change dramatically affects the lifelong health of each individual patient. Preventive health messages stated by a health care provider can be powerful, and they are a strong predictor of change in health behaviors (Nisbeth et al, 2000; Thomas et al, 2002; Tresch & Aronow, 1996; Winslow et al, 1996). Currently, however, preventive health messages are delivered to a relatively small number of patients by their health care providers. Thus lifestyle recommendations should be delivered as a holistic management priority to *every* patient, in a structured, conscious manner

comparable to the precision of a prescribed treatment program. The cumulative time the physical therapist spends with each patient over days, weeks, and years translates into hundreds of teachable moments. Multiplying this time spent annually in teachable moments by the number of physical therapists in the world indicates that the potential for having a societal impact and making a global assault on the diseases of civilization is enormous.

Sending a patient home with a brochure on exercise or telling a patient not to smoke has a low probability of producing lasting results or any results at all. The educational needs of the patient, in terms of receptivity to new information and to the styles of teaching and learning that are being used, must be established; otherwise, both the clinician and the patient are wasting their time. Educational needs are multifactorial; they include health beliefs, self-efficacy, readiness to change, and motivation. The transtheoretical model (Prochaska & DiClemente, 1982) of readiness to change (see Boxes 1-3 and 1-4) is valuable in demonstrating how to determine the patient's stage through appropriate questions and how to devise strategies for moving a patient from one stage to the next in a progression toward preparation, action, and maintenance. Self-efficacy is an important determinant of readiness to change and of one's capacity to effect and maintain a behavioral change (Meland et al, 1999). If the stage of readiness to change is considered when promoting healthy lifestyles, health coaching can be successful even if brief (Steptoe et al, 2001). The level of importance a person ascribes to a behavior and that person's sense of confidence that she or he can effect the change are the main determinants in whether the person will achieve the threshold level and make the change. Factors that contribute to this decision

TABLE 1-3

Health Behavior Change: Decision Balance Analysis

CHANGE	NO CHANGE
Benefits	Benefits
1.	1.
2.	2.
3.	3.
4.	4.
Costs	Costs
1.	1.
2.	2.
3.	3.
4.	4.

The individual is asked to weigh the benefits and costs of changing a given lifestyle behavior as opposed to. not changing that behavior at that point in time.
Modified from Marcus, B., Rossi, J., Selby, V., Miaura, R., & Adams, D. (1992). The stages and processes of exercise adoption and maintenance in a worksite sample. Health Psychology 11:386-395; Rollnick, S., Mason, P., & Butler, C. (2002). Health behavior change: a guide for practitioners. Philadelphia: Churchill Livingstone.

should be integral components of the assessment; they can be examined systematically, as outlined in Table 1-3. Decision balance analysis involves having the patient identify the benefits and costs of making a lifestyle change and of not making the change. This information is useful to the practitioner in directing and planning interventions that will effect changes in health behavior in an individual.

People in need of care, such as hospitalized patients, are a receptive and captive audience. They present prime opportunities to find teachable moments. These individuals, even if older, are motivated to better understand their risk factors and to change their lifestyles (Gariballa et al, 1996).

The impact of the physical therapist as an agent of change may reflect her or his capacity to serve as a role model. Physicians who exercise, for example, are more likely to recommend that their patients exercise, as well as to advocate other health behaviors (Abramson et al, 2000; Wells et al, 1984). Thus, practicing what one preaches can have a powerful effect and can increase adherence by patients to lifestyle change and health recommendations.

EVIDENCE-BASED PRACTICE

Evidence-based practice has become a major thrust in the physical therapy profession; it ensures that our practice has both a physiologic and a scientific basis. An important source of evidence that has shaped cardiovascular and pulmonary physical therapy over the past 50 years has been systematic, methodologically rigorous studies in the physiologic and clinical sciences.

BOX 1-5

Basis for Clinical Recommendations Based on Levels of Evidence and Grading of Recommendations

Level of Evidence	Type of Evidence
I	Evidence is obtained from metaanalysis of multiple, well-designed, controlled studies. Randomized trials with low false-positive and low false-negative errors (high power). Evidence is obtained from at least one well-designed experimental study.
II	Randomized trials with high false-positive and/or negative errors (low power).
III	Evidence is obtained from well-designed, quasiexperimental studies, such as nonrandomized, controlled single group, pre-post, cohort, time, or matched case-control series.
IV	Evidence is from well-designed, nonexperimental studies such as comparative and correlational descriptive and case studies.
V	Evidence from case reports and clinical examples.
Grade	**Grading of Recommendations**
A	There is evidence of type I or consistent findings from multiple studies of types II, III, or IV.
B	There is evidence of types II, III, or IV and findings are generally consistent.
C	There is evidence of types II, III, or IV but findings are inconsistent.
D	There is little or no systematic empirical evidence.

From Cook, D.J., Guyatt, G.H., Laupacis, A., & Sackett, D.L. (1992). Rules of evidence and clinical recommendations on the use of antithrombotic agents. Chest 102(4 Suppl):305S-311S.

Putting Knowledge into Practice

With the advent of Sackett's rules of evidence (Sackett et al, 2000) and schemes for grading the quality of scientific studies and critical-appraisal topics (Maher et al, 2003), physical therapists have had to learn to be discriminating consumers of research. In addition, systematic reviews and metaanalyses have emerged to examine areas of practice where there are discrepancies in the literature regarding a treatment's effect and to answer specific clinical questions. The levels of evidence and the grading recommendations for the quality of studies are shown in Box 1-5.

In becoming an evidence-based practitioner, the physical therapist needs to know what is not known in the field as well as what is known. The therapist must distinguish this knowledge from what is known inconclusively and from areas in which no studies have been done. The physical therapist must be comfortable with uncertainty when applying interventions and receptive to integrating new information as it emerges.

The effectiveness of exercise-based interventions in the prevention and remediation of the diseases of civilization has been documented for the components of such interventions and at the highest levels of evidence. Physical therapy has to ensure that its practices are based on the literature and that the profession assumes a leadership role in promoting exercise for the development and maintenance of health, for the prevention of disease and disability, and for the remediation of illness and injury.

PHYSICAL THERAPISTS AS AGENTS OF CHANGE

Physical therapists are health care professionals well qualified to bridge the gap between knowledge and practice in heath care and its delivery. Our role is to increase the number of people at low risk for the diseases of civilization rather than to focus primarily on high-risk individuals. The biomedical model is being replaced by a broader health model that views the individual in the context of his or her life and culture.

Strategies of behavioral change such as the transtheoretical model (Prochaska & DeClemente, 1982) are being adopted with increasing frequency for the purpose of promoting healthy lifestyle change. Implementation of such a program in the workplace has been shown to increase physical activity in previously sedentary adults, to reduce the number of reported barriers to such activity, and to increase muscle endurance, predicted $\dot{V}O_2$, and flexibility (White & Ransdell, 2003).

Refocusing and Expanding the Clinical Repertoire of Physical Theapists

Today's health care system is complex, and multiple forces drive the direction of types of services and their delivery. The reductionist perspective of the human body in the biomedical model persists as a major model underlying illness care. (Reductionism is the belief that the whole can be understood by the examination of small parts, that is, that treatment focuses on the disease rather than the mind and body as a whole.) Such illness care has been increasingly influenced by economic forces and directed care based on economic factors, such as drug prescription, rapid discharge from the hospital, and focus on process and functional outcomes (Guilmette et al, 2001). The absence of health promotion and wellness initiatives on a patient-by-patient basis before hospital discharge results from economic priorities and is a lost window of opportunity at a time when an individual may be receptive to information relating to changes in health behaviors—the teachable moment (Guilmette et al, 2001). Preventive information about nutrition, exercise, smoking cessation, and alcohol control is not receiving the attention it deserves from health care providers or from patients.

As noninvasive practitioners, physical therapists are positioned professionally to be leaders in effecting health behavior change. Knowledge of physiology, pathophysiology, and clinical medicine and surgery is insufficient for the physical therapist to be able to address complex, contemporary, population-wide health problems. To implement effective prevention and interventions with sustainable outcomes, the physical therapist has to consider the interface of treatments and recommendations for each individual. Establishing rapport, exploring the patient's perception of the importance of change in health behavior, building confidence, exchanging information, and reducing resistance are key interpersonal skills needed to promote sustainable health-behavior change (Rollnick et al, 1992, 1997, 2002).

The medical literature abounds with consensus statements of policies and procedures for treating specific conditions. Physical therapy has the expertise to develop parallel guidelines for noninvasive interventions, which in many cases should be considered first, before invasive interventions, or at least concurrently with them. The medical literature supports invasive care, so often it is not balanced with noninvasive interventions. For example, the report of the Sixth American College of Chest Physicians Consensus Conference on Antithrombotic Therapy has been cited in recommendations for patients following total hip arthroplasty (Krotenberg, 2004). Physical therapy has a primary perioperative role in the prophylaxis and management of the potentially lethal effects of thrombosis after surgery. This perspective is relatively obscure in the position statement, compared with the emphasis on drug cocktails and other options, yet it is highly efficacious, has an excellent cost-benefit ratio, and results in minimal side effects compared with the systemic risks of antithrombotic therapy.

It is time for a call to action within the physical therapy profession concerning the ill health that plagues our village. It is time to take a leadership role in the prevention of the diseases of civilization and in their remediation. In the pursuit of health and participation for all, physical therapists have a primary role in health care policy making, including the health of communities and countries, and should become involved in urban and environmental health initiatives, in community health planning (Bean et al, 2004; Campbell, 2003; Jones et al, 2004), and in health and wellness programs, as well as continuing to provide vital one-on-one care to people. Physical therapists can be leaders in promoting community-based programs for healthy people, such as community-based t'ai chi programs (Jones et al, 2004) and programs for individuals with physical challenges, including stroke (Ada et al, 2003; Eng et al, 2003). Community-based programs have been shown to be effective if they are well planned and supervised. In addition, they are accessible, so they are likely to be well used, and they have demonstrated the sustainability of their effect over time.

Translating sustainable health behavior from the hospital or clinic to the home cannot be assumed; rather, it is a unique skill that must be based on psychosocial teaching and learning factors. Although center- and clinic-based care is convenient for the health care provider, transitioning to home and community is fundamental to the process. The closer-to-home philosophy allows skills to be generalized from one setting to another. Closer-to-home health care delivery has attracted interest largely for economic reasons. However, the fact that better care and longer lasting sustainable health behaviors may result is also a major reason to promote such care. Cardiac rehabilitation, for example, when initiated in the home environment in low-risk individuals, shows more sustainable physical and psychosocial benefits over time than when initiated in a facility (Smith et al, 2004). Community-based programs have to be adapted to the cultural and socioeconomic conditions of that community to promote optimal buy-in from the participants and to maximize their success (Clark et al, 2002; Dundas et al, 2001).

Continuing Professional Education

With the ongoing need to be up to date, physical therapists have to accrue continuing education credits. With the plethora of opportunities in the open marketplace, courses and workshops must be stringently evaluated regarding the evidence base of their content and the qualifications of their instructors.

Practice evolves dynamically. Physical therapists can expect that what they learn in school will be challenged and refined over time, with the advancement of knowledge. The practitioner must identify where the research gaps are and help to support research activity, even if not engaged in research. Being receptive to changes in practice and serving as an agent of change are characteristics of the contemporary physical therapist. The work of clinicians and scientists has to be closely interwoven and ongoing partnerships must exist between them. Only in this way can clinically important questions be addressed and practice changed on the basis of advances and discoveries. This approach is subsumed in so-called participatory action research, which aims to unite the needs of the researchers and the stake-holders (patients and clinicians).

Another component of staying up-to-date through continuing education is reading the professional literature. Knowing what to read and how to read is as important to the clinician as clinical skills, and they both have to be refined throughout the practitioner's career. Box 1-6 shows the levels of quality of common publications and reading materials accessed by clinicians. Box 1-7 identifies important factors that should be considered when reading so as to enhance professional expertise. Journal clubs in the profession have become a popular means of sharing and discussing published information.

The role of the physical therapist as a health coach for every patient could be one of the most rewarding activities for the contemporary physical therapist in terms of having an impact on population health, one patient at a time.

EVERY PATIENT IS A CASE STUDY

The randomized controlled clinical trial (RCCT) has become the gold standard for assessing clinical interventions. Despite

---

BOX 1-6

Sources of Health Information and Quality Rating

Information Source	Quality Rating
Scientific/Professional journals	Usually externally peer-reviewed (blind or nonblinded); although not infallible, information in journals has the highest probability of containing credible information, compared with other sources
Monographs	May or may not be peer reviewed
Books	Usually not peer reviewed
Professional newsletters	Typically not reviewed
Magazines	Highly variable
Newspapers	Highly variable
Television and radio	Highly variable
Internet	Highly variable

BOX 1-7

Factors to Consider When Reading to Enhance Professional Expertise

Clinical Studies: Extracting Information and Translating the Findings into Practice

What is the source of the information and its credibility?
Was the work reviewed objectively by leaders in the field?
Are the reviewers unbiased and free of any conflict of interest in reviewing the work (no financial or other gain from reviewing the work favorably or unfavorably)?
Is the information based on a sound study?
Is the research question derived from the existing literature appropriately?
Is the study designed appropriately to address the question?
What type of clinical trial? Is there a control group?
Are subjects randomly selected and randomly assigned to groups?
Do the methods control for all confounding variables?
Are the methods standardized?
How valid and reliable are the measures?
Is the statistical analysis appropriate for the research design and research question?
Is the sample size appropriate?
Could the outcomes have been influenced by the outcome testers? Are the testers blind to the intervention group that each subject is assigned to?
Are the results appropriately interpreted (neither over or under stated)?
Do the results support the hypotheses or answer the research questions?
Is the interpretation of the results and their clinical implications stated appropriately?

Physiologic Studies: Extracting Information and Translating the Findings into Practice

How sound is the physiologic rationale?
Are the methods rigorous and sound?
How credible is the generalization to patient populations in the clinical setting?

the scientific rigor involved, the limitations of the RCCT should be appreciated by clinicians. Because of these limitations, Simon (2001) has argued that the clinical relevance of the RCCT may be overestimated and would be better described as a "silver standard." The designs of RCCTs and their statistical analyses are based on probability theory. Because of this, the results can be generalized only to comparable groups, not to an individual—the focus of the clinical situation. The results of RCCTs homogenize the outcomes for individuals who responded to treatment, failed to respond, or had negative outcomes. As clinical practitioners, we are interested in knowing how a particular individual with a given presentation will respond to a given treatment. The clinician needs to exercise a high level of clinical reasoning and judgment in determining the probability of a favorable response to a given treatment regimen in a given individual, based on studies of groups. Thus the therapist must understand the differences between the responders (favorable and unfavorable) in an RCCT and the nonresponders. This information is seldom detailed in published articles.

Another limitation of RCCTs is that in the real world, individuals seen by the physical therapist have multiple comorbidities. In the interest of experimental control, conditions that confound the patient's presentation and treatment response are selectively eliminated, or the groups are randomized so that they are relatively equivalent in this dimension. Nonetheless, rarely can the findings of a study that compares groups be applied perfectly to a given clinical situation.

The clinical decision-making process is iterative and time limited (APTA, 2001). Physical therapy diagnoses are derived from detailed histories and assessments. Clinical hypotheses are formulated, and the physical therapist systematically evaluates them to home in on the causes of the complaints. The physical therapist selects valid and reliable measures and outcomes and conducts them in a standardized manner. The patient's treatment response and prognosis are predicted so as to establish a timeline for treatment. Based on the assessment, each treatment intervention is prescribed (e.g., in exercise, the type, intensity, duration, frequency, and course). Periodic reevaluations are conducted to determine whether the patient has achieved the treatment objective and may be discharged or whether the prescriptions should be modified. The relevant outcomes are identified at the start of treatment, and the treatment responses are evaluated over time until the predetermined outcomes are achieved within the predetermined time frame.

Aligning practice with research (Dean, 1983) requires that the physical therapist apply research tools in practice, or at least have an understanding of them and their impact on drawing conclusions about the effect of treatment. For example, patients improve spontaneously with time. This phenomenon is called regression toward the mean. Physical therapy often involves an eclectic treatment approach involving multiple interventions. Because of this, individual treatment effects cannot be isolated. Rather, the physical therapist has to conclude that treatments A, B, and C may have resulted in

some improvement; however, the effect of spontaneous improvement with time can be determined only in a controlled clinical trial or on the basis of a prolonged unchanging baseline in the patient's symptoms. Confounding variables such as medications and improvement with time must be isolated so that it is possible to say that they may have contributed to the outcome, even if they cannot be ruled out. Confounding variables, which result from inadequate experimental control, cloud the interpretation of cardiopulmonary physical therapy studies (Dean, 1994). The effect of placebo also plays a major role in treatment outcome. This effect reflects such factors as patient expectancy. Once maligned and considered a characteristic of the hypochondriac, the placebo effect is now known to be a potent and clinically important self-healing effect that should be promoted. To date, there is little scientific evidence about how to exploit the power of the placebo effect systematically to promote self-healing.

An example of an individual with comorbidities is the person with acute back pain who is also overweight, has high blood pressure, and has a family history of heart disease. In such cases the physical therapist may have to introduce interventions in a stepwise manner. Even though immediate relief must be provided for the acute back discomfort, the comorbidities, as well as the low back pain, contribute significantly to the state of the individual's health and well-being. Thus for maximal and sustainable health, a lifelong health program must be implemented. To do this effectively, the practitioner needs a stepwise, paced approach. The first goal is to provide physical relief of acute pain. Then a weight-reduction and exercise program plan is introduced commensurate with the individual's needs and wants. Weight reduction, improved core and general strength, and aerobic conditioning may eliminate the cause of the low back pain or may attenuate it significantly over the long term. Follow-up is implemented to monitor progress and maintain psychosocial supports so as to ensure the long-term sustainability and success of the lifestyle changes. Such a regimen overcomes the limitations of a conventional course of analgesia and musculoskeletal physical therapy. Although the latter may produce short-term results, it does not necessarily address the underlying problem or eliminate the likelihood of recurrence of the primary problem and related health risks over time.

The contemporary physical therapist must be a culturally competent practitioner who can adapt communication style, assessments, and treatments to the unique needs of a given individual. Differences in people with respect to culture, traditions, and religion have to be appreciated because these factors can affect health, illness, health reporting, beliefs and expectations about treatment intervention, and adherence to the treatment program. The holy month of Ramadan, for example, creates special challenges for Muslims with respect to maintaining participation in exercise programs. During Ramadan, Muslims are required to fast from dawn to dusk, and the fast includes abstinence from water as well as from food. Sedentary people show greater adverse physiologic effects during this period, both when at rest and during exercise, than do active people (Ramadan et al, 1999). Body weight drops in a predictable manner. The respiratory exchange ratio decreases during exercise, reflecting increased fat metabolism. Serum iron and platelets decrease, particularly in sedentary people, and fluid balance is better maintained in active people. Exercise, particularly whole-body exercise, may have to be curtailed or modified during fasting. This is especially true when Ramadan falls during the hot summer months.

Adapting lifestyle and treatment recommendations to the needs of the people physical therapists serve is fundamental to a successful outcome. The parameters of exercise prescription for optimal health benefits have been well documented (see Chapter 18). Prolonged adherence to physical activity and exercise programs, however, is poor. Understanding the factors that sustain health behaviors is as critical as the physiological basis for them. One study compared the effects of conventional aerobic training with the effects of a program designed to increase strength, endurance, and mind-body coordination but designed also for "comfort," so that the program would be more appealing to people unused to exercise. After training, participants in the latter group had superior endurance compared with those in the conventional group, and they reported more comfort and less exertion. This preliminary study supported the idea that an exercise program modified for comfort and enjoyment still resulted in a greater capacity to adapt to increased physiologic demands. Such programs should be extended so that adherence over time can be evaluated. In addition, readiness to change as described in the transtheoretical model must be considered in studies of long-term lifestyle change (Prochaska & DiClementi, 1982).

Physical Therapy's Role: Participation in Health Promotion and Prevention

In addition to promoting health and wellness one on one, physical therapists need to present a high profile in health promotion and illness prevention by developing and writing physical therapy publications throughout the various levels of their professional associations. They can participate in consensus groups within these associations to issue physical therapy position statements, broadcast television and radio public service announcements, and set up information booths in shopping malls, community centers, and other strategic places within the community. Innovative wellness and prevention programs such as heart camps and retreats should be established (Sung & Lee, 2001). Such active leadership and participation by physical therapists enables them to exploit a range of avenues for effective communication and education strategies directed to the general public in addition to one-on-one contact with patients.

Capitalizing on public health and disease-of-the-week and disease-of-the-month initiatives can reinforce existing community, state or province, national, and global health initiatives. The physical therapist should be proactive and function as a role model for health as a community leader by

acknowledging these important initiatives and arranging activities to support them. Formal acknowledgment of the initiatives strengthens the profession's identity and its responsibility regarding the conditions being addressed. It also educates the public and reinforces physical therapy's role in the prevention and primary management of these conditions in the minds of the public, insurers, health care policy makers, health care colleagues, legislators, and others. To address the serious pandemic of type 2 diabetes, the state of Tennessee has initiated statewide action. Schools and communities have been selected as primary prevention targets for the promotion of healthy food choices and activity programs (Bailey et al, 2003). The initiative is multidisciplinary and multisectorial, and health profession organizations, government, churches, schools, and employers across the state are participating. The World Health Organization has several important annual health markers, including May 31 of each year, which is World No Smoking Day. These occasions should be publicized and supported collectively by the global physical therapy community.

Physical Therapy's Role: Participation in Population-wide Health Initiatives

As primary health care professionals, physical therapists are uniquely positioned to develop, support, and promote innovative health programs, thereby strengthening the health of communities en masse as well as doing so one person at a time in the clinic. Several excellent resources are available on the subject of building healthy neighborhoods and communities; they are highly recommended to physical therapists as bases for practicing at village and community, as well as the individual, levels (Kawachi & Berkman, 2003; Minkler, 2002).

Multicomponent, multidisciplinary wellness and preventive health programs have been proposed to be components of each hospital department, including the emergency department. Hospital-based programs can be successfully implemented in diverse geographic areas and can be focused on each region's needs (Koertge et al, 2003). Despite the compelling benefits of home- and community-based care, their efficacy cannot be assumed. Programs must be judiciously targeted, with due consideration given to the purpose of care, the target population, the congruence of the care and individuals' needs and wants, and outcomes at the individual and societal levels (Smith et al, 2002).

The Groningen Active Living Model is an example of a behavior change model that has been developed to encourage sedentary adults to be physically activity (Stevens et al, 2003). The variables that were examined to determine program success included perceived fitness, social support, self-efficacy, and enjoyment. The outcomes were program adherence and physical activity. With respect to adherence, task self-efficacy was an important mediating variable in this cohort, followed by self-efficacy in overcoming barriers, in social support, and in enjoyment. Perceived physical ability and fitness were relatively less important mediators.

The Hearts for Life community-based program has shown positive outcomes with respect to risk reduction and improvement of knowledge (Kirk-Gardner & Steven, 2003). The Choose to Move physical activity program for women provides an important model for public health and participatory research organizations of targeted, low-cost self-help programs that support the Healthy People 2010 objectives for physical activity, nutrition, and cardiovascular health (Koffman et al, 2001). Women who completed the program increased their physical activity, reduced their consumption of high-fat foods, and increased their knowledge and awareness of cardiovascular risk and its symptoms. Schools and workplaces are also sites for innovative health programs in the community. Preventive cardiology programs for children such as HeartPower! show some success in nutritional domains (Skybo & Ryan-Wenger, 2002). Such programs, however, would benefit from the expertise of a physical therapist in developing, coordinating, integrating, and evaluating a physical activity and an exercise component. Low-income families in particular have an increased risk for inactivity and obesity. A school program for children of low-income families used the Internet, videos, provision of health snacks, and participation in a gym lab to promote exercise and healthy food choices (Frenn et al, 2003). This program resulted in reduced fat intake and increased physical activity by the children.

One medium in which a physical therapist can assume the role of health coach has been through telerehabilitation. Telerehabilitation has come of age and is a major vehicle that can be exploited by physical therapists for targeted education of patients in the community (Lai et al, 2004) and for general preventive health. Home-based education about nutrition and exercise has been reported as a means of targeting individuals with obstructive sleep apnea and promoting lifestyle change (Oki et al, 1999).

Marketing research methods have been investigated as a means of improving population health outcomes and making their success rates comparable to those that have been well established in business marketing. Mass media promotion has been used to communicate an innovative physical activity and exercise resource called Small Steps (Poscente et al, 2002). Callers responded to a mass publication campaign to promote Small Steps. People phoned toll free to a call-in center where trained screeners recruited members of the public into a controlled trial, identified their stage of readiness to change based on a few structured questions, and sent out the Small Steps kit, which provided information about being physically active and exercising as well as a workbook. More than 80% of the callers were women. The prospect of making small steps toward improving their health was as compelling for men as for women. At 3-month follow-up, self-reported current levels of physical activity (main outcome) had significantly changed. Thus the results supported the idea that with the use of mass media, people who are in the preparation stage of being more physically active can shift to the action stage. Long-term studies are needed to establish the long-term benefits of this program and its translation into health outcomes. The reasons given for calling the resource center included the appeal of taking small steps when undertaking health behavior changes, improving nutrition, becoming more active, learning new things, and assisting others to improve their diets and activity levels.

Implications of Epidemiology and Health Care Trends for Physical Therapy Practice

In the 21st century the impact of noninvasive physical therapy outcomes will be reflected in the number of individuals who are encouraged to quit smoking, lose weight, eat better foods, exercise, and manage life stress (including moderate use of alcohol) most effectively, irrespective of the patients' primary diagnoses. Addressing these priorities first can also address musculoskeletal and neuromuscular problems or at least potentially offset their consequences (such as low back pain) and can reduce the energy cost of walking in individuals with stroke, heart disease, or lung disease. Furthermore, addressing these priorities reduces the need for use of the health care system (doctor- and hospital-based care) and helps to avoid or minimize the need for drugs and surgery. The physical therapist has a primary role in addressing these priorities in every patient. Such a strategy will enable the profession collectively to address the leading population-wide health priorities of our time one patient at a time and to affect health globally.

Implications of Epidemiology and Health Care Trends for Physical Therapy Professional Education

Physical therapy professional curricula have to be continuously reviewed with respect to their congruence with epidemiology and health care trends and to the provision of evidence-based practice in the context of evidence-based planning. In high-income and increasingly in low-income countries, the diseases of civilization are pandemic; they are largely preventable with a healthy lifestyle. Noninvasive interventions include targeted and specific educational strategies and encouragement of regular physical activity and exercise and optimal nutrition. The physical therapist requires a high level of expertise in these areas, specifically in education (including smoking cessation), nutrition, and the prescription of exercise. Education should be based on assessment of learning styles and readiness to change and should include setting and prioritizing goals, delivering health information, evaluating outcomes, and promoting lifelong behavior changes. Physical therapists' capacities to teach and promote learning should be formally evaluated just as are their capacities to prescribe exercise or other physical therapy interventions. A cross-sectional study of health care providers and their provision of health information to patients reported considerable disparities among providers. The provider's gender and that of the patient influenced whether education was attempted and, if so, what type. Female providers included health education more often than did their male counterparts.

THE MAGIC BULLET AND THE FOUNTAIN OF YOUTH

A magic bullet and a fountain of youth exist, and they are not to be found in a pill or in surgery. Education and exercise have been, for several decades, the hallmarks of physical therapy (Colsen, 1958; Gardner, 1969; Tidy, 1952) and the elixir that adds years to life and life to years. These "drugs" have been at the core of the practice of the physical therapist, who is distinguished from invasive-medicine practitioners primarily by the use of noninvasive "drugs," as opposed to the invasive interventions of pharmacotherapy and surgery. In addition to providing preventive health benefits, such lifestyle changes as smoking cessation, optimal nutrition, and exercise can enhance the quality of life (Hellenius et al, 1995) and increase the probability of long-term health.

Given the epidemiologic changes in global health, this is physical therapy's moment on the world health care stage, a time to promote health and wellness in every patient and to prevent and manage the diseases of civilization that are disabling and killing the world's population by the millions annually. The profession is uniquely and strategically positioned to lead the assault on the diseases of civilization. If a drug could offer the benefits of physical therapy's noninvasive strategies, including physical activity and exercise and healthy lifestyle, and similarly improve public health, it would be heralded as nothing short of a miracle remedy.

SUMMARY

This chapter describes the pivotal role of the noninvasive practitioner, namely, the physical therapist, within the contemporary framework of health and within an evolving health versus biomedical care delivery system. With the pandemic of the diseases of civilization, physical therapists need to consider the underlying risk factors for these diseases in every individual, irrespective of their own specialties or areas of practice and irrespective of the primary reasons for the consultation. A patient's low back pain or tennis elbow may be mere inconvenience compared with his or her smoking, excessive body weight, inactivity, high blood pressure, high cholesterol, or high blood sugar levels. Physical therapists are uniquely qualified professionally and are strategically well positioned to address the leading health problems of our time by using the profession's primary "drugs"—education and exercise—in diverse settings, one individual at a time or in groups. In addition to addressing these lurking killers, the physical therapist must identify risk factors so that she or he can prescribe optimal treatment, including exercise, for any indication of underlying risk factors and monitor the patient for therapeutic and safety reasons. Physical therapists pride themselves on their communication skills, which are fundamental to effecting lifelong behavior change in each individual. This expertise can be exploited because physical therapists not only spend more time with people during visits than most health professionals, but also see them for repeat visits. As effective agents of change, physical therapists can exert considerable influence on their patients over time, given the potential teachable moments available to them. In the 21st century, physical therapy's impact will be reflected in outcomes associated with prevention as well as management of the diseases of civilization, over and above the conventional practice of physical therapists in all clinical areas and settings.

Review Questions

1. Describe the diseases of civilization.
2. How do the diseases of civilization affect every patient seen by the physical therapist? Relate your answer to the World Health Organization's International Classification of Function.
3. Distinguish physical therapy's role in the promotion of health and wellness versus prevention, 'cure,' and management.
4. Describe the physical therapist in her or his role as a consumer of research.
5. Describe the concept of evidence-based practice in the context of evidence-based planning.
6. Describe how you, as a physical therapist, are an agent of change.
7. Describe how the profession of physical therapy is uniquely positioned to assume a leadership role in addressing the leading health problems of our time.
8. Describe the power of noninvasive practice as opposed to invasive practice.
9. Reference is made in the chapter to the "magic bullet" and the "fountain of youth." Describe these fabled constructs in the context of contemporary physical therapy.

REFERENCES

Abraham, W.T. (2004). Preventing cardiovascular events in patients with diabetes mellitus. American Journal of Medicine 116(Suppl 5A):39S-46S.

Abramson, S., Stein, J., Schaufele, M., Frates, E., & Rogan, S. (2000). Personal exercise habits and counseling practices of primary care physicians: a national survey. Clinical Journal of Sports Medicine 10:40-44.

Ada, L., Dean, C.M., Hall, J.M., Bampton, J., & Crompton, S. (2003). A treadmill and overground walking program improves walking in persons residing in the community after stroke: a placebo-controlled, randomized trial. Archives of Physical Medicine and Rehabilitation 84:1486-1491.

AHCPR Supported Clinical Practice Guidelines. (2000). Smoking cessation: brief clinical interventions. www.ncbi.nlm.nih.gov; retrieved January 2005.

American Cancer Society. (2004). When smokers quit. http://www.cancer.org/downloads/COM/WhenSmokersQuit.pdf; retrieved Januray 2005.

American Heart Association. (2005). Blood pressure guidelines. www.americanheart.org; retrieved January 2005.

American Lung Association. Quit Smoking. http://www.lungusa.org/site/pp.asp?c=dvLUK9O0E&b=22938; retrieved January 2005.

American Physical Therapy Association. (2001). Guide to physical therapist practice, ed 2. Physical Therapy 81:1-746.Washington, DC: American Physical Therapy Association.

Anderson, L.M., Scrimshaw, S.C., Fullilove, M.T., Fielding, J.E., & Normand, J. (2003). Culturally competent healthcare systems: a systematic review. American Journal of Preventive Medicine 24:68-79.

Anonymous. (2000). Obesity: preventing and managing the global epidemic. Report of a WHO consultation. World Health Organization Technical Report Series 894:i-xii 1-253.

Anonymous. (2003). Your heart attack risk: inflammation counts. Harvard Women's Health Watch 10:1-3.

Anonymous. (2004). Overcoming the threat of anger: more than type A behavior, hostility raises health risks. Heart Advisor 7:6.

Astrup, A., Larsen, T.M., & Harper, A. (2004). Aktins and other low-carbohydrate diets: hoax or an effective tool for weight loss? Lancet 364:897-899.

Azjen, I. (1983). From intention to actions: a theory of planned behavior. In Kuhl, J., Beckman, J. (Eds). Action control: from cognition to behavior. Heidelberg, Germany: Springer.

Bailey, J.E., Gibson, D.V., Jain, M., Connelly, S.A., Ryder, K.M., & Dagogo-Jack, S. (2003). QSource quality initiative: reversing the diabetes epidemic in Tennessee. Tennessee Medicine 96:559-563.

Baxter, A.P., Milner, P.C., Hawkins, S., Leaf, M., Simpson, C., Wilson, K.V., Owen, T., Higginbottom, G., Nicholl, J., & Cooper, N. (1997). The impact of heart health promotion on coronary heart disease lifestyle risk factors in school children: lessons learnt from a community-based project. Public Health 111: 231-237.

Bean, J.F., Vora, A., & Frontera, W.R. (2004). Benefits of exercise for community-dwelling older adults. Archives of Physical Medicine and Rehabilitation 85(Suppl 3):S31-S42.

Bauman, A.E. (2004). Updating the evidence that physical activity is good for health: an epidemiological review 2000-2003. Journal of Science in Medicine and Sport 7(1 Suppl):6-19.

Bergman, E., & Bertero, C. (2001). You can do it if you set your mind to it: a qualitative study of patients with coronary artery disease. Journal of Advances in Nursing 36:733-741.

Bijnen, F.C., Caspersen, C.J., & Mosterd, W.L. (1994). Physical inactivity as a risk factor for coronary artery disease: a WHO and International Society and Federation of Cardiology position statement. Bulletin World Health Organization 72:1-4.

Billings, J.H. (2000). Maintenance of behavior changes in cardiorespiratory risk reduction: a clinical perspective from the Ornish Program for reversing coronary heart disease. Health Psychology 19(1 Suppl):70-75.

Bond, V., Stephens, Q., Adams, R.G., Vaccaro, P., Demeersman, R., Williams, D., Obisesan, T.O., Franks, B.D., Oke, L.M., Coleman, B., Blakely, R., & Millis, R.M. (2002). Aerobic exercise attenuates an exaggerated exercise blood pressure response in normotensive young adult African-American men. Blood Pressure 11:229-234.

Blair, S.N., Cheng, Y., & Holder, J.S. (2001). Is physical activity or physical fitness more important in defining health benefit? Medicine and Science in Sports and Exercise 33(6 Suppl): 379-399.

Bradberry, J.C. (2004). Peripheral arterial disease: pathophysiology, risk factors, and role of antithrombotic therapy. Journal of the American Pharmacy Association 44(2 Supp 1):S37-S44.

Brod, S.A. (2000). Unregulated inflammation shorts human functional longevity. Inflammation Research 49:561-570.

Burkman, R.T. Jr. (1991). Strategies for reducing cardiovascular risk in women. Journal of Reproductive Medicine 36(3 Suppl): 238-246.

Caballero, B. (2001). Early nutrition and risk of disease in the adult. Public Health and Nutrition 4:1335-1336.

Cabrera, C., Wilhelmson, K., Allebeck, P., Wedel, H., Steen, B., & Lissner, L. (2003). Cohort differences in obesity-related indicators of 70-year-olds, with special reference to gender and education. European Journal of Epidemiology 18:883-890.

Calverley, P.M., & Walker, P. (2003). Chronic obstructive pulmonary disease. Lancet 362:1053-1061.

Campbell, I. (2003). The obesity epidemic: can we turn the tide? Heart 89(Suppl 2):ii22-24.

Carlsson, C.M., & Stein, J.H. (2002). Cardiovascular disease and the aging woman: overcoming barriers to lifestyle changes. Curr Women's Health Rep 2:366-372.

Centers for Disease Control and Prevention. (2002). Recent trends in mortality rates for four major cancers, by sex and race/ethnicity—United States, 1990-1998. MMWR Weekly 51:49-53. www.cdc.gov/mmwr; retrieved January 2005.

Current Women' Health Report 2:366-372.

Chakravarthy, M.V., & Booth, F.W. (2004). Eating, exercise, and "thrifty" genotypes: connecting the dots toward an evolutionary understanding of modern chronic disease. Journal of Applied Physiology 96:3-10.

Chalmers, J., & Chapman, N. (2001). Challenges for the prevention of primary and secondary stroke: the importance of lowering blood pressure and total cardiovascular risk. Blood Pressure 10:344-351.

Charkoudian, N., & Joyner, M.J. (2004). Physiologic considerations for exercise performance in women. Clinics in Chest Medicine 25:247-255.

Chatila, W.M., Wynkoop, W.A., Vance, G.G., & Criner, G.J. (2004). Smoking patterns in African Americans and whites with advanced COPD. Chest 125:15-21.

Cheng, A., Braunstein, J.B., Dennison, C., Nass, C., & Blumenthal, R.S. (2002). Reducing global risk for cardiovascular disease: using lifestyle changes and pharmacotherapy. Clinical Cardiology 25:205-212.

Cheng, T.O. (2001). Price of the modernization of China. Circulation 103:E131-E133.

Chobanian, A.V., Bakris, G.L., Black, H.R., Cushman, W.C., Green, L.A., Izzo, J.L., Jones, D.W., Materson, B.J., Oparil, S., Wright, J.T., & Roccella, E.J. (2003). Seventh report of the joint national committee on prevention, detection, evaluation, and treatment of high blood pressure. Hypertension 42: 1206-1252.

Clark, A.M., Barbour, R.S., & McIntyre, P.D. (2002). Preparing for change in the secondary prevention of coronary heart disease: a qualitative evaluation of cardiac rehabilitation within a region of Scotland. Journal of Advances in Nursing 39:589-598.

Cleeland, C.S., Gonin, R., Baez, L., Loehrer, P., & Panya, K.J. (1997). Pain and treatment of pain in minority patients with cancer. The Eastern Co-operative Oncology Group Minority Outpatient Pain Study. Annals of Internal Medicine 127:813-816.

Clini, E., Costi, S., Lodi, S., & Rossi, G. (2003). Non-pharmacological treatment for chronic obstructive pulmonary disease. Medical Science Monitor 9:300-305.

Cohen, J.A., Estacio, R.O., Lundgren, R.A., Esler, A.L., & Schrier, R.W. (2003). Diabetic autonomic neuropathy is associated with an increased incidence of strokes. Autonomic Neuroscience 108:73-78.

Colson, J.R.C. (1958). Progressive exercise therapy in rehabilitation and physical education. Bristol, UK: John Wright & Sons Ltd.

Cook, D.J., Guyatt, G.H., Laupacis, A., & Sackett, D.L. (1992). Rules of evidence and clinical recommendations on the use of antithrombotic agents. Chest 102(4 Suppl):305S-311S.

Costa, F.V. (2002). Non-pharmacological treatment of hypertension in women. Journal of Hypertension 20(Suppl 2):S57-S61.

Cox, K.L., Gorely, T.J., Puddey, I.B., Burke, V., & Beilin, L.J. (2003). Exercise behavior change in 40- to 65-year-old women: the SWEAT Study (Sedentary Women Exercise Adherence Trial). British Journal of Health Psychology 8(Pt 4):477-495.

Critchley, J.A., Capewell, S., & Unal, B. (2003). Life-years gained from coronary artery disease mortality reduction in Scotland: prevention or treatment? Journal of Clinical Epidemiology 56:583-590.

Cucchiara, B.L., & Kasner, S.E. (2002). Atherosclerotic risk factors in patients with ischemic cerebrovascular disease. Current Treatment Options in Neurology 4:445-453.

Cupples, M.E., & McKnight, A. (1999). Five year follow up of patients at high cardiovascular risk who took part in randomized control trial of health promotion. British Medical Journal 319:687-688.

Dean, E. (1983). Research: the right way. Clinical Management in Physical Therapy 3:29-33.

Dean, E. (1985). A psychobiologic adaptation model of physical therapy practice. Physical Therapy 65:158-161.

Dean, E. (1994). Invited commentary on "Are incentive spirometry, intermittent positive pressure breathing, and deep breathing exercises effective in the prevention of postoperative pulmonary complications after upper abdominal surgery?" A systematic overview and meta-analysis. Physical Therapy 74:10-15.

Demarais, A., & Robichaud-Ekstrand, S. (1998). McEwen's conceptual model in cardiac rehabilitation. Canadian Nurse 94:40-46. (English abstract).

Doyle, J., & Creager, M.A. (2003). Pharmacotherapy and behavioral intervention for peripheral arterial disease. Reviews in Cardiovascular Medicine 4:18-24.

Dubbert, P.M., Carithers, T., Sumner, A.E., Barbour, K.A., Clark, B.L., Hall, J.E., & Crook, E.D. (2002). Obesity, physical inactivity, and risk for cardiovascular disease. American Journal of Medical Science 324:116-126.

Dundas, R., Morgan, M., Redfern, J., Lemic-Stojcevic, N., & Wolfe, C. (2001). Ethnic differences in behavioural risk factors for stroke: implications for health promotion. Ethnicity and Health 6:95-103.

Ebrahim, S. (2000). Cost-effectiveness of stroke prevention. British Medical Bulletin 56:557-570.

Ebrahim, S., & Smith, G.D. (2001). Exporting failure? Coronary heart disease and stroke in developing countries. International Journal of Epidemiology 30:201-205.

Eckel, R.H., & Krauss, R.M. (1998). American Heart Association call to action: obesity as a major risk factor for coronary artery disease. AHA Nutrition Committee. Circulation 97:2099-2100.

Egan, F. (1999). Cardiac rehabilitation in the new millennium. Intensive Critical Care Nursing 15:163-168.

Egusa, G., Watanabe, H., Ohshita, K., Fujikawa, R., Yamane, K., Okubo, M., & Kohno, N. (2002). Influence of the extent of westernization of lifestyle on the progression of preclinical atherosclerosis in Japanese subjects. Journal of Atherosclerosis and Thrombosis 9:299-304.

Endres, M., Gertz, K., Lindauer, U., Katchanov, J., Schultze, J., Schrock, H., Nickenig, G., Kuschinsky, W., Dirnagl, U., & Laufs, U. (2003). Mechanisms of stroke protection by physical activity. Annals of Neurology 54:582-590.

Eng, J.J., Chu, K.S., Kim, C.M., Dawson, A.S., Carswell, A., & Hepburn, K.E. (2003). A community-based group exercise program for persons with chronic stroke. Medicine and Science in Sports and Exercise 35:1271-1278.

Everson, S.A., Lynch, J.W., Kaplan, G.A., Lakka, T.A., Sivenius, J., & Salonen, J.T. (2001). Stress-induced blood pressure reactivity and incident stroke in middle-aged men. Stroke 32:1263-1270.

Felmeden, D.C., Spencer, C.G., Blann, A.D., Beevers, D.G., & Lip, G.Y. (2003). Physical activity in relation to indices of endothelial function and angiogenesis factors in hypertension: a substudy of the Anglo-Scandinavian Cardiac Outcomes Trial (ASCOT). Journal of Internal Medicine 253:81-91.

Ferreira, S.R., Lerario, D.D., Gimeno, S.G., Sanudo, A., & Franco, L.J. (2002). Obesity and central adiposity in Japanese immigrants: role of the Western dietary pattern. Journal of Epidemiology 12:431-438.

Feskanich, D., Willett, W., & Colditz, G. (2002). Walking and leisure-time activity and risk of hip fractures in postmenopausal women. Journal of the American Medical Association 288:2300-2306.

Fletcher, G.F., Balady, G., Blair, S.N., Blumenthal, J., Caspersen, C., Chaitman, B., Epstein, S., Sivarjan, Froelicher, E.S., Froelicher, V.F., Pina, I.L., & Pollock, M.L. (1996). Statement on exercise: benefits and recommendations for physical activity programs for all Americans. A statement for health professionals by the Committee on Exercise and Cardiac Rehabilitation of the Council on Clinical Cardiology, American Heart Association. Circulation 94:857-862.

Foss, M., & Keteyian, S. (1998). Fox's physiologic basis for exercise and sport. Boston: McGraw-Hill.

Franklin, B.A. (2001). The downside of our technological revolution? An obesity-conducive environment. American Journal of Cardiology 87:1093-1095.

Frayne, K.N. (2002). Insulin resistance, impaired postprandial lipid metabolism and abdominal obesity: a deadly triad. Medical Principles and Practice 11(Suppl 2):31-40.

Frenn, M., Malin, S., Bansal, N., Delgado, M., Greer, Y., Havice, M., Ho, M., & Schweizer, H. (2003). Addressing health disaparities in middle school students' nutrition and exercise. Journal of Community Health Nursing 20:1-14.

Gardner, M.D. (1969). The principles of exercise therapy, ed 3. London: G. Bell & Sons, Ltd.

Gariballa, S.E., Peet, S.M., Fotherby, M.D., Parker, S.G., & Castledon, C.M. (1996). The knowledge of hospital patients about vascular disease and their risk factors. Postgraduate Medical Journal 72:605-608.

Giannuzzi, P., Mezzani, A., Saner, H., Bjornstad, H., Fioretti, P., Mendes, M., Cohen-Solal, A., Dugmore, L., Hambrecht, R., Hellemans, I., McGee, H., Perk, J., Vanees, L., & Veress, G. (2003). Physical activity for primary and secondary prevention: position paper of the Working Group on Cardiac Rehabilitation and Exercise Physiology of the European Society of Cardiology. Journal of Cardiovascular Risk 10:19-27.

Gibbons, L.W., & Clark, S.M. (2001). Exercise in the reduction of cardiovascular events: lessons from epidemiologic trials. Cardiology Clinics 19:347-355.

Gidding, S.S. (1999). Preventive pediatric cardiology: tobacco, cholesterol, obesity, and physical activity. Pediatric Clinics of North America 46:253-262.

Giles, P.D., Ramachandran, S., Whitaker, A.J., Phillips, A.W., Fell, S.J., Mitchell, A., & Coleman, T.D. (1996). The one-stop coronary cholesterol clinic: a multidisciplinary approach to implementing evidence-based treatment. Postgraduate Medicine Journal 72:744-748.

Glassman, S.J., Rashbaum, I.G., & Walker, W.C. (2001). Cardiopulmonary rehabilitation and cancer rehabilitation. 1. Cardiac rehabilitation. Archives of Physical Medicine and Rehabilitation 82(3 Suppl 1):S47-S51.

Goel, M.S., McCarthy, E.P., Phillips, R.S., & Wee, C.C. (2004). Obesity among US immigrant subgroups by duration of residence. Journal of the American Medical Association 292:2860-2867.

Gordon, N.F., Gulanick, M., Costa, F., Fletcher, G., Franklin, B.A., Roth, E.J., & Shepherd, T. (2004). Physical activity and exercise recommendations for stroke survivors: an American Heart Association scientific statement from the Council on Clinical Cardiology, Subcommittee on Exercise, Cardiac Rehabilitation, and Prevention; the Council on Cardiovascular Nursing; the Council on Nutrition, Physical Activity, and Metabolism; and the Stroke Council. Circulation 109:2031-2041.

Graves, K.D., & Miller, P.M. (2003). Behavioral medicine in the prevention and treatment of cardiovascular disease. Behavior Modification 27:3-25.

Greenland, K.J., Giles, W.H., Keenan, N.L., Croft, J.B., & Mensah, G.A. (2002). Physician advice, patient actions, and health-related quality of life in secondary prevention of stroke through diet and exercise. Stroke 33:565-570.

Gregg, E.W., Mangione, C.M., Cauley, J.A., Thompson, T.J., Schwartz, A.V., Ensrud, K.E., & Nevitt, M.C. (2002). Diabetes and incidence of functional disability in older women. Diabetes Care 25:61-67.

Grundy, S.M. (2002). Obesity, metabolic syndrome, and coronary atherosclerosis. Circulation 105:2696-2698.

Guilmette, T.J., Motta, S.I., Shadel, W.G., Mukand, J., & Niaura, R. (2001). Promoting smoking cessation in the rehabilitation environment. Archives of Physical Medicine and Rehabilitation 80:560-562.

Guiese, B.J. (2000). Behavioral medicine strategies for heart disease prevention: the example of smoking cessation. Preventive Cardiology 3:10-15.

Gunnarsson, O.T., & Judge, J.O. (1997). Exercise in midlife: how and why to prescribe it for sedentary patients. Geriatrics 52:71-2, 77-80.

Hambrecht, R., Walther, C., Mobius-Winkler, S., Gielen, S., Linke, A., Conradi, K., Erbs, S., Kluge, R., Kendziorri, K., Sabri, O., Sick, P., & Schuler, G. (2004). Percutaneous coronary angioplasty compared with exercise training in patients with stable coronary artery disease: a randomized trial. Circulation 109:1371-1378.

Hamilton, B.P., & Hamilton, J.H. (1997). Hypertension in elderly persons. Endocrine Practice 3:29-41.

Hannan, E.L., Kilburn, H., & O'Donnel, J.F. (1990). Adult open heart surgery in New York State: an analysis of risk factors and hospital mortality rates. Journal of the American Medical Association 264:1768-1774.

Hart, R.G., & Halperin, J.L. (1999). Atrial fibrillation and thromboembolism: a decade of progress in stroke prevention. Annals of Internal Medicine 131:688-695.

Haskell, W.L. (2003). Cardiovascular disease prevention and life-style interventions: effectiveness and efficacy. Journal of Cardiovascular Nursing 18:245-255.

Haskell, W.L., Alderman, E.L., Fair, J.M., Maron, D.J., Mackey, S.F., Superko, H.R., Williams, P.T., Johnstone, I.M., Champagne, M.A., Krauss, R.M., & Farquhar, J.W. (1994). Effects of intensive multiple risk factor reduction on coronary atherosclerosis and clinical cardiac events in men and women with coronary artery disease. The Stanford Coronary Risk Intervention Project (SCRIP). Circulation 89:975-990.

Health Canada. Office of Nutrition Policy and Promotion. Revision of Canada's Food Guide to Health Eating. www.hc-sc.gc.ca; retrieved January 2005.

Heart and Stroke Foundation Canada (2005). www.heartandstroke.ca; retrieved January 2005.

Henrichon, C., & Robichaud-Ekstrand, S. (2002). Adaptive strategies and adaptation after participation in an education program after a first coronary event. Recherche et Soins Infirmiere 70:39-65. (English abstract).

Holund, U., Thomassen, A., Boysen, G., Charles, P., Eriksen, E.F., Overvad, K., Peterssen, B., Sandstrom, B., & Vittrup. M. (1997). Importance of diet and sex in prevention of coronary artery disease, cancer, osteoporosis, and overweight or underweight: a study of attitudes and practices of Danish primary care physicians. American Journal of Clinical Nutrition 65:2004S-2006S.

Heart and Stroke Foundation of Canada. (2003). The growing burden of heart disease and stroke in Canada. HSFC Publication No. 1-896242-30-8. Ottawa, Ontario: Heart and Stroke Foundation of Canada.

Hellenius, M.L., Dahlof, C., Aberg, H., Krakau, I., de Faire, U. (1995). Quality of life is not negatively affected by diet and exercise intervention in healthy men with cardiovascular risk factors. Quality of Life Research 4:13-20.

Hu, F.B. (2003). Overweight and obesity in women: health risks and consequences. Journal of Women's Health 12:163-172.

Hu, F.B., Stampfer, M.J., Solomon, C., Liu, S., Colditz, G.A., Speizer, F.E., Willett, W.C., & Manson, J.E. (2001). Physical activity and risk for cardiovascular events in diabetic women. Annals of Internal Medicine 134:96-105.

Hu, G., Barengo, N.C., Tuomilehto, J., Lakka, T.A., Nissinen, A., & Jousilahti, P. (2004). Relationship of physical activity and body mass index to the risk of hypertension: a prospective study in Finland. Hypertension 43:25-30.

Jakes, R.W., Day, N.E., Khaw, K.T., Luben, R., Oakes, S., Welch, A., Bingham, S., & Wareham, N.J. (2003). Television viewing and low participation in vigorous recreation are independently associated with obesity and markers of cardiovascular disease risk: EPIC-Norfolk population-based study. European Journal of Clinical Nutrition 57:1089-1096.

Jones, A.Y.M., Dean, E., & Scudds, R. (2004). Effectiveness of a community-based Tai Chi program and implications for public health initiatives. Archives of Physical Medicine and Rehabilitation 86:619-625.

Joseph, L.N., Babikian, V.L., Allen, N.C., & Winter, M.R. (1999). Risk factor modification in stroke prevention: the experience of a stroke clinic. Stroke 30:16-20.

Kannel, W.B. (1990). Influence of multiple risk factors on the hazards of hypertension. Journal of Cardiovascular Pharmacology 16(Suppl 5):S53-S57.

Kannel, W.B., Wilson, P.W., Nam, B.H., & D'Agostino, R.B. (2002). Risk stratification of obesity as a coronary risk factor. American Journal of Cardiology 90:697-701.

Katz, D. (2003). The basic (care) and feeding of homosapiens: consensus, controversy, and cluelessness. Proceedings of the Canadian Cardiovascular Congress, Toronto, Ontario.

Katzmarzyk, P.T., Gledhill, N., & Shepherd, R.J. (2000). The economic burden of physical inactivity in Canada. Canadian Medical Association Journal 163:1435-1440.

Kavanagh, T. (2001). Exercise in the primary prevention of coronary artery disease. Canadian Journal of Cardiology 17:155-161.

Kawachi, I., & Berkman, L.F. (Eds). (2003). Neighborhoods and health. New York: Oxford University Press.

Keller, C., Fleury, J., & Mujezinovic-Womack, M. (2003). Managing cardiovascular risk reduction in elderly adults: by promoting and monitoring healthy lifestyle changes, health care providers can help older adults improve their cardiovascular health. Journal of Gerontological Nursing 29:18-23.

Keller, K.B., & Lemberg, L. (2003). Obesity and the metabolic syndrome. American Journal of Critical Care 12:167-170.

Khattab, M.S., Abolfotouh, M.A., Alakija, W., Al-Humaidi, M.A., & Al-Wahat, S. (1999). Risk factors of coronary artery disease: attitude and behaviour in family practice in Saudi Arabia. Eastern Mediterranean Health Journal 5:35-45.

Kingsbury, K. (1998). Taking AIM: how to teach primary and secondary prevention effectively. Canadian Journal of Cardiology 14(Suppl)22A-26A.

Kingsley, C.M., & Gupta, S.C. (1992). How to reduce the risk of coronary artery disease: teaching patients a healthy life-style. Postgraduate Medicine 91:147-50, 153-4, 157-60.

Kirk-Gardner, R., & Steven, D. (2003). Hearts for Life: a community program on health promotion. Canadian Journal of Cardiovascular Nursing 13:5-10.

Kirshner, H.S. (2003). Medical prevention of stroke, 2003. Southern Medical Journal 96:354-358.

Koertge, J., Weidner, G., Elliott-Edler, M., Scherwitz, L., Merritt-Worden, T.A., Marlin, R., Lipsenthal, L., Guarneri, M., Finkel, R., Saunders, D.E. Jr., McCormac, P., Scheer, J.M., Collins, R.E., & Ornish, D. (2003). Improvement in medical risk factors and quality of life in women and men with coronary artery disease in the Multicenter Lifestyle Demonstration Project. American Journal of Cardiology 91:1316-1322.

Koffman, D.M., Bazzarre, T., Mosca, L., Redberg, R., Schmid, T., & Wattigney, W.A. (2001). An evaluation of Choose to Move 1999: an American Heart Association physical activity program for women. Archives of Internal Medicine 161:2193-2199.

Kok, F.J., Matroos, A.W., van den Ban, A.W., & Hautvast, J.G. (1982). Characteristics of individuals with multiple behavioral risk factors for coronary artery disease: the Netherlands. American Journal of Public Health 72:986-991.

Krill, J.J., & Halliday, G.M. (2001). Alzheimer's disease: its diagnosis and pathogenesis. International Review of Neurobiology 48: 167-217.

Krotenberg, R. (2004). Current recommendations for extended out-of-hospital thromboprophylaxis following total hip arthroplasty. American Journal of Orthopedics 33:180-184.

Kromhout, D., Menotti, A., Keseloot, H., & Sans, S. (2002). Prevention of coronary heart disease by diet and lifestyle: evidence from prospective cross-cultural, cohort, and intervention studies. Circulation 105:893-898.

Kurl, S., Laukkanen, J.A., Rauramaa, R., Lakka, T.A., Sivenius, J., & Salonen, J.T. (2003). Cardiorespiratory fitness and the risk of stroke in men. Archives of Internal Medicine 163: 1682-1688.

Kurl, S., Tuomainen, T.P., Laukkanen, J.A., Nyyssonen, K., Lakka, T., Sivenius, J., & Salonen, J.T. (2002). Plasma vitamin C modifies the association between hypertension and risk of stroke. Stroke 33:1568-1573.

Kurth, T., Kase, C.S., Berger, K., Schaeffner, E.S., Buring, J.E., & Gaziano, J.M. (2003). Smoking and the risk of hemorrhagic stroke in men. Stroke 34:1151-1155.

Lai, J.C., Woo, J., Hui, E., & Chan, W.M. (2004). Telerehabilitation—a new model for community-based stroke rehabilitation. Journal of Telemedicine and Telecare 10:199-205.

LaMonte, M.J., Eisenman, P.A., Adams, T.D., Shultz, B.B., Ainsworth, B.E., & Yanowitz, F.G. (2000). Cardiorespiratory fitness and coronary heart disease risk factors: the LDS Hospital Fitness Institute cohort. Circulation 102:1623-1628.

Larsen, C.S. (2003). Animal source foods and human health during evolution. Journal of Nutrition 133(11 Suppl 2): 3893S-3897S.

Lau-Walker, M. (2004). Cardiac rehabilitation: the importance of patient expectations—a practitioner survey. Journal of Clinical Nursing 13:177-184.

Lee, C.D., & Blair, S.N. (2002). Cardiopulmonary fitness and stroke mortality in men. Medicine and Science in Sports and Exercise 34:592-595.

Leng, G.C., Papacosta, O., Whincup, P., Wannamethee, G., Walker, M., Ebrahim, S., Nicolaides, A.N., Dhanjil, S., Griffin, M., Beclaro, G., Rumley, A., & Lowe, G.D. (2000). Femoral atherosclerosis in an older British population: prevalence and risk factors. Atherosclerosis 152:167-174.

Liu, S., & Manson, J.E. (2001). What is the optimal weight for cardiovascular health? British Medical Journal 322:631-632.

Liu, S., Manson, J.E., Lee, I.M., Cole, S.R., Hennekens, C.H., Willett, W.C., & Buring, J.E. (2000a). Fruit and vegetable intake and risk of cardiovascular disease: the Women's Health Study. American Journal of Clinical Nutrition 72:922-928.

Liu, S., Manson, J.E., Stampfer, M.J., Rexrode, K.M., Hu, F.B., Rimm, E.B., & Willett, W.C. (2000b). Whole grain consumption and risk of ischemic stroke in women: a prospective study. Journal of the American Medical Association 284:1534-1540.

Lloyd, T., Petit, M.A., Lin, H.M., & Beck, T.J. (2004). Lifestyle factors and the development of bone mass and bone strength in young women. Journal of Pediatrics 144:776-782.

Luedemann, J., Schminke, U., Berger, K., Piek, M., Willich, S.N., Doring, A., John, U., & Kessler, C. (2002). Association between behavior-dependent cardiovascular risk factors and asymptomatic carotid atherosclerosis in a general population. Stroke 33: 2929-2935.

Luepker, R.V. (2001). Cardiovascular disease among Mexican Americans. American Journal of Medicine 110:147-148.

Macken, L.C., Yates, B., & Blancher, S. (2000). Concordance of risk factors in female spouses of male patients with coronary artery disease. Journal of Cardiopulmonary Rehabilitation 20:361-368.

Maher, C.G., Sherrington, C., Herbert, R.D., Moseley, A.M., & Elkins, M. (2003). Reliability of the PEDro scale for rating quality of randomized controlled trials. Physical Therapy 83: 713-721.

Maltais, F., & Bourbeau, J. (1995). Medical management of emphysema. Chest Surgery Clinics of North America 5:673-689.

Mann, J.I. (2002). Diet and risk of coronary heart disease and type 2 diabetes. Lancet 360:783-789.

Manson, J.E., Tosteson, H., Ridker, P.M., Satterfield, S., Hebert, P., O'Connor, G.T., Buring, J.E., & Hennekens, C.H. (1992). The primary prevention of myocardial infarction. New England Journal of Medicine 326:1406-1416.

Marcus, B., Rossi, J., Selby, V., Miaura, R., & Adams, D. (1992). The stages and processes of exercise adoption and maintenance in a worksite sample. Health Psychology 11:386-395.

Marota Montero, J.M., & Velasco Rami, J.A. (1995). Cardiac rehabilitation and secondary prevention in ischemic cardiopathy. Revista Espanda de Cardiologia 48(Suppl 1):85-89.

McBurney, M.L. (2001). Candidate foods in the Asia-Pacific region for cardiovascular protection: relevance of grains and grain-based foods to coronary artery disease. Asia Pacific Journal of Clinical Nutrition 10:123-127.

McCreadie, R.G. (2003). Diet, smoking and cardiovascular risk in people with schizophrenia: descriptive study. British Journal of Psychiatry 183:534-539.

McCrindle, B.W. (2001). Cardiovascular risk factors in adolescents: relevance, detection, and intervention. Adolescent Medicine 12:147-162.

McCullough, M.L., Feskanich, D., Rimm, E.B., Giovannucci, E.L., Ascherio, A., Variyam, J.N., Spiegelman, D., Stampfer, M.J., & Willett, W.C. (2000a). Adherence to the Dietary Guidelines for Americans and risk of major chronic disease in men. American Journal of Clinical Nutrition 72:1223-1231.

McCullough, M.L., Feskanich, D., Stampfer, M.J., Rosner, B.A., Hu, F.B., Hunter, D.J., Variyam, J.N., Colditz, G.A., & Willett, W.C. (2000b). Adherence to the Dietary Guidelines for Americans and risk of major chronic disease in women. American Journal of Clinical Nutrition 72:1214-1222.

McDaniel, A.M. (1999). Assessing the feasibility of a clinical practice guideline for inpatient smoking cessation intervention. Clinical Nurse Specialist 13:228-235.

McKeown, N.M., Meigs, J.B., Liu, S., Wilson, P.W.F., & Jacques, P.F. (2002). Whole-grain intake is favorably associated with metabolic risk factors for type 2 diabetes and cardiovascular disease in the Framingham Offspring Study. American Journal of Clinical Nutrition 76:390-398.

McPherson, R. (2000). Coronary artery disease and women: applying the guidelines for risk factor management. Canadian Journal of Cardiology 16(Suppl A):5A-10A.

Meland, E., Maeland, J.G., & Laerum, E. (1999). The importance of self-efficacy in cardiovascular risk factor change. Scandinavian Journal of Public Health 27:11-17.

Mengden, T., Chamontin, B., Phong Chau, N., Luis Palma Gamiz, J., & Chanudet, X. (2000). User procedure for self-management of blood pressure. First International Consensus Conference on Self Blood Pressure Measurement. Blood Pressure Monitoring 5:111-129.

Merchant, A.T., Pitiphat, W., Rimm, E.B., & Joshipura, K. (2003). Increased physical activity decreases periodontal risk in men. European Journal of Epidemiology 18:891-898.

Messinger-Rapport, B.J., & Sprecher, D. (2002). Prevention of cardiovascular diseases: coronary artery disease, congestive heart failure, and stroke. Clinical Geriatric Medicine 18:463-483.

Minkler, M. (Ed.). (2002). Community organizing and community building for health. New Brunswick, NJ: Rutgers University Press.

Misra, A. (2000). Risk factors for atherosclerosis in young individuals. Journal of Cardiovascular Risk 7:215-229.

Mitani, H., Hashimoto, H., Isshiki, T., Kurokawa, S., Ogawa, K., Matsumoto, K., Miyake, F., Yoshino, H., & Fukuhara, S. (2003). Health-related quality of life of Japanese patients with chronic heart failure: assessment using the Medical Outcome Study Short Form 36. Circulation Journal 67:215-220.

Mokdad, A.H., Marks, J.S., Stroup, D.F., & Gerberding, J.L. (2004). Actual causes of death in the United States, 2000. Journal of the American Medical Association 291:1238-1245.

Mozaffarian, D., Fried, L.P., Burke, G.L., Fitzpatrick, A., & Siscovick, D.S. (2004). Lifestyles of older adults: can we influence cardiovascular risk in older adults? American Journal of Geriatric Cardiology 13:153-160.

Mozaffarian, D., Kumanyika, S.K., Lemaitre, R.N., Olson, J.L., Burke, G.L., Siscovick, D.S. (2003). Cereal, fruit, and vegetable fiber intake and the risk of cardiovascular disease in elderly individuals. Journal of the American Medical Association 289:1659-1666.

Musaiger, A.O. (2002). Diet and prevention of coronary heart disease in the Arab Middle East countries. Medical Principles and Practice 11(Suppl 2):9-16.

Nakamura, J., Amano, W., Araki, Y., Ishii, K., Uchida, Y., Kon, T., Sato, Y., Shiozaki, M., Takada, K., Naito, H., Nagaiwa, J., Nakajima, K., Yoshida, K., Watanabe, Y., Tomaru, T., & Aoyagi, T. (2003). Coronary risk factor management in primary practice in Shibuya, Tokyo. Journal of Cardiology 42:207-212. (English abstract).

Naslund, G.K., Fredrikson, M., Hellenius, M.L., & de Faire, U. (1996a). Effect of diet and physical exercise intervention programmes on coronary artery disease risk in smoking and non-

smoking men in Sweden. Journal of Epidemiology and Community Health 50:131-136.

Naslund, G.K., Fredrikson, M., Hellenius, M.L., & de Faire, U. (1996b). Determinants of compliance in men enrolled in a diet and exercise intervention trial: a randomized, controlled study. Patient Education and Counseling 29:247-256.

National Cancer Institute. Cancer facts. http://cancerweb.ncl.ac.uk/cancernet/600813.html; retrieved January 2005.

National Institutes of Health. (2004). Average blood pressure on the rise among American children/teenagers. Washington, DC: U.S. Department of Health and Human Services.

National Vital Statistics Reports. (2004). Estimated life expectancy at birth in years, by race and sex. 53:6.

Nesto, R.W. (2003). The relation of insulin resistance syndromes to risk of cardiovascular disease. Reviews in Cardiovascular Medicine 4(Suppl 6):S11-S18.

New York Heart Association Functional Classification. http://encyclopedia.thefreedictionary.com; retrieved November 2004.

Niebauer, J., Hambrecht, R., Velich, T., Hauer, K., Marburger, C., Kalberer, B., Weiss, C., von Hodenberg, E., Schlierf, G., Schuler, G., Zimmerman, R., & Kubler, W. (1997). Attenuated progression of coronary artery disease after 6 years of multi-factorial risk intervention: role of physical exercise. Circulation 96:2534-2541.

Nisbeth, O., Klausen, K., & Andersen, L.B. (2000). Effectiveness of counseling over 1 year on changes in lifestyle and coronary heart disease risk factors. Patient Education and Counseling 40:121-131.

Nguyen, M.N., Beland, F., & Otis, J. (1998). Is the intention to quit smoking influenced by other heart-healthy lifestyle habits in 30- to 60-year-old men? Addiction and Behavior 23:23-30.

Nguyen, M.N., Beland, F., Otis, J., & Potvin, L. (1996). Diet and exercise profiles of 30- and 60-year-old male smokers: implications for community heart health programs. Journal of Community Health 21:107-121.

North, K.E., Howard, B.V., Welty, T.K., Best, L.G., Lee, E.T., Yeh, J.L., Fabsitz, R.R., Roman, M.J., & MacCluer, J.W. (2003). Genetic and environment contributions to cardiovascular disease risk in American Indians: the Strong Heart Family Study. American Journal of Epidemiology 157:303-314.

Nyenhuis, D.L., Gorelick, P.B., Easley, C., Garron, D.C., Harris, Y., Richardson, D., Raman, R., & Levey, P. (2003). The black Seventh-day Adventist exploratory health study. Ethnicity and Disease 13:208-212.

Ockene, I.S., & Miller, N.H. (1997). Cigarette smoking, cardiovascular disease, and stroke: a statement for healthcare professionals from the American Heart Association. American Heart Association Task Force on Risk Reduction, Circulation 96:3243-3247.

Oki, Y., Shiomi, T., Sasanable, R., Maekawa, M., Hirota, I., Usui, K., Hasegawa, R., & Kobayashi, T. (1999). Multiple cardiovascular risk factors in obstructive sleep apnea syndrome patients and an attempt at lifestyle modification using telemedicine-based education. Psychiatry and Clinical Neuroscience 53:311-313.

Ornish, D. (1998). Avoiding revascularization with lifestyle changes: The Multicenter Lifestyle Demonstration Project. American Journal of Cardiology 82:72T-76T.

Ornish, D., Scherwitz, L.W., Billings, J.H., Brown, S.E., Gould, K.L., Merritt, T.A., Sparler, S., Armstrong, W.T., Ports, T.A., Kirkeeide, R.L., Hogeboom, C., & Brand, R.J. (1998). Intensive lifestyle change for reversal of coronary heart disease. Journal of the American Medical Association 280:2001-2007.

Orozco-Valero, M. (2002). Large therapeutic studies in elderly patients with hypertension. Journal of Human Hypertension 16(Suppl 1):S38-S43.

Owens, P.L., Bradley, E.H., Horwitz, S.M., Viscoli, C.M., Kernan, W.N., Brass, L.M., Sarrel, P.M., & Horwitz, R.I. (2002). Clinical assessment of function among women with a recent cerebrovascular event: a self-reported versus performance-based measure. Annals of Internal Medicine 136:802-811.

Panagiotakos, D.B., Pitsavos, C., Chrysohoou, C., Stefanadis, C., & Toutouzas, P. (2002). Risk stratification of the coronary heart disease in Greece: final results from the CARDIO2000 Epidemiological Study. Preventive Medicine 35:548-556.

Park, S.K., Park, J.H., Kwon, Y.C., Yoon, M.S., & Kim, C.S. (2003). The effect of long-term aerobic exercise on maximal oxygen consumption, left ventricular function and serum lipids in elderly women. Journal of Physiologic Anthropology and Applied Human Science 22:11-17.

Paterno, C.A. (2003). Coronary risk factors in adolescence. The FRICELA study. Revista Espanda de Cardiologia 56:452-458. (English abstract).

Peto, R., Lopez, A.D., Boreham, J., Thun, M., & Heath, C. Jr. (1992). Mortality from tobacco in developed countries: indirect estimation from national vital statistics. Lancet 339:1268-1278.

Pierson, D.J. (2004). Translating new understanding into better care for the patient with chronic obstructive pulmonary disease. Respiratory Care 49:99-109.

Piravej, K., & Wiwatkul, K. (2003). Risk factors for stroke in Thai patients. Journal of the Medical Association of Thailand 86:S291-S298.

Pitsavos, C., Panagiotakos, D.B., Chrysohoou, C., Kokkinos, P.F., Menotti, A., Singh, S., Dontas, A.; Seven Countries Study (the Corfu Cohort). (2004). Physical activity decreases the risk of stroke in middle-age men with left ventricular hypertrophy: 40-year follow-up (1961-2001) of the Seven Countries Study (the Corfu Cohort). Journal of Human Hypertension 18:495-501.

Pitsavos, C., Panagiotakos, D.B., Chrysohoou, C., Kokkinos, P.F., Skoumas, J., Papaioannou, I., Stefanadis, C., & Toutouzas, P. (2002). The effect of the combination of Mediterranean diet and leisure time physical activity on the risk of developing acute coronary syndromes, in hypertensive subjects. Journal of Human Hypertension 16:517-524.

Polidori, M.C. (2003). Antioxidant micronutrients in the prevention of age-related diseases. Journal of Postgraduate Medicine 49:229-235.

Poscente, N., Rothstein, M., & Irvine, M.J. (2002). Using marketing research methods to evaluate a stage-specific intervention. American Journal of Health Behavior 26:243-251.

Prochaska, J.O., & DiClemente, C.C. (1982). Transtheoretical therapy: toward a more integrative model of change. Psychotherapy: Theory, Research and Practice 19:276-288.

Racette, S.B., Deusinger, S.S., & Deusinger, R.H. (2003). Obesity: overview of prevalence, etiology, and treatment. Physical Therapy 83:276-288.

Ramadan, J., Telahoun, G., Al-Zaid, N.S., & Barac-Nieto, M. (1999). Responses to exercise, fluid, and energy balances during Ramadan in sedentary and active males. Nutrition 15:735-739.

Rashbaum, I.G., Walker, W.C., & Glassman, S.J. (2001). Cardio-pulmonary rehabilitation and cancer rehabilitation. 2. Cardiac rehabilitation in disabled populations. Archives of Physical Medicine and Rehabilitation 82(3 Suppl 1):S52-S55.

Rausch, M., & Turkoski, B. (1999). Developing realistic treatment standards in today's economic climate: stroke survivor education. Journal of Advances in Nursing 30:329-334.

Rimmer, J.H., Riley, B., Creviston, T., & Nicola, T. (2000). Exercise training in a predominantly African-American group of stroke survivors. Medicine and Science in Sports and Exercise 32:1990-1996.

Rollnick, S., Butler, C.C., & Stott, N. (1997). Helping smokers make decisions: the enhancement of brief intervention for general medical practice. Patient Education and Counseling 31:191-203.

Rollnick, S., Heather, N., & Bell, A. (1992). Negotiating behaviour change in medical settings: the development of brief motivational interviewing. Journal of Mental Health 1:25-37.

Rollnick, S., Mason, P., & Butler, C. (2002). Health behavior change: a guide for practitioners. Philadelphia: Churchill Livingstone.

Sackett, D.L., Straus S.E., Richardson, W.C., Rosenberg, W., & Haynes, R.B. (2000). Evidence-based medicine. Philadelphia: Churchill Livingstone.

Sato, Y. (2000). Diabetes and life-styles: role of physical exercise for primary prevention. British Journal of Nutrition 84(Suppl): S187-S190.

Sakakibara, H., Fujii, C., & Naito, M. (2004). Plasma fibrinogen and its association with cardiovascular risk factors in apparently healthy Japanese students. Heart Vessels 19:144-148.

Sanders, T.A. (2003). High- versus low-fat diets in human diseases. Current Opinions in Clinical Nutrition and Metabolic Care 6:151-155.

Savage, P.D., Brochu, M., & Ades, P.A. (2004). Gender alters the high-density lipoprotein cholesterol response to cardiac rehabilitation. Journal of Cardiopulmonary Rehabilitation 24:248-254.

Scott, C.L. (2003). Diagnosis, prevention, and interventions for the metabolic syndrome. American Journal of Cardiology 92:35-42.

Scott, I.A., Denaro, C.P., Flores, J.L., Bennett, C.J., Hickey, A.C., & Mudge, A.M. (2002). Quality of care of patients hospitalized with acute coronary syndromes. Internal Medicine Journal 32:502-511.

Sebregts, E.H., Falger, P.R., & Bar, F.W. (2000). Risk factor modification though nonpharmacological interventions in patients with coronary artery disease. Journal of Psychosomatic Research 48:425-441.

Shaper, A.G. (1996). Obesity and cardiovascular disease. Ciba Foundation Symposium 201:90-103.

Shapiro, J.S. (2000). Primary prevention of coronary artery disease in women through diet and lifestyle. New England Journal of Medicine 343:16-22.

Shaw, M., Mitchell, R., & Dorling, D. (2000). Time for a smoke? One cigarette reduces your life by 11 minutes. British Medical Journal 36:297-298.

Shike, M. (1999). Diet and lifestyle in the prevention of colorectal cancer: an overview. American Journal of Medicine 106: 11S-15S.

Shinton, R. (1997). Lifelong exposures and the potential for stroke prevention: the contribution of cigarette smoking, exercise, and body fat. Journal of Epidemiology and Community Health 51:138-143.

Simon, S.D. (2001). Is the randomized clinical trial the gold standard of research? Journal of Andrology 22:938-943.

Simonds, A.K. (2003). Ethics and decision making in end-stage lung disease. Thorax 58:272-277.

Singleton, J.R., Smith, A.G., Russell, J.W., & Feldman, E.L. (2003). Microvascular complications of impaired glucose tolerance. Diabetes 52:2867-2873.

Skybo, T.A., Ryan-Wenger, N. (2002). A school-based intervention to teach third-grade children about the prevention of heart disease. Pediatric Nursing 28:223-229, 235.

Slama, M., Susic, D., & Frolich, E.D. (2002). Prevention of hyper-tension. Current Opinions in Cardiology 17:531-536.

Sleight, P. (1991). Cardiovascular risk factors and the effects of intervention. American Heart Journal, 121:990-994.

Smith Jr., S.C. (1998). Need for a paradigm shift: the importance of risk factor reduction therapy in treating patients with cardiovascular disease. American Journal of Cardiology 82:10T-13T.

Smith, K.M., Arthur, H.M., McKelvie, R.S., & Kodis, J. (2004). Differences in sustainability of exercise and health-related quality of life outcomes following home or hospital-based cardiac rehabilitation. European Journal of Cardiovascular Prevention and Rehabilitation 11:313-319.

Smith, B.J., McElroy, H.J., Ruffin, R.E., Frith, P.A., Heard, A.R., Battersby, M.W., Esterman, A.J, Del Fante, P., & McDonald, P.J. (2002). The effectiveness of coordinated care for people with chronic respiratory disease. The Medical Journal of Australia 177:481-485.

Song, R., & Lee, H. (2001). Managing health habits for myocardial infarction (MI) patients. International Journal of Nursing Studies 38:375-380.

Sorenson, M. (1992). Herbivorous by design. In Mega health. Ivins, Utah: National Institute of Fitness.

Sorrentino, M.J. (2000). Cholesterol reduction to prevent CAD: what do the data show? Postgraduate Medicine 108:40-42, 45-46, 49-52.

Squires, R.W. (1996). Preventive rehabilitation cardiology: the Mayo Clinic approach. Medical Interface 9:62-68.

Srinath, U., Jonnalagadda, S.S., Naglak, M.C., Champagne, C., & Kris-Etherton, P.M. (1995). Diet in the prevention and treatment of atherosclerosis: a perspective for the elderly. Clinical Geriatric Medicine 11:591-611.

Steptoe, A., Kerry, S., Rink, E., & Hilton, S. (2001). The impact of behavioral counseling on stage of change in fat intake, physical activity, and cigarette smoking in adults at increased risk of coronary artery disease. American Journal of Public Health 91:265-269.

Steptoe, A., Wardle, J., Cui, W., Bellisle, F., Zotti, A.M., Baranyai, R., & Sanderman, R. (2002). Trends in smoking, diet, physical exercise, and attitudes toward health in European university students from 13 countries, 1990-2000. Preventive Medicine 35:97-104.

Stevens, M., Lemmink, K.A., van Heuvelen, M.J., de Jong, J., & Rispens, P. (2003). Groningen Active Living Model (GALM): stimulating physical activity in sedentary older adults' validation of the behavioral change model. Preventive Medicine 37:561-570.

Stewart, R., Richards, M., Brayne, C., & Mann, A. (2001). Vascular risk and cognitive impairment in an older, British, African-Caribbean population. Journal of the American Geriatric Society 49:263-269.

Storey, M., Stevens, J., Himes, J., Stone, E., Holy Rock, B., Ethelbah, B., & Davis, S. (2003). Obesity in American-Indian children: prevalence, consequences, and prevention. Preventive Medicine 37(Suppl)S3-S12.

Stretcher, V.J.R. & Rosenstock, I.M. (1997). The health belief model. In Glanz, K., Lewis, F.M., & Rimer, B.K., (Eds). Health behavior and health education: theory, research and practice. San Francisco: Jossey-Bass.

Suh, I., Oh, K.W., Lee, K.H., Psaty, B.M., Nam, C.M., Kim, S.I., Kang, H.G., Cho, S.Y., & Shim, W.H. (2001). Moderate dietary fat consumption as a risk factor for ischemic heart disease in a population with a low fat intake: a case-control study in Korean men. American Journal of Clinical Nutrition 73:722-727.

Sumanen, M., Koskenvuo, M., Immonen-Raiha, P., Suominen, S., Sundell, J., & Mattila, K. (2004). Secondary prevention of coronary artery disease is disappointing among patients of working age. Family Practice 21:304-306.

Svendsen, A. (2003). Heart failure: an overview of consensus guidelines and nursing implications. Canadian Journal of Cardiovascular Nursing 13:30-34.

Tanaka, K., & Nakanishi, T. (1996). Obesity as a risk factor for various diseases: necessity of lifestyle changes for healthy aging. Applied Human Science 15:139-148.

Ten, S., & MacLaren, N. (2004). Insulin resistance syndrome in children. Journal of Clinical Endocrinology and Metabolism 89:2526-2539.

Teri, L., Gibbons, L.E., McCurry, S.M., Logsdon, R.G., Buchner, D.M., Barlfow, W.E., Kukull, W.A., LaCroix, A.Z., McCormick, W., & Larson, E.B. (2003). Exercise plus behavioral management in patients with Alzheimer disease: a randomized controlled trial. Journal of the American Medical Association 290:2015-2022.

Tidy, N.M. (1958). Massage and remedial exercise, ed 9. Bristol, UK: John Wright & Sons.

The stages of readiness to change. internetrd.com/content. print%20change%20readiness.htm; retrieved Januaary 2005.

Thomas, R.J., Kottke, T.E., Brekke, M.J., Brekke, L.N., Brandel, C.L., Aase, L.A., & DeBoer, S.W. (2002). Attempts at changing dietary and exercise habits to reduce risk of cardiovascular disease: who's doing what in the community? Preventive Cardiology 5:102-108.

Todd, K.H., Samaroo, N., & Hoffman, J.R. (1993). Ethnicity as a risk factor for inadequate emergency department analgesia. Journal of the American Medical Association 269:1537-1539.

Toobert, D.J., Glasgow, R.E., & Radcliffe, J.L. (2000). Physiologic and related behavioral outcomes from the Women's Lifestyle Heart Trial. Annals of Behavioral Medicine 22:1-9.

Trakas, K., Oh, P.I., Singh, S., Risebrough, N, & Shear, N.H. (2001). The health status of obese individuals in Canada. International Journal of Obesity 25:662-668.

Tresch, D.D., & Aronow, W.S. (1996). Smoking and coronary artery disease. Clinics in Geriatric Medicine 12:23-32.

Tudor-Locke, C., & Bassett D.R. Jr. (2004). How many steps/day are enough? Preliminary pedometer indices for public health. Sports Medicine 34:1-8.

Turtle, J.R. (2000). The economic burden of insulin resistance. International Journal of Clinical Practice (Suppl):23-8.

Twardella, D., Kupper-Nybelen, J., Rothenbacher, D., Hahmann, H., Wusten, B., & Brenner, H. (2004). Short-term benefit of smoking cessation in patients with coronary artery disease: estimates based on self-reported smoking data and serum cotinine measurements. European Heart Journal 25:2101-2108.

Twisk, J.W., Snel, J., Kemper, H.C., & van Mechelen, W. (1999). Changes in daily hassles and life events and the relationship with coronary heart disease risk factors: a 2-year longitudinal study in 27-29-year-old males and females. Journal of Psychosomatic Research 46:229-240.

Twisk, J.W., Kemper, H.C., van Mechelen, W., & Post, G.B. (1997). Which lifestyle parameters discriminate high- from low-risk participants for coronary heart disease risk factors: longitudinal analysis covering adolescence and young adulthood. Journal of Cardiovascular Risk 4:393-400.

Uppaluri, C.R., Schumm, L.P., & Lauderdale, D.S. (2001). Self-reports of stress in Asian immigrants: effects of ethnicity and acculturation. Ethnicity and Disease 11:107-114.

United States Department of Health and Human Services, Consumer Information Center. The food guide pyramid. www.usda.gov; retrieved January 2005.

United States Department of Health and Human Services. Reducing tobacco use: a report of the surgeon general—2000. www.cdc. gov/tobacco; retrieved January 2005.

Varo Cenarruzabeita, J.J., Martinez Hernandez, J.A., & Martinez-Gonzalez, M.A. (2003). Benefits of physical activity and harms of inactivity. Medical Clinics (Barcelona) 121:665-672.

van Rooyen, J.M., Huisman, H.W., Eloff, F.C., Laubscher, P.J., Malan, L., Steyn, H.S., & Malan, N.T. (2002). Cardiovascular reactivity in black South-African males of different age groups: the influence of urbanization. Ethnicity and Disease 12:69-75.

Vuori, I.M. (2001). Health benefits of physical activity with special reference to interaction with diet. Public Health Nutrition 4:517-528.

Wahlqvist, M.L. (2002a). Asian migration to Australia: food and health consequences. Asia Pacific Journal of Clinical Nutrition 11:S562-S568.

Wahlqvist, M.L. (2002b). Chronic disease prevention: a life-cycle approach which takes account of the environmental impact and opportunities of food, nutrition and public health policies—the rationale for an eco-nutritional disease nomenclature. Asia Pacific Journal of Clinical Nutrition 11(Suppl):S759-S762.

Wannamethee, S.G., Shaper, A.G., & Perry, I.J. (2001). Smoking as a modifiable risk factor for type 2 diabetes in middle-aged men. Diabetes Care 24:1590-1595.

Ware, J.E. Jr., & Sherbourne, C.D. (1992). The MOS36-item short-form health survey (SF-36): conceptual framework and item selection. Medical Care 30:473-483.

Weintraub, W.S., Jones, E.L., Morris, D.C., King, S.B., Guyton, R.A., & Craver, J.M. (1997). Outcome of reoperative coronary bypass surgery versus coronary angioplasty after previous bypass surgery. Circulation 95:868-877.

Wells, K.B., Lewis, C.E., Leake, B., & Ware, J.E. Jr.. (1984). Do physicians preach what they practice? A study of physicians' health habits and counseling practices. Journal of the American Medical Association 252:2846-2848.

Wenche, D.B., Holmen, J., Kruger, O., & Midthjell, K. (2004). Leisure-time physical activity and change in body mass index: an 11-year follow-up study of 9357 normal weight healthy women 20-49 years old. Journal of Women's Health 13:55-62.

Wessel, T.R., Arant, C.B., Olson, M.B., Johnson, B.D., Reis, S.E., Sharaf, B.L., Shaw, L.J., Handberg, E., Sopko, G., Kelsey, S.F., Pepine, C.J., & Bairey Merz, C.N. (2004). Relationship of physical fitness vs body mass index with coronary artery disease and cardiovascular events in women. Journal of the American Medical Association 292:1179-1187.

White, J.L., & Ransdell, L.B. (2003). Worksite intervention model for facilitating changes in physical activity, fitness, and psychological parameters. Perceptual and Motor Skills 97:461-466.

Whitt, M., Kumanyika, S., & Bellamy, S. (2003). Amount and bouts of physical activity in a sample of African-American women. Medicine and Science in Sport and Exercise 35:1887-1893.

Wilbur, J., Chandler, P.J., Dancy, B., & Lee, H. (2003a). Correlates of physical activity in urban Midwestern African-American women. American Journal of Preventive Medicine 25:45-52.

Wilbur, J., Chandler, P.J., Dancy, B., & Lee, H. (2003b). Correlates of physical activity in urban Midwestern Latinas. American Journal of Preventive Medicine 25:69-76.

Wierenga, M.E., & Oldham, K.K. (2002). Weight control: a lifestyle-modification model for improving health. Nursing Clinics of North America 37:303-313.

Williams, M.A., Fleg, J.L., Ades, P.A., Chaitman, B.R., Miller, N.H., Mohiuddin, S.M., Ockene, I.S., Taylor, C.B., & Wenger, N.K. (2002). Secondary prevention of coronary heart disease in the elderly (with emphasis on patients > or = 75 years of age): an American Heart Association scientific statement from the Council on Clinical Cardiology Subcommittee on Exercise, Cardiac Rehabilitation, and Prevention. Circulation 105:1735-1743.

Wilson, P.W., & Kannel, W.B. (2002). Obesity, diabetes, and risk of cardiovascular disease in the elderly. American Journal of Geriatric Cardiology 11:119-123, 125.

Winslow, E., Bohannon, N., Brunton, S.A., & Mayhew, H.E. (1996). Lifestyle modification: weight control, exercise, and smoking cessation. American Journal of Medicine 101:25S-31S.

Woo, J. (2000). Relationships among diet, physical activity and other lifestyle factors and debilitating diseases in the elderly. European Journal of Clinical Nutrition 54(Suppl 3):S143-S147.

Woo, J., Ho, S.C., & Yu, A.L. (2002). Lifestyle factors and health outcomes in elderly Hong Kong Chinese aged 70 years and over. Gerontology 48:234-240.

Wood, D. (2001). Asymptomatic individuals—risk stratification in the prevention of coronary artery disease. British Medical Journal 59:3-16.

World Health Organization. (1998). Obesity: preventing and managing the global epidemic. Geneva, Switzerland: World Health Organization.

World Health Organization. Annual Health Reports 1999-2003. Geneva, Switzerland: World Health Organization.

World Health Organization. (2002). International Classification of Functioning, Disability and Health, 2002. www.sustainable-design.ie/arch/ICIDH-2PFDec-2000.pdf; retrieved December 2004.

World Health Organization. (2003). Technical Report Series. Geneva, Switzerland: World Health Organization 916:i-vii1-149.

World Health Organization. Definition of health. www.who.int/about/definition; retrieved November 2004.

Wright, L., Murcer, S., Adams, K., Welch, S., & Paris, D. (1994). The factor analysis structure of seven physical CHD risk factors: a replication study. Journal of Clinical Psychology 50:216-219.

Xu, H., Barnes, G.T., Yang, Q., Tan, G., Yang, D., Chou, C.J., Sole, J., Nichols, A., Ross, J.S., Tartaglia, L.A., & Chen, H. (2003). Chronic inflammation in fat plays a crucial role in the development of obesity in the development of obesity-related insulin resistance. Journal of Clinical Investigation 112:1821-1830.

Yohannes, A.M., & Hardy, C.C. (2003). Treatment of chronic obstructive pulmonary disease in older patients: a practical guide. Drugs and Aging 20:209-228.

Zafari, A.M., & Wenger, N.K. (1998). Secondary prevention of coronary heart disease. Archives of Physical Medicine and Rehabilitation 79:1006-1017.

CHAPTER 2

Oxygen Transport: The Basis of Cardiopulmonary Physical Therapy

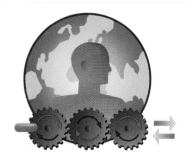

Elizabeth Dean

KEY TERMS　　Cellular respiration　　　　　　　　Gravitational stress
　　　　　　　　　　Exercise stress　　　　　　　　　　Oxygen transport pathway

Oxygen transport is essential to life, activity, and participation in life consistent with the International Classification of Function (World Health Organization, 2000). Maximizing the efficiency of the oxygen transport pathway promotes optimal mobility and independence, which are the cornerstones of quality of life and well-being. Attention to oxygen transport—its deficits and threats to it—is the concern of physical therapists, irrespective of the primary clinical area of their practice. This is particularly true given the trend toward physical therapists' direct access to patients and the prevalence of the diseases of civilization, all of which affect oxygen transport either directly or indirectly.

Cardiopulmonary physical therapy is an essential non-invasive medical intervention that can reverse or mitigate insults to oxygen transport. It can eliminate, delay, or reduce the need for medical interventions, such as supplemental oxygen, intubation, mechanical ventilation, suctioning, bronchoscopy, chest tubes, surgery, and medications. A comprehensive understanding of oxygen transport and the factors that determine and influence it is therefore essential for the comprehensive assessment of oxygen transport and optimal treatment prescription to effect these outcomes.

This chapter details the oxygen transport system, including the pathway and its component steps, which provides a conceptual basis for cardiopulmonary physical therapy practice. Oxygen transport is the basis of life. Treatment of impaired or threatened oxygen transport (i.e., cardiopulmonary dysfunction) is a physical therapy priority.

In a healthy person, the oxygen transport system is perturbed by movement and activity, changes in body position, and emotional stress. In a person with pathology, disruption of or threat to this system is a medical priority because of the threat to life or the impairment of functional capacity.

The fundamental steps in the oxygen transport pathway, as well as their function and interdependence, are described first. Special attention is given to cellular respiration and the use of oxygen during metabolism at the cellular level in muscle. Second, the factors that perturb oxygen transport in health are described, namely, gravitational stress secondary to changes in body position, exercise stress secondary to increased oxygen demand of the working muscles, and emotional stress and arousal. A thorough understanding of the effects of those factors that normally perturb oxygen transport is essential to accurately assess and treat deficits in oxygen transport.

OXYGEN TRANSPORT

Oxygen transport refers to the delivery of fully oxygenated blood to peripheral tissues, cellular uptake of oxygen, use of oxygen within the tissue, and the return of partially desaturated blood to the lungs. The oxygen transport pathway consists of multiple steps, ranging from the ambient air to the perfusion of peripheral tissues with oxygenated arterial blood (Figure 2-1). Oxygen transport has become the basis for conceptualizing cardiopulmonary function and diagnosing and managing cardiopulmonary dysfunction (Dantzker, 1985,

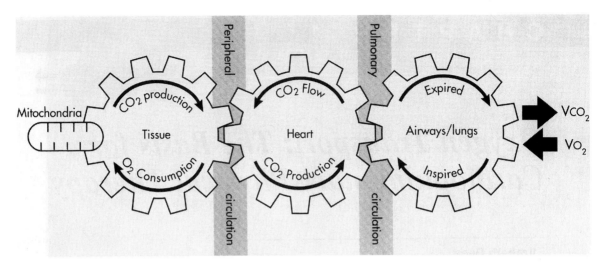

FIGURE 2-1 Scheme of components of ventilatory-cardiovascular-metabolic coupling underlying oxygen transport. *(Modified from Wasserman, K., et al. [1987]. Principles of exercise testing and interpretation. Philadelphia: Lea & Febiger.)*

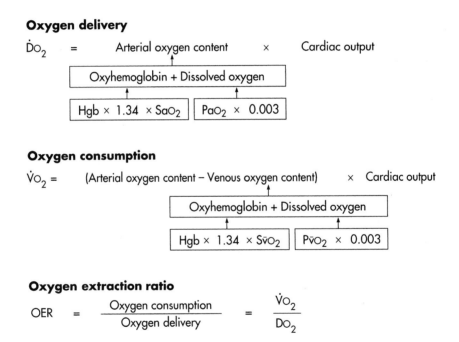

FIGURE 2-2 Formulas for determining oxygen delivery (DO_2), oxygen consumption ($\dot{V}O_2$), and oxygen extraction ratio (OER). *(Modified from Epstein, C.D., Henning R.J. [1993]. Oxygen transport variables in the identification and treatment of tissue hypoxia. Heart Lung 22:328-348.)*

1993; Dantzker et al, 1991; Dean, 1994a; Dean & Ross 1992a; Goldring, 1984; Ross & Dean, 1989; Weber et al, 1983).

Oxygen transport variables include oxygen delivery (DO_2), oxygen consumption ($\dot{V}O_2$), and the oxygen extraction ratio (OER), the utilization coefficient. Oxygen demand is the amount of oxygen required by the cells for aerobic metabolism. Oxygen demand is usually reflected by $\dot{V}O_2$; however, in cases of severe cardiopulmonary dysfunction and compromise to oxygen transport, $\dot{V}O_2$ can fall short of the demand for oxygen. Oxygen transport variables, including the components of DO_2, $\dot{V}O_2$ and the OER, are shown in Figure 2-2. DO_2 is determined by arterial oxygen content and cardiac output, $\dot{V}O_2$ by the arterial and venous oxygen content difference and cardiac output, and oxygen extraction by the ratio of DO_2 to $\dot{V}O_2$.

Measures and indexes of oxygen transport that reflect the function of the component steps of the oxygen transport pathway are shown in Box 2-1.

BOX 2-1

Measures and Indexes of the Function of the Steps in the Oxygen Transport Pathway

Control of Ventilation

- PO.1 (central drive to breathe)
- Ventilatory responses of hypoxia and hypercapnia
- PaO_2 and SaO_2 responses to exercise

Inspired Gas

- Alveolar oxygen pressure
- Alveolar carbon dioxide pressure
- Alveolar nitrogen pressure

Hematological Variables

- Hemoglobin
- Plasma proteins and their concentrations
- Red blood cells and count
- White blood cells and count
- Platelets
- Clotting factors
- Clotting times
- Hematocrit
- PaO_2
- $PaCO_2$ (end tidal CO_2)
- $P(A-a)O_2$
- CaO_2
- $C\bar{v}O_2$
- $C(a-\bar{v})O_2$ difference
- HCO_3
- SaO_2
- pH
- PaO_2/PAO_2
- PaO_2/FiO_2
- Serum lactate

Pulmonary Variables

- Minute ventilation
- Tidal volume
- Respiratory rate
- Dead space volume
- Alveolar volume
- Alveolar ventilation
- Distribution of ventilation
- Static and dynamic lung compliance
- Airway resistance
- Functional residual capacity
- Closing volume
- Vital capacity
- Forced expiratory volumes and flows
- Other pulmonary volumes, capacities, and flow rates
- Inspiratory and expiratory pressures
- Work of breathing
- Respiratory muscle strength and endurance

Pulmonary Hemodynamic Variables

- Cardiac output
- Total perfusion
- Distribution of perfusion

- Anatomical shunt
- Physiological shunt
- Systolic and diastolic pulmonary artery pressures
- Pulmonary capillary blood flow
- Pulmonary capillary wedge pressure
- Pulmonary vascular resistance
- Pulmonary vascular resistance index

Systemic Hemodynamic Variables

- Heart rate
- Electrocardiogram (ECG)
- Systemic blood pressure
- Mean arterial blood pressure
- Systemic vascular resistance
- Systemic vascular resistance index
- Central venous pressure
- Pulmonary artery pressure
- Wedge pressure
- Blood volume
- Cardiac output
- Cardiac index
- Stroke volume
- Stroke index
- Shunt fraction
- Ejection fraction
- Left ventricular work
- Right ventricular work
- Fluid balance
- Renal output
- Creatinine clearance and blood urea nitrogen (BUN)

Diffusion

- $D(A-a)O_2$
- Diffusing capacity
- Diffusing capacity/alveolar volume

Gas Exchange

- Oxygen consumption ($\dot{V}O_2$)
- Carbon dioxide production ($\dot{V}CO_2$)
- Respiratory exchange ratio ($\dot{V}CO_2/\dot{V}O_2$)
- Ventilation and perfusion matching
- PaO_2/PAO_2
- $P(A-a)O_2$

Oxygen Extraction and Use

- Oxygen extraction ratio ($\dot{V}O_2/DO_2$)
- $C(a-\bar{v})O_2$ difference
- $P(a-\bar{v})O_2$ difference
- $S\bar{v}O_2$
- Metabolic enzymes at the cellular level
- Oxyhemoglobin dissociation

Adequacy of Tissue Perfusion and Oxygen Transport

- Tissue oxygenation
- Tissue pH

Energy Transfer and Cellular Oxidation

Cellular metabolism and survival depend on the continuous synthesis and degradation of adenosine triphosphate (ATP), the major source of energy for biological work. Work is performed in biological systems for contraction of skeletal, cardiac, and smooth muscle (e.g., exercise, digestion, glandular secretion, and thermoregulation) and for nerve impulse transmission (Box 2-2). These processes require a continuous supply of ATP, which is made available primarily by aerobic (oxygen-requiring) processes. In the event that oxygen delivery is inadequate, nonaerobic (anaerobic, or non–oxygen-requiring) energy-transferring processes can also supply ATP. Supplying energy anaerobically, however, is more costly metabolically; that is, it is not efficient, is limited, and cannot be sustained because of the disruptive effects of lactate (a cellular by-product of anaerobic metabolism) on physiological processes in general. Metabolic acidosis is a consequence of lactate accumulation. In patients who are critically ill, the presence of metabolic acidosis secondary to anaerobic metabolism can be life threatening. Prolonged anaerobic metabolism is lethal in two respects. First, the patient is increasingly dependent on anaerobic metabolism because of inadequate DO_2 to peripheral tissues, and second, acidosis interferes with normal cellular processes and homeostasis, which require an optimal pH of 7.40.

The ATP molecule consists of an adenine and a ribose molecule with three phosphates attached. The splitting of the terminal phosphate bond or the two terminal phosphate bonds generates a considerable amount of energy. This energy is used to power various chemical reactions associated with metabolism. These metabolic processes take place in specialized organelles in the cells called mitochondria. The primary pathways that are responsible for the formation of ATP are the Krebs cycle and the electron transfer chain.

The Krebs cycle and the electron transfer chain are the biochemical pathways in the mitochondria of the cell responsible for harnessing oxygen for aerobic metabolism and ensuring a continuous supply of oxygen for this process. Initially, glucose is phosphorylated to produce two molecules of ATP (glycolysis). Glucose is oxidized to produce two molecules of pyruvic acid, yielding a net gain of two molecules of ATP per molecule of glucose. The two pyruvate molecules enter the Krebs cycle, where they are oxidized to CO_2 and water. This process yields 30 ATP molecules. Hydrogen ions released in the process are transferred to the electron transfer chain, yielding 4 ATP molecules for cellular metabolism. Electrons are removed from hydrogen and funneled down the electron transport chain by specialized electron carrier molecules, cytochromes 1 to 5. Only the last of these cytochromes, cytochrome oxidase, can reduce molecular oxygen to water. This process is driven by a gradient of high-to-low potential energy. This energy, transferred as electrons, is passed from H_2 to O_2 and is trapped and conserved as high-energy phosphate bonds. Oxygen is involved in these metabolic pathways only at the end of the electron transfer chain, where oxygen is the final electron acceptor and combines with H_2 to form H_2O. More than 90% of ATP synthesis takes place through the electron transfer chain by means of the oxidative reactions associated with oxidative phosphorylation. An individual's peak aerobic capacity is determined by the availability of oxygen at the end of the electron transport chain.

For each molecule of glucose that is metabolized, 36 molecules of ATP are produced: 4 molecules by substrate phosphorylation (anaerobic) and 32 by oxidative phosphorylation (aerobic). The low ATP yield from anaerobic metabolism explains why anaerobic metabolism can serve only as a short-term energy source.

The complex, enzymatically controlled chemical reactions of metabolism are designed to form and conserve energy through the Krebs cycle and the electron transfer chain and then use this energy for biological work (Ganong, 2003; Shephard, 1985). Carbohydrates, fats, and proteins ingested from foodstuffs in the diet are oxidized to provide the energy for phosphorylation of adenosine diphosphate (ADP) (i.e., the formation of ATP by combining ADP with phosphate). These substances are broken down, and they access the Krebs cycle at the pyruvic acid or acetyl coenzyme A (CoA) levels (Figure 2-3). Some amino acids can enter the Krebs cycle directly.

The Krebs cycle degrades acetyl CoA to carbon dioxide (CO_2) and hydrogen (H_2) atoms. The primary purpose of this cycle is to generate hydrogen ions for the electron transfer chain by two principal electron acceptors, nicotinamide adenine dinucleotide (NAD) and flavin adenine dinucleotide (FAD). Many acids catalyze the numerous reactions of the Krebs cycle.

Cellular oxidation, or respiration, refers to the function of the electron transfer chain to release energy in small amounts and to conserve energy in the formation of high-energy bonds. It is this process that ensures a continual energy supply to meet the needs of metabolism (Figure 2-4).

Three major systems of energy transfer exist to supply energy during all-out exercise over varying durations (McArdle et al, 2000). Although these systems are discrete, they overlap. Cellular ATP and creatine phosphate (CP) are immediate energy sources for the first 10 seconds of exercise. From 30 to 60 seconds, glycolysis provides a short-term energy source. The ATP-CP system and the glycolytic system

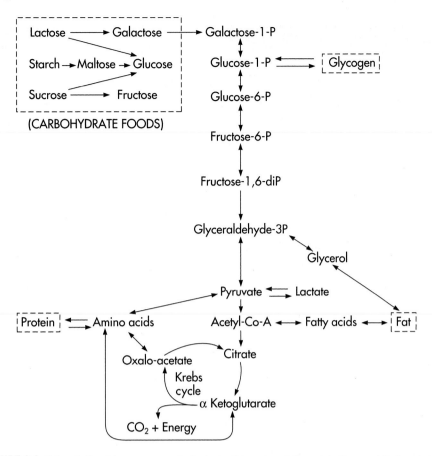

FIGURE 2-3 Interrelationships among carbohydrate, fat, and protein metabolism and their points of entry into the Krebs cycle. *(From Shepard, R.J. [1985]. Physiology and biochemistry of exercise. Philadelphia: Praeger Scientific.)*

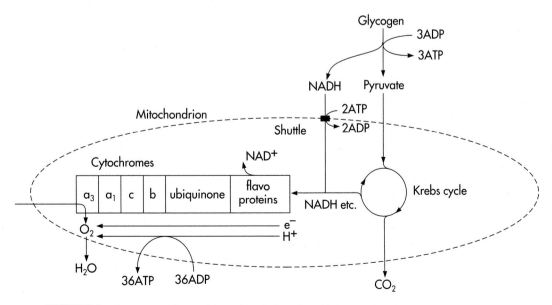

FIGURE 2-4 Electron transfer chain and its relationship with the Krebs cycle. *(From Shepard R.J. [1985]. Physiology and biochemistry of exercise. Philadelphia: Praeger Scientific.)*

are anaerobic processes. As exercise persists for several minutes, the long-term aerobic system predominates. Thus, for sustained physical activity and exercise, energy is provided primarily by aerobic metabolism. For this process, oxygen is provided by the oxygen transport pathway. Carbon compounds that enter the body in the form of carbohydrate, fat, and protein undergo oxidative metabolism in the form of aerobic glycolysis in the mitochondria in the cytoplasm of cells.

Muscle Contraction and Metabolism

The basic mechanism for muscle contraction is excitation contraction coupling (Kirchberger, 1991; Tortora & Anagnostakos, 2003). Action potentials mediated centrally or through the spinal cord depolarize the muscle cell membrane (the sarcolemma) and stimulate the release of calcium from the lateral sacs of the sarcoplasmic reticulum. The sarcoplasmic reticulum is an extensive network of invaginations and tubular channels encasing the muscle fibers (myofibrils). The calcium floods over the myofilaments of the myofibrils. Myofilaments consist of thin actin fiber and thick myosin fiber protein, which interdigitate with each other, giving the typical striated appearance to skeletal muscle (Figures 2-5 and 2-6). Actin is a helical molecule with tropomyosin intertwined along its length. Tropomyosin normally inhibits the interaction of actin and myosin. Calcium causes a conformational change of the tropomyosin molecule that enables troponin, also distributed along the actin molecule, to combine with calcium. The combining of calcium and troponin triggers the interdigitation of actin and myosin (the sliding-filament theory of muscle contraction). Contraction involves myosin heads (cross bridges) attaching to and detaching from actin in a cyclical manner that causes the actin and myosin filaments to slide past each other. In this way, the muscle is shortened without shortening of the myofilaments.

The energy for muscle contraction in the form of ATP is generated within the mitochondria of the myofibrils (Shephard, 1985). Myosin ATPase splits ATP so that the transfer of this energy can be used for muscle contraction. Specifically, the enzyme ATPase is activated when actin and myosin are joined. ATP is then available to bind with the cross bridge, causing it to detach from actin. Relaxation occurs with the cessation of electrical excitation and the rapid removal or sequestration of calcium into the lateral sacs of the sarcoplasmic reticulum.

The specific metabolic properties of muscle depend on the constituent muscle fiber types (Foss & Keteyian, 1998). The three primary muscle fiber types are fast-twitch fibers, slow-twitch fibers, and intermediate fibers, which have the properties of both. The fast-twitch fibers (fast glycolytic fibers) are recruited during short-term, sprint-type exercise that relies mainly on anaerobic metabolism. These fibers are well adapted for rapid, forceful contractions because they have large amounts of myosin ATPase, rapid calcium release and uptake, and a high rate of cross bridge cycling. Slow-

twitch fibers (slow oxidative fibers) are recruited during prolonged aerobic exercise. These fibers have large amounts of myoglobin, mitochondria, and oxidative enzymes. Compared with the fast-twitch fibers, slow-twitch fibers are fatigue resistant. The intermediate fibers have both anaerobic and aerobic metabolic enzymes, which makes these fibers capable of both types of muscle work. Although the characteristics of the fiber types are distinct, activity and exercise recruit both types of fibers. Depending on the particular activity or exercise, one fiber type may be preferentially recruited over the others.

Principles of Oxygen Transport

Individuals need a continuous supply of oxygen to meet moment-to-moment demands for oxygen commensurate with changing metabolic demands for energy at the cellular level, as well as basal metabolic demands (Dantzker et al, 1997; Samsel & Schumacker, 1991). Oxygen transport occurs by convection or diffusion. Convection of oxygen refers to the movement of oxygen from the alveoli to the tissue capillaries and is determined primarily by hemoglobin concentration, oxygen saturation, and cardiac output. The diffusion of oxygen refers to the movement of oxygen from the capillaries to the mitochondria and is determined by metabolic rate, vascular resistance, capillary recruitment, and tissue oxygen consumption and extraction.

Normally, DO_2 is regulated by tissue metabolism and the overall demand for oxygen. At rest, DO_2 is three to four times greater than oxygen demand, and $\dot{V}O_2$ is not directly dependent on DO_2. In a healthy individual the increased metabolic demands of exercise constitute the greatest challenge to the oxygen transport system. The $\dot{V}O_2$ can increase 20 times. In response to increased muscle metabolism, blood flow increases to the peripheral muscles through vasodilation and capillary recruitment, thereby increasing the availability of oxygen to working tissues and its extraction from the arterial blood. As DO_2 and $\dot{V}O_2$ increase, venous return, stroke volume, and heart rate also increase, thereby increasing cardiac output (CO). The CO can increase by more than five times during strenuous exercise.

At rest, regional differences in the proportion of CO normally delivered to the body organs reflect differences in organ functions and are not necessarily matched to the metabolic rate (Guyton, 2000). For example, the distribution of CO to the kidneys is 20% and to the mesenteric, splenic, and portal tissues, 20% to 30%. Comparatively, muscle at rest receives 10% and the brain and myocardium receive less than 5% each.

Oxygen Content of the Blood

The majority of oxygen is transported in arterial blood to the tissues in combination with hemoglobin (98%), compared with a relatively minimal amount of oxygen that is dissolved in the blood (2%). The oxyhemoglobin dissociation curve

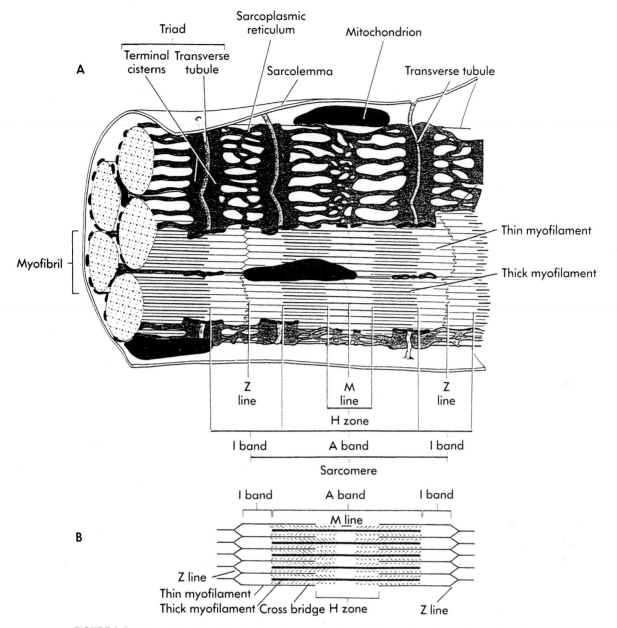

FIGURE 2-5 Schematic of the ultrastructure of a muscle fiber. **A,** View of muscle membrane structure and myofibril arrangement. **B,** A single functional unit (sarcomere) of a myofibril showing the interdigitation of the actin and myosin filaments. *(From Tortora, G.J., & Anagnostakos, N.P. [2003]. Principles of anatomy and physiology. New York: Harper & Row.)*

represents the relationship between the affinity of hemoglobin for oxygen and the arterial oxygen tension. The affinity of hemoglobin for oxygen depends on the tissues' oxygen demand. In a healthy individual, exercising muscle increases the demand for oxygen. The heat of the working muscles and the acidic environment during exercise result in reduced oxyhemoglobin affinity and increased oxygen release. This is reflected by a shift to the right of the oxyhemoglobin dissociation curve (see Chapter 4). The affinity of hemoglobin and oxygen is increased with the cessation of exercise, which is reflected by a leftward shift of the curve.

Oxygen Delivery to the Tissues

The final steps in oxygen transport involve the dissociation of oxygen from hemoglobin and the diffusion of oxygen from the capillaries to the cells (Schumacker & Samsel, 1989). Diffusion depends on the quantity and rate of blood flow, the difference in capillary and tissue oxygen pressures, the capillary surface area, capillary permeability, and diffusion distance (West, 2004). With increased metabolic demand by the tissues, capillary dilation and recruitment increase capillary surface area and reduce vascular resistance to flow, diffusion

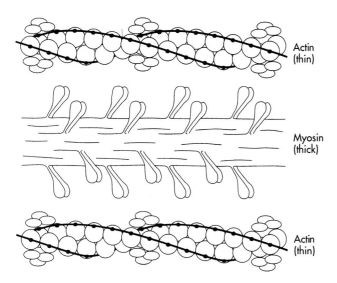

FIGURE 2-6 Arrangement of the thick and thin myofilaments. *(From Hasson, S. [1994]. Clinical exercise physiology. St. Louis: Mosby.)*

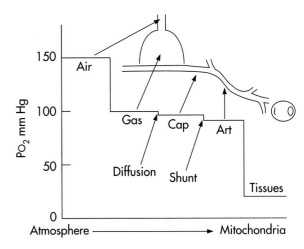

FIGURE 2-7 Scheme of oxygen partial pressures from air to tissue. The cascade reflects the removal of oxygen by the pulmonary capillary blood and the tissues. Depressions caused by the effects of diffusion and shunt are also illustrated. *(From West, J.B. [2004]. Respiratory physiology—the essentials, ed 5. Baltimore: Williams & Wilkins.)*

distance is decreased, the movement of oxygen into the cell is facilitated, and the tissue oxygen tension is increased.

Two diffusion gradients determine effective oxygen transport: one occurs between the pulmonary capillaries and the alveoli; the other occurs between the peripheral capillaries and the tissue cells. Diffusion of oxygen occurs as the blood moves from the aorta to the arterioles. The mean oxygen tension in the aorta is about 95 mm Hg and in the arterioles is 70 to 80 mm Hg. The oxygen gradient between the arterioles and the cells is the steepest. The mean oxygen pressure is less than 50 mm Hg in the capillaries. The oxygen tension in the capillaries determines the rate of diffusion to the cells. An optimal diffusion gradient maintains the oxygen tension in the cell at between 1 and 10 mm Hg; oxygen tension is less than 0.5 mm Hg in the mitochondria (Guyton, 2000). This decremental PaO_2 profile down the oxygen transport pathway, from the airways to the tissues, is termed the oxygen cascade (Figure 2-7).

Cardiac Output

In addition to arterial oxygen content, CO is a primary determinant of DO_2 (Dantzker et al, 1997). The transport of oxyhemoglobin to the tissues is dependent on convective blood flow by way of CO. The CO is the volume of blood pumped from the right or left ventricle per minute. The components of CO are stroke volume (SV) and heart rate (HR) (i.e., CO = SV × HR). Stroke volume is the amount of blood ejected from the left ventricle during each ventricular systole or heartbeat and is determined by the preload, myocardial distensibility, myocardial contractility, and afterload. The DO_2 is optimized in patients by increasing CO through the therapeutic manipulation of preload, myocardial contractility, afterload, and heart rate.

Preload

Preload is the end-diastolic muscle fiber length of the ventricles before systolic ejection, and on the left side it reflects the left ventricular end-diastolic volume (LVEDV). The LVEDV is dependent on venous return, blood volume, and left atrial contraction. An increase in ventricular volume stretches the myocardial fibers and increases the force of myocardial contraction (the Starling effect) and stroke volume. This effect is limited by the physiologic limits of distension of the myocardium. Excessive stretching, as in fluid overload of the heart, leads to suboptimal overlap of the actin and myosin filaments, thus impairing rather than enhancing contractility.

Afterload

Afterload is the resistance to the ejection of blood during ventricular systole. Afterload of the left ventricle is determined primarily by four factors: the distensibility of the aorta, the vascular resistance, the patency of the aortic valve, and the viscosity of the blood.

Myocardial Contractility

Myocardial contractility reflects actin-myosin coupling during contraction and is assessed by the ejection fraction, the rate of circumferential muscle fiber shortening, the pressure-volume relationships, and the rate of change of ventricular pressure over time.

Oxygen Debt

Tissue oxygen debt, or recovery oxygen consumption, is the difference between oxygen demand and oxygen consumption.

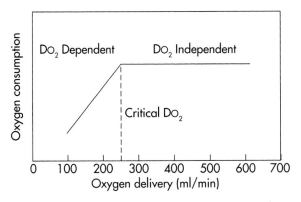

FIGURE 2-8 Relationship between oxygen consumption ($\dot{V}O_2$) and oxygen delivery (DO_2). The DO_2-independent phase represents the normal metabolic state. The DO_2-dependent phase represents the dependency of $\dot{V}O_2$ on DO_2 when DO_2 falls below the critical DO_2. *(Modified from Phang, P.T., and Russell, J.A. [1993]. When does $\dot{V}O_2$ depend on DO_2? Respiratory Care 38:618-630.)*

In healthy individuals, oxygen debt can be sustained for short periods during intense exercise. Anaerobic metabolism is stimulated to produce ATP under these conditions. In patients who are critically ill, the degree of oxygen debt is correlated with survival (Mizock & Falk, 1992).

Oxygen Extraction Ratio or Utilization Coefficient

The OER, or utilization coefficient, reflects the proportion of oxygen delivered to that consumed. The OER is calculated by dividing $\dot{V}O_2$ by DO_2. Normally, the OER is 23% at rest.

Supply-Dependent Oxygen Consumption

Normally, a decrease in DO_2 does not reduce $\dot{V}O_2$ (Phang & Russell, 1993). With a decrement in DO_2, the tissues extract a commensurate amount of oxygen from the blood. In patients who are critically ill, the DO_2 may be limited to the point where basic metabolic needs for oxygen (300 ml/min/M^2) are not met (Fenwick, 1990; Lorente et al, 1991; Myles et al, 1996; Phang & Russell, 1993). The critical level at which $\dot{V}O_2$ falls is associated with tissue anaerobic metabolism and the development of lactic acidosis and decreased pH (Figure 2-8) (Mizock & Falk, 1992; Schumaker & Cain, 1987). Serum lactates correspondingly increase and provide a valid index of anaerobic metabolism in patients with multiorgan system failure. When oxygen transport data are analyzed, the effect of sedation may suggest a dependency between DO_2 and $\dot{V}O_2$, so the impact of medication in this relationship must be considered (Boyd et al, 1992).

Oxygen Transport Pathway

Oxygen transport is dependent on several interconnecting steps, ranging from inhalation of oxygen-containing air through

the nares to oxygen extraction at the cellular level in response to metabolic demand (see Figure 2-1). These steps provide the mechanism for ventilatory, cardiovascular, and metabolic coupling. In addition, blood is responsible for transporting oxygen within the body; thus its constituents and consistency directly affect this process.

Quality and Quantity of Blood

Although not considered a discrete step in the oxygen transport pathway, blood is the essential medium for transporting oxygen. To fulfill this function, blood must be delivered in an adequate yet varying amount, proportional to metabolic demands, and must have the appropriate constituents and consistency. Thus consideration of the characteristics of the circulating blood volume is essential to any discussion of oxygen transport.

Blood volume is compartmentalized within the intravascular compartment such that 70% is contained within the venous compartment, 10% in the systemic arteries, 15% in the pulmonary circulation, and 5% in the capillaries (Sandler, 1986). The large volume of blood contained within the venous circulation permits adjustments to be made as CO demand changes. The veins constrict, for example, when CO needs to be increased. When blood volume is normal and body fluids are appropriately distributed between the intravascular and extravascular compartments, fluid balance is considered normal. When they are disrupted, a fluid balance problem exists. In addition, fluid imbalance affects the concentration of electrolytes, particularly sodium, which is present in the highest concentration in the extracellular fluid. Four primary fluid problems that have implications for oxygen transport are water deficit, water excess, sodium deficit, and sodium excess (see Chapter 16). Other ions that are affected often in fluid and electrolyte imbalance deficits include potassium, chloride, calcium, and magnesium (see Figure 2-8). These electrolyte disturbances also contribute to impaired oxygen transport by affecting the electrical and mechanical behavior of the heart and blood vessels, hence CO and the distribution of oxygenated arterial blood to the periphery.

Blood is a viscous fluid composed of cells and plasma. Because 99% of blood comprises red blood cells, the white blood cells play almost no role in determining the physical characteristics of blood.

Hematocrit refers to the proportion of red blood cells in the plasma. The normal hematocrit is 38% for women and 42% for men. Blood is several times more viscous than water, which increases the difficulty with which blood is pumped through the heart and flows through vessels; the greater the number of cells, the greater the friction between the layers of blood, which results in increased viscosity. Thus the viscosity of the blood increases significantly with increases in hematocrit. An increase in hematocrit, as in polycythemia, increases blood viscosity several times. The concentration and types of protein in the plasma can also affect viscosity, but to a lesser extent.

In adults, red blood cells are produced in the marrow of the membranous bones, such as the vertebrae, sternum, ribs, and pelvis. The production of red blood cells at these sites diminishes with age. Tissue oxygenation is the basic regulator of red blood cell production. Hypoxemia stimulates red blood cell production through erythropoietin production in bone (Guyton, 2000).

Viscosity of the blood has its greatest effect in the small vessels. Blood flow is considerably reduced in small vessels, which results in aggregates of red blood cells adhering to the vessel walls. This effect is not offset by the tendency of the blood to become less viscous in small vessels (a result of the alignment of the blood cells flowing through them, which minimizes the frictional forces between layers of flowing blood cells). In small capillaries, blood cells can become stuck, particularly where the nuclei of endothelial cells protrude and momentarily obstruct blood flow.

The major function of the red blood cells is to transport hemoglobin, which in turn carries oxygen from the lungs to the tissues. Red blood cells also contain a large quantity of carbonic anhydrase, which catalyzes the reaction between CO_2 and H_2O. The rapidity of this reaction makes it possible for blood to react with large quantities of CO_2 to transport it from the tissues to the lungs for elimination.

Hemoglobin is contained within red blood cells in a concentration of up to 34 g/dl of cells. Each gram of hemoglobin is capable of combining with 1.34 ml of oxygen (see Figure 2-2). In healthy women, 19 ml of oxygen and in healthy men, 21 ml of oxygen can be carried in the blood (given that the whole blood of women contains an average of 14 g/100 ml of blood and the whole blood of men 16 g/dl).

The clotting factors of the blood are normally in a proportion that does not promote clotting. Factors that promote coagulation (procoagulants) and factors that inhibit coagulation (anticoagulants) circulate in the blood. In the event of a ruptured blood vessel, prothrombin is converted to thrombin, which catalyzes the transformation of fibrinogen to fibrin threads. This fibrin mesh captures platelets, blood cells, and plasma to form a blood clot.

The extreme example of abnormal clotting is disseminated intravascular coagulation, when both hemorrhage and coagulation occur simultaneously. The acute form of this syndrome occurs in patients who are critically ill and undergoing multiorgan system failure. The mechanism appears to involve tissue factors, factors that damage the blood vessel walls, and factors that increase platelet aggregation (Green & Esparaz, 1990). The chronic form of the syndrome occurs in chronic conditions such as neoplastic disease.

Plasma is the extracellular fluid of the blood and contains 7% proteins, namely albumin, globulin, and fibrinogen. The primary function of albumin and, to a lesser extent, globulin and fibrinogen, is to create osmotic pressure at the capillary membrane and to prevent fluid leaking into the interstitial spaces. Globulins transport substances in the blood and provide immunity as the antibodies that fight infection and toxicity. Fibrinogen is fundamental to blood clotting. Most blood proteins, including hemoglobins, are also excellent acid-base buffers and are responsible for 70% of all the buffering power of whole blood.

Blood flow (Q) depends on a pressure gradient (P) and vascular resistance (R) (i.e., $Q = P/R$). Thus blood flow equals the pressure gradient divided by resistance. The length of a given blood vessel and the viscosity of the blood are also determinants of blood flow.

The average blood volume is 5000 ml. Approximately 3000 ml of this is plasma and 2000 ml is red blood cells. These values vary according to gender, weight, and other factors. Normally, changes in blood volume reflect fluid imbalances (deficits and excesses) created by losses through the skin and respiratory tract, as well as through urinary, sweat, and fecal losses. Exercise and hot weather are major challenges to fluid balance in health.

Plasma contains large quantities of sodium and chloride ions and small amounts of potassium, calcium, magnesium, phosphate, sulfate, and organic acid ions. Plasma also contains a large amount of protein. The large ionic constituents of plasma are responsible for regulating intracellular and extracellular fluid volumes and the osmotic factors that cause shifts of fluid between the intracellular and extracellular compartments.

Oxyhemoglobin Dissociation

Demand for oxygen at the cellular level changes from moment to moment. The properties of oxyhemoglobin dissociation ensure that there is a continuous supply of oxygen at the cellular level. Oxygen combines with hemoglobin molecules in the pulmonary circulation and then is released in the tissue capillaries in response to a reduced arterial oxygen tension. The S-shaped oxyhemoglobin dissociation curve (see Chapter 4) shifts to the right in response to reduced tissue pH, increased CO_2, increased temperature, and increased diphosphoglycerate (DPG), a constituent of normal blood cells.

Blood delivery and its ability to effectively transport oxygen are central to all steps in the oxygen transport pathway and must be considered at each step in clinical problem solving and decision making.

Steps in the Oxygen Transport Pathway
Step One: Inspired Oxygen and Quality of the Ambient Air

In healthy individuals, the concentration of inspired oxygen is relatively constant at 21%. If an individual is at a high altitude, the fraction of inspired oxygen is reduced as elevation increases.

Atmospheric air consists of 79% nitrogen, 20.97% oxygen, and 0.03% CO_2. Because nitrogen is an inert gas and is not absorbed in the lungs, it has a crucial role in keeping the alveoli open. The constituents of the air have become an increasingly important social, environmental, and health issue because of environmental hazards, pollution, and the thinning of the ozone layer, which result in deterioration of air quality, an increase in toxic oxygen free radicals, and a reduction in atmospheric oxygen pressure.

Many factors influence air quality: geographical region, season, urban versus rural area, high versus low elevation, home environment, work environment, indoor versus outdoor ambience, level of ventilation, presence of air conditioning, buildings that are closed, areas with high particulate matter, areas with gaseous vapors and toxic materials that can be inhaled, and smoke-filled versus smoke-free environments. Poor air quality may overwhelm the filtering ability of the upper respiratory tract and the airway's sensitivity and cause lung damage, both acutely and over time. Chronic irritation of the lungs by poor air quality can lead to allergies, chronic inflammatory reactions, fibrosis, and alveolar capillary membrane thickening. At the alveolar level, the inspired air is saturated with water vapor. In dry environments, however, the upper respiratory tract may become dehydrated, lose its protective mucous covering, become eroded, and provide a portal for infection even though the air is adequately humidified by the time it reaches the lower airways and alveoli.

Step Two: Airways

The structures of the airways throughout the respiratory tract change according to their functions. The main airway, the trachea, consists of cartilaginous rings, connective tissue, and small amounts of smooth muscle. This structure is essential to provide a firm and relatively inflexible conduit for air to pass from the nares through the head and neck to the lungs while avoiding airway collapse. As the airways become smaller and branch throughout the lung tissue, they consist primarily of smooth muscle. Airway narrowing, or obstruction, and the resulting increased resistance to airflow can be caused by a variety of factors, including edema, mucus, foreign objects, calcification, particulate matter, and space-occupying lesions, as well as by hyperreactivity of bronchial smooth muscle. The airways are lined with cilia, fine, microscopic, hairlike projections that are responsible for wafting debris, cells, and microorganisms away from the lungs into larger airways to be removed and evacuated. The airways are also lined with mucus, which consists of two layers, the upper gel layer and the lower sol layer, with which the cilia communicate.

Step Three: Lungs and Chest Wall

Air entry into the lungs depends on the integrity of the respiratory muscles, in particular the diaphragm, the lung parenchyma, and the chest wall. The contraction and descent of the diaphragm generate a negative intrapleural pressure that inflates the lungs. The distribution of ventilation is determined primarily by the negative intrapleural pressure gradient down the lungs. The negative intrapleural pressure gradient results in uneven ventilation down the lungs and in interregional differences (see Chapter 4). There are, however, other factors that contribute to uneven ventilation within regions of the lung. These intraregional differences reflect regional differences in lung compliance and airway resistance (Ross & Dean, 1992). In patients with partially obstructed airways, reduced

lung compliance and increased airway resistance increase the time needed for alveolar filling. Gas exchange is compromised if there is inadequate time for alveolar filling or emptying (i.e., increased time constants) (West, 2004). Different time constants across lung units contribute to uneven patterns of ventilation during inspiration. A lung unit with a long time constant is slow to fill and empty and may continue filling when surrounding units are emptying. Another factor that contributes to uneven ventilation is altered diffusion distance. In diseases in which diffusion distance is increased, ventilation among lung units is uneven.

The lungs and the parietal pleura are richly supplied with thin-walled lymphatic vessels (Guyton, 2000). Lymphatic vessels have some smooth muscle and thus can actively contract to propel lymph fluid forward. This forward motion is augmented by valves along the lymphatic channels. The rise and fall of the pleural pressure during respiration compress lymphatic vessels with each breath, which promotes a continuous flow of lymph. During expiration and increased intrapleural pressure, fluid is forced into the lymphatic vessels. The visceral pleura continuously drains fluid from the lungs. This creates a negative pressure in the pleural space, which keeps the lungs expanded. This pressure exceeds the elastic recoil pressure of the lung parenchyma that counters the tendency of elastic recoil to collapse the lungs.

The peritoneal cavity of the abdomen consists of a visceral peritoneum containing the viscera and a parietal peritoneum lining the abdominal cavity. Numerous lymphatic channels interconnect the peritoneal cavity and the thoracic duct; some arise from the diaphragm. With cycles of inspiration and expiration, large amounts of lymph are moved from the peritoneal cavity to the thoracic duct. High venous pressures and vascular resistance through the liver can interfere with normal fluid balance in the peritoneal cavity. This leads to the transudation of fluid with high protein content into the abdominal cavity. Such an accumulation of fluid is referred to as ascites. Large volumes of fluid can accumulate in the abdominal cavity and significantly compromise cardiopulmonary function secondary to increased intraabdominal pressure on the underside of the diaphragm.

Optimal diaphragmatic excursion requires a balance between thoracic and intraabdominal pressures. Increases in abdominal pressure secondary to factors such as fluid accumulation can impair diaphragmatic descent and chest wall expansion. Other factors include gas entrapment, gastrointestinal obstruction, space-occupying lesions, and paralytic ileus.

Step Four: Diffusion

Diffusion of oxygen from the alveolar sacs to the pulmonary arterial circulation depends on four factors: the area of the alveolar capillary membrane, the diffusing capacity of the alveolar capillary membrane, the pulmonary capillary blood volume, and the ventilation and perfusion ratio (Ganong, 2003). The transit time of blood at the alveolar capillary membrane is also an important factor that determines diffusion. The blood remains in the pulmonary capillaries for 0.75 second at rest. Within 0.25 second, one third of that time, the blood is completely saturated. This provides a safety margin during exercise or other conditions in which CO is increased and pulmonary capillary transit time is reduced. The blood can normally be fully oxygenated even with reduced transit time.

Step Five: Perfusion

The distribution of blood perfusing the lungs is primarily gravity dependent, so the dependent lung fields are perfused to a greater extent than are the nondependent lung fields. In upright lungs the bases are better perfused than the apices (see Chapter 4). Ventilation and perfusion matching is optimal in the midzones of upright lungs (West, 2004). In healthy individuals the ventilation-to-perfusion ratio is a primary determinant of arterial oxygenation. In upright lungs this ratio is 0.8 in the midzone.

Step Six: Myocardial Function

Optimal myocardial function and CO depend on the synchronized coupling of electrical excitation of the heart and mechanical contraction. The sinoatrial node, located in the right atrium, is the normal pacemaker for the heart and elicits the normal sinus rhythm with its multiple-component P-QRS-T configuration (see Chapter 12). This wave of electrical excitation spreads throughout the specialized neural conduction system of the atria, the interventricular septum, and the ventricles and is followed by the contraction of the atria and then of the ventricles. The contraction of the right and left ventricles ejects blood into the pulmonary and systemic circulations, respectively.

CO depends on several factors in addition to the integrity of the conduction system and the adequacy of myocardial depolarization (dromotropic effect). The amount of blood returned to the heart (preload) determines the amount ejected (the Starling effect). The distensibility of the ventricles to accommodate this blood volume must be optimal—neither too stiff nor too compliant. The force and contractility of the myocardial muscle must be sufficient to eject the blood (inotropic effect and chronotropic effect, respectively). CO is determined by the aortic pressure needed to overcome peripheral vascular resistance and the capacity of the ventricles to eject blood into the pulmonary and systemic circulations (afterload).

The pericardial cavity, like the pleural and peritoneal cavities, is a potential space containing a thin layer of fluid. The space normally has a negative pressure. During expiration, pericardial pressure is increased and fluid is forced out of the space into the mediastinal lymphatic channels. This process is normally facilitated by increased volumes of blood in the heart and each ventricular systole.

Step Seven: Peripheral Circulation

When oxygenated blood is ejected from the heart, the peripheral circulation provides a conduit to supply this blood to metabolically active tissue. Blood vessels throughout the body are arranged both in series and in parallel. The arteries and capillaries are designed to advance blood and thus perfuse the tissues with oxygenated blood. The architecture of the vasculature is such that the proximal large arteries have a higher proportion of connective tissue and elastic elements than the distal medium and small arteries, which have a progressively higher proportion of smooth muscle. This structure enables the large proximal arteries to withstand high pressure when blood is ejected during ventricular systole. Considerable potential energy is stored within the elastic walls of these blood vessels as the heart contracts. During diastole the forward propulsion of blood is facilitated by the elastic recoil of these large vessels. The thin-walled muscular arterioles serve as the stopcocks of circulation and regulate blood flow through regional vascular beds and maintain peripheral vascular resistance to regulate systemic blood pressure. Blood flow through these regional vascular beds is determined by neural and humoral stimulation (exogenous) and by local tissue factors (endogenous). Blood pressure control is regulated primarily by neural stimulation of the peripheral circulation and regional vascular beds.

Microcirculation consists of the precapillary arteriole, capillary, and venule. The Starling effect governs the balance of hydrostatic and oncotic pressures within the capillary and surrounding tissue. The balance of these pressures is 0.3 mm Hg; its net effect is a small outward filtration of fluid from the microvasculature into the interstitial space (see Chapter 4). Any excess fluid or loss of plasma protein is drained into the surrounding lymphatic vessels, which usually has a small negative pressure, as does the interstitium. Integrity of the microcirculation is essential to regulate the diffusion of oxygen across the tissue capillary membrane and removing CO_2 and waste products.

The greater the muscular component of blood vessels, the greater their sensitivity to both exogenous neural stimulation and endogenous stimulation by circulating humoral neurotransmitters such as catecholamines and local tissue factors. This sensitivity is essential for the moment-to-moment regulation of the peripheral circulation with respect to tissue perfusion and oxygenation, commensurate with tissue metabolic demands and control of total peripheral resistance and systemic blood pressure.

Step Eight: Tissue Extraction and use of Oxygen

Perfusion of the tissues by oxygenated blood is the principal goal of the oxygen transport system (Dantzker, 1993). Oxygen is continuously being used by all cells in the body; thus it diffuses out of the circulation and through cell membranes rapidly to meet metabolic needs. Diffusion occurs down a gradient from areas of high to low oxygen pressure. The distances between capillaries and cells are variable, so a significant safety factor is required to ensure adequate arterial oxygen tensions. Intracellular P_{O_2} ranges from 5 to 60 mm Hg, with an average of 23 mm Hg (Guyton, 2000). Given that only 3 mm Hg of oxygen pressure is needed to support metabolism, 23 mm Hg of oxygen pressure provides an adequate safety margin. These mechanisms ensure an optimal oxygen supply over a wide range of oxygen demands during healthy functioning and in the event of impaired oxygen delivery because of illness. Normally the rate of oxygen extraction by the cells is regulated by the oxygen demand of cells (i.e., the rate at which ADP is formed from ATP) and not by the availability of oxygen.

The adequacy of quality and quantity of mitochondrial enzymes required for the Krebs cycle and electron transfer chain, and the availability of myoglobin, may be limiting factors in the oxygen transport pathway secondary to nutritional deficits and muscle enzyme deficiencies. Myoglobin is a protein comparable to hemoglobin and is localized within muscle mitochondria. Myoglobin combines reversibly with oxygen to provide an immediate source of oxygen when there are increased metabolic demands and to facilitate oxygen transfer within the mitochondria.

Normally the amount of oxygen extracted by the tissues at rest is 23% (i.e., the ratio of oxygen consumed to oxygen delivered). This ratio ensures that considerably greater amounts of oxygen can be extracted during periods of increased metabolic demand. To detect tissue hypoxia, particularly in patients who are critically ill, regional assessments such as gastric mucosal PCO_2 and pH show promise of being superior to global assessment of $\dot{V}O_2$ and DO_2 (Baigorri & Russell, 1996). Regional measures of oxygenation are a relatively new area of interest; they help to enhance the specificity of treatment based on tissue indicators (Maizes et al, 2000).

Step Nine: Return of Partially Desaturated Blood and CO2 to the Lungs

Partially desaturated blood and CO_2 are removed from cells via venous circulation to the right side of the heart and lungs. CO_2 diffuses across the alveolar capillary membrane and is eliminated from the body through the respiratory system, and deoxygenated venous blood is reoxygenated. The oxygen transport cycle repeats and is sensitively tuned to adjust to changes in the metabolic demand of the various organ systems, such as digestion in the gastrointestinal system and cardiac and skeletal muscle work during exercise.

Factors that interfere with tissue oxygenation and the capacity of the tissue to use oxygen include abnormal oxygen demands, reduced hemoglobin and myoglobin levels, edema, and poisoning of the cellular enzymes (Kariman & Burns, 1985).

FACTORS THAT NORMALLY PERTURB OXYGEN TRANSPORT

Basal metabolic rate (BMR) reflects the rate of metabolism for an individual in a completely rested state: no food intake within several hours, a good night's sleep, no arousing or distressing emotional stimulation, and a comfortable ambient temperature. Normally the BMR is constant within and between individuals if measured under standardized conditions. BMR reflects the energy expended by the body's cells to maintain resting function and includes the work of breathing; heart, renal, and brain function; and thermoregulation.

Normally, over the course of the day, the human body is exposed to fluctuations in ambient temperature and humidity, ingestion states, activity and exercise levels (exercise stress), body positions and body position changes (gravitational stress), emotional states (emotional stress), and states of arousal. These factors significantly influence $\dot{V}O_2$ and energy expenditure from moment to moment and thus increase rate of metabolism.

Several factors related to disease can significantly increase oxygen consumption and metabolic rate over and above the BMR. Such factors include fever, the disease process itself, the process of healing and recovery from injury or disease, thermoregulatory disturbance, reduced arousal, increased arousal resulting from anxiety or pain, sleep loss, medical and surgical interventions, fluid imbalance, and medications (Dean, 1994). These factors may contribute to a systemic increase in the BMR or may reflect local changes in tissue metabolism. Autoregulation of the regional vascular beds promotes increased regional blood flow in accordance with their local tissue metabolic demand.

Because gravitational stress and exercise stress are fundamental to normal cardiopulmonary function and oxygen transport, the effects of gravity and exercise are highlighted. These two factors augment arousal through stimulation of the reticular activating system in the brainstem and the autonomic nervous system (ANS), which, when depressed, significantly compromises oxygen transport. Emotional stress also has a marked effect on the stimulation of the ANS (the fight-or-flight response) and hence on oxygen transport. These concepts and their clinical implications are described in detail in Chapters 18 and 19.

Gravitational Stress

Humans are designed to function in a 1-*g* gravitational field. Given that 60% of the body weight is fluid contained within the intravascular and extravascular compartments and that this fluid has considerable mass, changes in body position result in significant instantaneous fluid shifts that can threaten hemodynamic stability (Dean & Ross, 1992a, 1992b). To maintain consciousness and normal body function during changes in body position, the heart and peripheral vasculature are designed to detect these fluid shifts and accommodate quickly to avoid deleterious functional consequences (e.g., reduced stroke volume, CO, circulating blood volume, and cerebral perfusion). The preservation of the fluid-regulating mechanisms is essential to counter the hemodynamic effects of changing body position. This capacity is impaired with recumbency, which is the primary cause of bed rest deconditioning in patient and older populations (Chase et al, 1966; Winslow, 1985). Restoration of adaptation to gravitational stress by upright positioning of a patient is the *only* means by which these fluid-regulating mechanisms can be maintained and orthostatic intolerance and its short- and long-term sequelae averted.

Exercise Stress

Exercise constitutes the greatest perturbation to homeostasis and oxygen transport in humans. CO can increase by five times to adjust to the metabolic demands of exercise stress. All steps in the oxygen transport pathway are affected by exercise stress. Ventilation is increased, and ventilation and perfusion matching is optimized to maximize oxygenation of blood. Heart rate and stroke volume are increased to effect greater CO of oxygenated blood to the tissues. At the tissue level, oxygen extraction is enhanced.

Emotional Stress

The body responds to emotional stress much as it does to exercise stress—by undergoing the sympathetic stress reaction (the fright-fight-flight reaction). Perceived threat, the basis of emotional stress, can also trigger the fright-fight-flight reaction and a series of sympathetically mediated physiological responses. This reaction, which prepares the body for fight or for flight, includes an increase in circulating stress hormones, heart rate, blood pressure, CO, blood glucose, muscle strength, mental alertness, cellular metabolism, and local blood flow to specific muscle groups, as well as inhibition of involuntary function.

SUMMARY

This chapter describes the oxygen transport system, a system that is essential to life, activity, and social participation. Its component steps and their interdependence are highlighted. This framework provides a conceptual basis for the practice of cardiopulmonary physical therapy.

The oxygen transport system is designed to deliver oxygen from the ambient air to every cell in the body to support cellular respiration (i.e., metabolic use of oxygen at the cellular level). Blood is the essential medium in which cellular and noncellular components transport oxygen from the cardiopulmonary unit to the peripheral tissues. The fundamental components in the oxygen transport pathway are described. These components include the quality of the ambient air, the airways, lungs, chest wall, pulmonary circulation, lymphatics, heart, peripheral circulation, and peripheral tissues of the organs of the body.

In healthy individuals the most significant factors that perturb oxygen transport are changes in gravitational stress secondary to changes in body position, exercise stress secondary to the increased oxygen demand of working muscles, arousal, and emotional stress. A thorough understanding of the normal effects of gravitational and exercise stress and arousal is essential to understanding deficits in oxygen transport. Numerous factors can impair and threaten oxygen transport, including underlying pathophysiology, restricted mobility, recumbency, factors related to the patient's care, and factors related to the individual (see Chapter 17). The physical therapist needs a detailed understanding of these concepts to diagnose such deficits, to understand their impact on activity and participation, and to prescribe efficacious treatments.

Review Questions

1. Describe the clinical implications of limitations of oxygen transport at three levels: structure and function, activity, and participation (consistent with the International Classification of Function).
2. Describe the oxygen transport pathway, its steps, and their interdependence.
3. Describe the physiological processes of energy transfer and cellular oxidation.
4. Explain oxygen transport with respect to oxygen delivery, uptake and extraction, and the interrelationship among these processes.
5. Outline the factors that perturb oxygen transport in health.

REFERENCES

Baigorri, F., & Russell, J.A. (1996). Oxygen delivery in critical illness. Critical Care Clinics 12:971-994.

Boyd, O., Grounds, M., & Bennett, D. (1992). The dependency of oxygen consumption on oxygen delivery in critically ill postoperative patients is mimicked by variations in sedation. Chest 101:1619-1624.

Chase, G.A., Grave, C., & Rowell, L.B. (1966). Independence of changes in functional and performance capacities attending prolonged bed rest. Aerospace Medicine 37:1232-1237.

Dantzker, D.R. (1985). The influence of cardiovascular function on gas exchange. Clinical Chest Medicine 4:149-159.

Dantzker, D.R., Boresman, B., & Gutierrez, G. (1991). Oxygen supply and utilization relationships. American Review of Respiratory Disorders 143:675-679.

Dantzker, D.R. (1993). Adequacy of tissue oxygenation. Critical Care Medicine 21:S40-S43.

Dantzker, D.R., Scharf, S.M., & Fletcher, J. (1997). Cardiopulmonary critical care, ed 3. Philadelphia: Elsevier.

Dean, E. (1994). Oxygen transport: a physiologically based conceptual framework for the practice of cardiopulmonary physiotherapy. Physiotherapy 80:347-355.

Dean, E. (2002). Physiotherapy skills: positioning and mobilization of the patient. In: Pryor, J.A., & Ammani, P.S. (Eds). Physiotherapy for respiratory and cardiac problems: adults and paediatrics, Edinburgh: Churchill Livingstone.

Dean, E., & Ross, J. (1992a). Discordance between cardiopulmonary physiology and physical therapy. Chest 101:1694-1698.

Dean, E., & Ross, J. (1992b). Oxygen transport: the basis for contemporary cardiopulmonary physical therapy and its optimization with body positioning and mobilization. Physical Therapy Practice 1:34-44.

Epstein, C.D. & Henning, R.J. (1993). Oxygen transport variables in the identification and treatment of tissue hypoxia. Heart Lung 22:328-348.

Fenwick, J.C. (1990). Increased concentrations of plasma lactate predict pathologic dependence of oxygen consumption on oxygen delivery in patients with adult respiratory distress syndrome. Journal of Critical Care 5:81-86.

Foss, M.L., & Keteyian, S.J. (Eds) (1998). Fox's physiological basis for exercise and sport, ed 6. Madison, Wis.: Brown & Benchmark.

Ganong, W.F. (2003). Review of medical physiology, ed 21. New York: McGraw-Hill Professional Publishing.

Goldring, R.M. (1984). Specific defects in cardiopulmonary gas exchange. American Review of Respiratory Disorders 129:S57-S59.

Green, D., & Esparaz, B. (1990). Coagulopathies in the critically-ill patient. In Cane, R.D., Shapiro, B.A., & Davidson, R. (Eds). Case studies in critical care medicine, ed 2. Chicago: Year Book.

Guyton, A.C., & Hall, J.E. (2000). Textbook of medical physiology, ed 10. Philadelphia: Elsevier.

Hasson, S.M. (Ed) (1994). Clinical exercise physiology. Philadelphia: Mosby.

Kariman, K., & Burns, S.R. (1985). Regulation of tissue oxygen extraction is disturbed in adult respiratory distress syndrome. American Review of Respiratory Diseases 132:109-114.

Kirchberger, M.A. (1991). Excitation and contraction of skeletal muscle. In West, J.B. (Ed). Best and Taylor's physiological basis of medical practice. Baltimore: Williams & Wilkins.

Lorente, J.A., Renes, E., Gomez-Agunaga, M.A., Landin, L., de la Morena, J., & Liste, O. (1991). Oxygen delivery–dependent oxygen consumption in acute respiratory failure. Critical Care Medicine 19:770-775.

Maizes, J.S., Murtuza, M., & Kvetan, V. (2000) Oxygen transport and utilization. Respiratory Care Clinics in North America 6:473-500.

McArdle, W.D., Katch, F.I., & Katch, V.L. (2000). Essentials of exercise physiology, ed 2. Philadelphia: Lippincott Williams & Wilkins.

Mizock, B.A., & Falk, J.L. (1992). Lactic acidosis in critical illness. Critical Care Medicine 20:80-93.

Myles, P.S., McRae, R., Ryder, I., Hunt, J.O., & Buckland, M.R. (1996). Association between oxygen delivery and consumption in patients undergoing cardiac surgery. Is there supply dependence? Anaesthesiology and Intensive Care Medicine 24:651-657.

Phang, P.T., & Russell, J.A. (1993). When does $\dot{V}O_2$ depend on DO_2? Respiratory Care 38:618-630.

Ross, J., & Dean, E. (1989). Integrating physiological principles into the comprehensive management of cardiopulmonary dysfunction. Physical Therapy 69:255-259.

Ross, J., & Dean, E. (1992). Body positioning. In Zadai, C.C. (Ed). Clinics in physical therapy. Pulmonary management in physical therapy. New York: Churchill Livingstone.

Samsel, R.W., & Schumacker, P.T. (1991). Oxygen delivery to tissues. European Respiratory Journal 4:1258-1267.

Sandler, H. (1986). Cardiovascular effects of inactivity. In Sandler, H., & Vernikos, J. (Eds). Inactivity physiological effects. Orlando, Fla.: Academic Press.

Schumaker, P.T., & Cain, S.M. (1987). The concept of critical oxygen delivery. Intensive Care Medicine 13:223-229.

Schumaker, P.T., & Samsel, R.W. (1989). Oxygen delivery and uptake by peripheral tissues: physiology and pathophysiology. Critical Care Clinics 5:255-269.

Shephard, R.J. (1985). Physiology and biochemistry of exercise. Philadelphia: Praeger Scientific.

Tortora, G.J., & Anagnostakos, N.P. (2003). Principles of anatomy and physiology, ed 8. Boston: Addison-Wesley Education.

Wasserman, K., Hansen, J.E., Sue, O.V., Stringer, W.W., & Whipp, B.J. (2004). Principles of exercise testing and interpretation: including pathophysiology and clinical applications, ed 4. Philadelphia: Lippincott Williams & Wilkins.

Weber, K.T., Janicki, J.S., Shroff, S.G., & Likoff, M.J. (1983). The cardiopulmonary unit: the body's gas exchange system. Clinics Chest Medicine 4:101-110.

West, J.B. (1985). Ventilation, blood flow and gas exchange, ed 4. Oxford: Blackwell Scientific.

West, J.B. (2004). Respiratory physiology—the essentials, ed 7. Philadelphia: Lippincott Williams & Wilkins.

Winslow, E.H. (1985). Cardiovascular consequences of bed rest. Heart Lung 14:236-246.

World Health Organization. (2000). International Classification of Functioning, Disability and Health. www.sustainable-design.ie/arch/ICIDH-2PFDec-2000.pdf; retrieved January, 2005.

C H A P T E R 3

Cardiopulmonary Anatomy

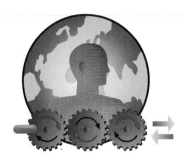

Elizabeth Dean

KEY TERMS

Cardiopulmonary unit
Heart
Heart-lung interdependence
Lymphatic circulation
Parenchyma

Peripheral circulation
Pulmonary circulation
Respiratory muscles
Thoracic cavity
Tracheobronchial tree

The heart lies in series with the lungs, constituting the cardiopulmonary unit, the central component of the oxygen transport pathway (Scharf & Cassidy, 1989; Weber et al, 1983). Virtually all the blood returned to the right side of the heart passes through the lungs and is delivered to the left side of the heart for ejection into the systemic, coronary, and bronchopulmonary circulations. Because of this interrelationship, changes in lung function can exert changes in heart function and vice versa. A detailed understanding of the anatomy of the heart and lungs and how these organs work synergistically is essential to the practice of cardiopulmonary physical therapy.

This chapter presents the anatomy of the cardiopulmonary system, including the skeletal features of the thoracic cavity; muscles of respiration; anatomy of the tracheobronchial tree; lung parenchyma; basic anatomy of the heart; and peripheral, pulmonary, and lymphatic circulations (Berne & Levy, 2000; Burton, 1997; Cheitlin, 2004; Ganong, 2003; Guyton & Hall, 2000; Katz, 2000; Murray, 1986; Murray & Nadel, 2000; Nunn, 1999; West, 2004; Williams et al, 1989).

THORAX

The bony thorax covers and protects the principal organs of respiration and circulation as well as the liver and the stomach (Figures 3-1 and 3-2). The anterior surface is formed by the sternum and the costal cartilage. The lateral surfaces are formed by the ribs. The posterior surface is formed by the 12 thoracic vertebrae and the posterior part of the 12 ribs. At birth, the thorax is nearly circular, but during childhood and adolescence it becomes more elliptical. In adulthood the transverse diameter of the chest wall is greater than the anteroposterior diameter.

Sternum

The sternum, or breastbone, is a flat bone with three parts: manubrium, body, and xiphoid process. The manubrium is the widest and thickest bone of the sternum. Its upper border is scalloped by a central jugular notch, which can be palpated, and by two clavicular notches that house the clavicles. Its lower border articulates with the upper border of the body at a slight angle, the sternal angle or angle of Louis. This angle can be easily palpated, is a landmark located between thoracic vertebrae T4 and T5, and is on a level with the second costal cartilages. The bifurcation of the trachea into the right and left main stem bronchi also occurs at the sternal angle. The manubrium and body are joined by fibrocartilage, which may ossify in later life.

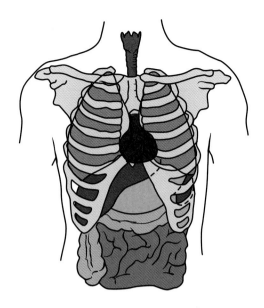

FIGURE 3-1 The relationship of the bony thorax and lungs to the abdominal contents (anterior view).

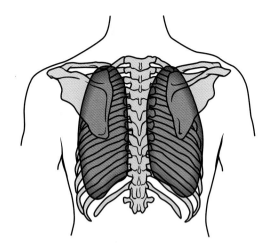

FIGURE 3-2 The relationship of the lungs to the bony thorax (posterior view).

The body of the sternum is twice as long as the manubrium. It is a relatively thin bone and can be easily pierced by needles for bone marrow aspirations. The heart is located beneath and to the left of the lower third of the body of the sternum. Although it is attached by cartilage to the ribs, this portion of the sternum is flexible and can be depressed without breaking. This maneuver is used, with care, in closed cardiac massage to artificially circulate blood to the brain and extremities. The lower margin of the body is attached to the xiphoid process by fibrocartilage. This bone is the smallest of the three parts of the sternum and usually fuses with the body of the sternum in later life.

Ribs

A large portion of the bony thoracic cage is formed by 12 ribs located on either side of the sternum. The first seven ribs connect posteriorly with the vertebral column and anteriorly through costal cartilages with the sternum. These are known as the true ribs. The remaining five ribs are known as the false ribs. The first three have their cartilage attached to the cartilage of the rib above. The last two are free, or floating, ribs. The ribs increase in length from the first to the seventh rib and then decrease to the twelfth rib. They also increase in obliquity until the ninth rib and then decrease in obliquity to the twelfth rib.

Each rib has a small head and a short neck that articulate with two thoracic vertebrae. The shaft of the rib curves gently from the neck to a sudden sharp bend, the angle of the rib. Fractures often occur at this site. A costal groove is located on the lower border of the shaft of the ribs. This groove houses the intercostal nerves and vessels. Chest tubes and needles are inserted above the ribs to avoid these vessels and nerves. The ribs are separated from each other by the intercostal spaces that contain the intercostal muscles.

MOVEMENTS OF THE THORAX

The frequency of movement of the bony thorax joints is greater than that of almost any other combination of joints in the body. Two types of movements have been described: the pump-handle movement and the bucket-handle movement (Figure 3-3) (Cherniack & Cherniack, 1983). The upper ribs are limited in their ability to move. Each pair swings like a pump handle, with elevation thrusting the sternum forward. This forward movement increases the anteroposterior diameter and the depth of the thorax and is called the pump-handle movement. In the lower ribs, there is little anteroposterior movement. During inspiration, the ribs swing outward and upward, each pushing against the rib above during elevation. This bucket-handle movement increases the transverse diameter of the thoracic cage. Thus, during inspiration, the thorax increases its volume by increasing its anteroposterior and transverse diameters.

MUSCLES OF RESPIRATION
Inspiration

Inspiration is an active movement involving the contraction of the diaphragm and intercostal muscles. Additional muscles may come into play during exertion by a healthy person. In disease, the role of these accessory muscles of inspiration may have an important role, even at rest. The accessory muscles include the sternocleidomastoids, scalenes, serratus anterior, pectoralis major and minor, trapezius, and erector spinae. The degree to which these accessory muscles are used by the patient is dependent on the severity of cardiopulmonary distress (Clemente, 1985; Murray & Nadel, 2000; Williams et al, 1989).

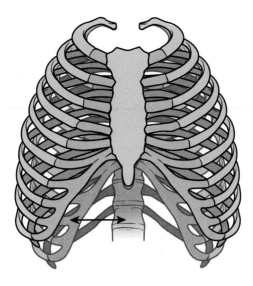

FIGURE 3-3 The movements of the ribs. **A,** "Bucket handle," lower rib. **B,** "Pump handle," first rib.

Diaphragm

The diaphragm is the principal muscle of respiration. During quiet breathing, the diaphragm contributes approximately two thirds of the tidal volume in the sitting or standing positions and approximately three fourths of the tidal volume in the supine position. Approximately two thirds of the vital capacity in all positions is contributed by the diaphragm.

The diaphragm is a large, dome-shaped muscle that separates the thoracic and abdominal cavities. Its upper surface supports the pericardium (with which it is partially blended), heart, pleurae, and lungs. Its lower surface is almost completely covered by the peritoneum and overlies the liver, kidneys, suprarenal glands, stomach, and spleen (Figure 3-4). This large muscle can be divided into right and left halves. Each half is made up of three parts: sternal, lumbar, and costal. These three parts insert into the central tendon, which lies just below the heart. The sternal part arises from the back of the xiphoid process and descends to the central tendon. On each side is a small gap, the sternocostal triangle, which is located between the sternal and costal parts. It transmits the superior epigastric vessels and is often the site of diaphragmatic hernias. The costal parts form the right and left domes. They arise from the inner surfaces of the lower four ribs and the lower six costal cartilages and interdigitate and transverse the abdomen to insert into the anterolateral part of the central tendon, the central part of the diaphragm. The lumbar part arises from the bodies of the upper lumbar vertebrae and extends upward to the central tendon. The central tendon is a thin, strong aponeurosis situated near the center of the muscle, somewhat closer to the front of the body. It resembles a trefoil leaf, with its three divisions, or leaflets. The right leaflet is the largest, the middle is the next largest, and the left leaflet is the smallest.

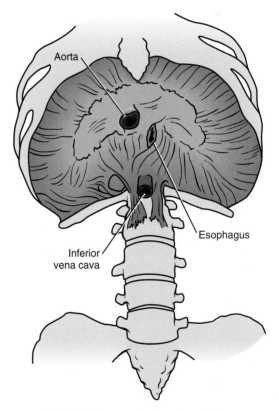

FIGURE 3-4 The diaphragm from below.

Major vessels traverse the diaphragm through one of three openings (see Figure 3-4). The vena caval opening is located to the right of the midline in the central tendon and contains branches of the right phrenic nerve and the inferior vena cava. The esophageal opening is located to the left of the midline

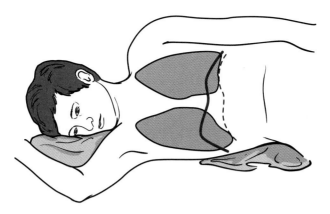

FIGURE 3-5 When the patient is lying on his or her side, the dome of the diaphragm on the lower side rises farther in the thorax than the dome on the upper side.

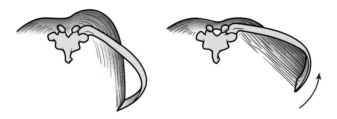

FIGURE 3-6 Contraction of the costal fibers of the diaphragm causes rib eversion and elevation.

and contains the esophagus, the vagal nerve trunks, and branches of the gastric vessels. The aortic opening is located in the midline and contains the aorta, the thoracic duct, and sometimes the azygos vein. The diaphragm is also pierced by branches of the left phrenic nerve, small veins, and lymph vessels.

The position of the diaphragm and its range of movement vary with posture, the degree of distention of the stomach, size of the intestines, size of the liver, and obesity. Average movement of the diaphragm in quiet respiration is 12.5 mm on the right and 12 mm on the left. This can increase to a maximum of 30 mm on the right and 28 mm on the left during increased ventilation. An individual's posture determines the position of the diaphragm. In the supine position, the resting level of the diaphragm rises. The greatest respiratory excursions during normal breathing occur in this position; however, the lung volumes are decreased because of the elevated position of the abdominal organs within the thoracic cavity. In a sitting or upright position, the dome of the diaphragm is pulled down by the abdominal organs, allowing a larger lung volume. For this reason, individuals who are short of breath are more comfortable sitting than reclining. In a side-lying position, the dome of the diaphragm on the lower side rises farther into the thorax than the dome on the upper side (Figure 3-5). The abdominal organs tend to be displaced forward in a side-lying

position, allowing greater excursion of the dome on the lower side. In contrast, the upper side moves little with respiration. On radiograph, the position of the diaphragm can indicate whether the film was taken during inspiration or expiration, and may also indicate pathology in the lungs, pleurae, or abdomen.

Each half of the diaphragm is innervated by a separate nerve—the phrenic nerve on that side. Although the halves contract simultaneously, it is possible for half of the muscle to be paralyzed without affecting the other half. Generally the paralyzed half remains at the normal level during rest. With deep inspiration, however, the paralyzed half is pulled up by the negative pressure in the thorax. A special radiograph, moving fluoroscopy, is used to determine paralysis of the diaphragm.

Contraction of the diaphragm increases the thoracic volume vertically and transversely. The central tendon is drawn down by the diaphragm as it contracts. As the dome descends, abdominal organs are pushed forward as far as the abdominal walls will allow. When the dome can descend no farther, the costal fibers of the diaphragm contract to increase the thoracic diameter of the thorax. This occurs because the fibers of the costal part of the diaphragm run vertically from their attachment at the costal margin. Thus contraction of these fibers elevates and everts the ribs (Figure 3-6). If the diaphragm is

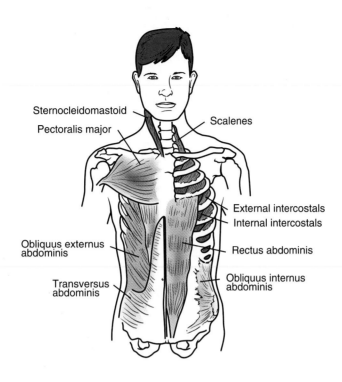

FIGURE 3-7 Respiratory muscles (anterior view).

in a low position, it will change the angle of pull of the muscle's costal fibers. Contraction of these fibers creates a horizontal pull, which causes the lateral diameter to become smaller as the ribs are pulled in toward the central tendon.

As the diaphragm descends, it compresses the abdominal organs, increasing intraabdominal pressure. At the same time, the intrathoracic pressure decreases as the lung volume is increased by the descending diaphragm. Inspiratory airflow occurs as a result of this decrease in intrathoracic pressure (see Chapter 4). The pressure gradient between the abdominal and thoracic cavities also facilitates the return of blood to the right side of the heart.

Movement of the diaphragm can be controlled voluntarily, to some extent. Vocalists spend years learning to manipulate their diaphragms so they can produce controlled sounds when singing. The diaphragm momentarily ceases movement when a person holds his or her breath. The diaphragm is involuntarily involved in parturition, bearing down in bowel movements, and laughing, crying, and vomiting. Hiccups are spasmodic, sharp contractions of the diaphragm that may indicate disease (e.g., a subphrenic abscess) if they persist.

Intercostals

The external intercostals extend down and forward from the tubercles of the ribs (above) to the costochondral junction

of the ribs (below) where they become continuous with the anterior intercostal membrane (Figure 3-7). This membrane extends the muscle forward to the sternum. There are 11 external intercostal muscles on each side of the sternum. They are thicker posteriorly than anteriorly, and thicker than the internal intercostal muscles. They are innervated by the intercostal nerves, and contraction draws the lower rib up and out toward the upper rib. This action increases the volume of the thoracic cavity.

There are 11 internal intercostals on each side. These are considered primarily expiratory in function. The intercartilaginous or parasternal portion of the internal intercostals contracts with the external intercostals during inspiration to help elevate the ribs. In addition to their respiratory functions, the intercostal muscles contract to prevent the intercostal spaces from being drawn in or bulged out during respiratory activity.

Sternocleidomastoid

The sternocleidomastoid (SCM) muscles are strong neck muscles arising from two heads, one from the manubrium and one from the medial part of the clavicle (see Figure 3-7). These two heads fuse into one muscle mass that inserts behind the ear into the mastoid process. It is innervated by the accessory nerve and the second cervical nerve. There are two of these muscles, one on each side of the neck. When one SCM contracts, it tilts the head toward the shoulder of the same side and rotates the face toward the opposite shoulder. If the two SCM muscles contract together, they pull the head forward into flexion. When the head is fixed, they assist in elevating the sternum, increasing the anteroposterior diameter of the thorax.

The SCMs are the most important accessory muscles of inspiration. Their contractions can be observed in all patients during forced inspiration and in all patients who are dyspneic. These muscles become visually predominant in patients who are chronically dyspneic (see Chapter 5).

Scalenes

The anterior, medial, and posterior scalenes are three separate muscles that are considered a functional unit. They are attached superiorly to the transverse processes of the lower five cervical vertebrae and inferiorly to the upper surface of the first two ribs (see Figure 3-7). They are innervated by their corresponding cervical spinal nerves. These muscles are primarily supportive neck muscles, but they can assist in respiration through reverse action. When their superior attachment is fixed, the scalenes act as accessory respiratory muscles and elevate the first two ribs during inspiration.

Serratus Anterior

The serratus anterior arises from the outer surfaces of the first eight or nine ribs. It curves backward, forming a sheet of muscle that inserts into the medial border of the scapula. It is innervated by the long thoracic nerve (cervical nerves C5, C6, and C7). There are two of these muscles, one on each side of the body. Normally they assist in forward pushing of the arm (as in punching). When the scapulae are fixed, serratus anterior act as accessory respiratory muscles and elevate the ribs to which they are attached.

Pectoralis Major

The pectoralis major is a large muscle arising from the clavicle, the sternum, and the cartilages of all the true ribs (see Figure 3-7). This muscle spreads across the anterior chest and inserts into the intertubercular sulcus of the humerus. It is innervated by the lateral and medial pectoral nerves and cervical nerves C5, C6, C7, C8, and T1. There are two of these muscles, one on each side of the body. This muscle rotates the humerus medially and draws the arm across the chest. In climbing and pull-ups, it draws the arms toward the trunk. During forced inspiration when the arms are fixed, it draws the ribs toward the arms, thereby increasing thoracic diameter.

Pectoralis Minor

The pectoralis minor is a thin muscle originating from the outer surfaces of the third, fourth, and fifth ribs near their cartilages. It inserts into the coracoid process of the scapula. It is innervated by the pectoral nerves (cervical nerves C6, C7, and C8). There are two of these muscles, one on each side of

the body. They contract with the serratus anterior to draw the scapulae toward the chest. During deep inspiration, they contract to elevate the ribs to which they are attached.

Trapezius

The trapezius consists of two muscles that form an extensive diamond-shaped sheet extending from the head down the back and out to both shoulders (Figure 3-8). Its upper belly originates from the external occipital protuberance, curves around the side of the neck, and inserts into the posterior border of the clavicle. The middle part of the muscle arises from a thin diamond-shaped tendinous sheet, the supraspinous ligaments and the spines of the upper thoracic region, runs horizontally, and inserts into the spine of the scapula. Its lower belly arises from the supraspinous ligaments and the spines of the lower thoracic region, runs upward, and inserts into the lower border of the spine of the scapula. This large muscle is innervated by the external or spinal part of the accessory nerve and cervical nerves C3 and C4. Its main function is to rotate the scapulae during arm elevation and control gravitational descent of the arms. It also braces the scapulae and raises them, as in shrugging the shoulders. Its ability to stabilize the scapulae makes it an important accessory muscle in respiration. This stabilization enables the serratus anterior and pectoralis minor to elevate the ribs.

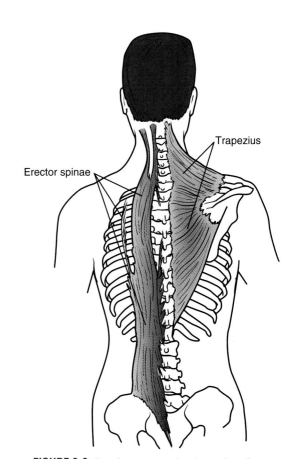

FIGURE 3-8 Respiratory muscles (posterior view).

Erector Spinae

The erector spinae is a large muscle extending from the sacrum to the skull (see Figure 3-8). It originates from the sacrum, the iliac crest, and the spines of the lower thoracic and lumbar vertebrae. It separates into a lateral iliocostalis, an intermediate longissimus, and a medial spinalis column. This muscle mass inserts into various ribs and vertebral processes all the way up to the skull. It is innervated by the corresponding spinal nerves. These muscles extend, laterally flex, and rotate the vertebral column. They are considered accessory respiratory muscles through their extension of the vertebral column. In deep inspiration, these muscles extend the vertebral column, allowing further elevation of the ribs.

Expiration

Expiration is a passive process that occurs when the intercostals and diaphragm relax. Relaxation of the intercostals and diaphragm allows the ribs to drop to their preinspiratory position and the diaphragm to rise. These activities compress the lungs, which raises intrathoracic pressure above atmospheric pressure and contributes to air flow out of the lungs.

Rectus Abdominis

The rectus abdominis rises from the pubic crest, extends upward, and inserts into the xiphoid process and the costal margin of the fifth, sixth, and seventh costal cartilages (see Figure 3-7). It is innervated by corresponding spinal nerves, and its action is considered within the context of the other abdominal muscles.

Obliquus Externus Abdominis

The obliquus externus abdominis arises in an oblique line from the fifth costal cartilage to the twelfth rib (see Figure 3-7). Its posterior fibers attach in an almost vertical line with the iliac crest. The other fibers extend down and forward and attach to the front of the xiphoid process, the linea alba, and the pubic symphysis. It is innervated by the lower six thoracic spinal nerves.

Obliquus Internus Abdominis

The obliquus internus abdominis originates from the lumbar fascia, the anterior two thirds of the iliac crest, and the lateral two thirds of the inguinal ligament (see Figure 3-7). Its posterior fibers run almost vertically upward and insert into the lower borders of the last three ribs. The other fibers join an aponeurosis attached to the costal margin above, the linea alba in the midline, and the pubic crest below. It is innervated by the lower six thoracic nerves and the first lumbar spinal nerves.

Transversus Abdominis

The transversus abdominis arises from the inner surface of the lower six costal cartilages, the lumbar fascia, the anterior two thirds of the iliac crest, and the lateral one third of the inguinal ligament (see Figure 3-7). It runs across the abdomen horizontally and inserts into the aponeurosis, extending to the linea alba. It is innervated by the lower six thoracic nerves and the first lumbar spinal nerves.

Action of the Abdominal Muscles

The four muscles of the abdomen work together to provide a firm but flexible wall to keep the abdominal viscera in position. The abdominal muscles exert a compressing force on the abdomen when the thorax and pelvis are fixed. This force can be used in defecation, urination, parturition, and vomiting. In forced expiration, the abdominal muscles help force the diaphragm back to its resting position and thus force air from the lungs. If the pelvis and vertebral column are fixed, the obliquus externus abdominis aids expiration further by depressing and compressing the lower part of the thorax. Patients with chronic obstructive pulmonary disease (COPD) have difficulty in exhalation, which causes them to trap air in their lungs. The continued contraction of the abdominal muscles throughout exhalation helps them force this air from the lungs. The abdominal muscles also play an important role in coughing. First, a large volume of air is inhaled, and the glottis is closed. The abdominal muscles then contract, raising intrathoracic pressure. When the glottis opens, the large difference in intrathoracic and atmospheric pressure causes the air to be expelled forcefully at tremendous flow rates (tussive blast). Individuals with weak abdominal muscles (from neuromuscular diseases, paraplegia, quadriplegia, or extensive abdominal surgery) often have ineffective coughs (see Chapters 28 and 33).

The four abdominal muscles have many other nonrespiratory functions, both individually and as a group; these are not discussed here.

Internal Intercostals

There are 11 internal intercostal muscles on each side of the thorax. Each muscle arises from the floor of the costal groove and cartilage, passes inferiorly and posteriorly and inserts on the upper border of the rib below. These internal intercostals extend from the sternum anteriorly, around the thorax to the posterior costal angle. They are generally divided into two parts: the interosseous portion, located between the sloping parts of the ribs, and the intercartilaginous portions, located between costal cartilages. The intercartilaginous portions are considered inspiratory in function. Contraction of the interosseous portions of the intercostals depresses the ribs and may aid in forceful exhalation. These muscles are innervated by the adjacent intercostal nerves.

OVERVIEW OF THE PROCESS OF BREATHING

During quiet inspiration, the diaphragm, external intercostals, and intercartilaginous portions of the internal intercostals are the primary muscles that contract. The diaphragm contracts first and then descends, enlarging the thoracic cage vertically. When abdominal contents prevent further descent of the diaphragm, the costal fibers of the diaphragm contract, which causes the lower ribs to swing up and out to the side (bucket-handle movement). This lateral rib movement is assisted by the external intercostals and the intercartilaginous portion of the internal intercostals. The transverse diameter of the thorax is increased by this bucket-handle movement. Finally, the upper ribs move forward and upward (pump-handle movement), also through contraction of their external intercostals and the intercartilaginous portions of the internal intercostals. This increases the anteroposterior diameter of the thorax. The epigastric area protrudes, then the ribs swing up and out laterally, and finally the upper ribs move forward and upward.

Quiet expiration is passive and involves no muscular contraction, although some electrical activity can be detected with electromyography. The inspiratory muscles relax, which raises intrathoracic pressure as the ribs and diaphragm return to their preinspiratory positions and compress the lungs. This increased pressure allows air flow from the lungs.

During forced inspiration, an additional number of accessory muscles may contract along with the muscles involved in quiet inspiration. The erector spinae contract to extend the vertebral column. This extension permits greater elevation of the ribs during inspiration. Various back muscles (e.g., erector spinae, trapezius, rhomboids) contract to stabilize the vertebral column, head, neck, and scapulae. This enables accessory respiratory muscles to assist inspiration through reverse action. The SCM raises the sternum. The scalenes elevate the first two ribs. The serratus anterior, pectoralis major, and pectoralis minor assist bilateral elevation of the ribs. All these accessory muscles tend to elevate the ribs, thus increasing the anteroposterior diameter but not the transverse diameter of the thorax. (The transverse diameter does increase slightly as a result of the increased strength of the contraction of the normal inspiratory muscles.) The marked increase in antero-posterior diameter in relation to transverse diameter creates an impression of en bloc breathing in a patient using accessory muscles.

During forced expiration, the interosseous portion of the internal intercostals and the abdominal muscles contract to force air out of the lungs. Forced expiration can be slow and prolonged (as in patients with COPD) or rapid and expulsive (as in a cough). If the abdominal contractions are strong enough, the trunk flexes during exhalation. This flexion further compresses the lungs, forcing more air from them.

UPPER AIRWAYS
Nose

Noses vary in size and shape among individuals and nationalities. The nose is composed of bony and cartilaginous parts. The upper one third is primarily bony and contains the nasal bones, the frontal processes of the maxillae, and the nasal part of the frontal bone. Its lower two thirds are cartilaginous and contain the septal, lateral, and major and minor alar nasal cartilages. The nasal cavity is divided into right and left halves by the nasal septum. This cavity extends from the nostrils to the posterior apertures of the nose in the nasopharynx. The

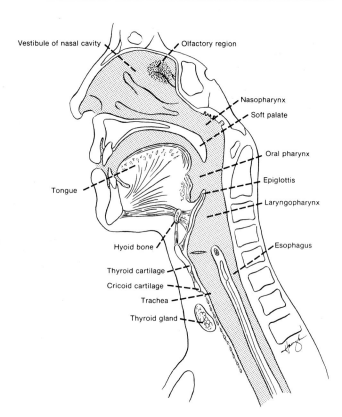

FIGURE 3-9 Sagittal section of the head and neck.

lateral walls of the cavity are irregular as a result of projecting superior, middle, and inferior nasal chonchae. There is a meatus located beneath or lateral to each choncha through which the sinuses drain. The chonchae increase the surface area of the nose for maximum contact with inspired air. The superior chonchae and adjacent septal wall are referred to as the olfactory region. They are covered with a thin, yellow olfactory mucous membrane that consists of bipolar nerve cells that are olfactory in function. Only a portion of inspired air reaches the olfactory region to provide a sense of smell. When people smell something specific, they sniff. This action lifts the inspired air so that more of it comes into contact with the olfactory region.

The anterior portion (vestibule) of the nasal cavity (Figure 3-9) is lined with skin and coarse hairs (vibrissae) that entrap inhaled particles. The rest of the cavity and sinuses (with the exception of the olfactory region) is lined with respiratory mucous membrane. This membrane is composed of pseudostratified columnar ciliated epithelium (Figure 3-10). It contains goblet cells, as well as mucous and serous glands that produce mucus and serous secretions. These secretions entrap foreign particles and bacteria. This mucus is then swept to the nasopharynx by the cilia at a rate of 5 to 15 mm/min, where it is swallowed or expectorated. The mucous membrane is vascular, with arterial blood supplied by branches of the internal and external carotid arteries. Venous drainage occurs through the anterior facial veins. The mucous membrane is thickest over the chonchae. As air is inhaled, it

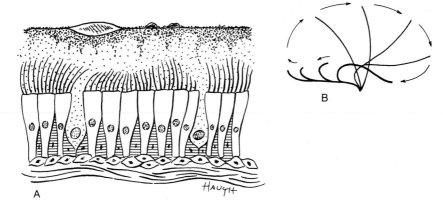

FIGURE 3-10 A, Pseudostratified columnar ciliated epithelium. **B,** Normal movements of cilia.

passes around and over the chonchae, whose vascular moist surfaces heat, humidify, and filter the inspired air. The mucous membrane may become swollen and irritated due to upper respiratory infections and may secrete copious amounts of mucus. Because this membrane is continuous with sinuses, auditory tubes, and lacrimal canaliculi, people with colds often complain of sinus headaches, watery eyes, earaches, and other symptoms. Secretions are often so copious that the nasal passages become completely blocked.

Pharynx

The pharynx is an oval fibromuscular sac located behind the nasal cavity, mouth, and larynx. It is approximately 12 to 14 cm long and extends from the base of the skull to the esophagus below, at the level of the cricoid cartilage opposite the sixth cervical vertebra. Anteriorly it opens into the nasal cavity (nasopharynx), mouth (oropharynx), and larynx (laryngopharynx). The pharyngeal walls are lined with ciliated respiratory mucous membrane in the nasal portion and with stratified squamous membrane in the oral and laryngeal parts.

The nasopharynx is a continuation of the nasal cavities (see Figure 3-9). It lies behind the nose and above the soft palate. With the exception of the soft palate, its walls are immovable, so its cavity is never obliterated as are the oropharynx and laryngopharynx. The nasopharynx communicates with the nasal cavity anteriorly through the posterior apertures of the nose. It communicates with the oropharynx and laryngopharynx through an opening, the pharyngeal isthmus, which is closed by elevations of the soft palate during swallowing.

The oropharynx extends from the soft palate to the epiglottis (see Figure 3-9). It opens into the mouth anteriorly through the oropharyngeal isthmus. Its posterior walls lie on the bodies of the second and third cervical vertebrae. Laterally, two masses of lymphoid tissue—the palatine tonsils—may be seen. These tonsils form part of a circular band of lymphoid tissue surrounding the opening into the digestive and respiratory tracts.

The laryngopharynx lies behind the larynx and extends from the epiglottis above to the inlet of the esophagus below (see Figure 3-9). The fourth to sixth cervical vertebrae lie behind the laryngopharynx. In front of the laryngopharynx are the epiglottis, the inlet of the larynx, and the posterior surfaces of the arytenoid and cricoid cartilages.

Larynx

The larynx is a complex structure composed of cartilages and cords moved by sensitive muscles (Figure 3-11). It is located between the trachea and laryngopharynx, for which it forms an anterior wall. With its rapid closure it acts as a sphincteric valve, preventing food, liquids, and foreign objects from entering the airway. It controls airflow and at times closes so that thoracic pressure may be raised and the upper airways cleared by a propulsive cough when the larynx opens. Expiratory airflow vibrates as it passes over the contracting vocal chords, producing the sounds used for speech. (The larynx is not essential for speech. Humans can speak by learning to dilate the upper part of the esophagus so that air vibrates as it passes over that area; this is called esophageal speech.)

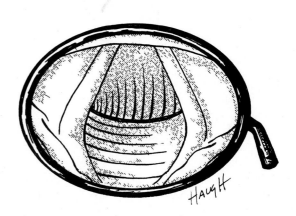

FIGURE 3-11 Visualization of the larynx via a laryngoscope.

In adult men, the larynx is situated opposite the third, fourth, and fifth cervical vertebrae; it is situated somewhat higher in women and children. The larynx is essentially the same in children, but at puberty, the male larynx increases in size considerably until its anteroposterior diameter has almost doubled. All the cartilages enlarge, and the thyroid cartilage becomes prominent anteriorly.

Vocal cord adductor contraction results in approximation of the vocal cords and narrowing of the glottis. The adductors of the cords are important in protecting the lower airways. Their contraction prevents fluids, food, and other substances from being aspirated. All the intrinsic laryngeal muscles are innervated by the recurrent laryngeal nerve (a branch of the vagus nerve), with the exception of the cricothyroid muscle, which is supplied by the external branch of the superior laryngeal nerve (also a branch of the vagus nerve).

LOWER AIRWAYS
Trachea

The trachea is a semirigid cartilaginous tube approximately 10 to 11 cm long and 2.5 cm wide. It lies in front of the esophagus and descends with a slight inclination to the right from the level of the cricoid cartilage (Figure 3-12; see also Figure 3-11). It travels behind the sternum into the thorax to the sternal angle (opposite the fifth thoracic vertebra) where it

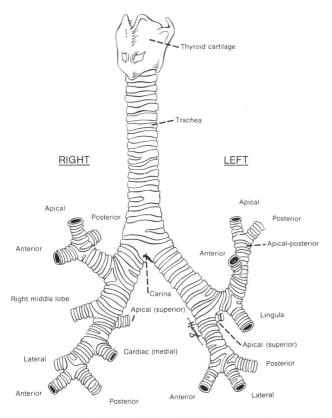

FIGURE 3-12 Tracheobronchial tree (a three quarter view, rotated toward the right side).

divides to form the right and left main stem bronchi. The tracheal wall is strengthened by 16 to 20 horseshoe-shaped cartilaginous rings. The open parts of the tracheal rings are completed by fibrous and elastic tissue and unstriated transverse muscle. This highly flexible part of the ring is positioned posteriorly. It indents or curves inward during coughing, which increases the velocity of expelled air. The cartilaginous rings lie horizontally one above the other, separated by narrow bands of connective tissue. The trachea is lengthened during hyperextension of the head; during swallowing, which raises the trachea; and during inspiration, when the lungs expand and pull the trachea downward. Its cross-sectional area becomes smaller with contraction of the unstriated transverse muscle fibers that complete the tracheal rings.

The mucous membrane of the trachea contains columnar ciliated epithelium and goblet cells. Each ciliated epithelial cell contains approximately 275 cilia. These structures beat rapidly in a coordinated and unidirectional manner, propelling a sheet of mucus toward the head, from the lower respiratory tract to the pharynx, where it is swallowed or expectorated. The cilia beat in this layer of mucus with a forceful forward stroke followed by an ineffective backward stroke that returns the cilia to their starting position. Mucociliary escalator, propelling of mucus by the cilia, is essential. When cilia are paralyzed by smoking, alcohol, dehydration, anesthesia, starvation, or hypoxia, mucus begins to accumulate in distal, gravity-dependent airways, causing infiltrates and eventually localized areas of lung collapse referred to as atelectasis.

The number of mucus-containing goblet cells is approximately equal to the number of ciliated epithelial cells. Reserve cells lie beneath the ciliated and goblet cells. These reserve cells can differentiate into either goblet cells or ciliated cells. Beneath the reserve cells lie the gland cells. There are approximately 40 times more gland cells than goblet cells. Mucus is composed of 95% water, 2% glycoprotein, 1% carbohydrate, trace amounts of lipid, deoxyribonucleic acid (DNA), dead tissue cells, phagocytes, leukocytes, erythrocytes, and entrapped foreign particles. Mucus lines the airways from the trachea to the alveoli. Two separate layers have been observed: the sol layer, which lies on the mucosal surface and contains high concentrations of water, and the gel layer, which is more superficial and viscous because of its lower concentration of water.

The right main stem bronchus is an extension of the trachea and is wider, shorter, and more vertical than the left main stem bronchus. Greater width and more vertical course cause a majority of aspirated foreign material to pass through the right main stem bronchus. The azygos vein arches over the right main stem bronchus; the right pulmonary artery lies beneath it. The right main stem bronchus divides to form the right upper lobe bronchus, the right middle lobe bronchus, and the right lower lobe bronchus. The right upper lobe divides into three segmental bronchi: apical, posterior, and anterior. The apical bronchus runs almost vertically toward the apex of the lung. The posterior bronchus is directed posteriorly in a horizontal direction, and the anterior bronchus is directed anteriorly in an almost horizontal direction. The right middle lobe bronchus divides about 10 mm below the right upper lobe bronchus and descends anterolaterally. The right lower lobe bronchus divides into five segmental bronchi. The apical or superior bronchus runs almost horizontally, posteriorly. The medial or cardiac bronchus descends medially toward the heart. The anterior basal bronchus descends anteriorly. The lateral basal bronchus descends laterally, and the posterior bronchus descends posteriorly. Each segment describes its anatomical position.

The left main stem bronchus is narrower and runs more horizontally than the right main stem bronchus. The aortic arch passes over it and the esophagus, descending aorta, and thoracic duct lie behind it. The left pulmonary artery lies anteriorly and above the left main stem bronchus. The left main stem bronchus has two major divisions: the left upper lobe bronchus and the left lower lobe bronchus. The left upper lobe bronchus has three major segmental bronchi. The anterior bronchus ascends at approximately a 45-degree angle. The apical-posterior bronchus has two branches; one runs vertically and the other posteriorly toward the apex of the left lung. The lingular bronchus descends anterolaterally, much like the right middle lobe bronchus of the right lung. The right lower lobe bronchus divides into four segmental bronchi. The superior or apical bronchus runs posteriorly in a horizontal direction. The anterior bronchus descends anteriorly. The lateral bronchus descends laterally, and the posterior bronchus descends posteriorly. The segments describe their anatomical position.

The bronchi of the airways continue to divide until there are approximately 23 generations (Table 3-1). The main, lobar, and segmental bronchi are made up of the first four generations. The walls contain U-shaped cartilage in the main bronchi. This cartilage becomes less well defined and more irregularly shaped as the bronchi continue to divide. In the segmental bronchi, the walls are formed by irregularly shaped helical plates with bands of bronchial muscle. The mucous membrane in these airways is essentially the same as that in the trachea, but the cells become more cuboidal in the lower divisions.

The subsegmental bronchi extend from the fifth to the seventh generation. Although the diameter of these airways becomes progressively smaller, the total cross-sectional area increases because of the increased number of divisions. The mucous membrane is essentially the same, and helical cartilaginous plates and cilia become sparser. These changes continue throughout the eighth to eleventh generations, which are referred to as bronchioles.

The terminal bronchioles extend from the twelfth to the sixteenth generation. The diameter of these airways is approximately 1 mm. Cartilage is no longer present to provide structural rigidity. The airways are embedded directly in the lung parenchyma, and it is the elastic properties of this parenchyma that keep these lower airways open. Strong helical muscle bands are present and their contraction forms longitudinal folds in the mucosa that sharply decrease the diameter of the airways. The epithelium of the terminal bronchioles is cuboidal and no longer ciliated. The cross-sectional area of the airways increases sharply at this level. All the airways to this level (1 to 16 generations) are considered conducting airways because their purpose is to transport gas to the respiratory bronchioles and alveoli, where gas exchange occurs. The conducting airways receive their arterial blood from the bronchial circulation (branches of the descending aorta). Airways below this point receive their arterial blood from the pulmonary arteries.

The respiratory bronchioles extend from the seventeenth to the nineteenth generation. They are considered a transitional zone between bronchioles and alveoli. Their walls contain cuboidal epithelium interspersed with some alveoli. The number of alveoli increases with each generation. The walls of the bronchioles are also buried in the lung parenchyma. The airways depend on traction of this parenchyma to maintain their lumen. Muscle bands are also present between alveoli.

Alveolar ducts extend from the twentieth to the twenty-second generation. Their walls are composed entirely of alveoli, which are separated from one another by their septae. Septae contain smooth muscle, elastic and collagen fibers, nerves, and capillaries.

Alveolar sacs comprise the twenty-third generation of air passages. They are essentially the same as alveolar ducts, except that they end as blind pouches. Communication occurs between blind pouches in the form of the pores of Kohn, which are channels in alveolar walls, and the Lambert canals, which are communications between bronchioles and alveoli. These communications are thought to be responsible for the rapid spread of lung infection. They also provide collateral ventilation to alveoli, whose bronchi are obstructed. Although this ventilation does little to arterialize blood, it does help prevent collapse of these alveoli. Each alveolar sac contains approximately 17 alveoli. There are about 300 million alveoli in an adult man, 85% to 95% of which are covered with pulmonary capillaries. Alveolar epithelium is composed of two cell types. Type I cells, squamous pneumocytes, have broad thin extensions that cover about 95% of the alveolar surface. Type II cells, the granular pneumocytes, are more numerous than type I cells but occupy less than 5% of the alveolar surface. This is because of their small, cuboidal shape. These cells are responsible for the production of surfactant, a phospholipid that lines the alveoli. Surfactant keeps alveoli expanded by lowering their surface tension. Type II cells have been shown to be the primary cells involved in repair of the alveolar epithelium. Type III cells, alveolar brush cells, are rare and found only occasionally in humans.

An additional type of cell, the alveolar macrophage, is found within the alveoli. These cells are thought to originate from stem cell precursors in the bone marrow and reach the lung through the blood stream. They are large, mononuclear, ameboid cells that roam in the alveoli, alveolar ducts, and alveolar sacs. Macrophages contain lysosomes, which are capable of killing engulfed bacteria. They are especially

TABLE 3-1

Structural Characteristics of the Air Passages

	GENERATION (MEAN)	NUMBER	MEAN DIAMETER (mm)	AREA SUPPLIED	CARTILAGE	MUSCLE	NUTRITION	PLACEMENT	EPITHELIUM
Trachea	0	1	18	Both lungs	U-shaped		Links open end of cartilage		
Main bronchi	1	2	13	Individual lungs				Within connective tissue sheath alongside arterial vessels	Columnar ciliated
Lobar bronchi	2 → 3	4 → 8	7 → 5	Lobes	Irregular shape and helical plates	Helical bands	From the bronchial circulation		
Segmental bronchi	4	16	4	Segments					
Small bronchi	5 → 11	32 → 2,000	3 → 1	Secondary lobules					
Bronchioles and terminal bronchioles	12 → 16	4,000 → 65,000	1 → 0.5			Strong helical muscle bands		Embedded directly in the lung parenchyma	Cubiodal
Respiratory bronchioles	17 → 19	130,000 → 500,000	0.5	Primary lobes	Absent	Muscle band between alveolar			Cubiodal to flat between the alveoli
Alveolar ducts	20 → 22	1,000,000 → 4,000,000	0.3	Alveoli		Thin bands in alveolar septa	From the pulmonary circulation	Forms the lung parenchyma	Alveolar epithelium
Alveolar sacs	23	8,000,000	0.3						

From Weibel, E.R. (1963). Morphometry of the human lung. New York: Springer. Used with permission.

effective in neutralizing inhaled gram-positive organisms. They also engulf foreign matter and are transported to the lymphatic system or migrate to the terminal bronchioles where they attach themselves to the mucus. Macrophages are carried by the mucus to larger airways and eventually to the pharynx. Because cilia are not present below the eleventh generation of air passages, clearance of foreign matter and bacteria from these areas is largely dependent on macrophages.

Other cells located in the distal airways that are important in the defense of the lung are the lymphocytes and polymorphonuclear leukocytes. Immunoglobulins (IgA, IgG, and IgM) in the blood serum enhance the engulfing activity of the macrophages. Two types of lymphocytes are found in the lung: the B-lymphocyte and the T-lymphocyte. The B-lymphocytes produce gamma globulin antibodies to fight lung infections, whereas the T-lymphocytes release a substance that attracts macrophages to the site of the infection. The polymorphonuclear leukocytes are important in engulfing and killing blood-borne gram-negative organisms.

LUNGS

Two lungs, each covered with its pleurae—the visceral pleura and the parietal pleura—lie within the thoracic cavity. Each lung is attached to the heart and the trachea by its root and the pulmonary ligament. They are otherwise free in the thoracic cavity. The lungs are light, soft, spongy organs whose color darkens with age as they become impregnated with inhaled air pollutants. They are covered with the visceral pleura, a thin, glistening serous membrane that covers all surfaces of the lungs. The visceral pleura extends to the mediastinum and inner thoracic wall, where it becomes known as the parietal pleura. The space between the two pleurae maintains a negative pressure at all times and is therefore termed a potential space. This negative pressure maintains lung inflation. A small amount of pleural fluid lubricates the two pleurae as they slide over each other during breathing. In disease, fluid, tumor cells, or air can invade the pleural space and collapse the underlying lung.

Each lung has an apex, a base, and three surfaces (costal, medial, and diaphragmatic). There are also three borders (anterior, inferior, and posterior). Each lung is divided by fissures into separate lobes. In the right lung, the oblique fissure separates the lower lobe from the middle, whereas the horizontal fissure separates the upper lobe from the middle. The right lung is heavier and wider than the left lung. It is also shorter because of the location of the right lobe of the liver. The left lung is divided into upper and lower lobes by the oblique fissure. It is longer and thinner than the right lung because the heart and pericardium are located in the left thorax. Numerous structures enter the lung at the hilus, or root of the lung, including the main stem bronchus, the pulmonary artery, pulmonary veins, bronchial arteries and veins, nerves, and lymph vessels. The root, or hilus, of the lungs lies opposite the bodies of the fifth, sixth, and seventh thoracic vertebrae. The lungs are connected to the upper airways by the trachea and main stem bronchi.

Surface Markings

Surface markings of the lungs can be outlined on the chest with a basic knowledge of bony landmarks and of the gross anatomy of each lung (Table 3-2 and Figures 3-13, 3-14, 3-15). The apices of both lungs extend 2 or 3 cm above the clavicles at the medial ends. The anteromedial border of the right lung runs from the sternoclavicular joint to the sternal angle and downward to the xiphisternum. The inferior border runs from the xiphisternum laterally to the sixth rib in the midclavicular line, the eighth rib in the midaxillary line, and the tenth rib in the midscapular line. The midscapular line runs downward from the inferior angle of the scapula with the arm at rest. The inferior border joins the posterior medial border of the lung 2 cm lateral to the tenth thoracic vertebra. The posterior medial border runs 2 cm lateral to the vertebral column from the seventh cervical vertebra to the tenth thoracic vertebra.

The left lung is generally smaller than the right and accommodates the position of the heart. The medial border on the anterior aspect runs from the sternoclavicular joint to the middle of the sternal angle, down the midline of the sternum to the fourth costal cartilage. A lateral indentation of about 2 to 3 cm forms the cardiac notch at the level of the fifth and sixth costal cartilages. The courses of the inferior and medial borders on the posterior aspect are similar in the left and right lungs. In the left lung, however, the inferior border crosses at the level of the tenth thoracic vertebra, not the twelfth, as is observed in the right lung.

The position of the fissures of the lungs can be outlined over the chest wall. In both lungs, the oblique fissure begins between the second to fourth thoracic vertebrae. This can be roughly estimated by following a line continuous with the medial border of the abducted scapula around the midaxillary line at the fifth rib and terminating at the sixth costal cartilage anteriorly. The horizontal fissure of the right lung originates from the oblique fissure at the level of about the fourth intercostal space in the midaxillary line and courses medially and slightly upward over the fourth rib anteriorly. The left lung has no horizontal fissure.

Bronchopulmonary Segments

The bronchopulmonary segments lie within the three lobes of the right lung and the two lobes of the left lung. There are 10 bronchopulmonary segments on the right and eight on the left. Brief anatomic descriptions of the position of each lobe are provided in Table 3-2. Figure 3-13 illustrates the surface markings on the anterior view of the lungs and the position of the various bronchopulmonary segments within the major anatomic divisions provided by the fissures. Figure 3-14 shows some of these features from the lateral views. Figure 3-15 illustrates the surface markings and bronchopulmonary segments of the posterior aspect of the lungs.

TABLE 3-2

Anatomical Arrangement of the Bronchopulmonary Segments

LOBE	RIGHT LUNG: BRONCHOPULMONARY SEGMENTS	LOBE	LEFT LUNG: BRONCHOPULMONARY SEGMENTS
Upper	Apical—extends above the clavicle anteriorly; smaller area posteriorly	Upper	Apical posterior—extends above the clavicle anteriorly; occupies area comparable to the apical and posterior segments of the right lung
	Anterior—occupies area between the clavicle and horizontal fissure		Anterior—occupies area between the clavicle and the border of the lingula (line comparable to the horizontal fissure of the right lung)
	Posterior—remainder of upper lobe on the posterior aspect down to the oblique fissure	(Lingula)‡	Superior—occupies upper half of the lingula
Middle	Lateral—extends medially from junction of the two fissures at the third intercostal space to occupy one third of the anterior surface of the lobe		Inferior—occupies lower half of the lingula
	Medial—occupies the remaining anterior surface of the lobe		
Lower (Base)	Anterior—occupies basal area beneath the oblique fissure anteriorly	Lower (Base)	Anterior—occupies area inferior to the oblique fissure anteriorly
	Superior—occupies half the area ffrom the oblique fissure downward* on the posterior aspect		Superior—occupies one third of the basal area posteriorly from the oblique fissure downward
	Lateral—extends from the junction of the middle lobe over the midaxillary area to occupy one third the area inferior to the superior segment on the posterior aspect		Lateral—occupies the lateral half of the remaining two thirds of the left lower lobe beneath the superior segment on the posterior aspect
	Posterior—occupies two thirds of the area posteriorly beneath the superior segment		Posterior—occupies the medial portion of the remaining two thirds of the left lower lobe beneath the superior segment on the posterior aspect
	Medial—occupies a space on the inner aspect of the right base†		

*This segment is best drained when the patient lies prone. Superior segments also called apical segments.

†Medial basal segment has no direct exposure to the chest wall; therefore, it cannot be directly auscultated. This segment is best drained when the patient is positioned for the left lateral basal segment because of the comparable angle of its bronchus.

‡Lingula is not an area that is anatomically distinct from the right middle lobe; rather, it is anatomically part of the left upper lobe.

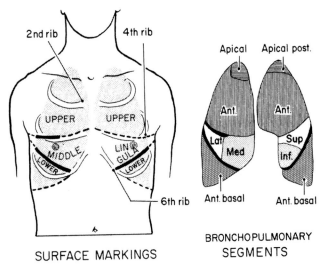

FIGURE 3-13 Surface markings of the lungs (anterior aspect). The underlying bronchopulmonary segments are also shown. *(From Cherniak, R.M., & Cherniack, L. [1983]. Respiration in health and disease, ed 3. Philadelphia: WB Saunders.)*

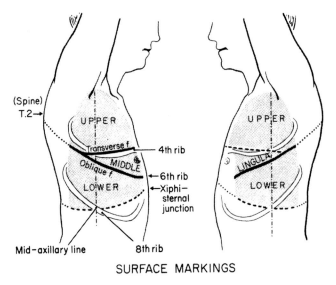

FIGURE 3-14 Surface markings of the lungs (lateral aspect). *(From Cherniak, R.M., & Cherniack, L.[1983]. Respiration in health and disease, ed 3. Philadelphia: WB Saunders.)*

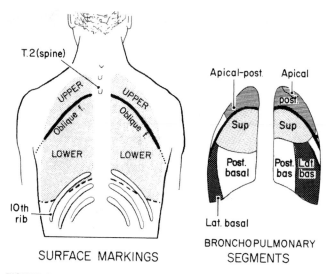

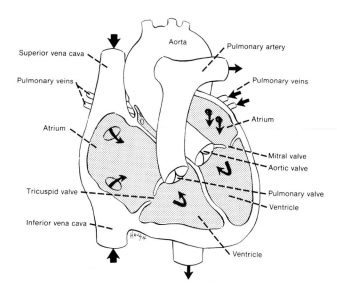

FIGURE 3-15 Surface markings of the lungs (posterior aspect). The underlying bronchopulmonary segments are also shown. *(From Cherniak, R.M., & Cherniack, L. [1983]. Respiration in health and disease, ed 3. Philadelphia: WB Saunders.)*

FIGURE 3-16 Blood flow of the heart.

HEART

The heart is a conical, hollow muscular pump enclosed in a fibroserous sac, the pericardium. Its size is closely related to body size and corresponds remarkably to the size of an individual's clenched fist. It is positioned in the center of the chest behind the lower half of the sternum. The largest portion of the heart lies to the left of the midsternal line; the apex is found approximately 9 cm to the left, in the fifth intercostal space.

The surface markings of the heart can be traced by joining four points over the anterior chest wall. On the right, the heart extends from the third to the sixth costal cartilage at a distance of about 10 to 15 mm from the sternum. On the left, the heart extends from the second costal cartilage to the fifth intercostal space, 12 to 15 mm and 9 cm from the left sternal border, respectively. Joining the two points on the left side outlines the left atrium and ventricle. The heart is rotated to the left in the chest, so the right side of the heart is foremost. Joining the two uppermost points outlines the level of the atria, and joining the two lower points represents the margin of the right ventricle.

The heart as a whole is freely movable within the pericardial cavity and changes position during both contraction and respiration. During contraction, the apex moves forward, strikes the chest and imparts the chest-and-apex beat, which may be felt and seen. Abnormal positioning of the apex beat can indicate cardiac enlargement or displacement. During breathing, the movements of the diaphragm determine the position of the heart. This is because of the attachment of the central tendon of the diaphragm to the pericardium. Changes in position during quiet breathing are hardly noticeable, but with deep inspirations, the downward excursion of the diaphragm causes the heart to descend and rotate to the right.

The opposite occurs during expiration. Pathology of the lungs can also change the position of the heart. Atelectasis shifts the heart to the same side. In tension pneumothorax, where air enters the chest (usually through an opening in the chest wall) and cannot escape, the positive pressure shifts the heart away from the side of the pathology.

The heart is enclosed by the pericardium, whose two surfaces can be visualized by visualizing the heart as a fist plunged into a large balloon. The outer surface, a tough fibrous membrane, is called the fibrous pericardium. It encases the heart as well as the organs and terminations of the great vessels. This membrane is so unyielding that when fluid accumulates rapidly in the pericardial cavity, it can compress the heart and impede venous return. When this occurs often, a window is cut in the pericardium, allowing the fluid to escape. The inner surface, the serous pericardium, is a serous membrane that lines the fibrous pericardium. Between 10 and 20 ml of clear pericardial fluid separates and moistens the two pericardial surfaces. The pericardium with its fluid minimizes friction during contraction. It also holds the heart in position and prevents dilation. The serous pericardium consists of an outer layer, the parietal layer, and an inner layer, the visceral layer or epicardium.

The heart is divided into right and left halves by an obliquely placed longitudinal septum (Figure 3-16). Each half has two chambers: the atrium, which receives blood from veins, and the ventricle, which ejects blood into the arteries. The superior vena cava, inferior vena cava, and intrinsic veins of the heart deposit venous blood into the right atrium. Blood then passes through the tricuspid valve to the right ventricle. The right ventricle ejects the blood through the pulmonary valve into the pulmonary arteries, which are the only arteries in the body that contain deoxygenated blood. Pulmonary veins return the blood to the left atrium and from there it passes through the mitral valve to the left ventricle. From the

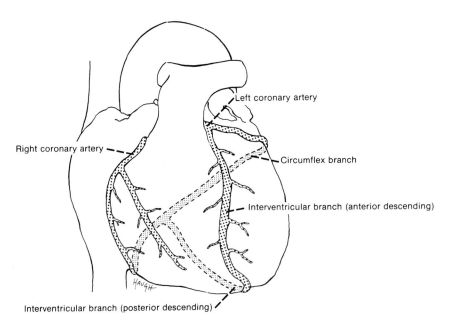

FIGURE 3-17 Blood supply of the heart.

left ventricle it is ejected through the aortic valve into the main artery of the body, the aorta.

The heart is divided into three layers: the epicardium, myocardium, and endocardium. The outermost layer, the epicardium, is visceral pericardium and is often infiltrated with fat. The coronary blood vessels that nourish the heart run in this layer before entering the myocardium. The myocardium consists of cardiac muscle fibers. The thickness of the layers of cardiac muscle fibers is directly proportional to the amount of work they perform. The ventricles do more work than the atria, hence their walls are thicker. The pressure in the aorta is higher than that in the pulmonary trunk. This requires greater work from the left ventricle, so its walls are twice as thick as those of the right ventricle. The innermost layer, the endocardium, is the smooth endothelial lining of the interior of the heart.

Heart Valves

The four valves of the heart, although delicate in appearance, are designed to withstand repetitive closures against high pressures (see Figure 3-16). Normally they operate for more than 80 years without need of repair or replacement. The tricuspid and mitral valves function differently from the other valves of the heart. Being located between the atria and ventricles, they must effect a precise closure within a contracting cavity.

During diastole, the two leaflets or cusps of the mitral valve and the three cusps of the tricuspid valve relax into the cavities of the ventricles, allowing blood to flow between the two chambers. As the ventricular chambers fill with blood, the cusps of the valves are forced up into a closed position. Fibrous cords, the chordae tendinae, are located on the

ventricular surfaces of these cusps. These cords connect the cusps of the valve with the papillary muscles of the ventricular walls. As pressure builds in the ventricular chambers, contraction of these muscles prevents the cusps from being forced up into the atria. Dysfunction or rupture of the chordae tendinae or the papillary muscles may undermine the support of one or more valve cusps, producing regurgitation from the ventricles to the atria.

The pulmonic and aortic valves are similar in appearance but the aortic cusps are slightly thicker than the pulmonic cusps. Each valve has three fibrous cusps, the bases of which are firmly attached to the root of the aorta or the pulmonary artery. The free edges of these valves project into the lumen of the vessels. At the end of systole, blood in the aorta and pulmonary artery forces the cusps of the valves shut. These valves are attached in such a manner that they cannot be everted into the ventricles by increased pressure in the vessels. During diastole, the cusps support the column of blood filling the ventricles. Contraction of the ventricles during systole increases pressure within the ventricular chambers, forcing the cusps to open and allow blood flow into the vessels.

The arterial supply of the heart muscle is derived from the right and left coronary arteries, which arise from the aortic sinuses (Figure 3-17). The left coronary artery (LCA) divides into the anterior descending artery and the left circumflex artery. These arteries supply most of the left ventricle, the left atrium, most of the ventricular septum and, in 45% of people, the sinoatrial (SA) node. The right coronary artery (RCA) supplies most of the right ventricle, the atrioventricular (AV) node and, in 55% of people, the SA node. Infarction of these arteries or their branches can cause interruption or cessation of the conduction system and death of the myocardial muscle in the area supplied by the artery. The severity of the infarction

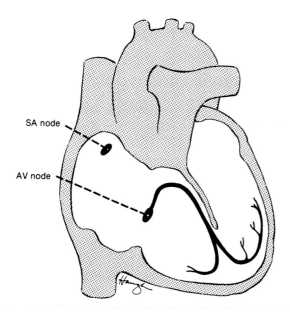

FIGURE 3-18 Electrical conduction of the heart.

is dependent on the size of the artery and the importance of the area it supplies.

The heart is drained by a number of veins. Most of the veins of the heart enter the coronary sinus, which then empties into the right atrium. A small portion of veins, the thebesian veins, empty directly into the right and left ventricles.

Innervation

Innervation of the heart involves a complex balance between its intrinsic automaticity and extrinsic nerves (Figure 3-18). The SA and AV nodes provide the heart with an inherent ability for spontaneous rhythmic initiation of the cardiac impulse. The rate of this impulse formation is regulated by the autonomic nervous system (ANS), which also influences other phases of the cardiac cycle. It controls the rate of spread of the excitation impulse and the contractility of both atria and ventricles.

The ANS extends its influence to the heart via the vagus nerve (parasympathetic) and upper thoracic nerves (sympathetic). These nerves mingle around the root and arch of the aorta near the tracheal bifurcation, forming the cardiac plexus. Extensions from the cardiac plexus richly supply the SA and AV nodes. They are so well mingled that scientists are unable to determine which nerves supply which parts of the heart. Stimulation of the sympathetic nervous system causes acceleration of the discharge rate in the SA node, an increase in AV nodal conduction, and an increase in the contractile force of both atrial and ventricular muscles. Stimulation of the vagus nerve causes cardiac slowing and decreased AV nodal conduction. Thus the parasympathetic system decelerates heart rate and the sympathetic system accelerates heart rate.

Intrinsic innervation of the heart centers around the SA node, which lies near the junction of the superior vena cava

and the right atrium. It is the normal pacemaker of the heart, sending concentric waves of excitation throughout the atrium. Without neural influence, impulse formation from this node would be greater than 100 beats per minute. Vagal influence, however, decreases the impulse formation to 60 to 90 beats per minute. The SA node paces the heart as long as it generates impulses at a faster rate than any other part of the myocardium and as long as these impulses are rapidly conducted from the atria to the ventricles. Normal impulse formation may be interrupted by vascular lesions (occlusion of the coronary arteries) or by cardiac disease (pericarditis). The SA node is especially susceptible to pericarditis and all other surface cardiac diseases because of its superficial position immediately beneath the epicardium.

The muscle fibers of the heart are self-excitatory, which enables the heart to contract rhythmically and automatically. The normal pacemaker of the heart, the SA node, is located in the posterior wall of the right atrium. The concentric waves of excitation sent out by the SA node must travel through the AV node to reach the ventricles. This node is located in the floor of the right atrium, just above the insertion of the tricuspid valve. Its main function is to cause a 0.04-second delay in impulse transmission. This delay is good for two reasons: it postpones ventricular excitation until the atria have had time to eject their contents into the ventricles, and it limits the number of signals that can be transmitted by the AV node. The AV node also has its own inherent rhythmicity, firing at a much slower rate than the SA node (40 to 60 beats per minute). Its main pathology is a result of occlusion of the right coronary artery, which supplies the AV node in 90% of cases. From the AV node arises a triangular group of fibers known as the AV bundle, or bundle of His. This bundle divides in the ventricular septum into two branches: the left bundle branch and the right bundle branch. Each of these bundles continues to divide into many fine nerve fibers that spread throughout the ventricles and terminate in the Purkinje fibers, which are continuous with the cardiac muscle. The waves of excitation pass through the bundle of His, down the bundle branches, and through the Purkinje fibers, which permeate the ventricles and cause them to contract. This wave of depolarization gives rise to the normal P-QRS-T configuration of the electrocardiogram (ECG) tracing (Figure 3-19) (see Chapter 12). The P wave indicates atrial depolarization, the QRS complex indicates ventricular depolarization, and the T wave indicates ventricular repolarization. There is no wave indicating atrial repolarization because atrial repolarization is embedded in the QRS complex (Kinney & Packa, 1995; Wagner, 2001) (see Physiology of the Electrical Excitation of the Heart and ECG Interpretation, Chapter 12; Dubin, 2000; Marriott and Conover, 1998; Wagner, 2001).

SYSTEMIC CIRCULATION

The systemic vascular system is a complex series of branching blood vessels throughout the body. It provides nutrition and oxygen to and removes waste products from all tissues of the

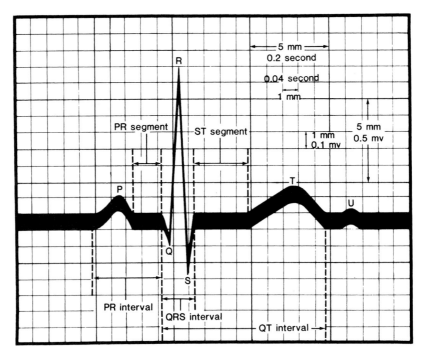

FIGURE 3-19 A normal ECG showing characteristic waves, intervals, and segments.

body. The driving force for this system is the heart. The vascular system has two major components: the peripheral and the pulmonary circulations (Fuster et al, 2004).

Blood vessels are designed to forward oxygenated blood from the heart during systolic ejection from the left ventricle, perfuse the vascular beds commensurate with their metabolic needs, and remove metabolic waste. Anatomically, the proximal vessels have a higher proportion of connective tissue and elastin so as to withstand high pulse pressures (e.g., the aorta, which carries blood to the head, viscera, and limbs). In addition, potential energy is stored in the walls of the larger vessels during systole. During diastole, the elastic recoil of these vessels maintains the forward motion of the blood between ventricular systoles. The medium-size blood vessels have proportions of connective tissue and elastin comparable to smooth muscle. As the blood vessels become smaller, smooth muscle predominates. The arterioles are primarily smooth muscle, so their diameter can alter significantly. They regulate the blood flow to regional tissue beds and are also responsible for regulating total peripheral resistance and systemic blood pressure. They are called the stopcocks of the circulation. Many factors (e.g., nervous impulses, hormonal stimulation, drugs, oxygen, and carbon dioxide concentrations) determine the degree of contraction of vascular smooth muscle and whether contraction occurs locally or throughout the entire body.

Arterioles branch to form the smallest vessels, capillaries, which consist of a single layer of endothelial cells forming lumen just large enough for red blood cells to pass. The capillary bed is enormous, with a capacity far exceeding 5 L. In active tissue like muscle and brain, the capillary network is finer and denser; the network is less dense in less active tissue such as tendon. Gas exchange occurs in the capillary bed, where red blood cells give up their oxygen and blood plasma transudes capillary walls, carrying nutrition to tissue.

The microcirculation specifically consists of the metarterioles, the capillary bed, and the venules. The capillary wall is a semipermeable membrane that is responsible for the transfer of oxygen, nutrients, and waste between the circulation and tissue via the interstitial fluid (see Chapters 2 and 4). The capillary pores selectively allow molecules of different size to pass through them. This is an essential feature that regulates the movement of fluid in and out of the intravascular and extravascular compartments. This process is fundamental to maintaining and regulating normal hemodynamics.

Capillaries give rise to the venules, which are the smallest veins. These veins branch and become increasingly larger. Blood flow through the veins is largely dependent on muscular or visceral action or pressures. These pressures are intermittent and, were it not for double-cusp valves located within the veins, blood would flow backward with fluctuation in the pressure gradient and cessation of flow. In the extremities, muscular contractions move blood into the trunk. In the pelvic and abdominal region, blood flow is dependent on intra-abdominal pressure exceeding intrathoracic pressure. Veins in the trunk become increasingly larger until they finally enter the superior and inferior vena cavae.

PULMONARY CIRCULATION

The vena cavae empty directly into the right atrium. Blood flow from the right side of the heart through the lungs is known as pulmonary circulation. The quantity of blood flowing through pulmonary circulation is approximately equal to that flowing through systemic circulation. Blood flows from the right ventricle into the pulmonary artery, which divides into right and left branches 4 cm from the ventricle. These branches then separate, one to each lung, where they continue to divide into smaller arteries. The pulmonary arteries and arterioles are much shorter, have thinner walls and larger diameters, and are more distensible than their systemic counterparts. This gives the pulmonary system compliance as great as that of the systemic arterial system, thereby allowing the pulmonary arteries to accommodate the stroke volume output of the right ventricle. Pulmonary vascular resistance and arterial pressure are one sixth that of the systemic system (pulmonary arterial pressure is 20/10 mm Hg compared with 120/80 mm Hg systemically).

Pulmonary capillaries are short and arise abruptly from larger arterioles. They form a dense network over the walls of the alveoli to minimize the distance over which gas exchange occurs. The pulmonary veins are also very short but have distensibility characteristics similar to those of veins in the systemic system. Unlike systemic veins, however, pulmonary veins have no valves. Pulmonary veins act as a capacitance vessel, or a blood reservoir, for the left atrium. Contraction of smooth muscle in the veins makes the reservoir constrict. This increases blood volume in relation to the internal volume of the vessels. The pulmonary veins become larger until they converge into two veins from each lung, which then carry oxygenated blood to the left atrium.

LYMPHATIC CIRCULATION

The lymphatic circulation provides an additional route for fluid to be returned from the interstitium to the systemic circulation and thus has a central role in the regulation of interstitial fluid dynamics. Lymph, the fluid that flows in the lymphatic channels, is interstitial fluid with a composition similar to that of tissue fluid. The vessels of the lymphatic system move excess fluid, large proteins, and other large molecules away from the interstitial spaces. Although relatively little protein leaks from the capillaries into the surrounding tissue, the absence of its immediate removal is life-threatening.

Virtually all areas of the body drain into a network of lymphatic channels. From the lower portion of the body and from the left head and neck, excess tissue fluid and protein drain into the thoracic duct, which empties into the venous circulation at the junction of the left internal jugular vein and the subclavian vein. Lymph from the right side of the head, neck, arm, and parts of the right thorax drain into the right lymph duct, which empties into the venous circulation at the junction of the right internal jugular vein and the subclavian vein. Lymph from the lower part of the body drains into the inguinal and abdominal lymphatic channels. The pressure in the lymphatic system is usually slightly negative, which helps to keep the interstitium "dry." The lymph vessels are thin-walled and have some smooth muscle, so they can contract to propel their contents. In addition, lymph vessels have valves to facilitate forward motion and minimize retrograde movement of lymph.

SUMMARY

This chapter reviews the anatomy of the cardiopulmonary system. The anatomic features of the respiratory pump are described with respect to the structures of the bony thorax; of the muscles of respiration associated with the chest wall; and of the diaphragm. The upper and lower respiratory tracts are described, as is the relationship of the tracheobronchial tree to the lung parenchyma. The lung parenchyma is defined anatomically in terms of discrete bronchopulmonary segments contained within three major divisions of each lung. The specific surface markings defined by the lung fissures and the landmarks of the bronchopulmonary segments are outlined. The basic anatomy of the heart is described. The structures of the peripheral and pulmonary circulations are also presented. Special reference is made to the lymphatic circulation and its central role in the regulation of capillary fluid dynamics. A detailed understanding of cardiopulmonary anatomy is fundamental to the knowledge base underlying the assessment and management by physical therapists of cardiopulmonary dysfunction and impaired oxygen transport.

Review Questions

1. Describe the cardiopulmonary unit and why it is a more useful classification than describing either the heart or lungs separately.
2. Describe the thorax and its movements.
3. Describe the respiratory muscles and their functions.
4. Explain the pathway of oxygen from the atmosphere to the alveolar capillary membrane.
5. Describe the movement of blood returning from the periphery through the heart to the pulmonary and peripheral circulations.
6. Describe the movement of deoxygenated blood from the periphery back to the heart.
7. Explain the role of the lymphatic circulation and its physiologic significance.
8. Describe the interdependence between the lungs and the heart in relation to its clinical implications.

REFERENCES

Berne, R.M., & Levy, M.N. (2000). Cardiovascular physiology, ed 8. Philadelphia: Elsevier.

Burton, G.G. (1997). Respiratory care: a guide to clinical practice, ed 4. Philadelphia: Lippincott Williams & Wilkins.

Cheitlin, M.D. (2004). Clinical cardiology, ed 7. Stamford: Appleton & Lange.

Cherniack, R.M., & Cherniack, L. (1983). Respiration in Health and Disease, ed 3. Philadelphia: WB Saunders.

Clemente, C.D. (Ed) (1985). Gray's anatomy of the human body, ed 30. Philadelphia: Lippincott Williams & Wilkins.

Dubin, D. (2000). Rapid interpretation of EKGs: a programmed course, ed 6. Tampa, Fla.: Cover Publishing.

Fuster, V., Alexander, W.R., O'Rourke, R.A., Roberts, R., King, S.B. Prystowsky, E.N., &, Nash, I. (2004). Hurst's the heart, ed 11. New York: McGraw-Hill.

Ganong, W.F. (2003). Review of medical physiology, ed 21. New York: McGraw-Hill Professional Publishing.

Guyton, A.C., & Hall, J.E. (2000). Textbook of medical physiology, ed 10. Philadelphia: Elsevier.

Katz, A.M. (2000). Physiology of the heart, ed 3. Philadelphia: Lippincott Williams & Wilkins.

Kinney, M.R., & Packa, D.R. (1995). Andreoli's comprehensive cardiac care, ed 8. Philadelphia: Elsevier.

Marriott, H.J.L., & Conover, M.B. (1998). Advanced concepts in arrhythmias, ed 3. Philadelphia: Elsevier.

Murray, J.F. (1986). The normal lung, ed 2. Philadelphia: Elsevier.

Murray, J.F., & Nadel, J.A. (2000). Textbook of respiratory medicine, ed 3. Philadelphia: Elsevier.

Nunn, J.F. (1999). Applied respiratory physiology, ed 5. San Diego: Elsevier.

Scharf, S.M., & Cassidy, S.S. (Eds) (1989). Heart-lung interactions in health and disease. New York: Marcel Dekker.

Wagner, G.S. (2001). Marriott's practical electrocardiography, ed 10. Philadelphia: Lippincott Williams & Wilkins.

Weber, K.T., Janicki, J.S., Shroff, S.G., & Likoff, M.J. (1983). The cardiopulmonary unit: the body's gas transport system. Clinics in Chest Medicine 4:101-110.

Weibel, E.R. (1963). Morphometry of the human lung. New York: Springer-Verlag.

West, J.B. (2004). Respiratory physiology—the essentials, ed 7. Baltimore: Williams & Wilkins.

Williams, P.L., & Bannister, L.H. (Eds) (1989). Gray's anatomy: the anatomical basis of medicine and surgery, ed 38. Philadelphia: Elsevier.

CHAPTER 4

Cardiopulmonary Physiology

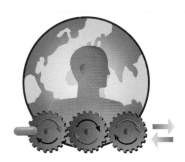

Elizabeth Dean

This chapter reviews the basics of cardiopulmonary physiology. A thorough understanding of normal physiology provides a basis for understanding the deficits in cardiopulmonary function (in the context of limitation of activity and social participation as well as structure and function) and the adaptations to changing physiological and pathophysiological demands. This knowledge provides the foundation for conducting a thorough assessment and prescribing treatment (Bates, 1989; Berne & Levy, 2000; Ganong, 2003; Goldberger, 1990; Guyton & Hall, 2000; Katz, 2000; Murray & Nadel, 2000; Nunn, 1999; Scharf & Cassidy, 1989; Fuster et al, 2004; and West, 2004).

CONTROL OF BREATHING

The act of breathing is a natural process to which most of us give little thought. Breathing unconsciously adjusts to various degrees of activity, maintaining optimum arterial levels of Po_2 and Pco_2, whether we are resting or physically active. Sighing, yawning, hiccoughing, laughing, and vomiting are all involuntary acts that use respiratory muscles. Breathing can also be done under voluntary control. A person can stop breathing momentarily by breath holding or increase breathing by rapidly panting until he or she faints (from cerebral vascular constriction due to a decrease in arterial Pco_2). Exhalation is used in singing, speaking, coughing, and blowing, whereas

inspiration is used for sniffing and sucking. Parturition, defecation, and the Valsalva maneuver are all performed while voluntarily holding one's breath. These activities are regulated by control centers located in the brain. The centers integrate a multitude of chemical, reflex, and physical stimuli before transmitting impulses to the respiratory muscles. The cerebral hemispheres control voluntary respiratory activity, whereas involuntary respiratory activity is controlled by centers located in the pons and medulla of the midbrain (Figure 4-1).

Medullary and Pontine Respiratory Centers

The respiratory center in the medulla is in the reticular formation. It contains the minimum number of neurons necessary for the basic sequence of inspiration and expiration. Although this center is capable of maintaining some degree of respiratory activity, these respirations are not normal in character.

The apneustic center is in the middle and lower pons. If uncontrolled by the pneumotaxic center, prolonged inspiratory gasps (apneustic breathing) occur.

The pneumotaxic center is in the upper one third of the pons. It maintains the normal pattern of respiration, balancing inspiration and expiration by inhibiting either the apneustic center or the inspiratory component of the medullary center.

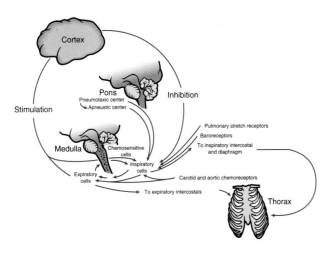

FIGURE 4-1 Control of breathing.

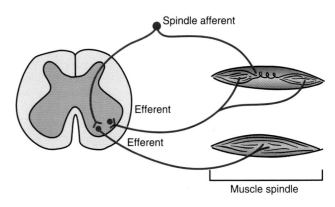

FIGURE 4-2 Stretch reflex.

REFLEXES
Hering-Breuer Reflex

In the late 1800s, Hering and Breuer noted that distention of anesthetized animal lungs caused a decrease in the frequency of inspiration and an increase in expiratory time. Receptors for this reflex are thought to lie in the smooth muscle of airways from the trachea to the bronchioles. More than 800 ml of lung volume above functional residual capacity are needed to activate the reflex and delay the next breath.

Cough Reflex

Mechanical or chemical stimuli to the larynx, trachea, carina, and lower bronchi result in a reflex cough and bronchoconstriction. The high velocity created by the cough sweeps mucus and other irritants up toward the pharynx (see Chapter 23).

Stretch Reflex

The intercostal muscles and the diaphragm contain sensory muscle spindles that respond to elongation. A signal is sent to the spinal cord and anterior horn motor neurons. These neurons signal more muscle fibers to contract (recruitment) and thus increase the strength of the contraction. Theoretically, such a stretch reflex may be useful when there is an increase in airway resistance or a decrease in lung compliance. Stretching the ribs and the diaphragm may activate the stretch reflex and help the patient take a deep breath. The fundamental pathways of the stretch reflex are shown in Figure 4-2. Research is needed, however, to establish the therapeutic role of proprioceptive neurofacilitation techniques based on stretch reflex theory in altering pulmonary function.

Joint and Muscle Receptors

Peripheral joints and muscles of the limbs are believed to have receptors that respond to movement and enhance ventilation in preparation for activity. Ventilation has also been shown to

Central Chemoreceptors

Central chemoreceptors are located on the ventral lateral surfaces of the upper medulla. They are bathed in the cerebrospinal fluid (CSF), which is separated from blood by the blood-brain barrier. Although this barrier is relatively impermeable to hydrogen (H^+) and bicarbonate (HCO_3) ions, carbon dioxide (CO_2) diffuses through the barrier. Increased stimulation of central chemoreceptors by a rising arterial P_{CO_2} results in increased depth and rate of ventilation.

Peripheral Chemoreceptors

Peripheral chemoreceptors are located in the carotid bodies, which lie in the bifurcations of the common carotid artery and the aortic bodies above and below the aortic arch. These bodies receive blood from small branches of the vessels on which they are located. The peripheral chemoreceptors respond to an increase in arterial P_{CO_2} by increasing ventilation, but their response to P_{CO_2} is much less important than that of the central chemoreceptors.

The main role of the peripheral chemoreceptors is to respond to hypoxemia by increasing ventilation. If arterial P_{CO_2} is normal, the P_{O_2} must drop to 50 mm Hg before ventilation increases. A rising P_{CO_2} causes the peripheral chemoreceptors to respond more quickly to a decreasing P_{O_2}. In some patients with severe lung disease, this response to hypoxemia (the hypoxic drive) becomes very important. These patients often have a permanently elevated P_{CO_2} (CO_2 retention). The CSF in these patients compensates for a chronically elevated arterial P_{CO_2} by returning the pH of the CSF to near normal values. When these patients have lost the ability to stimulate ventilation in response to an elevated P_{CO_2}, arterial hypoxemia becomes the major stimulus to ventilation (hypoxic drive).

be stimulated by a similar reflex in humans and anesthetized animals in response to passive movement of the limbs. The precise pathways for these reflexes have not been well established.

Mechanoreceptors

Changes in systemic blood pressure cause corresponding changes in pressure receptors in the carotid and aortic sinuses. Increase in blood pressure causes mechanical distortion of the receptors in these sinuses, producing reflex hypoventilation. Conversely, a reduction in blood pressure can result in hyperventilation.

MECHANICAL FACTORS IN BREATHING

The flow of air into the lungs is a result of pressure differences between the lungs and the atmosphere. In normal breathing, inspiration occurs when alveolar pressure is less than atmospheric pressure. Muscular contraction of the respiratory muscles lowers alveolar pressure and enlarges the thorax. The decreased pressure causes air to flow from the atmosphere into the lungs. Patients who are unable to create adequate negative pressure may have to be mechanically ventilated. The ventilators create a positive pressure (greater than atmospheric pressure) that forces air into the lungs, where there is atmospheric pressure. The iron lung used during the poliomyelitis epidemic of the 1950s assisted ventilation by using cycles of negative pressure to inflate the lungs.

Exhalation occurs when alveolar pressure is greater than atmospheric pressure. At the cessation of inspiration, the respiratory muscles return passively to their resting positions. The diaphragm rises, compressing the lungs and thereby increasing alveolar pressure. As the intercostals relax, the ribs resume their preinspiratory position, further compressing the lungs and increasing alveolar pressure. The increased alveolar pressure contributes to air flowing from the lungs. Normally expiration is a passive process reflecting the elastic recoil of the lung parenchyma.

Resistance to Breathing
Compliance

The inner wall of the thorax, which is lined with parietal pleura, and the parenchyma of the lung, which is enclosed in visceral pleura, lie in close proximity to one another. The pleurae are separated by a potential space containing a small amount of pleural fluid. Muscular contraction of the intercostals and the diaphragm mechanically enlarges the thorax. The lungs are enlarged at this time because of their close proximity to the thorax. The healthy lung resists this enlargement and tries to pull away from the chest wall. The ease with which the lungs are inflated during inspiration is known as compliance and is defined as the volume change per unit of pressure change. Normal lungs are very distensible, or compliant. They can become more rigid and less compliant

due to diseases that cause alveolar, interstitial, or pleural fibrosis, or alveolar edema. Compliance increases with age and in emphysema, due to loss of elastin.

The elastic recoil, or compliance, of the lung is also dependent on a surface fluid called surfactant, which lines the alveoli. This fluid increases alveolar compliance by lowering the surface tension, thereby reducing the muscular effort necessary to ventilate the lungs and keep them expanded. It is a complex lipoprotein that is produced in the type II alveolar cells (see Chapter 2). A decrease in surfactant causes the alveoli to collapse. Reexpanding these alveoli requires a tremendous amount of work on the part of the patient. The patient may become fatigued and need mechanical ventilation. This occurs in respiratory distress syndrome in premature infants (previously called hyaline membrane disease) and in acute respiratory distress syndrome in adults. In another disease, alveolar proteinosis, there is excessive accumulation of protein in the alveolar spaces. This may be because of excessive production of surfactant or deficient removal of surfactant by alveolar macrophages.

The elastic properties of the lung tend to collapse the lung if not counterbalanced by external forces. The tissues of the thoracic wall also have elastic recoil, which causes them to expand considerably if unopposed. These two forces oppose each other, keeping the lungs expanded and the thoracic cage in a neutral position. If these forces are interrupted (as in pneumothorax), the lung collapses and the thoracic wall expands (Figure 4-3). Similarly, the overinflated, barrel-shaped chest of a patient with chronic obstructive pulmonary disease (COPD) is caused by the elastic tension of the chest wall's being unopposed by the usual elastic forces of the lungs, which have been damaged by disease.

Pressure-Volume Relationships

Pressure-volume curves help define the elastic properties of the chest wall and lungs. The elasticity of the respiratory system as a whole is the sum of its two major components, the lungs and the chest wall. The so called relaxation pressure curve is shown in Figure 4-4. The curve illustrates the static pressure of the lungs and chest wall and the combination of the two measured at given lung volumes. Functional residual capacity (FRC) reflects the balance of elastic forces exerted by the chest wall and the lungs and has significant implications for the clinical presentation and management of patients with cardiopulmonary dysfunction.

The relaxation pressure curve represents static pressure measurements. This means that the respiratory muscles are inactive, and the volume in the lungs at a given point in the respiratory cycle is determined by the balance of forces between the chest wall and the lungs. The chest wall and lungs exert elastic forces that oppose each other. The chest wall attempts to pull the lung out and the lungs attempt to recoil and pull the chest wall in. The curves labeled *lung* and *chest wall* are theoretical and illustrate the elastic force exerted by each when it is permitted to act unopposed by

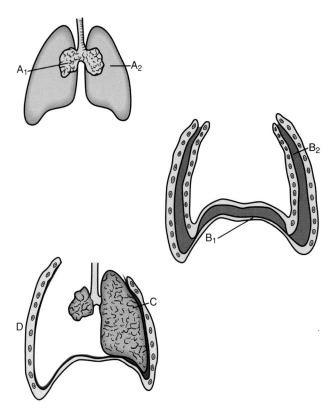

FIGURE 4-3 Various relationships between the lungs and the thorax. **A1,** The size the lungs would assume if they were not acted on by the elastic recoil of the thoracic wall. **A2,** The normal size of lungs within the thorax. **B1,** The size the thorax would assume if it were not acted on by the elastic recoil of the lungs. **B2,** The normal position of the chest wall when acted on by the elastic recoil of the lungs. **C,** The normal relationship of lungs to thorax. **D,** The positions assumed by the lungs and thorax in a tension pneumothorax.

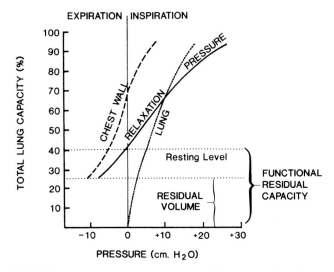

FIGURE 4-4 The relaxation pressure curve. The pressure in the lungs at any volume reflects the elastic forces of the lungs and chest wall.

the other. Normally these two forces are exerted together, producing the pressure volume relaxation curve. At FRC, these forces are in equilibrium; therefore, this capacity constitutes the resting volume of the respiratory system.

In lung disease, the balance between chest wall and lung forces is disrupted (West, 2004). More work and energy are required to sustain the respiratory effort (Jones et al, 2003). The patient is less able to rely on normal elastic recoil of the chest wall, lungs, or both. Therefore, the patient must expend more energy to effect equivalent respiration. The limits of respiratory excursion are determined by both elastic and muscular forces. At total lung capacity, the elastic forces of the respiratory system are balanced by the inspiratory muscle force. At residual volume, the elastic forces of the chest wall are balanced by the maximum expiratory muscle force. This volume excursion from total lung capacity to residual volume reflects vital capacity.

Although the curves representing the elastic forces of the lungs and chest wall are theoretical, they are helpful in understanding the effect of lung dysfunction on pulmonary function and on the clinical presentation of the patient (West, 2003). For example, in individuals with COPD, the characteristic barrel chest reflects the unopposed elastic forces of the chest wall as it succeeds in increasing the excursion of the chest as a result of reduced elastic recoil of the lungs. At the other extreme is the effect on the chest wall of a puncture wound, which disrupts the intrapleural pressure gradient that normally keeps the lung expanded and the chest wall contained. The result of such a puncture is to produce a pneumothorax in which the lung collapses down to the hilum and the chest wall springs outward (see Figure 4-3).

Airway Resistance

The flow of air into the lungs depends on pressure differences and on the resistance to flow in the airways. Resistance is defined as the pressure difference required for one unit flow change. The air passages are divided into upper and lower airways (see Chapter 3). The upper airways are responsible for 45% of airway resistance. The resistance to airflow by the lower airways depends on many factors and is therefore difficult to predict. The branching of the lower airways is irregular, and the diameter of the lumen may vary because of external pressures and because of the contraction or relaxation of bronchial or bronchiolar smooth muscle. The lumen diameter may also decrease as a result of edema or mucus. Any of these changes in the airway diameter may cause an increase in airway resistance. Flow of air through these airways can be either laminar or turbulent (Figure 4-5). Laminar flow is a streamlined flow in which resistance occurs mainly between the sides of the tubes and the air molecules. It tends to be cone-shaped, with the molecules in contact with the walls of the tubes moving more slowly than the molecules in the middle of the tube. Turbulent flow occurs when there are frequent molecular collisions in addition to the resistance of the sides of the tubes. This type of flow occurs at high flow rates and in airways where there are irregularities caused by

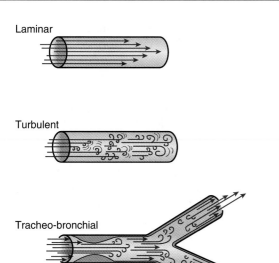

Laminar

Turbulent

Tracheo-bronchial

FIGURE 4-5 The different types of airflow seen within the tracheobronchial tree.

mucus, exudate, tumor, or other obstructions. In normal lungs, airflow is a combination of laminar and turbulent flow and is known as tracheobronchial flow.

The airways are distensible and compressible and thus susceptible to outside pressures. As these pressures compress the airways, they alter airway resistance. Transmural pressure is the difference between pressures in the airways and pressures surrounding the airways. In erect humans, there is a higher transmural pressure at the apices of the lungs than at the bases. This expands the alveoli at the apices relative to those at the bases. Although the alveoli in the apices have a greater volume at end expiration, the alveoli in the bases are better ventilated. This is because the alveoli in the bases operate at lower transmural pressures and can therefore accommodate a greater volume during inspiration than those at higher pressures.

Airway resistance decreases during inspiration as a result of the widening of the airways. During expiration, airways narrow, thus increasing resistance. The positive alveolar pressure that occurs during expiration partially compresses the airways. If these airways have lost their structural support as a result of disease, they may collapse and trap air distally (as in emphysema).

VENTILATION

Ventilation is the process by which air moves into the lungs. The volume of air inhaled can be measured with a spirometer. The various lung capacities and volumes are defined in Chapter 9.

Regional differences in ventilation exist throughout the lung. Studies using radioactive inert gas with a radiation counter over the chest wall have shown that when the gas is inhaled by an individual in the seated position and measurements are

taken, radiation counts are greatest in the lower lung fields, intermediate in the midlung fields, and lowest in the upper lung fields. This effect is position or gravity dependent. In the supine position, the apices and bases are ventilated comparably, and the lowermost lung fields are better ventilated than the uppermost lung fields. Similarly, in the lateral, or side-lying, position, the lower lung fields are preferentially ventilated compared with the upper lung fields (see Chapter 19).

The causes of regional differences in ventilation can be explained in terms of the anatomy of the lung and the mechanics of breathing. An intrapleural pressure gradient exists down the lung. In the upright position, intrapleural pressure tends to be more negative at the top of the lung and becomes progressively less negative toward the bottom of the lung. This pressure gradient is thought to reflect the weight of the suspended lung. The more negative intrapleural pressure at the top of the lung results in relatively greater expansion of that area and a larger resting alveolar volume. The expanding pressure in the bottom of the lung, however, is relatively small, so there is a smaller resting alveolar volume in the bottom. This distinction between the upper and lower lung fields is fundamental to understanding differences in regional ventilation. Regional differences in resting alveolar volume should not be confused with regional differences in ventilation volume. Ventilation refers to volume change as a function of resting volume. The relatively higher resting volume in the upper lung fields renders them stiffer, or less compliant, than the lower lung fields, where there are low lung volumes and greater compliance. The lower lung fields, therefore, exhibit a greater volume change in relation to resting volume, and that effects greater overall ventilation, compared with the upper lung fields. Ventilation is favored in the lowermost lung fields, regardless of body position.

DIFFUSION

Once air has reached the alveoli, it must cross the alveolar-capillary (A-C) membrane (Figure 4-6). Gases, specifically oxygen entering the lungs and carbon dioxide leaving the lungs, must cross through the surfactant lining, the alveolar epithelial membrane, and the capillary endothelial membrane. Oxygen then has to travel through a layer of plasma, the erythrocyte membrane, and intracellular fluid in the erythrocyte, until it encounters a hemoglobin molecule. This distance is actually small in normal lungs, but in disease states it may increase. The alveolar wall and the capillary membrane often become thickened. Fluid, edema, or exudate may separate the two membranes. These conditions are often first detected when arterial P_{O_2} becomes chronically lower than normal. Oxygen diffuses slowly through the A-C membrane in comparison to CO_2 diffusion. As a result, patients with diffusion problems frequently have hypoxemia with a normal P_{CO_2}. Sarcoidosis, berylliosis, asbestosis, scleroderma, and pulmonary edema are some diseases that decrease the diffusing capacity of the gases. The capacity may also decrease in emphysema because of a decrease in total surface area for gas exchange.

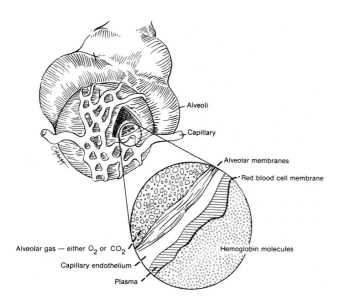

FIGURE 4-6 The components of the alveolar-capillary membrane.

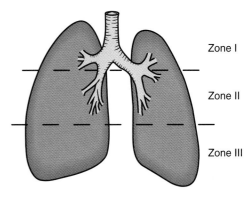

FIGURE 4-7 The perfusion of the lungs is dependent on posture. In the upright position, three areas can be seen. Zone III has perfusion in excess of ventilation. In zone II, perfusion and ventilation are fairly equal. In zone I, ventilation occurs in excess of perfusion.

PERFUSION

Perfusion of the lung refers to the blood flow of the pulmonary circulation available for gas exchange. The pulmonary circulation operates at relatively low pressures compared to the systemic circulation. For this reason, the walls of the blood vessels in the pulmonary circulation are significantly thinner than comparable vessels in the systemic circulation. Compared to the systemic circulation, the lungs have little requirement for significant regional differences in perfusion.

Hydrostatic pressure has a significant effect on the perfusion of the lower lobes. Hydrostatic pressure reflects the effect of gravity on the blood and tends to favor perfusion of the lower lung fields. This fact has been substantiated using radioactive tracers in the pulmonary circulation and measuring radiation counts over the lung fields. The non-uniformity of perfusion reflects the interaction of alveolar, arterial, and venous pressures down the lung. Normally blood flow is determined by the arteriovenous pressure gradient. In the lungs there are regional differences in alveolar pressure that can exert an effect on the arteriovenous pressure gradient. For example, in the upper lung fields, alveolar pressure approximates atmospheric pressure, which overrides the arterial pressure and effectively closes the pulmonary capillaries. In the lower lung fields, the opposite occurs. The relatively low volume of air in the alveoli is overridden by the greater capillary hydrostatic pressure. Thus the capillary pressure effectively overcomes the alveolar pressure.

Pulmonary blood vessels constrict in response to low arterial pressures of oxygen. This is termed hypoxic vaso-constriction. Hypoxic vasoconstriction in the lung is believed to serve as an adaptive mechanism for diverting blood away from underventilated or poorly oxygenated lung areas.

Although hypoxic vasoconstriction may have an important role in improving the efficiency of the lungs as a gas exchanger, it may be potentially deleterious to a patient who has reduced arterial oxygen pressure secondary to pulmonary pathology.

The acid-base balance of the blood also affects pulmonary blood flow. A low blood pH, or acidemia, for example, potentiates pulmonary vasoconstriction. Thus impaired ventilatory function can disturb blood-gas composition and, in turn, acid-base balance. This effect can be amplified because of the cyclical reaction of pH on pulmonary vasoconstriction. Consideration of these basic physiologic mechanisms is tantamount to optimize physical therapy intervention.

Ventilation and Perfusion Matching

As discussed previously, gravity tends to pull blood into the dependent positions of the lung (Figure 4-7). In erect humans, therefore, there is greater blood flow at the bases of the lung. In places, the arterial blood pressure exceeds the alveolar pressure and causes compression or collapse of the airways (Figure 4-8). Blood flow to the apices is decreased because of gravity. Alveoli in this region are more fully expanded as a result of high transmural pressures and may further decrease blood flow by compressing blood vessels. It follows that the areas of optimal gas exchange occur where there is the greatest amount of perfusion and ventilation. This occurs toward the base of the lungs in erect humans. Changes in posture cause changes in perfusion and ventilation. Generally, greater air exchange occurs toward the gravity-dependent areas. In side-lying, there is greater gas exchange in the dependent lung (Figure 4-9).

In normal lungs there is an optimal ratio, or matching of gas and blood. This ratio of ventilation to perfusion (V/Q) is 0.8 to maintain normal blood gas values of Po_2 and Pco_2. Therefore, the lungs must be able to supply four parts ventilation to about five parts perfusion. When the ratio is not uniform throughout the lung, the arterial blood cannot contain normal blood-gas values. Regions with low ratios (perfusion in excess of ventilation) act as shunts, whereas regions with high ratios (ventilation in excess of perfusion) act as dead space (Figure 4-10). Hypoxemia results if regions of abnormal V/Q predominate. An elevation in arterial P_{CO_2} may also occur unless the patient increases ventilation.

Physical therapists who are positioning patients with cardiopulmonary pathology may find that their patients experience greater distress when placed in certain positions. Such position-dependent distress can be explained by ventilation-perfusion inequalities that cause poor gas exchange in the dependent lung.

The relationship of ventilation and perfusion in the lung is summarized in the following figures. Figure 4-11 shows increases in ventilation and perfusion down the upright lung. When optimal ventilation and perfusion match, V/Q occurs in the midlung zones. In the upright position, ventilation is in excess of perfusion in the apices, and perfusion is in excess of ventilation in the bases. Figure 4-12 illustrates the effects of shunt and physiological dead space on V/Q matching in the upright lung and shows their effect on alveolar gas. Specifically, Figure 4-12 shows a schematic representation of regional differences in ventilation and perfusion in the upper, middle, and lower zones of the upright lung. These gradients are reflected in the alveolar P_{O_2} and P_{CO_2} levels associated with alveolar dead space in the apices, appropriate V/Q matching in the midlung, and shunt in the bases.

CARDIAC REFLEXES

The heart behaves automatically and is therefore termed a functional syncytium. Three primary reflexes enable the heart

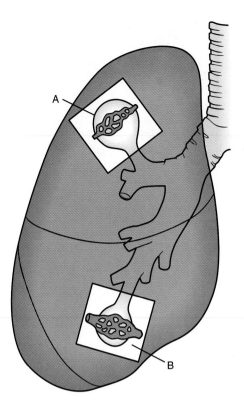

FIGURE 4-8 The relationship between the size of the airways and the amount of perfusion in the area when lungs are in the upright position. **A,** Perfusion is decreased in the apices because of gravity. This enables the alveoli to expand fully. This expansion may compress blood vessels and thereby further decrease blood flow. **B,** Perfusion is increased in the bases of the lungs because of gravity. The enlarged vessels prevent full expansion of alveoli and may, in fact, compress them to a smaller size.

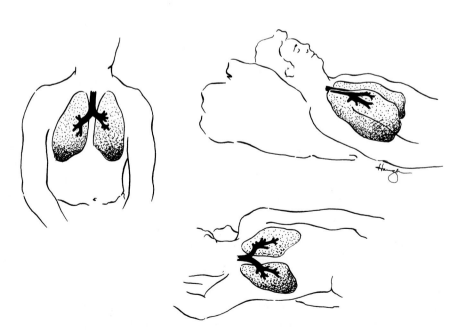

FIGURE 4-9 The effect of positioning on the perfusion of the lung. Note that gravity-dependent segments have the greatest amount of perfusion.

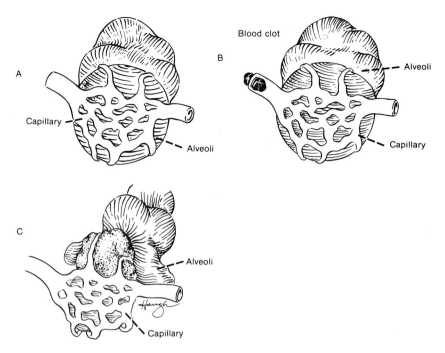

FIGURE 4-10 **A**, Normal alveolus. **B**, Dead space. **C**, Shunt.

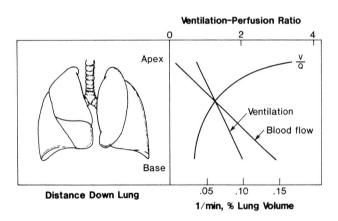

FIGURE 4-11 The effect of gravity on ventilation, perfusion, and ventilation-perfusion matching (V/Q ratio).

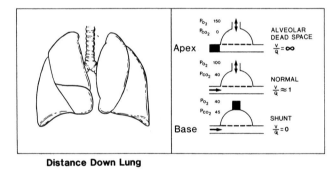

FIGURE 4-12 Schemata showing the effect of gravity on ventilation and perfusion down the upright lung.

to increase stroke volume and cardiac output with moment-to-moment changes in myocardial demand.

The first reflex is the Starling effect, which refers to the increased force of contraction that occurs with increased venous return (preload). The second reflex, the Anrep effect, refers to the increase in ventricular contractile force as a result of an increase in aortic pressure (afterload). The third reflex, the Bowdich effect, refers to the corresponding increase in heart rate when myocardial contractile force increases. The integrated function of these three reflexes ensures that cardiac output adjusts as demands on the heart change (i.e., in healthy

individuals, primarily in response to exercise, body position, and emotional stress).

COORDINATION OF CARDIAC EVENTS

The mechanical activity of the heart is precisely regulated in accordance with the electrical activity of the heart to effect optimal cardiac output to the organs of the body (Dubin, 2000; Kinney & Packa, 1995). The electrical activity of the heart, based on electrocardiography, in both health and pathology, is described in detail in Chapter 12. The electrical

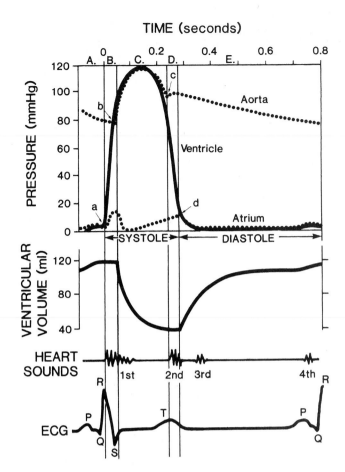

TIME (seconds)

FIGURE 4-13 Summary of electrical and mechanical events of the heart. *A*, Atrial systole. *B*, Isovolumetric contraction. *C*, Ejection. *D*, Isovolumetric relaxation. *E*, Rapid inflow, diastasis, and active rapid filling. Note the relationship between ventricular pressure and volume: *a*, closure of the atrioventricular valves; *b*, opening of the semilunar valves; *c*, closure of the semilunar valves; *d*, opening of the atrioventricular valves.

and mechanical events of the cardiac cycle are summarized in Figure 4-13. These events include the spread of the wave of electrical excitation throughout the myocardium; the resulting sequence of contraction of the atria and ventricles, followed by dynamic changes in blood pressure and volume in the heart chambers; the heart sounds; and the timing of these events. The cardiac cycle takes 0.8 second in a heart beating at 75 beats per minute. Ventricular systole or ejection takes about one third of this time. Its onset and termination are marked, respectively, by the closing and opening of the atrioventricular valves (mitral and tricuspid). Diastole, or the period between successive ventricular systoles, in which the ventricles fill with blood, takes two thirds of the 0.8 second of each cardiac cycle.

Phases of Systole and Diastole

Ventricular systole normally has three phases: the isovolumetric contraction period, the rapid ejection period, and the slower ejection period. Ventricular diastole also has three phases: the passive rapid-filling phase, the slower filling phase (diastasis), and the active rapid-filling phase.

Heart Sounds

The heart sounds are described as a low-pitched, long-duration sound (S_1) followed by a higher pitched, slower duration sound (S_2) that resembles the phonic sounds of LUB-dub. S_1 is associated with the closure of the atrioventricular valves. S_2 is associated with the closure of the semilunar valves. In inspiration, the aortic valve closes several milliseconds before the pulmonic valve, resulting in a splitting of the second heart sound, S_2. During inspiration, intrathoracic pressure becomes more negative, and venous return and right heart volume increase; hence, pulmonary ejection is prolonged in this situation, and closure of the pulmonary valve is delayed. Other variations in splitting of S_2 occur with pathology. The presence of a third (S_3) or fourth (S_4) heart sound is usually considered abnormal. S_3 is usually associated with the passive rapid-filling phase and S_4 with the active rapid-filling phase.

Volume and Pressure Changes

Changes in the ventricular volume curve and aortic pressure wave reflect changes in atrial and ventricular pressures during systole and diastole. The sequence of events appears in a flow chart in Figure 4-14. Pressure gradients within the heart are responsible for the opening and closing of the valves. Coordinated valve opening and closure are important to promote the forward movement of blood and prevent mechanical inefficiency of the heart pump resulting from valvular regurgitation of blood during ventricular contraction. Regurgitation of blood in the retrograde direction gives rise to heart murmurs that are audible on auscultation of the heart.

Peripheral Circulation

The purpose of the peripheral circulation, including the microcirculation at the tissue level, is to provide saturated oxygenated blood and remove partially desaturated blood. The microcirculation within each organ regulates the blood flow both exogenously, via the neurologic system, and endogenously, via the humoral system, commensurate with the metabolic needs of that tissue bed (see Chapter 3). The four principal factors that determine the movement of fluid in the microcirculation are the following:

1. The capillary hydrostatic pressure from the blood pressure, which tends to move blood across the capillary membrane and out of the circulation into the interstitium
2. The capillary oncotic pressure from the proteins within the blood vessels, which tends to retain fluid in the circulation
3. The interstitial hydrostatic pressure, which tends to move fluid back into the circulation

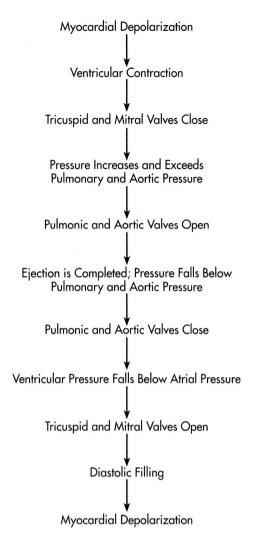

Myocardial Depolarization

↓

Ventricular Contraction

↓

Tricuspid and Mitral Valves Close

↓

Pressure Increases and Exceeds
Pulmonary and Aortic Pressure

↓

Pulmonic and Aortic Valves Open

↓

Ejection is Completed; Pressure Falls Below
Pulmonary and Aortic Pressure

↓

Pulmonic and Aortic Valves Close

↓

Ventricular Pressure Falls Below Atrial Pressure

↓

Tricuspid and Mitral Valves Open

↓

Diastolic Filling

↓

Myocardial Depolarization

FIGURE 4-14 The sequence of pressure changes in the heart during the cardiac cycle.

TABLE 4-1

Balance of Forces Moving Fluid In and Out of the Capillary

MEAN FORCES MOVING FLUID OUT OF CAPILLARY	mm Hg
Mean capillary pressure	17.0
Negative interstitial pressure	6.3
Oncotic interstitial pressure	5.0
Total outward pressure	28.3
Mean forces moving fluid into capillary	
Plasma oncotic pressure	28.0
Total inward pressure	28.0
Outward pressure – inward pressure = net outward pressure	0.3

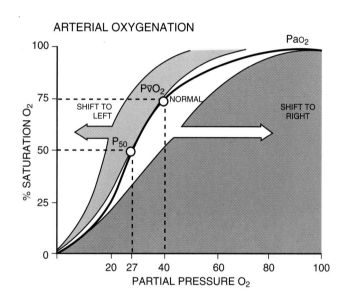

FIGURE 4-15 The oxyhemoglobin dissociation curve.

4. The interstitial oncotic pressure, which tends to draw fluid out of the circulation and into the interstitium.

The net forces acting on the capillary fluid are nearly in equilibrium, with a slight tendency for fluid to be filtered out of the systemic circulation into the interstitium. Table 4-1 illustrates the mean pressures that determine normal fluid dynamics across capillary membranes.

TRANSPORT OF OXYGEN BY THE BLOOD

Once oxygen reaches the blood it rapidly combines with hemoglobin to form oxyhemoglobin. A small proportion of oxygen is dissolved in the plasma. The use of the hemoglobin molecule as an oxygen carrier allows for greater availability and efficiency of oxygen delivery to the tissues in response to metabolic demand. Saturation of the oxygen-carrying sites on the hemoglobin molecule is curvilinearly related to the partial pressure of oxygen in the tissues. This relationship is called the oxyhemoglobin dissociation curve and is a sigmoid, or S-shaped, curve (Figure 4-15). The hemoglobin of arterial blood is 99%, or almost completely saturated with oxygen. Under normal circumstances, arterial blood is mixed with a small proportion of venous blood from the coronary and pulmonary circulation, resulting in arterial saturation slightly less than 100%. The graph shows a range of partial pressures of oxygen that may exist in the tissues. At relatively high arterial oxygen pressures, the oxygen saturation is high. This reflects high association or low dissociation between oxygen and hemoglobin. Saturation does not fall significantly until the partial pressure of oxygen falls below 80 mm Hg. Even at Po_2 levels of 40 to 50 mm Hg, arterial saturation is still 75%. This suggests that the oxyhemoglobin dissociation system has an enormous capacity to meet the varying needs of different tissues without severely compromising arterial saturation. A Po_2 of less than 50%, for example, has a profound effect on arterial saturation. This demonstrates an adaptive response of hemoglobin dissociation to respond to low oxygen tissue pressures by greater dissociation of oxygen from hemoglobin as the need arises. As Po_2 improves with increased supply of oxygen or decreased demand, the affinity between oxygen and hemoglobin increases, and arterial saturation increases. Thus oxygen is not released unless there is a need for greater oxygen delivery to the tissues.

Various conditions can increase or decrease hemoglobin's affinity for oxygen and thereby cause a shift in the oxyhemoglobin dissociation curve (see Figure 4-15). A shift to the right results in decreased oxygen affinity and greater dissociation of oxygen and hemoglobin. In this instance, for any given partial pressure of oxygen, there is a lower saturation than normal. This means that there is more oxygen available to the tissues. Shifts in the curve to the right occur with increasing concentration of hydrogen ions (i.e., decreasing pH), increasing Pco_2, increasing temperatures, and increasing levels of 2,3-DPG (diphosphoglycerate), a byproduct of red blood cell metabolism. West (2004) suggests that "A simple way to remember these shifts is that an exercising muscle (increased metabolic demand), is acid, hypercapnic and hot, and it benefits from increased unloading of oxygen from its capillaries."

A shift of the curve to the left results in increased oxygen affinity. Thus for any given partial pressure of oxygen, there is a higher saturation than normal. This means that there is less oxygen available to the tissues. This occurs in alkalemia, hypothermia, and decreased 2,3-DPG.

Anemia (reduced red blood cell count and hemoglobin) and polycythemia (excess red blood cell count and hemoglobin) produce changes in the oxygen content of the blood as well as in its saturation. Anemia shifts the curve to the right and lowers the maximal saturation achievable. Polycythemia has the opposite effect. The curve is shifted to the left, and maximal saturation approaches 100%.

TRANSPORT OF CARBON DIOXIDE

CO_2 is an acid produced by cells as a result of cell metabolism. It is carried in various forms by venous blood to the lungs, where it is eliminated. Most of the CO_2 added to plasma diffuses into the red blood cells, where it is buffered and returned to the plasma to be carried to the lungs. The buffering mechanism is so effective that large changes in dissolved CO_2 can occur with small changes in blood pH.

The transport of CO_2 has an important role in the acid-base status of the blood and maintenance of normal homeostasis. The lung excretes 10,000 mEq of carbonic acid per day. (Carbonic acid is broken down into water and CO_2. The CO_2 is buffered and eliminated through the lungs.) The kidney can excrete only 100 mEq of acid per day. Therefore, alterations in alveolar ventilation can have profound effects on the body's

acid-base status. A decrease in the lung's ability to ventilate causes a sharp rise in Pco_2 and a drop in pH. This causes acute respiratory acidosis. If this change occurs gradually, the pH will remain within normal limits while the Pco_2 is elevated. This is known as a compensated respiratory acidosis. Hyperventilation or excessive ventilation causes rapid elimination of CO_2 from the blood. This results in a decreased Pco_2 and an increased pH and is known as acute respiratory alkalosis. Again, if the change occurs gradually, the pH remains within normal limits even though the Pco_2 is decreased. This is a compensated respiratory alkalosis.

SUMMARY

This chapter presents an overview of cardiopulmonary physiology with respect to breathing control and the central and peripheral mechanisms, such as muscle, joint, and lung and chest wall stretch receptors, involved in the regulation of respiration. The mechanical factors of breathing, chest wall and lung compliance, and airway resistance are described. The elastic properties of the respiratory system (i.e., chest wall and lungs) are reflected in the pressure-volume relaxation curve. This curve has important implications for the clinical presentation of a patient with cardiopulmonary dysfunction and, in particular, the efficiency and energy requirement of the respiratory system. Ventilation and perfusion matching is the basis of gas exchange and the adequacy of lung function. Many factors in addition to disease, however, can affect ventilation and perfusion matching, including age, body position, exercise, breathing at low lung volumes, and smoking history. The function of the heart is to provide adequate cardiac output, hence, adequate oxygen delivery to the vital organs and peripheral tissues. The optimal coupling of electrical and mechanical events in the heart to effect cardiac output is described.

Arterial Po_2 and Pco_2 are normally maintained within certain prescribed limits. In healthy individuals, oxyhemoglobin dissociation ensures adequate oxygen delivery to the tissues once oxygen has diffused through the alveolar capillary membrane into the circulation. Transport of CO_2 and its buffering mechanisms are central to acid-base balance and normal homeostasis.

Review Questions

1. Describe the control of breathing.
2. Explain respiratory mechanics with respect to airway resistance and lung compliance.
3. Describe the distributions of ventilation, perfusion, and diffusion.
4. Explain the determinants of ventilation and perfusion matching.
5. Describe electromechanical coupling in the heart.
6. Describe oxyhemoglobin dissociation and the oxyhemoglobin dissociation curve.

REFERENCES

Bates, D.V. (1989). Respiratory function in disease, ed 3. Philadelphia: WB Saunders.

Berne, R.M., & Levy, M.N. (2000). Cardiovascular physiology, ed 8. St Louis: Mosby.

Dubin, D. (2000). Rapid interpretation of EKGs: a programmed course, ed 6. Tampa, Fla.: Cover Publishing.

Fuster, V., Alexander, W.R., O'Rourke, R.A., Roberts, R., King, S.B. Prystowsky, E.N., &, Nash, I. (2004). Hurst's The heart, ed 11. New York: McGraw-Hill.

Ganong, W. F. (2003). Review of medical physiology, ed 21. New York: McGraw-Hill Professional Publishing.

Goldberger, E. (1990). Essentials of clinical cardiology. Philadelphia: JB Lippincott.

Guyton, A.C., & Hall.J.E. (2000). Textbook of medical physiology, ed 10. Philadelphia: WB Saunders.

Jones, A.Y.M., Dean, E., & Chow, C.C.S. (2003). Comparison of the oxygen cost of breathing exercises and spontaneous breathing in patients with chronic obstructive pulmonary disease. Physical Therapy, 83:424-431.

Katz, A.M. (2000). Physiology of the heart, ed 3. New York: Raven Press.

Kinney, M.R., & Packa, D.R. (1995). Andreoli's comprehensive cardiac care, ed 7. Philadelphia: Elsevier.

Murray, J.F., & Nadel, J.A. (2000). Textbook of respiratory medicine. Philadelphia: WB Saunders.

Nunn, J.F. (1999). Applied respiratory physiology, ed 5. London: Butterworths.

Scharf, S.M., & Cassidy S.S. (Eds.) (1989). Heart-lung interactions in health and disease. New York: Marcel-Dekker.

West, J.B. (2004). Respiratory physiology: the essentials, ed 7. Baltimore: Williams & Wilkins.

West, J.B. (2003). Pulmonary pathophysiology: the essentials, ed 6. Philadelphia: Lippincott Williams and Wilkins.

C H A P T E R   5

Cardiopulmonary Pathophysiology

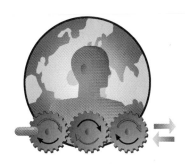

Willy E. Hammon III and Elizabeth Dean

KEY TERMS

Acute coronary syndromes
Anemia
Angina
Athletic heart syndrome
Bronchiectasis
Chronic bronchitis
Coronary artery disease
Drug-related restrictive lung disease
Emphysema

Hypertension
Lung cancer
Myocardial infarction
Noncardiopulmonary conditions
Obstructive lung disease
Restrictive lung disease
Scleroderma
Syncope
Tuberculosis

Because cardiovascular and pulmonary conditions are among the leading causes of morbidity and mortality, they present clinically to the physical therapist as both secondary and primary diagnoses. In addition, patients commonly have one or more risk factors for one or both of these broad categories of conditions. Lifestyle and environmental factors are primary causes and contributors (see Chapter 1).

Smoking is a principal contributor to cardiovascular disease and the primary cause of chronic obstructive lung disease worldwide. Abstinence from smoking is the *only* intervention that can prevent the majority of cases of chronic obstructive pulmonary disease (COPD), and smoking cessation is the only intervention to retard its progression. Thus cessation of smoking is a primary health care goal at the communal, societal, and individual levels (Dhala et al, 2004; Kamholz, 2004), and it should be a primary intervention by the physical therapist in any patient who smokes (see Chapter 1).

Risk factors for cardiovascular and pulmonary diseases should be assessed in every patient, irrespective of the reason for physical therapy referral or management. An individual with an overt history of cardiovascular or pulmonary disease is managed based on the related signs and symptoms. If, however, a patient comes to the physical therapist with dysfunction of the musculoskeletal, neuromuscular, or other system and happens to have a secondary diagnosis of cardiovascular or pulmonary disease, this diagnosis must be considered in overall management and the interventions modified accordingly. A secondary diagnosis of cardiovascular or pulmonary disease may be more clinically important for the physical therapist to manage (because it is life-threatening) than the primary diagnosis (e.g., low back pain, osteoarthritis, or Parkinson syndrome).

Recent advances in understanding the pathophysiology of cardiovascular and pulmonary conditions have highlighted a common denominator: inflammation of the endothelium of the blood vessels and the epithelium of the airways. With increasing severity of disease, proteins alter their structure, and repair is required to maintain their essential structure and

85

function with the upregulation of reparative proteins (Sartori & Scherrer, 2003). Activation of this defense system is triggered by ischemia, hypoxemia, and inflammation.

Myopathic changes have been observed in the peripheral muscles of people with chronic cardiovascular disease and lung disease (see Chapter 24). People with chronic lung disease, for example, have increased muscle fibrosis compared with age-matched people without the disease, and the cross-sectional area of type IIX muscle fibers is smaller (Gosker, 2003).

Some common causes underlying COPD have been proposed. The Dutch hypothesis explaining the development of both asthma and chronic obstructive lung disease proposes that environmental factors (e.g., smoking and air pollutants) are superimposed upon and interact with allergic and airway hyperresponsiveness components (genetic components). Smoking and airway hyperresponsiveness are common risk factors for these conditions (Postma & Boezen, 2004).

It has been reported that gender plays a role in susceptibility, severity, and response to management of cardiovascular and pulmonary dysfunction, and this is reflected in the finding that women with COPD have an almost three-fold greater death rate than men. Specifically, women are more susceptible to the long-term adverse effects of smoking. Compared to men, they develop pathological changes more readily and have more severe symptomatology for a given long-term exposure to tobacco (Chapman, 2004).

The Global Initiative for Chronic Obstructive Lung Disease has proposed universal guidelines for the classification of COPD (Global Initiative for Chronic Obstructive Lung Disease, 2002) on the basis of both spirometry and clinical symptoms to define stage of disease. Mild COPD is defined as having a predicted $FEV_1/FVC < 70\%$ and an $FEV_1 \geq 80\%$. Moderate COPD is defined as a predicted $FEV_1/FVC < 70\%$ and an $FEV_1 < 50\%$ to 80%. Severe COPD is defined as a predicted $FEV_1/FVC < 70\%$ and an $FEV_1 < 30\%$. Serum or tissue markers are being sought to provide a basis for an objective diagnosis and a refinement of intervention strategies (Pauwels et al, 2004).

Objective measures of limitations of structure and function or impairments associated with cardiovascular and pulmonary disease are not necessarily closely associated with health-related quality of life. Outcome measures of health-related quality of life and life satisfaction are supplemental to structure and function outcomes and are now being included in the overall clinical assessment of people with these conditions (Tomas & Varkey, 2004). Thus management programs focus on interdisciplinary rehabilitation consisting of multiple components to address the complexity of the limitations associated with these conditions rather than traditional primary focus on limitations of structure and function (World Health Organization, 2002; see Chapters 1 and 17).

This chapter describes common pathophysiology of the cardiovascular and pulmonary systems and some common conditions that affect these systems secondarily. The two

classic types of lung pathophysiology (obstructive and restrictive) are presented, followed by the two classic types of heart pathology (acquired and congenital). Interdependent pathophysiology affecting both organs is described in Chapters 6 and 31, and in Chapters 15, 34, and 36, which are related to critical care. The structure and function of the cardiovascular and pulmonary systems are interdependent (Meyer et al, 2003; see Chapters 2, 3, and 4). Dysfunction in one system can impact the function of the other.

Obstructive pulmonary conditions are characterized by a reduced expiratory airflow rate due to increased airway resistance. Restrictive pulmonary conditions are characterized by the reduced inspiratory capacity of the lungs. Often, however, there is overlap between the two categories.

The second part of this chapter, beginning with atherosclerosis and coronary artery disease (CAD), describes the pathophysiology of common cardiovascular conditions. CAD is manifested in various clinical syndromes and results from atherosclerosis in the coronary arteries, which ultimately affects heart performance (i.e., stroke volume and heart rate) and, hence, cardiac output. The causes of clinical syndromes associated with CAD and the medical management and prognoses are briefly reviewed. Hypertension, anemia, type 2 diabetes mellitus, metabolic syndrome, syncope, and the athletic heart syndrome are also addressed.

OBSTRUCTIVE LUNG DISEASE

COPD is also known as chronic obstructive lung disease (COLD), chronic obstructive airway disease (COAD), and chronic airway or airflow obstruction (CAO) (American Thoracic Society, 2004). Exacerbations characterize these conditions and contribute largely to their associated morbidity and mortality (Sethi & Murphy, 2004).

COPD is common worldwide and contributes to major disability as well as economic and social burdens. More than 30 million Americans have COPD (Evans & Scanlon, 2003). In 2002, health care cost for COPD was $32.1 billion. Deaths from COPD numbered 118,744 in 2001. It remains the fourth leading cause of death in the United States, with an age-adjusted death rate of 42.2 per 100,000. The most important change in the rate of death resulting from COPD in recent years has been among women. Over the past 20 years, their death rate has increased almost three-fold, from 20.1 per 100,000 in 1980 to 56.7 per 100,000 in 2000, whereas for men the death rate increased less dramatically, from 73.0 to 82.6 per 100,000 (American Thoracic Society, 2005).

The first part of this chapter describes chronic bronchitis, emphysema, asthma, and bronchiectasis. A patient usually presents with more than one of these conditions. Most people with COPD have a combination of chronic bronchitis, emphysema, and airway hyperactivity. The typical presentation includes episodic wheezing along with a variable degree of chronic bronchitis and emphysema (Murray & Nadel, 2000). A radiograph shows hyperinflated lungs, flattened diaphragms, and an enlarged right ventricle as a result of hypoxemia and increased pulmonary artery pressure. Other findings vary from patient to patient, depending on the predominant disease process contributing to the COPD.

Inflammation of the bronchial wall is typically present through the course of the disease, with increasing inflammation during exacerbations. In addition to destruction of the lung parenchyma in emphysema, small airways are affected (obstructive bronchiolitis). Chronic inflammation leads to the remodeling and narrowing of the small airways. The destruction of lung parenchyma and the inflammation cause loss of elasticity. The two principal theories about COPD include oxidative stress and an imbalance between proteinases and antiproteinases. Chronic inflammation of the lung parenchyma associated with COPD can be associated with systemic inflammation and further chronic degenerative dysfunction Because of the prominence of inflammation in the underlying pathophysiology in COPD, there has been considerable interest in the use of inflammatory markers in clinical assessment (Andreassen & Vestbo, 2003; Oudijk et al, 2003).

The symptoms of individuals with COPD can be accentuated during sleep. The mechanisms can originate centrally as well as peripherally (i.e., in lower airways and the chest wall) (McNicholas, 2003). Adverse effects include hypoventilation, dysrhythmias, and pulmonary hypertension, all of which can predispose an individual to nocturnal death. Evaluation of sleep is therefore an essential component of the overall assessment.

Chronic Bronchitis

Chronic bronchitis is a condition associated with chronic swelling and inflammation of the bronchi and bronchioles. The diagnosis is based upon report of a cough producing sputum on most days for 3 months during 2 consecutive years when other conditions have been ruled out (American Thoracic Society, 2005). The degree of airway narrowing is assessed with spirometry.

Pathologically there is an increase in the size of the tracheobronchial mucous glands (increased Reid index) and goblet cell hyperplasia (Crapo et al, 2004). Mucous cell metaplasia of bronchial epithelium results in a decreased number of cilia. Ciliary dysfunction and disruption of the continuity of the mucous blanket are common. In the peripheral airways, bronchiolitis, bronchiolar narrowing, and increased amounts of mucus are observed (Cosio, 1987; Wright et al, 1992).

Chronic bronchitis results from long-term irritation of the tracheobronchial tree. The most common cause of irritation is cigarette smoking (U.S. Department of Health and Human Services, 2000). Regular exposure to the inhaled toxic particles and gases in cigarette smoke causes inflammation in the epithelium of the central airways (larger than 4 mm in internal diameter). This inflammatory process is associated with an increased production of mucus by the goblet cells and mucous glands. Smoking inhibits ciliary action and destroys cilia. The hypersecretion of mucus and the loss and impairment of cilia

lead to a chronic productive cough. The fact that smokers secrete an abnormal amount of mucus predisposes them to respiratory infection and prolonged recovery from such infection. The irritation of smoke in the tracheobronchial tree causes bronchoconstriction. Although smoking is the most common cause of chronic bronchitis, other triggers include air pollution, bronchial infections, and occupations in which air quality is affected.

Patients with chronic bronchitis were formerly referred to as "blue bloaters" because they are often stocky and appear "blue" as a result of hypoxemia; however, the clinical usefulness of this term has been questioned (Bates, 1989). Although many patients have a high arterial partial pressure of carbon dioxide ($PaCO_2$), the pH is normalized by renal retention of bicarbonate (HCO_3). The bone marrow compensates for chronic hypoxemia by increasing the production of red blood cells, leading to polycythemia (Murray & Nadel, 2000). Polycythemia increases blood viscosity and the work required by the heart to pump and circulate the blood through the lungs and systemic vasculature. Long-term hypoxemia leads to hypoxic pulmonary vasoconstriction, increased pulmonary artery pressure and, potentially, right ventricular hypertrophy.

Individuals with bronchitis often expectorate mucoid sputum. In an exacerbation, usually from infection, they have an even greater amount of purulent sputum. Ventilation-perfusion abnormalities are common, and they increase hypoxemia and $PaCO_2$ retention. The respiratory rate increases, as does the use of accessory muscles. Oxygen demand by these muscles and production of carbon dioxide (CO_2) increase beyond the capacity of the ventilatory system. The work of breathing increases disproportionately. This contributes to a further decrease in the arterial partial pressure of oxygen (PaO_2) and an increase in $PaCO_2$. The hypoxemia and respiratory acidemia increase pulmonary artery constriction, which further increases pulmonary artery pressure and right ventricular strain. During an exacerbation, these patients are usually treated with intravenous fluids, antibiotics, bronchodilators, and low-flow oxygen. Corticosteroids may be administered. Diuretics and digitalis are used to treat right ventricular failure.

Emphysema

Emphysema is defined as "a condition of the lung characterized by abnormal permanent enlargement of airspaces distal to the terminal bronchiole, accompanied by destruction of their walls" (National Heart, Lung, and Blood Institute, 2003). There are two main types of emphysema: centrilobular and panlobular (Hogg & Senior, 2002). Centrilobular emphysema is 20 times more common than panlobular emphysema, although both types often coexist in the same patient.

Centrilobular emphysema is characterized by inflammation, edema, thickened bronchiolar walls, and destruction of the respiratory bronchioles. These changes are common and are marked in the upper lobes and the superior segments of the lower lobes (Hogg, 2004). Centrilobular emphysema is more common in men than in women, is rare in nonsmokers, and is common in patients with chronic bronchitis.

Panlobular emphysema, characterized by destructive enlargement of the alveoli, affects primarily the lower lobes (Figure 5-1). This type of emphysema is characteristic of alpha$_1$-antitripsin deficiency, which involves an imbalance

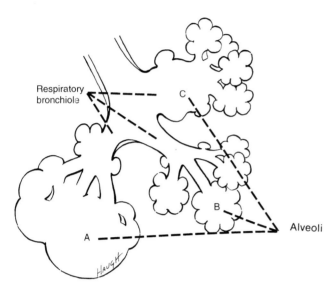

FIGURE 5-1 **A**, Panlobular emphysema is characterized by a destructive enlargement of the alveoli. **B**, A normal respiratory bronchiole and alveoli. **C**, Centrilobular emphysema is characterized by a selective enlargement and destruction of the respiratory bronchiole.

between the elastin and elastase in the lung parenchyma. The emphysematous lung develops secondary to loss of radial traction on the bronchioles and loss of the elastic recoil of the alveoli. When individuals without pulmonary dysfunction inhale, the airways are stretched open by the enlarging elastic lung. In exhalation, the airways are narrowed as a result of the decreasing stretch of the lung. The lungs of people with panlobular emphysema have decreased elasticity because of the destruction of surrounding alveolar walls. Thus the bronchioles lack tethering and support, which exposes them to collapse, even during normal exhalation.

Bullae, emphysematous spaces larger than 1 cm in diameter, are commonly present in patients with emphysema (Figure 5-2) (Celli, 1999; Thurlbeck & Wright, 1998). Bullae develop from a coalescence of adjacent areas of emphysematous lung or because of an obstruction of the conducting airways that permits the flow of air into the alveoli during inspiration but impedes the outflow of air during expiration. The alveoli become hyperinflated and eventually the walls are damaged, leading to an enlarged air space in the lung parenchyma. These bullae can exceed 10 cm in diameter and they compromise the function of the remaining lung tissue (Figure 5-3). Surgical intervention to remove bullae may be indicated. Pneumothorax, a serious complication, can result from their rupture.

There are several long-term structural and functional changes in the lungs of people with emphysema. The diagnosis is based on these changes. Chronic airflow obstruction reflects both the effect of chronic inflammation of the small airways (contributing to obstructive bronchiolitis) and parenchymal destruction (emphysema). The latter contributes to the loss of

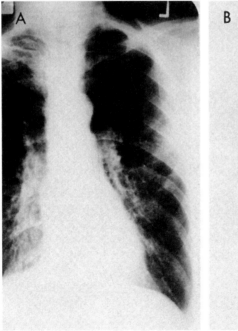
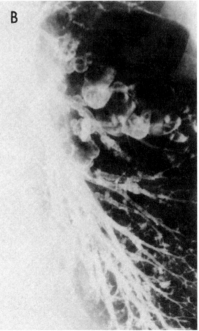

FIGURE 5-2 **A**, AP chest film reveals bullous emphysema with multiple, thin, rounded fibrotic lucencies. **B**, The spot film bronchogram of the left midlung field shows intact bronchi and distal emphysematous blebs. *(Courtesy of T. H. Johnson, M.D.)*

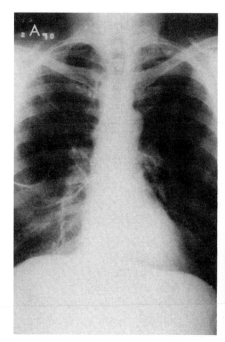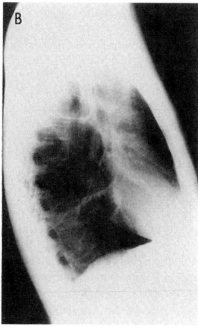

FIGURE 5-3 **A**, AP view, and **B**, lateral view, of the chest of a patient with advanced bullous emphysematous changes. Note the bullae in the upper lung fields. The lateral film reveals an increased AP diameter of the thorax, a flattening of the diaphragm, and an increased anterior clear space. *(Courtesy of T. H. Johnson, M.D.)*

alveolar tethering and attachment, resulting in increased lung compliance (reduced elastic recoil) of the affected lung regions. The airways lose their ability to remain open during expiration, resulting in dynamic airway compression.

Shortness of breath is the most common complaint of a person with emphysema, and it reflects psychological factors as well as pulmonary impairment (De Peuter et al, 2004). Dyspnea is persistent (present daily) and worsens with exertion and during respiratory infections. These patients appear thin and have elevated shoulders and an increased anteroposterior chest diameter. They tend to breathe with the accessory muscles of respiration. These patients tend to lean forward when distressed, resting their forearms on their knees or sitting with their arms extended at their sides and pushing down against the bed or chair, to elevate their shoulders and improve the efficiency of the accessory muscles to support breathing. They may breathe through pursed lips during the expiratory phase of breathing.

In the past, these patients were referred to as "pink puffers" because of the increased respiratory work needed to maintain relatively normal blood gases (Bates, 1989). This term, like "blue bloaters," is no longer considered clinically useful.

On auscultation, breath sounds are reduced throughout most or all lung fields. Radiographs show overinflated lungs, flattened hemidiaphragms, and elongated hearts (Figure 5-4). Pulmonary function tests show decreased vital capacity, FEV_1, maximum voluntary ventilation, and diffusing capacity. The total lung capacity increases due to greater anatomic dead space caused by hyperinflation, whereas the residual volume

and functional residual capacity increase even more. Arterial blood gases reflect a mildly or moderately low PaO_2, a normal or slightly elevated $PaCO_2$, and a normal pH. At the end stage of disease, these patients develop heart failure (Figure 5-5).

COPD is often associated with sodium retention leading to massive edema and the development of right heart failure (de Leeuw & Dees, 2003). Cardiac output can remain remarkably normal, suggesting that the pathology is related to fluid overload. Underfilling of the arterial side of the circulation has been proposed for stimulating the sodium-retaining mechanism in right heart failure.

Exacerbations of the disease are more frequent and severe with increased severity of lung pathology and impairment of baseline pulmonary function (Wouters, 2004). The principal cause of an acute exacerbation of COPD is infection, which may be of viral or bacterial origin. The infection causes an inflammatory response, which causes an increased production of mucus and airflow obstruction. If hospitalization is required, treatment usually includes IV fluids, antibiotics, and low-flow oxygen (Murray & Nadel, 2000). Some patients also may receive bronchodilators, corticosteroids, diuretics, and digitalis. Theophylline is often prescribed as a bronchodilator in COPD, but it also has other important benefits. Theophylline has been shown to improve respiratory muscle strength and endurance, mucociliary clearance, respiratory drive, and cardiac function (Saint et al, 1985; Sutherland & Martin, 2000; Ziment, 1987). Pursed-lip breathing can relieve dyspnea and improve arterial blood gases in some people with COPD (Dechman & Wilson, 2004). The majority of people with COPD also report

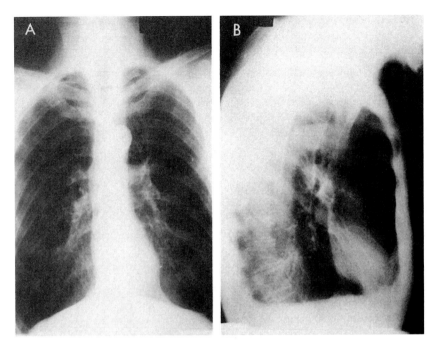

FIGURE 5-4 A, AP chest film reveals the increased lucency of lung fields and the flattening of the diaphragm in emphysema. The vascular structures are crowded medially. **B**, Lateral chest film reveals an increased AP diameter and flattening of the diaphragms. There is an increase in the anterior clear space. These are all findings in emphysema. *(Courtesy of T. H. Johnson, M.D.)*

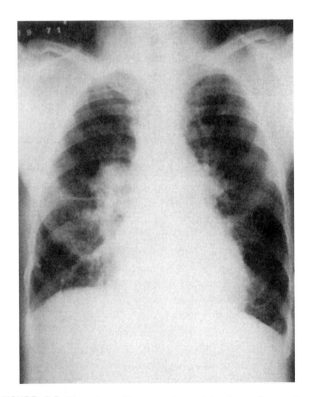

FIGURE 5-5 The chest film reveals peripheral emphysematous lucency. The hilar areas are tremendously enlarged by the pulmonary arteries in a typical cor pulmonale configuration. Cardiomegaly is also present. *(Courtesy of T. H. Johnson, M.D.)*

symptoms consistent with asthma, bronchitis, or both, which explains why inhaled corticosteroids reduce symptoms and improve survival in some patients (Mapel, 2004; Scuirba, 2004; Sutherland & Martin, 2003).

Individuals with COPD who are hypoxemic when awake become more hypoxemic during sleep, with desaturation most marked during REM sleep (Weitzenblum & Chaouat, 2004). The mechanism is thought to reflect alveolar hypoventilation and ventilation perfusion mismatch. Diminished ventilation during sleep also increases the risk of cardiac dysrhythmias (McNicholas, 2003). If COPD is associated with obstructive sleep apnea, patients have increased risk for respiratory insufficiency and failure. During acute exacerbations, these effects can be augmented, thus contributing to nocturnal death.

Risk factors for emphysema include smoking, a history of chronic bronchitis, and increasing age (American Thoracic Society, 2005). The risk for developing COPD is 30 times greater in smokers than in nonsmokers (Hogg & Senior, 2002; Hogg, 2004). The relatively rare form of inherited emphysema, alpha$_1$-antitrypsin deficiency, develops fairly early in life and is unrelated to smoking history (Anthonisen, 1989). Repeated lower respiratory tract infections can play a role.

COPD is associated with extrapulmonary effects, including peripheral skeletal muscle dysfunction, muscle wasting, and osteoporosis (Andreassen & Vestbo, 2003). Recent literature supports the theory that chronic lung and heart disease share a common myopathy (Polla et al, 2004; Troosters et al, 2004; Warburton & Mathur, 2004) (see Chapters 24 and 31). Both muscle wasting and altered muscle protein metabolism have been implicated in the muscle adaptation to COPD (Jogoe & Engelen, 2003). This finding has important implications for rehabilitation (see Chapter 24).

Respiratory muscle weakness and fatigue are associated with the severity of COPD (Orozco-Levi, 2003). Muscle weakness results from structural ventilatory impairments, adaptations to the chronic mechanical load imposed by the underlying pathology, and deconditioning. A delicate balance exists between respiratory muscle overload and adaptation. Respiratory muscle strength and endurance are fundamental to assessment, evaluation, treatment prescription, and prognosis.

Venous thromboembolism poses major risk to individuals with COPD, particularly during acute exacerbations, when blood volume may be relatively reduced in the presence of normally elevated hematocrit and the individuals are more physically inactive (Ambrosetti et al, 2003). Even though pharmacologic prophylaxis has been advocated for high-risk patients, the physical therapist should institute prophylactic measures for all patients.

For comprehensive evaluation of the functional status of individuals with chronic lung disease, exercise testing provides an integrated perspective of organ-system function and can be used to prescribe physical activity and a structured exercise program (see Chapter 24). Exercise testing data provide supplemental information in the assessment because resting pulmonary function is not necessarily closely associated with functional capacity.

COPD progresses from respiratory insufficiency to failure. The two categories include lung failure resulting in hypoxemia and pump failure resulting in alveolar ventilation and hypercapnia (Roussos & Koutsoukou, 2003). These two conditions are managed differently, depending on their underlying pathophysiological mechanisms.

Prognosis of Chronic Bronchitis and Emphysema

Without cessation of smoking and with chronic respiratory irritation, progressive loss of lung function and worsening of symptoms will progress in people with chronic bronchitis and emphysema (Keller, 2003).

Smoking cessation is the only effective intervention for preventing or reducing the life-threatening effects of COPD (Willemse et al, 2004). The decline in pulmonary function (FEV_1) is decelerated, supporting the theory that inflammation and remodeling of the airways are positively affected. Histopathological studies, however, support the idea that inflammation can persist after cessation of smoking. Longitudinal studies are needed to identify the time course and other factors that may contribute to this negative sequela and its remediation.

Individuals with COPD are at risk for tissue catabolism and associated weight loss. Poor nutrition is associated with increased morbidity. Diets are optimized, and nutritional supplements are recommended on the basis of consultation with a nutritionist. The physical therapist pays particular attention to nutrition because interventions that include

exercise impose energetic demands. Diet and exercise confer considerable benefits to the functional status of people with COPD that cannot be duplicated by pharmacological interventions (Berry & Baum, 2004).

The life-threatening complications of COPD are associated with prolonged hypoxemia leading to oxidative stress on the individual, which is manifested by ischemia affecting the organ systems; that causes dysfunction of the brain, heart, kidneys, and lungs. The most common causes of death in patients with COPD are congestive heart failure (CHF), respiratory failure, pneumonia, bronchiolitis, and pulmonary embolism. The basic mechanism underlying acute respiratory dysfunction is ventilation perfusion mismatching with increased anatomical and physiological dead space that leads to hypercapnia and acidosis (Calverley, 2003).

With increasing severity of disease, the load on the heart increases due to several factors. COPD leads to sodium retention, volume overload, edema, and right heart dysfunction (de Leeuw & Dees, 2003). Cardiac output, however, can remain relatively normal. Total peripheral vascular resistance falls with reduced effective circulating blood volume.

An individual with end-stage COPD is severely compromised and may be unable to engage in much meaningful activity. Lung-volume reduction surgery has demonstrable long-term (at least 5 years) objective and subjective benefits in selected patients with disease of the upper lobes and impaired exercise tolerance (Martinez et al, 2003; Trow, 2004).

Asthma

Asthma is a chronic inflammatory condition of the airways that is characterized by an increased responsiveness of the airway smooth muscle to various stimuli. It is manifested by widespread narrowing of the airways that reverses either spontaneously or as a result of treatment (Peters, 2003; Tarlo et al, 1998; Wagner, 2003). During an asthma attack, the lumens of the airways are narrowed or occluded by a combination of bronchial smooth muscle spasm, inflammation of the mucosa, and overproduction of viscous mucus (Minoguchi & Adachi, 1999; Rodrigo et al, 2004; Rogers, 2004). Specifically, eosinophilic inflammation is prevalent, and airway remodeling of the bronchial airways occurs over time (Cohn et al, 2004; Wenzel, 2003). Clinically, peak expiratory flow rates are sensitive to subtle changes in airway status, which may be detected before the onset of symptoms (Lung & Lung, 2003). This early objective sign can be useful in anticipating an asthma attack.

Asthma is a widespread condition that affects 5% to 10% of the population of the United States (Bowler, 2004). Asthma is prevalent in individuals under 25 years of age, where estimates of prevalence vary from 5% to 15% (Kamp, 2003). Approximately 80% of children with asthma do not have asthma after 10 years of age.

Asthma that begins before the age of 35 is usually allergic or extrinsic. Asthma attacks are precipitated when an individual comes into contact with a substance to which she or he is

BOX 5-1

Factors That Can Precipitate an Asthma Attack

Allergic or extrinsic asthma

Pollen (especially ragweed)
Animals
Feathers
Molds
Household dust
Food

Nonallergic or intrinsic asthma

Inhaled irritants

Cigarette smoke
Dust
Pollution
Chemicals

Weather

High humidity
Cold air

Respiratory infections

Common cold
Bacterial bronchitis

Drugs

Aspirin

Emotions

Stress

Exercise

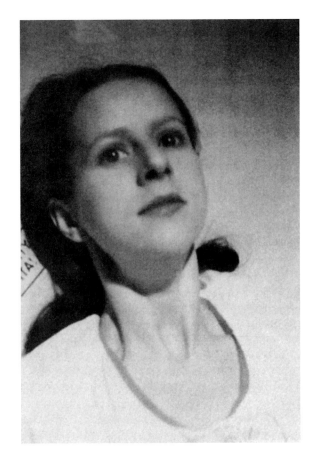

FIGURE 5-6 A patient in respiratory distress during an acute asthma attack. Note the marked use of the sternocleidomastoids and other accessory muscles during inspiration.

sensitive, such as pollens or household dust (Box 5-1). Commonly, people with asthma are allergic to multiple allergens (Tarlo et al, 1998).

Exercise-induced asthma (EIA) is prevalent in school children as well as in competitive athletes. EIA appears to result from hyperosmolar changes or exposure to temperature changes in the airways (Storms, 2003). The condition can often be well controlled medically.

If a person's first asthma attack occurs after 35 years of age, there is usually evidence of chronic airway obstruction with intermittent episodes of acute bronchospasm. These individuals, whose attacks are not triggered by specific substances, are referred to as having nonallergic or intrinsic asthma (see Box 5-1). Chronic bronchitis is commonly found in this group, and this type of individual is often seen in the hospital setting.

Individuals with acute asthma attacks often report being awakened at night or early in the morning with one or more symptoms, including cough, dyspnea, wheezing, and chest tightness (Crapo et al, 2004). Waking at night is so common in the patient with asthma that its absence from the history may cast doubt on its diagnosis (Turner-Warwick, 1988). The patient has a rapid rate of breathing and is using the accessory respiratory muscles (Figure 5-6). The expiratory phase of breathing is prolonged, with audible wheezing. As the lungs become increasingly hyperinflated, however, the breath sounds diminish (Bates, 1989). The patient may cough often, though unproductively, and may complain of chest tightness. Radiologically, the lungs may appear hyperinflated or may show small atelectatic areas caused by retained secretions. Tachypnea, hyperinflation, accessory muscle use, sitting upright, and pulsus paradoxus (difference in systolic blood pressure during inspiration and expiration) are useful guides for determining the severity of airway obstruction present (Brenner et al, 1983; Rodrigo et al, 2004; Woolcock, 2000). Early in the attack, arterial blood gases reflect slight hypoxemia and a low $PaCO_2$ (from hyperventilation). As the attack progresses, the PaO_2 continues to fall and the $PaCO_2$ increases. As obstruction becomes severe, deterioration of the patient occurs, evidenced by a high $PaCO_2$, a low PaO_2, and a pH below 7.30. Optimal monitoring of the patient's status is based on flow-volume loops and clinical judgment (Brand & Roorda, 2003).

The goals of medical management of acute asthma include maintenance of adequate arterial oxygen saturation, relief of airway obstruction, and reduction of airway inflammation

(Rodrigo et al, 2004). Patients who are hospitalized usually require intravenous fluids, bronchodilators, supplemental oxygen, and corticosteroids.

A severe asthma attack that persists for hours and is unresponsive to medical management is referred to as status asthmaticus. The patient may appear dehydrated, cyanotic, and near exhaustion due to labored breathing. In contrast to the audible wheezing heard early in the attack, the lung sounds can be greatly diminished or absent. Status asthmaticus has a significant death rate, so it is a medical emergency. Bilateral manual lower chest compression can assist expiration and may have value as an emergency treatment of asthma (Fisher et al, 1989; Watts, 1989). Patients in respiratory failure require mechanical ventilation. Averting the adverse consequences of dynamic hyperinflation is the goal (Shapiro, 2002).

On autopsy, the lungs of people with asthma are hyperinflated and fail to deflate when the thorax is opened (Saetta et al, 1991). The airway mucosa is inflamed and edematous, and the basement membrane is thickened. The mucous glands are enlarged, and the number of goblet cells is increased. Bronchospasm is evidenced by airway smooth muscle hypertrophy. The lumens of the bronchioles are filled with viscous, sticky mucus, which can precipitate death by asphyxiation (Figure 5-7). Secretions in the tracheobronchial tree of a patient with asthma are a combination of mucus, secreted by the mucous glands, and an exudate from the dilated capillaries beneath the basement membrane (Kuyper et al, 2003). Cilia fail to sweep the mucoserous fluid as effectively as they sweep mucus alone. In addition, sheets of ciliated epithelium can be shed into the bronchial lumens, further contributing to airway obstruction. Although the alveoli are overinflated, the permanent destructive changes associated with emphysema are not present.

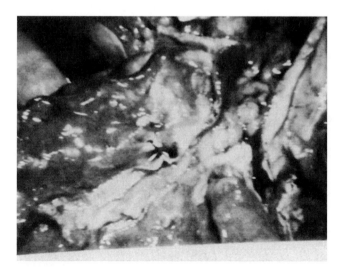

FIGURE 5-7 Gross specimen of lung showing large mucus plug within the bronchial tree of a patient who died of status asthmaticus. *(Courtesy of J. J. Coalson, Ph.D.)*

Prognosis of Asthma

In 2001 there were more than 4200 asthma-related deaths in the United States. Early detection of the severity of an exacerbation of asthma is imperative. Mortality has been attributed to the failure to detect severity early (Rodrigo et al, 2004). As a chronic disease of inflammation, asthma may result in irreversible lung damage if untreated (DeKorte, 2003). Antiinflammatory medications such as inhaled corticosteroids have a role in controlling mild to moderate cases of asthma. In severe disease that requires heavier doses, the adverse effects of long-term corticosteroid use become prevalent, namely, osteoporosis and glaucoma.

Bronchiectasis

Bronchiectasis is defined as an abnormal dilation of medium-sized bronchi and bronchioles (about the fourth to ninth generations) and generally associated with a previous, chronic necrotizing infection within these airways. Ordinarily there is sufficient cartilage within the walls of the larger bronchi to protect them from dilation.

The airway deformities can be classified into three types (Murray & Nadel, 2000). Cylindrical (or longitudinal) bronchiectasis is the most common type, with a uniform dilation of the airways. Varicose bronchiectasis refers to a greater dilation than in cylindrical bronchiectasis, causing the bronchial walls to resemble varicose veins (Figure 5-8). Saccular (or cystic) bronchiectasis refers to airways that have intermittent spherical ballooning (Figure 5-9).

Bronchiectasis is usually localized to a few segments or an entire lobe of one lung and has a predilection for the basal segments of the lower lobes. Some 40% to 50% of cases are bilateral. When the left lower lobe is involved, it is not unusual to find bronchiectasis in the lingula of the left upper lobe as well. It is interesting to note that bronchiectasis of the right middle lobe is relatively common in older adults and can contribute to both hemoptysis and repeated infections of this lobe. Upper lobe bronchiectasis generally involves the apical and posterior segments and is usually caused by tuberculosis or bronchopulmonary aspergillosis.

Pathologically the mucosa appears edematous and ulcerated. Destruction of the elastic and muscular structures of the airway walls is evident, with resultant dilation and fibrosis. The walls are lined with hyperplastic, nonciliated, mucus-secreting cells that have replaced the normal ciliated epithelium. This change is significant because it interrupts the mucociliary blanket and causes the pooling of infected secretions, which further damages and irritates the bronchial walls (Barker, 2002).

The cause of bronchiectasis is related to obstruction of the airways and respiratory infections (Barker 2002; Murray & Nadel, 2000). Some 60% of cases of bronchiectasis are preceded by acute respiratory infections. The infection involves the bronchial walls. Portions of the mucosa are destroyed and replaced by fibrous tissue. The radial traction of the lung parenchyma on the damaged bronchi causes the

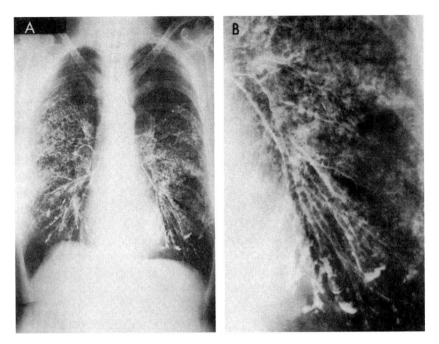

FIGURE 5-8 A, AP chest film of a bronchogram with cylindrical and varicose bronchiectasis in the lower lung fields. **B**, Close-up view of cylindrical and varicose bronchiectatic changes in the left lower lobe. *(Courtesy of T. H. Johnson, M.D.)*

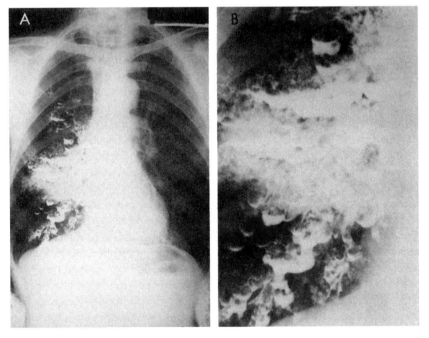

FIGURE 5-9 A, AP chest film of a bronchogram shows saccular bronchiectasis. **B**, Close-up view of bronchiectatic areas with grapelike saccular bronchiectasis. *(Courtesy of T. H. Johnson, M.D.)*

involved airways to become permanently dilated and distorted (Barker, 1988). These areas, devoid of normal ciliated cells, contain secretions that eventually become chronically infected.

Obstruction can cause bronchiectasis by collapsing lung tissue (atelectasis) distal to the obstruction (Barker, 2002).

The increased negative pressure in the chest (resulting from the collapsed lung) increases the traction on the airways, causing them to expand and become distorted. Secretions are retained, and if the obstruction is prolonged, infection may destroy the walls of the bronchi. Infection control with antibiotics has markedly decreased the incidence of bronchiectasis.

Sputum volume during a 24-hour period can be used as an indicator of severity of disease to categorize patients with bronchiectasis. Those producing less than 10 ml per day have been categorized as having mild bronchiectasis, 10 to 150 ml as having moderate bronchiectasis, and more than 150 ml as having severe bronchiectasis.

It is now relatively uncommon for people to have severe, diffuse, long-standing bronchiectasis. Those who do have it appear physically emaciated, and as many as 25% of them may have clubbed fingers. A chronic cough, with expectoration of unpleasant-tasting, purulent sputum, is typical in these patients. When this sputum is collected and allowed to stand, it may separate into three distinct layers: the uppermost layer is frothy, the middle layer is serous or mucopurulent, and the lowest layer is purulent and may contain small grayish or yellowish plugs (Dittrich plugs). Changes in body position while sleeping or on arising often stimulate coughing as secretions drain from the small peripheral to the large central airways. These individuals may have right heart failure due to fibrosis that extends into and involves the pulmonary capillary bed. Patients with widespread bronchiectasis appear dyspneic and must work hard to breathe because of hypoxemia and hypercapnia due to ventilation-perfusion mismatching. Anastomosis of the bronchial and pulmonary vascular systems causes shunting of the systemic blood from the hypertrophied bronchial arteries (Bates, 1989; West, 2003).

Most patients have a chronic productive cough. Some patients complain of relatively few symptoms except during a respiratory infection, when they have increased cough and sputum production. The amount of sputum expectorated and the severity of the cough vary from patient to patient, according to the amount of involvement. Hemoptysis does occur in about half of the older patients, evidently because of the erosion of enlarged bronchial arteries that accompany the dilated bronchi. Other common symptoms include dyspnea, wheezing, and pleuritic chest pain (Barker, 2002).

Pulmonary function tests of patients with localized bronchiectasis show few or no abnormalities. In more widespread disease, however, there is a reduction in the FEV_1, maximum midexpiratory flow rate, maximal voluntary ventilation (MVV), and diffusing capacity and an increase in the residual volume (Crapo et al, 2004; Murray & Nadel, 2000).

Prognosis of Bronchiectasis

Before the era of antibiotics, the prognosis for individuals with bronchiectasis was poor. Infection was usually the precipitating cause of death. Today, with advances in medical management, the prognosis for patients is much better (Barker, 2002). Most patients can lead relatively normal lives. Right-sided heart failure, a complication of diffuse, long-standing bronchiectasis, can lead to death. Pneumonia and hemorrhage are less common causes of death. Repeated bronchopulmonary infections can contribute to worsening

pulmonary function and an earlier death. Before the antimicrobial era, most patients with untreated, widespread, severe bronchiectasis died within 25 years. Prognosis depends on the extent of the disease process at the time of diagnosis and on optimal medical management. Patients with moderate, localized disease, with timely intervention, can expect a relatively normal life expectancy.

RESTRICTIVE LUNG DISEASE

Environmental factors play a major role in the etiology of primary restrictive lung conditions. Recently, smoking, which has been largely implicated in COPD and has been associated with all-cause cancer, has been reported to have an associated restrictive pulmonary component in some people (Flaherty & Martinez, 2004). Primary restrictive lung disease is characterized by stiffening of the lung parenchyma, which prevents the lungs from expanding fully. Normally, as the diaphragm descends during inspiration, the dimensions of the chest wall increase and the alveoli expand. A decrease in the compliance of the lung parenchyma, as in interstitial fibrosis, sarcoidosis, pneumoconiosis, and scleroderma, can produce this defect. Pleural abnormalities such as pleural effusion due to alveolar compression prevent the lungs from expanding fully. Thoracic changes such as kyphoscoliosis and ankylosing spondylitis restrict lung expansion due to restriction of chest wall movement. Obesity and ascites restrict lung expansion by limiting diaphragmatic displacement.

The pulmonary function of individuals with intersititial lung dysfunction has characteristic features (Chetta et al, 2004). Vital capacity, inspiratory capacity, and total lung capacity are reduced. Residual volume can be normal or reduced. If the restriction is pulmonary in origin, the lung compliance and diffusing capacity are reduced. Reduced exercise tolerance is associated with marked arterial desaturation (Chung & Dean, 1989).

Common restrictive lung conditions are described below. Multisystem conditions that can predispose an individual to restrictive lung dysfunction are common and are presented in Chapter 6.

Diffuse Interstitial Pulmonary Fibrosis

Pulmonary fibrosis is a common response to various types of lung injuries (American Thoracic Society, 2000a). Numerous acute and chronic lung conditions are associated with fibroproliferation, inflammation, or both, predisposing an individual to fibrosis. These are collectively known as interstitial lung disease.

The hypothesis that inflammation causes the development of interstitial pulmonary fibrosis is being challenged by a growing body of evidence that suggests there is an abnormal wound-healing response to multiple microscopic sites of acute alveolar injury that progress to fibrosis (Kamp, 2003; Selman, 2001). The resolution of the fibroproliferation response to irritation and injury is essential to patient survival. More than

130 types of interstitial lung disease have been described. Diffuse interstitial pulmonary fibrosis represents a common histological response to a wide variety of insults (Garantziotis et al, 2004). Initially, an insult or injury to the pulmonary parenchyma causes an influx of inflammatory and immune cells, resulting in a diffuse inflammatory process distal to the terminal bronchiole (alveolitis) (Thannickal et al, 2004). This can progress to subacute interstitial disease with the presence of acute and chronic inflammatory cells. Chronic disease is manifest by thickened alveolar walls and progression to fibrosis and scarring. A role for circulating cells of hematopoietic origin has been proposed as a causal factor (Garantziotis et al, 2004). In addition, apoptosis has been implicated in the pathophysiology of pulmonary fibrosis (Kuwano et al, 2004).

The known causes of pulmonary fibrosis include occupational or environmental exposure to inorganic dusts (e.g., silica and coal), toxic gases, and certain drugs or poisons (Higenbottam et al, 2004; Panos & King, 1999). In addition, interstitial lung disease is associated with rheumatoid arthritis and systemic sclerosis (Strange & Highland, 2004). Twins, siblings, and other family members have been reported to have a higher incidence of diffuse interstitial pulmonary fibrosis, which supports the idea that there is a genetic link. Less commonly, interstitial pulmonary fibrosis has been reported in individuals with Raynaud's phenomenon and ulcerative colitis.

Idiopathic pulmonary fibrosis (IPF), or cryptogenic fibrosing alveolitis, is a chronic, progressive, irreversible disease of unknown cause (American Thoracic Society, 2000a; Selman, 2001). The median survival time after diagnosis is approximately 3 years. Idiopathic interstitial pneumonia is associated with idiopathic pulmonary fibrosis and is a type of chronic fibrosing interstitial pneumonia with the histologic appearance of usual interstitial pneumonia (UIP) (American Thoracic Society, 2000). It is a condition that occurs primarily in individuals over 50 years of age. Risk factors include cigarette smoking, use of antidepressants, chronic aspiration, and exposure to metal and wood dusts.

The most common early symptoms of IPF are fatigue, dyspnea on exertion, and chronic unproductive cough. As the disease progresses, the patient becomes more dyspneic and cyanotic. On auscultation, crackles are noted, chest expansion is reduced, and clubbing of the fingers may be present.

Chest radiograph usually indicates diffuse reticular markings that show prominently in the lower lung fields. High resolution computerized tomography is often used because it is more sensitive than a radiograph; it usually reveals patchy, predominantly peripheral reticular abnormalities in the bases. It is used to evaluate the extent of parenchymal involvement and to monitor disease progression.

Pulmonary function tests show reduced lung volumes and capacities, maintained flows, and abnormal gas exchange (Khalil & O'Connor, 2004). Compliance is markedly reduced to less than half of the predicted value. Reduced diffusing capacity is the earliest and most consistent change. Initially arterial PaO_2 may be normal at rest but decrease markedly with exercise. $PaCO_2$ is reduced as a result of hyperventilation, and pH is maintained by renal compensation. Later the PaO_2 is greatly reduced because of the thickened alveolar membrane and ventilation-perfusion mismatching.

Bronchoalveolar lavage (BAL) may be used to assess the amount of inflammation and the accumulation of immune effector cells and proteins in the alveoli (Kavuru, 2002). The technique consists of wedging a fiberoptic bronchoscope into a sublobar airway, then infusing 20 to 50 ml aliquots of saline into the peripheral airway. The saline is immediately aspirated by syringe. A total of 150 to 300 ml is instilled and recovered. The fluid and cells are analyzed. High-intensity alveolitis is defined by the presence of 10% or more polymorphonuclear granulocytes (PMNs) in BAL cell differential counts; low-intensity alveolitis consists of 10% PMNs or less (Reynolds, 1987).

Lung biopsies that demonstrate an abundance of inflammatory cells suggest early disease, whereas a prevalence of fibrosis is indicative of advanced disease. A distinct category of IPF has been described and may be clinically useful (Panos & King, 1999). Desquamous interstitial pneumonitis (DIP) is characterized by the intraalveolar accumulation of mononuclear cells, relatively intact alveolar walls without destruction or fibrinous exudates (numerous inflammatory cells with little or no fibrosis). This pattern has correlated with a more benign course and a better response to corticosteroids. Because a pattern of DIP is commonly seen with UIP and IPF, DIP may represent an earlier, more easily reversible stage of IPF.

Cortiocosteroids are the mainstay of treatment for diffuse interstitial pulmonary fibrosis (Panos & King, 1999; Raghu & Chang, 2004), although their efficacy is being questioned for IPF because the favorable response rate is only 25% to 30% and there is a high incidence of adverse effects (Douglas et al, 2000; Flaherty et al, 2001). However, a trial of immunosuppressive therapy is usually prescribed for a short period. Objective measures such as blood counts, erythrocyte sedimentation rate, pulmonary function testing, exercise tests with measurement of arterial oxygen desaturation and diffusing capacity, BAL fluid analysis, and the patient's symptoms should demonstrate improvement or the medication should be discontinued. A composite clinical roentgenographic physiological (CRP) score of eight variables may be used to quantify the patient's clinical course and response to therapy (Watters et al, 1986).

Individuals who are not responsive to corticosteroids may be placed on antiinflammatory medications such as colchicines (Douglas et al, 2000) or immunosuppressive drugs such as cyclophosphamide, azathioprine, or penicillamine (American Thoracic Society, 2000a; Flaherty et al, 2001; Reynolds & Matthay, 2005). Penicillamine is more effective in patients with connective tissue diseases and interstitial fibrosis other than IPF.

Patients should stop smoking. Supplemental oxygen is important, along with exercise, as there is a characteristic significant fall in arterial oxygen tension (PaO_2) (Chung & Dean, 1989; Reynolds & Matthay, 2005). Individuals who require more than a 4 L flow per minute by nasal prongs may prefer direct administration of oxygen into the trachea. In addition to supplying higher concentrations of oxygen to the lungs, many patients prefer not to wear conspicuous nasal prongs.

Patients who have refractory restrictive lung disease may be candidates for single or double lung transplantation. Outcomes of transplantation surgery have been improving (see Chapter 40).

Most individuals with acute interstitial pneumonia and diffuse alveolar damage die within 6 months (American Thoracic Society, 2000a). Patients with the chronic form who are treated with steroids can survive for years. Untreated, these patients commonly die within 1 to 4 years. The cause of death is usually related to respiratory or heart failure, but some die of adenocarcinoma and undifferentiated or alveolar cell carcinoma of the lung.

Pulmonary Infiltrates with Eosinophilia

Eosinophils are commonly present in lung tissue as part of the body's cellular response to a variety of agents and systemic immunological diseases (Crapo et al, 2000). They are present in the airways and lung tissue of patients with idiopathic pulmonary fibrosis. In interstitial lung disease that appears to have an allergic component (e.g., hypersensitivity pneumonitis, drug-induced lung syndromes, and sarcoidosis), eosinophils are minor components of the tissue reaction. In certain primary or systemic diseases, however, eosinophils can be the most conspicuous inflammatory cell present in the lung. These conditions can be grouped together and referred to as eosinophilic syndromes. Considerable overlapping exists among these syndromes because their causes and pathogenesis remain poorly understood (Reynolds & Matthay, 2005).

Simple Pulmonary Eosinophilia

Simple pulmonary eosinophilia is a self-limiting disease in which chest radiographs demonstrate migratory, fleeting areas of pulmonary infiltrates located in the periphery of the lungs, along with minimal respiratory symptoms and blood eosinophilia. Certain drugs such as sulfonamides have been implicated as a cause (Reynolds & Matthay, 2005). This disease is also referred to as Loeffler pneumonia and as the PIE syndrome (peripheral infiltrates with blood eosinophilia). If the disease is related to an allergic response to microfilaria, human parasites (e.g., *Ascaris lumbriocoides, Strongyloides stercoralis*), or cat and dog parasites (ascarids) that produce visceral larva migrans, it is termed tropical eosinophilia.

Prolonged Pulmonary Eosinophilia

Prolonged pulmonary eosinophilia is more chronic than the simple form and is associated with a more severe symptom complex. Over time, it can eventually result in a form of diffuse interstitial pulmonary fibrosis that reveals honeycombed lung changes on chest radiograph and a restrictive pattern on pulmonary function tests.

The condition is more common in women. Symptoms include an acute respiratory illness with fever, night sweats, weight loss, and dyspnea. Prolonged pulmonary eosinophilia can be confused with tuberculosis, but patients with prolonged pulmonary eosinophilia deteriorate when treated with anti-tuberculosis drugs. This disease must also be differentiated from eosinophilic granuloma and the desquamative form of idiopathic interstitial pneumonitis. Dense infiltrates located in the periphery of the lung on chest radiographs provide an important clue. Often a lung biopsy is necessary to confirm the diagnosis. Corticosteroids markedly improve the patient's symptoms and the appearance of the chest radiograph within weeks. Months or years of treatment may be required (Panos & King, 1999).

Eosinophilic Granuloma

Eosinophilic granuloma (or histiocytosis X) can be either a unifocal disease affecting the lungs only or a multifocal disease involving the bones of the skull, mandible, vertebrae, pelvis, ribs, and extremities (Marcy & Reynolds, 1985). Lung involvement is characterized by an interstitial granuloma composed of moderately large, pale histiocytes and eosinophils, and arteriolitis with eosinophils. The histiocytic process with eosinophils then involves bronchioles, alveolar ducts, and alveolar septae, which leads to their destruction. The proliferative endarteritis causes necrosis.

This disease most commonly affects men in their 30s or 40s. They usually have symptoms of fatigue, malaise, weight loss, a nonproductive cough, dyspnea on exertion, and chest pain, sometimes related to a pneumothorax or rib lesions. The chest radiograph often indicates a diffuse micronodular and interstitial infiltrate initially involving the middle and lower lung fields. In more advanced disease, small cystic areas develop in the infiltrate, producing a honeycomb pattern. Spontaneous pneumothorax is a complication in approximately 25% of cases.

The course of the disease varies (Panos & King, 1999). Spontaneous regression with residual symptoms occurs in 10% to 25% of cases. In many patients, the disease stabilizes or "burns out," leaving them with a moderate pulmonary impairment as a result of fibrosis, cystic lung changes, and a restrictive defect on pulmonary function tests. Dyspnea on exertion is common. Some patients have persistent bronchitis. Corticosteroids are not particularly effective. Treatment is mainly symptomatic, with judicious use of antibiotics and bronchodilators. Occasionally progressive pulmonary disease leads to right heart failure and respiratory failure.

Pulmonary Alveolar Proteinosis

Pulmonary alveolar proteinosis (PAP) is an uncommon condition of unknown origin that is characterized by alveoli filled with lipid-rich "proteinaceous" material (i.e., surfactant phospholipids) in the absence of defects of the alveolar wall, interstitial spaces, conducting airways, or pleural surfaces. Most commonly, men between the ages of 30 and 50 are

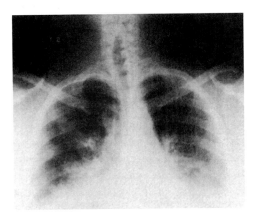

FIGURE 5-10 Pulmonary alveolar proteinosis. AP chest film demonstrates an irregular, patchy, poorly defined confluence of acinar shadows that are symmetrical in both lower lung fields. The appearance is very similar to that of pulmonary edema. *(Courtesy of T. H. Johnson, M.D.)*

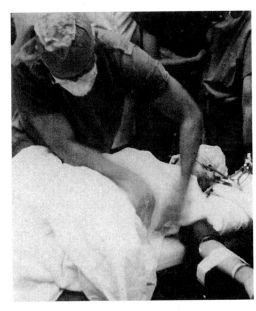

FIGURE 5-11 A patient with pulmonary alveolar proteinosis in the operating room undergoing bronchial alveolar lavage of her left lung. Percussion is done over the left lung as the saline runs out, increasing the amount of proteinaceous material removed during this procedure.

affected, although people of all ages and both sexes can be affected. There are three clinical types of PAP. The most common type (>90%) is acquired PAP, which is considered an autoimmune response. Hemoatopoietic growth factor (granulocyte-macrophage colony stimulating factor [GM-CSF]) is essential for local regulation of surfactant homeostasis in the lungs. People with acquired PAP have a circulating, neutralizing GM-CSF antibody. The remaining two types are congenital PAP and secondary PAP; the latter is associated with environmental factors, immunological disorders, malignancies, and hematopoietic disorders (Venkateshiah et al, 2004).

The most common symptoms are progressive dyspnea and weight loss, with cough; hemoptysis and chest pain are reported less frequently (Claypool et al, 1984). Chest radiographs reveal diffuse bilateral (commonly perihilar) opacities (Figure 5-10). Physical findings may include fine inspiratory crackles, dullness to percussion and, in the later stages, cyanosis and finger clubbing. Pulmonary function studies show reduced vital capacity, functional residual capacity, and diffusing capacity. Arterial blood gases indicate a low PaO_2, especially during exercise, with normal $PaCO_2$, and pH (Crapo et al, 2004).

The treatment of choice for patients with moderate to severe dyspnea on exertion due to alveolar proteinosis is whole-lung lavage (Seymour & Presnelli, 2002). In the operating room, after general anesthesia and the placement of a double-lumen tube (which isolates each lung), the patient is turned into the lateral decubitus position, with the lung to be lavaged lowermost. The double-lumen tube enables the patient to be ventilated to functional residual capacity by the uppermost lung while the lower lung is filled with saline. An additional 300 to 500 ml saline is alternately allowed to run in and out of the lung in response to gravity. As the saline flows out, manual percussion is performed over the lavaged lung, which increases the amount of proteinaceous material washed

from the affected lung (Figure 5-11). The effectiveness of mechanical percussion, manual vibration, and manual percussion in removing material from involved lungs has been compared, and manual percussion has been found to be superior (Hammon et al, 1993; Perez & Rogers, 2004). In this procedure the affected lung is lavaged with 20 to 70 L saline. The patient may be positioned prone during the administration of the final 10 to 15 L of the lavage. After the procedure, the patient is transported to the recovery room and, once stabilized, to the ward. After a few days the procedure may be repeated in the opposite lung.

Most patients show significant clinical improvement after whole-lung lavage, including improved PaO_2, diffusing capacity and vital capacity (Perez & Rogers, 2004; Seymour & Presnelli, 2002). Many also show an improved radiograph. After lavage, patients must be followed-up because the material may reaccumulate over time. Some patients do have spontaneous remissions without undergoing lavage.

The use of limited lobar lavage through a bronchoscope has shown some benefit (Cheng et al, 2002). Half of patients who have acquired PAP with subcutaneous GM-CSF show improvement, but they show a lower rate of improvement than is seen after whole-lung lavage (Claypool et al, 1984; Seymour & Presnelli, 200).

Before whole-lung lavage became standard treatment, almost all children with alveolar proteinosis died and 20% to 25% of adults died within a few years, usually because of respiratory failure, right heart failure, or uncontrolled infection. The majority now improves greatly or recovers (Seymour & Presnelli, 2002).

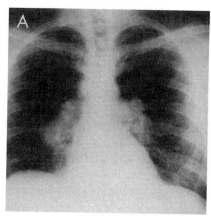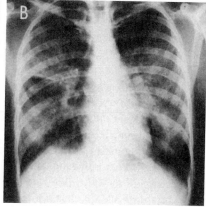

FIGURE 5-12 A, Sarcoidosis in its first stage is manifested by bilateral hilar adenopathy. Usually there are no significant physical symptoms. **B,** Disseminated sarcoidosis (third stage) reveals widespread parenchymal changes with scarring. The hilar adenopathy is usually decreased. *(Courtesy of T. H. Johnson, M.D.)*

Sarcoidosis

Sarcoidosis is one of the most common causes of interstitial pulmonary disease (Baughman, 2004; Crapo et al, 2004). It is a granulomatous disorder of unknown origin that can affect multiple organ systems (Wu & Schiff, 2004). Initial findings can include bilateral hilar adenopathy, pulmonary infiltration, and skin or eye lesions (Sharma, 1997). The lungs are the organs most often involved, and in such cases, 20% to 50% of patients seek medical attention because of respiratory symptoms. African Americans are affected 10 to 20 times more often than Caucasians, and women are affected twice as often as men. It usually occurs in the third or fourth decade of life.

The intrathoracic changes can be classified into four stages (Crapo et al, 2004). In the first stage, the patient is asymptomatic, with the chest radiograph showing bilateral hilar adenopathy and right paratracheal adenopathy (Figure 5-12, *A*). In the second stage, a diffuse pulmonary infiltration is found along with the bilateral hilar adenopathy. Interstitial infiltration or fibrosis, without hilar adenopathy, characterizes the third stage (Figure 5-12, *B*). In the fourth stage, emphysematous changes, cysts, and bullae occur.

In 60% to 90% of people with hilar adenopathy, the disease spontaneously regresses over 1 to 2 years. About one third of people with sarcoidosis involving the lungs have spontaneous regressions with some residual fibrosis. The remaining two thirds have progressive pulmonary impairment along with a variable degree of impairment to the heart, liver, spleen, lymph nodes, muscles, bones, and central nervous system.

Most people with sarcoidosis need no treatment. Corticosteroids, although controversial, have shown benefit (Turner-Warwick et al, 1986).

Rheumatoid Arthritis

Rheumatoid arthritis (RA) is a systemic disease that involves the joints but can affect the lungs, pleurae, and heart. The most common thoracic complication in RA is pleuritis, with or without pleural effusions. Although RA occurs twice as often in women, pleuritis has a striking predilection for men (Reynolds & Matthay, 2005). Pleural disease is one manifestation of RA, occasionally causing fibrothorax and restrictive lung disease that requires decortication.

Interstitial lung disease, indicated by abnormal pulmonary function tests demonstrating a restrictive ventilatory impairment and a reduced ventilatory capacity, is evident in about 40% of people with RA (Frank et al, 1973). It is also more prevalent in men. The chest radiograph shows diffuse interstitial infiltrates, especially in the lung bases. Pulmonary nodules, which are pathologically identical to the subcutaneous nodules found in RA, may also occur and may cavitate (Strange & Highland, 2004).

Coal miners with RA may have chest radiographs that demonstrate rounded densities that evolve rapidly and undergo cavitation (Caplan syndrome) in contrast to the massive fibrosis found in coal miners' pneumoconiosis (Caplan, 1953).

Systemic Lupus Erythematosus

Although systemic lupus erythematosus (SLE) is a systemic collagen vascular disease, 50% to 90% of patients have pleural or pulmonary involvement (Hunninghake & Fauci, 1979). Pleuritic chest pain often signals polyserositis associated with SLE. Pleural effusions are a manifestation of polyserositis and are present in 40% to 60% of individuals with SLE. Often they are bilateral.

Chronic interstitial pneumonitis is found in 3% to 13% of people with SLE, and acute lupus pneumonitis occurs in 1% to 4% (Keane & Lynch, 2000). Patients with pulmonary involvement have dyspnea on exertion and cough productive of mucoid sputum (Strange & Highland, 2004). Although rare, complaints of supine dyspnea suggest diaphragmatic paresis or a diffuse myopathy of the diaphragm (Keane & Lynch, 2000). The chest radiograph usually indicates patchy, non-specific densities, basilar linear or platelike atelectasis, or both. Pleural effusions and pulmonary infiltrates are common, whereas diffuse interstitial fibrosis is rare (Hunninghake & Fauci, 1979). Pulmonary function tests often indicate a restrictive pattern with a decreased diffusing capacity and reduced arterial oxygen saturation.

Progressive Systemic Sclerosis (Scleroderma)

Progressive systemic sclerosis (scleroderma) is an uncommon condition that causes thickening and fibrosis of the connective tissue throughout the body and replacement of many elements of the connective tissue by colloidal collagen. Although the skin is most often involved, the lungs, heart, kidney, bones, and other parts of the body can also be affected. Approximately two thirds of people with progressive systemic sclerosis have pulmonary involvement (Reynolds & Matthay, 2005; Strange & Highland, 2004).

Many of these patients with pulmonary involvement are asymptomatic, although symptoms can include weight loss, progressive dyspnea, low-grade fever, and cough (sometimes producing mucoid sputum). Chest radiographs shows a characteristic fibrosis of the middle and lower lung fields. Auscultation often reveals bibasilar crackles. Pulmonary function tests reveal a restrictive defect with impaired diffusion.

The form of treatment for pulmonary involvement in patients with progressive systemic sclerosis is controversial, but usually involves corticosteroids, cyclophosphamide, or both (Strange & Highland, 2004).

The prognosis for patients with only skin and joint involvement is much better than for those with involvement of the heart, lungs, and kidneys. Those with kidney involvement have a poor prognosis and a survival rate of only several years. Women have a poorer prognosis than men.

Tuberculosis

Tuberculosis (TB), a highly infectious bacterial disease, was prominent in the first half of the 1900s. With improved sanitation and medical care, TB was largely controlled. A recent resurgence of the disease has been documented, however, probably resulting from the migration patterns of people globally and the poor becoming poorer in high-income countries. TB affects many organ systems, including the lungs, and is more prevalent in people living in poor sanitary conditions with poor health. Myobacterium tuberculosis is highly contagious but responds well to medication (American Thoracic Society, 2000b; 2003). The resurgence of tuberculosis in high-income countries has been raised as a public health concern.

Lung Cancer

Lung cancer is by far the leading cause of death due to cancer in both men and women (American Cancer Society, 2000). The growth and division of cells is regulated by the DNA within every cell. When the DNA is damaged, which is estimated to be due to lifestyle behaviors and environmental factors at least 50% of the time, cell division becomes uncontrolled. Cancer-causing agents, carcinogens, related to lung disease include oxygen radicals and toxins in cigarette smoke. Although lung cancer is associated primarily with smoking, the occurrence of many other cancers is also higher in smokers. Thus the risk of cancer in general is increased in smokers. A physical therapist must understand the pathophysiology of all cancers, particularly lung cancer, and their medical and surgical management as well as the impact of their natural history and the stages of cancer on an individual's health-related quality of life. Lung cancer, as all cancers, tends to have multisystem consequences that must be understood by the physical therapist and considered during management. The physical therapist has a primary role in cancer prevention, in its early detection (by recognizing the seven warning signs of cancer), and in its management during conservative and surgical phases of care and over the long term.

End-Stage Lung Disease

Lung transplantation may be indicated in end-stage lung disease. Bronchiolitis obliterans syndrome is a serious complication of lung transplantation, but its cause is uncertain (Corris, 2003).

CORONARY ARTERY DISEASE
Hypercholesterolemia

Although hypercholesterolemia is a primary risk factor for the development of atherosclerosis, increased cholesterol affects cardiac function independently in the absence of atherosclerosis and primary ischemic heart disease (Saini et al, 2004). Elevated cholesterol levels change the structure and function of cell membranes which, in turn, affects myocardial contractility, excitability, and conduction properties. In addition, smooth muscle and endothelial dysfunction occurs, and enzyme activity and cation transporters are disrupted throughout the cardiovascular system. Thus the consequences of hypercholesterolemia are pervasive and warrant assessment even in the absence of overt atherosclerosis and ischemic heart disease.

Atherosclerosis
Pathophysiology

Atherosclerosis is triggered by trauma to the intima of the arterial wall. The trauma may be related to various primary cardiac risk factors, such as high blood pressure and cigarette smoking. Oxidative stress has been identified as the common denominator for atherogenesis, acute myocardial infarction (MI), and heart failure (Molavi & Mehta, 2004). Healthy endothelium is central to optimal vascular control.

High blood pressure has been identified as a trauma inducer because increased pressure and turbulence can damage the endothelial cells of the intima of the blood vessel wall, thus exposing the media to the circulation. The media, which consists primarily of smooth muscle, is thought to be the origin of the atherosclerotic lesion.

Cigarette smoking has also been identified as a potential inducer of trauma in the blood vessel wall. The hypothesized mode of injury appears to be different from that observed with increased blood pressure. Cigarette smoke is high in carbon monoxide and hydrocarbons that are carried by the red blood cells and the plasma. The hydrocarbons and carbon monoxide are thought to bind to the endothelial cells, causing damage to and possibly death of these cells.

Diabetes is another risk factor for cardiovascular disease of the myocardium and of the peripheral arteries (Belke & Dillmann, 2004). The reduced contractility of the heart in people with diabetes is attributed to reduced calcium handling in the sarcoplasmic reticulum of muscle.

Once the media is exposed to the circulation, the process of atherosclerosis is initiated and this predisposes an individual to thromboembolic events, in even mild cases. Platelets aggregate at the injury site and release substances that induce endothelial and smooth muscle cell replication. It is at this site that fatty streaks and fibrous plaques develop. The cause of fatty-streak development is the deposition of low-density lipoproteins (LDLs) into the smooth muscle of the media. Why this occurs is unknown, but it appears to be related to smooth muscle cell proliferation and perhaps to increased energy demands. The initial fatty streaks are generally only slightly raised and do not impede circulation. When a fibrous plaque develops, however, impingement on the vessel lumen occurs. The plaque is relatively hard and consists of connective "scar-like" tissue, smooth muscle, and fat. Finally, the plaque may undergo calcification or may lead to hemorrhaging if the vessel wall necroses. The result is decreased blood flow (ischemia) and oxygenation (hypoxia), or complete lack of blood flow and oxygen (anoxia) to the target organ.

Atherothrombosis is a generalized and diffuse progressive process affecting multiple vascular beds (Foresta et al, 2004; Munger & Hawkins, 2004). The clinical consequences include the acute coronary syndromes, ischemic stroke, and peripheral arterial disease. Thus these conditions can be viewed as diverse manifestations of a common underlying pathology. The time course of these conditions is unpredictable, yet they can be life-threatening.

Thyroid is an important regulator of cardiac function and cardiovascular hemodynamics (Danzi & Klein, 2004). The effects of the physiologically active form of thyroid hormone triiodothyronine (T_3) on the systemic vasculature include relaxation of the vascular smooth muscle, hence, reduced resistance and diastolic blood pressure. In hypothyroidism, cardiac contractility and cardiac output are decreased and systemic vascular resistance is increased, whereas the opposite occurs in hyperthyroidism. Cardiac dysfunction is associated with low levels of T_3.

Because of the current appreciation and understanding of the involvement of inflammation and endothelial injury in cardiovascular dysfunction, endothelial function biomarkers have been proposed as a sensitive means of evaluating cardiovascular disease (Szmitko et al, 2003; Verma et al, 2003).

Risk Factors

As described earlier, high blood pressure, cigarette smoking, and hyperlipidemia are direct or primary risk factors for atherosclerosis. Secondary risk factors include age, gender, race, obesity, stress, and activity level. Modifiable risk factors include hypertension, hyperlipidemia, smoking, obesity, abnormal glucose tolerance and diabetes, stress level, and activity level. Homocysteine levels have a strong relationship with atherothrombotic disease and venous thromboembolism, and elevated levels may indicate thrombotic tendencies in individuals, particularly those who are younger, in the absence of other established risk factors (Kaira, 2004). Homocysteine levels can be reduced and regulated through diet by increasing fruit and vegetable intake. Recently the tendency to panic has been implicated as a risk factor for cardiovascular disease (Katerndahl, 2004), and depression can result in a worse outcome (Kemp et al, 2003).

Vascular calcification is an established marker of atherosclerosis, which leads to increased arterial stiffness and reduced compliance and increased pulse pressure. Vascular calcification is highly correlated with mortality resulting from cardiovascular disease, particularly if diabetes or renal disease complicates the clinical presentation (Giachelli, 2004; Verma et al, 2004). The three primary risk factors—diet, hypertension, and smoking—are modifiable by the individual, and altering the diet alone can reduce the probability of CAD five- to ten-fold (Ornish, 1998; Ornish et al, 1990, 1998).

A proposed and potentially underestimated risk factor for cardiovascular disease is related to circadian rhythms (Young, 2003). It has been well established that people with heart failure have a higher rate of mortality in the early morning hours. This probably reflects diurnal variations in neurohumoral factors, including the activity of the sympathetic nervous system. The cardiac circadian clock synchronizes the response of the heart to the diurnal variations in the environment. Impairment of this mechanism could contribute to the pathogenesis of cardiovascular disease.

Aging has been implicated in lowering the threshold for the manifestation of cardiovascular disease (Oxenham & Sharpe, 2003). Stiffening of the arteries increases afterload and alters left ventricular architecture. Left ventricular diastolic function changes, whereas systolic function remains unchanged.

Angina Pectoris

Angina pectoris is defined as chest pain that is related to ischemia of the myocardium. Ischemic pain, however, may be referred to the left shoulder, neck, jaw, or between the shoulder blades. In fact, pain anywhere above the umbilicus could be related to coronary ischemia. Angina can be classified as stable, unstable, or variant. People with chest pain but normal coronary arteries on angiography tend to be women, and this presentation is not as benign as previously believed (Bugiardini et al, 2005). With the advent of the ability to assess endothelial function, those at risk may be more readily identified and managed.

Stable Angina

Stable angina generally occurs during physical effort but may be related to stress. The individual is able to describe what type and intensity of activity causes the angina. Stable angina is characterized by substernal, usually nonradiating pain lasting between 5 and 15 minutes after relief from the initiating trigger, such as a given physical or psychological stressor. Sublingual nitrates and cessation of the activity causing the angina are indicated. Usually the angina subsides completely with treatment. Angina brought about by emotional stress is more difficult to treat because stress cannot be stopped as easily as exercise.

Unstable Angina

Unstable angina occurs during physical exertion or psychological stress. The major difference between stable and unstable angina is the frequency, duration, and intensity of the pain. In unstable angina, the episodes are more frequent and the duration of each event is usually greater than 15 minutes. In addition, the intensity of the pain may be more severe. Unstable angina is usually an indicator of the progression of coronary artery disease. Individuals with unstable angina are at increased risk of MI. Unstable angina is less responsive to treatment with rest and sublingual nitrates. Often the individual needs to be hospitalized and treated with intravenous nitrates.

Variant Angina

Variant angina occurs while the individual is at rest, usually during waking and at the same hour. Exertion does not influence variant angina. This type of angina may benefit from rest and sublingual nitrates. Like unstable angina, the pain is intense and prolonged and can lead to infarction. In addition, dysrhythmias occur more commonly in individuals who have variant angina than in those with exertional angina (i.e., stable and unstable angina). Stable and unstable angina reflect progressive arterial stenosis and ischemia. Variant angina is caused by a combination of stenosis and coronary artery spasm and is successfully treated with calcium channel blockers.

Prognosis of Angina

Individuals do not die of angina per se. The progression of atherosclerosis of the coronary arteries is reflected in the clinical changes that occur between the experience of angina and an MI. Even though there is no risk of mortality as a result of angina, an individual's lifestyle can change drastically. People with angina may be fearful of being active and may deny that they are having exertional chest pain. Denial, depression, anger, and hostility are common psychosocial correlates (Beckham et al, 1994). Depression and further reduction in physical activity can be associated with angina (diagnosed or undiagnosed and denied). Although restricted activity is an important component of initial treatment, low levels of activity can modify several risk factors and arrest the progression of atherosclerosis (Niebauer et al, 1995). In addition, diet and exercise have been documented to reverse atherosclerosis (Ornish, 1998; Ornish et al, 1998; Schuler et al, 1992).

Obstructive Sleep Apnea Syndrome

Obstructive sleep apnea (OSA) has a greater incidence in individuals with atherosclerosis, cardiac dysrhythmias, and hypertension than in those without (Shamsuzzaman et al, 2003). This has been explained in part by the presence of proinflammatory and prothrombotic factors (Parish & Somers, 2004). OSA is characterized by the repetitive closing and opening of the posterior pharynx that are synchronized with breathing while sleeping, usually when recumbent. Apneic periods and arterial desaturation are also common to the syndrome. Additional pathologies common to OSA and atherosclerosis include endothelial dysfunction, increased C-reactive protein, fibrinogen, reduced fibronolytic activities, and increased platelet activity and aggregation. OSA is now considered a risk factor for cardiovascular disease. The complications of sleep apnea syndrome are exacerbated by autonomic dysfunction as well. Sleep apnea often coexists undiagnosed in people with cardiovascular disease, activates mechanisms known to aggravate and advance cardiovascular injury, and contributes to resistance to therapeutic interventions (Shamsuzzaman et al, 2003).

Myocardial Infarction

MI is defined as necrosis of a portion of the myocardium. The death of the myocardium occurs as a result of ischemia and anoxia. The vessels affected by occlusion are the right and left coronary arteries and their anterior and posterior descending branches. The right coronary artery supplies the posterior section and portions of the inferior section of the left ventricle. The left coronary artery branches and forms the circumflex and anterior descending arteries. The circumflex supplies the lateral portion of the left ventricle, and the anterior descending artery supplies the anterior portion. In addition, the right coronary artery supplies the right atrium atrioventricular bundle and the right ventricle. The left coronary artery supplies the left atrium and the primary portion of the conduction pathway. Generally the clinical symptoms are similar to those of angina, with emphasis on extreme pressure as well as tightness over the sternal region. In addition, pain can radiate to the jaw, upper back, and shoulders (on the left more often than on the right).

MIs are categorized by location, size, and degree of involvement of the myocardial wall. The terms *small* and *large* are often used to describe MIs. Degrees of complication are also used in conjunction with size. MIs can be described as uncomplicated and complicated, based on the size of the MI and the patient's recovery. Location indicates the area of the heart involved and the coronary artery or branches that are involved. The anatomic areas of the heart are differentiated as anterior, posterior, lateral, and inferior. Finally, MIs are classified by the extent of damage to the wall. A transmural (or full-wall) infarct extends from the endocardium to the epicardium, whereas only some involvement of the ventricle wall may occur, for example, just beneath the epicardium (subepicardial) or just beneath the endocardium (subendocardial).

Silent ischemia is particularly prevalent in patients with high cardiac risk and is associated with a poor outcome (Solomon & DeBusk, 2004). Silent MIs can be detected when a patient has undergone ECG investigation or imaging for other problems.

Uncomplicated Myocardial Infarction

An uncomplicated MI is described as a small infarction with no complications during recovery. Usually the result is full recovery without a significant decrease in cardiac performance at rest and during minimal to moderate activity (Cahalin, 1994). Location and the extent of the MI are critical with respect to outcome. MIs located in the inferior portion of the heart are considered the least clinically significant, and partial-wall-thickness MIs are less significant than transmural MIs.

Treatment. Initially the treatment of a patient with an uncomplicated MI is comparable to that of a patient with a complicated MI, so the patient is cared for in a coronary care unit. The medical treatment is designed to decrease myocardial work and oxygen demand. Patients receive supplemental oxygen and are administered coronary vasodilators (nitroglycerin) to increase myocardial blood flow and analgesics to reduce ischemic pain. In addition, calcium channel blockers or beta blockers are administered to reduce the contractility and work of the myocardium. Antidysrhythmia medication may be prescribed if an aberrant cardiac rhythm is present or likely to occur.

Because the clinical course is uncomplicated, a patient's stay in the coronary care unit may be only a couple of days, with a total hospital stay of 3 to 5 days. Once the patient's condition is stabilized, management is oriented toward increasing physical activity and educating the patient and family with respect to risk factor reduction (Wenger, 1984; see Chapters 29, 30, and 31). This process is described as cardiac rehabilitation, phase I (see Chapter 30).

Complicated Myocardial Infarction

A complicated MI is distinct from an uncomplicated case because the patient may have one, a combination, or all four of the following complications: dysrhythmia, heart failure, thrombosis, and damage to heart structures.

Dysrhythmias. Dysrhythmias occur in 95% of patients with MIs. The type and severity of the dysrhythmia is dependent on the location and extent of the myocardial damage. Imbalance in autonomic regulation has been implicated in dysrhythmogenesis and sudden cardiac death (Sztajel, 2004). Blunted heart rate variability has been established as a marker of sympathovagal imbalance and can serve as an indicator of cardiac risk.

The risk of serious or frequent dysrhythmias is lower in a patient with an uncomplicated MI because a small area of the myocardium is involved. Dysrhythmias that are life-threatening include complete AV heart block, ventricular-paced dysrhythmia, and ventricular tachycardia including ventricular flutter and fibrillation. In these conditions, either heart rate (comprising stroke volume, ejection fraction, and overall cardiac output) is too slow and cardiac output is impaired, or heart rate is too fast. Treatment of these conditions is immediate and requires drugs. If refractory to conservative management, cardioversion or electric shock (for flutter and fibrillation) is indicated. If a normal rhythm cannot be restored and maintained by the patient's own inherent pacemaker, an artificial pacemaker may have to be implanted.

Dysrhythmias may be present in the absence of overt myocardial ischemia or heart damage. Common dysrhythmias are presented in Chapter 4, and their clinical implications are presented in Chapter 12. One conduction abnormality that is receiving increasing attention is atrial fibrillation (Waldo, 2004). This dysrhythmia warrants management, given its association with thromboemboli and stroke (see Chapter 1). Furthermore, atrial fibrillation is the most common dysrhythmia associated with cardiac surgery (25% to 60%), and it leads to increased postoperative morbidity and mortality and to associated health care costs (Knotzer et al, 2004; Palin et al, 2004). Atrial fibrillation has been reported not only to be more common in men but also to be better tolerated by them than by women (Peters & Gold, 2004).

Heart failure. Another complication after MI is cardiac insufficiency and failure. Heart failure is a condition in which the heart is weakened by myocardial damage and is unable to provide cardiac output to meet the body's metabolic needs for oxygen, nutrition, and removal of waste products. When the heart experiences ischemia, the myocardium contracts with less force and conduction abnormalities may alter the mechanics of the contraction. If an area of the heart is infarcted, the affected myocardium does not contract, thus affecting overall cardiac output. Another type of heart failure not directly related to ischemia and infarction is congestive heart failure (described in the next section).

Recent terminology regarding the classification of heart failure differentiates diastolic and systolic heart failure (Banerjee et al, 2004; Gutierrez & Blanchard, 2004; Paul, 2003; Thohan, 2004). Diastolic heart failure refers to the presence of the symptoms of heart failure in the absence of left ventricular dysfunction, the hallmark of systolic heart failure. Diastolic heart failure in which the left ventricle is stiff (reduced compliance and impaired relaxation resulting in increased end diastolic pressure) has been estimated to account for 40% to 50% of all cases of heart failure (Khouri et al, 2004). Diastolic dysfunction has been of increasing interest in nonprimary heart disease such as systemic sclerosis, and it appears to be more common than previously thought (Steen, 2004). The two types of heart failure must be distinguished on the basis of Doppler echocardiography because their signs and symptoms are comparable. Both types are associated with marked morbidity and mortality.

Immediately post-MI, cardiac output is markedly reduced. The compensatory response of the body is to increase sympathetic and renin-angiotensin-aldosterone stimulation, resulting in increased heart rate and myocardial contractility. The result of this compensation is to normalize cardiac output to normal resting values. If myocardial damage is extensive, the kidneys compensate by retaining sodium and water to improve circulatory volume and venous return. Depending on the amount of myocardial tissue death, the individual may survive, but with resulting chronic congestive heart failure through persistent fluid retention and hypotension. If more than 40% of the left ventricle is infarcted, the result is usually cardiogenic shock followed by the death of the individual. Renin-angiotensin-aldosterone activation contributes to left ventricular remodeling, which is further augmented by vascular endothelial dysfunction, resulting in decreased nitric oxide bioavailability (Bauersachs & Schafer, 2004).

Diabetic cardiomyopathy leads to heart failure independent of underlying coronary artery disease (Hayat et al, 2004). Both structural and functional abnormalities associated with diabetic cardiomyopathy have been linked to an underlying metabolic disorder. Other factors include myocardial fibrosis due to an inflammatory process, small blood vessel pathology, cardiac autonomic neuropathy, and insulin resistance (Fang et al, 2004).

Thrombosis. Deep vein thrombosis (DVT) and related pulmonary emboli are largely preventable clinical complications, and when they do occur, their diagnosis may be missed in hospitalized patients (Goldhaber & Elliott, 2003; Tapson, 2004). These life-threatening complications are serious and warrant early detection. Mortality resulting from thrombi that migrate to the lungs (pulmonary emboli) is greatest initially after an acute MI. DVTs can be challenging to detect because of the lack of specificity of their clinical presentation. Another complication is increased incidence of thrombosis originating in deep leg veins and in the damaged heart itself. Thrombosis that starts in deep leg veins occurs because of lower limb inactivity and circulatory stasis. This is a complication that can be observed in patients after surgery. Emboli from a deep leg vein thrombus usually cause pulmonary complications. If the emboli are large or numerous, the result can be pulmonary tissue infarction and death. The incidence of pulmonary emboli has been reduced because patients now are usually ambulated soon after a medical event or surgery. Nonetheless, a pulmonary embolus must be considered a distinct possibility in all patients after an MI, surgery, or major trauma.

Heart, or mural wall, thrombosis can lead to an embolus lodging in the brain, intestine, kidney, artery to the extremities, or any location in the systemic arterial circulation. Usually mural thrombi do not affect the pulmonary system because the small fragments become lodged in the capillaries and fail to access the venous system.

Structural damage. Structural damage to the myocardium is another serious complication of MI. If the neural conduction pathway (bundle branch) located primarily within the septum is damaged, dysrhythmias result. In addition, papillary muscles that regulate heart valve closure can be infarcted. Valve incompetence leads to regurgitation and retrograde flow of blood from the ventricles, thus impeding the forward movement of blood through the heart and decreasing cardiac output. Full-thickness damage to the myocardial wall significantly compromises normal cardiac function. Heart wall damage can result in ventricular aneurysms or ventricular wall rupture. Ventricular aneurysm, or the bulging of the weakened ventricular wall, occurs in transmural (full-wall thickness) infarcts. Ventricular wall rupture, which can occur acutely after transmural infarction but is more common in the first to second week post-MI after an aneurysm, is usually fatal. Therefore, after an MI, it is critical to determine whether an aneurysm has occurred within the myocardium so that appropriate surgical intervention can be performed.

Risk factors for cardiac rupture include being female, being older, having hypertension, and experiencing the first cardiac event (Wehrens & Doevendans, 2004). Clinical signs of rupture include syncope, chest pain, and jugular venous distention. In addition, defective ventricular remodeling may predispose the heart to rupturing.

Treatment. The treatment of a complicated MI is initially like that of an uncomplicated MI, where the patient is cared for in the coronary care unit. Similarly, medical treatment is designed to decrease myocardial work and oxygen demand. Patients receive supplemental oxygen and coronary vasodilators (nitroglycerin) to increase myocardial blood flow and analgesics to help further reduce ischemic pain. Myocardium calcium channel blockers or beta blockers are administered to reduce contractility. Finally, antidysrhythmia medication is prescribed to stabilize the electrical conduction system of the heart or if an aberrant cardiac rhythm is present.

Patients with complicated MIs require longer stays in the coronary care unit, and their total hospital stay times are longer than those of patients with uncomplicated MIs. The time in coronary care and total hospital stay are dependent on the complications that occur after the MI. Individuals with heart failure, thrombolytic events, or structural damage requiring surgery may be in the coronary care unit for a couple of weeks. Total hospital-stay times for patients with complicated MIs may exceed this length of time. Treatment after discharge from the intensive care unit, however, is similar to that of the patient with an uncomplicated MI; the goal is to increase physical activity and educate the patient and family in risk-factor reduction. The major difference in phase I cardiac rehabilitation for patients with complicated rather than uncomplicated

MIs is the intensity, duration, and frequency of the initial exercise workload (i.e., a much lighter workload is prescribed for a patient with a complicated MI) (Rowe, 1989). This patient also requires closer monitoring. Progression is more conservative because after a complicated MI, a patient is at higher risk than a patient whose MI was uncomplicated (Rowe, 1989).

Prognosis After a Myocardial Infarction

After an MI, the prognosis is dependent upon many factors. Compared with the patient's premorbid status, cardiovascular performance is reduced unless the structural damage to the ventricle is minor (as in the case of many patients with uncomplicated MIs). The most important factor is the extent of ventricular damage. With early detection of transmural infarction and improvement in surgical intervention and coronary care, however, the number of acute post-MI deaths has been reduced (Wenger, 1984). Other critical factors include remaining cardiac capacity and cardiac status and risk factors. Even though CAD mortality has declined in the United States, the disease remains the leading cause of death in adults.

Severe infarction can necessitate emergency or elective revascularization surgery. Emergency surgery for an acute MI complicated by cardiogenic shock is associated with satisfactory long-term survival; however, perioperative risk is high (Vitali et al, 2004).

Congestive Heart Failure

Congestive heart failure is a leading cause of hospitalization and death. It is characterized by the inability of the heart to maintain adequate cardiac output. The incidence of congestive heart failure appears to be increasing because of the prevalence of injurious lifestyle behaviors, aging, and improved survival after acute cardiac episodes (Murray-Thomas & Cowie, 2003).

Almost half of all patients with congestive heart failure are women (Pijna & Buchter, 2003). Smoking, diabetes, and high blood pressure are stronger risk factors for congestive heart failure in women than men. Peripartum cardiomyopathy, which is unique to women in their child-bearing years, occurs either in the late stages of pregnancy or within several months after giving birth.

The causative factors of heart failure are usually ischemia and MI secondary to ischemic heart disease. For the heart to maintain optimal blood flow to the pulmonary and systemic circulations, heart rate and stroke volume must be adequate. Provided heart rate is regular and within an acceptable range, stroke volume is the critical factor for maintaining adequate cardiac output. Stroke volume is a function of the amount of blood in the left ventricle at the end of diastole (preload); the amount of pressure and resistance the heart must overcome to eject blood into the systemic circulation (afterload); and myocardial contractility, which is the amount of force the left ventricle can apply to the blood within the chamber. If any one of these three variables is adversely affected, cardiac output is reduced. Progressive deterioration of myocardial contractility and dilation as well as fluid overload precipitate heart failure.

Dyspnea is the primary complaint of people with congestive heart failure. It can be challenging to distinguish between dyspnea resulting from congestive heart failure and dyspnea resulting from pulmonary causes. B-Type natriuretic peptide (BNP) is synthesized, stored, and released in the ventricular myocardium, and it is stimulated by changes in ventricular wall tension and stretch (Maisel & McCullough, 2003). The use of BNP holds some promise as a marker for congestive heart failure and a guide to clinical management.

Congestive heart failure is a major contributor to progressive renal dysfunction and anemia (Silverberg et al, 2004). Anemia is observed in one third of all patients with congestive heart failure. Conversely, chronic renal dysfunction can cause severe cardiac injury and is often associated with anemia. Thus congestive heart failure, chronic renal insufficiency, and anemia create a vicious circle that warrants aggressive medical management to attenuate the progression of the three conditions.

Acute Heart Failure

If an individual has a significant MI, the contractility and pumping ability of the heart is immediately reduced. The initial result is decreased cardiac output and the damming of blood in the veins. (The damming of blood in the pulmonary circulation leads to congestive heart failure, as discussed earlier). The result is increased systemic venous pressure. This acute phase, which may reduce cardiac output to 40% of normal resting values, is short-lived, lasting only a few seconds before the sympathetic nervous system is stimulated, and the parasympathetics become reciprocally inhibited. Sympathetic innervation causes an increase in the contractility of viable myocardial tissue, and the increase in cardiac output may be 100%. In addition, sympathetic innervation also increases venous return because the tone of blood vessels is increased. The result is increased systemic filling pressure and, thus, increased preload. The sympathetic reflex after MI becomes maximally operational within 30 seconds; therefore, except for some pain and fainting, individuals experiencing mild MIs may not know they have suffered a heart attack. The sympathetic response can continue if cardiac output is maintained at an adequate level at rest. Ischemic pain, however, may persist and warrants treatment.

Chronic Heart Failure

After an MI, several physiological responses occur along with sympathetic reflex compensation. The kidneys retain fluid almost immediately after an MI. A decrease in glomerular pressure secondary to decreased cardiac output is implicated. In addition, there is an increase in renin output and therefore an increase in angiotensin production. Angiotensin promotes reabsorption of water and salt from the renal tubules. The effect of moderate fluid retention is an increase in blood volume and venous return. This increases preload, hence cardiac output. If the MI was severe, however, the result can be excessive fluid retention. This results in systemic edema and overstretching of the heart due to excessive blood volume and venous return. In the chronic state, this condition is termed chronic heart failure (CHF).

Recovery of the damaged myocardium occurs after MI. New collateral arteries are formed to supply the peripheral portions of the infarcted region. This revascularization can assist marginally active cells to become fully functional again. In addition, the unaffected myocardial cells hypertrophy. In a mild to moderate MI, such recovery can result in major improvement in cardiac function and can take 6 weeks to several months, depending on extent of injury.

Gas transfer across the alveolar-capillary membrane is impeded in CHF. This may be explained by the pressure and volume overloading, which injures the alveolar blood-gas barrier; hence, the impairment of diffusion of blood across it (Guazzi, 2003). In the short term these changes may be reversible. If the membrane is chronically challenged, however, the anatomical and physiological integrity of the membrane is remodeled. These changes have been associated with worsened symptoms and exercise tolerance. Further, these changes may be prognostic.

Cardiac remodeling is a central feature of heart-failure progression (Sharpe, 2004). Remodeling refers to the alteration of the structure and geometry of the heart in response to myocardial insult or pressure or volume overload. Such remodeling reflects the adaptation that is needed to maintain adequate heart function with changing conditions. Increased muscle mass is one of the primary adaptations, and it usually involves left ventricular hypertrophy (Titcomb, 2004). Adaptive hypertrophy of the left ventricle is clinically important in that it is associated with increased morbidity and mortality rates (Maron et al, 2003). A further consequence of adaptive cardiac hypertrophy is the potential for reduced responsiveness to the metabolic and functional effects of insulin, which further contributes to the heart's hypoeffectiveness (Allard et al, 2000). Pharmacological studies have been conducted to examine the role of drugs on the remodeling process in individuals with heart failure. Studies of the role of non-pharmacological interventions, including exercise, in cardiac remodeling have not been made.

A reciprocal relationship between CHF and diabetes has been well established (Tenenbaum & Fisman, 2004). People with CHF may be at increased risk for diabetes due to reduced physical activity, cellular metabolic defects, reduced muscle perfusion, and poor nutrition. The increased sympathetic stimulation associated with CHF increases insulin resistance and decreases insulin release from the beta cells of the pancreas. Both factors contribute to glucose intolerance and diabetes, which in turn lead to hyperglycemia and increased risk for cardiovascular and metabolic complications.

Even in patients with chronic heart failure, regular exercise may be associated with a protective metabolic phenotype (Burelle et al, 2004). This effect of exercise could explain why fit people have less severe MIs than nonfit people.

Compensated and Decompensated Heart Failure

Compensated heart failure is the final stage after the acute, then chronic, physiological compensation for cardiac dysfunction. In this state the heart can pump blood effectively but at a reduced cardiac output compared with the pre-MI condition. The individual's cardiac reserve, that is, the difference between maximum and resting cardiac output, is greatly reduced. With even small increases in metabolic demand through exercise, symptoms of acute failure reappear because the limits of compensation are exceeded. These symptoms include rapid heart rate, pallor, and diaphoresis.

Decompensated heart failure affects 5 million Americans and is associated with a 5-year mortality rate of almost 50% (Peacock et al, 2003). Decompensated failure occurs when the heart is so severely damaged or weakened that normal cardiac output cannot be attained. This type of failure is defined as a sustained deterioration of at least one New York Heart Association functional class, usually with evidence of sodium retention (Mills & Hobbs, 2001). Cardiac output is insufficient to maintain normal renal function. Fluid continues to accumulate so the heart is stretched and weakened further, permitting only moderate to low quantities of blood to be pumped. In unilateral heart failure, the left ventricle may fail while the right ventricle continues to pump vigorously. Blood volume and pulmonary capillary pressure increase. If this occurs, fluid filters into the interstitial spaces of the alveoli, resulting in pulmonary edema, impaired gas exchange, and suffocation. As the heart weakens, not only is systemic blood flow compromised, so is the coronary system. The area most affected is the subendocardial region. As these cells become infarcted, the heart weakens further until other regions of the heart also become ischemic and infarcted.

Prognosis

End-stage cardiac disease without effective pharmaceutical or surgical intervention, including revascularization or heart transplantation, results in death. Intermediate measures to avert deterioration have emerged, including cardiac resynchronization therapy through biventricular pacing (Gura & Foreman, 2004). The addition of implantable cardioverter defibrillators may help to minimize the occurrence of sudden death in people with CHF. Left-ventricle assistance devices may be used to support the function of the failing heart until it responds to conservative management or until surgery is scheduled (Hirsch & Cooper, 2003). Surgical ventricular restoration holds some promise for reversing inappropriate remodeling of the myocardium after infarction and restoring its normal elliptical shape (Conte, 2004). The primary pharmaceutical interventions used to mitigate heart failure include diuretics to reduce fluid overload and cardiac glycosides such as digitalis to improve myocardial contractility.

These interventions are combined with modification of salt and fluid intake. Other factors can predict a poor outcome. Sleep apnea syndrome, for example, is common in people with CHF and is associated with a poor prognosis. As ejection fraction is decreased, the risk of thrombus formation and stroke increase (Pulerwitz et al, 2004).

In cases where the heart has compensated poorly and remains weak and the cardiac output is minimal, heart transplant is the only recourse. Because organ donors are not readily available, the number of individuals who need new hearts far exceeds the available donor organs. Posttransplant prognosis is related to the recipient's surgical suitability and the health of the donor organ. The prognosis will also reflect the amount of cardiac reserve.

Valvular Heart Disease

Heart valve incompetence is classified as being either congenital or acquired (i.e., after a bacterial or viral infection of the heart valves) and can affect any one of the four heart valves. Surgical repair or replacement of defective mitral valves, tricuspid valves, and aortic valves constitutes a significant proportion of cardiac surgeries. Mitral and aortic valve disease is particularly common in people over 65 years of age (Segal, 2003a, 2003b). In this age group, symptoms can be masked by such comorbidities as cardiovascular disease, pulmonary disease, and hypertension. Surgical repair is associated with favorable short- and long-term outcomes. Some valve defects are benign and treatment is not indicated. Some people can tolerate heart valve defects as children, but they become symptomatic with age. Currently these types of valve defects are often corrected at birth or early in life.

One common valve defect is prolapse of the mitral valve, which is more common in women than in men and may warrant repair.

Cardiac defects may be present as secondary diagnoses in an individual being managed by a physical therapist. Such defects need to be considered in terms of an individual's capacity to respond to exercise and how the condition impacts an individual's life overall. Exercise limitation secondary to heart valve disease may mask limitations due to other causes, or vice versa.

Systemic Hypertension

Systemic hypertension, or wide pulse pressure hypertension, has become increasingly prevalent and is implicated in multiorgan dysfunction, not only in cardiac dysfunction and failure (see Chapter 1). Systolic hypertension syndrome refers to a complex of hemodynamic maladaptations, including stiff central arteries, normal peripheral arteries, arteriolar constriction, metabolic abnormalities, cardiac hypertrophy, and increased blood pressure variability (Izzo, 2004). In addition to the conventional measures of hemodynamic status, measures of arterial mechanics, including arterial compliance, elastic modulus, impedence, pulse wave velocity,

and pulse pressure amplification, are used for diagnosis and management.

Hypertension is strongly implicated in cardiovascular disease and stroke (Mayet & Hughes, 2003). When systemic hypertension syndrome advances to heart disease, the prognosis is poor (Kostis, 2003).

Obesity is considered a primary risk factor for hypertension as well as for heart disease, stroke, and renal dysfunction. Mechanisms that have been proposed for obesity-related hypertension include insulin resistance, hyperinsulinemia, dyslipidemia, increased sympathetic activity, sodium and water retention, cardiac dysfunction, and endothelial dysfunction (Sharma, 2004). To adapt to an increasing workload, the heart enlarges. When it can no longer adequately compensate, the heart begins to fail, and that is usually coupled with respiratory failure. Myocardial hypertrophy is considered an independent risk factor for cardiovascular disease in people who are obese and is a strong predictor of heart failure.

The occurrence and clinical implications of myocardial fibrosis in people with hypertension are well established (Moncrieff et al, 2004). The rennin-angiotensin-aldosterone system and contributions of mineralocorticoids and endothelin have been implicated in the development of myocardial fibrosis.

Thyroid hormone has well-documented effects on cardiovascular function, including blood pressure (Danzi & Klein, 2003). In hyperthyroidism, pulse pressure is increased, whereas in hypothyroidism, pulse pressure is narrowed. Adaptations of the cardiovascular system alter blood pressure to accommodate new demands on the system. The effects of thyroid hormone on blood pressure, therefore, are mediated both directly and indirectly.

Pulmonary Hypertension

Pulmonary hypertension is increasingly recognized as a pathology that can occur secondary to some other pulmonary condition or with no apparent cause (idiopathic pulmonary hypertension). By definition, pulmonary hypertension exists when the mean pulmonary pressure is greater than 25 mm Hg at rest and greater than 30 mm Hg during exercise (World Health Organization, 2003). Pulmonary blood pressure can increase in response to increased pulmonary vascular resistance, blood flow, and pulmonary artery wedge pressure. The cause of pulmonary hypertension has shifted from being attributed to vasoconstrictive dysfunction to being attributed to angio-proliferative dysfunction (Voekel & Cool, 2004). Endothelial dysfunction has been implicated (Budhiraja et al, 2004). Although the prognosis is variable, with some people surviving months and others decades, guidelines have been recommended to assess the prognosis for individuals with pulmonary artery hypertension and to institute appropriate intervention expeditiously (McLaughlin et al, 2004).

Anemia

Anemia usually results from blood loss or from acute or

chronic dysfunction of red blood cell production. The adaptive responses of the oxygen transport system involve the cardiovascular system and an increase in cardiac output and redistribution of blood flow to favor coronary and cerebral circulations at the expense of the splanchnic vascular beds (Hebert et al, 2004). These adaptations can maintain tissue oxygenation with hematocrit levels as low as 21% (Morisaki & Sibbald, 2004).

Anemia is also commonly seen clinically in patients after orthopedic surgery, in renal failure, and in patients undergoing chemotherapy for cancer. Patients may be treated with blood transfusion or erythropoietin. Mild anemia may be managed by dietary measures and over-the-counter vitamin and mineral tablets alone. Moderate anemia may require mineral supplements. Anemia compromises recovery. Optimal management augments responses to rehabilitation and recovery, reduces fatigue, and improves exercise capacity, muscle strength, and performance of the activities of daily living (Carson et al, 2003). Whether there is a critical hemoglobin level that allows for optimal participation and activity performance is unclear. The presence of CAD may mitigate hemodynamic compensation to blood loss and other causes of anemia and may attenutate treatment responses (Nappi, 2003).

Sickle cell anemia is a genetic condition that is common in African Americans and characterized by an abnormal shape of the red blood cell that impedes its movement through the capillary beds. Patients with sickle cell anemia have a low anaerobic threshold in the presence of a high heart rate reserve, but they have no gas exchange abnormalities (Callahan et al, 2002). Patients may have restrictive lung pathology, increased alveolar dead space, and hypoxemia (Pianosi et al, 1991). Increased dead space may reflect impaired pulmonary capillary perfusion due to the sickle cells. Exercise hyperventilation is thought to be associated with increased anaerobiosis.

Type 2 Diabetes Mellitus

Type 2 diabetes mellitus is increasing in prevalence worldwide (see Chapter 1). Insulin resistance and glucose intolerance result from the additive effect of poor diets and inactivity. Diabetes is a multisystem condition; however, cardiovascular disease is the leading cause of morbidity and mortality in people with diabetes (Candido et al, 2003). Organ system dysfunction results from hyperglycemia and the deposition of sorbitol on cell membranes. The toxicity of sorbitol leads to the vascular and neurological complications of this life-threatening condition. Recent evidence supports the theory that the metabolic defects associated with diabetes (impaired glucose tolerance, insulin resistance, and proinflammatory and prothrombotic states) lead to endothelial dysfunction and acceleration of atherosclerosis (Nesto, 2004). Hyperglycemia is associated with changes in the myocardium that lead to diabetic cardiomyopathy and heart failure. These changes can occur even in the absence of hyperglycemia, which has been linked with cardiovascular remodeling (Giles, 2003). Erectile dysfunction in men has been associated with atherosclerosis

and with high fasting blood sugar (Foresta et al, 2004). A diagnosis of erectile dysfunction can lead to the detection of diabetes. Adequate control of diabetes is essential to minimize these consequences.

Metabolic Syndrome

People with metabolic syndrome are at increased risk for cardiac, pulmonary, and metabolic dysfunction and diabetes. The syndrome results from deleterious body weight, inactive lifestyle, atherogenic diet, or some combination thereof (Wagh & Stone, 2004). The assessment is based on elevated triglycerides, low high-density lipoprotein cholesterol, elevated fasting blood glucose, elevated blood pressure, and increased abdominal circumference. At least three of these findings must be present for a diagnosis of metabolic syndrome.

Syncope

Syncope is a syndrome hallmarked by a short period of loss of consciousness due to transient reduction of blood flow to the brain. Although systemic hypotension is the most common cause, it may result from a combination of factors. Syncope occurs mostly in people with cardiovascular dysfunction and in older people. Cardiovascular-related causes include orthostatic syncope related to position change, cardiac dysrhythmia, and structural cardiac and pulmonary causes (Benditt et al, 2004). Less common causes include neurally mediated reflex syncope and syncope resulting from cerebrovascular disorders. A patient complaining of light-headedness, dizziness, grayouts, blackouts, or fainting episodes needs a thorough multisystem assessment to establish and manage the precise causes.

Cardiac Dysfunction in Noncardiac Conditions

Cardiopulmonary consequences of noncardiopulmonary conditions are described in Chapter 6. Although their affect can be subtle, cardiopulmonary manifestations of these conditions can be serious and even life-threatening. These consequences need to be addressed by the physical therapist during the assessment to guide and modify management. Tools such as ECG are essential in detecting ECG abnormalities at rest and during exercise in patients with noncardiopulmonary conditions such as electrolyte disturbance, pulmonary embolism, esophageal disorders, drug-related conditions, and neuromuscular conditions (Van Mieghem et al, 2004).

The connective tissue disorders, including systemic sclerosis, have cardiovascular consequences (Steen, 2004). Because the heart is significantly involved, scleroderma can manifest as myocardial dysfunction, conduction abnormalities, and pericardial disease. The cardiovascular system can also be involved secondarily due to involvement of the lungs and kidneys.

Myocardial and cardiovascular dysfunction is well recognized as a leading cause of morbidity and mortality in people with neuromuscular conditions, and it can be a major complication in their management (Bhakta & Groh, 2004; Pathak & Senard, 2004). Early detection and management of such dysfunction is key to lifelong health in this cohort of individuals, reduced incidence and severity of associated morbidity, and modification of rehabilitation.

Obesity is an independent risk factor for heart failure (Coviello & Nystrom, 2003). The cellular changes reflect the increased metabolic strain mediated by increased mechanical strain and work of the heart.

Renal disease can lead to heart failure or result from it. In addition, anemia is implicated in both conditions. The triad of these conditions has been termed the cardiorenal anemia syndrome (Silverberg et al, 2003). Anemia increases the severity of CHF and mortality, and renal disease causes anemia. Both renal dysfunction and anemia worsen heart complications. Epoetin (recombinant human erythropoietin), which is used to correct anemia associated with renal dysfunction, also decreases the compensatory increase in left ventricular muscle mass, thereby reducing associated cardiac morbidity and mortality (London, 2003).

Athletic Heart Syndrome

Although physical fitness is associated with innumerable health benefits (see Chapters 1 and 18), cardiovascular adaptation to intense exercise in athletes (athletic heart syndrome) can mimic disease processes associated with cardiovascular disease (Vasamreddy et al, 2004). Sudden cardiac death in athletes is often associated with cardiac hypertrophy, dysrhythmias, or both. In addition, cardiac episodes in athletes may reflect the manifestation of congenital abnormalities in electrical activity or mechanical function of the heart. Thus screening athletes for cardiovascular adaptation is warranted. Physical therapists involved with sports teams need to be vigilant regarding risk factors associated with the athletic heart syndrome to detect and avoid untoward events.

SUMMARY

Knowledge of the pathophysiology of primary and secondary cardiovascular and pulmonary dysfunction is essential to the practitioner for relating the underlying pathophysiology to the clinical signs and symptoms and to the appropriate treatment goals and interventions. The cardiovascular and pulmonary systems are interdependent anatomically and physiologically. The physical therapist must distinguish the contribution of cardiovascular or pulmonary pathology to an individual's limitations on participation in life and ability to perform life's requisite activities. In addition, this knowledge is essential in prescribing interventions and appropriately monitoring the patient.

This chapter first distinguishes the pathophysiology related to the structure and function of obstructive and restrictive lung conditions. Obstructive conditions are characterized by

decreased airflow during expiration (as a result of increased airway resistance), airway obstruction, and hyperinflation of the lungs. Restrictive conditions are characterized by increased lung stiffness or chest wall rigidity that limits inspiration. Both types of lung pathology progressively limit functional capacity. Second, the essential pathophysiological features of atherosclerosis, ischemic heart disease, and coronary artery disease and related syndromes are described. Hypertension, diabetes mellitus, anemia, and syncopy are highlighted. Cardiac dysfunction secondary to noncardiac conditions is addressed and linked to discussion of this topic covered elsewhere.

Review Questions

1. Describe the role of smoking in the incidence of cardiovascular and pulmonary conditions. If smoking were unknown, what would be the epidemiological impact on cardiovascular and pulmonary disease?
2. Describe how lung dysfunction can lead to cardiac dysfunction and provide examples.
3. Describe how cardiac dysfunction can lead to lung dysfunction and provide examples.
4. Distinguish obstructive from restrictive pulmonary pathology and how each manifests clinically.
5. Obstructive and restrictive lung pathology seldom exist alone. Describe how these types of pathology can coexist.
6. Describe tuberculosis and why it must be a concern to the contemporary physical therapist.
7. Describe the process of atherosclerosis and the ways in which it is injurious to life.
8. Evaluate the relative contributions of acquired cardiovascular disease and congenital cardiovascular disease to your role as a physical therapist.
9. Describe the pathophysiological progression of cardiac insufficiency to failure and death. Describe how lifestyle changes recommended by the physical therapist as part of comprehensive management could stall such progression.
10. Describe the implications of hypertension, anemia, diabetes mellitus, and syncope on your practice as a physical therapist across clinical settings, including the community and working with healthy seniors.
11. What is meant by the term *athletic heart syndrome*? What are the implications in terms of your role as a physical therapist with a sports team?

ACKNOWLEDGMENT

We appreciate the contribution of Scott Hasson as a coauthor of this chapter in the previous edition.

REFERENCES

Allard M.F., Wambolt, R.B., Longnus, S.L., Grist, M., Lydell, C.P., Parsons, H.L., Rodrigues, B., Hall, J.L., Stanley, W.C., & Bond, G.P. (2000). Hypertrophied rat hearts are less responsive to the metabolic and functional effects of insulin. American Journal of Endocrinology and Metabolism, 279:E487-E493.

Ambrosetti, M., Ageno, W., Spanevello, A., Salerno, M., & Pedretti, R.F. (2003). Prevalance and prevention of venous thromboembolism in patients with acute exacerbations of COPD. Thrombosis Research 112:203-207.

American Cancer Society. (2000). Cancer facts and figures. Atlanta: American Cancer Society.

American Thoracic Society. (2000a). Idiopathic pulmonary fibrosis: diagnosis and treatment. International Consensus Statement. American Thoracic Society and the European Respiratory Society. American Journal of Respiratory and Critical Care Medicine 161:646-664.

American Thoracic Society. (2000b). Official statement of the American Thoracic Society and the Centers for Disease Control and Prevention adopted by the ATS Board of Directors. Diagnostic Standards and Classification of Tuberculosis in Adults and Children. American Journal of Respiratory and Critical Care Medicine 161:1376-1395.

American Thoracic Society. (2003). American Thoracic Society/ Centers for Disease Control and Prevention/Infectious Diseases Society of America: Treatment of Tuberculosis. Journal of Respiratory and Critical Care Medicine 167:603-662.

American Thoracic Society. (2005). Epidemiology, risk factors and natural history. www.thoracic.org/COPD/epidemiology.asp.

Andreassen, H., & Vestbo, J. (2003). Chronic obstructive pulmonary disease as a systemic disease: an epidemiological perspective. European Respiratory Journal 46(Suppl):2S-4S.

Anthonisen, N. (1989). Prognosis in chronic obstructive pulmonary disease: results from multicenter clinical trials. American Review of Respiratory Disease 140:595-599.

Banajee, P., Clark, A.L., Nikitin, N., & Cleland, J.G. (2004). Diastolic heart failure: paroxysmal or chronic? European Journal of Heart Failure 6:427-431.

Barker, A.F. (2002). Bronchiectasis. New England Journal of Medicine 346:1383-1393.

Barnes, P. (1993). Asthma. In Bone, R. (Ed). Pulmonary and critical care medicine. St. Louis: Mosby.

Bates, D.V. (1989). Respiratory function in disease, ed 3, Philadelphia: WB Saunders.

Bauersachs, J., & Schafer, A. (2004). Heart failure, platelet activation and inhibition of the rennin-angiotensin-aldosterone system. Archives des Maladies du Coeur et des Vaisseaux 97:889-893.

Baughman, R.P. (2004). Pulmonary sarcoidosis. Clinics of Chest Medicine 25:521-530.

Beckham, J.C., et al. (1995). Pain coping strategies in patients referred for evaluation of angina pectoris. Journal of Cardiopulmonary Rehabilitation 15:173-180.

Belke, D.D., & Dillmann, W.H. (2004). Altered cardiac calcium handling in diabetes. Current Hypertension Report 6:424-429.

Benditt, D.G., van Dijk, J.G., Sutton, R., Wieling, W., Lin, J.C, Sakaguchi, S., & Lu, F. (2004). Syncope. Current Problems in Cardiology 29:152-229.

Berry, J.K., & Baum, C. (2004). Reversal of chronic obstructive pulmonary disease-associated weight loss: are there pharmacological treatment options? Drugs 64:1041-1052.

Bhakta, D., & Groh, W.J. (2004). Cardiac function tests in neuromuscular diseases. Neurology Clinics 22:591-617.

Bowler, R.P. (2004). Oxidative stress in the pathogenesis of asthma. Current Allergy and Asthma Reports 4:116-122.

Brand, P.L., & Roorda, R.J. (2003). Usefulness of monitoring lung function in asthma. Archives of Diseases in Children 88:1021-1025.

Brenner, B., Abraham, E., & Simmon, R. (1983). Position and diaphoresis in acute asthma. American Journal of Medicine 74:1005-1009.

Budihiraja, R., Tuder, R.M., & Hassoun, P.M. (2004). Endothelial dysfunction in pulmonary hypertension. Circulation 109:159-165.

Bugiardini, R., & Bairey Merz, C.N. (2005). Angina with "normal" coronary arteries: a changing philosophy. Journal of the American Medical Association 293:477-484.

Burelle, Y., Wambolt, R.B., Grist, M., Parsons, H.L., Chow, J.C.F., Antler, C., Bonen, A., Keller, A., Dunaway, G.A., Popov, K.M., Hochachka, P.W., & Allard, M.F. (2004). Heart and circulatory physiology, American Journal of Physiology 287:H1055-H1063.

Cahalin, L.P. (1994). Exercise tolerance and training for healthy persons and patients with cardiovascular disease. In Hasson, S. (Ed).Clinical exercise physiology, St. Louis: Mosby.

Callahan, L.A., Woods, K.F., Mensah, G.A., Ramsey, L.T., Barbeau, P., & Gutin, B. (2002). Cardiopulmonary responses to exercise in women with sickle cell anemia. American Journal of Respiratory and Critical Care Medicine 165:1309-1316.

Calverley, P.M. (2003). Respiratory failure in chronic obstructive pulmonary disease. European Respiratory Journal 47(Suppl): 26S-30S.

Candido, R., Srivastava, P., Cooper, M.E., & Burrell, L.M. (2003). Diabetes mellitus: a cardiovascular disease. Current Opinions and Investigations and Drugs 4:1088-1094.

Caplan, A. (1953). Certain unusual radiological appearances in chest of coal miners suffering from rheumatoid arthritis. Thorax 8:29-37.

Carson, J.L., Terrin, M.L., & Jay, M. (2003). Anemia and postoperative rehabilitation. Canadian Journal of Anaesthesiology 50(Suppl):S60-S64.

Celli, B.R. (1999). Pathophysiology of chronic pulmonary disease. In Cherniack, N.S., Altose, M.D., & Homma, I. (Eds). Rehabilitation of the patient with respiratory disease, New York: McGraw-Hill.

Chapman, K.R. (2004). Chronic obstructive pulmonary disease: are women more susceptible than men? Clinics in Chest Medicine 25:331-341.

Cheng, S.L., Chang, H.T., Lau, H.P., Lee, L.N., & Yang, P.C. (2002). Pulmonary alveolar proteinosis: treatment by bronchofiberoptic lobar lavage. Chest 122:1480-1485.

Chetta, A., Marangio, E., & Olivieri, D. (2004). Pulmonary function testing in interstitial lung diseases. Respiration 71:209-213.

Chung, F., & Dean, E. (1989). Pathophysiology and cardiorespiratory consequences of interstitial lung disease: review and clinical implications. Physical Therapy 69:956-966.

Claypool, W., Rogers, R., & Matuschak, G. (1984). Update on the clinical diagnosis, management and pathogenesis of pulmonary alveolar proteinosis (phospholipidosis). Chest 85:550-558.

Cohn, L., Elias, J.A., & Chupp, G.L. (2004). Asthma: mechanisms of disease persistence and progression. Annual Reviews in Immunology 22:789-815.

Conti, J.V. (2004). Surgical ventricular restoration: techniques and outcomes. Congestive Heart Failure 10:248-251.

Corris, P.A. (2003). Lung transplantation. Bronchiolitis obliterans syndrome. Chest Surgery Clinics of North America 13:543-557.

Cosio, M. (1987). The relations between structural changes in small airways and pulmonary function tests. New England Journal of Medicine 298:1277-1281.

Coviello, J.S., & Nystrom, K.V. (2003). Obesity and heart failure. Journal of Cardiovascular Nursing 18:360-366.

Crapo, J.D., Glassroth, J., Karlinsky, J., & King, T.E., Jr. (Eds) (2004). Baum's textbook of pulmonary diseases, ed 7, Philadelphia: Lippincott Williams & Wilkins

Currie, D.C., Pavia, D., Agnew, J.E., Lopez-Vidriero, M.T., Diamond, P.D., Cole, P.J., & Clarke, S.W. (1987). Impaired tracheobronchial clearance in bronchiectasis. Thorax 42:126-130.

Danzi, S., & Klein, I. (2003). Thyroid hormone and blood pressure regulation. Current Hypertension Report 513-520.

De Leeuw, P.W., & Dees, A. (2003). Fluid homestasis in chronic obstructive lung disease. European Respiratory Journal 46(Suppl):33S-40S.

De Peuter, S., Van Diest, I., Lemaigre, V., Verleden, G., Demedts, M., & Van den Bergh, O. (2004). Dyspnea: the role of psychological processes. Clinical Psychological Review 24:557-581.

Dechman, G., & Wilson, C. (2004). Evidence underlying breathing retraining in people with stable chronic obstructive pulmonary disease. Physical Therapy 84:1189-1197.

DeKorte, C.J. (2003). Current and emerging therapies for the management of chronic inflammation in asthma. American Journal of Health Systems in Pharmacy 60:1949-1959.

Dhala, A., Pinsker, K., & Prezant, D.J. (2004). Respiratory health consequences of environmental tobacco smoke. Medical Clinics of North America 88:1535-1552.

Douglas, W.M., Ryu, J.H., & Shroeder, D.R. (2000). Idiopathic pulmonary fibrosis: impact of oxygen and colchicine, prednisone or no therapy on survival. American Journal of Respiratory and Critical Care Medicine 161:1172-1178.

Evans, S.E., & Scanlon, P.D. (2003). Current practice in pulmonary function testing. Mayo Clinical Proceedings 78:758-763.

Fang, Z.Y., Prins, J.B., & Marwick, T.H. (2004). Diabetic cardiomyopathy: evidence, mechanisms, and therapeutic implications. Endocrine Review 25:543-567.

Fisher, M., Bowery, C., & Ladd-Hudson, K. (1989). External chest compression in acute asthma: a preliminary study. Critical Care Medicine 17:686-687.

Flaherty, K.R., & Martinez, F.J. (2004). Cigarette smoking in interstitial lung disease: concepts for the internist. Medical Clinics of North America 88:1643-1653.

Flaherty, K.R., Toews, G.B., Lynch, J.P. 3rd, Kazerooni, E.A., Gross, B.H., Strawderman, R.L., Hariharan, K., Flint, A., & Martinez, F.J. (2001). Steroids in idiopathic pulmonary fibrosis: a prospective assessment of adverse reactions, response to therapy and survival. American Journal of Medicine 110:278-282.

Foresta, C., Caretta, N., Aversa, A., Bettocchi, C., Corona, G., Mariani, S., & Rossato, M. (2004). Erectile dysfunction: symptom or disease? Journal of Endocrinological Investigation 27:80-95.

Frank, S.T., Weg, J.G., Harkleroad, L.E., & Fitch, R.F. (1973). Pulmonary dysfunction in rheumatoid disease. Chest 63:27-34.

Garantziotis, S., Steele, M.P., & Schwartz, D.A. (2004). Pulmonary fibrosis: thinking outside of the lung. Journal of Clinical Investigation 114:319-321.

Giachelli, C.M. (2004). Vascular calcification mechanisms. Journal of the American Society of Nephrology 15:2959-2964.

Giles, T.D. (2003). The patient with diabetes mellitus and heart failure: at-risk issues. American Journal of Medicine 115(Suppl 8A):107S-110S.

Global Initiative for Chronic Obstructive Pulmonary Disease. GOLD Patient Guide. May 2002. http:/www.goldcopd.com; retrieved January 2005.

Goldhaber, S.Z., & Elliott, C.G. (2003). Acute pulmonary embolism: part 1: epidemiology, pathophysiology, and diagnosis. Circulation 108:2726-2729.

Gosker, H.R. (2003). Myopathological features in skeletal muscle of patients with chronic obstructive pulmonary disease. European Respiratory Journal 22:280-285.

Guazzi, M. (2003). Alveolar-capillary membrane dysfunction in heart failure: evidence of pathophysiologic role. Chest 124:1090-1102.

Guidelines and Protocols Advisory Committee. (2003). Diagnosis and Management of Asthma. www.healthservices.gov.bc.ca/msp/protoguides/gps/asthma.pdf; retrieved March 2005.

Gura, M.T., & Foreman, L. (2004). Cardiac resynchronization therapy for heart failure management. American Academy of Cardiac Nurses Clinical Issues 15:326-339.

Gutierrez, C., & Blanchard, D.G. (2004). Diastolic heart failure: challenges of diagnosis and treatment. American Family Physician 69:2609-2616.

Hammon, W., McCaffree, D., & Cucchiara, A. (1993). A comparison of manual to mechanical chest percussion for clearance of alveolar material in patients with pulmonary alveolar proteinosis (phospholipidosis). Chest 103:1409-1412.

Hayat, S.A., Patel, B., Khattar, R.S., & Malik, R.A. (2004). Diabetic cardiomyopathy: mechanisms, diagnosis and treatment. Clinical Science (London) 107:539-557.

Hebert, P.C., Van der Linden, P., Biro, G., & Hu, L.Q. (2004). Physiologic aspects of anemia. Critical Care Clinics 20:187-212.

Higenbottam, T., Kuwano, K., Nemery, B., & Fujita, Y. (2004). Understanding the mechanisms of drug-associated interstitial lung disease. British Journal of Cancer 91(Suppl 2):S31-S37.

Hirsch, D.J., & Cooper, J.R. Jr. (2003). Cardiac failure and left ventricular assist devices. Anesthesiology Clinics in North America 21:625-638.

Hogg, J.C. (2004). Pathophysiology of airflow limitation in chronic obstructive pulmonary disease. Lancet 364:709-721.

Hogg, J.C., & Senior, R.M. (2002). Chronic obstructive pulmonary disease 2: pathology and biochemistry of emphysema. Thorax 57:830-834.

Hunninghake, G., & Fauci, A. (1979). Pulmonary involvement in the collagen vascular diseases (state of the art). American Review of Respiratory Diseases 119:471-480.

Izzo, J.L. Jr. (2004). Arterial stiffness and the systolic hypertension syndrome. Current Opinions in Cardiology 19:341-352.

Jogoe, R.T., & Engelen, M.P. (2003). Muscle wasting and changes in muscle protein metabolism in chronic obstructive pulmonary disease. European Respiratory Journal 46(Suppl):52S-63S.

Kaira, D.K. (2004). Homocysteine and cardiovascular disease. Current Atherosclerosis Report 6:101-106.

Kamholz, S.L. (2004). Pulmonary and cardiovascular consequences of smoking. Medical Clinics of North America 88:1415-1430.

Kamp, D.W. (2003). Idiopathic pulmonary fibrosis: the inflammatory hypothesis revisited. Chest 12:1187-1189.

Katerndahl, D. (2004). Panic plaques: panic disorder and coronary artery disease in patients with chest pain. Journal of the American Board of Chest Physicians 17:114-126.

Kavuru, M. (2002). Therapeutic whole lung lavage: a stop-gap therapy for alveolar proteinosis. Chest 122:1123-1124.

Keane, M., & Lynch, J. (2000). Pleuropulmonary manifestations of systemic lupus erythematosus. Thorax 55:159-166.

Keller, C.A. (2003). Pathophysiology and classification of emphysema. Chest Surgery Clinics in North America 13:589-613.

Kemp, D.E., Malhotra, S., Franco, K.N., Tesar, G., Bronson, D.L. (2003). Heart disease and depression: don't ignore the relationship. Cleveland Clinic Journal of Medicine 70:749-754.

Khalil, N., & O'Connor, R. (2004). Indiopathic pulmonary fibrosis: current understanding of the pathogenesis and the status of treatment. Canadian Medical Association Journal 171:153-160.

Khouri, S.J., Maly, G.T., Suh, D.D., & Walsh, T.E. (2004). A practical approach to the echocardiographic evaluation of diastolic function. Journal of the American Society of Echocardiography 17:290-297.

Knotzer, H., Dunser, M.W., Mayr, A.J, & Hasibeder, W.R. (2004). Postbypass arrhythmias: pathophysiology, prevention, and therapy. Current Opinions in Critical Care 10:330-335.

Kostis, J.B. (2003). From hypertension to heart failure: update on the management of systolic and diastolic dysfunction. American Journal of Hypertension 16:18S-22S.

Kuwano, K., Hagimoto, N., & Nakanishi, Y. (2004). The role of apoptosis in pulmonary fibrosis. Histology and Histopathology 19:867-881.

Kuyper, L.M., Pare, P.D., Hogg, J.C., Lambert, R.K., Ionescu, D., Woods, R., & Bai, T.R. (2003). Characterization of airway plugging in fatal asthma. American Journal of Medicine 115:6-11.

London, G.M. (2003). Left ventricular hypertrophy: why does it happen? Nephrology, Dialysis, and Transplantation 18(Suppl 8): viii2-6.

Lung, C.L., & Lung, M.L. (2003). General principles of asthma management: symptom monitoring. Nursing Clinics of North America 38:585-596.

Maisel, A.S., & McCullough, P.A. (2003). Cardiac natriuretic peptides: a proteomic window to cardiac function and clinical management. Review of Cardiovascular Medicine 4(Suppl 4): S3-S12.

Mapel, D.W. (2004). Treatment implications on morbidity and mortality in COPD. Chest 126(Suppl 2):150S-158S.

Marcy, T., & Reynolds, H. (1985). Pulmonary histiocytosis. Lung 163:129-150.

Maron, B.J., McKenna, W.J., Danielson, G.K., Kappenberger, L.J., Kuhn, H.J., Seidman, C.E., Shah, P.M., Spencer, W.H. 3rd, Spirotto, P., Ten Cate, F.J., & Wigle, E.D. (2003). A Report of the American College of Cardiology Foundation Task Force on Clinical Expert Consensus Documents and the European Society of Cardiology Committee for Practice Guidelines. Journal of the American College of Cardiology 42:1687-1713.

Martinez, F.J., Flaherty, K.R., & Iannettoni, M.D. (2003). Patient selection for lung volume reduction surgery. Chest Surgery Clinics in North America 13:669-685.

Mayet, J., & Hughes, A. (2003). Cardiac and vascular pathophysiology in hypertension. Heart 89:1104-1109.

McLaughlin, V.V., Presberg, K.W., Doyle, R.L., Abman, S.H., McCrory, D.C., Fortin, T., & Ahearn, G. (2004). Prognosis of pulmonary arterial hypertension: ACCP evidence-based clinical practice guidelines. Chest 126(Suppl 1):78S-92S.

McNicholas, W.T. (2003). Impact of sleep on ventilation and gas exchange in chronic lung disease. Monaldi Archives of Chest Diseases 59:212-215.

Meyer, F.J., Schoene, A.M., & Borst, M.M. (2003). Pathophysiological aspects of cardiopulmonary interaction. Clinical Nephrology 60(Suppl 1): S75-S80.

Mills, R.M., & Hobbs, R.E. (2001). Drug treatment of patients with decompensated heart failure. American Journal of Cardiovascular Drugs 1:119-125.

Minoguchi, K., Adachi, M. (1999). Pathophysiology of asthma. In Cherniak, N.S., Altose, M.D., & Homma, I. (Eds). Rehabilitation of the patient with respiratory disease, New York: McGraw-Hill.

Molavi, B., & Mehta, J.L. (2004). Oxidative stress in cardiovascular disease: molecular basis of its deleterious effects, its detection, and therapeutic considerations. Current Opinions in Cardiology 19:488-493.

Moncrieff, J., Lindsay, M.M., & Dunn, F.G. (2004). Hypertensive heart disease and fibrosis. Current Opinions in Cardiology 19:326-331.

Morisaki, H., & Sibbald, W.J. (2004). Tissue oxygen delivery and the microcirculation. Critical Care Clinics 20:213-223.

Munger, M.A., & Hawkins, D.W. (2004). Atherothrombosis: epidemiology, pathophysiology, and prevention. Journal of the American Pharmaceutical Association 44(2 Suppl 1):S5-S12.

Murray, J.F., & Nadel, J.A. (2000). Textbook of respiratory medicine, Philadelphia: WB Saunders.

Murray-Thomas, T., & Cowie, M.R. (2003). Epidemiology and clinical aspects of congestive heart failure. Journal of the Renin Angiotensin Aldosterone System 4:131-136.

Nappi, J. (2003). Anemia in patients with coronary artery disease. American Journal of Health-System Pharmacy 60(14 Suppl 3): S4-S8.

National Heart, Lung, and Blood Institute, Division of Lung Diseases (2003). National Emphysema Treatment Trial (NETT): Evaluation of lung volume reduction surgery for emphysema: What is emphysema? http://www.nhlbi.nih.gov/health/prof/lung/ nett/lvrsweb.htm#emphysema; retrieved March 2005.

Nesto, R.W. (2004). Correlation between cardiovascular disease and diabetes mellitus: current concepts. American Journal of Medicine 116(Suppl 5A):11S-22S.

National Heart, Lung, and Blood Insititute. (2003). The definition of emphysema. Report of a National Heart, Lung, and Blood Institute Division of Lung Diseases Workshop. American Review of Respiratory Disease 132:182-185.

Niebauer, J., Hambrecht, R., Schlierf, G., Marburger, C., Kalberer, B., Kubler, W., & Schuler, G. (1995). Five years of physical exercise and low fat diet: effects on progression of coronary artery disease. Journal of Cardiopulmonary Rehabilitation 15:47-64.

Ornish, D., Brown, S.E., Scherwitz, L.W., Billings, J.H., Armstrong, W.T., Ports, T.A., McLanahan, S.M., Kirkeeide, R.L., Brand, R.J., & Gould, K.L. (1990). Can lifestyle changes reverse coronary heart disease? The Lifestyle Heart Trial. Lancet 336:129-133.

Ornish, D. (1998). Avoiding revascularization with lifestyle changes: The Multicenter Lifestyle Demonstration Project. American Journal of Cardiology 82:72T-76T.

Ornish, D., Scherwitz, L.W., Billings, J.H., Brown, S.E., Gould, K.L., Merritt, T.A., Sparler, S., Armstrong, W.T., Ports, T.A., Kirkeeide, R.L., Hogeboom, C., & Brand, R.J. (1998). Intensive lifestyle change for reversal of coronary heart disease. Journal of the American Medical Association 280:2001-2007.

Orozco-Levi, M. (2003). Structure and function of the respiratory muscles in patients with COPD: impairment or adaptation? European Respiratory Journal 46(Suppl):41S-51S.

Oudijk, E.J., Lammers, J.W., & Koenderman, L. (2003). Systemic inflammation in chronic obstructive pulmonary disease. European Respiratory Journal 46(Suppl):5S-13S.

Oxenham, H., & Sharpe, N. (2003). Cardiovascular aging and heart failure. European Journal of Heart Failure 5:427-434.

Palin, C.A., Kailasam, R., & Hogue, C.W. Jr. (2004). Atrial fibrillation after cardiac surgery: pathophysiology and treatment. Seminars in Cardiothoracic and Vascular Anesthesia 8:175-183.

Panos, R.J., & King, T.E. (1999). Pathophysiology of interstitial lung disease. In Cherniack, N.S., Altose, M.D., & Homma, I. (Eds). Rehabilitation of the patient with respiratory disease, New York: McGraw-Hill.

Parish, J.M., & Somers, V.K. (2004). Obstructive sleep apnea and cardiovascular disease. Mayo Clinic Proceedings 79:1036-1046.

Pathak, A., & Senard, J.M. (2004). Pharmacology of orthostatic hypotension in Parkinson's disease: from pathophysiology to management. Expert Review of Cardiovascular Therapy 2:393-403.

Paul, S. (2003). Diastolic dysfunction. Critical Care Nursing Clinics in North America 15:495-500.

Pauwels, R., Calverley, P., Buist, A.S., Rennard, S., Fukuchi, Y., Stahl, E., & Lofdahl, C.G. (2004). COPD exacerbations: the importance of a standard definition. Respiratory Medicine 98:99-107.

Peacock, W.F., Allegra, J., Ander, D., Collins, S., Diercks, D., Emerman, C., Kirk, J.D., Starling, R.C., Silver, M., & Summers, R. (2003). Management of acute decompensated heart failure in the emergency department. Congestive Heart Failure Sept-Oct (Suppl 1):3-18.

Perez, A., & Rogers, R. (2004). Enhanced alveolar clearance with chest percussion therapy and positional changes during whole-lung lavage for alveolar proteinosis. Chest 125:2351-2356.

Peters, R.W., & Gold, M.R. (2004). The influence of gender on arrhythmias. Cardiology in Review 12:97-105.

Peters, S.P. (2003). Heterogeneity in the pathology and treatment of asthma. American Journal of Medicine 115(Suppl 3A): 49S-54S.

Pianosi, P., D'Souza, S.J., Esseltine, D.W., Charge, T.D., & Coates, A.L. (1991). Ventilation and gas exchange during exercise in sickle cell anemia. American Review of Respiratory Disease 143:226-230.

Pijna, I.L., & Buchter, C. (2003). Heart failure in women. Cardiology in Review 11:337-344.

Polla, B., D'Antona, G., Bottinelli, R., & Reggiani, C. (2004). Respiratory muscle fibers: specialization and plasticity. Thorax 59:808-817.

Postma, D.S., & Boezen, H.M. (2004). Rationale for the Dutch hypothesis: allergy and airway hyperresponsiveness as genetic factors and their interaction with environment in the development of asthma and COPD. Chest 126(2 Suppl):96S-104S.

Pulerwitz, T., Rabbani, L.E., & Pinney, S.P. (2004). A rationale for the use of anticoagulation in heart failure management. Journal of Thrombosis and Thrombolysis 17:87-93.

Raghu, G., & Chang, J. (2004). Idiopathic pulmonary fibrosis: current trends in management. Clinics in Chest Medicine 25:621-636.

Reynolds, H. (1987). Bronchoalveolar lavage. American Review of Respiratory Disease 135:250-263.

Reynolds, H., Matthay, R. (2005). Diffuse interstitial and alveolar inflammatory disease. In George, R.B., Light, R.W., Matthay, M.A., & Matthay, R.A. (Eds). Chest medicine: essentials of pulmonary and critical care medicine, ed 5, Philadelphia: Lippincott Williams & Wilkins.

Rodrigo, G., Rodrigo, C., & Hall, J. (2004). Acute asthma in adults: a review. Chest 125:1081-1102.

Rogers, D.F. (2004). Airway mucus hypersecretion in asthma: an undervalued pathology? Current Opinions in Pharmacology 4:241-250.

Roussos, C., & Koutsoukou, A. (2003). Respiratory failure. European Respiratory Journal 47(Suppl):3S-14S.

Rowe, M.H. (1989). Effect of rapid mobilization on ejection fractions and ventricular volumes after myocardial infarction. American Journal of Cardiology 63:1037-1041.

Saetta, M., Di Stefano, A., Rosina, C., Thiene, G., & Fabbri, L.M. (1991). Quantitative structural analysis of peripheral airways and arteries in sudden fatal asthma. American Review of Respiratory Disease 143:138-143.

Saini, H.K., Arneja, A.S., & Dhalla, N.S. (2004). Role of cholesterol in cardiovascular dysfunction. Canadian Journal of Cardiology 20:333-346.

Saint, S., Bent, S., Vittinghoff, E., & Grady, D. (1985). Antibiotics in chronic obstructive pulmonary disease exacerbation: a meta-analysis. Journal of the American Medical Association 273: 957-960.

Sartori, C., & Scherrer, U. (2003). Turning up the heat in the lungs: a key mechanism to preserve their function. Advances in Experimental Medical Biology 543:263-275.

Schuler, G., Hambrecht, R., Schlierf, G., Grunze, M., Methfessel, S., Hauer, K., & Kuble, W. (1992). Myocardial perfusion and regression of coronary artery disease in patients on a regimen of intensive physical exercise and low fat diet. Journal of the American College of Cardiology 19:34-42.

Sciurba, F.C. (2004). Physiologic similarities and differences between COPD and asthma. Chest 126(Suppl):117S-124S.

Segal, B.L. (2003a). Valvular heart disease, part 1: diagnosis and surgical management of aortic valve disease in older adults. Geriatrics 58:31-35.

Segal, B.L. (2003b). Valvular heart disease, part 2: mitral valve disease in older adults. Geriatrics 58:26-31.

Selman, M. (2001). Idiopathic pulmonary fibrosis: challenges for the future. Chest 120:8-10.

Sethi, S., & Murphy, T.F (2004). Acute exacerbations of chronic bronchitis: new developments concerning microbiology and pathophysiology: impact on approaches to risk stratification and therapy. Infectious Disease Clinics of North America 18:861-882.

Seymour, J., & Presnelli, J. (2002). Pulmonary alveolar proteinosis: progress in the first 44 years. American Journal of Respiratory and Critical Care Medicine 166:215-235.

Shamsuzzaman, A.S., Gersh, B.J., & Somers, V.K. (2003). Obstructive sleep apnea: implications for cardiac and vascular disease. Journal of the American Medical Association 290:1906-1914.

Shapiro, J.M. (2002). Management of respiratory failure in status asthmaticus. American Journal of Respiratory Medicine 1:409-416.

Sharma, A.M. (2004). Is there a rationale for angiotensin blockade in the management of obesity hypertension? Hypertension 44:12-19.

Sharma, O.P. (1997). A clinical picture of sarcoidosis: treatment and prognosis. Resident and Staff Physician 23:123.

Sharpe, N. (2004). Cardiac remodeling in coronary artery disease. American Journal of Cardiology 93:17B-20B.

Silverberg, D., Wexler, D., Blum, M., Schwartz, D., & Iaina, A. (2004). The association between congestive heart failure and chronic renal disease. Current Opinions in Nephrology and Hypertension 13:163-170.

Silverberg, D., Wexler, D., Blum, M., Wollman, Y, & Iaina, A. (2003). The cardio-renal anaemia syndrome: does it exist? Nephrology, Dialysis and Transplantation 18(Suppl 8):viii7-12.

Solomon, H., & DeBusk, R.F. (2004). Contemporary management of silent ischemia: the role of ambulatory monitoring. International Journal of Cardiology 96:311-319.

Steen, V. (2004). The heart in systemic sclerosis. Current Rheumatology Reports 6:137-140.

Storms, W.W. (2003). Review of exercise-induced asthma. Medicine and Science in Sports and Exercise 35:1464-1470.

Strange, C., & Highland, K. (2004). Interstitial lung disease in the patient who has connective tissue disease. Clinics in Chest Medicine 25:549-559.

Sutherland, E., & Martin, R. (2000). COPD: combination therapy. In Martin, R., & Kraft, M. (Eds). Combination therapy for asthma and chronic obstructive pulmonary disease, New York: Marcel Dekker.

Sutherland, E.R., & Martin, R.J. (2003). Airway inflammation in chronic obstructive pulmonary disease: comparisons with asthma. Journal of Allergy Clinical Immunology 112:819-827.

Szmitko, P.E., Wang, C.H., Weisel, R.D., Jeffries, G.A., Anderson, T.J, & Verma, S. (2003). Biomarkers of vascular disease linking inflammation to endothelial activation: part II. Circulation 108:2041-2048.

Sztajel, J. (2004). Heart rate variability: a noninvasive electro-cardiographic method to measure the autonomic nervous system. Swiss Medical Weekly 134:514-522.

Tapson, V.F. (2004). Acute pulmonary embolism. Cardiology Clinics 22:353-365.

Tarlo, S.M., Boulet, L., Cartier, A., Cockcroft, D., Côté, J., Hargreave, F.E., Holness, L., Liss,G., Malo, J., & Chan-Yeung, M. (1998). Canadian Thoracic Society Guidelines for occupational asthma. Canadian Respiratory Journal 5:289-300.

Tenenbaum, A., & Fisman, E.Z. (2004). Impaired glucose metabolism in patients with heart failure: pathophysiology and possible treatment strategies. American Journal of Cardiovascular Drugs 4:269-280.

Thannickal, V.J., Toews, G.B., White, E.S., Lynch, J.P. 3rd, & Martinez, F.J. (2004). Mechanisms of pulmonary fibrosis. Annual Reviews in Medicine 55:395-417.

Thohan, V. (2004). Prognostic implications of echocardiography in advanced heart failure. Current Opinions in Cardiology 19:238-249.

Thurlbeck, W.M., & Wright, J.L. (1998). Thurlbeck's chronic airflow obstruction, ed 2, Hamilton: BC Decker.

Titcomb, C.P. Jr. (2004). LVH: consequences associated with cardiac remodeling. Journal of Insurance in Medicine 36:42-46.

Tomas, L.H., & Varkey, B. (2004). Improving health-related quality of life in chronic obstructive pulmonary disease. Current Opinions in Pulmonary Medicine 10:120-127.

Troosters, T., Gosselink, R., & Decramer, M. (2004). Chronic obstructive pulmonary disease and chronic heart failure: two muscle diseases? Journal of Cardiopulmonary Rehabilitation 24:137-145.

Trow, T.K. (2004). Lung-volume reduction surgery for severe emphysema: an appraisal of its current status. Current Opinions in Pulmonary Medicine 10:128-132.

Turner-Warwick, M. (1988). Epidemiology of nocturnal asthma. American Journal of Medicine 85:6-8.

Turner-Warwick, M., & Haslam, P. (1987). The value of serial bronchoalveolar lavages in assessing the clinical progress of patients with cryptogenic fibrosing alveolitis. American Review of Respiratory Disease 135:26-34.

Turner-Warwick, M., McAllister, W., Lawrence, R., Britten, A., & Haslam, P.L. (1986). Corticosteroid treatment in pulmonary sarcoidosis: do serial lavage lymphocyte counts, serum angiotensin converting enzyme measurements, and gallium-67 scans help management? Thorax 41:903-913.

United States Department of Health and Human Services. Reducing Tobacco Use. A Report of the Surgeon General: 2000. www.cdc.gov/tobacco.

Van Mieghem, C., Sabbe, M, & Knockaert, D. (2004). The clinical value of the ECG in noncardiac conditions. Chest 125:1561-1576.

Vasamreddy, C.R., Ahmed, D., Gluckman, T.J., & Blumenthal, R.S. (2004). Cardiovascular disease in athletes. Clinics in Sports Medicine 23:455-471.

Venkateshiah, S.B, Thomassen, M.J., & Kavuru, M.S. (2004). Pulmonary alveolar porteinosis: clinical manifestations and optimal treatment strategies. Treatments in Respiratory Medicine 3:217-227.

Verma, S., Buchanan, M.R., & Anderson, T.J. (2003). Endothelial function testing as a biomarker of vascular disease. Circulation 108:2054-2059.

Verma, S., Szmitko, P.E., & Anderson, T.J. (2004). Endothelial function: ready for prime time? Canadian Journal of Cardiology 20:1335-1339.

Vitali, E., Colombo, T., Garatti, A., Tarelli, G., Bruschi, G., & Ribera, E. (2004). Surgical treatment of acute myocardial infarction. Italian Heart Journal 5(Suppl 6):92S-99S.

Voelkel, N.F., & Cool, C. (2004). Pathology of pulmonary hypertension. Cardiology Clinics 22:343-351.

Wagh, A., & Stone, N.J. (2004). Treatment of metabolic syndrome. Expert Review of Cardiovascular Therapy 2:213-228.

Wagner, C.W. (2003). Pathophysiology and diagnosis of asthma. Nursing Clinics of North America 38:561-570.

Waldo, A.L. (2004). Mechanisms of atrial fibrillation. Journal of Cardiovascular Electrophysiology 14(12 Suppl):S267-S274.

Warburton, D.E.R., & Mathur, S. (2004). Skeletal muscle training in people with chronic heart failure or chronic obstructive pulmonary disease. Physiotherapy Canada 56:143-157.

Watters, L.C., King, T.E., Schwarz, M.I., Waldron, J.A., Stanford, R.E., & Cherniack, R.M. (1986). A clinical, radiological and physiological scoring system for the longitudinal assessment of patients with idiopathic pulmonary fibrosis. American Review of Respiratory Disease 133:97-103.

Watts, J. (1989). Thoracic compression for asthma. Chest 86:505.

Wehrens, X.H., & Doevendans, P.A. (2004). Cardiac rupture complicating myocardial infarction. International Journal of Cardiology 95:295-392.

Weitzenblum, E., & Chaouat, A. (2004). Sleep and chronic obstructive pulmonary disease. Sleep Medical Review 8:281-294.

Wenger, N. (1984). Early ambulation physical activity: myocardial infarction and coronary artery bypass surgery. Heart & Lung: The Journal of Critical Care 1:14-17.

Wenzel, S. (2003). Mechanisms of severe asthma. Clinical Experimental Allergy 33:1622-1628.

West, J.B. (2003). Pulmonary pathophysiology: the essentials, ed 6, Philadelphia: Lippincott Williams and Wilkins.

Willemse, B.W., Postma, D.S., Timens, W., & Hacken, N.H. (2004). The impact of smoking cessation on respiratory symptoms, lung function, airway hyperresponsiveness and inflammation. European Respiratory Journal 23:464-476.

Woolcock, A. (2000). Asthma. In Murray, J., & Nadel, J. (Eds). Textbook of respiratory medicine, ed 3, Philadelphia: Elsevier.

World Health Organization. International Classification of Functioning, Disability and Health. (2002). www.sustainable-design.ie/arch/ICIDH-2PFDec-2000.pdf; retrieved December 2004.

World Health Organization (2003). Venice Classification of Pulmonary Artery Hypertension.

Wouters, E.F. (2004). Management of severe COPD. Lancet 364:883-895.

Wright, J.L., Cagle, P., Churg, A., Colby, T.V., Myers, J. (1992). Diseases of the small airways. American Review of Respiratory Disease 146:240-262.

Wu, J.J., & Schiff, K.R. (2004). Sarcoidosis. American Family Physician 70:312-322.

Young, M.E. (2003). Circadian rhythms in cardiac gene expression. Current Hypertension Report 5:445-453.

Ziment, I. (1987). Theophylline and mucociliary clearance. Chest 92:385S-435S.

C H A P T E R   6

Cardiopulmonary Manifestations of Systemic Conditions

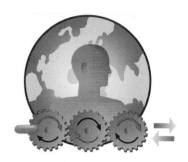

Elizabeth Dean

KEY TERMS

Connective tissue dysfunction
Endocrine dysfunction
Gastrointestinal dysfunction
Hematological dysfunction
Hepatic dysfunction
Immunological dysfunction

Malnutrition
Musculoskeletal dysfunction
Neurological dysfunction
Obesity
Renal dysfunction
Systemic disease

This chapter describes the cardiopulmonary consequences of systemic diseases. Systemic diseases can significantly affect oxygen transport, either directly or in combination with primary cardiopulmonary dysfunction. Although these effects can be as catastrophic as those resulting from primary cardiopulmonary dysfunction, their presentation is often subtle and may elude detection until significant impairment is apparent. The pulmonary and pleural complications of cardiac disease and the cardiac complications of pulmonary disease are described first. The cardiopulmonary complications of conditions involving the following systems are then described: musculoskeletal, connective tissue, neurological, gastrointestinal (GI), hepatic, renal, hematological, endocrine, and immunological. Finally, the cardiopulmonary manifestations of nutritional disorders, specifically obesity and starvation (anorexia nervosa), are presented.

To maximize the efficacy of their treatment prescriptions, physical therapists need to be able to predict the impact of systemic disease on oxygen transport in a given patient. Complications due to systemic disease are increasingly prevalent. This may reflect both the aging of the population and the improved survival rate and prognosis of patients with multisystem disease. In addition, physical therapists are treating an increasing number of patients without referral and thus may not be alerted by a referring practitioner to the presence and significance of underlying systemic disease. In their role as clinical exercise physiologists, physical therapists must be able to identify all factors that compromise or threaten oxygen transport so that treatment interventions can be prescribed most effectively and with minimal risk.

DIAGNOSIS AND ASSESSMENT

A comprehensive assessment of all factors that affect or threaten oxygen transport is essential, particularly in patients who are not obviously at risk (i.e., those without overt cardiopulmonary disease). The physical therapist must be able to "red-flag" a patient with an underlying problem for which physical therapy may be contraindicated or an untoward treatment response anticipated. Alternatively, treatment may have to be modified or treatment responses monitored more often.

Specific diagnosis of the factors that contribute to or threaten cardiopulmonary and cardiovascular dysfunction is tantamount to efficacious treatment across all physical therapy specialties. The overall capacity of the oxygen transport system

BOX 6-1

Systems and Systemic Conditions that Affect the Cardiopulmonary System and Oxygen Transport

Cardiopulmonary system
Musculoskeletal system
Connective tissue conditions
Collagen vascular conditions
Neurological system
Gastrointestinal system
Hepatic system
Renal system
Hematological system
Endocrine system
Immunological system
Nutritional disorders

should be established to ensure that it can adequately respond to changes in metabolic demand, including those imposed by physical therapy treatment. Even though cardiopulmonary dysfunction may not be the primary problem, it is essential to identify whether cardiopulmonary dysfunction can limit a patient's response to treatment, whether treatment should be modified to avert an incident, or whether treatment is contraindicated all together.

Oxygen transport can be significantly affected by dysfunction in the major organ systems of the body (Box 6-1). The pulmonary and pleural complications of heart disease and the cardiac complications of pulmonary disease are usually predictable and therefore are most readily detected clinically. The cardiopulmonary complications of conditions affecting other organ systems, however, can be more subtle, if not more devastating.

CARDIAC CONDITIONS

The pulmonary complications of heart disease and the cardiac complications of pulmonary disease are well known (Scharf & Cassidy, 1989). A mechanically inefficient heart disrupts the normal forward propulsion of deoxygenated and oxygenated blood to and from the lungs. Because the right and left sides of the heart are in series, a problem on one side inevitably has some effect, which can lead to a problem, on the other side. For these reasons the heart and lungs should be thought of as a single functioning unit. Disruption of the cardiopulmonary circuit leads to the backlogging of blood and an increased volume of blood in the capacitance vessels, or the veins. Right heart failure contributes to increased central venous pressure (i.e., right atrial pressure), and if sufficiently severe leads to bilateral peripheral edema in the dependent body parts. Because blood is not forwarded to the lungs adequately, hypoxemia can result. In turn, hypoxic vasoconstriction of the pulmonary circulation leads to increased pulmonary vascular resistance and, hence, to increased right ventricular afterload and work. Left heart failure can result in inadequate forward movement of blood through the left heart, resulting in backlogging in the pulmonary circulation and cardiogenic pulmonary edema. Pulmonary edema alters lung mechanics and lymphatic drainage and, in turn, these effects contribute to an increased risk for infection secondary to impaired macrophage function and bacterial growth. Excess pulmonary fluid around the alveolar capillary membrane creates a diffusion defect. If fluid accumulation is extreme, backlogging may be transmitted to the right side of the heart and to the periphery. Comparable to excess fluid in the lungs, backup of fluid in the peripheral circulation can impair tissue perfusion. Other cardiovascular conditions such as systemic hypertension increase systemic afterload, which, in turn, increase the work of the heart, thereby reducing its mechanical efficiency.

Pulmonary function can be significantly altered in cardiac disease (Bates, 1989). Left heart failure, for example, is associated with accumulation of fluid in the pulmonary interstitium. This leads to reduced caliber of the airways and early airway closure, air trapping, and increased residual volume. The fluid can produce reflex constriction of bronchial smooth muscle, leading to the syndrome of cardiac asthma. The combination of airway collapse and bronchoconstriction decreases total lung capacity, flow rates, and forced expiratory volumes. Ventilation and perfusion abnormalities are also associated with cardiac disease. Ventilation of underperfused lung zones contributes to increased ventilatory dead space, and perfusion of underventilated lung zones leads to a right-to-left shunt. In left heart failure, reduced lung compliance may contribute to inhomogeneous ventilation and perfusion.

In left heart failure, the normal pattern of increased ventilation to the bases may be reversed (i.e., the apices of the lungs may be better ventilated) (James et al, 1971). If pulmonary edema complicates the clinical picture, the alveoli become flooded, resulting in reduced ventilation and significant ventilation and perfusion mismatching. The alveolar-arterial oxygen (A-aO_2) gradient is then increased, diffusing capacity is decreased, and arterial partial pressure of oxygen (PaO_2) is decreased. Lung compliance is inversely related to pulmonary artery pressures and interstitial fluid accumulation (Saxton et al, 1956). The net effect of these abnormalities is both obstructive and restrictive pathophysiological patterns of lung dysfunction (i.e., reduced forced expiratory volumes and vital capacity and an overall increase in the work of breathing).

Pleural effusions can result from heart disease, in particular, congestive heart failure (CHF). Changes in intravascular pressures lead to transudative pleural effusions, and cardiac injury leads to exudative effusions. Comparable to fluid balance in other parts of the circulation, fluid balance in the lung is dependent on Starling forces (i.e., hydrostatic and oncotic pressures). In healthy individuals, several liters of fluid a day are absorbed from the pleural space, so when the balance of these forces is disrupted in disease, considerable fluid can accumulate in the pleural space. Impaired alveolar expansion due to pleural effusions is of clinical concern. Small effusions displace rather than compress the lung (Anthonisen & Martin, 1977).

PULMONARY CONDITIONS

Lung disease can contribute to cardiac dysfunction in several ways. Lung disease invariably threatens oxygen transport by its effects on respiratory mechanics and ventilation-perfusion matching. To compensate, the heart attempts to increase cardiac output, which produces a corresponding increase in cardiac work. Overall, ventilation and oxygen transport is less efficient. Hypoxemia secondary to inadequate ventilation-perfusion matching may predispose the patient to cardiac dysrhythmias.

Pleural complications can arise from lung disease as well as from heart disease. Both heart and lung function can be compromised by altered fluid balance in the pleurae. Fluid balance in the pleural space is comparable, in terms of its regulation, to that in the alveolar space. Both are determined by Starling forces. Specifically, hydrostatic pressure pushes fluid into the pleural space while oncotic pressure counters the effect of the hydrostatic forces. The net effect of these filtration and absorption forces is a minimal net filtration pressure. When the balance of these forces is disrupted, heart and lung function can be threatened. Excessive fluid floods the space, usually reflecting both excessive hydrostatic pressure and diminished oncotic pressure. The lymphatic vessels become overwhelmed and are unable to keep the pleural space dry. Pleural fluid accumulates and either displaces lung tissue (in small to moderate effusions) or restricts the opening of adjacent alveolar sacs, causing atelectasis (severe effusions) (Brown et al, 1978), which, if sufficiently severe, may restrict cardiac filling. Pleural fluid accumulation poses a unique threat to oxygen transport as a result of its direct physical effect on the lungs, heart, or both, so it warrants special attention by physical therapists.

Pulmonary lymphatics control fluid balance within the lung parenchyma. Lymphatic vessels arise within the pleurae and not within the alveolar capillary space. They drain fluid from the interlobular septae and subpleural areas into the hilar vessels and the primary tracheobronchial lymph nodes. Problems arising within the heart or lungs can contribute to imbalances in the major lymphatic inflow and outflow channels. This contributes to fluid accumulation, stagnation, and physical compression of the myocardium and lungs (Guyton & Hall, 2000).

Both heart and lung disease can produce deleterious hematological changes to compensate for hypoxemia. Increases in the number of red blood cells raise the hematocrit and viscosity of the blood. This phenomenon increases the work of the heart further. In addition, viscous blood increases the probability of thromboemboli. This risk is superimposed on the existing risk of thromboemboli in hypoeffective hearts.

A thorough understanding of the interrelationship of the heart and lungs is essential for diagnosis and optimal management. In addition, the cardiopulmonary and cardiovascular manifestations of other primary organ systems must be recognized and anticipated, particularly in patients with multi-system disease.

BOX 6-2

Cardiopulmonary Manifestations of Musculoskeletal Conditions

General Manifestations

↓ *Alveolar ventilation*

Altered respiratory mechanics
Chest wall rigidity
↓ Chest wall excursion

Impaired mucociliary transport

Airflow obstruction
Pulmonary restriction
Atelectasis
Inspissated secretions

↑ *Work of breathing*

Inefficient breathing pattern

↑ *Work of the heart*

Inefficient breathing pattern
Constrictive pericarditis

↓ *Aerobic capacity*

Manifestations in Specific Conditions

Rheumatoid arthritis

Pleuritis
Diffuse interstitial pneumonitis and fibrosis
Pulmonary arteritis
Bronchiolitis
Pleural effusions

Ankylosing spondylitis

Upper lobe fibrobullous disease
Chest wall restriction

MUSCULOSKELETAL CONDITIONS

Musculoskeletal conditions impact cardiopulmonary function secondary to their effects on muscle (in particular the diaphragm, muscles of the chest wall, oropharynx, larynx, and abdomen) and bones and joints (e.g., arthritis, ankylosing spondylitis, kyphoscoliosis, and the deformity secondary to neuromuscular diseases and chronic lung diseases) (Box 6-2). Additional effects are imposed by inactivity (i.e., muscle wasting, joint rigidity, and deformity). Increased joint rigidity limits the amount of physical activity a patient may perform, which contributes to cardiopulmonary compromise, in addition to the local effect of increased chest wall rigidity and compromised bucket-handle and pump-handle motions. The normal three-dimensional movement of the chest wall and normal pulmonary circulation and lymphatic function are compromised (Chapter 23). The cardiopulmonary manifestations of musculoskeletal conditions are summarized in Box 6-2.

The cardiopulmonary deficits associated with musculoskeletal disorders of the chest wall include reduced and potentially asymmetric lung volumes consistent with pulmonary

---

BOX 6-3

Cardiopulmonary Manifestations of Connective Tissue/Collagen Vascular Conditions

General Manifestations

Acute injury to the alveolar-capillary unit
Alveolar hemorrhage
Interstitial pneumonitis
Interstitial pulmonary fibrosis
Pulmonary hypertension
Respiratory muscle dysfunction
Pulmonary edema
Pulmonary infection
Abnormal diffusing capacity
Chest wall restriction

Specific Manifestations in Scleroderma

Restrictive ventilatory impairment
↓ Diffusing capacity
Diaphragmatic dysfunction
Gastroesophageal reflux and aspiration

---

restriction, reduced flow rates, reduced inspiratory and expiratory pressures, increased atelectasis, increased dynamic airway compression, ventilation-perfusion mismatching, inefficient breathing pattern, impaired cough and gag reflexes, increased risk for aspiration, increased risk for obstruction secondary to impaired mucociliary clearance, restricted mobility, compression of mediastinal structures and heart, and impaired lymphatic drainage, which depends on normal expiratory and inspiratory cycles (Bates, 1989).

CONNECTIVE TISSUE CONDITIONS

Connective tissue, or collagen, vascular disorders (e.g., scleroderma and systemic lupus erythematosus) invariably affect the cardiopulmonary system (Bagg & Hughes, 1979) (Box 6-3). Inflammation and tissue injury can affect the airway, lung parenchyma, pulmonary vasculature, pleurae, respiratory muscles, heart, and pericardium. Shrinking-lung syndrome associated with chronic connective tissue changes is a feature of advanced disease and is characterized by a significant loss of alveolar surface area, diffusion capacity, and lung volumes. Fibrotic changes increase the elasticity of the lung parenchyma and reduce lung compliance, thereby increasing the work of breathing. These changes are comparable to those in idiopathic pulmonary fibrosis. Both the electrical conduction system of the heart and its mechanical behavior are adversely affected by systemic connective tissue changes (Goldman & Kotler, 1985). Furthermore, connective tissue changes in the skin can lead to chest wall restriction. The cardiopulmonary manifestations of connective tissue conditions are summarized in Box 6-3.

NEUROLOGICAL CONDITIONS

Cardiopulmonary consequences of neurological disease reflect the specific pathophysiological mechanisms involved (Griggs & Donohoe, 1982). There are three basic patterns of pathology: involvement of the central nervous system (CNS), involvement of the peripheral nervous system, and involvement of the autonomic nervous system. The cardiopulmonary manifestations of neurological conditions are summarized in Box 6-4.

Involvement of the CNS

The primary centers for breathing control and control of the heart are seated in the midbrain. The generator for breathing control produces a regular respiratory rate through modulation of inspiratory and expiratory inhibitory and excitatory neurons.

Activity of the central generator is affected by arousal and the general alerting reaction of the reticular activating system. In addition, breathing control is influenced by the hypothalamus, orbital cortex, forebrain, and amygdala (Hitchcock & Leece, 1967).

Insult to the CNS can result in cardiovascular responses that precipitate neurogenic pulmonary edema. Such responses include systemic hypertension, pulmonary hypertension, intracranial hypertension, and bradycardia. The medulla is believed to mediate the cardiovascular responses associated with neurogenic pulmonary edema. Marked sympathetic stimulation, catecholamine release, and vagotonia appear to precipitate neurogenic pulmonary edema and the resulting leaking of the alveolar capillary membrane and alveolar flooding (Colice, 1985). The possibility of a primary pulmonary endothelial permeability abnormality has been suggested, however (Peterson et al, 1983).

Cortical disturbances may have a direct effect on cardiopulmonary function. Among the most common disturbances seen clinically are cortical infarction and seizures. Hemispheric infarction can lead to contralateral weakness of the diaphragm and other respiratory muscles. Epileptic seizures disrupt breathing, which causes hypoxemia, respiratory acidosis, and a metabolic acidosis secondary to extreme muscle contraction and lactate accumulation. The associated increase in sympathetic stimulation can precipitate cardiac dysrhythmias and pulmonary edema.

Demyelinating diseases such as multiple sclerosis result in progressive deterioration of neuromuscular function. The muscles of respiration become increasingly involved, resulting in respiratory insufficiency due to weakness (Cooper et al, 1985). In addition, with increasing debility, cardiopulmonary conditioning is reduced. Weakness of the pharyngeal musculature contributes to loss of airway protection in addition to the loss of cough and gag reflexes. Aspiration is problematic for these patients as the disease advances.

Patients with stroke may have central involvement that affects cardiopulmonary regulation and function, including reduced electrical activity of the respiratory muscles or peripheral involvement such that weakness, spasticity, impaired

---

BOX 6-4

Cardiopulmonary Manifestations of Neurological Conditions

General Manifestations

Impaired mucociliary transport

↓ Physical mobility
Cilia dyskinesia
↑ Mucus accumulation
↓ Cough and gag reflexes
Impaired airway protection
↑ Airway resistance
↑ Risk of airway obstruction
Impaired glottic closure
↑ Risk of aspiration

Impaired alveolar ventilation

↓ Lung volumes and capacities, as well as flow rates
Weakness of pharyngeal and laryngeal structures
Respiratory muscle weakness
↓ Respiratory muscle endurance

↑ Work of breathing

↓ Aerobic capacity and deconditioning

Manifestations in Specific Conditions

Multiple sclerosis

Respiratory muscle weakness
Impaired ventilation secondary to spasm
↑ Oxygen consumption secondary to spasm
↑ Oxygen consumption secondary to impaired posture and gait
Impaired gag and cough reflexes
Ineffective cough

Cerebral palsy

↑ Oxygen consumption secondary to increased muscle tone
↓ Mobility and activity
Impaired movement economy
Impaired swallowing
Impaired saliva control
↓ Gag and cough reflexes
Impaired coordination of thoracic and abdominal motion during respiration
Ineffective cough and airway clearance mechanisms

Stroke

↓ Movement economy
Spasticity and increased oxygen demands
Flaccidity of respiratory muscles
Impaired respiratory muscle strength
Impaired pulmonary function
Asymmetric chest wall
Weak and ineffective cough

Parkinson syndrome

↑ Oxygen consumption secondary to increased muscle tone
↓ Movement economy
Chest wall restriction and impaired pulmonary function
Ineffective cough

---

biomechanics, and gait directly affect respiratory muscle function and chest wall excursion (DeTroyer et al, 1981). Hemiparesis of the diaphragm on the affected side can occur. Abdominal muscle weakness contributes to impaired cough effectiveness. Pharyngeal weakness contributes to sleep apnea in these patients. The common clinical presentation of unilateral involvement leads to a posture listing to the affected side when recumbent or sitting, and during ambulation. This posture impairs ventilation and chest wall expansion on the affected side. Abdominal muscle involvement directly affects intraabdominal pressure and the efficiency of diaphragmatic descent during contraction (i.e., should the abdominal muscles become flaccid, the efficiency of diaphragmatic contraction is significantly reduced). Lung volumes and flow rates are reduced proportionately, causing a restrictive pattern of lung function. Muscle spasticity contributes to chest wall restriction and increased metabolic cost. Reduced activity and exercise around the time of the stroke contribute to reduced cardiopulmonary conditioning and capacity of the oxygen transport system. A high proportion of patients with strokes are hypertensive and older, a population with a higher prevalence of heart disease and atherosclerosis (Chimowitz & Mancini, 1991).

Cerebral palsy is associated with significantly increased muscle tone, which correspondingly increases basal and exercise oxygen consumption, resulting in increased oxygen demands. Even though the demands are increased in this condition, oxygen delivery is compromised. For example, thoracic deformity and spasm of the muscles of the chest wall and abdomen impair the breathing pattern and its efficiency (Fullford & Brown, 1976). The airways of patients with cerebral palsy are vulnerable to obstruction because of poor gag, cough, and swallowing reflexes. In addition, these patients often have poor saliva control, which further increases the risk of aspiration. Mental retardation often complicates the presentation of cerebral palsy and prevents these patients from responding adequately to their hydration needs and being able to cooperate with life-preserving treatments (Bates, 1989). These patients harbor numerous microorganisms, which adds further to their general risk for infection.

Patients with Parkinson syndrome also exhibit significant cardiopulmonary deficits (Mehta et al, 1978). Oxygen demand is increased commensurate with increased muscle tone. Patients with Parkinson syndrome have reduced cardiopulmonary conditioning levels as a result of compromised agility and ability to be independently mobile. These patients have a restrictive pattern of lung disease in which most lung volumes and capacities are reduced. Chest wall rigidity impairs the normal pump-handle and bucket-handle movements, so breathing efficiency is reduced. The energy cost of breathing is correspondingly increased. Respiratory insufficiency in Parkinson syndrome likely reflects increases in tone of the respiratory muscles, chest wall rigidity, and parasympathetic tone and resulting airway obstruction.

Patients with a history of poliomyelitis, with or without cardiopulmonary complications at onset, may exhibit pulmonary limitation several decades later (Dean et al, 1991; Steljes et al, 1990). These individuals are at risk for developing respiratory insufficiency as a result of respiratory and abdominal muscle weakness, chest wall deformity, minor infection, and periods of relative immobility; or secondary to medical interventions, such as anesthesia and sedation. Further, because of prolonged reduced physical activity, patients with chronic poliomyelitis may be overweight.

Diseases and lesions involving the brainstem can lead to various abnormal breathing patterns. Some common breathing aberrations are Cheyne-Stokes respiration, central neurogenic hyperventilation, apneustic breathing, and ataxic breathing. Cerebellar and basal ganglia lesions may produce respiratory muscle discoordination and dyspnea (Hormia, 1957; Neu et al, 1967).

Spinal cord lesions have a variable effect on cardiopulmonary function, depending on the level of the lesion. Cervical lesions result in a high mortality rate due to cardiopulmonary complications. All lung volumes are diminished with the exception of total lung capacity (TLC), which over time returns to normal; tidal volume (TV), which is usually preserved (10% of TLC); and residual volume (RV), which is significantly increased (Estenne & DeTroyer, 1987; Fugl-Meyer, 1971). Patients with quadriplegia tend to have a greater diaphragmatic contribution to tidal ventilation than healthy people (Estenne & DeTroyer, 1985). In addition, these patients have impaired cough as a result of the loss of innervation and paresis of the diaphragm, in some cases, and of abdominal and intercostal muscles. The contribution of accessory muscle activity to ventilation varies considerably (McKinley et al, 1969). In quadriplegia in which only the accessory muscles and diaphragm have been spared, platypnea (increased dyspnea when upright) may occur (Dantzker et al, 1997). In the upright position, the diaphragm is flattened and less efficient when moved downward by reduced abdominal pressures.

Thoracic lesions tend to have less effect on pulmonary function (vital capacity and forced expiratory volumes in particular) than cervical lesions, and the significance of this effect is reduced as the level of the lesion is reduced. Lumbar lesions may have minimal or no effect on pulmonary function; however, involvement of the abdominal muscles may limit cough effectiveness.

Involvement of the Peripheral Nervous System

Disorders of the peripheral nervous system include those of the motor neuron, peripheral nerve, neuromuscular junction, and muscle. Neuromuscular disorders of the larynx, pharynx, and tongue can lead to upper airway obstruction and increased airway resistance and can interfere with maintaining a clear airway. Aspiration is a common and serious problem associated with impaired motor control of the larynx, pharynx, and tongue.

Involvement of the Autonomic Nervous System

Cardiopulmonary consequences of disorders of the autonomic nervous system have been documented. Of those diseases with an autonomic component, autonomic neuropathies, diabetes, and alcoholism have been the most thoroughly studied. Multiple-system atrophy accompanies autonomic failure affecting multiple systems. Because of the anatomic proximity of the autonomic, respiratory, and hypnogenic neurons and the degeneration of these structures in this condition, dysfunction of the respiratory control mechanisms parallels autonomic and somatic dysfunction. The respiratory dysrhythmias that are seen in multiple-system atrophy include central and upper airway obstruction; irregular rate, rhythm, and amplitude of respiration, with or without oxygen desaturation; transient uncoupling of the intercostal and diaphragmatic muscle activity; prolonged periods of apnea; Cheyne-Stokes respiration; inspiratory gasps; and transient sudden respiratory arrest (Bannister & Mathais, 2002).

Patients with diabetes and autonomic neuropathies exhibit variable cardiopulmonary dysfunction. Postural hypotension is a complication of diabetic autonomic neuropathy and efferent sympathetic vasomotor denervation. Norepinephrine levels are generally reduced in these patients. The splanchnic and peripheral circulations fail to constrict in response to standing, so cardiac output falls. The postural effect is exacerbated by reduced cardiac acceleration in patients with diabetes. Insulin has been associated with cardiovascular effects, including reduced plasma volume, increased peripheral blood flow secondary to vasodilation, and increased heart rate. In the presence of autonomic neuropathies, insulin can induce postural hypotension. Diabetic diarrhea secondary to abnormal gut motility can contribute to fluid loss and its sequelae. Cardiopulmonary changes associated with autonomic neuropathy secondary to diabetes include altered ventilatory responses to hypoxia and hypercapnia, altered respiratory pattern and apneic episodes during sleep, altered bronchial reactivity, and impaired cough (Bannister & Mathais 2002; Montserrat et al, 1985). Impaired peripheral perfusion and tissue nutrition are also consequences of diabetes and autonomic neuropathies, which will be described later in this chapter under the heading Endocrine Conditions.

GASTROINTESTINAL CONDITIONS

The cardiopulmonary manifestations of gastrointestinal (GI) dysfunction are summarized in Box 6-5. Inflammatory bowel disease and pancreatitis are principal examples of GI dysfunction that affects cardiopulmonary function. Aspiration is a significant cause of morbidity and mortality in patients with GI dysfunction, so it should be prevented or detected

---

BOX 6-5

Cardiopulmonary Manifestations of GI Conditions

Risk of aspiration

Gastroesophageal reflux

↑ **Airway resistance**

Bronchospasm

↓ **Lung volumes**

Elevated hemidiaphragms
Compression atelectasis

Arterial hypoxemia

Alveolar capillary leak and V/Q mismatch
Alveolar hemorrhage and consolidation worsen shunt
↑ Pulmonary vascular resistance

BOX 6-6

Cardiopulmonary Manifestations of Liver Conditions

Intrapulmonary vascular dilation
Pulmonary hypertension
Expiratory airflow obstruction
Chest wall deformity
Pleural effusions
Panacinar emphysema
Pleuritis
Bronchitis
Bronchiectasis
Hypoxic vasoconstriction
Interstitial pneumonitis
Pulmonary fibrosis

---

early. The pathophysiology, management, and outcome depend on the nature of the aspirate. Several predisposing factors produce aspiration pneumonia, including a decreased level of consciousness, disorders of pharyngeal and esophageal motility, altered anatomy, disorders of gastric and intestinal motility, and iatrogenic factors such as surgery, nasogastric intubation, and general anesthesia.

Inflammatory bowel disease can lead to the following cardiopulmonary pathologies: vasculitis, fibrosis, granulomatous disease, and pulmonary thromboembolism. Bronchitis and bronchiectasis have also been associated with inflammatory bowel disease; however, their occurrence is not related to disease severity or therapy. Biopsy specimens have shown basement membrane thickening, thickening of the epithelium, and infiltration of the underlying connective tissue with inflammatory cells (Higenbottam et al, 1980).

The pulmonary manifestations of pancreatitis are among the most important sequelae of this disease. Of the deaths that occur in the first week of hospitalization, 60% are associated with respiratory failure (Renner et al, 1985). Problems include elevated hemidiaphragms, particularly on the right side; basal atelectasis; diffuse pulmonary infiltrates that appear more commonly on the right side than on the left side; pleural effusions that occur more commonly on the left side than on the right side; and pneumonitis. These findings are not specific for pancreatitis and are probably secondary to localized peritonitis, subphrenic collections, ascites, pain, and abdominal distension. In chronic pancreatitis, abdominal symptoms may be reduced and thoracic symptoms such as dyspnea, chest pain, and cough may predominate. Chronic effusions may result in pleural thickening.

LIVER CONDITIONS

Both acute and chronic liver conditions can predispose a patient to cardiopulmonary and cardiovascular complications (Box 6-6). Hepatic dysfunction can lead to hypoxemia secondary to intrapulmonary vascular dilation and noncardiogenic

pulmonary edema. Hepatopulmonary syndrome, hallmarked by intrapulmonary vascular dilation, produces both diffusion and perfusion defects in the lungs and is the principal reason for severe hypoxemia (Sherlock, 1988). The origin of pulmonary edema is secondary to hepatic encephalopathy and cerebral edema (Trewby et al, 1978).

With respect to chronic liver conditions, cardiopulmonary manifestations have been associated with cirrhosis and hepatitis. The most common pulmonary abnormalities associated with these conditions are intrapulmonary vascular dilation with and without shunt, pulmonary hypertension, airflow obstruction, chest wall deformity, pleural effusions, panacinar emphysema, pleuritis, bronchitis, bronchiectasis, hypoxic vasoconstriction, interstitial pneumonitis, and fibrosis. Hypoxemia results from shunting, ventilation-perfusion mismatching, and diffusion abnormalities.

Pleural effusions and ascites interfere with diaphragm function and present unique problems in a patient with liver disease. Rich lymphatic connections exist between the abdominal and thoracic cavities, so ascitic fluid can flow into the pleural space. This effect is enhanced during inspiration, when the intraabdominal pressure is relatively positive and the intrapleural space is negative (Crofts, 1954).

The liver is a primary organ for the production of procoagulants and anticoagulants in the blood, both of which are carefully regulated to maintain optimal balance. Liver dysfunction can disrupt the production of these complementary agents and lead to a tendency to bleed or clot. Disseminated intravascular coagulation refers to an extreme imbalance between these vasoactive agents in which bleeding and clotting problems occur simultaneously, resulting in serious consequences to the patient. With respect to central involvement, recently impaired myocardial contractility has been reported in patients with cirrhosis (Laffi et al, 1997).

RENAL CONDITIONS

Cardiopulmonary complications can result from renal dysfunction and from the category of disorders referred to as renal-pulmonary syndromes (Box 6-7) (Matthay et al, 1980;

BOX 6-7

Cardiopulmonary Manifestations of Renal Conditions

Alveolar hemorrhage
Airway obstruction
↓ Lung volumes
↓ Diffusing capacity

BOX 6-8

Cardiopulmonary Manifestations of Hematological Conditions

General Cardiopulmonary Manifestations

Hemorrhage
Edema
Polycythemia
Anemia
Infection

Abnormalities of the Fluid Portion of the Blood

Abnormal blood volume
Abnormal fluid balance (water excesses and deficits)
Abnormal electrolytes
Abnormal plasma proteins
Abnormal procoagulants and anticoagulants
Abnormal clotting times

Abnormalities of the Cellular Portion of the Blood

Abnormal red blood cell count
Abnormal red blood cells
Abnormal deformability of the red blood cells
Abnormal hemoglobin
Abnormal oxyhemoglobin dissociation (e.g., carbon monoxide poisoning)
Abnormal white blood cells and antibodies
Blood dyscrasias

Rankin & Matthay, 1982). The pathophysiological characteristics of these disorders include alveolar hemorrhage, interstitial and alveolar inflammation, and involvement of the pulmonary vasculature. Pulmonary function testing may detect both obstructive and restrictive abnormalities as a result of bronchial complications and as a result of inflammation and hemorrhage, respectively.

In systemic illness, pathology of the lungs and kidneys often coexist. Physical therapy warrants being aggressive, given the course of the renal-pulmonary syndromes and the potential for relapses and irreversible organ damage.

HEMATOLOGICAL CONDITIONS

Hematological disorders that can manifest cardiopulmonary symptoms include abnormalities of the fluid and cellular components of the blood, and coagulopathies (Bromberg & Ross, 2000). Cardiopulmonary manifestations of hematological conditions are summarized in Box 6-8. The primary underlying mechanisms by which these conditions disrupt gas exchange include hemorrhage, infection, edema, anemia, fibrosis, and malignancies.

Abnormalities related to red blood cells and their ability to transport hemoglobin and oxygen may produce signs resembling pulmonary pathology, (e.g., tachypnea, dyspnea, and cyanosis). Abnormalities of the deformability of red blood cells alter blood viscosity and pulmonary blood flow. The interstitium can be disrupted by such factors as hemorrhage and malignancies. Coagulopathies disrupt the normal hemostasis and clotting mechanisms of the blood. Pulmonary hemorrhage and hemoptysis are common sequelae. The most common causes of pulmonary hemorrhage include vitamin-K deficiency, hemophilia, hepatic failure, and disseminated intravascular coagulation. Pharmacological agents such as platelet inhibitors and anticoagulants can also result in pulmonary hemorrhage. Pulmonary thromboemboli are common events; symptoms include pleuritic chest pain, dyspnea, and hemoptysis.

Of the erythrocyte disorders, sickle cell anemia is probably the most common. Acute chest infection and thrombosis leading to pulmonary infarction may occur with clinical symptoms such as fever, pleuritic chest pain, cough, and pulmonary infiltrates. The pulmonary function of patients with sickle cell anemia is abnormal; there is likely to be a reduction in TLC, vital capacity, diffusing capacity, arterial oxygen tensions, and exercise capacity (Femi-Pearse et al, 1970).

The hematological malignancy disorders that can affect pulmonary function include the leukemias and Hodgkin disease. The three primary mechanisms by which these disorders can affect pulmonary function include direct infiltration, increased risk of opportunistic infection, and secondary effects of treatment, such as interstitial pneumonitis and fibrosis.

Disorders of plasma proteins can have significant effects on the Starling forces that maintain normal fluid balance within the tissue vascular beds. Depending on the amount of plasma protein, particularly albumin, fluid is retained in or lost from circulation. With reduced protein and oncotic pressure within the vasculature, more fluid is filtered out of the circulation into the interstitium. In catabolic states in which protein is broken down in the body, more protein leaks through the capillaries and takes water with it, thus leading to edema.

ENDOCRINE CONDITIONS

Endocrine and metabolic disorders can be associated with cardiopulmonary complications (Box 6-9) (Guyton & Hall, 2000; Kirby et al, 1996). Disorders of the thyroid gland, pancreas (diabetes mellitus), and adrenal glands are examples that are often seen clinically. Thyroid hormone influences surfactant synthesis and the central drive to breathe. Hypothyroidism can lead to sleep apnea, pleural effusions

---

BOX 6-9

Cardiopulmonary Manifestations of Endocrine Conditions

Thyroid Disorders

Hypothyroidism

Hypometabolism
Fatigue and excessive sleeping
↓ Aerobic conditioning
↓ Vital capacity secondary to muscle weakness
Sleep apnea
↓ Heart rate
↓ Cardiac output
↓ Blood volume
Pleural effusions
Pericardial effusions

Hyperthyroidism

Hypermetabolism
↓ Vital capacity and diffusing capacity
Fluid loss (diarrhea)
Respiratory muscle weakness
Fatigue and inability to sleep
↓ Aerobic conditioning

Pancreatic Disorders (Diabetes)

↑ Pulmonary endothelial thickness
↓ TLC

↓ Vital capacity and forced expiratory volumes
↓ Airway vagal tone
↑ Risk of aspiration
Possible reduced elastic recoil
Impaired hypoxic and hypercapnic responses
Impaired ventilatory response to exercise
Defective neutrophil production
Colonization with gram-negative bacilli
Pleural effusions and pulmonary edema with diabetic
   nephropathy
↑ Sensitivity to increases in inspiratory resistive loading
Accelerated atherosclerotic vascular and cardiac changes
↑ Ischemic heart disease
Cardiomyopathy
↑ Risk of infection

Adrenal Insufficiency

Orthostatic symptoms
↓ Aerobic capacity secondary to anorexia, weakness and
   fatigue
Impaired breathing mechanics secondary to GI symptoms
↑ Tendency to retain fluid

---

secondary to altered capillary permeability, and pericardial effusions. Decreases in vital capacity have also been reported secondary to muscle weakness. Individuals with hypothyroidism have exercise intolerance (Kahaly et al, 2002). Hyperthyroidism increases cellular oxidative metabolism (the metabolic rate), leading to an increase in oxygen consumption and CO_2 production and an overall increase in minute ventilation (Kahaly et al, 2002). Vital capacity, lung compliance, and diffusion capacity can be reduced. In addition, maximal inspiratory and expiratory pressures can be reduced secondary to muscle weakness. In thyroid dysfunction, cardiorespiratory function can be normal at rest but dysfunction can be unmasked during exercise stress.

Individuals with diabetes are prone to aspiration and respiratory infections. Late complications of diabetic neuropathy include renal failure, which may be accompanied by pleural effusions and pulmonary edema. Autonomic neuropathy may affect vagal activity and airway tone and the vasomotor tone of the blood vessels. Ischemic heart disease and cardiomyopathies are common in patients with diabetes and may cause CHF and cardiogenic pulmonary edema. Patients with diabetes have been reported to have reduced sensitivity to inspiratory loading (O'Donnell et al, 1988), which may impair their subjective responses to exercise. Peripheral perfusion can be compromised, resulting in diabetes. Limbs are endangered by reduced perfusion and reduced sensation. Severe cases result in limb ischemia, gangrene, and surgical amputation. Infection rates are high in patients with diabetes.

Adrenal insufficiency can also compromise oxygen transport (Kirby et al, 1996). Reduced aerobic capacity results from symptoms of weakness and fatigue and associated muscle and joint complaints. Orthostatic intolerance primarily reflects reduced inotrophic capacity of the heart and reduced systemic vascular resistance.

IMMUNOLOGICAL CONDITIONS

Congenital and acquired defects in the immunological status of the lungs lead to cardiopulmonary dysfunction, including inflammation and infection. In addition, patients who are immunodeficient have an increased risk for pulmonary malignancies (Shackleford & McAlister, 1975).

Acquired immunodeficiency syndrome (AIDS), an example of a primary disorder of cell-mediated immunity, has reached epidemic proportions over the past 20 years. This syndrome leads to lymphocyte death. The most serious pulmonary infection associated with AIDS is *Pneumocystis carinii* pneumonia (Murray et al, 1984). The fact that a patient with the human immunodeficiency virus (HIV) is likely to have recurrent pneumonia suggests that the infecting organisms persist in the lung despite treatment (Shelhamer et al, 1984). The clinical presentation includes diffuse pulmonary infiltrates, cough, dyspnea, and hemoptysis. These patients can also have symptoms of upper airway obstruction.

NUTRITIONAL DISORDERS

The two most common nutritional disorders seen in Western countries are obesity and anorexia nervosa, which is akin to starvation. Two thirds of the population is now categorized as being overweight and at risk for its sequelae. Obesity contributes in several ways to impaired oxygen transport (Alexander, 1985; Bates, 1989). Alveolar hypoventilation and impaired PaO_2 and gas exchange result from chest wall restriction. Systemic and pulmonary blood pressures are increased. In addition, large abdomens and abdominal contents impinge on diaphragmatic motion and can restrict diaphragmatic descent. This can lead to compression of the dependent lung fields. Recumbency can induce respiratory insufficiency (positional respiratory failure). Individuals who are obese have a higher incidence of snoring and obstructive sleep apnea secondary to weakness and increased compliance of the postpharyngeal structures. In addition, these patients often have weak, ineffectual coughs resulting from expiratory muscle weakness and the mechanical inefficiency of these muscles. The work of breathing is markedly increased. Furthermore, in chronic cases, reactive pulmonary vasoconstriction in response to chronic hypoxemia contributes to right ventricular insufficiency and increased work of the heart and cardiomegaly. Individuals who are obese tend to be less active and aerobically deconditioned, with reduced efficiency of oxygen transport overall and increased risk for thromboemboli. Hypertension is also a serious sequela of obesity.

The major cardiopulmonary manifestations of anorexia nervosa relate to generalized weakness and reduced endurance of all muscles, including the respiratory muscles. Cough effectiveness is correspondingly compromised. Oxygen transport reserve is minimal. Because of poor nutrition and fluid intake, the patient is at significant risk for anemia, fluid and electrolyte imbalances, and cardiac dysrhythmias (Kasper et al, 2004). Common manifestations of nutritional disorders are summarized in Box 6-10.

SUMMARY

This chapter describes the cardiopulmonary consequences of common systemic conditions. Oxygen transport, the purpose of the cardiopulmonary system, can be significantly affected by dysfunction in virtually all organ systems of the body. The pathophysiological consequences of conditions of the following systems of oxygen transport are presented: cardiac, pulmonary, musculoskeletal, connective tissue/collagen vascular, neurological, gastrointestinal, hepatic, renal, hematological, endocrine, and immunological. In addition, the cardiopulmonary manifestations of nutritional disorders, including obesity and anorexia nervosa, are described.

Knowledge of these effects is essential to the practice of physical therapy across all specialties because of the prevalence of systemic conditions either singly or in combination. The presentation of the cardiopulmonary consequences of systemic conditions is often subtle or obscured

---

BOX 6-10

Cardiopulmonary Manifestations of Nutritional Disorders

Obesity

Alveolar hypoventilation
Obstructive sleep apnea
↓ Outward recoil of the chest wall
↑ Abdominal contents
↑ Mass of the abdominal wall
↓ Functional residual capacity
↓ Expiratory reserve volume
↓ Lung volumes, arterial oxygen tension (PaO_2) and saturation (SaO_2) in recumbency
Basal airway closure and resulting ↓ PaO_2
Marked pulmonary abnormalities during sleep
↓ Ventilatory responses to CO_2
Cardiomegaly
Rotation and horizontal position of the heart
Axis deviation on ECG
↓ Myocardial pumping efficiency
↓ Aerobic conditioning and oxygen transport reserve capacity

Starvation or Anorexia Nervosa

Generalized weakness, debility, ↓ cardiopulmonary conditioning
Impaired mucociliary transport
Ineffective cough
Fluid and electrolyte disturbances
Cardiac dysrhythmias
Respiratory muscle weakness

---

and is associated with a poor prognosis, so early detection and appropriate management are essential.

Physical therapists need to be able to diagnostically distinguish cardiopulmonary manifestations of systemic conditions in order to appropriately identify indications for physical therapy, contraindications, side effects, and unusual treatment responses. In addition, detailed assessment of the patient's problems ensures that problems amenable to physical therapy are appropriately treated and that those that are not are referred back to a physician. These skills are particularly important given the advent of direct-access practice and that a high proportion of patients being treated by physical therapists have systemic conditions as secondary diagnoses as well as primary diagnoses. Further, cardiopulmonary manifestations of systemic diseases may not have been previously diagnosed, but rather identified on the physical therapy assessment or manifested by the patient during exercise stress.

Review Questions

Describe the cardiopulmonary manifestations and clinical implications when a patient has one or more of the following types of dysfunction:

1. Musculoskeletal dysfunction (chest wall and peripheral)
2. Connective tissue dysfunction

3. Neurological dysfunction
4. Hepatic dysfunction
5. Renal dysfunction
6. Hematological dysfunction
7. Endocrine dysfunction
8. Obesity
9. Malnutrition (e.g., anorexia nervosa)

REFERENCES

Alexander, J.K. (1985). The cardiomyopathy of obesity. Progress in Cardiovascular Disease 27:325-334.

Anthonisen, N.R, & Martin, R.R. (1977). Regional lung function in pleural effusions. American Review of Respiratory Diseases 116:201-206.

Bagg, L.R., & Hughes, D.T. (1979). Serial pulmonary function tests in progressive systemic sclerosis. Thorax 34:224-228.

Bannister, R., & Mathais, C.J. (2002). Autonomic failure, ed 4. New York: Oxford University Press.

Bates, D.V. (1989). Respiratory function in disease, ed 3. Philadelphia: WB Saunders.

Bromberg, P.A., & Ross, D.W. (2000). The lungs and hematologic disease. In Murray, J.F., & Nadel, J. (Eds). Textbook of respiratory medicine, ed 3. Philadelphia: WB Saunders.

Brown, N.E., Zamel, N., & Aberman, A. (1978). Changes in pulmonary mechanics and gas exchange following thoracentesis. Chest 74:540-542.

Chimowitz, M.I., & Mancini, G.B.J. (1991). Asymptomatic coronary artery disease in patients with stroke. Current Concepts of Cerebrovascular Diseases and Stroke 26:23-27.

Colice, G.L. (1985). Neurogenic pulmonary edema. Clinics in Chest Medicine 6:473-489.

Cooper, C.B., Trend, P.S., & Wiles, C.M. (1985). Severe diaphragm weakness in multiple sclerosis. Thorax 40:631-632.

Crofts, N.F. (1954). Pneumothorax complicating therapeutic pneumoperitoneum. Thorax 9:226-228.

Dantzker, D.R., Schay, S.M., & Fletcher, J. (1997). Cardiopulmonary critical care, ed 3. Philadelphia: Elsevier.

Dean, E., Ross, J., Road, J.D., Courtenay, L., & Madill, K. (1991). Pulmonary function in individuals with a history of poliomyelitis. Chest 100:118-123.

DeTroyer, A., De Beyl, D.Z., & Thirion, M. (1981). Function of the respiratory muscles in acute hemiplegia. American Review of Respiratory Diseases 123:631-632.

Estenne, M., & DeTroyer, A. (1985). Relationship between respiratory muscle electromyogram and rib cage motion in tetraplegia. American Review of Respiratory Diseases 132:53-59.

Estenne, M., & DeTroyer, A. (1987). Mechanism of the postural dependence of vital capacity in tetraplegic subjects. American Review of Respiratory Diseases 135:367-371.

Femi-Pearse, D., Gazioglu, K.M., & Yu, P.N. (1970). Pulmonary function and infection in sickle cell disease. Journal of Applied Physiology 28:574-577.

Fugl-Meyer, A.R. (1971). A model for treatment of impaired ventilatory function in tetraplegic patients. Scandinavian Journal of Rehabilitation Medicine 3:168-177.

Fullford, F.E., & Brown, J.K. (1976). Position as a cause of deformity in children with cerebral palsy. Developmental Medicine in Child Neurology 18:305-314.

Goldman, A.P., & Kotler, M.N. (1985). Heart disease in scleroderma. American Heart Journal 110:1043-1046.

Griggs, R.C., & Donohoe, K.M. (1982). Recognition and management of respiratory insufficiency in neuromuscular disease. Journal of Chronic Diseases 35:497-500.

Guyton, A.C., & Hall, J.E. (2000). Textbook of medical physiology, ed 10. Philadelphia: Elsevier.

Higenbottam, T., Cochrane, G.M., Clark, T.J.H., Turner, D., Millis, R., & Seymour, W. (1980). Bronchial disease in ulcerative colitis. Thorax, 35: 581-5.

Hitchcock, E., & Leece, B. (1967). Somatotopic representation of the respiratory pathways in the cervical cord of man. Journal of Neurosurgery 27:320-329.

Hormia, A.L. (1957). Respiratory insufficiency as a symptom of cerebellar ataxia. American Journal of Medical Science 233:635-640.

James, A.E., Cooper, M., White, R.I., & Wagner, H.N. (1971). Perfusion changes on lung scans in patients with congestive heart failure. Radiology 100:99-106.

Kahaly, G.J., Kampmann, C., & Mohr-Kahaly, S. (2002). Cardiovascular dynamics and exercise tolerance in thyroid disease. Thyroid 12:473-481.

Kasper, D.L., Braunwald, E., Fauci, A., Hauser, S., Longo, D., Jameson, J.L., & Wilson, J.D. (Eds) (2004). Harrison's principles of internal medicine, ed 16. St. Louis: McGraw-Hill.

Kirby, R.R., Taylor, R.W., & Civetta, J.M. (1996). Handbook of critical care, ed 2. Philadelphia: Lippincott Williams & Wilkins.

Laffi, G., Barletta, G., La Villa, G., Del Bene, R., Riccardi, D., Ticali, P., Melani, L., Fantini, F., & Gentilini, P. (1997). Altered cardiovascular responsiveness to active tilting in nonalcoholic cirrhosis. Gastroenterology 113:891-898.

Matthay, R.A., Bromberg, S.I., & Putman, C.E. (1980). Pulmonary renal syndromes: a review. Yale Journal of Biology and Medicine 53:497-523.

Mehta, A D., Wright, W.B., & Kirby, B. (1978). Ventilatory function in Parkinson's disease. British Medical Journal 1:1456-1457.

McKinley, C.A., Auchincloss, J.H., Gilbert, R., & Nicholas, J. (1969). Pulmonary function, ventilatory control, and respiratory complications in quadriplegic subjects. American Review of Respiratory Diseases 100:526-532.

Montserrat, J.M., Cochrane, G.M., Wolf, C., Picado, C., Roca, J., & Agustividal, A. (1985). Ventilatory control in diabetes mellitus. European Journal of Respiratory Disease 67:112-117.

Murray, J.F., Felton, C.P., Garay, S.M., Gottlieb, M.S, Hopewell, P.C., Stover, D.E., & Teirstein, A.S. (1984). Pulmonary complications of the acquired immunodeficiency syndrome. New England Journal of Medicine 310:1682-1688.

Neu, H.C., Connolly, J.J., Schwertley, F.W., Ladwig, H.A., & Brody, A.W. (1967). Obstructive respiratory dysfunction in Parkinsonian patients. American Review Respiratory Diseases 95:33-47.

O'Donnell, C.R., Friedman, L.S., Russomanno, J.H., & Rose, R.M. (1988). Diminished perception of inspiratory-resistive loads in insulin-dependent diabetics. New England Journal of Medicine 319:1369-1373.

Peterson, B.T., Ross, J.C., & Brigham, K.L. (1983). Effect of naloxone on the pulmonary vascular responses to graded levels of intracranial hypertension in anesthetized sheep. American Review of Respiratory Diseases 128:1024-1029.

Rankin, J.A., & Matthay, R.A. (1982). Pulmonary renal syndromes. II. Etiology and pathogenesis. Yale Journal of Biology and Medicine 55:11-26.

Renner, I.G., Savage, W.T., Pantoja, J.L., & Renner, V.J. (1985). Death due to acute pancreatitis: a retrospective analysis of 405 autopsy cases. Digestive Diseases and Sciences 30:1005-1008.

Saxton, G.A., Rabinowitz, W., Dexter, L., & Haynes, F. (1956). The relationship of pulmonary compliance to pulmonary vascular pressures in patients with heart disease. Journal of Clinical Investigation 35:611-618.

Shackleford, M.D., & McAlister, W.H. (1975). Primary immunodeficiency diseases and malignancy. American Journal of Roentgenology, Radium Therapy & Nuclear Medicine 123:144-153.

Scharf, S.M., & Cassidy, S.S. (1989). Heart-lung interactions in health and disease. New York: Marcel Dekker.

Shelhamer, J.H., Ognibene, F.P., Macher, A.M., Tuacon, C., Steiss, R., Longo, D., Kovacs, J.A., Parker, M.M., Natanson, C., & Lane, H.C. (1984). Persistence of *Pneumocystis carinii* in lung tissue of acquired immunodeficiency syndrome patients treated for pneumocystis pneumonia. American Review of Respiratory Diseases 130:1161-1165.

Sherlock, S. (1988). The liver lung interface. Seminars in Respiratory Medicine 9:247-253.

Steljes, D.G., Kryger, M.H., Kirk, B.W., & Millar, T.W. (1990). Sleep in postpolio syndrome. Chest 98:133-140.

Trewby, P.N., Warren, R., Contini, S., Crosbie, W.A., Wilkinson, S.P., Laws, J.W., & Williams, R. (1978). Incidence and pathophysiology of pulmonary edema in fulminant hepatic failure. Gastroenterology 74:859-865.

PART II

Cardiopulmonary Assessment

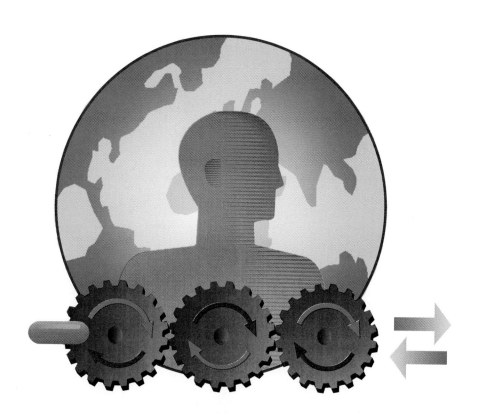

C H A P T E R 7

Measurement and Documentation

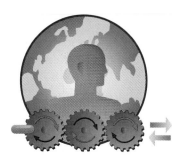

Claire Peel

Documentation
HIPAA Guidelines
Measurement

Reliability
Validity

Measurement and documentation are critical components in the process of providing patient care. Measurements form the basis for deciding treatment strategy and therefore influence patient response to therapeutic interventions. Measurements are also used during treatment sessions to determine rate of progression and appropriateness of exercise prescriptions. Typically therapists make a series of measurements and, in combination with those made by other health care professionals, form an impression of the client. The impression includes both physical and psychosocial aspects. If parts of the impression are incorrect because of inaccurate measurements, the course of treatment may be misdirected, which can result in treatment that is either not effective or unsafe. Consequently, knowledge of the qualities of measurements that relate to the cardiovascular and pulmonary systems is essential for quality patient care.

Documentation of the results of measurements, interpretation of the results, and the patient care plan are important not only for reimbursement but also to assure communication among health care team members. Timely and appropriate sharing of information on physiological responses to activity is often critical for optimal medical management. Documentation needs to be written clearly and concisely and include objective findings that will facilitate efficient and continuous care from all members of the health care team.

This chapter provides a discussion of types and characteristics of measurements that are common to cardiopulmonary physical therapy, followed by a discussion of the process of selecting, performing, and interpreting measurements. A discussion of the purposes and recommended terminology for documentation follows, including suggestions for providing objective and outcome-oriented information.

CHARACTERISTICS OF MEASUREMENTS

The purpose of performing a measurement is to assess or evaluate a characteristic or attribute of an individual. The characteristic to be measured first must be defined, and the purpose of performing each measurement must be clear. Therapists then can select the most appropriate method of measurement given the available resources and their clinical skills.

Levels or Types of Measurements

Measurements can be described according to their type or level of measurement. There are four levels of measurements: nominal, ordinal, interval and ratio (Rothstein & Echternach, 1993). Recognizing the level of measurement aids understanding and interpretation of the result.

BOX 7-1

Common Causes for the Development of Heart Failure

Myocardial infarction (MI) or ischemia
Cardiac arrhythmias
Renal insufficiency
Cardiomyopathy
Heart valve abnormalities
Pericardial effusion or myocarditis
Pulmonary embolism or pulmonary hypertension
Spinal cord injury
Congenital abnormalities
Aging

From Cahalin, L.P. (1994). Cardiac muscle dysfunction. In Hillegass, E.A., & Sadowsky, H.S. (Eds). Essentials of cardiopulmonary pulmonary physical therapy. Philadelphia: WB Saunders.

BOX 7-2

Angina Scale

Grade 1: Light—The discomfort is established, but just established
Grade 2: Light-moderate—Discomfort from which one can be distracted by a noncataclysmic event; it can be pain but usually is not
Grade 3: Moderate-severe—Discomfort or pain that prevents distraction by a beautiful woman, handsome man, television show, or other consuming interest; only a tornado, earthquake or explosion can distract one from a grade 3 discomfort or pain
Grade 4: Severe—Discomfort that is the most excruciating pain experienced or imaginable

---

Nominal

Objects or people are often placed in categories according to specific characteristics. If the categories have no rank or order, then the measurement is considered nominal. An example of a nominal measurement is the classification of patients with pulmonary dysfunction into those with obstructive lung disease, restrictive lung disease, or a combination of both types of dysfunction. The categories are mutually exclusive (i.e., all patients fit into one and only one category).

The categories of a nominal measurement scale are defined using objective indicators that are universally understood. For example, the classification of patients with heart failure could be based on the primary cause for the development of the condition (Box 7-1). In each case, the cause could be determined by diagnostic testing such as angiography or echocardiography. Clear descriptions of the criteria for inclusion in each category facilitate clinicians' agreement on the assignment of patients to categories. A high percentage of agreement indicates high interrater reliability.

Ordinal

Ordinal measurements are similar to nominal measurements with the exception that the categories are ordered or ranked. The categories in an ordinal scale indicate more or less of an attribute. The scale for rating angina is an example of an ordinal scale (Pollock et al, 1978) (Box 7-2). Each category is defined and a rating of grade 1 angina is less than a rating of grade 4. In an ordinal scale, the differences between consecutive ratings are not necessarily equal. The difference between grade 1 angina and grade 2 is not necessarily the same as between grade 3 and grade 4 angina. Consequently, if numbers are assigned to categories, they can be used to represent rank but cannot be subjected to mathematical operations. Averaging angina scores is incorrect because averaging assumes that there are equal intervals between categories.

Categorical measurements are considered ordinal if being assigned to a specific category is considered better than or worse than another category. For example, patients with angina could be classified as having either stable or unstable angina. This measurement would be considered ordinal, because stable angina usually is considered a better condition to have compared to unstable angina (Hurst, 1990).

Ratio

Ratio measurements have scales with units that are equal in size and have a zero point that indicates absence of the attribute being measured. Examples of ratio measurements that are used in cardiopulmonary physical therapy include vital capacity, cardiac output, and oxygen consumption. Ratio measurements are always positive values and can be subjected to all arithmetic operations. For example, an aerobic capacity of 4 L/min is twice as great as an aerobic capacity of 2 L/min.

When deciding whether a measurement is a ratio, the attribute that is being measured is defined. If the zero point indicates absence of the attribute, then the scale would be considered ratio. For example, cardiac output can be defined as the amount of blood in liters ejected from the left ventricle over a 1-minute period. A measurement of zero cardiac output would be absence of the characteristic, or no blood ejected from the left ventricle.

Interval

Interval measurements have units on a scale with equal distance between consecutive measurements and are differentiated from ratio measurements because the zero point is arbitrary rather than absolute. An arbitrary zero point is one that does not mean an absence of the characteristic that is being measured. Temperature, for example, can be measured using either an interval or a ratio scale. The Celcius temperature scale (interval measurement) assigns the zero point to the temperature at which water freezes, whereas the Kelvin scale (ratio measurement) assigns the zero point to an absence of heat.

Measuring force production using an isokinetic dynamometer is an example of an interval measurement commonly used in physical therapy. Patients may generate muscle tension and move an extremity but register a score of zero because they cannot move as fast as the dynamometer. Interval measurements can have negative values and can be subjected to some arithmetic operations. Adding and subtracting values is logical. A patient who generates 10 ft-lbs of torque at one session and 20 ft-lbs at the following session increased her torque production by 10 ft-lbs. Interval values cannot be subjected to division or multiplication. It cannot be stated that the patient generated twice as much torque on the second session compared to the first session because it cannot be assumed that a reading of zero indicates no torque production.

Reliability

Reliability is defined as the consistency or reproducibility of a measurement. Ideally, when attempting to measure a specific attribute, the value of the measurement should change only when the attribute changes. All measurements, however, have some element of error that contributes to the variability of the measurement. When the error is relatively high, the value of the measurement can change even when the attribute does not change. Believing that a change has occurred when it has not can result in an inaccurate clinical decision related to treatment planning or progression.

Many factors contribute to variability in the results of measurements. The characteristic being measured may demonstrate a certain degree of variability. Blood pressure and heart rate vary depending on mental and physical factors such as body position, hydration level, anxiety, and time of day. For these attributes, multiple measurements often are used to provide the best estimate of the patient's true heart rate and blood pressure.

Another factor that contributes to the variability of a measurement is changes in the testing instrument. Testing instruments may vary in their readings because of changes in environmental conditions or malfunction of instrument parts. Instruments should be calibrated (i.e., compared with a known standard) on a regular basis to assure accuracy of the readings. Some instruments are relatively easy to calibrate. For example, values obtained using aneroid blood pressure devices can easily be compared with values obtained using mercury manometers. Values obtained using either palpation or a heart rate monitor can be compared with values obtained from electrocardiograph (ECG) recordings. The mercury manometer and the ECG would be considered the standard method of measurement. Other devices, such as cycle ergometers, are more difficult to calibrate, and the usual approach is to rely on the manufacturer's specifications regarding the accuracy of the work rate readings.

A third factor contributing to measurement variability is the difference in the methods therapists use to make measurements. If a result is consistent when the same therapist repeats a measurement, the measurement is said to have high intrarater reliability. Measurements that are consistent when multiple therapists perform the measurement under the same conditions are said to have high interrater reliability. Often, measurements have high intrarater reliability but lower interrater reliability because of variations in the specific methods used by therapists to attain the same measurement. For example, a slight variation in the anatomical site used for measuring skinfold thickness can produce relatively large differences in percent fat estimates (Ruiz et al, 1971). Interrater reliability is important in clinical settings where a patient may be evaluated and treated by more than one therapist. If the interrater reliability of a measurement is low, changes in the patient over time may not be accurately reflected.

Validity

Valid measurements are those that provide meaningful information and accurately reflect the characteristic for which the measurement is intended. For a measurement to be useful in a clinical setting, the measurement must possess a certain degree of validity. Measurements can be reliable but not valid. For example, measurements made using bioelectrical impedance analyses have been shown to be valid for the estimation of total body water, but uncertainty exists as to the validity of estimates of percent body fat made with this device (Kusher & Schoeller, 1986).

There are various types of validity. Of importance in clinical practice are concurrent, predictive, and prescriptive validity. Concurrent validity is when a measurement accurately reflects measurements made with an accepted standard. Comparing bioelectrical impedance measurements for estimating percent body fat with estimates made from hydrostatic weighing is an example of determining concurrent validity. In this example, hydrostatic weighing would be considered the gold or accepted standard. Measurements with predictive validity can be used to estimate the probability of occurrence of a future event. Screening tests often involve measurements that are used to predict future events. For example, identifying people with risk factors for coronary artery disease (CAD) leads to a prediction that their likelihood of developing CAD is higher than normal. Measurements with prescriptive validity provide guidance to the direction of treatment. The categorical measurement of determining a person's risk for a future coronary event is a measurement that would need to have prescriptive validity. By classifying patients into high- versus low-risk categories on the basis of results of a diagnostic exercise test, the intensity and rate of progression of treatment is determined.

Accuracy of various types of exercise tests often is described by reporting sensitivity and specificity. Sensitivity is the ability of a test to identify individuals who are positive, or who have the characteristic that is being measured. Specificity is the ability of a test to identify individuals who are negative, or who do not have the characteristic. If a test produces a high number of false-positive results, then the sensitivity will be low. A false-positive result means that the test result was positive but the characteristic was absent. Young women often have positive stress test results but do not have CAD. The consequence of a false-positive test result could be unnecessary treatment. A high number of false-negative results would produce a low specificity. A false-negative result has a negative test result even though the disease or characteristic is present. The consequence of a false-negative test result is not receiving treatment when it is indicated.

Objective and Subjective Measurements

Measurements vary in degree of subjectivity versus objectivity. Subjective measurements are those that are affected in some way by the person taking the measurement (i.e., the measurer must make a judgment as to the value assigned). The assessment of a patient's breath sounds is influenced by many factors including the therapist's choice of terminology for describing the findings, perception of normal breath sounds, and hearing acuity. The grading of functional skills may be influenced by the therapist's interpretation of what constitutes minimal versus moderate assistance. Because of the influence of the person performing the measurement, subjective measurements usually have lower interrater reliability compared to objective measurements (Rothstein & Echternach, 1993).

Objective measurements are not affected by the person performing the measurement (i.e., these measurements do not involve judgement of the measurer). Heart rate measured by a computerized ECG system is an example of an objective measurement. Other examples include measurement of blood pressure using an intraarterial catheter and oxygen consumption using a metabolic system. Objective measurements are not necessarily accurate but usually have high interrater reliability (Rothstein & Echternach, 1993).

Most measurements cannot be classified as either objective or subjective. The quality of a measurement can be placed on a continuum based on the degree of reliability, as shown in Figure 7-1. The attribute or characteristic that is being measured

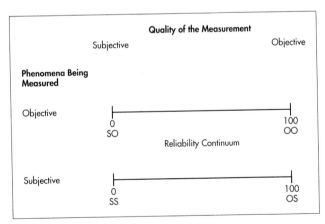

FIGURE 7-1 Illustration of the relationship between the quality of a measurement being either subjective or objective and the phenomenon being measured. The scales indicate that the objectivity of a measurement, or reliability, lies along a continuum. For example, a subjective phenomenon may be measured subjectively (subjective sign [SS]) or objectively (objective sign [OS]). *(From Rothstein JM. [1989]. On defining subjective and objective measurements. Phys Ther 69:577-579.)*

also can be viewed as a subjective or objective phenomena (Rothstein, 1989). A subjective attribute such as pain can be measured in either a subjective manner with a low degree of reliability or in an objective manner with a high degree of reliability.

SELECTING MEASUREMENTS

At the initial session with a client, how do therapists decide on the measurements to be performed? What additional measurements need to be performed during the course of treatment and at follow-up evaluations? Many factors influence the therapist's choice, including information obtained from the medical record and patient interview and knowledge of available treatment options. Therapists also must strive for efficiency and not repeat tests that have been performed by other health care professionals. Characteristics or qualities of measurements, such as reliability and validity, also influence the therapist's decision.

Medical and personal information about the client are primary factors that guide the selection of measurements. For example, appropriate measurements differ for a patient with an acute MI compared to a patient who is 3 weeks post-MI. Other factors to consider include the size of the infarction and associated complications such as arrhythmias, heart failure, or angina. Information collected during the patient interview also may guide the selection. For example, for a patient who displays anxiety when discussing walking on a treadmill, another mode of exercise may be prudent. Measurements need to be selected that are appropriate to the specific pathology, severity of the condition, and other characteristics unique to the patient.

Another important factor to consider in selecting measurements is the application of the information. Every measurement should contribute to the therapist's decisions regarding course and progression of treatment. Measurements that do not contribute to assessment of the patient result in an inefficient use of the therapist's time and add unnecessary costs to health care.

Another factor that influences the selection of measurements is the risk-benefit ratio. How do risks of conducting a test or measurement relate to the value of the information gained? Subjecting a patient to a symptom-limited exercise test during the acute stage post-MI could provide information to formulate an exercise prescription; however, the risks of performing this procedure at this time in the recovery period may outweigh the benefits.

PERFORMING MEASUREMENTS

When performing measurements, care must be taken to use procedures that can be replicated for future comparisons. Time must be taken to ensure that conditions are optimal and that the patient is informed of his or her part in the activity. For example, measuring blood pressure in a noisy treatment area immediately when the patient arrives for an appointment may not provide an accurate measurement of resting or baseline blood pressure. Documenting the conditions in which a measurement was made is also important. Conditions may include, but are not limited to, time of day, room temperature, recent activities performed by the patient, and type of measuring device.

Measurements should be made with an objective and open mind (i.e., without anticipating the result of the measurement). A measurement that is approached with a preconceived idea of the outcome may be affected by the therapist's expectations. Having confidence in the results of one's measurements is important and develops as clinical skills develop.

In clinics where more than one therapist is likely to evaluate or treat a patient, written procedures for performing measurements are needed. Therapists also need to review the written procedures on a regular basis and practice performing the measurements as a group. Practicing together is especially important for therapists who are new to the clinic. Interrater reliability for commonly used measurements then can be determined. If the reliability is low, written procedures may need to be revised to assure optimal consistency of measurement.

INTERPRETING MEASUREMENTS

Interpreting the results of measurements often is a difficult task. Usually patients' problems are understood not by reviewing results of a single measurement but by viewing relationships between results of several measurements. For example, the finding that blood pressure does not increase with activity may not be considered abnormal by itself if the activity level is low and the patient is taking a beta-receptor antagonist medication. The finding of no increase in blood pressure with signs and symptoms of exercise intolerance during moderate-level activity in another patient may be indicative of inadequate cardiac output.

Knowledge of what is "normal" is important to interpret the results of tests. For some measurements, normal values are well-defined. Measurements of resting blood pressure, cholesterol, and blood glucose have defined categories of normal, borderline, and elevated. For other measurements, population normative standards are not well-defined. For example, what is the normal increase in heart rate when walking at 3.5 mph on a level surface? Values for individuals differ depending on age, medications, fitness level, and walking efficiency. Results need to be interpreted by considering these factors and pathological conditions, if present. Each individual has their own "normal" or usual response, and variations from this value could be considered abnormal.

Interpreting the results of tests is similar to putting the pieces of a puzzle together to create a picture of the patient and his limitations. Information is collected from several sources, including the medical record, patient interview, and physical therapy examination. Measurements performed and interpreted by other health care professionals can be obtained from the medical record and include results such as chest x-ray, blood analyses, and echocardiograph. During an interview, the patient reports information about his current and past medical problems. It is important to be sensitive to the patient's feelings about his condition, noting his stage of emotional recovery. Detecting attitudes related to changing lifestyle habits also is important. After the interview, the therapist should have a sense of the patient as a person and begin to plan a strategy for optimizing his physical function.

Measurements made during the physical examination may include physiological responses to activity, breathing patterns, ventilatory capacity, and breath sounds. The results of these measurements are integrated with results collected during the chart review and viewed in the context of the patient's personal goals. Therapists develop a picture of the severity of the cardiopulmonary condition, stage of recovery, and presence of coexisting conditions. A treatment plan is developed on the basis of the composite of findings. The plan is implemented and continuously checked for appropriate direction by measurements made during treatment sessions. Because of the dynamic nature of many of the conditions that affect the cardiovascular and pulmonary systems, each treatment session can be viewed as a reassessment.

PURPOSES OF DOCUMENTATION

To be useful, measurements need to be recorded or documented in a concise and organized manner. Measurements that remain in the mind of the evaluator often are forgotten or not remembered accurately. Documentation is becoming more important to assist and to maximize reimbursement, as well as to facilitate efficiency of care through communication between health care professionals.

Documentation includes information about results of the examination, assessment of the patient's condition, and the plan of care. Reasons for documentation include the following.

1. To provide information for other therapists, assistants, or aides who may evaluate and/or treat the client
2. To communicate with the referring physician and other health care professionals
3. To provide data to determine treatment effectiveness and efficiency through collection of information on the results or outcomes of various types of care
4. To verify services for payers

GUIDELINES FOR CONTENT AND ORGANIZATION

Writing notes in a clear and concise format is important so that information is conveyed accurately. Examples of unclear notes are those that contain typographical errors, illegible handwriting, or vague statements that can be interpreted in more than one way. Concise notes are more likely to be read by other health care professionals. Most clinicians do not have time in their schedules to read through extensive patient information that may not be relevant. A concise note includes only essential information in a clear communication style free of unnecessary phrases. Another important rule is to use only standard or accepted abbreviations. Facilities have lists of approved abbreviations for their facility. The list should be available to those who write, read, and review records. Notes also need to clearly demonstrate the need for professional skills if a physical therapist is performing the evaluation and/or treatment. Activities that can be performed by physical therapist assistants, aides, nursing personnel, or family members need to be delegated to the appropriate individual. In addition, patients can be instructed in those activities that they can perform independently.

Documentation is essential when an unusual or adverse event occurs. For example, abnormal responses to activity that may appear relatively benign are important to record. Abnormal responses include dizziness, anginal or musculoskeletal pain, or arrhythmias. An unusually high or low heart rate or blood pressure response also should be noted. Combined with findings noted by the patient or other health care professionals, these results may indicate significant changes in the patient's cardiopulmonary status.

The organization of documentation varies between facilities. The following section presents an overview of a format for documentation using terminology described in the *Guide to Physical Therapist Practice* (APTA, 2001).

Examination

The examination includes obtaining a patient's history and administering tests and measurements to gather data that will be used to determine appropriate interventions. The patient's perception of his or her cardiac or pulmonary condition is important, as are descriptions of pain or discomfort that may be associated with either a cardiac event or a pulmonary complication. The history may include information from the medical record if it is relevant to the patient's current condition. To be relevant, the information should have potential impact on the direction of the examination and intervention: current medications and results of diagnostic tests, for example. The history also will indicate why the patient is being seen by a physical therapist and what the patient and/or family would like to accomplish.

As a result of the patient interview, the therapist selects tests and measurements to identify the patient's problems, which will be addressed by physical therapy. Tests can be categorized as measuring either impairments or functional limitations. An impairment is an abnormality of physiological function or anatomical structure at the tissue, organ, or body system level (Jette, 1994). Examples of impairments include decreases in muscle strength or range of motion, and abnormal heart rate and blood pressure values. A functional limitation is a restriction in performance at the level of the whole person (Jette, 1994). Functional limitations can be attributed to physical, social, cognitive, or emotional factors. Examples of functional limitations include the inability to dress, transfer, ambulate, or climb stairs. Improvements in functional status

usually are of primary interest to patients and families and to those who reimburse for health care. Measurements of impairments are important because they assist therapists in deciphering the causes or reasons for limitations in function.

When examining patients with cardiopulmonary disorders, therapists often assess responses to activity. Specific information on the activity, or exercise stress, and on the physiological responses is needed, including the following.

1. Mode of activity (corridor or track walking, lower extremity cycling)
2. Work level or rate (mph, percent grade, estimated MET level)
3. Duration of activity at each work level

The description of the activities should be written clearly so that the workload can be reproduced. The responses to activity include changes in heart rate and rhythm, blood pressure, respiratory rate, oxygen saturation levels, and heart and breath sounds from preactivity to either during or immediately after activity. Signs of exercise intolerance, such as changes in skin color, decrease in coordination, and sweating, also need to be documented. Whether the patient used oxygen during treatment or required physical assistance should be noted. By objectively recording the activity performed and the physiological responses, therapists can estimate the patient's activity tolerance.

Tests and measures are selected to rule in or out impairments or functional limitations. Tests and measures should be limited to those that are necessary to establish a clinical hypothesis, make decisions about appropriate interventions, and determine the effectiveness of the intervention.

Evaluation

The evaluation process involves using the results of the examination to make clinical judgments. Therapists state their "clinical hypothesis," or explanation of reasons for functional deficits. Whether the patient needs to be referred to other health care professionals or to community services is indicated.

The patient's problems that physical therapy will address are identified by the results of the interview, chart review, and tests and measures. Problems can be listed in order of priority and stated in functional terms. For example, it is recommended to state "patient unable to climb stairs because of abnormal ECG responses and dizziness," rather than "abnormal ECG response during activity."

Plan of Care and Prognosis

After identifying the patient's problems and determining a diagnosis for physical therapy, a plan of care that includes prognosis is developed. The plan of care includes goals and anticipated outcomes, specific interventions to be used and the recommended frequency and duration of the interventions. The prognosis is the predicted level of improvement and the amount of time needed to reach that level.

Goals are the outcomes to be achieved by participating in a physical therapy program and are generated by the therapist and patient in consultation. Goals are stated in functional terms and concern what the patient will be able to do at discharge. "Patient will be able to carry one 25-lb bag a distance of 50 feet with appropriate heart rate and rhythm responses, within 2 weeks," for example.

To determine whether a goal has been met, the therapist must be able to observe or measure the activity. Therapists also estimate the time it will take to achieve the outcome. In a discharge or follow-up note, it is stated whether each goal has been met. If a goal has not been achieved, an explanation is provided.

The plan provides a description of the approach that will be taken to assist the patient in achieving the stated goals. The plan may include a description of treatment that can be provided, education for the patient and/or family, and referrals to other services. Descriptions of home or ward programs should be included in the plan. The plan of care also includes discharge planning.

Intervention

Interventions are physical therapy procedures and techniques designed to produce changes in the patient's condition. Procedures typically used by therapists treating patients with cardiopulmonary disorders include therapeutic exercise, functional training (work hardening or work conditioning), and airway clearance techniques. The specific intervention selected by the therapist will be influenced by the severity of the cardiopulmonary disorder and the presence of complications. Patient and family and/or caregiver education is a part of all physical therapy interventions. Communication with other health care disciplines involved in the patient's care is essential to assure efficient and effective health care. For example, for a patient who is being discharged from the hospital after cardiac surgery, the therapist may need to coordinate with the social worker to assure that the patient receives home services that he or she needs for assistance with activities of daily living.

Documenting is an essential part of intervention. It is important to record the patient's responses to interventions, including changes in heart rate, blood pressure, and heart and lung sounds, recovery time after exercise, and feelings of angina, dyspnea, or fatigue. A description of the intervention is recorded so that another therapist or physical therapist assistant can continue the program. In addition to the medical record, the therapist also may be required to provide documentation to other sources such as home health or insurance agencies.

Reexamination and Outcomes Assessment

Throughout the course of treatments, therapists routinely perform reexaminations to determine whether patients are progressing. For patients with cardiopulmonary disorders, for example, the therapist may reexamine the patient at every session to determine whether physiological responses to activity are appropriate or whether the patient's lungs are clearing. Results of reexamination are used to modify or redirect interventions.

As the patient approaches discharge from physical therapy services, the therapist assesses the outcomes of the intervention. The therapist measures the impact of physical therapy services on the patient's impairments, functional limitations, and disabilities. The therapist relates the assessment of outcomes to the original goals established by the therapist and patient. As a result of the outcomes assessment, the therapist may refer the patient back to the physician or to another health care professional. A systematic review of medical records from a group of patients with similar diagnoses can be performed to determine outcomes of selected physical therapy interventions.

HIPAA GUIDELINES

The Health Insurance Portability and Accountability Act (HIPAA) includes federal guidelines that protect the confidentiality of health information. Health information is to be shared only with persons authorized to view the information (i.e., professionals involved in providing health care). Facilities assume the responsibility of designing systems to assure that health information is protected and kept confidential. All health care professionals are bound by these guidelines. Therapists must assure that discussions involving patients' health information occur in secure locations.

SUMMARY

Measurement and documentation are important components in the process of providing patient care. Therapists select measurements because they reveal information about patient characteristics that is needed to determine appropriate directions for intervention. Performing measurements in a consistent way allows comparison of patient characteristics at varied points in time. The recording, or documentation, of the results of measurements and other information about the patient serves as a legal record. Although documentation formats vary between facilities, information from records can be organized to include the following topics: examination, evaluation, plan of care and prognosis, interventions and reexamination. Documentation can be viewed as a way to assist therapists in organizing their findings, reflect on the significance of the findings, and generate an efficient and comprehensive care plan.

Review Questions

1. Describe and give examples of nominal, ordinal, ratio and interval measurements.
2. Identify three factors that contribute to the variability of measurements.

3. Define sensitivity and specificity of tests.
4. Differentiate between objective and subjective measurements.
5. Identify four purposes for documenting the results of examination and interventions.

REFERENCES

Guide to physical therapist practice, ed 2. Phys Ther 2001;81:9-744.

Hurst, J.W. (1990). The recognition and treatment of four types of angina pectoris and angina equivalents. In Hurst, J.W., Schlant, R.C., Rackley, C.E., Sonnonblick, E.H., & Wenger, N.K. (Eds.). The heart, ed 7. New York: McGraw-Hill.

Jette, A.M. (1994). Physical disablement concepts for physical therapy research and practice. Physical Therapy 74:380-386.

Kusher, R.F. & Schoeller, D.A. (1986). Estimation of total body water by bioelectrical impedance analysis. American Journal of Clinical Nutrition 44:417-424.

Pollock, M.L., Wilmore, J.H., & Fox, S.M. (1978). Health and fitness through physical activity. New York: John Wiley and Sons.

Rothstein, J.M. (1989). On defining subjective and objective measurements. Physical Therapy 69:577-579.

Rothstein, J.M., & Echternach, J.L. (1993). Primer on measurement: an introductory guide to measurement issues. Alexandria, VA: American Physical Therapy Association.

Ruiz, L., Colley, J.R.T., & Hamilton, P.J.S. (1971). Measurement of triceps skinfold thickness: an investigation of sources of variation. British Journal of Preventive and Social Medicine 25:165-167.

CHAPTER 8

History

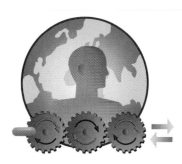

Willy E. Hammon III

KEY TERMS   Cough   History

                           Dyspnea   Pain

The value of a history depends in large part on the skill of the interviewer. When eliciting the history from a patient, the physical therapist must be alert to recognize the symptoms that are indicative of cardiac and pulmonary disease. This information is then used in the decision-making process to select the most appropriate intervention for the individual.

THE INTERVIEW

Obtaining a thorough and accurate patient history is truly an art. One important goal of history taking is to establish a good patient-therapist rapport. The patient must be allowed to explain the history in his or her own words and at a comfortable pace (Hurst et al, 1990). If the therapist appears hurried, distracted, preoccupied, irritated, or uncaring; is often interrupted; or fails to be an attentive listener, the patient-therapist relationship will likely suffer.

The interviewer must be careful not to allow personal feelings about the patient's grooming, appearance, demeanor, or behavior during the interview to unduly question the validity of the chief complaints (Birdwell, 1993). By the time the patient is referred for physical therapy, he or she may have seen one or more physicians, have been subjected to a number of noninvasive or invasive studies, or have been prescribed oral or inhaled medications with variable or unsatisfactory alleviation of symptoms. The patient is likely to manifest a degree of anxiety and frustration. Therefore, the therapist's approach, history-taking, and interviewing style are important for gaining the patient's confidence and cooperation.

The patient history interview can be divided into the data-gathering and interpretative sections (Snider, 1994). The data-gathering segment begins with asking why the patient has sought medical attention and has been referred for physical therapy services. In other words, what is the patient's chief complaint—the symptom that caused the patient to seek help?

Each chief complaint should be carefully explored. Supplementary questions should be nonleading, using words the patient can easily understand. This allows the interviewer to determine the significance of the complaint. An in-depth knowledge of cardiopulmonary pathophysiology allows the therapist to almost simultaneously gather data about the patient's symptoms and to interpret the likely type of cardiopulmonary dysfunction that exists. This in turn serves as a basis for the therapist to begin to select the appropriate assessment and treatment modalities for the individual.

It is important to remember that patient satisfaction is greatest if the patient is allowed to fully express major concerns without being interrupted. In addition, the risk of missing what is really of greatest concern to the patient is reduced if the patient is allowed sufficient time to describe it in his or her own words. Studies have shown that this usually takes only 1 to 3 minutes.

The patient's view of what is the problem and his or her suggestions for addressing the problem should be included in

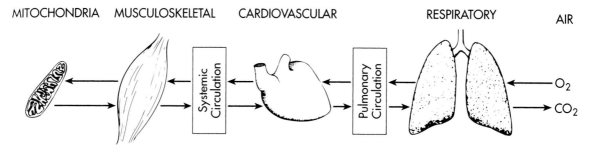

FIGURE 8-1 Schematic illustration of the oxygen transport system, which involves the interaction between the respiratory, cardiovascular, and musculoskeletal systems. *(Reprinted with permission from Mahler, D. [1987]. Dyspnea: diagnosis and management. Clinical Chest Medicine 8:215-230.)*

the interview. Patient satisfaction is improved by his or her involvement in the interview as well as in the establishment of short- and long-term goals.

The depth of the history taken by the physical therapist can vary according to the following factors:

1. Whether the individual is an inpatient or an outpatient. Many inpatients have detailed medical records available for the therapist to review. This significantly reduces the amount of information the physical therapist needs to obtain from the patient during an interview. If the information in the chart is scant, or if the individual is an outpatient with only a treatment referral and few or no medical records available, the physical therapist should obtain a more detailed history.
2. Whether the treatment order is narrow or broad in scope.
3. The acuteness of the patient's illness, level of consciousness, and ability to provide accurate information.

This chapter presents a comprehensive approach to history taking. Physical therapists may find part or all of this information applicable, depending on the particular circumstances.

QUESTIONNAIRES

Printed symptom or medical questionnaires can be beneficial or detrimental to the patient-therapist relationship, depending on how they are used. Questionnaires can expedite the data-gathering portion of the initial visit by allowing the patient to note in advance all symptoms, medical conditions, surgeries, occupations, medications, and other factors that may influence physical therapy intervention. They can reduce the amount of nontreatment time therapists may otherwise spend inquiring about irrelevant symptoms and conditions. Printed questionnaires also allow patients sufficient time to recall relevant information and respond more accurately than they often do in an interview setting (Miller, 1980). Used in this way, a printed questionnaire can be a valuable tool for expediting a comprehensive evaluation of cardiopulmonary patients.

However, if questionnaires are used improperly, they can depersonalize the history-taking portion of the initial visit

(Hurst et al, 1990). If the physical therapist allows the printed form to become a substitute for interaction with the patient, patient satisfaction will be low and the patient-therapist relationship will suffer.

DYSPNEA

Dyspnea, breathlessness or shortness of breath, can be defined as the sensation of difficulty in breathing (George, 1990). It is one of the most common reasons for patients to seek medical attention. Dyspnea is difficult to quantitate because it is subjective and at times is normal (i.e., at high altitudes and during or following vigorous exercise). Also, patients of different backgrounds use different descriptors for their breathlessness (Mahler, 1990). Dyspnea is a symptom of cardiac and pulmonary diseases as well as of other conditions.

When a patient complains of shortness of breath or breathlessness, it should be noted that this complaint is often unrelated to the patient's arterial oxygen level (PaO_2). Many times, it appears that altered mechanical factors during breathing contribute to the sensation of breathlessness (Mahler, 1987). Numerous receptors that have a role in sensing dyspnea have been identified; they include vagal receptors (e.g., irritant, stretch, and J-receptors), chemoreceptors, proprioceptive receptors (e.g., tendon organs, muscle spindles, joint and skin receptors), and upper airway receptors (Snider, 1994).

Analyzing the oxygen transport system (Figure 8-1) can help the physical therapist to determine the likely cause of each patient's dyspnea and the most appropriate physical therapy intervention. The delivery of oxygen from ambient air to the mitochondrion within the cell depends on the intact interaction of the respiratory, cardiovascular, and muscular systems. Also, carbon dioxide (CO_2) is eliminated in the opposite direction. Dyspnea can be caused by dysfunction in any of the systems.

Dyspnea commonly occurs when the body's requirement for breathing (ventilation) exceeds the body's capacity to provide it (Snider, 1994). In other words, the symptom varies directly with the body's demand for ventilation and, inversely, with the body's ventilatory capacity.

There are three basic causes of dyspnea: (1) an increased awareness of normal breathing, (2) an increase in the work of breathing, and (3) an abnormality in the ventilatory system itself (George, 1990).

An increased awareness of normal breathing is usually related to anxiety (Miller, 1980). The patient commonly complains of "not getting a deep enough breath," a feeling of "smothering," or "not getting air down in the right places" (Szidan and Fishman, 1988). These sensations have been designated as psychogenic dyspnea. The patient's breathing pattern is irregular, with frequent sighs. When severe, it is associated with tingling of the hands and feet, circumoral numbness, and lightheadedness. Coaching the patient to hyperventilate and to reproduce the symptoms may help the patient better understand the cause of these symptoms and how to control them (Miller, 1980). The hyperventilation syndrome is properly diagnosed only after organic causes have been excluded and pulmonary function tests indicate normal respiratory mechanics and PaO_2.

The second cause of dyspnea is an increase in the work of breathing. Greater inspiratory pressures must be generated by the respiratory muscles to move air in and out of the lungs when the mechanical properties of the lungs have changed. This may be related to an increase in lung water resulting from cardiac disease or the high cardiac output of anemia. A loss of compliance (increased lung stiffness) because of diffuse inflammatory or fibrotic lung disease often causes shortness of breath. Small or large airway obstruction as a result of bronchoconstriction, sputum, inflammation, and other effects commonly produces dyspnea.

The third cause of dyspnea is an abnormality in the ventilatory apparatus or pump. The ventilatory apparatus consists of the thoracic cage, respiratory muscles, and nerves. Any of these may become dysfunctional. Thoracic cage abnormalities include kyphoscoliosis, extreme obesity, and large pleural effusions. Diseases of the respiratory muscles include polymyositis and muscular dystrophy. Neurological abnormalities include spinal cord injuries, phrenic nerve injuries, brachial plexus neuropathy, ascending polyneuritis (Guillain-Barré syndrome), myasthenia gravis, amyotrophic lateral sclerosis, poliomyelitis, neurotoxins, and exposure to paralytic agents.

The time course of the appearance and progression of dyspnea should be identified (Mahler, 1998; Sharf, 1989). Acute dyspnea is common in pulmonary embolism, pneumothorax, acute asthma, pulmonary congestion related to congestive heart failure (CHF), pneumonia, and upper airway obstruction. Most of these conditions require immediate physician evaluation of the acute problem before physical therapy intervention. Subacute or chronic progression of dyspnea generally presents, over time, as increasingly severe dyspnea with exertion. It occurs with emphysema, restrictive lung disorders such as pulmonary fibrosis, chest wall deformities, respiratory muscle dysfunction, occupational lung diseases, chronic CHF, and large pleural effusions.

Dyspnea may also be related to body position (Mahler, 1998). Therefore, when evaluating dyspnea, the physical therapist should ask the patient whether he or she has difficulty breathing when reclining horizontally. Is it necessary to be propped up on several pillows to sleep at night (orthopnea)? Does she have more difficulty breathing when reclining on one side (trepopnea)? Does he ever wake up at night short of breath and need to sit up or walk around the room to "catch his breath" (paroxysmal nocturnal dyspnea)?

Acute Dyspnea

A patient who has acute dyspnea requires a rapid and thorough history and physical assessment. The physical therapist should ask several important questions to address the possible causes of acute dyspnea (Mahler, 1987):

1. Are you short of breath at rest? If the answer is yes, it suggests a severe physiological dysfunction. The patient likely needs prompt evaluation by a physician if this is of recent onset and the patient has not had a medical workup.
2. Do you have chest pain? If so, what part of your chest? Unilateral localized chest pain raises the possibility of spontaneous pneumothorax, pulmonary embolism, or chest trauma.
3. What were you doing immediately before or at the time of the onset of shortness of breath? Approximately 75% of spontaneous pneumothoraces occur during sedentary activity, 20% during some strenuous activity, and 5% are related to coughing or sneezing. A history of immobilization of a lower extremity, recent surgery, bed rest, travel requiring prolonged sitting, obesity, CHF, and venous disease of the lower extremities are all risk factors for pulmonary embolism. If the patient's symptoms are related to chest trauma, the fact that a fall, a blow, or an accident occurred can usually be quickly established.
4. Do you have any major medical or surgical conditions? Cystic fibrosis, chronic obstructive pulmonary disease (COPD), interstitial lung disease, and malignancies are important causes of secondary spontaneous pneumothorax.

Acute dyspnea in cardiac patients is difficult to assess because the signs and symptoms are so similar to those caused by pulmonary disease. It is most often due to arrhythmias and acute coronary ischemia with associated left ventricular dysfunction, but it can be caused by any cardiac disorder (Mahler, 1998).

If the therapist strongly suspects pneumothorax, pulmonary emboli, or an acute cardiac disorder on the basis of the history and physical assessment, the patient should be referred for immediate medical evaluation.

Dyspnea on Exertion

Dyspnea on exertion is a common complaint of patients with cardiopulmonary dysfunction. Dyspnea during exercise or exertion usually precedes dyspnea at rest (Wasserman, 1982).

TABLE 8-1
Disorders Limiting Exercise Performance, Pathophysiology, and Discriminating Measurements*

DISORDERS	PATHOPHYSIOLOGY	MEASUREMENTS THAT DEVIATE FROM NORMAL
Pulmonary		
Airflow limitation	Mechanical limitation to ventilation mismatching of V_A/Q, hypoxic stimulation to breathing	V_E max/MVV, expiratory flow pattern, V_D/V_T; VO_2 max, V_E/VO_2 VE response to hypoeroxia, (A-a)PO_2
Restrictive	Mismatching V_A/Q, hypoxic stimulation to breathing	
Chest wall	Mechanical limitation to ventilation	V_E max/MVV, $PaCO_2$ VO_2 max
Pulmonary circulation	Rise in physiologic dead space as fraction of V_T, exercise hypoxemia	V_D/V_T, work-rate-rrelated hypoxemia VO_2 max, V_E/VO_2, (a-ET)PCO_2, O_2-pulse
Cardiac		
Coronary	Coronary insufficiency	Electrocardiogram (ECG), VO_2 max, anaerobic threshold O_2, V_E/VO_2 O_2-pulse, blood pressure (BP) (systolic, diastolic, pulse)
Valvular	Cardiac output limitation (decreased effective stroke volume)	
Myocardial	Cardiac output limitation (decreased ejection fraction and stroke volume)	
Anemia	Reduced O_2 carrying capacity	O_2-pulse, anaerobic threshold VO_2, VO_2 max, V_E/VO_2
Peripheral circulation	Inadequate O_2 flow to metabolically active muscle	Anaerobic threshold VO_2, VO_2 max
Obesity	Increased work to move body; if severe, respiratory restriction and pulmonary insufficiency	VO_2-work rate relationship, PaO_2, $PaCO_2$, VO_2-max
Psychogenic	Hyperventilation with precisely regular respiratory rate	Breathing pattern, PCO_2
Malingering	Hyperventilation and hypoventilation with irregular respiratory rate	Breathing pattern, PCO_2
Deconditioning	Inactivity or prolonged bed rest; loss of capability for effective redistribution of systemic blood flow	O_2-pulse, anaerobic threshold VO_2, VO_2 max

*V_A, Alveolar ventilation; Q, pulmonary blood flow; *MVV*, maximum voluntary ventilation; V_D/V_T, physiologic dead space/tidal volume ratio; O_2, oxygen; VO_2, O_2 consumption; *(A-a)PO_2*, alveolar-arterial PO_2 difference; *(a-ET)PCO_2*, arterial-end tidal PCO_2 difference. (*Reprinted with permission from Wasserman, K. [1982]. Dyspnea on exertion: is it the heart or lungs? Journal of the America Medical Association, 2 2039-43.*)

It most often is a result of chronic pulmonary disease or CHF. Some causes of dyspnea during exertion or exercise are listed in Table 8-1.

It is important to establish the amount of activity required to produce dyspnea. Various scales (Borg, 1982; Mahler, 2000) have been developed to categorize the level of dyspnea and impairment present in patients (Figures 8-2 and 8-3 and Table 8-2). The patient should be asked about daily activity and what activities produce breathlessness (Constant, 1993). Does the patient become short of breath climbing a flight of stairs or walking uphill? Is the patient able to walk and talk simultaneously? Does walking more slowly affect the individual's dyspnea?

In addition, the time at which the patient began to notice an increase in shortness of breath should be noted. A recent onset of dyspnea is more characteristic of heart failure than of chronic lung disease, which has a longer, more insidious onset. Acute pulmonary problems such as pneumothorax, atelectasis, pneumonia, and other conditions superimposed on chronic lung disease can also explain a recent intensification of symptoms.

FIGURE 8-2 The visual analogue scale is a vertical line 100 mm in length. The patient is asked to make a mark along this line that represents his level of breathlessness. The distance of the patient's mark above zero represents the measurement of dyspnea. (*Reprinted with permission from Mahler, D. [1987]. Dyspnea: diagnosis and management. Clinical Chest Medicine 8:215-230.*)

Is wheezing present with the dyspnea on exertion? Has there been an associated weight gain? Does the patient have a positive smoking history and sputum production? If a positive response is received, these suggest that COPD is the primary cause of symptoms (Constant, 1993).

The basic defect that cardiac diseases produce during exertion is a limited cardiac output, which is caused primarily by a reduced stroke volume (Wasserman, 1982). To compensate for the relatively low stroke volume, the patient develops a rapid heart rate and a wide arteriovenous O_2 difference (decreased capillary Po_2) at an inappropriately low work rate. Therefore, the exercising muscles (both skeletal and myocardial) have increased difficulty getting an adequate oxygen supply to perform the necessary work: this results in dyspnea, fatigue, or pain. The lactic acidosis that results from the low level of oxygen delivery to the muscles can be measured by either invasive or noninvasive gas-exchange

0	Nothing at all
0.5	Very, very slight (just noticeable)
1	Very slight
2	Slight
3	Moderate
4	Somewhat severe
5	Severe
6	
7	Very severe
8	
9	Very, very severe (almost maximal)
10	Maximal

FIGURE 8-3 The Borg category scale for rating breathlessness. (Reprinted with permission from Borg, G. [1982]. Psychophysical bases of perceived exertion. Medicine of Science and Sports Exercise 14:377-381.)

methods during exercise testing. The functional and therapeutic capacity of the patient with heart disease can be estimated on the basis of the history and symptoms (Box 8-1).

Dyspnea in patients with cardiac disorders is usually related to metabolic acidosis-induced hydrogen ion stimulus. Also, increased pressure in the right side of the heart and pulmonary circulation during exertion may stimulate mechanoreceptors that increase ventilation and induce dyspnea.

Diseases that involve the lungs or thoracic cage generally prevent external respiration (ventilation) from keeping pace with internal respiration (in the cells) (Wasserman, 1982). In other words, patients outwalk or outrun their lungs during activities or exertion. The primary symptom that limits exercise in patients with pulmonary disorders is dyspnea, which occurs because of the difficulty they have eliminating the CO_2 produced by metabolism. Some individuals, such as those with pulmonary fibrosis and some of those with COPD, do experience a decrease in Po_2 with exercise. Hence, dyspnea on exertion in pulmonary patients is usually related to hypoxic or hypercapnic stimuli.

Dyspnea in Cardiac Patients

The cause of dyspnea in cardiac patients is determined by whether an associated stiffness of the lungs (a loss of compliance) is also present (Szidan, 1988). Dyspnea is the primary symptom of a decompensating left ventricle (Mahler, 1998; Marriott, 1993). As the ventricle fails to eject the normal volume of blood, it produces chronic pulmonary venous hypertension, congestion, and pulmonary edema, resulting in stiff or less compliant lungs. This, along with modest hypoxemia that augments the respiratory drive, increases ventilation and the work of breathing. Tachypnea is often seen at rest. Exercise exaggerates the pulmonary congestion and edema and promotes arterial and mixed venous hypoxemia, which also increase the amount of dyspnea and tachypnea manifested. Fatigue, resulting from low cardiac output, also affects the respiratory muscles, further increasing the sensation of breathlessness.

Dyspnea in cardiac patients without stiff lungs is seen primarily during exertion or exercise (Szidan, 1988). In uncomplicated pulmonic stenosis, it is probably related to an

TABLE 8-2

American Thoracic Society Dyspnea Scale

GRADE	DEGREE	
0	None	Not troubled with breathlessness except with strenuous exercise
1	Slight	Troubled by shortness of breath when hurrying on the level or walking up a slight hill
2	Moderate	Walks slower than people of the same age on the level because of breathlessness or has to stop for breath when walking at own pace on the level
3	Severe	Stops for breath after walking about 100 yards or after a few minutes on the level
4	Very severe	Too breathless to leave the house or breathless when dressing or undressing

Reprinted with permission from Brooks, S.M., (1982). Surveillance for respiratory hazards. ATS News 8:12-16.

BOX 8-1

Functional and Therapeutic Classification of Patients with Heart Disease

Functional Classification

Class I

Patients with cardiac disease but without resulting limitations of physical activity; ordinary physical activity does not cause undue fatigue, palpitation, dyspnea, or anginal pain.

Class II

Patients with cardiac disease resulting in slight limitation of physical activity; they are comfortable at rest. Ordinary physical activity results in fatigue, palpitation, dyspnea, or anginal pain.

Class III

Patients with cardiac disease resulting in marked limitation of physical activity; they are comfortable at rest. Less than ordinary physical activity causes fatigue, palpitation, dyspnea, or anginal pain.

Class IV

Patients with cardiac disease resulting in inability to carry on any physical activity without discomfort; symptoms of cardiac insufficiency or of the anginal syndrome may be present even at rest. If any physical activity is undertaken, discomfort increases.

Therapeutic Classification

Class A

Patients with cardiac disease whose physical activity need not be restricted in any way.

Class B

Patients with cardiac disease whose ordinary physical activity need not be restricted but who should be advised against severe or competitive efforts.

Class C

Patients with cardiac disease whose ordinary activity should be moderately restricted and whose more strenuous efforts should be discontinued.

Class D

Patients with cardiac disease whose ordinary activity should be markedly restricted.

Class E

Patients with cardiac disease who should be at complete rest, confined to bed or chair.

Reprinted with permission from the New York Heart Association. (1964). Diseases of the heart and blood vessels; nomenclature and criteria for diagnosis, ed 6. Boston: Little, Brown.

inadequate cardiac output during exercise. Patients with tetralogy of Fallot and other forms of cyanotic heart disease experience both dyspnea and fatigue during exercise when the arterial oxyhemoglobin saturation has fallen appreciatively below the resting level.

Orthopnea

Orthopnea is dyspnea that occurs when the patient is in the recumbent position (Hurst, 1990). The patient may state the need for two or three pillows under the head to rest at night. This symptom is commonly associated with CHF but may also be associated with severe chronic pulmonary disease.

Paroxysmal Nocturnal Dyspnea

Paroxysmal nocturnal dyspnea (PND) is an important type of shortness of breath. This symptom has strong predictive value as a sign of CHF (Hurst, 1990). The patient usually falls asleep in the recumbent position, and 1 or 2 hours later, awakens from sleep with acute shortness of breath. The patient sits upright on the side of the bed or goes to an open window to breathe "fresh air" and get relief from shortness of breath.

The mechanism of PND is the transfer of fluid from extravascular tissues into the blood stream (or intravascularly) during sleep (Constant, 1993). The intravascular volume of fluid gradually increases until the compromised left ventricle can no longer manage it. The left atrial pressure rises when the rate of lymphatic drainage from the lungs is unable to keep up with the increased volume of fluid. The increased atrial pressure leads to a sufficiently elevated pulmonary capillary pressure to produce interstitial edema. Patients who are light sleepers awaken early with dyspnea. Deep sleepers may not awaken until they develop alveolar edema.

Classic PND cannot usually be eliminated by only elevating the trunk without lowering the legs. The patient must pool blood in the extravascular tissues of the legs to get adequate relief, which usually takes at least 30 minutes. This is why the patient must sit up or stand up and ambulate.

The patient should be asked about the amount of exercise or work performed during the day before an attack of PND. A true episode of left ventricular failure in PND is more likely to occur after a day of unusual exertion, which causes an increased amount of extravascular fluid to accumulate in the legs. If the patient is participating in an exercise or rehabilitation program, the level of exercise may have to be reduced to prevent PND.

Platypnea

Platypnea is the onset of dyspnea when the patient assumes the sitting position from the supine position (Sharf, 1989; Mahler, 1998). This unusual phenomenon is commonly found in patients with basilar pulmonary fibrosis or basilar arteriovenous malformation. It can be related to the redistribution of blood flow to the lung bases when assuming the sitting position and the resultant ventilation-perfusion mismatching and hypoxemia.

Trepopnea

Trepopnea refers to dyspnea in one lateral position but not the other (Snider, 1994). It is caused by the positional mismatching of ventilation to perfusion in unilateral respiratory system pathology such as lung disease, pleural effusion, or airway obstruction (Mahler, 1998; Remolina, 1981; Zack, 1974). It also is commonly seen in patients with mitral stenosis (Constant, 1993). Occasionally, it may be the result of a fall in blood pressure when the patient is in the left lateral decubitus position. If the patient has ischemic heart disease, the reduction in coronary perfusion can cause either angina or dyspnea.

Functional Dyspnea

Functional dyspnea is defined as shortness of breath at rest but not during exertion (Sharf, 1989). It is most commonly seen in young women who complain of the need to take a deep breath or to sigh, and they interpret this sensation as shortness of breath. The physical examination and pulmonary function tests are negative. Reassurance is usually all that is necessary.

WHEEZING

Patients who complain of wheezing associated with dyspnea may have pulmonary or cardiac disease. This symptom, if first reported in patients over the age of 40, is often related to heart failure (Hurst et al, 1990). When it has been confirmed that the wheezing results from heart disease, the patient is said to have cardiac asthma. Wheezing in cardiac patients is a manifestation of narrowed airways and thickened bronchial walls as a result of pulmonary edema (Szidan and Fishman, 1988). However, if patients have a history of episodes of wheezing and dyspnea since childhood, COPD or asthma is the likely cause. Other pulmonary conditions, such as eosinophilic pneumonia, bronchopulmonary aspergillosis, allergic granulomatosis, and others can cause wheezing (Miller, 1980). Wheezing must be differentiated from stridor, which is commonly caused by laryngotracheal narrowing due to a tracheostomy scar, trauma of intubation, laryngeal paralysis, epiglottitis, or tumors. Chronic pulmonary patients may also develop heart conditions, so it is good to remember that patients who complain of wheezing may have both cardiac and pulmonary disease.

COUGH

Cough is a common symptom of pulmonary disease. The cough mechanism consists of three phases: (1) an inspiratory phase, (2) a compressive phase, and (3) an expiratory phase (Irwin, 1977).

Numerous cough-irritant receptors are located on the mucosa of the larynx, trachea, bronchi, pleura, and external auditory canal. These receptors are most sensitive at the glottis and carina and diminish rapidly beyond the fourth-generation bronchi. A cough follows stimulation of these mucosal receptors by any of a number of factors including inflammation, sputum, foreign bodies, noxious gases or odors, chemical substances, endobronchial tumors, and extrabronchial pressure on the trachea or bronchi (Sharf, 1989).

A productive cough is beneficial for clearing the airways of sputum and foreign material and generally should not be inhibited. However, a dry, hacking cough is usually of no value and can have a self-perpetuating irritant effect on the respiratory mucosa. A dry cough may be the initial symptom of certain interstitial lung diseases such as allergic alveolitis, sarcoidosis, and pulmonary fibrosis. Some causes and characteristics of coughs are listed in Table 8-3.

Cough may be the only presenting symptom of asthma and is a common cause of chronic cough (Dicpinigaitis, 2004; Morice, 2003). In individuals with asthma, cough is precipitated by inhaling cold air and by exercising, and the cough is dry. Cough can precipitate an asthma attack in sensitive patients; in that instance, it is known as cough-induced bronchospasm.

It is important to determine the length of time cough has been present (Sharf, 1989). The most common cause of an acute cough is a viral respiratory infection, which generally resolves within a few days or 2 to 3 weeks. Exposure to noxious gases also precipitates acute coughing.

A cough that has persisted for more than 3 weeks can be termed chronic (Snider, 1994). The most common cause of chronic cough is chronic bronchitis, which is present in up to 30% of cigarette smokers. The next most common cause is the postnasal discharge syndrome. Patients describe a sensation of secretions dripping from the back of the nose into the throat, prompting throat clearing or coughing. Gastroesophageal disorders are present in 10% to 40% of patients with chronic cough and may contribute to coughing due to microaspiration or irritation of cough receptors in the lower esophagus (Fontana, 2003; Irwin, 2000; Morice, 2003).

Various cardiac conditions may stimulate receptors in the bronchi and provoke coughing (Goldberger, 1990). Because the bronchial veins empty into the pulmonary veins (leading to the left side of the heart), the systemic veins, and the superior vena cava (leading to the right side of the heart), venous congestion and coughing may occur with either right- or left-side CHF. It is more common, however, in left-sided CHF. The onset of a cough in a patient with paroxysmal tachycardia or acute myocardial infarction (MI) is often an early symptom of acute left-side heart failure.

Coughing may be caused by other cardiovascular conditions, such as a large left atrium displacing the left main-stem bronchus upward, aortic aneurysms placing pressure on the bronchi, and a double aortic arch compressing the trachea.

A specific diagnosis can be made in 80% of cases of chronic cough by an appropriate history alone (Stulberg, 1985). Determining the precipitating causes or the time of onset points the clinician to a probable diagnosis. For example, does the patient cough primarily at night? If so, it points to heart failure, esophageal problems, bronchiectasis, or asthma as the potential cause. An early-morning cough is more common in bronchitis and in individuals with postnasal drip. Cough following meals suggests esophageal disease. Cough precipitated by exertion or deep breathing suggests asthma or interstitial lung disease. Allergens or irritant fumes at home or

TABLE 8-3	
Some Causes and Characteristics of Coughs	
CAUSE	**CHARACTERISTICS**
Acute infections of lungs	
Tracheobronchitis	Cough associated with sore throat, running nose and eyes
Lobar pneumonia	Cough often preceded by symptoms of upper respiratory infection; cough dry, painful at first; later becomes productive
Bronchopneumonia	Usually begins as acute bronchitis; dry or productive cough
Mycoplasma and viral pneumonia	Paroxysmal cough, productive of mucoid or blood-stained sputum associated with influenza-like syndrome
Exacerbation of chronic bronchitis	Cough productive of mucoid sputum becomes purulent
Chronic infections of lungs	
Bronchitis	Cough productive of sputum on most days for more than 3 consecutive months and for more than 2 successive years; sputum mucoid until acute exacerbation, when it becomes mucopurulent
Bronchiectasis	Cough copious, foul, purulent, often since childhood; forms layer on standing
Tuberculosis or fungus	Persistent cough for weeks to months, often with blood-tinge sputum
Parenchymal inflammatory processes	
Interstitial fibrosis and infiltrations	Cough nonproductive, persistent; depends on causes
Smoking	Cough usually associated with injected pharynx; persistent, most marked in morning, usually only slightly productive unless succeeded by chronic bronchitis
Tumors	
Bronchogenic carcinoma	Nonproductive to productive cough for weeks to months; recurrent small hemoptysis common
Alveolar cell carcinoma	Cough similar to bronchogenic carcinoma, except in occasional instance when large quantities of watery, mucoid sputum are produced
Benign tumor in airways	Cough nonproductive, occasionally hemoptysis
Mediastinal tumor	Cough, often with breathlessness, caused by compression of trachea and bronchi
Aortic aneurysm	Brassy cough
Foreign bodies	
Immediate, while still in upper airway	Cough associated with progressive evidence of asphyxiation
Later, when lodged in lower airway	Nonproductive cough, persistent, associated with localizing wheeze
Cardiovascular sources	
Left ventricular failure	Cough intensifies while body is supine; aggravation of dyspnea
Pulmonary infarction	Cough associated with hemoptysis, usually with pleural effusion

Reprinted with permission from Szidon, J., Fishman, A. (1988). Approach to the pulmonary patient with respiratory signs and symptoms. In: Pulmonary diseases and disorders. Fishman, A., Ed. New York: McGraw-Hill.

at work may be a cause of cough. Postviral cough may be present for weeks following a viral illness.

Some medications can elicit coughing. Beta blockers prescribed to treat hypertension, migraine headaches, cardiovascular disease (CVD), or glaucoma may precipitate asthma. Many drugs, including chemotherapeutic agents, can cause interstitial lung disease and coughing.

Cough and wheezing may result from COPD, asthma, or early left heart failure. Early left heart failure predisposes the patient to respiratory infections and may be responsible for chronic bronchitis.

Cough Complications

One of the more common complications of cough is syncope. Tussive, or cough-induced, syncope, which is more common in men than in women, can be recognized through accurate history taking (Miller, 1980). It is typically reported by middle-aged men who "smoke hard, eat hard, drink hard, and

cough hard." They experience fainting or near-fainting following cough paroxysms. The cause is obscure but may be related to vagus-induced cardiac slowing or vasodilation or to high intrathoracic pressures that impair venous return, decrease cardiac output, increase intracranial pressure, and result in a reduced cerebral blood flow. Cough syncope is often resolved by smoking cessation.

Complications of cough include headache, back pain, muscular tears, hematomas, and rib fractures (along the posterior axillary line); occasionally vertebral compression fractures (in osteopenic patients), urinary incontinence (UI) (in women), and inguinal hernias (in men) may occur (Braman, 1987).

CHEST PAIN

Taking an accurate history is crucial to the proper evaluation of chest pain (Snider, 1994). Although the definitive cause of chest pain cannot be fully established without diagnostic medical tests, it is usually possible to determine whether the pain originates in the pleurae, chest wall, or thoracic organs by means of careful history taking.

Chest pain can be divided into two basic types: chest wall pain and visceral pain (George, 1990). The first arises from involved thoracic-cage structures and tends to be superficial and welllocalized. The latter arises from the heart, pericardium, aorta, mediastinum, bronchi, or esophagus. It is described as deep and difficult to localize.

Pleuritic

Pleuritic chest pain originates from the parietal pleura or endothoracic fascia but not the visceral pleura, which have no pain receptors. The patient can usually identify it as being close to the thoracic cage (Szidan, 1988). Pleuritic chest pain worsens sharply with inspiration as the inflamed parietal pleura are stretched with chest wall motion. Deep breathing, coughing, and laughing are extremely painful, requiring the patient to apply pressure over the involved area to control the pain.

Pleuritic chest pain is ordinarily found in patients who have other signs of respiratory illness, such as cough, fever, chills, and malaise. Inflammation of the central portion of the diaphragmatic pleura produces ipsilateral shoulder pain by way of the phrenic nerve (Miller, 1980). Outer portions of the diaphragmatic pleura are innervated by the seventh through twelfth intercostals nerves. Irritation of these pleura causes referred pain in the lower thorax or upper abdomen (Fraser, 1999).

The onset of pleuritic chest pain varies according to its cause (Snider, 1994). Sudden severe pleuritic chest pain suggests a spontaneous pneumothorax, pulmonary embolism, or infarct. Pulmonary embolism is usually accompanied by sudden dyspnea, hemoptysis, tachycardia, cyanosis, hypotension, anxiety, and agitation (Marriott, 1993).

Cardiac

Three cardinal features are characteristic of cardiac chest pain. The patient should be asked the following questions (Marriott, 1993):

1. Does the pain have maximal intensity from the onset or does it build up for several seconds? Ischemic cardiac pain, or angina, is caused by the myocardium's contracting in the absence of an adequate oxygen supply. The same type of pain can be produced by placing a blood pressure cuff around the upper arm and inflating it until the brachial pulse can no longer be palpated at the wrist. If a patient opens and closes a fist, pain will gradually appear and escalate in the forearm. The causal mechanism of this pain is the same as that of myocardial pain: continuing muscular contraction in the absence of an adequate oxygen supply. This type of pain requires several contractions of the myocardium to reach its maximal intensity. In other

words, there is a characteristic buildup, or escalation, of angina pain.
2. Can you point to the area of pain with one finger? Anginal pain is characteristically demonstrated by patients' using their entire hand or closed fist against the anterior chest wall. It is described as a sign of angina because it is so typical (Marriott, 1993). By contrast, any pain that can be localized by pointing with a fingertip is unlikely to be angina.
3. Is the pain deep inside your chest or does it seem as though it is close to the surface? Anginal pain is visceral pain that may be referred superficially but always has a deep internal component.

Myocardial ischemia may be completely painless (silent ischemia). Angina may, in fact, not be painful but rather may be described as discomfort, pressure, squeezing, a tight band, heaviness, burning, or indigestion. It usually is located substernally and radiates into one or both arms, the neck, the jaw, or the back.

Angina is not limited to patients with coronary artery disease (CAD) (Marriott, 1993). Individuals who have normal coronary arteries but an insufficient oxygen supply for a given cardiac workload can also experience angina. These include individuals with anemia, hypertension, tachycardia, and thyrotoxicosis. Hypertrophic and dilated cardiomyopathy can produce typical angina pain, although the latter tends to be intermittent, usually occurring with episodes of CHF. Aortic valve disease can cause angina as a result of impairment of adequate coronary artery blood flow.

Angina is usually precipitated by exertion, such as walking uphill, against the wind, or in cold weather (Marriott, 1993). It is more likely to be brought on after a meal or by emotional stress. The rapid resolution of chest pain by rest or sublingual nitroglycerin strongly suggests a cardiac origin. The pain produced by MI is longer, persisting more than 20 minutes; it occurs at rest and is accompanied by nausea, diaphoresis, hypotension, and dyspnea.

Pulmonary Hypertension

Chest pain related to pulmonary hypertension may mimic angina pectoris. It is usually found in patients with mitral stenosis or Eisenmenger syndrome (pulmonary hypertension related to an interventricular septal defect, a patent ductus arteriosus, or an atrial septal defect). This type of chest pain usually is absent at rest, occurs during exertion, and is invariably associated with dyspnea (Hurst, 1990). It is believed to result from dilation of the pulmonary artery or from right ventricular ischemia. The pain is not relieved by nitrates. Primary pulmonary hypertension may be accompanied by syncope and the Raynaud phenomenon (Sharf, 1989).

Pericardial

Pericardial chest pain is also midline, but because of its anatomic relationship with the mediastinal pleura, it has features that suggest pleural involvement (Snider, 1994). Deep breathing, coughing, swallowing, movement, and lying down may make it worse. If the central tendon of the diaphragm is involved, the pain may be referred to the left shoulder or scapular area (Marriott, 1993). The patient may report that each heartbeat affects the pain. Sitting up and leaning forward or lying on the right side often relieves the pain.

Esophageal

Diffuse esophageal spasm or esophageal colic is a common cause of chest pain. It is often confused with cardiac pain because it is located substernally, has a squeezing or aching quality, and may radiate into one or both arms (George, 1990). Furthermore, diffuse esophageal spasm may be relieved by sublingual nitroglycerin as a result of its generalized function as a smooth-muscle relaxant.

Pain that radiates through the chest to the back, pain that decreases with a change in position from supine to upright, or relief induced by ingesting antacids all suggest an esophageal origin (Snider, 1994). Also, diffuse esophageal spasm is often associated with pain on swallowing (odynophagia), dysphagia, and regurgitation of stomach contents. Swallowing hot or cold liquids and emotional stress tend to precipitate this type of chest pain.

Chest Wall

Chest wall pain is the most common type of chest pain. Clues in the patient's history to this type of pain include intermittent occurrence, variable intensity, and local tenderness (Miller, 1980). Because it is commonly located on the anterior chest wall, many patients believe it is heart pain. However, an important differentiation from cardiac pain is that it does not occur during but rather following exertion. It may worsen with inspiration, but its association with trunk motions (flexion, extension, rotation) distinguish it from pleuritic chest pain.

Localized anterior chest pain as a result of costochondritis of the second to fourth costosternal articulations (Tietze syndrome) is described as tender to touch (George, 1990). A complaint of rib tenderness together with a history of trauma, fall, long-term steroid use, coughing, or upper extremity exertion suggests rib fracture.

Degenerative disk disease and arthritis of the cervical or thoracic spine, thoracic outlet syndrome, spondylitis, fibromyalgia, kyphoscoliosis, and herpes zoster can all produce chest wall pain (Epstein, 1979; Miller, 1980; Pellegrino, 1990; Snider, 1994; Wise et al, 1992). Primary lung cancer that invades the adjoining chest wall, ribs, or spine produces severe, persistent, localized pain (Snider, 1994). Another possible cause of chest wall pain is the Pancoast syndrome (superior sulcus tumor), in which a primary lung tumor located in the extreme apex of the lung invades the brachial plexus and produces pain in the shoulder, scapular region, or medial aspect of the arm and hand.

Chest wall pain may be caused, rarely, by thrombosis of a superficial vein on the chest wall (Mondor's disease). It is a self-limited condition of unknown origin and can last several weeks (Snider, 1994). The only physical finding is a subcutaneous cord that can be palpated along the lateral chest wall.

HEMOPTYSIS

Hemoptysis is defined as coughing up blood. It can vary in amount from being blood-streaked sputum to being virtually all blood. The bleeding site may be anywhere in the upper or lower respiratory tract.

The timing and frequency of hemoptysis, as determined in the history, can offer clues about its cause. A history of nosebleeds is significant because blood may be aspirated during sleep at night and expectorated the following morning. Intermittent bouts of hemoptysis are characteristic of respiratory infections such as bronchiectasis, tuberculosis, fungus infections, or broncholithiasis (Miller, 1980). Persistent expectoration of blood-streaked sputum on a daily basis is highly suggestive of bronchogenic neoplasm.

The lung receives its blood supply in two ways: the pulmonary arteries (a low-pressure system) and the bronchial arteries (a high-pressure system) off the aorta (Sharf, 1989). The appearance of hemoptysis may vary according to which blood supply is involved. If the bronchial vessels are the source, there tend to be large amounts of bright-red blood. This is often the site of bleeding in bronchiectasis, because bronchial arteries undergo enlargement and extensive anastomosis with the pulmonary artery system. In mitral stenosis, where there is increased pulmonary vascular resistance, hemoptysis arises from passively engorged submucosal bronchial veins (Szidan and Fishman, 1988).

Hemoptysis sourced in the low-pressure pulmonary artery system tends to occur in small amounts and is composed of dark or clotted venous blood (Snider, 1994). It may arise from the pulmonary parenchyma, as in the case of the highly vascular granulation tissue found in the walls of lung abscesses. These abscesses may be caused by infections, such as tuberculosis, anaerobic bacteria, staphylococci, or chronic irritation bya fungus ball in an abscess cavity. If a blood vessel ruptures in an abscess cavity, hemorrhage tends to be massive, even exsanguinating.

Cardiovascular conditions, such as mitral stenosis, pulmonary infarction, Eisenmenger physiology, and aortic aneurysm, are also associated with hemoptysis (Hurst et al, 1990). Pink frothy sputum is commonly found with acute pulmonary edema. Physical therapists should carefully evaluate complaints of hemoptysis and be certain of its cause before cautiously conducting treatment.

FATIGUE AND WEAKNESS

There are multiple causes of fatigue and weakness (Hurst et al, 1990). Physical therapists should not conclude too quickly that they are related to physical inactivity and decreased muscular strength in sedentary cardiopulmonary patients. The most common causes of complaint of fatigue and weakness are depression, anxiety, and emotional stress. They often accompany anemia, hypothyroidism, and chronic disease states.

Fatigue is commonly associated with CHF. In this condition, it is probably related to cardiac output insufficient to perfuse the entire body adequately, including the skeletal muscles. Generally, fatigue caused by cardiac disease is related to exertion, but fatigue related to anxiety tends to be continuous (Hurst et al, 1990).

Diuretics used to treat CHF can cause potassium depletion and hypokalemia with resultant weakness. Antihypertensive medications can produce weakness through postural hypotension.

PEDAL EDEMA

CHF is a common cause of bilateral pedal edema (Marriott, 1993). However, 10 to 20 pounds of fluid generally accumulate in the body before foot and ankle swelling is evident. Therefore, weight gain is an even earlier indication of fluid retention due to CHF. Occasionally, patients may complain only about an increase in abdominal girth, which results from ascites. When caused by CHF, the onset of ascites virtually always occurs after pedal edema is present. If the amount of ascites is disproportionate to that of pedal edema, restrictive cardiomyopathy or constrictive pericarditis should be a consideration.

It is important to determine whether the patient had dyspnea on exertion before the onset of lower-extremity edema. If the edema is a result of a poorly functioning left ventricle, mitral stenosis, or cor pulmonale, it usually follows dyspnea on exertion.

Patients with CHF and altered renal function commonly report edema of the ankle and lower legs while upright during the day, but indicate a decrease during the night (Hurst et al, 1990). This is a result of local hydrostatic factors related to the upright position.

Edema may be present in nephrosis or starvation, when the total blood protein falls below 5 g/100 ml (hypoproteinemia). Other causes of pedal edema include liver disease, kidney disease, and anemia. Edema of one leg ordinarily occurs because of local factors such as thrombophlebitis or varicose veins.

HOARSENESS

Hoarseness (abnormal vocal cord motion during phonation) is a symptom of laryngeal dysfunction (Miller, 1980). It is usually associated with upper respiratory tract infections or allergies and resolves in 1 to 2 weeks (Sharf, 1989). Trauma following intubation, laryngeal polyps, or tumors are other common causes of hoarseness. However, this symptom is also related to cardiopulmonary conditions. Because the recurrent laryngeal nerves pass through the upper thorax, intrathoracic

pathology that involves one of these nerves can cause unilateral vocal cord paralysis, resulting in hoarseness (Sharf, 1989). These include lung or mediastinal tumors, granulomatous disease, enlarged mediastinal lymph nodes, and pericardial or mediastinal adhesions.

Several cardiovascular conditions can produce hoarseness because the left recurrent laryngeal nerve loops under the arch of the aorta and above the pulmonary artery as it returns to the neck (Hurst et al, 1990). Therefore, an aneurysm of the arch of the aorta, a dilated pulmonary artery or atrium resulting from an atrial septal defect, or mitral stenosis can cause hoarseness (Goldberger, 1990).

Hence, if a patient manifests hoarseness, it is necessary to inquire about the length of time it has been present, the patient's smoking history, and any history of cardiac or pulmonary diseases.

OCCUPATIONAL HISTORY

Taking an occupational history is particularly important for pulmonary patients who arrive for physical therapy with little or no accompanying medical information. The internal surface of the lung measures 50 to 100 m^3 and is in constant contact with the environment (Miller, 1980). Jobs that involve exposure to silica or silicates (e.g., miners, sandblasters, foundry workers, stone cutters, brick layers, and quarry workers) or other inorganic substances place workers at risk for combinations of obstructive and restrictive lung disease (e.g., silicosis). Construction workers, shipyard workers, pipefitters, and other industrial workers exposed to asbestos are at increased risk for developing a restrictive lung disease such as asbestosis (Varkey, 1983). Benign pleural plaques may be found on the diaphragmatic pleurae and bilaterally between the sixth and tenth ribs on the anterolateral or posterolateral chest wall. Progressive pleural thickening rarely occurs. These individuals have an increased incidence of malignant neoplastic diseases such as bronchogenic carcinoma and malignant mesothelioma. Some firefighters, iron workers, and other rescuers working at the World Trade Center disaster site following September 11, 2001, have developed respiratory symptoms and disorders (Feldman et al, 2004; Skloot et al, 2004).

Coal workers are exposed to coal mine dust. About 10% have simple pneumoconiosis, whereas a smaller proportion develop the complicated form—progressive massive pulmonary fibrosis (Brandstetter, 1982).

A history of paroxysmal coughing, chest tightness, or dyspnea that is worse during the week but remits on weekends strongly suggests occupational asthma (Brandstetter, 1982). This condition is difficult to diagnose because symptoms commonly occur several hours after exposure to the provoking agent. Causal agents include grain dusts, wood dusts, formalin, enzyme detergents, ethanolamines (in spray paints and soldering flux), and nickel and hard metals (tungsten carbide). Workers exposed to cotton flax and hemp dusts may develop byssinosis, an obstructive lung disease. In the early stages, it is reversible, but long-term exposure over a number of years causes chronic irreversible obstructive lung disease.

A history of fever, cough, shortness of breath, and recurrent pneumonias in farmers in the northern United States suggests farmer's lung (Brandstetter, 1982). This is the most common hypersensitive pneumonitis; it is caused by inhaling fungal agents such as thermophilic actinomycetes. Long-term exposure can lead to pulmonary fibrosis. There are numerous occupations that expose workers to factors that cause hypersensitive pneumonitis.

SMOKING HISTORY

The patient should be asked about his or her tobacco-smoking history (Snider, 1994). The number of pack-years of cigarettes smoked may be calculated (average number of packs per day to number of years smoked) as a relative risk for lung cancer and COPD. Regular smoking of marijuana is more damaging to the lungs than cigarette smoking.

FAMILY HISTORY

The family history is useful in evaluating the possibility of hereditary pulmonary diseases, such as alpha$_1$-antitrypsin deficiency, cystic fibrosis, allergic asthma, hereditary hemorrhagic telangiectasia, and others (Miller, 1980; Sharf, 1989). A family history of diabetes, hypertension, CAD, or rheumatic fever raises the possibility that these conditions might exist in the patient as well (Marriott, 1993).

PRIOR TREATMENT

It is important to determine what treatment(s) the patient has received for his or her condition. Specifically, has the patient ever received physical therapy for this or any other condition? What types of treatments were done? Were they helpful in improving or resolving the condition? In this way it is possible to determine what treatment modalities have been used, which of them the patient believes may have merit, and which the patient finds objectionable or lacks confidence in, thus avoiding alienating the patient by repeating what he or she believes to be ineffective therapy.

SUMMARY

Obtaining an accurate and thorough history is the cornerstone of the physical therapy evaluation process. The probable cause and severity of many cardiopulmonary symptoms can be determined by careful history taking. This information enables therapists to select the most appropriate evaluation and treatment techniques. When properly performed, accurate history taking gains the patient's confidence and cooperation and provides the basis for a good patient-therapist relationship.

Review Questions

1. What are the basic causes of dyspnea?
2. What questions can be asked of a patient with dyspnea so as to determine the likely cause?
3. What scales have been developed to quantitate dyspnea?
4. What are the principal features of chest pain that originates in the pleurae? The chest wall? The thoracic organs?
5. What are the cardinal features of cardiac chest pain?
6. What occupations can place workers at risk for respiratory disease?

REFERENCES

Birdwell, B., Herbers, J., & Kroenke, K. (1993). Evaluating chest pain: the patient's presentation style alters the physician's diagnostic approach. Archives of Internal Medicine 153: 1991-1995.

Brog, G. (1982). Psychophysical bases of perceived exertion. Medical Science of Sports and Exercise 14:377-381.

Braman, S., & Corrao, W. (1987). Cough: differential diagnosis and treatment. Clinical Chest Medicine 8:177-188.

Brandstetter, R., & Sprince, N. (1982). Occupational lung disease. Medical Times 110:56-63.

Constant, J. (1993). The evolving checklist in history-taking. In: Bedside cardiology. Boston: Little, Brown.

Dicpinigaitis, D.V. (2004). Cough in asthma and eosiniphilic bronchitis. Thorax 59:71.

Epstein, S., Gerber, L., & Borer, J. (1979). Chest wall syndrome: a common cause of unexplained cardiac pain. JAMA 241: 2793-2797.

Feldman, D.M., Baron, S.L., Bernard, B.P., Lushniak B.D., Banauch, G., Arcentales, N., Kelly, K.J., & Prezant, D.J. (2004). Symptoms, respirator use, and pulmonary function changes among New York City firefighters responding to the World Trade Center disaster. Chest 125:1256-1264.

Fontana, G.A., Pistolesi, M. (2003). Chronic cough and gastro-oesophageal reflux. Thorax 58:1092-1095.

Fraser, R.S., Muller, N.L., & Colman, N.C. (1999). The clinical history and physical examination. In Fraser, R.S., Muller, N.L., Colman, N.C., & Pare, P.D. (Eds). Diagnosis and diseases of the chest. Philadelphia: WB Saunders.

George, R. (1990). History and physical examination. In: George, R. (Ed). Chest medicine: essentials of pulmonary and critical care medicine. Baltimore: Williams and Wilkins.

Goldberger, E. (1990). Symptoms referable to the cardiovascular system. In Goldberger, E. (Ed). Essentials of clinical cardiology. Philadelphia: JB Lippincott.

Hurst, J., Morris, D.C., Crawley, I.S., & Dorney, E.R. (1990). The history: past events and symptoms related to cardiovascular disease. In Hurst, J., Schlant, R.C., Rackley, C.E., Sonnenblick, E.H., & Wenger, N.K. (Eds). The heart. New York: McGraw-Hill.

Irwin, R., Rosen, M., & Braman, S. (1977). Cough: a comprehensive review. Archives of Internal Medicine 137:1186-1191.

Irwin, R.S., & Madison, M. (2000). The diagnosis and treatment of cough. New England Journal of Medicine 343:1715-1721.

Mahler, D. (1987). Dyspnea: diagnosis and management. Clinical Chest Medicine 8:215-230.

Mahler, D. (1998). Diagnosis of dyspnea. In Mahler, D. (Ed). Dyspnea. New York: Marcel Dekker.

Mahler, D., & Harver, A. (1990). Clinical measurements of dyspnea. In Mahler, D. (Ed). Dyspnea. Mount Kisco, NY: Futura.

Mahler, D., & Harver, A. (2000). Do you speak the language of dyspnea? Chest 117:928-929.

Marriott, H. (1993). Taking the history. In Marriott, H. (Ed). Bedside cardiac diagnosis. Philadelphia: JB Lippincott.

Miller, D. (1980). The medical history. In Sackner, M. (Ed). Diagnostic techniques in pulmonary disease. New York: Marcel Dekker.

Morice, A.H., & Kastelik, .JA. (2003). Chronic cough in adults. Thorax 58:901-907.

Pellegrino, M. (1990). Atypical chest pain as an initial presentation of primary fibromyalgia. Archives of Physical Medicine Rehabilitation 71:526-528.

Remolina, C., Khan, A.U., Santiago, TV, & Edelman, N.H. (1981). Positional hypoxemia in unilateral lung disease. New England Journal of Medicine 304:523-525.

Sharf, S. (1989). History and physical examination. In Baum, G., & Wolinski, E., (Ed). Textbook of pulmonary diseases, ed 4. Boston: Little, Brown.

Skloot, G., Goldman, M., Fischler, D., Goldman, C., Schechter, C., Levin, S., & Teirstein, A. (2004). Respiratory symptoms and physiologic assessment of ironworkers at the World Trade Center disaster site. Chest 125:1248-1255.

Snider, G. (1994). History and physical examination. In Baum, G., & Wolinski, E. (Eds). Textbook of pulmonary diseases, ed 5. Boston: Little, Brown.

Stulberg, M. (1985). Evaluating and treating intractable cough—Medical Staff Conference, University of California, San Francisco. Western Journal of Medicine 143:223-228.

Szidan, P., & Fishman, A. (1988). Approach to the pulmonary patient with respiratory signs and symptoms. In Fishman, A. (Ed). Pulmonary diseases and disorders, ed 2. New York: McGraw-Hill.

Varkey, B. (1983). Asbestos exposure: an update on pleuro-pulmonary hazards. Postgraduate Medicine 74:93-103.

Wasserman, K. (1982). Dyspnea on exertion: is it the heart or the lungs? JAMA 248:2039-2043.

Wise, C., Semble, E., & Dalton, C. (1992). Musculoskeletal chest wall syndromes in patients with noncardiac chest pain: a study of 100 patients. Archives of Physical Medicine Rehabilitation 73:147-149.

Zack, M.B., Pontoppidan, H., & Kazemi, H. (1974). The effect of lateral positions on gas exchange in pulmonary disease. American Review of Respiratory Diseases 110:49-55.

CHAPTER 9

Pulmonary Function Tests

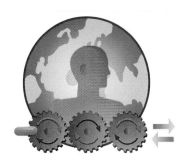

Donna Frownfelter

KEY TERMS

Dead space
Expiratory reserve volume
Functional residual capacity
Inspiratory capacity
Inspiratory reserve volume
Lung capacities
Lung volume

Obstructive component
Predicted values
Restrictive component
Residual volume
Tidal volume
Total lung capacity
Vital capacity

Pulmonary function tests (PFTs) help in the evaluation of the mechanical function of the lungs (Cherniak et al, 1992). They are based on researched norms, taking into account sex, height, and age. For example, there are predicted values for a male, age 65, who is 6 feet tall (Morris et al, 1971; Zelenik, 2003). Race and ethnic differences also play roles in the reference values and need to be taken into account for diagnostic and research purposes (Aelony, 1991; Cruz-Merida, 2004; Hankinson, 1999).

When the patient performs the test, actual results (observed) are compared with the predicted value expected of a person of that gender, height, and age to see if he or she falls within the "normal" range or has a restrictive or obstructive component, based on the tests. If the patient is not within the normal range, a bronchodilator is given, and the test is repeated to see whether there is significant improvement with medication. Basically, the pulmonary function tests are categorized as volume, flow, or diffusion studies. Diagnosis of pulmonary disease or dysfunction and improvement with treatment are evaluated after interpreting a patient's pulmonary function tests.

PREOPERATIVE PULMONARY EVALUATION

Preoperative pulmonary evaluation can predict postoperative pulmonary complications (Kocabas et al, 1996; Smetana, 1999; Wang, 2004). As people are living longer lives, more elderly individuals will be candidates for surgery. From 1980 to 1995 the rates of cardiovascular surgical procedures in patients over 65 tripled (Kozak et al, 1999). In 1997 the performance of ten of the most common surgical procedures in the United States totaled 1 in 350,0000 operations in the 65- to 84-year-old age group (HCUPnet.2001). Considering the comorbidities of an aging population and the concern about complications in the elderly, a thorough preoperative pulmonary screening is recommended (Smetana, 2003).

Risk factors that contribute to postoperative complications include smoking, older age, obesity, poor health, and chronic obstructive pulmonary disease (Smetana, 1999). Additional procedure-related risk factors include the site of surgery (abdominal, chest wall versus extremity, duration of surgery, and type of anesthesia or neuromuscular blockage) (Trayner & Celli, 2001).

OFFICE SPIROMETRY TO IMPROVE EARLY DETECTION OF CHRONIC OBSTRUCTIVE PULMONARYISEASE DISEASE

The National Lung Health Education Program has recommended that office spirometry be used to screen for subclinical lung disease in adult smokers. Spirometric measurements can be considered another vital sign, along with blood pressure and cholesterol levels, in routine physical examinations in adults, beginning at age 40, who are smokers and in patients with unexplained dyspnea, cough, wheezing, or excessive mucous (Petty, 1999, 2001).

In a study of 35- to 70-year-old patients visiting their general practitioners, people were given a questionnaire on symptoms of obstructive lung disease (Buffels et al, 2004). Spirometry was performed in patients with positive answers to the questions and in a random sample of 10% of the group. It was found that 42% of the newly diagnosed cases of obstructive disease would not have been detected without spirometry. The researchers concluded that office spirometry is essential in general practice and can be done by general practioners with training in the performance and in interpretation of the pulmonary function tests. There is a concern that there be good quality assurance and good training when these tests are performed in a general practitioner's office. Studies have shown variability between the results of pulmonary function tests done in the office versus those done in a lab, so the results should not be considered interchangeable (Eaton, 1999; Schermer, 2003).

Respiration: Effect of Anatomical and Physiological Dead Space

The most important function of the lungs is to supply the body with oxygen and to the remove carbon dioxide (CO_2) that is produced as a waste product of metabolism. As this continuous gas exchange takes place, sufficient ventilation is needed to move the gases to the alveoli. There is a series of conducting airways in the lungs, from the trachea down to the terminal bronchi, that do not participate in respiration but only move the gases to the alveoli. This is the volume known as anatomical dead space. Generally, the anatomical dead space is proportional to the adult body weight. For example, in a 150-pound person, there is an anatomical dead space of approximately 150 ml. A normal tidal volume (TV), the breath normally taken, has to be large enough to reach the alveoli well past the anatomical dead space. In a normal adult, the TV is generally 450 to 600 ml. The anatomical dead space would thus represent about one third of the TV volume. The rest of the breath would reach the alveoli and be considered "alveolar ventilation." In many neurologically impaired patients who have limited TVs, it is important to note that little alveolar ventilation may be taking place when the patient is breathing in a rapid and shallow pattern. For example, if a patient's TV is 200 ml, 150 ml would be anatomical dead space, and only 50 ml of each breath would be alveolar ventilation.

Many diseases and conditions can alter the volume of dead space that requires ventilation. In some cases the dead space decreases, as in a pneumonectomy, when it is physically removed, or in asthma, when bronchospasm may narrow the airways. In other conditions such as pulmonary emboli, dead space increases when ventilated areas of lung cease to be perfused. The alveoli continue to receive fresh gas, but there is no blood available for gas exchange. This type of dead space is known as physiological dead space.

When dead space is increased, a larger percentage of the tidal volume is ventilating the dead space, leaving a smaller percentage for alveolar ventilation. The patient must work harder to get enough air to the functioning alveoli. This causes increased work of breathing and may result in patient fatigue. Work of breathing, or minute ventilation (MV), is defined as the TV times the respiratory rate (RR): (MV = TV × RR): an MV of 8 L per minute = 500 ml × 16 breaths per minute. When the ventilatory rate increases, the TV decreases; thus the effective alveolar ventilation decreases.

Neurological and neuromuscular weakness may result in the inability to reach a normal TV. Similarly, surgical procedures or pain caused by fractured ribs can also compromise a patient's ability to take a breath. Patients given a thoracolumbosacral orthosis (TLSO), or a corset for low back pain, may find their pulmonary function compromised by the restriction of the rib cage and abdomen. As the TV drops, a large percentage of the breath is anatomical dead space. This results in increased work of breathing for the patient and may ultimately result in respiratory failure if the patient is unable to provide effective alveolar ventilation.

LUNG VOLUMES

The lung has four volumes: TV; inspiratory reserve volume (IRV); expiratory reserve volume (ERV); and residual volume (RV) (Figure 9-1).

- TV is the normal breath.
- IRV is the maximum amount of air that can be inhaled above a normal inspiration.
- ERV is the maximum amount of air that can be expired after a normal exhalation.
- RV is the volume of gas that remains in the lungs at the end of a maximum expiration.

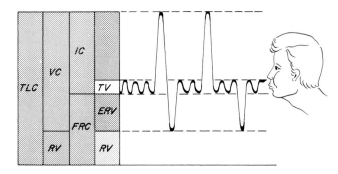

FIGURE 9-1 A spirogram (pulmonary function testing).

Changes in RV can help in the diagnosis of certain medical conditions. An increase in RV means that even with maximum effort, the patient cannot exhale excess air from the lungs. This results in hyperinflated lungs and indicates that certain changes have occurred in the pulmonary tissue, which in time may cause mechanical changes in the chest wall (e.g., increased [AP] diameter, flattened diaphragm). These changes may be reversible in patients with partial bronchial obstruction, such as young asthmatics, or irreversible, as in patients with advanced emphysema. Restrictive lung disease can cause a decrease in residual volume, as can cancer of the lung, microatelectasis, or musculoskeletal impairment (Smith & Dickson, 1994).

LUNG CAPACITIES

A lung capacity is two or more volumes added together (see Figure 9-1). The capacities include total lung capacity (TLC), vital capacity (VC), inspiratory capacity (IC), and functional residual capacity (FRC).

TLC is the amount of gas the lung contains at the end of a maximum inspiration. It is made up of all four lung volumes. An increased TLC is seen with hyperinflation such as emphysema. A decrease in TLC may be seen in restrictive lung disease, such as pulmonary fibrosis, atelectasis, neoplasms, pleural effusions, and hemothorax, as well as in restrictive musculoskeletal problems such, as spinal cord injury and kyphoscoliosis, and as secondary to morbid obesity or pregnancy.

VC is the maximum amount of gas that can be expelled from the lungs by forceful effort after a maximum inspiration. It contains the IRV, TV, and ERV. A decrease in VC can occur as a result of absolute reduction in distensible lung tissue. This is seen in pneumonectomy, atelectasis, pneumonia, pulmonary congestion, occlusion of a major bronchus by a tumor or foreign object, and restrictive lung disease, due to either a primary cause such as pulmonary fibrosis or a secondary cause such as the application of a TLSO.

A decrease in VC may also be seen without primary lung disease or airway obstruction. In neuromuscular or musculoskeletal dysfunction, VC can be compromised (as in Guillain-Barré syndrome, spinal cord injury, drug overdose, motor vehicle accident with fractured ribs, severe scoliosis, pectus excavatum, and kyphoscoliosis). Additional contributing factors, such as morbid obesity, pregnancy, enlarged heart, and pulmonary effusion, may involve limitation of expansion of the lungs.

IC is the maximum amount of air that can be inspired when starting at the resting expiratory level. It contains the IRV and the TV.

FRC is the volume of air remaining in the lungs at the resting expiratory level. It contains the ERV and the RV.

The FRC prevents large fluctuations in Pao_2 with each breath. An increase in FRC represents hyperinflation of the lungs. It causes the thorax to be larger than normal, which results in muscular inefficiency and some mechanical dis-

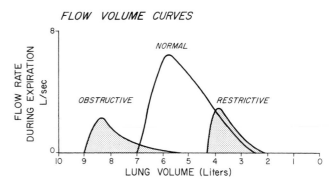

FIGURE 9-2 Comparison of flow volume curves in the normal patient and in the patient with obstructive and restrictive lung disease.

advantage. Patients on mechanical ventilators may increase their FRC with positive pressure and by additional modes such as positive end-expiratory pressure (PEEP). Spontaneously breathing patients can also be on continuous positive airway pressures (CPAP and BIPAP), which keep the lungs at a positive airway pressure to improve ventilation and oxygenation.

AIR-FLOW MEASUREMENTS

Forced Expiration

When a patient performs a VC maneuver, it can either be slow or fast. During exhalation, the amount of air exhaled over time can be measured. In a slow VC, a patient with emphysema can take a great deal of time to empty his or her lungs. In a forced VC, a normal individual can exhale 75% of the VC in the first second of exhalation (FEV_1). Patients with emphysema often have greatly decreased VCs, only 40% of which are predicted. Some pulmonary function laboratories also offer an FEV_6, which measures the flow at six seconds rather than just at one second.

Flow Volume Curve

The flow volume curve is helpful in diagnosing lung disease because it is independent of effort. The curve in Figure 9-2 demonstrates that flow rises to a high value and then declines over most of expiration (Rahn et al, 1946). In restrictive lung disease, the maximum flow rate is reduced, as is the total volume exhaled. In obstructive lung disease, the flow rate is low in relation to lung volume, and a scooped-out appearance is often seen (see Figure 9-2).

Another diagnostic test that uses forced expiration is the flow volume loop. It is a graphic analysis of the flow generated during a forced expiratory volume maneuver followed by a forced inspiratory volume maneuver (Figure 9-3). This graph offers a pictorial representation of data from many individual tests (e.g., peak inspiratory and expiratory flow rates, FVC,

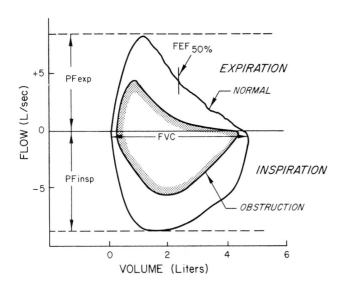

FIGURE 9-3 Comparison of flow volume loops in the normal patient and in the patient with obstructive lung disease.

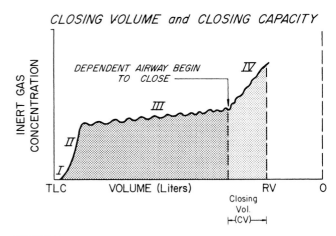

FIGURE 9-4 The single-breath nitrogen washout test to assess airway closure.

and FEV). The shape of the graph may also be helpful in diagnosing disease, because again there is a more scooped-out appearance in cases of obstructive disease.

CLOSING VOLUME AND AIRWAY CLOSURE

The assessment of closing volume is used to help diagnose small-airway disease. A test called the single-breath nitrogen (N_2) washout is used for assessing closing volume and closing capacity of the small airways. In this test, the patient takes a single VC breath of 100% oxygen. During complete exhalation, the N_2 concentration can be measured. The characteristic tracing of N_2 concentration can be measured. The characteristic tracing of N_2 concentration versus lung volume reflects the sequential emptying of differentially ventilated lung units, resulting in different expiratory concentrations of N_2. Four phases can be identified (Figure 9-4). Phase I contains pure dead space and virtually none of the potential N_2 from the RV. Phase II is associated with an increasing N_2 concentration of a mixture of gas from the dead space and alveoli. The plateau in N_2 concentration observed in phase III reflects pure alveolar gas emanating from the base and middle lung zones. Phase IV occurs toward the end of expiration and is characterized by an abrupt increase in N_2 concentration. This high N_2 concentration reflects the closure of airways at the base of the lungs and the expiration of gas from the upper lung zones, because in the single breath of 100% oxygen, less oxygen was initially directed to this area.

Closing volume is the lung volume at which the inflection of phase IV, the marked increase in N_2 concentration after the plateau, is observed. Closing capacity refers to closing volume and RV. The same characteristic tracing of the single-breath nitrogen washout test can be obtained with by the inhalation of a bolus of tracer gas (e.g., argon, helium, xenon 133).

The closing volume is 10% of the vital capacity in young, healthy individuals. It increases with age and is 40% of the vital capacity at age 65. Closing volume is used as an aid in the diagnosis of small-airway disease and as a means of evaluating treatment and drug response.

MAXIMUM VOLUNTARY VENTILATION

Maximum voluntary ventilation measures the maximum breathing capacity of the patient. It reflects strength and endurance of the respiratory muscles. The patient is asked to pant for 15 seconds into the spirometer tubing. The results are commonly examined preoperatively with the other results to determine a patient's prognosis for success after surgery, such as his or her ability to cough, to take deep breaths, and to enhance airway clearance.

DIAGNOSIS OF RESTRICTIVE AND OBSTRUCTIVE LUNG DISEASE

Physicians use the results of pulmonary function tests to diagnose lung disease or characteristic components of lung disease such as bronchospasm. A restrictive component describes conditions that limit the amount of volume coming into the lungs (restriction to inspiration). An obstructive component generally relates to problems in exhalation air flows and characteristic patterns of obstruction, such as in the first second of expiration FEV_1 measurement. Patients do not commonly have only one primary disease process but may have overlapping lung conditions (Clausen, 1984). A diagnosis may read, "PFTs consistent with moderate emphysema with bronchospastic component; good response to bronchodilators." A patient with an abnormal PFT is given a bronchodilator and retested. If there is a 15% to 20% increase in the PFT after bronchodilators are administered, they will be a recommended part of the patient's medications. However, some patients are given a trial of bronchodilators, even if there is not such a dramatic response on PFTs.

NORMAL   OBSTRUCTIVE   RESTRICTIVE

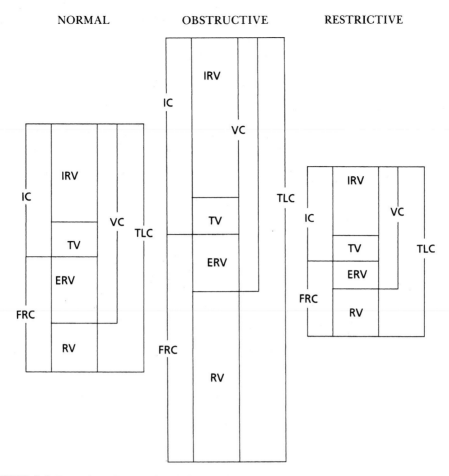

FIGURE 9-5 Examples of proportional changes in lung volumes and capacities characteristic of obstructive and restrictive lung diseases.

A pictorial demonstration of the differences in obstructive and restrictive lung disease is shown in Figure 9-5. Disease has a marked effect on pulmonary function, yet TV usually remains 10% of total lung capacity until the disease is relatively severe. Physiological pulmonary reserves in both disease processes are limited and generally affect a patient's response to exercise. Exercise is limited by the ventilatory status rather than by a cardiac end point. As obstructive lung disease progresses, TLC, FRC, and RV are markedly increased. In severe COPD, the increased FRC can compromise the VC. More energy is expended to breathe than that expended by a normal individual. This effect can be disproportionally increased with minimal amounts of activity. In restrictive lung disease, restriction of the chest wall or lung tissue can produce a decrease in TLC. A VC of 80% or less of predicted values for a patient is considered a diagnostic feature. A residual decline in FRC potentiates airway closure.

The phenomenon of closing volume in the lungs is particularly significant to physical therapists who prescribe breathing exercises and body positioning and can thereby alter pulmonary mechanics and gas exchange. These treatment interventions may have pronounced effects on lung volumes

and airway closure (Dean, 1985). At low lung volumes (e.g., breathing at FRC, in the Trendelenberg position, and in lung disease) intrapleural pressures are generally less negative, and the pressure of dependent lung regions may equal or exceed atmospheric pressure. Intrapleural pressure is less negative because the lungs are less expanded and elastic recoil is decreased. As a result, airway closure is potentiated. In young individuals, closure is evident at RV; however, in older individuals, closure is observed at higher lung volumes, such as at FRC. Premature closure of the small airways results in uneven ventilation and impaired gas exchange with a given lung unit. Airway closure occurs more readily in chronic smokers and in patients with lung disease.

Aging has a significant effect on airway closure. With aging, a loss of pulmonary elastic recoil results in a loss of intrapleural negative pressure. In older individuals, therefore, airway closure occurs at higher lung volumes. For example, closure has been reported to occur at the age of 65 in the upright lung during normal breathing. In the supine position, where FRC is reduced, closure occurs at a significantly younger age (about age 44). In addition to the often compounding effect of age, the lung volume at which airway closure occurs increases with chronic smoking and lung disease and is changed with the alterations in body position (Berry et al, 1990; Zadai, 1985).

SUMMARY

Pulmonary functions change as a patient's condition gets better or worse (Emery et al, 1991; Emerson et al, 1994). There are normal declines in volumes and flows with aging as well as with disease processes. Basic bedside spirometry is often done to assess a patient's breathing mechanical ability and screen preoperatively to predict possible postoperative complications, especially in high-risk patients. Bedside screening can detect improvement or decline in a clinical status. In a patient with Guillain-Barré syndrome, as breathing becomes labored, the VC is monitored to determine whether a ventilator is needed. On the other hand, in a patient with obstructed airways, such as a patient with cystic fibrosis, the pulmonary function tests will improve (Versteegh et al, 1986). In a patient with spinal cord injury or neuromuscular weakness, as strength improves, vital capacity increases. However, because of the lack of abdominal muscles, the flows may be reduced.

Review Questions

1. What effect will an obstructive or restrictive component have on exercise performance?
2. Why is it important to compare the patient's predicted values with the actual observed values in a pulmonary function test?
3. What response should you see to determine whether bronchodilators have a positive effect on pulmonary function?
4. How can pulmonary function tests be used to assess patient improvement or decline over a period of time?
5. What is the value of using pulmonary function tests as a "vital sign"?

REFERENCES

Aelony, Y. (1991). Ethnic norms for pulmonary function tests. Chest 99:1051.

Berry, R., Pai, U., & Fairshter, R. (1990). Effect of age on changes in flow rates and airway conductance after a deep breath. Journal of Applied Physiology 68:635-643.

Buffels, J., Degryse, J., Hetman, J., & Decramer, M. (2004). Office spirometry significantly improves early detection of COPD in general practice. Chest 125:1394-1399.

Cherniak, R.M. (1992). Evaluation of respiratory function in health and disease. Disease-a-month 38:505-576.

Clausen, J.L. (1984). Pulmonary function testing guidelines and controversies. London: Grune and Stratton.

Crapo, R.O. (1994). Pulmonary function testing. New England Journal of Medicine 331:25-30.

Cruz-Merida, A.J., Soto-de la Fuente, A.E., Mendez-Vargas, M.M., & Mendez-Ramirez, I. (2004). Prediction equations for spirometric parameters in Mexican adult population. Archives of Medical Research 35:446-449.

Dean, E. (1985). The effect of body position on pulmonary function. Physical Therapy 65:613-618.

Eaton, T., Withy, S., Garrett, J.E., Mercer, J., Whitlock, R.M., & Rea, H.H. (1999). Spirometry in primary care practice: the importance of quality assurance and the impact of spirometry workshops. Chest 116:416-423.

Emerson, C.L., Lukens, T.W., & Effron, D. (1994). Physician estimation of FEV_1 in acute exacerbation of COPD. Chest 105:1709-1712.

Emery, C.E. (1991). Psychological outcome of a pulmonary rehab program. Chest 100:613-617.

Hankinson, J., Odencrantz, J., & Fedan, K., (1999). Spirometrical reference values from a sample of the general US population. American Journal of Respiratory Critical Care Medicine 159:179-187

HCUPnet. (2001). Healthcare cost and utilization project, agency for healthcare research and quality. Rockville, MD: http:www.ahrq.gov/data/hcup/hcupnet.htm.

Kocabas, A., Kara, K., Ozgur, G., Sonmez, H., & Burgut, R. (1996). Value of preoperative spirometry to predict postoperative complications. Respiratory Medicine 90:25-33.

Kozak, L.J., McCarthy, E., & Pokras, R. (1999). Changing patterns of surgical care in the United States 1980-1995. Health Care Finance Review 21:31-49.

Morris, J., Koski, A., & Johnson, L. (1971). Prediction nomograms (BTPS) spirometric values in normal males and females. American Review of Respiratory Diseases 163:57-67.

Petty, T. (1999). Testing patients' lungs: spirometry as part of the physical examination. Clinical Therapy 21:1908-1922.

Petty, T. (2001). Simple office spirometry. Clinical Chest Medicine 22:845-859.

Rahn, H. (1946). The pressure-volume diagram of the thorax and lung. American Journal of Physiology 146:161.

Schermer, T., Jacobs, J.E., Chavannes, N.H., Hartman, J., Folgering, H.T., Bottema, B.J., & van Weel, C. (2003). Validity of spirometric testing in a general population of patients with COPD. Thorax 58:861-866.

Smetana, G. (1999). Preoperative pulmonary evaluation. New England Journal of Medicine 340:937-944.

Smith, R.M., & Dickson, R.A. (1994). Changes in residual volume relative to vital capacity and total lung capacity after arthrodesis of the spine in patients who have idiopathic scoliosis. Bone and Joint Surgery of America 76:153.

Trayner, E., & Celli, B. (2001). Postoperative pulmonary complications. Medical Clinics of North America 85:1129-1139.

Versteegh, F.G.A., Neijens, H.J., Bogaard, J.M., Stam, H., Robijn, R.J., & Kerrebijn, K.F. (1986). Relationship between pulmonary function, O_2 saturation during sleep and exercise with cystic fibrosis. Advanced Cardiology 35:151-155.

Wang, J.S. (2004). Pulmonary function test in preoperative pulmonary evaluations. Respiration Medicine 98:598-605.

Williams-Russe, P., Charlson, M.E., MacKenzie, C.R., Gold, J.P., & Shires, G.T. (1992). Predicting postoperative complications: is it a real problem? Archives of Internal Medicine 152:1209-1213.

Youtsey, J.W. (1990). Basic pulmonary function measurement. In Scanlon, C.L., Spearman, C.B., & Sheldan, R.L. (Eds). Egan's fundamentals of respiratory care, ed 5. St. Louis: Mosby.

Zadai, C. (1985). Pulmonary physiology of aging: the role of rehabilitation. Topics in Geriatric Rehabilitation 1:49-56.

Zelenik, J. (2003). Normative aging of the respiratory system. Clinical Geriatric Medicine19:1-18.

C H A P T E R   1 0

Arterial Blood Gases

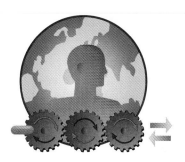

Donna Frownfelter

An arterial blood gas is a physiological assessment tool that measures a patient's acid-base balance, and alveolar and oxygenation status (Cherniak, 1992). It is a valuable resource for information, from respiratory monitoring in the intensive care unit to follow-up of outpatients to evaluate the therapy for and progress of their diseases.

The purpose of this chapter is to help the clinician evaluate and interpret arterial blood gases more effectively and to integrate the information into treatment planning and the progress of the patient. Blood gases give a picture of a given time and patient condition and are important in the management of acutely ill, unstable patients.

Noninvasive monitoring has become more readily available and is used to measure expired carbon dioxide (Pet CO_2) and transcutaneous CO_2 (T CO_2) in pediatric patients. Pulse oximetry has been used to measure trends in oxygen saturation in patients who are stable and during exercise. These measures have resulted in fewer invasive arterial sticks and in the ability to monitor patients in an ongoing manner; they have made it possible to improve the care of patients with cardiovascular and pulmonary illness and to administer the most appropriate ventilation and oxygenation support.

ACID-BASE BALANCE

Normal body metabolism consists of the consumption of nutrients and the excretion of acid metabolites. Acid metabolites must be kept from accumulating in large amounts because the body's cardiovascular and nervous systems operate in a relatively narrow free hydrogen ion (H^+) range (narrow pH). Free H^+ concentration is discussed as pH ($-\log$ [H^+]). The maintenance of body systems requires an appropriate acid-base balance (Shapiro, 1994).

Approximately 98% of normal metabolites exist in the form of CO_2, which reacts readily with water to form carbonic acid.

$$CO_2 + H_2O \oslash'' H_2CO_3$$

Carbonic acid can exist as either a liquid or a gas. Because carbonic acid can change to CO_2, much of the acid content can be excreted through the lungs during respiration.

The Henderson-Hasselbach equation demonstrates how the H^+ concentration results from the dissociation of carbonic acid and the interrelationship of the blood acids, bases, and buffers.

$$H_2O + CO_2 \oslash'' H_2CO_3\ H^+ + HCO_3^-$$

Renal Buffering Mechanisms

The kidneys are the main route of excretion of the normal metabolic acids. H^+ is excreted in the urine and also resorbed by bicarbonate into the blood. In this manner, the kidneys can respond when there is an acid-base imbalance and return the body to normal homeostasis.

PARTIAL PRESSURE OF GASES

To better understand blood gases, it is important to remember the properties of gases. The earth's surface consists of gas molecules that have mass and are attracted to the earth's center of gravity. At the surface, this atmospheric weight exerts a pressure that can support a column of mercury 760 mm high.

Dalton's law states that in a mixture of gases, the total pressure is equal to the sum of the partial pressures of the separate gases. Oxygen is 20.9% of the atmosphere, so it has a partial pressure of 159 (760 × 20.9% = 159). Nitrogen is 79% of the atmosphere, so it has a partial pressure of 600 (760 × 79% = 600). Other gases make up 0.1% of the atmosphere.

The diffusion of gases across semipermeable membranes shows gradients from higher concentrations to lower concentrations. Each gas moves independently from the others.

During respiration, oxygen and CO_2 exchange across the alveolar capillary membrane. Special situations may affect the normal progress of respiration and gas exchange.

Normally, alveolar units ventilate and capillary units bring oxygenated blood to the tissues, excreting CO_2 back into the alveoli to be removed through the lungs. Some abnormal situations may occur, however, such as shunts and dead-space units. In a shunt unit, the alveoli have collapsed, but blood flow continues and is unable to pick up oxygen. An example of this is atelectasis, in which a lung segment or part of a segment has retained secretions and lung tissue distal to the mucous plug collapses. Circulation continues but oxygenation does not occur, and the Po_2 decreases. On the other hand, a dead-space unit can have ventilation but not perfusion. This occurs with pulmonary embolism, when a blood clot obstructs the circulation. The oxygen is available in the ventilated alveoli, but with no circulation, a dead unit is credited. Figure 10-1 demonstrates the regional differences seen in respiratory units.

Normal Blood Gas Values

The acid-base balance is denoted by the pH scale; it ranges from 1 to 14, where 1 is the most acidic and 14 the most basic. The arterial pH values are normally 7.35 to 7.45. If the pH is below 7.35, the patient is considered to be in a more acidotic state. If the pH is above 7.45, the patient is considered to be in a more alkalotic state.

Alveolar ventilation is reflected in the partial pressure of carbon dioxide (Pco_2). Normal Pco_2 values are 35 to 45 mm Hg. If the Pco_2 is below 35 mm Hg, the patient is said to be hyperventilating (having increased ventilation, blowing off more CO_2 than normal). If the Pco_2 is above 45 mm Hg, the patient is hypoventilating (having decreased alveolar ventilation, not blowing off enough CO_2 to maintain normal alveolar ventilation).

Arterial oxygen is measured as Po_2, the partial pressure of oxygen. Normal values are 80 to 100 mm Hg. If the Po_2 is below 80 mm Hg in someone younger than 60 years of age, the patient is hypoxemic. A value of 60 to 80 mm Hg is

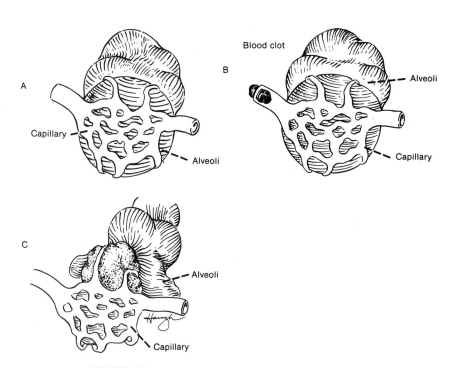

FIGURE 10-1 A, Normal alveolus. **B**, Dead space. **C**, Shunt.

considered mild hypoxemia; 40 to 60 mm Hg is considered moderate hypoxemia, and less than 40 mm Hg is severe hypoxemia (Cherniak, 1992).

Base Excess/Base Deficit

The blood normally has the capacity to buffer acid metabolites. The normal level of base HCO_3 in the blood is 22 to 26 millimoles per liter (mmol/L). This buffering capacity diminishes in the presence of acidemia or alkalemia. Acidosis is an abnormal acid-base balance in which the acids dominate. Alkalemia is an abnormal acid-base balance in which the bases dominate. When there is a decrease in HCO_3^-, it is seen in a negative base excess and referred to as a base deficit, which is usually seen as a negative number on the blood gas report, such as −3.

As one looks at the base excess and the base deficit (BE/BD), it is helpful to determine whether the patient's condition is acute or chronic. This state can also be thought of as uncompensated (acute); partially compensated; or completely compensated (chronic). The pH is the key to making this determination. If the pH is not in the normal 7.35 to 7.45 range, then the patient is in an acute state. As the balance progresses back toward normal, it may be partially compensated. When a normal pH exists, it is compensated, or chronic. The interpretation comes from looking at the BE/BD and then at the pH. Having a series of arterial blood gases for comparison is helpful, for example, in a patient with respiratory failure and on a ventilator; the patient's improvement can be documented.

Another example is that of a patient in the chronic state who has chronic obstructive pulmonary disease (COPD) and is retaining CO_2 at a level of 55 mm Hg. If the pH reads 7.25, this would be considered an acute state. As the body retains base, the pH will rise back toward the normal numbers. If the pH is 7.32 with a PCO_2 of 55 and +3 base excess, the reading would be partially compensated. If the pH is within normal limits, with a PCO_2 of 55 and a pH of 7.35, the reading would be compensated or chronic. This is a means of identifying people who are chronic CO_2 retainers.

Hemoglobin

Hemoglobin (Hgb) is the main component of the red blood cell. It is crucial for oxygen transport. The normal Hgb range is 12 to 16 g/100 ml blood. In patients who have lost blood through surgical procedures or disease, the decreased hemoglobin can account for their extreme weakness as a result of decreased total oxygen transport capacity. Some of the patients at highest risk are those who have just undergone joint replacement in which there has been much blood loss. Often their Hgb levels are only 8, and because they are considered "orthopedic" patients, it is thought that the low levels can be overlooked. In addition, patients with advanced COPD can at times desaturate (pulse oximetry below 90%) with exercise when the PO_2 is low (i.e., PO_2 55-60). Pulse oximetry is essential for monitoring the exercise of patients with low PO_2, low Hgb, or both.

Cyanosis, the presence of a bluish color to the skin, mucous membranes, and nail beds, is indicative of an abnormal amount of reduced Hgb concentration, usually greater than 5 g of reduced Hgb. The presence of cyanosis suggests a high probability of hypoxemia; however, hypoxemia can occur without cyanosis. Two examples may be cited, one in which an anemic patient with hypoxemia can have little cyanosis, and the other in which a patient with polycythemia can have cyanosis with minimal hypoxemia.

There is a predictable relationship between the arterial oxygen saturation of the Hgb and the PO_2. It is represented in the oxyhemoglobin dissociation curve as follows. When oxygen saturation is monitored during exercise, saturation is kept at or above 90%. As the curve denotes at a level of approximately 60 mm Hg, the saturation is about 90%. As the PO_2 drops at the sharp part of the curve, there is a marked decrease in oxygen saturation for every mm Hg PO_2 (Guyton, 1986).

Chemoreceptor Response to Hypoxemia

The peripheral chemoreceptors, the carotid, and the aortic bodies are located at the bifurcation of the internal and external carotid arteries and the arch of the aorta. These receptors are nervous tissue that have a high metabolic rate and an abundant oxygen supply. When tissue PO_2 decreases, their response to the brain is to increase ventilation and cardiac output. When that is not sufficient to affect a normal PO_2, supplemental oxygen or increased mechanical assistance such as continuous positive airway pressure (CPAP) is given (Tarpy & Farber, 1994).

BLOOD GAS INTERPRETATION

The norms for the pH, PCO_2, PO_2, and base have been established for a given patient, and they should be considered first. Is the current value normal or not? Is the patient acute (uncompensated), partially compensated, or fully compensated (chronic)?

A stepwise interpretation can be helpful. To perform the assessment in the same order each time provides a comprehensive and standard overview.

1. Look at the PCO_2 to determine whether there is normal alveolar ventilation.
2. Look at the pH to see if there is a normal acid-base balance or whether it is acute or chronic.
3. Look at the PO_2 to see if there is normal oxygenation or if there is hypoxemia and to what degree.
4. Look at the BE/BD.

In addition, it is important to note other clinical considerations. Is the patient receiving oxygen or mechanical ventilation? If the patient is on forced inspiratory oxygen

(FIO_2) of 40% and the PO_2 is not close to acceptable levels, it is more of a concern than if the patient is on a low FIO_2 and the PO_2 is within normal limits. Similarly, if the patient is on mechanical ventilation, the blood gases should be close to normal. The exception would be a patient who is a chronic CO retainer; that patient would be ventilated to his or her normal level (i.e., at the PCO_2 level where the pH becomes closer to normal).

Acceptable Ranges of Arterial Blood Gases

At times, for many medical reasons, an acceptable range of blood gases will be used, rather than trying to get an ideal reading. The following ranges may be acceptable, depending on the physician and the circumstances of the patient.

- pH 7.30 to 7.50
- PCO_2 30 to 50 mm Hg
- pH 7.45 alkalemia
- pH 7.35 acidemia

A relationship between the pH and the PCO_2 exists also. There is a predictable change caused by variation in carbonic acid.

- For every 20 mm Hg increase in PCO_2, the pH decreases by 0.10 (PCO_2 60, pH 7.25)
- For every 10 mm Hg decrease in PCO_2, the pH increases by 0.10 (PCO_2 25, pH 7.50)

There is also a relationship between the PCO_2 and the plasma bicarbonate.

- For every increase of 10 mm Hg in the PCO_2, there is a decrease of 1 mmol/L of plasma bicarbonate
- For every 10 mm Hg PCO_2, there is a decrease in plasma bicarbonate of 2 mmol/L

By knowing these guidelines, it can be determined whether the changes in the arterial blood gases are in line with respiratory problems as opposed to metabolic problems such as acidosis due to diabetic ketoacidosis, in which the base deficit can be very low, and the pH can be low (acidemic), but the PCO_2 can be within normal limits (Shapiro, 1994; Shapiro et al, 1994).

RESPIRATORY FAILURE

Respiratory failure is defined as the failure of the pulmonary system to meet the metabolic demands of the body (i.e., ventilation and oxygenation) (Shapiro et al, 1994). The blood gases usually have a pH below 7.30 and a PCO_2 above 50. Generally the patient is also hypoxemic.

During the acute phase the kidneys have not started to compensate and the base HCO_3^- is within normal limits. Later, a base excess can be noted as the kidneys try to compensate for the acidotic pH. Chronic respiratory failure

can be noted by an increased PCO_2, a pH within normal limits, and a low PO_2.

In assessing the PO_2, the following ranges are used: mild hypoxemia, less than 80 mm Hg; moderate hypoxemia, 60 to 80 mm Hg; and severe hypoxemia, below 40 mm Hg.

Positional changes can affect the oxygenation status. For example, unilateral right lower lobe atelectasis with the patient lying on the right side causes increased blood flow to the right lung, which is collapsed. This causes increased shunting and a decrease in oxygenation (differential shunting). If the patient lies on the left side, the oxygenation will improve. When the patient lies in a supine position, a mixed PO_2 can be observed.

When hypoxemia is noted, treatment consists of oxygen therapy, CPAP or biphasic positive airway pressure, and alleviation of the cause of hypoxemia, if possible. This may be achieved by means of airway-clearance techniques or medication, in addition to the oxygen therapy or mechanical ventilation. Oxygen therapy treats the hypoxemia, decreases the patient's work of breathing, and decreases myocardial work.

FACTORS AFFECTING ARTERIAL BLOOD GASES

Many normal causes affect arterial blood gases, such as extremes of age, from neonatal to geriatric. The neonate has many changes going on in the initial life process; fetal circulation changes dramatically in the first hours and days of life. In the geriatric patient, decreases in cardiac output (CO), residual volume (RV) of the lungs, and maximal breathing capacity gradually lower PO_2 over the course of the life cycle. It is estimated that after 60 years of age, the PO_2 decreases by 1 mm Hg per year of age from 60 to 90 years.

Exercise or any increase in activity above rest may result in increased oxygen consumption in patients with cardiopulmonary dysfunction. In the normal population, the human body compensates by increasing oxygen consumption to meet the workload. Usually a plateau is reached and a constant oxygen consumption for that activity is achieved. In patients with cardiopulmonary dysfunction, oxygen consumption continues to increase, even at the same workload in untrained patients. It is important to monitor oxygen saturation to prevent desaturation in these patients (Guyton, 1986). During pregnancy, hormonal and mechanical factors have negative effects on cardiopulmonary function. During the last trimester, women commonly observe shortness of breath and difficulty in taking a deep breath because of hormonal issues and diaphragmatic encroachment.

During sleep there is a decrease in minute ventilation and a decreased responsiveness to CO_2 and hypoxemia. Many patients who have undergone spinal cord injuries or cerebrovascular accidents, who have COPD, or who are morbidly obese have been noted to have sleep apnea and hypoxemia during sleep. These possibilities should be considered in any patient with daytime somnolence who may complain of difficulty sleeping or staying awake during the day or who has trouble following directions or is mentally confused.

Low barometric pressure associated with high altitude significantly decreases the amount of oxygen available to an individual. As noted before, the partial pressure of oxygen is dependent on the total atmospheric pressure. When the total pressure is reduced, less O_2 is available. This is particularly important if a patient already has a decreased Po_2 and is traveling to an area with lower barometric pressure. Patients on oxygen need an oxygen prescription that is based on the area in which they are living.

Barometric pressure increases, such as in a hyperbaric oxygen chamber with higher barometric pressure, can help deliver increased oxygen for a select group of patients. Wound-healing needs and carbon monoxide poisoning are two such indications.

Increased temperature (a febrile state) can increase metabolism and therefore increase oxygen consumption, decrease Po_2 and, consequently, increase alveolar ventilation. Decreased temperatures can decrease oxygen consumption, as is seen in patients who have survived for several minutes in cold water and are then resuscitated.

On the arterial blood gas report it is important to note the status of the patient at the time the blood gas is drawn. Usually patients are at rest when the blood gas is drawn. If the Po_2 is low at rest (60 mm Hg), it is close to the sharp part of the oxyhemoglobin dissociation curve, and the patient may desaturate quickly with an increase in exercise.

If the patient is on supplemental oxygen and the Po_2 is only 55 mm Hg, the Po_2 is still inadequate because of the additional O_2 (Brunelli et al, 2003; Carpenter, 1991; Emtner et al, 2004). Any patient on oxygen at rest should be evaluated for appropriate oxygenation with exercise. Most patients' blood gases are drawn at rest, not with exercise. Similarly, if a patient is on mechanical ventilation, the blood gases should be within or near normal limits.

Noninvasive Monitoring

Noninvasive monitoring of respiratory function is convenient, accurate in showing trends, involves minimal complications, and causes little discomfort for the patient. The modalities are used as an ongoing examination, along with clinical monitoring. In this category are pulse oximetry, transcutaneous oxygen (Ptc O_2); transcutaneous Pco_2 (Ptc CO_2); and end-tidal CO_2 using capnography.

Pulse Oximetry

Pulse oximetry provides estimates of arterial oxyhemoglobin saturation (SaO_2) by utilizing selected wavelengths of light to noninvasively determine the saturation of oxyhemoglobin (SpO_2) (AARC, 1991).

Indications for Pulse Oximetry

There are several reasons to perform pulse oximetry.

1. To monitor the adequacy of arterial oxyhemoglobin saturation.

2. To evaluate the patient response to interventions and exercise.
3. To meet third-party payers' need to document desaturation and prescribe oxygen so as to meet regulations (Welch, 1990).

Contraindications for Pulse Oximetry

If a patient needs ongoing measurement of pH, $Paco_2$, and total Hgb, the presence of abnormal Hgbs may be a "relative" contraindication for pulse oximetry (AARC, 1991).

A probe is attached to the patient's finger, toe, or earlobe, and a measurement is made of the amount of light that is absorbed (i.e., relayed to a microprocessor that calculates SaO_2). It can be read intermittently or displayed continuously. In addition, a pulse reading is given.

A reading taken at rest as an additional vital sign, along with HR, BP, and RR, provides a baseline before exercise. When an exercise workload is given, the parameters can be compared to see if the patient has a normal or abnormal response to exercise. The recommendation is to keep the O_2 saturation above 90% during exercise. Supplemental oxygen can be titrated to keep the O_2 saturation within the appropriate range.

There are situations in which pulse oximetry may not yield accurate results: abnormal Hgb, jaundice, anemia, low perfusion (i.e., diabetes), the use of intravascular dye such as methylene blue, deeply pigmented skin, and dark nail polish (Schnapp & Cohen, 1990). In addition there can be movement artifacts, and highly lit fluorescent lights can have an effect on the readings. These concerns must be appreciated by therapists, especially during exercise, to ensure proper readings and correct evaluation of responses to exercise.

Documentation of patients' responses to exercise can be included with vital sign notations; ECG, HR, BP, RR, and SpO_2 may be recorded. The information taken at rest, during exercise, and at the end point of exercise is important, as is the time it takes for the patient to recover (to return to baseline). This information documents the physiological response to exercise.

Transcutaneous Oxygenation

To test for transcutaneous oxygenation (Pt co_2), a sensor is applied to the skin on the anterior chest or abdomen. The sensor is heated to produce localized erythema. This method is used primarily in the neonatal and pediatric intensive care units. There is an equilibration time of about 10 to 15 minutes, and the sensor must be calibrated to ensure accurate results. Inaccurate measurements may be caused by hypothermia, shock, severe anemia, edema, severe acidosis, and dislodgement of the sensor. Cases of thermal injury have occurred.

Transcutaneous Carbon Dioxide

Transcutaneous carbon dioxide (Pt co_2) measurements are used in the neonatal ICU, where continuous monitoring is indicated, especially if the baby is not intubated or being mechanically ventilated. It is also a skin sensor and is most effective in monitoring hemodynamically stable patients. The sensor must be calibrated and must be rotated frequently to prevent burns. There is a relatively close correlation between arterial P_{CO_2} and Pt_{CO_2}, and the latter has the additional benefit of requiring fewer needle sticks.

End Tidal Carbon Dioxide

Capnography uses infrared spectroscopy or mass spectrometry reading of expired CO_2 to analyze CO_2 content in a continuous reading. There is also a wave display of the breath-to-breath readings. The waveform can be divided into segments that represent various phases of the respiratory cycle. In the beginning of a normal exhalation, gas is expelled from the anatomical dead space and has a low CO_2 reading. As more alveoli empty, there is an increasing proportion of alveolar gas in relationship to dead space gas and thus a greater concentration of CO_2. A plateau level is reached when there is a nearly constant CO_2 concentration (alveolar plateau). At the alveolar plateau, the end tidal CO_2 concentrations closely approximate the arterial P_{CO_2}. Then with inspiration, the CO_2 concentration decreases rapidly to baseline.

The end tidal CO_2 readings help monitor changes in the ventilatory status and assist in determining the need for changes in the ventilator settings to improve alveolar ventilation. (Healey et al, 1987). Most notable is the ability to see trends in these readings and maintain an ongoing monitoring system that can allow for early detection of complications, such as pneumothorax, hypoventilation, pulmonary embolism, or fat embolism (any increase in dead space). The readings have also been used to determine the proper position of feeding tubes and endotracheal tubes (Ahrens et al, 1999; Burns et al, 2001).

SUMMARY

This chapter discusses the normal arterial blood gases and the meanings of their values. A guide to the interpretation of blood gases is suggested. The relationships between pH and P_{CO_2}; between P_{CO_2} and HCO_3^-; and between O_2 saturation and P_{O_2} are examined. Predictable changes that are caused by respiratory changes are described. In addition, it is noted that metabolic changes can have marked effects on blood gases. Oxygen therapy and airway-clearance techniques can improve hypoxemia, and position changes can be detrimental, causing differential shunting, or can improve the P_{O_2} by means of better ventilation-perfusion matching.

Noninvasive monitoring has been a great advance; it is now possible to see ongoing trends in a patient and assess complications early so patients can be moved forward more safely and efficiently.

As a physical therapist, it is necessary to be acutely aware of the respiratory monitors that can assess and progress patients safely to their optimal rehabilitation outcomes.

Review Questions

1. Which factors affect arterial blood gases?
2. What effect does an increased temperature have on the blood gases, and how does this relate clinically to treating a patient with an elevated temperature?
3. What is the benefit of noninvasive monitoring?
4. What parameters of the blood gas will guide you in determining whether the patient is a chronic CO_2 retainer?
5. What effect can body position have on blood gases, and how can this knowledge be used therapeutically?

REFERENCES

AARC. (1991). Clinical practice guidelines. Respiratory Care 36:1406-1409.

Ahrens, T., Wijeweera, H., & Ray, S. (1999). Capnography: a key underutilised technology. Critical Care Nursing Clinics of North America 11:49-62.

Brunelli, A., Al Refai, M., Monteverde, M., Borri, A., Salati, M., & Fianchini, A. (2003). Predictors of exercise oxygen desaturation following major lung resection. European Journal of Cardiothoracic Surgery 24:145-148.

Burns, S.B., Carpenter, R., & Truwit, J.D. (2001). Report on the development of a procedure to prevent placement of feeding tubes into the lungs using end-tidal CO_2 measurements. Critical Care Medicine 29:936-939.

Carpenter, K.D. (1991). Oxygen transport in the blood. Critical Care Nurse 11:20-33.

Cherniak, R.M. (1992). Evaluation of respiratory function in health and disease. Disease Monitor 38:505-576.

Emtner, M., Porszasz, J., Burns, M., Somfay, A., & Casaburi, R. (2003). Benefits of supplemental oxygen in exercise training in nonhypoxemic chronic obstructive pulmonary disease patients. American Journal of Respiratory Critical Care Medicine 168:1034-1042.

Guyton, A. (1986). Textbook of medical physiology, ed 7. Philadelphia: WB Saunders.

Healey, C.J., Fedullo, A.J., Swinburne, A.J., & Wahl, G.W. (1987). Comparison of noninvasive measurements of carbon dioxide tension during withdrawal from mechanical ventilation. Critical Care Medicine 15:764-768.

Kindopp, A.S., Crover, J.W., & Heyland, D.K. (2001). Capnography confirms correct feeding tube placement in intensive care unit patients. Canadian Journal of Anesthesia 48:705-710.

Schnapp, L.M., & Cohen, N.H. (1990). Pulse oximetry: uses and abuses. Chest 98:1244-1250.

Shapiro, B.A. (1994). Evaluation of blood gas monitors: performance criteria, clinical impact, and cost/benefit (editorial comment). Critical Care Medicine 22:546-548.

Shapiro, B.A., Peruzzi, W., & Templin, R. (1994). Clinical application of blood gases, ed 5. St. Louis: Mosby.

Tarpy, S.P., & Farber, H.W. (1994). Chronic lung disease: when to prescribe home oxygen. Geriatrics 49:27-8, 31-3.

Welch, J.P., DeCesare, M.S., & Hess, D. (1990). Pulse oximetry: instrumentation and clinical applications. Respiratory Care 35:584-601.

C H A P T E R 1 1

Imaging of the Chest

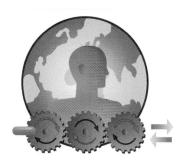

Patrick Knott

KEY TERMS

Aortic aneurism
Cardiac hypertrophy
Cardiac silhouette
Computed tomography
Consolidation
Hemothorax
Inspiratory effort
Ionizing radiation
Magnetic resonance imaging
Mediastinal widening

Nonionizing radiation
Pleural effusion
Pneumonia
Pneumothorax
Positron emission tomography
Radiolucent
Radionuclide imaging
Radiopaque
Ventilation-perfusion scans

Wilhelm Roentgen discovered the x-ray in 1895 and won the very first Nobel Prize in physics (1901) for this discovery. Since that time, radiography has been used in medicine to image the chest structures. Ionizing radiation has its disadvantages, however, as Thomas Edison learned when his laboratory assistant, Clarence Daley, became the first scientist to die of radiation exposure in the United States. By the 1940s, ultrasound was being used as a way to image the body using nonionizing radiation. Computed tomography (CT) was developed in the 1970s, and magnetic resonance imaging in the 1980s. All these methods have been used to image the chest, and each offers distinct advantages and disadvantages for the patient and the clinician.

Most imaging machines still use film to capture the image, but newer systems are using digital formats. In either case, the basic methods are similar: x-rays are generated when the anode of an x-ray tube is bombarded with electrons from the cathode of the tube. The collision gives off energy in the form of x-radiation, which travels out of the tube and through the

patient, then hitting the imaging cassette. The cassette contains film or a digital imaging sensor. The image is then processed by a digital processor or a film developer (Figure 11-1).

The film turns black (is exposed) if the x-rays pass through the patient and reach the film surface. If the x-rays are reflected or absorbed by the patient, they do not reach the film, and the resulting image stays white (unexposed). The patterns and shades of light and dark on the film reflect the differing densities present in the part of the human body being imaged.

The darkest images on a film (also called radiolucent areas) represent pockets of air within the body. Fat is the next densest tissue and produces a dark-gray image. Muscle and other soft tissues are more dense and produce a much lighter gray image. Finally, bone is most dense and produces a white image. Metallic objects are even more dense (also called radiopaque) than bone and produce a pure white image (Figure 11-2, *A-C*).

Figure 11-2, *A*, demonstrates all the different densities. This lateral view of the knee shows metal from a total knee

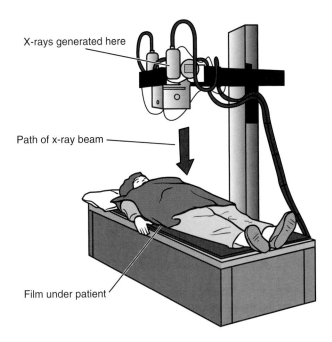

X-rays generated here

Path of x-ray beam

Film under patient

FIGURE 11-1 A typical x-ray machine.

replacement, bone, muscle, fat, and, on either side of the patient's knee, air.

The x-ray image is a summation of all the densities that the x-rays have passed through. The different layers of tissue that are on top of one another are flattened into a single two-dimensional image. Sometimes the various densities lie next to one another and are easily distinguished in the image. Other times the two densities overlap one another and are blurred together in the image. For this reason, the patient is usually positioned so that two or more images can be taken at a right angle to one another. This allows structures that are overlapping in one orientation to be seen side-by-side in another orientation.

EVALUATION OF A RADIOGRAPH

The first step in the evaluation of a radiograph it to check that the information identifying the patient has been properly provided on the image and that the image is indeed of the patient in question. Next, check that the part of the body in question is the part that was imaged, and that it was done

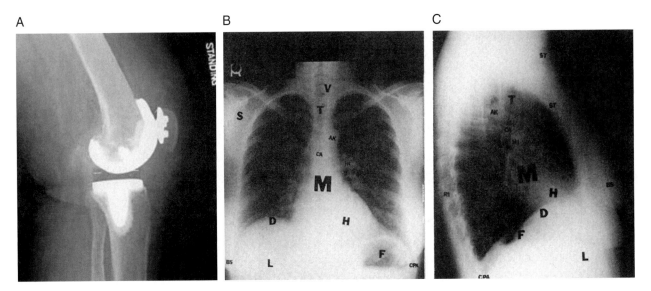

A   B   C

FIGURE 11-2 A, This radiograph of a knee with a total joint replacement shows the differences in density among air, fat, muscle, bone, cement, and titanium. **B,** PA radiograph, and **C,** lateral radiograph; these two views anatomically localize the basic structures that must be reviewed during the evaluation of chest radiographs. Some of the structures are seen in both views and others are seen in only one view. During evaluation, one should be able to see and identify the following basic anatomical structures.
Soft tissues and extrathoracic structures: soft tissues (*ST*), breast shadows, (*BS*), diaphragm (*D*), liver (*L*), and fundus of stomach (*F*)
Bony thorax: ribs (*RI*), vertebrae (*V*), scapulae (*S*, seen best on PA), clavicles (*C*, seen best on PA), and sternum (*S*, seen best on lateral)
Mediastinal structures: mediastinum (*M*), trachea (*T*), carina (*CA*), aortic knob (*AK*), heart (*H*), anterior clear space (*ACS*, seen best on lateral), and hilus of lungs (*HI*)
Lung fields: hilus of lungs (*HI*), pulmonary vessels (arise from hilus and branch outward), costophrenic angles (*CPA*), and lung apices (*LA*, seen best on PA)
There are many other structures that must be evaluated in addition to these basic ones, and pathologies must be identified.
(**A** *from GE Healthcare.*)

TABLE 11-1

Standard Radiograph Projections

AP (anteroposterior)	Frontal view, taken with the patient facing the x-ray tube, with the back toward the film.
PA (posteroanterior)	Looks the same as the AP, but the patient is positioned facing the film.
Right lateral	Side view, with the right side against the film.
Left lateral	Side view, with the left side against the film.
Oblique	A view taken at a 45-degree angle, between the AP and the lateral views.

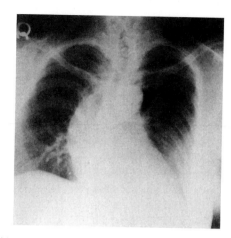

FIGURE 11-3 This chest radiograph of a patient with kyphoscoliosis reveals a markedly abnormal, reverse-S-shaped curve of the thoracic spine that is deforming the mediastinal structures and the ribs. This patient is breathing primarily with the diaphragm.

in at least two projections oriented 90 degrees apart (for example, one view from the front and one from the side). The left and right sides of the patient should be indicated on the films so that they can be viewed in proper orientation. A marker should also indicate what position the patient was in at the time of the radiograph. For instance, a frontal chest radiograph can be taken with the patient standing, sitting, or lying down.

Then check the overall exposure of the film. If all the structures are too dark, the film has been overpenetrated. It should be retaken using less radiation. If all the structures are too light, the film has been underpenetrated and should be retaken using more radiation.

Next, look at the different projections that have been taken. The most common projections are listed in Table 11-1.

There are also many special views that position the patient in such a way that a particular area of interest is oriented for optimal visualization. The standard chest radiograph is taken as a posteroanterior (PA) and a left lateral view, with the patient standing. These two views position the heart closest to the film. This is important because clinicians want to use the radiograph to judge the size of the heart, and the farther away from the film the heart is, the more it will appear magnified. This concept is easy to understand if you shine a light on your hand and view the resulting shadow on the wall. The closer your hand is to the wall, the more its size is true to life. The farther away it gets from the wall, the larger and fuzzier it appears. The evaluation of the heart and lungs is most accurate when these structures are positioned close to the film during imaging.

The next step in evaluating a chest radiograph is to do a quick scan of the entire image to look for obvious or life-threatening abnormalities. The general anatomy should be identified, including spine, sternum, clavicles and ribs; right and left diaphragms, and abdominal organs; heart, mediastinum, and great vessels; trachea, main bronchi, and lungs. Then a more thorough evaluation is begun.

The inspiratory effort should be evaluated. Patients are asked to take a deep breath at the time of the radiograph, and

this deep inspiration should make it possible to visualize 10 to 12 ribs within the thoracic cavity. If a radiograph is taken during expiration or during a poor inspiratory effort, the ribs will appear very close together and the lower ribs will be seen below the level of the diaphragm.

The bony skeleton (Figure 11-3) should be checked for signs of fracture, especially along the margins of the ribs. Fractures are seen as radiolucent lines within the bone or as disruptions of the smooth cortical line at the edges of the bone. Unexplained fragments of bone that are not in a normal anatomical position are another sign of fracture.

The position of the diaphragm should be noted. Its position, shape, and clarity and the appearance of the costophrenic angles are important. The costophrenic angles are where the diaphragm meets the chest wall. These thin, pointy areas at the base of the chest cavity are where blood or fluid inside the chest are seen on a standing film.

The lung fields should be evaluated next, to look for uniform density and vascular markings throughout. The hilar area, where the vascular and airway structures converge, is normally more dense; the peripheral lung fields, where the smallest vascular and airway structures are, appear the smoothest and least dense. Comparing them side by side for symmetry helps in the recognition of abnormal areas. Consolidation of lung tissue as a result of pneumonia, tumor, effusion, or other disease processes causes that tissue to become more dense than the rest of the lung fields (Figure 11-4).

Full expansion of the lung fields is also important to evaluate. A pneumothorax causes part of the lung to collapse, creating a less dense empty space in the chest cavity that is devoid of any pulmonary or vascular markings. Conversely, a hemothorax or pleural effusion fills the chest cavity with fluid that is denser than normal lung tissue. Both of these abnormalities are evident on chest radiographs (Figures 11-5 and 11-6).

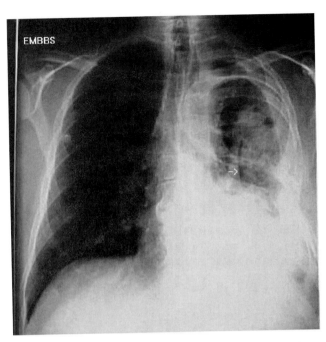

FIGURE 11-4 Left-sided empyema with consolidation of lung tissue. (*From EMBBS. Emergency Medicine and Primary Care Home Page.* www.embbs.com.)

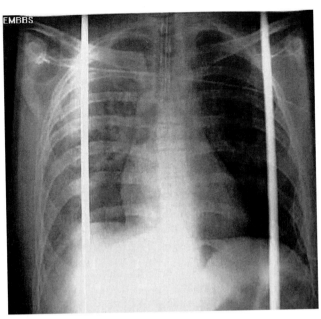

FIGURE 11-6 Right rib fractures with right hemothorax. (*From EMBBS. Emergency Medicine and Primary Care Home Page.* www.embbs.com.)

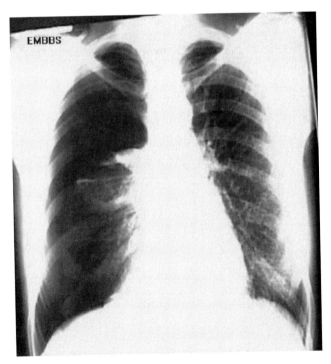

FIGURE 11-5 Right-sided pneumothorax. (*From EMBBS. Emergency Medicine and Primary Care Home Page.* www.embbs.com.)

Next, the heart size should be evaluated. Normally the heart is about as wide as one half of the chest cavity. Measuring the cardiac silhouette and then measuring the width of the hemithorax (from the center of the sternum to the outer edge of the ribs) for comparison helps to identify cardiac hypertrophy due to chronic or acute heart failure.

The width of the mediastinum is also important to evaluate. The mediastinal structures should be just wider than the thoracic spine. When the dense structures in this area are much wider than expected, an aortic aneurism should be suspected. As the aortic arch widens, it projects a higher density shadow over the upper left chest cavity that is visible on the radiograph (Figure 11-7).

Other common disease states can have typical findings on chest radiographs. The hyperinflation caused by an acute asthma attack may present as increased bronchial markings throughout the lung fields, a flattened diaphragm, and a maximally expanded chest cavity. Chronic obstructive pulmonary disease (COPD) causes similar effects, including a barrel-shaped chest (increased anteroposterior [AP] diameter), a flattened diaphragm, and an overall decreased density of the pulmonary markings.

OTHER IMAGING METHODS

CT scans of the chest can be a useful diagnostic tool for certain diseases. CT uses ionizing radiation as standard radiographs do, but it allows for rapid scanning in much more detail. The CT scan generates pictures that are "slices" through the patient in the axial plane. Although bone is visualized much

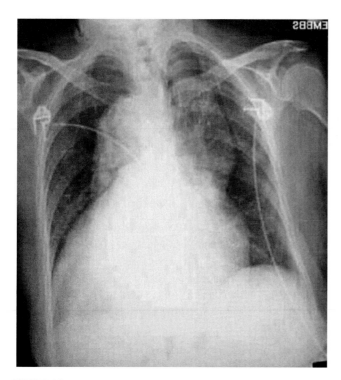

FIGURE 11-7 Thoracic aortic aneurism with widened mediastinum. (*From EMBBS. Emergency Medicine and Primary Care Home Page. www.embbs.com.*)

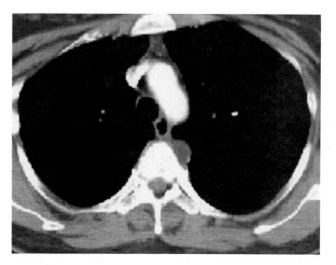

FIGURE 11-9 Chest CT showing spine, pulmonary spaces, and aortic arch. (*From GE Healthcare.*)

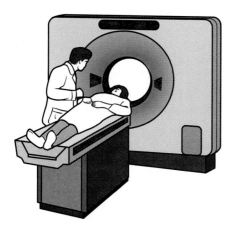

FIGURE 11-8 Computed tomography (CT) scanner. (To view a variety of CT scanners, go to the GE Healthcare Web site at http://www.gehealthcare.com/usen/index.html.)

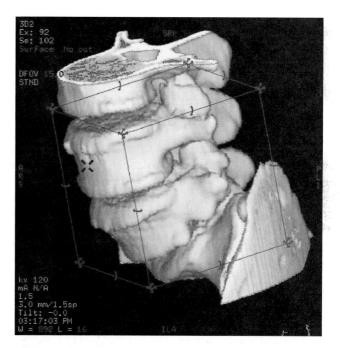

FIGURE 11-10 Three-dimensional reconstruction generated by a CT scanner. (*From GE Healthcare.*)

better than soft tissues, a CT scan can still provide excellent images of the lungs, vascular structures, and heart. New software can produce three-dimensional images that show the anatomy beautifully, and the sensitivity of these machines can allow for the detection of very small amounts of calcification in the coronary arteries, which can be an indication of early heart disease. Newer "ultrafast" CT scanners can see more subtle changes in the coronary arteries because they take a picture quickly, stopping the action and movement of the heart. This results in clearer pictures and the ability to discern small details more accurately (Figures 11-8, 11-9, and 11-10).

Magnetic resonance imaging (MRI) of the chest can be performed to evaluate the soft tissues of the chest cavity. MRI has the advantage of using magnetic energy rather than ionizing radiation, so there is no harmful exposure for the patient. These images provide much better quality views of soft tissues than CT scans offer, but the scans are more expensive and take nearly an hour to complete. A chest CT can be done in less than a minute, making it a better choice for evaluation of trauma (Figure 11-11).

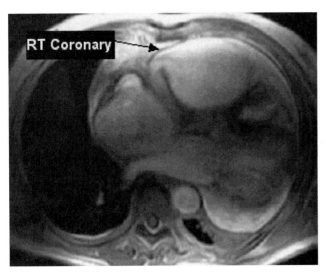

FIGURE 11-11 Cardiac MRI evaluating the coronary arteries. (*From GE Healthcare.*) (To view a variety of MRI scanners, go to the GE Healthcare Web site at http://www.gehealthcare.com/usen/index.html.)

A radionuclide ventilation-perfusion (VQ) scan is the primary test used to detect a pulmonary embolus. Radioactive isotopes are injected into the bloodstream and are also inhaled into the lungs. Scanning for the location of these isotopes is then able to determine the extent to which the lungs have been ventilated and perfused. A mismatch (for instance, an area that was perfused with gas but not perfused with blood) would indicate that a blood clot had become caught in the pulmonary vasculature. Research has found that a high number of these scans gave indeterminate results, however, and newer CT images have been found to be more accurate. A pulmonary angiogram is still the definitive test for a pulmonary embolism, but it is an invasive test that must be administered in the cardiac catheterization laboratory and involves injection of dye into the arterial vasculature.

Positron emission tomography (PET) scanning is a newer form of radionuclide imaging that also shows the function of organs rather than just their structure. The amount of radio-labeled glucose taken up by heart muscle cells, for instance,

can help clinicians determine whether the muscles have died after a myocardial infarction or whether they are still alive. If the cells are alive, they would benefit from bypass surgery. If they are dead, bypass surgery would not be worthwhile.

Ultrasound is an imaging modality commonly used in the abdomen, but because the sound waves bounce off bone, it is much less useful in the chest cavity. Ultrasound is sometimes used to identify pockets of fluid during thoracocentesis, but a CT scan is more commonly used whenever the precise placement of a needle in the chest is necessary.

SUMMARY

There are a variety of ways to image the chest. The standard chest radiograph is still an important way to gather information quickly, inexpensively, and at low risk for the patient. A physical therapist should be familiar with the basic techniques of reading a chest radiograph and should be able to identify common abnormalities viewable with this imaging technique.

Review Questions

1. What do the differing densities seen on a standard chest radiograph represent?
2. What are the basic steps in reading a chest radiograph?
3. What are the signs, visible on a chest radiograph, of the following disorders: pneumothorax, hemothorax, consolidation, and thoracic aneurism?
4. How does nuclear imaging give the clinician physiological and anatomical information about the patient?

REFERENCES

Johnson, T.R., & Steinbach, L.S. (2004). Essentials of musculoskeletal imaging. Rosemont, IL: American Academy of Orthopaedic Surgeons.

Novelline, R.A. (1999). Squire's fundamentals of radiology, ed 5. Cambridge: Harvard University Press.

Rothenberg, M.A. (1998). Understanding X-rays: a plain English approach. Eau Claire, WI: Professional Education Systems.

CHAPTER 12

Electrocardiogram Identification

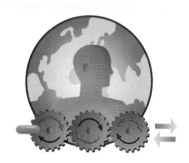

Christian Evans and Gary Brooks

KEY TERMS

Artifact
Bradycardia
Depolarization
Dysrhythmia
Ectopic focus

Electrocardiogram
Supraventricular
Syncytium
Tachycardia

Electrical signaling is a primary method of communication, control, and regulation in the human body and nowhere is this method employed with greater precision and elegance than in the heart. The rate, rhythm, and conduction of electrical signals are critical to cardiac function; it is these rhythmic electrical impulses that cause the mechanical contraction, or pumping of the heart muscle. This electrical current is detectable by electrodes that are placed on the surface of the skin. The flow of current during the cardiac cycle is then recorded as the characteristic waveforms of the electrocardiogram (ECG; sometimes also called EKG). Mechanical events such as the contraction and relaxation of the myocardium are inferred from the waveforms produced by the ECG.

The ECG is an essential tool for the diagnosis and medical management of patients with cardiac disease. Information provided by the ECG may also assist the physical therapist in the assessment of a patient's readiness for and response to physical activity. Physical therapists in many different practice environments have access to information afforded by the ECG. For example, in the intensive care unit or acute care setting or during cardiac rehabilitation, a patient's ECG may be continuously monitored via telemetry (a remote monitoring system in which ECG signals are sent via radio waves to a distant receiver) or by a bedside unit. In both the acute and

outpatient settings, past significant ECG recordings as well as an interpretation may be available in the medical record. Documentation accompanying a referral for outpatient physical therapy may also include a reference to the patient's ECG. It is therefore crucial that all physical therapists have a basic understanding of the uses and limitations of the ECG in their practices.

As an example of how an understanding of ECG interpretation may be useful for physical therapists, consider the following scenario. A physical therapist in a cardiac intensive care unit (CCU) initiates exercise for a patient recovering from open-heart surgery. The patient's ECG has been stable throughout the postoperative recovery phase, but the patient has not yet been challenged with moderate intensity activity or exercise. The therapist gets the patient up and begins an appropriate level of exercise; however, with this greater demand on the heart, the patient develops an exercise-induced dysrhythmia. This abnormal rhythm may be mild and fairly benign, but alternatively, it could be malignant or life-threatening. Depending on the physical therapist's abilities to interpret the ECG in this situation, this dysrhythmia may be caught and then referred to and treated by the physician, but if it is not recognized, a less favorable outcome may occur.

This chapter briefly reviews the basic anatomy and physiology of the myocardial conduction system as it relates to the ECG. The configuration of the normal ECG is presented and discussed along with several methods of quickly determining heart rate and rhythm from an electrocardiographic record, or "strip." Some of the more common dysrhythmias are examined, as are some other pathological features. Throughout the chapter, the uses and limitations of the ECG in physical therapy practice are highlighted.

PHYSIOLOGY AND ANATOMY OF THE CONDUCTION SYSTEM

Cardiac Action Potential

The cardiac action potential is generated by the flow of ions across myocardial cell membranes; it has a distinctive shape and five phases (phases 0 to 4) (Roden et al., 2002). In the cell's resting state, a negative membrane potential exists, based on the selective permeability of the cardiac cell membrane and the relative concentrations of sodium (Na^+), calcium (Ca^{2+}), and potassium (K^+) ions in the internal and external cellular environments. The relative time-sensitive ionic currents for each species are color-coded and labeled in Figure 12-1 and the cardiac action potential is superimposed over the individual currents that compose it. At rest, a typical ventricular cardiomyocyte membrane is primarily permeable only to K^+ ions, allowing the movement of K^+ out of the cell until the charge inside is approximately -90 mV, relative to the charge outside. This is the resting membrane potential of the cardiomyocyte and is close to the equilibrium potential for K^+. The membrane potential changes rapidly at the onset of depolarization, with the opening of Na^+ and Ca^{2+} channels, allowing these ions to cross the membrane and enter the cell. Calcium then becomes available for contraction of cardiac muscle myofibrils.

During depolarization, the membrane's potential becomes positive and the cell contracts. As in skeletal muscle, the Na^+ channels are fast-opening and fast-closing mechanisms, allowing Na^+ to rapidly enter the myocardial cell on depolarization (referred to as phase 0 of the cardiac action potential in Figure 12-1). Unlike skeletal muscle, however, cardiac muscle has a prolonged action potential as a result of the slower and extended opening of the Ca^{2+} channels. After initial depolarization, some K^+ channels remain open while others close, and repolarization begins (phase 1) due to outward K^+ current flowing through the open K^+ channels. A plateau phase (phase 2) of the action potential exists during which the outward flow of K^+ ions is balanced by an inward flow of Ca^{2+} ions. This prolongs depolarization and delays return to the resting membrane potential. Closure of the slow Ca^{2+} channels at onset of repolarization is accompanied by the opening of additional K^+ channels, causing a rapid outflow of K^+, which completes repolarization (phase 3 in Figure 12-1), restoring resting negative membrane potential. During the cell's resting phase (phase 4 of Figure 12-1), Na^+ and Ca^{2+} are actively pumped out of the cell, and K^+ is pumped into the

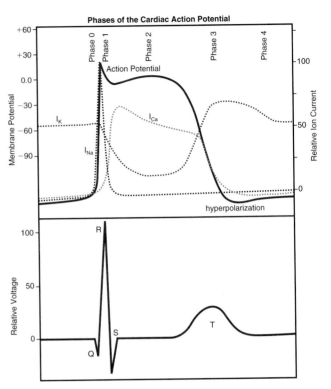

FIGURE 12-1 Relationship of an individual ventricular cardiomyocyte action potential to the ECG. **A,** The time-dependent ionic currents (IK, INa, and ICa,) of an individual ventricular cardiac cell that determine the shape, amplitude, and duration of the cell's action potential (shown in red). The action potential can be broken down into five distinct phases (0-4). **B,** The QRS complex and T wave of the ECG are temporally related to the cardiac action potential and the phases. However, the ECG also reflects the anatomical orientation of the wave of depolarization through the heart and the location of the recording electrodes.

cell, restoring the ionic gradients needed for repolarization (Berne & Levy, 2000; Guyton and Hall, 2000;, Roden et al., 2002).

Each cell has an absolute refractory period during depolarization, meaning that an additional stimulus will not cause an additional depolarization. A brief but important relative refractory period follows depolarization, during which a stimulus of greater than normal intensity is necessary to depolarize the cell again. The refractory period of atrial cells is significantly shorter than that of ventricular cells, allowing a more rapid intrinsic atrial rhythm than intrinsic ventricular rhythm. Therefore, atrial rhythms pace the heart, including the ventricles, given intact atrioventricular (AV) conduction.

From Figure 12-1 it can be seen that certain ionic currents contribute to particular phases of the cardiac action potential. The Na^+ current is the predominant factor in the initial depolarization, whereas the Ca^{2+} current is important in the plateau phase, and the K^+ currents are important in the duration of the action potential and in repolarization. Many of

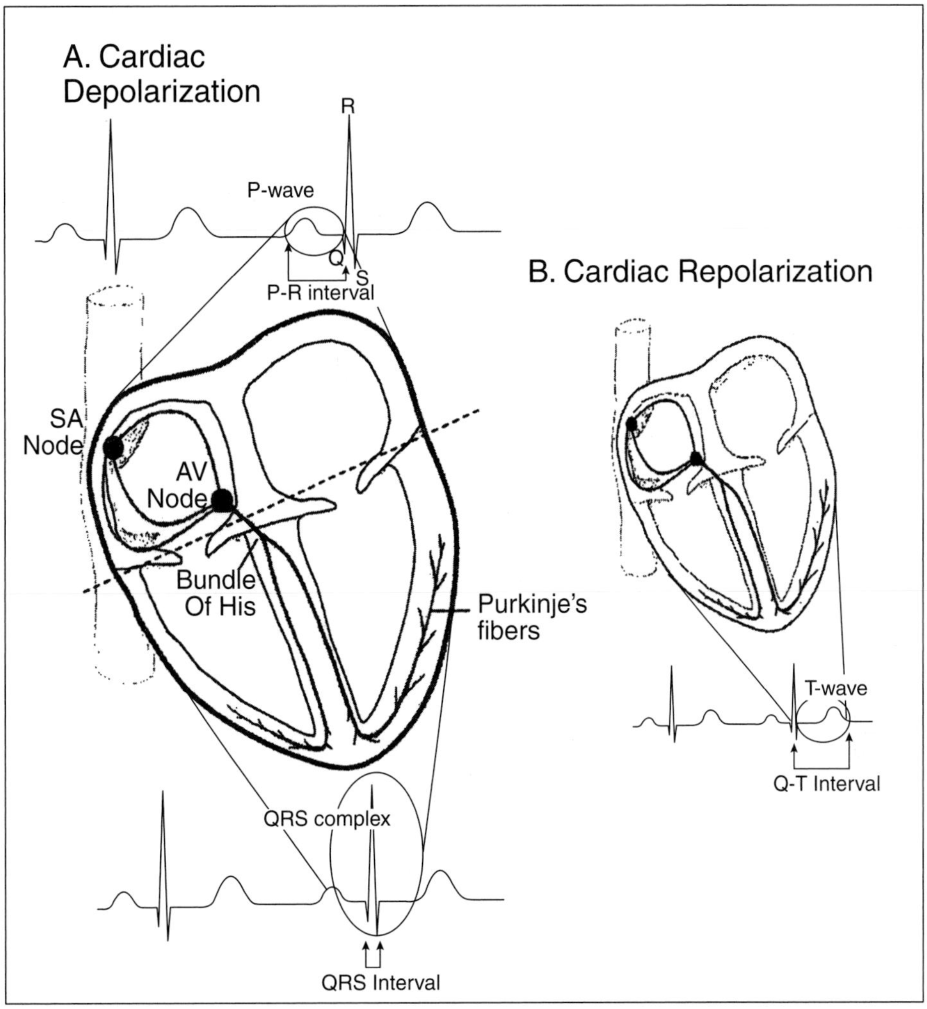

FIGURE 12-2 Relationship of ECG complex to conduction pathway. **A,** The sequence of events in depolarization: the wave of depolarization spreads from the SA node through the atria to the AV node. After a delay in the AV node, it travels through the bundle of His to the Purkinje fibers to the ventricular myocardium. The delay at the AV node accounts for the duration of the P-R interval. QRS duration is dependent on normal propagation from the atria and an intact ventricular conduction system. B, Ventricular repolarization.

the drugs used to treat dysrhythmias work on the channels for one or more of these three ions and affect their permeability. Furthermore, the electrical current produced by these ionic currents is transmitted through the conductive tissues surrounding the heart. The "wave" of depolarization that is propagated through the conduction system and contractile tissue of the heart, as well as repolarization, which takes place in a particular spatial manner, are detectable by the surface electrodes of the ECG.

Conduction System

It is the conduction system that initiates and rapidly transmits impulses to specific locations within the myocardium (the atria, apex, septum, and lateral wall), allowing for effective, coordinated myocardial contraction and pumping. The conduction system is composed of specialized cardiac muscle that contracts minimally because it contains few contractile myofibrils. Any portion of the conduction system is capable of self-excitation and may act as a pacemaker, generating action potentials. However, because of the intrinsically more rapid rate of spontaneous depolarization of the sinoatrial (SA) node, it normally acts as the heart's pacemaker. The rate of depolarization of the SA node determines the heart rate. In the absence of an impulse from the SA node, the AV node depolarizes spontaneously, taking over as pacemaker, with the important difference that the rate of depolarization is lower than that of the SA node.

Figure 12-2 displays the anatomical association of the cardiac electrical conduction system with its components on the ECG. Atrial depolarization is initiated by a spontaneously generated impulse that originates in the SA node. The impulse is then transmitted throughout the atrial muscle, resulting in atrial contraction. The event is recorded as the P wave of the ECG. The impulse is also transmitted, via rapidly conducting internodal pathways, to the AV node. Atrial repolarization is not recorded by the ECG because it occurs during ventricular depolarization.

Impulse conduction slows within the AV node considerably, resulting in a delaying of the impulse before it reaches the ventricular conduction system. The pause in impulse propagation allows the atria to contract and fill the ventricles with blood. The P-R interval of the ECG represents this period between the onset of atrial depolarization and the onset of ventricular depolarization. Normally the P-R interval lasts between 0.12 and 0.20 second (Huszar, 2002).

Following passage through the AV node, the impulse continues to the AV bundle (bundle of His) and then to Purkinje fibers, which transmit the impulse rapidly to the ventricular endocardium. Ventricular depolarization corresponds to phase 0 of the cardiac action potential (see Figure 12-1) and is represented in the ECG by the QRS complex. The depolarization wave propagates relatively slowly throughout the ventricular myocardium. The span of time elapsing during ventricular depolarization is reflected by the QRS interval, which normally ranges between 0.06 and < 0.12 second. Ventricular depolarization originates in the interventricular septum, creating the Q wave, which is normally small or absent, depending on the lead. The depolarization wave next spreads to the apex and then to the right and left ventricles, causing the R and S waves. Depolarization also propagates in an endocardial to epicardial direction within the ventricles (Berne & Levy, 2000; Guyton & Hall, 2000). A normal QRS duration indicates that the impulse originated in the SA node or a region above the AV node (supraventricular). A long QRS interval (≥ 0.12 second) suggests that the impulse arose from the ventricle or originated abnormally in supraventricular tissue. The normal sequence of depolarization is: SA node to AV node to bundle of His to Purkinje fibers to the ventricular myocardium. When this sequence is followed, the ECG correlates with the mechanical events of the cardiac cycle as shown in Figure 4-13.

After ventricular depolarization the ECG deflection returns to baseline, and this pause in electrical activity corresponds with the plateau phase (phase 2) of the cardiac action potential. Ventricular repolarization is represented by the T wave and corresponds to phase 3 of the cardiac action potential. The configuration of the S-T segment is an important marker of myocardial ischemia or infarction. Following the T wave, a U wave may also be present. The source of the U wave is not well understood (Surawicz, 1998). Although U-wave inversion may indicate ischemia involving the left ventricular wall (Kodame et al., 2000), it is not a unique marker and is not as sensitive as S-T segment changes in predicting ischemia; therefore, it is not a useful clinical marker (Ritseman van Eck et al., 2003).

Within the ventricle, individual cardiomyocytes are in direct communication with each other via gap junctions. This facilitates rapid spread of the wave of depolarization from cell to cell, allowing the right and left ventricular heart muscle to function as a syncytium, or a single pumping unit (Opie, 2004). Note that the ventricles remain in a state of contraction until slightly after repolarization. This period of contraction corresponds to the Q-T interval on the ECG. Diastole, therefore, begins subsequent to the end of the T wave and continues until the next ventricular depolarization. Note also that atrial depolarization and contraction occur during diastole.

ELECTROCARDIOGRAM

Recording the Electrocardiogram

Before examining the timing of the wave forms and the rhythms of the ECG, a basic understanding of the principles of electrocardiography is needed. A standard 12-lead configuration is used for the diagnosis and medical management of cardiac conditions. An example of a normal 12-lead ECG is shown in Figure 12-3: 6 leads record the electrical signals in the frontal plane, and 6 leads record signals in the transverse plane.

The placements of the 10 electrodes for a 12-lead ECG are shown in Figure 12-4. Note that 12 electrodes are not necessary because some leads serve a dual purpose. The frontal-plane leads include 3 standard bipolar limb leads, referred to as leads I, II, and III, and 3 augmented unipolar limb leads, referred to as aVR (right arm), aVL (left arm), and aVF (left leg). These two sets of leads share the same electrodes but view the electrical activity of the heart from different perspectives. The bipolar leads have a single positive and a single negative electrode and record the difference in electrical potential between them. The augmented limb leads have a single positive electrode and derive the negative electrode from the combination of the other electrodes. The standard limb leads form a triangle, known as the Einthoven triangle, around the heart that allows for advanced calculations related to the net vector of depolarization, or the axis of the heart (an index of the cardiac mass and position). If only a single lead is recorded, standard limb lead II is often chosen because all of the deflections are typically upright (Huszar, 2002).

The transverse-plane leads are referred to as the precordial, or chest, leads. These 6 leads form a semicircle around the anterior aspect of the heart; their placement is described in Figure 12-4. In addition to the 3 electrodes for the limb leads and the 6 electrodes for the chest leads, a 10th electrode that serves as a neutral ground must be used to reduce artifacts and stabilize the baseline. Imagine that each of the 12 leads "views" the heart from a different angle, therefore recording events in different locations of the heart in different ways. By convention, the waveform on the ECG is positive (upward) as current travels toward a positive electrode or lead and is negative (downward) when current travels away from a lead. Other lead configurations may be used for exercise testing (American College of Sports Medicine, 2000). Single-lead monitoring is commonly used during exercise training or in the acute care settings.

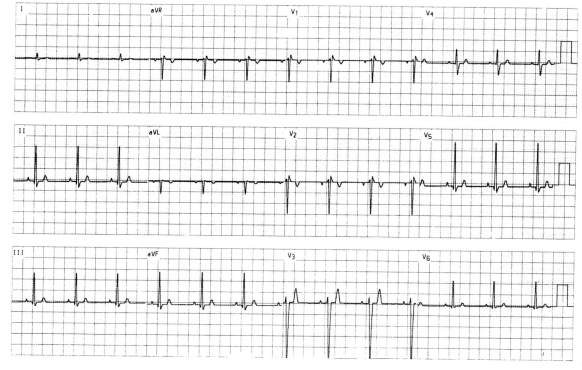

FIGURE 12-3 A normal 12-lead ECG.

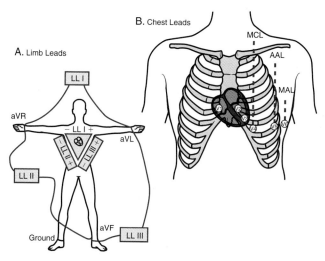

FIGURE 12-4 Anatomical placement of the 12-lead electrocardiogram electrodes. A, The placement of the electrodes for the three standard limb leads (LL), LL I, LL II, and LL III; and the placement for the augmented limb leads, aVR (right arm), aVL (left arm), and aVF (left leg). The standard limb leads are bipolar leads, whereas the augmented limb leads are unipolar. B, The placement of the six chest leads, or precordial leads, V1 to V6. Leads V1 and V2 are placed over the fourth intercostals spaces, on the left and right of the sternum, respectively. Typically, V4 is placed next on the midclavicular line (MCL) at the fifth intercostals space. V3 is placed midway between V2 and V4. V6 is placed next on the midaxillary line (MAL) on the same plane as V4. The V5 lead is placed at a point midway between V4 and V6, at the anterior axillary line (AAL). A 10th electrode must be attached (shown here attached to the right leg) to minimize artifact. Abbreviations: AAL, anterior axillary line; LL, standard limb lead; MAL, midaxillary line; MCL, midclavicular line.

Evaluating the ECG Strip

The evaluation of an ECG should be approached in a systematic fashion. The following questions are useful for appreciating the information that is relevant to current clinical practice (Cummins, 2003).

- What is the rate and pattern (regularity) of the rhythm? Is the R-R interval (the distance between successive R waves) equal for each beat? This indicates regularity of the beats.
- Does a P wave precede every QRS complex? This indicates that there is atrial activity.
- Is there a QRS complex after every P wave? This indicates conduction of impulses from the atria to the ventricles.
- What is the P-R interval? A P-R interval of 0.12 to 0.20 second indicates normal conduction from atria to ventricles. A P-R interval > 0.2 seconds indicates a conduction delay or block.
- Is the QRS complex of normal duration and morphology (shape)? A QRS complex greater than 0.12 second indicates either that an impulse arose within a ventricle or was conducted abnormally through the ventricular conduction system.

By answering each of these questions, the tendency to "eyeball" the rhythm and make a quick but inaccurate assessment is avoided.

Determination of Heart Rate

Several quick methods can be used to estimate heart rate. Most printed and displayed ECG recordings indicate a heart

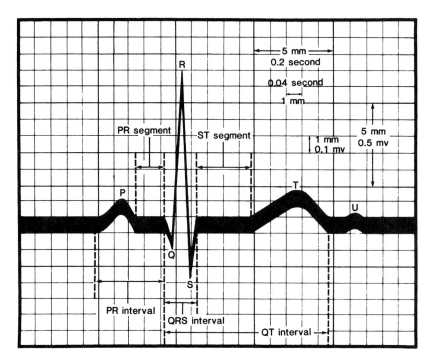

FIGURE 12-5 A normal ECG showing characteristic waves, intervals, and segments, and some of the features of the tracing paper.

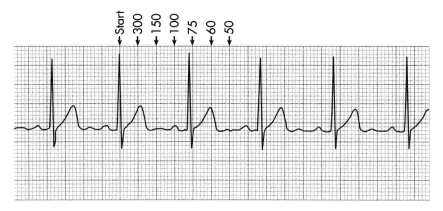

FIGURE 12-6 Count-off method of estimating heart rate.

rate. This must be interpreted with caution, however, because the presence of artifact (extraneous deflections of the waveform caused by movement or electrical interference) may render an automated heart rate calculation inaccurate. This is a common problem during activity or exercise, the circumstances during which many physical therapists monitor patients. It is possible to calculate or to estimate a heart rate on the basis of a printed ECG strip because, by convention, the recording paper is divided into 1-mm squares and larger 5-mm squares, which are defined by heavier lines (Figure 12-5). Also by convention, the standard paper speed for an ECG recording is a rate of 25 mm per second, and most recorders

mark each 3-second interval. Each millimeter of length then represents $\frac{1}{25}$th, or 0.04 second, and each 5-mm block represents $\frac{1}{5}$, or 0.20 second. Some monitor systems, however, place a mark on the recording paper at 25 mm, or 1-second intervals.

There are several methods of estimating heart rate from a printed ECG strip. On a printed ECG strip, find an R wave located on or near a heavy vertical line. Proceeding to the left of that R wave, for each subsequent heavy vertical line, assign the following numbers: 300 for the first heavy line encountered, 150 for the next, followed by 100, 75, 60, 50, and 42 (Figure 12-6). Stop at the first heavy vertical line following

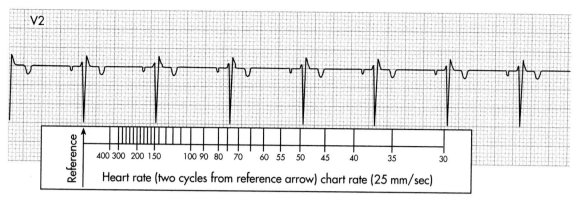

FIGURE 12-7 Using a rate-ruler to confirm heart rate.

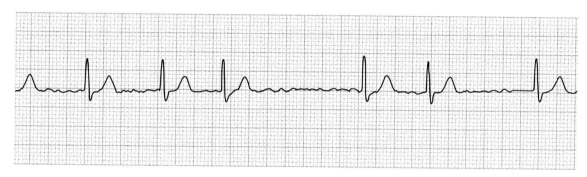

FIGURE 12-8 Heart rate estimation in an irregular rhythm (atrial fibrillation).

the next R wave that is encountered. The heart rate may be estimated as falling between the two most recently assigned values. In Figure 12-6, the rate would be estimated as falling between 100 and 75, or close to 80 beats per minute.

In many clinics, rulers are available that are calibrated so that heart rate may be estimated quickly by aligning markings on the ruler with features of the ECG strip. For example, after the arrow on the ruler is placed on an R wave, count two R waves to the left and read the number at that position on the ruler. In Figure 12-7, this method approximates the heart rate as 74 beats per minute.

It is important to note that the preceding two methods are useful *only* if the rhythm of the ECG strip is regular (i.e., the R waves are equally spaced, occurring at consistent intervals). Should the rhythm be irregular, with R waves appearing at varying intervals, another method must be employed to estimate the heart rate.

A common and easy method for estimating the heart rate is to count off the number of R waves in a 6-second strip. Depending on whether the ECG recorder makes a mark every 1, 3, or 6 seconds, one counts off the appropriate number of seconds to obtain a 6-second strip. The procedure is as follows: start at the mark corresponding to the beginning of the 6-second period and proceeding from left to right, count

the number of R waves within the 6-second recording. Now multiply by 10. That is the estimated heart rate, rounded down to the nearest 10 beats per minute. Several 6-second strips may be analyzed to document the heart rate range of an irregular rhythm. The rate of the irregular rhythm in Figure 12-8 is estimated at approximately 60 beats per minute.

Evaluation of Rhythms

Electrocardiographic monitoring is an important evaluation tool during the treatment of individuals with a history of, or potential for, acute myocardial infarction (MI) or myocardial ischemia. Most cardiac deaths are a result of lethal dysrhythmias, for which there is increased risk in the presence if infarction or ischemia. Rapid recognition of lethal dysrhythmias, or dysrhythmias that may deteriorate into lethal dysrhythmias, is essential for all health professionals involved in the care of individuals with cardiac disease. The dysrhythmias described in this chapter are those that must be recognized by providers of Advanced Cardiac Life Support as determined by the American Heart Association (Emergency Cardiac Care Committee and Subcommittees, 1992).

Normally, a cardiac impulse is generated by the SA node, causing atrial depolarization. This is followed by a slight

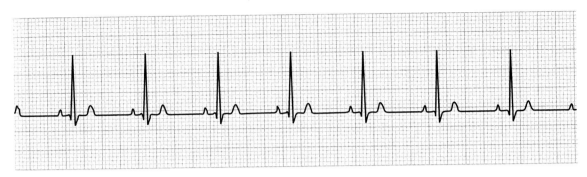

FIGURE 12-9 Normal sinus rhythm.

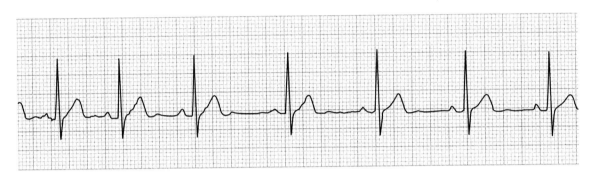

FIGURE 12-10 Sinus dysrhythmia.

delay in the AV node, after which the impulse is conducted to the ventricles, causing ventricular depolarization. These events are shown in Figure 12-9 in their normal spatial and temporal sequence and in normal sinus rhythm. A P wave precedes every QRS complex and every P wave is, in turn, succeeded by a QRS complex. This occurs within an interval of 0.12 to 0.20 second (one large box), as determined by the P-R interval. The QRS complexes occur within a range of 0.04 to 0.12 second, indicating that ventricular impulse conduction and depolarization is occurring in a normal interval. The positively deflected T wave indicates normal ventricular repolarization. Because the SA node spontaneously depolarizes at a rate of between 60 and 100 beats per minute, the rate of normal sinus rhythm must fall within these limits.

The identification of dysrhythmias affects clinical decision making, particularly with regard to a patient's readiness for or response to activity. The clinical significance of dysrhythmias range from benign to lethal. The clinical significance of a given dysrhythmia is determined by a number of considerations. Some of these considerations include the following: Is there evidence of hemodynamic compromise? Is the dysrhythmia a new or unusual finding? Might the dysrhythmia be a precursor to a more serious or perhaps lethal dysrhythmia? Is this an acute occurrence or a chronic dysrhythmia pattern? The clinical response to a patient with a dysrhythmia depends on the answers to these questions and the treatment setting.

DYSRHYTHMIA IDENTIFICATION

Supraventricular Dysrhythmias

Supraventircular dysrhythmias arise from an abnormality in impulse generation or conduction "above" the level of the ventricles. A sinus rhythm is any rhythm established by impulses from the SA node. Thus, depending on where the abnormality occurs—in the atria or at the level of the AV junction—a supraventricular dysrhythmia may be categorized as sinus, atrial, or junctional.

A cardiac rhythm may be a sinus rhythm but with an irregular or abnormally rapid or slow rate. Sinus dysrhythmia is an irregular sinus rhythm with varying R-R intervals (Figure 12-10). This is a normal variant that is associated with the individual's respiratory pattern. *Sinus bradycardia* is a sinus rhythm occurring at a rate of less than 60 beats per minute (Figure 12-11). This rhythm may significantly reduce cardiac output, causing hemodynamic compromise, manifested by hypotension or symptoms such as dizziness, lightheadedness, or syncope. On the other hand, individuals taking beta blockers, a group of medications that slow the heart, may exhibit this as their normal rhythm, as might individuals who achieve a high level of physical conditioning. *Sinus tachycardia* is a sinus rhythm occurring at a rate of greater than 100 beats per minute (Figure 12-12). Sinus tachycardia, or any other form of tachycardia, increases myocardial oxygen demand, or the

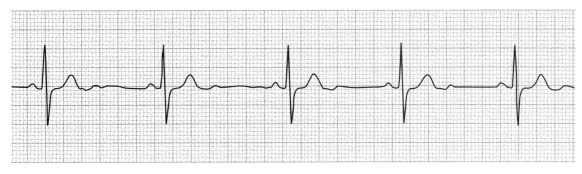

FIGURE 12-11 Sinus bradycardia.

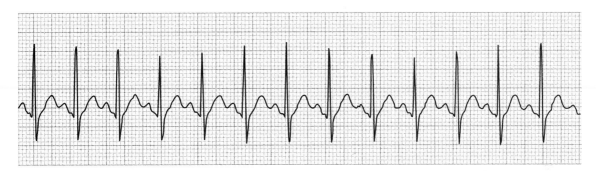

FIGURE 12-12 Sinus tachycardia.

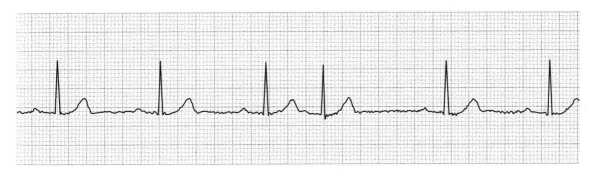

FIGURE 12-13 Premature atrial complex.

workload on the heart. This may initiate or exacerbate ischemia in the presence of coronary artery disease (CAD).

A beat or rhythm that does not originate in the SA node is considered to represent an ectopic focus or pacemaker. One common form of dysrhythmia is a "premature" complex (i.e., a beat that occurs sooner than expected given the established rhythm. A premature atrial complex, or PAC, is an early beat that has an ectopic atrial origin (Figure 12-13). An R wave appears closer to its preceding R wave than the other R waves in the established rhythm. The P wave of the odd beat may have a different shape or may be inverted relative to the normal P waves, indicating that it came from a focus other than the SA node, but the associated QRS complex is always preceded by a P wave, meaning that the impulse first depolarized the atria before being conducted to the ventricles.

Sometimes the AV junction may initiate an early beat, causing a premature junctional complex, or PJC. When this occurs, the R wave appears earlier; however, there may be no associated P wave, or there may be an unusual P wave, one that is inverted or follows the QRS complex. An inverted or late P wave indicates that the impulse was conducted in a retrograde (backwards) fashion. Clinically, a premature atrial or junctional complex may be palpated as a "skipped" or early beat during pulse taking, or the patient may perceive a palpitation or skipped beat. Otherwise, these dysrhythmias are usually of little clinical significance (Brown & Jacobson, 1988; Huszar 2002).

A more serious supraventricular dysrhythmia is supraventricular tachycardia, or SVT. In this dysrhythmia, the heart rate is rapid, exceeding 150 beats per minute. The tachycardia

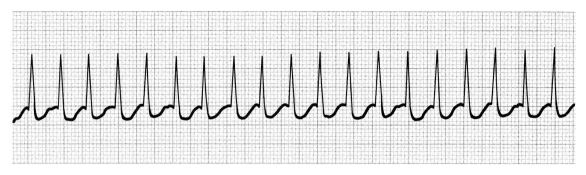

FIGURE 12-14 Supraventricular tachycardia.

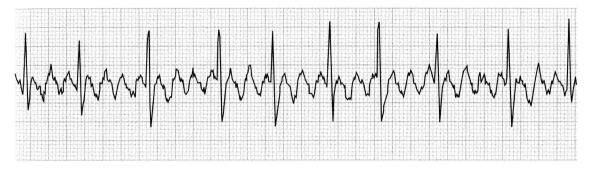

FIGURE 12-15 Atrial flutter.

may be sustained, lasting hours or even days, or it may be "paroxysmal" (PSVT), appearing abruptly and spontaneously reconverting to the previous rhythm within seconds or minutes. The P wave is often not visible, making assessment of atrial or junctional origin difficult, but the duration of the QRS complexes occurs within an appropriate interval. The R-R interval, however, is markedly shortened. Figure 12-14 demonstrates supraventricular tachycardia at a rate of 190 beats per minute. Other related forms of SVT include paroxysmal atrial tachycardia (PAT) and multifocal atrial tachycardia (MAT). Clinically, patients with SVT may perceive a "racing" heart rate, which may be quite distressing. At very rapid heart rates, for example, greater than 170 beats per minute, diastolic ventricular filling time is markedly reduced, which may cause hemodynamic compromise. Symptoms associated with inadequate cardiac output, such as dizziness, lightheadedness, and syncope may ensue. Some individuals with SVT remain asymptomatic, the rhythm being detected incidentally, for example, during routine pulse or telemetry monitoring.

Atrial fibrillation is the most common clinically encountered dysrhythmia; it is seen in approximately 0.4% of the general population but in more than 6% of patients over age 80 (American College of Cardiology & American Heart Association, 2004). Atrial fibrillation is characterized by inconsistent, irregular R-R intervals with an absence of true P waves (see Figure 12-8). P waves may be replaced by multiple, fibrillatory F waves of varying configurations. This dysrhythmia is characterized by the presence of many impulses simultaneously, generated from multiple locations within the atria. The atria, therefore, are not pumping effectively which, in turn, may impair ventricular contraction, resulting in a reduction in cardiac output of up to 25%. This is because of the loss of the additional ventricular filling supplied by atrial contraction. Impulses do conduct through the AV junction to the ventricles; however, this occurs inconsistently and results in the irregular R-R interval. The ventricular response to atrial fibrillation is important. A rapid ventricular response, resulting in tachycardia, may cause hemodynamic compromise with associated symptoms or poor activity tolerance. Of additional clinical significance is the association between atrial fibrillation and embolic cerebro-vascular accidents. Stasis of blood within the noncontracting atria may allow for thrombus formation. Figure 12-8 illustrates atrial fibrillation with a "controlled" (i.e., fewer than 100 beats per minute) ventricular response. Pulse monitoring of an individual in atrial fibrillation reveals an irregular pattern.

Another dysrhythmia that is characterized by abnormal atrial activity is atrial flutter, seen in Figure 12-15. In this rhythm, P waves are replaced by F waves that have a distinctive morphology often referred to as a saw-tooth or picket-fence appearance. Of clinical importance is the ratio of atrial to ventricular conduction and whether or not the patient is hemodynamically stable (Brown & Jacobson, 1988; Huszar, 2002).

Because the intrinsic rate of spontaneous depolarization of the AV node is less than that of the SA node, spontaneous AV node depolarization is normally prevented. However, in

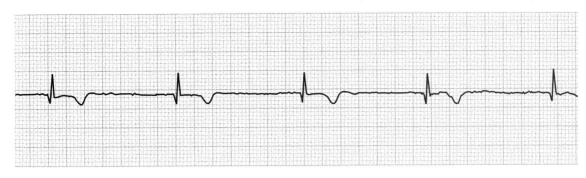

FIGURE 12-16 Junctional rhythm.

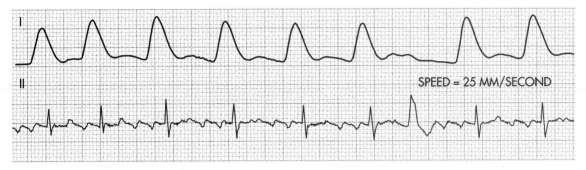

SPEED = 25 MM/SECOND

FIGURE 12-17 Diminished arterial pressure wave following a PVC.

the absence of an atrial impulse, the AV node depolarizes spontaneously and generates an impulse that then is conducted to the ventricles. Thus in junctional rhythm or nodal rhythm (Figure 12-16), the QRS complex is not preceded by a P wave. The AV node may generate an isolated "escape" beat, or it may take over as the heart's pacemaker. Sustained nodal or junctional rhythm is usually between 40 and 60 beats per minute, corresponding with the inherent rate of spontaneous AV node depolarization.

Ventricular Dysrhythmias

An ectopic pacemaker below the atria and outside the normal conduction system, such as a region in the ventricular myocardium, may give rise to a ventricular dysrhythmia. Ventricular dysrhythmias may be distinguished from supraventricular dysrhythmias in that the QRS duration of a ventricular dysrhythmia is longer than the normal 0.12 second. The appearance of ventricular dysrhythmias may be characterized as being "wide and weird." It is important to point out that not all rhythms with a QRS rhythms result from disturbance of impulse conduction within the ventricles, rather than from impulse generation within the ventricles.

The reason for the widening of the QRS complex resulting from ventricular impulse conduction disturbance or impulse generation is apparent when one considers the normal conduction of a sinus impulse within the ventricles. An impulse normally is rapidly conducted to ventricular myocardium via the Purkinje fibers. This ensures that the impulse reaches all regions of the ventricular myocardium in a timely fashion, with subsequent coordinated depolarization and contraction. Within the ventricular myocardium itself, however, propagation of the depolarization wave proceeds more slowly as a result of the syncytial arrangement of myocardial cells.

An impulse generated within the ventricles, outside the normal conduction pathways, initially depolarizes surrounding local myocardium. The depolarization wave then spreads outward from that focus, but it is propagated at a slower velocity. Ventricular contraction, in this case, is not coordinated; some regions contract well before the depolarization wave reaches regions remote from the ectopic focus. It follows that the ventricular ejection of blood is reduced during an ectopic beat (Figure 12-17). An ECG rhythm (Figure 12-17, bottom) is recorded simultaneously with the record of arterial blood pressure monitoring (top). The appearance of the wide and weird complex results in significant diminution of the corresponding arterial pressure wave.

The most common form of ventricular dysrhythmia is a premature ventricular complex, or PVC. In Figure 12-17 the wide and weird QRS complex appears early, interrupting the established rhythm. An electrical pause often follows a PVC, after which the established rhythm resumes. Clinically, a PVC may be perceived by a patient as a skipped beat or a palpitation. If a PVC occurs during a pulse monitoring, the examiner will likely sense a skipped, or irregular, beat.

PVCs sometimes happen in patterns, occurring at regular intervals. A PVC occurs in ventricular bigeminy on every second beat, in ventricular trigeminy on every third beat, and

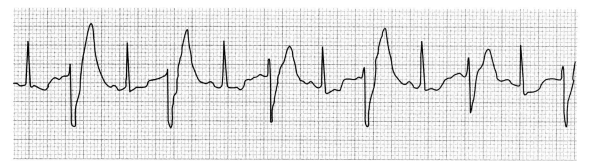

FIGURE 12-18 Ventricular bigeminy.

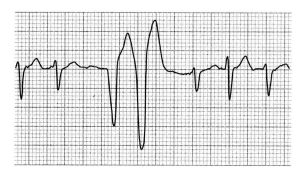

FIGURE 12-19 Ventricular couplet.

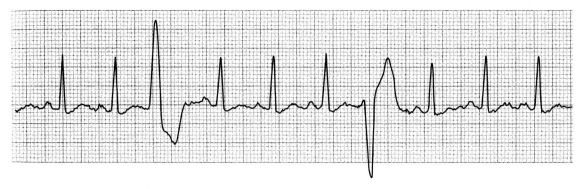

FIGURE 12-20 Multifocal PVCs.

in ventricular quadrigeminy on every fourth beat. Figure 12-18 illustrates ventricular bigeminy. With these rhythms, a regularly irregular pattern may be noted during pulse monitoring. PVCs may also occur twice in succession as a ventricular couplet, as seen in Figure 12-19.

PVCs that originate from more than one ectopic focus are termed multifocal PVCs. In this circumstance, the waveforms will have different morphologies according to the locations of the ectopic foci. Remember that the positive or negative deflection of the waveform depends on the direction of depolarization, as viewed by the lead used for monitoring. In Figure 12-20 the first PVC shown has an initial positive deflection, whereas the second PVC seen has an initial

negative deflection. Each of these PVCs comes from a different ectopic focus.

The physical therapist's decision-making process in response to observation of ventricular ectopic beats is complex and may not be grasped easily by the entry-level practitioner. Factors such as the presence or absence of symptoms, the acuity of the patient, and whether the rhythm is a new finding all influence a clinical response. The presence of a pattern such as bigeminy, couplets, or a multifocal pattern is also considered. Further elucidation of clinical responses to most dysrhythmias is beyond the scope of this chapter; however, some dysrhythmias demand an immediate response once they have been observed.

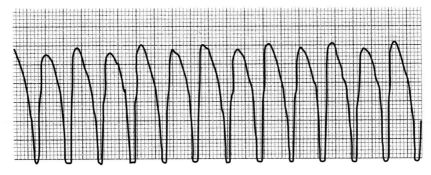

FIGURE 12-21 Ventricular tachycardia.

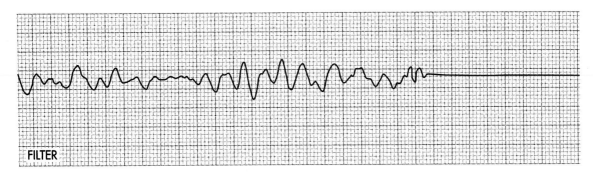

FIGURE 12-22 Ventricular fibrillation degenerating into asystole.

Ventricular tachycardia (v-tach, or VT) (Figure 12-21) is defined as three or more consecutive PVCs at a rate greater than 100 beats per minute (Akhtar, 1990; Samie & Jalife, 2001). This is a serious and potentially lethal dysrhythmia that requires that emergency measures be undertaken. During v-tach all complexes are ventricular in origin. V-tach sometimes occurs in runs of three or more ectopic complexes followed by reversion to the baseline rhythm, or it may be sustained. Effective circulation may be preserved, or it may be seriously compromised or absent in sustained v-tach. A patient may be asymptomatic, particularly if only a brief run of v-tach was experienced. If VT is sustained, the patient may be asymptomatic, symptomatic, or unconscious and pulseless. The physical therapist's response depends on the rhythm, regardless of whether it is sustained, and upon whether the patient is symptomatic or conscious. Clinical responses range from cessation of activity, ongoing patient monitoring and immediate notification of a physician to a full code.

Ventricular fibrillation (V-fib) is a lethal dysrhythmia accompanied by immediate loss of consciousness and loss of circulation (i.e., cardiac arrest). It is characterized by disorganized, simultaneous firing of multiple, ectopic ventricular foci; there is no organized rhythm (Figure 12-22). Effective ventricular contraction ceases and cardiopulmonary resuscitation is indicated until defibrillation is available. Death follows unless defibrillation with an automated external defibrillator (AED) or other device successfully restores an effective rhythm. Conditions that render the myocardium vulnerable to ventricular fibrillation include v-tach, myocardial ischemia or infarction, dilation of the heart, hyperkalemia, and electric shock (Guyton, 2000).

If not successfully treated, V-fib may further degenerate into asystole, which indicates complete absence of ventricular electrical activity (see Figure 12-22). Asystole may also occur as a primary event. This is known colloquially as flat-line rhythm. Like ventricular fibrillation, asystole requires that cardiopulmonary resuscitation begin immediately to save the patient's life.

Care must be taken to distinguish an apparent lethal dysrhythmia from lead disconnection or movement artifact. Unwary therapists have hastily summoned help upon observing V-fib or asystole, only to feel foolish when a lead is reattached to the patient and normal rhythm is restored. These dysrhythmias are always accompanied by loss of consciousness and pulse; a clinician should assess the patient before taking action. Similarly, during activity or exercise, movement artifact may easily be mistaken for v-tach. By assessing the patient and asking him or her to hold still, the issue may be quickly resolved.

Conduction Blocks

Conduction blocks are another type of ECG abnormality with which physical therapists should be familiar. The propagation

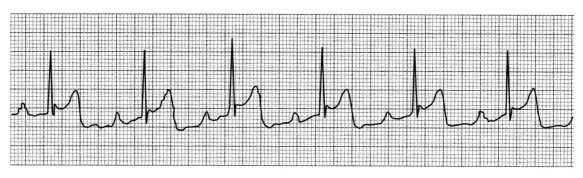

FIGURE 12-23 First-degree AB block.

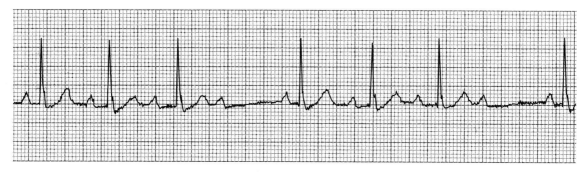

FIGURE 12-24 Second-degree AV block, Mobitz type 1.

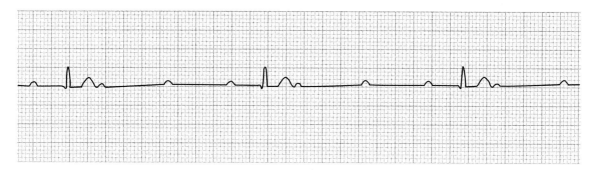

FIGURE 12-25 Second-degree AV block, Mobitz type 2.

of a cardiac impulse may be inhibited or terminated along the conduction pathway. Blockage can occur at the sinus node, between the atria and ventricles, or within the ventricular conduction system. Sinus block occurs if the impulse cannot propagate beyond the sinus node. In this case, the AV junction usually takes over as the pacemaker, and a junctional rhythm is seen with the absence of P waves.

More common are the AV blocks. They are ranked as first-, second-, or third-degree, depending on the extent of delay or obstruction of the cardiac impulse between the atria and ventricles. First-degree AV block is characterized by a prolongation of the P-R interval beyond its normal 0.2 second (Figure 12-23). Remember that the P-R interval is measured from the *beginning* of the P wave to the *beginning* of the QRS complex. Each impulse is delayed between the atria and ventricles, but each eventually reached the ventricular con-

duction system resulting in a normal QRS complex. Thus for each P wave, there is a QRS complex; therefore the conduction ratio is 1:1.

Second-degree AV block takes two forms, although in each form there are some sinus impulses that are not conducted to the ventricles. In second-degree block Mobitz type 1, also known as Wenckebach, the P-R interval lengthens progressively until a P wave fails to conduct to the ventricles (Figure 12-24). Notice how the first three P-R intervals lengthen until, after the fourth P wave, a QRS complex fails to appear. The cycle then repeats itself. Second-degree block Mobitz type 2 (Figure 12-25) is characterized by a fixed P-R interval with a "dropped" QRS following every second, third, or fourth P wave. The conduction ratio in Figure 12-25 is 3:1, or three P waves for each QRS complex. Both first- and second-degree AV blocks are considered to be incomplete heart blocks.

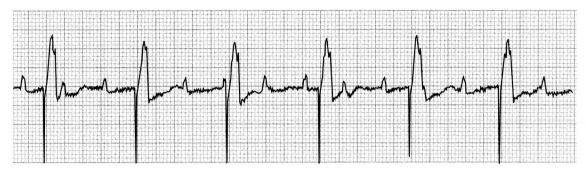

FIGURE 12-26 Third-degree AV block with ventricular pacing.

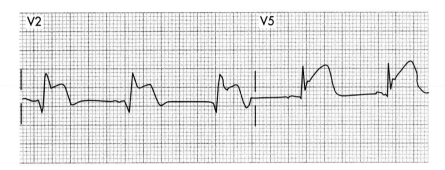

FIGURE 12-27 S-T segment elevation during myocardial infarction.

Third-degree AV block or complete heart block is also known as AV dissociation. In this rhythm (Figure 12-26), P waves are present, but there is no relationship between P waves and QRS complexes. P waves may be superimposed on QRS complexes, but none of the sinus impulses are conducted to the ventricles; the atria and ventricles are contracting independently of each other. In the absence of clinical intervention such as artificial pacing, ventricular depolarization is initiated by a junctional or ventricular pacemaker.

Clinically, AV blocks range in severity from benign, as is usually the case with first-degree AV block, to potentially lethal. Whether hemodynamic compromise occurs depends on the extent of impairment of cardiac output caused by too slow a rate of ventricular contraction (Huszar, 2002). Slow rates of ventricular contraction may cause lightheadedness or syncope. In most cases of third-degree block, treatment now includes the implantation of an artificial pacemaker. In Figure 12-26, the needle-like spikes indicate that an artificial pacemaker is depolarizing the ventricles at a rate of 60 beats per minute.

MYOCARDIAL ISCHEMIA OR INFARCTION

The ECG provides much more information than that gleaned from dysrhythmia analysis. Because physical therapists often treat patients with coronary heart disease, information regarding MI or myocardial ischemia is also of interest. Although physical therapists do not medically diagnose

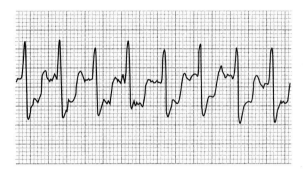

FIGURE 12-28 S-T segment depression during exercise.

myocardial ischemia or MI, they should have a working knowledge of its electrocardiographic evidence and the consequences of ischemia. During myocardial ischemia, blood flow to a portion of myocardium is compromised, resulting in alteration of myocardial metabolism. In MI, a portion of myocardium has died, but an adjacent zone of ischemic myocardial cells endures. These ischemic cells may remain leaky, and partially depolarized. A persistent current flows from the injured regions to the healthy regions (that are fully polarized), resulting in a current of injury, which is seen as a shift in the S-T segment above or below the isoelectric line (Guyton, 2000; Opie, 2004). S-T segment shifts have significant diagnostic value. For example, S-T segment elevation (Figure 12-27) is associated with transmural MI, whereas S-T segment depression (Figure 12-28) is associated with nontransmural or

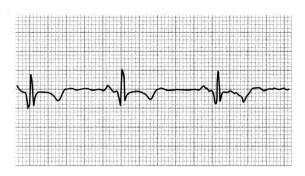

FIGURE 12-29 Significant Q wave.

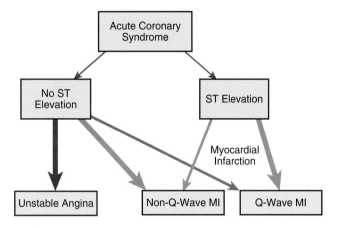

FIGURE 12-30 Algorithm for ECG diagnosis of ischemia or acute myocardial infarction. (Redrawn with permission of the American Heart Association [permission pending].)

subendocardial MI. Also, the onset of S-T segment depression during activity is often considered diagnostic of myocardial ischemia (American College of Cardiology & American Heart Association, 2002; American College of Cardiology & European Society of Cardiology, 2000). Figure 12-28 is an example of exercise-induced S-T segment depression observed in one lead during exercise.

The following is a brief discussion of other abnormalities of the ECG observed in coronary artery disease (CAD). A prominent, pathological Q wave is indicative of a transmural MI (American College of Cardiology & American Heart Association, 2002; Opie, 2004). Indeed, non-O is synonymous with nontransmural, in terms of MI. In addition, the presence of a prominent Q wave (Figure 12-29) does not distinguish between an old and an acute event. Figure 12-30 shows an algorithm for the classification of ischemia and MI based on the ECG (American College of Cardiology & European Society of Cardiology, 2000).

The T wave itself may also undergo changes during myocardial ischemia or MI. During ischemia, for example, the T wave may invert as a result of prolongation of repolarization (Guyton, 2000). Similarly, during MI, changes in the T wave may evolve with the infarct, at first becoming

indistinguishable within an elevated S-T segment, then inverting, then perhaps reverting to the original configuration after the passage of time. Although ST segment changes and the presence of a Q wave are compelling indicators for the diagnosis of ischemia or MI, it must be kept in mind that they are neither 100% sensitive nor 100% specific.

SUMMARY

Understanding the changes in the ECG during ischemia or MI may help physical therapists to integrate all available information so as to optimize patient evaluation. This knowledge, combined with astute recognition of dysrhythmia and assessment of symptoms, provides entry-level physical therapists with important tools for managing patients at risk for cardiopulmonary dysfunction.

CASES STUDIES

Case Study 1

An 81-year-old man is referred to physical therapy 2 days after angioplasty for treatment of coronary heart disease and blockages in the left circumflex and diagonal arteries. The patient has had an uncomplicated course and no cardiac arrhythmias since surgery. He is evaluated in the physical therapy gym and given a submaximal predictive treadmill test with electrocardiogram monitoring. The test consists of walking a 5% grade at 3 mph for 5 minutes. His ECG is normal at rest, but at 4 minutes of ambulation he complains of shortness of breath and requests that the test be stopped. The ECG in the last 6 seconds of ambulation is shown below (Figure 12-31). Answer the questions related to these findings. The answers can be found after the review questions.

1. Identify this dysrhythmia.
2. What are the hemodynamic and functional consequences of this dysrhythmia?
3. What action should be taken by the evaluating physical therapist?

Case Study 2

A 20-year-old basketball player is referred to a sports medicine clinic for a medical examination because of a knee injury. The physical examination shows mild tenderness and edema of the right knee but no other medical problems. During the examination by the physician, the athlete confides that he often experiences dizziness throughout the day. The physician performs a single-lead electrocardiogram and exercise test at that time. The test shows sinus bradycardia at rest and a normal response to exercise (Figure 12-32, A). The patient is sent home with a halter monitor (a device that records an ECG continuously over a 24-hour period. Analysis of the recording reveals that the pattern in Figure 12-32, B, is occurring sporadically approximately 25% of the time.

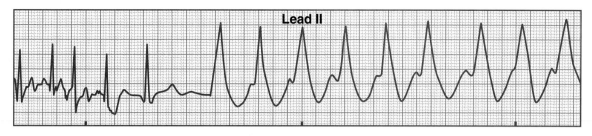

FIGURE 12-31 ECG tracing for case 1.

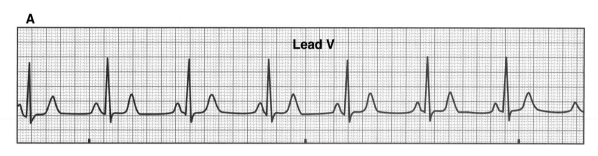

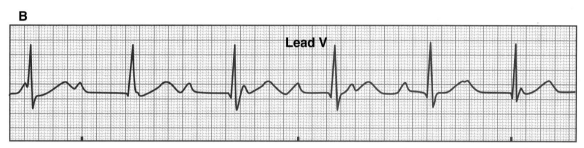

FIGURE 12-32 ECG tracing for case 2: **A,** normal ECG. **B,** typical dysrhythmia during 24-hour halter monitoring.

1. Identify this dysrhythmia and determine the patient's heart rate (3-second intervals are marked on the strip).
2. What are the possible hemodynamic consequences when this dysrhythmia occurs, and how could it lead to the patient's complaint of dizziness?

Review Questions

1. How may the following dysrhythmias be perceived by a clinician without the benefit of ECG monitoring? How may they be perceived by a patient?
   - Atrial fibrillation
   - Supraventricular tachycardia
   - Premature ventricular contractions
   - Third-degree AV block
   - Ventricular fibrillation
2. What determines the clinical significance of a dysrhythmia?
3. What property of the SA node allows it to pace the heart? Under what conditions do other portions of the conduction system act as pacemakers?

4. Does an impulse originating within the ventricular myocardium generate an effective myocardial contraction? If not, why not?
5. Why is ECG monitoring indicated after myocardial infarction?
6. What event is represented by each of the following:
   - P wave
   - QRS complex
   - T wave
   - U wave
7. What is the possible clinical significance of S-T segment depression, of S-T segment elevation? What symptoms might be anticipated in the presence of those conditions?

Answers to Case 1:

The ECG shows the beginning of a run of ventricular tachycardia with a rate of approximately 100 beats per minute. The consequences of this dysrhythmia range from asymptomatic to signs and symptoms of angina and acute heart failure to loss of consciousness and death. The physical therapist should get the patient to lie down as quickly, but as safely, as possible in a supine position and continue to observe and monitor him. Depending on the patient's symptoms and whether the v-tach is sustained, the therapist should wither notify the physician immediately and discuss the course of action or call a code.

Answers to Case 2:

Careful inspection of panel B in Figure 12-32 reveals that there is complete dissociation of the ventricular rhythm from the atrial rhythm, indicating third-degree or complete heart block. The rhythm strip shows that a regular atrial pattern (P waves) is superimposed on a regular ventricular rhythm (QRS complexes), but the QRS complexes do not follow the P waves. The heart rate is the ventricular rate and therefore approximately 40 beats per minute. Third-degree heart block results in asynchrony between the atrial ejection and the ventricular filling. In addition, the ventricular rate is typically very low and the combined effects of decreased filling and low heart rate may cause decreased blood pressure. The resulting hypotension, particularly during changes in position or movement, may lead to dizziness.

REFERENCES

Akhtar, M. (1990). Clinical spectrum of ventricular tachycardia. Circulation 82:1561-1573.

American College of Cardiology & American Heart Association. (2004). Key data elements and definitions for measuring the clinical management and outcomes of patients with atrial fibrillation: a report of the American College of Cardiology/ American Heart Association Task Force on Clinical Data Standards. http://www.acc.org/clinical/data_standards/atrial/pdf/atrial_clinicaldata.pdf; retrieved January 7, 2005.

American College of Cardiology & American Heart Association. (2002). Guideline update for the management of patients with unstable angina and on-ST-segment elevation myocardial infarction: a report of the American College of Cardiology/ American Heart Association task force on practice guidelines (Committee on the Management of Patients With Unstable Angina). http://qc.acc.org/clinical/guidelines/stemi/exec_summ/index.pdf; retrieved January 7, 2005.

American College of Cardiology & European Society of Cardiology. (2000). Myocardial infarction redefined—a consensus document of the Joint European Society of Cardiology/American College of Cardiology. http://www.acc.org/clinical/consensus/mi%5Fredefined/redefined.pdf; retrieved January 7, 2005.

American College of Sports Medicine. (2000). Guidelines for exercise testing and prescription, ed 6. Philadelphia: Lea and Febiger.

Berne, R.M., & Levy, M.N. (2000). Physiology, ed 4. St. Louis: Mosby Year Book.

Brown, K.R., & Jacobson, S. (1988). Mastering dysrhythmias: a problem-solving guide. Philadelphia: FA Davis.

Cummins, R.O. (Ed) (2003). Advanced cardiac life support: principles and practice (ACLS: the reference textbook). Dallas: American Heart Association.

Emergency Cardiac Care Committee and Subcommittees. (1992). Guidelines for cardiopulmonary resuscitation and emergency cardiac care, III: adult advanced cardiac life support. Journal of the American Medical Association 268:2199-2241.

Guyton, A.C. (2000). Textbook of medical physiology. Philadelphia: WB Saunders.

Huszar, R.J. (2002). Basic dysrhythmias, interpretation and management, ed 3. St. Louis: Mosby.

Kodma, K., Hiasa, G., Ohtsuka, T., Ikeda, S., Hashida, H., Kuwahara, T., Har, Y., Sigemastsu, Y., Hamada, M., Hiwada, K. (2000). Transient U wave inversion during treadmill exercise testing in patients with left anterior descending coronary artery disease. Angiology 51:581-589.

National Heart Lung and Blood Institute working group on atrial fibrillation. (1993). Atrial fibrillation: current understandings and research imperatives. Journal of the American College of Cardiologists 22:1830-1834.

Opie, L.H. (2004). Heart physiology, from cell to circulation, ed 4. Philadelphia: Lippincott Williams and Wilkins.

Ritsema van Eck, H.J., Kors, J.A., & Herpen, G. (2003). The elusive U wave: a simple explanation of its genesis. Journal of Electro-cardiology 36:133-137.

Roden, D.M., Balser, J.R., George, A.L., & Anderson, M.E. (2002). Cardiac ion channels. Annual Reviews in Physiology 64:431-475.

Samie, F.H., & Jalife, J. (2001). Mechanisms underlying ventricular tachycardia and its transition to ventricular fibrillation in the structurally normal heart. Cardiovascular Research 50:242-250.

Shih, H.T. (1994). Anatomy of the action potential in the heart. Texas Heart Institute Journal 21:30-41.

Surawicz, B. (1998). U wave: facts, hypotheses, misconceptions, and misnomers. Journal of Cardiovascular Electrophysiology 9:1217-1228.

CHAPTER 13

Multisystem Assessment and Laboratory Investigations

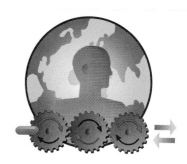

Elizabeth Dean

Blood
Endocrine function
Heart
Immune function
Kidneys

Liver
Lungs
Multisystem assessment
Peripheral vascular circulation

The purpose of this chapter is to describe the rationale for multisystem assessment in the patient managed for cardiopulmonary dysfunction and to dicuss some common laboratory tests related to multisystem assessment. The bases of tests that assess the function of the following organ systems are presented: blood, pulmonary, cardiac, peripheral vascular, renal, endocrine, liver, and immune systems. The information in this chapter is supplemental to the elements of cardiopulmonary and cardiovascular assessment and related laboratory investigations described in Part II.

The cardiopulmonary system affects and is affected by virtually every organ system in the body. The signs and symptoms of systemic disease can mimic other conditions, including cardiopulmonary dysfunction, treated by physical therapists. Therefore, the physical therapist must be able to differentiate among these presentations to determine what treatment, if any, is indicated, and what treatments may be contraindicated. Knowledge of multisystem function helps to confirm a diagnosis as well as to predict a patient's response to treatment and his or her recovery and prognosis. In addition, this information is crucial in refining and modifying treatment prescription. These abilities are particularly important in this era of professional accountability and with the advent of direct patient access.

RATIONALE FOR MULTISYSTEM ASSESSMENT

The cardiopulmonary system supports cellular respiration and life. Thus every system and every cell in the body is affected by the adequacy of oxygen transport, which is dependent on cardiopulmonary and cardiovascular function. In addition, these systems are affected by virtually every other system in the body. The cardiopulmonary physical therapist, therefore, needs thorough knowledge of multisystem function and of the interdependence of the organ systems, as well as the ability to assess multisystem function and to integrate this information into a comprehensive and progressive treatment plan.

The lungs and heart are anatomically and physiologically interdependent, and they function as a unit to transport oxygen via the peripheral circulation so as to perfuse and nourish tissues. Tissue homeostasis is dependent on the adequacy of the anatomy and physiology of the blood. The adequacy of peripheral perfusion determines the adequacy of the function of all organ systems in the body. Therefore, knowledge of the failure of the various organ systems can reflect impaired oxygen transport or may identify a threat to oxygen transport.

The elements of laboratory evaluation and testing, as well as the normal values, have been compiled from Bauer (1982); Dean (1987, 1999); Fischbach (2004); Guyton and Hall (2000);

TABLE 13-1

Common Tests of Multisystem Function and their Normal Values: Blood Tests

TEST	NORMAL VALUES (SI UNITS)
Red blood cell count (RBC)	
Men	2.09–2.71 nmol/L
Women	1.86–2.48 nmol/L
Hemoglobin (Hgb)	
Men	8.7–11.2 nmol/L
Women	7.4–9.9 nmol/L
Hematocrit (Hct)	
Men	40% to 54%
Women	37% to 47%
Platelet count	150,000–350,000/mm^3
Prothrombin time (PT)	10–14 seconds
Partial thromboplastin time (PTT)	60–85 seconds
White blood cell count (WBCC)	5–10^3/μL
(Differential WBCC includes counts of neutrophils, eosinophils, basophils, lymphocytes, and monocytes)	
Erythrocyte sedimentation rate (ESR)	
Men	0–15 mm/hr
Women	0–20 mm/hr
Proteins	
Albumin	38–50 g/L
Globulin	23–35 g/L
Fibrinogen	2.0–4.0 g/L
Lactate	
Venous	0.5–2.2 mmol/L
Arterial	0.5–1.6 mmol/L
Electrolytes (blood)	
Sodium (Na$^+$)	135–148 mmol/L
Potassium (K$^+$)	3.5–5.0 mmol/L
Calcium (Ca^{2+})	
Total	4.5–5.3 mmol/L
Ionized	2.1–2.6 mmol/L
Chloride (Cl$^-$)	98–106 mmol/L
Cholesterol	3.63–6.48 mmol/L
Creatine kinase	
Men	0.42–1.51 mmol/sec/L
Women	0.17–1.18 mmol/sec/L

Normal values may vary depending on the laboratory performing the measurement. Within-subject variation occurs as a result of are and variations in the pretest standardization procedures.

Jacobs et al (2001); Le Fever Kee (2000); Pagana and Pagana (2002); Siest et al (1985); and Wallach (2000).

ELEMENTS OF MULTISYSTEM ASSESSMENT
Blood

Some common blood tests are summarized in Table 13-1, along with their normal values.

The average blood volume consists of 5 L of blood—3 L of plasma and 2 L of cells. Plasma is the medium that suspends and transports blood cells. The complete blood count (CBC) is one of the most commonly ordered laboratory procedures. This basic screening test helps to establish the patient's diagnosis, treatment response, recovery, and prognosis. The CBC includes the red blood cell count (RBC), a variety of red blood cell indexes, differential white blood cell count (WBC), hematocrit (Hct), hemoglobin (Hgb), and platelet count.

Tests of coagulation and hemostasis reflect bleeding pathology, which often involves injury of blood vessels and cells. Damage to the blood vessel wall leads to constriction, a primary mechanism of hemostasis. Circulating platelets adhere to exposed subendothelial tissues, which can predispose thrombus formation.

The fluidity of the blood is regulated by the facilitation and the inhibition of thrombin formation. When these two processes are in balance, the blood has an optimal consistency; it is neither too thick nor too thin. This allows blood to flow optimally through the circulation without unduly affecting the work of the heart. Blood vessel injury can disrupt this balance and can promote coagulation.

Disseminated intravascular coagulation (DIC) results from an imbalance between the formation and deposition of fibrin, which leads to the formation of thrombi. The continuous production of thrombin causes depletion of the coagulation factors, and bleeding results. Tests used to assess bleeding capacity include thrombin time and fibrin clotting time (partial thromboplastin time [PTT]).

Proteins (amino acids) serve as regulators of metabolism. Much clinical information is obtained by examining and measuring proteins because proteins regulate many important physiologic functions in the body. Plasma proteins serve as a source of nutrition for the body tissues and function as buffers when combined with hemoglobin.

Albumin, a protein formed in the liver, maintains normal water distribution in the body (colloid osmotic pressure). It transports blood constituents such as ions, pigments, bilirubin, hormones, fatty acids, enzymes, and certain drugs. Approximately 55% of total protein is albumin. The remainder is globulin, which functions in antibody formation, and other plasma proteins (fibrinogen and prothrombin) involved with coagulation.

Lactic acid, a product of carbohydrate metabolism, is produced when cells receive inadequate oxygen in relation to oxygen demand (anaerobic metabolism). When the production of lactic acid exceeds its removal from the blood by the liver, lactic acid accumulates in the blood.

Cholesterol is used in the production of steroid hormones, bile acids, and cell membranes. Cholesterol is found in muscles, red blood cells, and cell membranes. Low-density and high-density lipoproteins (LDLs and HDLs) transport cholesterol in the blood. High levels of cholesterol, particularly LDLs and low HDLs, are associated with atherosclerosis and increased risk of coronary artery disease (CAD).

Electrolyte assessment is based on the electrolyte constituents of a blood or urine sample. Although present in minute quantities, electrolytes are essential in maintaining normal cellular function and homeostasis. The electrolytes that are routinely studied are sodium, potassium, chloride, calcium, phosphorus, and magnesium.

Pulmonary Function

See Chapters 9 and 15 for a detailed description of the assessment of the pulmonary system and its function.

Cardiac Function

A detailed description of the assessment of the cardiac system and its function appears in Chapters 12 and 15.

TABLE 13-2
Common Tests of Multisystem Function and their Normal Values: Tests of Peripheral Vascular Function

TEST	NORMAL VALUES
Skin temperature	Ranges from ambient temperature to 30°C
Ankle systolic pressures	97% of brachial pressure
Peripheral pulses	Apex heart rate
Capillary filling after quick pressure over the nail bed	Instantaneous filling

Peripheral Vascular Function

Assessment of the peripheral vascular circulation is essential to provide information regarding central and peripheral hemodynamic status as well as peripheral tissue perfusion. This assessment is essential to establishing the integrity of the patient's hemodynamic status at rest and during the physical and exercise stress that is associated with most physical therapy treatments. Laboratory tests include segmental blood pressure studies, skin temperature studies, pulse wave analysis, Doppler ultrasound studies, and arteriography. The physical examination corroborates the results of the laboratory investigations and includes the patient's history; inspection of the integrity of the peripheral circulation, particularly to the extremities; palpation to assess peripheral pulses; and auscultation, which can be helpful in detecting bruits or areas of turbulent blood flow associated with arterial stenoses.

Some common tests of peripheral vascular function are summarized in Table 13-2 along with their normal values.

Kidney Function

Urine consists of the end products of cellular metabolism and is produced by the large volumes of blood (approximately 25% of the cardiac output [CO]) that flow through the kidneys. When the kidneys are compromised, death can ensue within a few days. Although fluid is lost through several routes, the kidneys are primarily responsible for processing and regulating fluid balance in the body.

Urea, the major nonprotein nitrogenous end product of protein catabolism, is measured in the blood as blood urea nitrogen (BUN). The urea is then carried to the kidneys by the blood to be excreted in the urine.

Creatinine is a byproduct in the breakdown of muscle creatine phosphate resulting from energy metabolism. The production of creatinine is constant as long as muscle mass is constant. Kidney dysfunction reduces the excretion of creatinine, resulting in increased levels of blood creatinine. Analysis of urine for creatinine provides an index of kidney function.

Increased osmolality stimulates the secretion of antidiuretic hormone (ADH) that acts on renal tubules. This results in the

TABLE 13-3

Common Tests of Multisystem Function and their Normal Values: Tests of Renal Function

TEST	NORMAL VALUES (SI UNITS)
Blood urea nitrogen (BUN)	3.6-7.1 mmol/L
Creatinine	7.6-30.5 μmol/L

Normal values may vary depending on the laboratory performing the measurement. Within-subject variations occurs because of age and variations in the pretest standardization procedures.

reabsorption of water, more concentrated urine, and less concentrated serum.

Some common tests of renal function are summarized in Table 13-3, along with their normal values.

Endocrine Function

Endocrine glands are responsible for producing the substances and neuromediators responsible for maintaining homeostasis and enabling the body to adapt when physically and psychologically challenged or perturbed from a resting state. The key endocrine glands are the pancreas, the thyroid gland, and the adrenal glands. Endocrine glands regulate metabolism and are responsible for increasing blood flow and pressure and for reducing vascular resistance when metabolic demands increase.

Some common tests of endocrine function are summarized in Table 13-4, along with their normal values.

Pancreatic function and insulin production

Insulin, a hormone produced in the pancreas by the beta cells of the islets of Langerhans, regulates the metabolism of carbohydrates (as do the liver, adipose tissues, muscles, and other target cells) and is responsible for maintaining a constant level of blood glucose. The rate of insulin secretion is determined primarily by the level of blood glucose perfusing the pancreas and also by hormonal status, the autonomic nervous system, nutritional status, smoking, restricted mobility, physical stress such as traumatic insult to the body during illness and injury, and pharmacologic agents.

Amylase is an enzyme produced in the salivary glands, pancreas, and liver; it converts starch to sugar. Inflammation of the pancreas or salivary glands results in more of the enzyme entering the blood. The amylase test is used to diagnose and monitor the treatment of acute pancreatitis.

Thyroid

The function of the thyroid gland is to take iodine from the circulating blood, combine it with amino acid tyrosine, and convert it into the thyroid hormones thyroxine (T_4) and triiodothyronine (T_3). Thyroid hormones have a profound effect on metabolic rate. Increased metabolism causes more rapid use of oxygen than normal and causes greater quantities

TABLE 13-4

Common Tests of Multisystem Functions and their Normal Values: Tests of Endocrine Function

TEST	NORMAL VALUES (SI UNITS)
Thyroid Function	**Thyroid Function**
Total thyroxine (T4)	65-155 nmol/L
Total triiodothyronine (T3)	1.77-2.93 nmol/L
Adrenal Function	
Epinephrine	0.0-81.9 nmol/24 hr
Norepinephrine	0.0-591 nmol/24 hr
Cortisol	
Morning	138-635 nmol/L
Evening	82-413 nmol/L
Pancreatic Function	
Glucose tolerance test	
At 1 hr glucose	1.1-2.75 mmol/L
At 2 hr glucose	0.2-0.88 mmol/L
Insulin	
12 hr fasting	35-145 pmol/L
Amylase	
Blood level	25-125 units/L

Normal values may vary depending on the laboratory performing the measurement. Within-subject variation is dependent on age and variations in the pretest standardization procedures.

of metabolic end products to be released from the tissues. These effects cause vasodilation in most of the body tissues, thus increasing blood flow. An increase in the thyroid hormones increases cardiac output, heart rate, force of cardiac contraction, blood volume, arterial blood pressure, oxygen consumption, and carbon dioxide (CO_2) production; hence, there is an increase in the rate and depth of breathing and increased appetite, food intake, and gastrointestinal motility. The thyroid gland also stores T_3 and T_4 until they are released into the blood stream under the influence of thyroid stimulating hormone (TSH) from the pituitary gland.

Adrenal function

Catecholamines, epinephrine, and norepinephrine are produced by the adrenal medulla of the adrenal glands. Urine samples are used to test for these important vasoactive neurotransmitters in the investigation of various disorders. In addition to their vasoactive properties, the catecholamines are essential in stimulating the sympathetic response in the fight-or-flight mechanism.

Cortisol is produced by the adrenal cortex of the adrenal glands and is involved with metabolism of carbohydrate, protein, and fat. In addition, it inhibits the action of insulin and thus the uptake of glucose by the cells. The normal secretion of cortisol varies diurnally (i.e., it is high in the morning and low in the evening). In addition, cortisol is a stress hormone.

TABLE 13-5

Common Tests of Multisystem Function and their Normal Values: Tests of Liver Function

TEST	NORMAL VALUES (SI UNITS)
Alkaline phosphatase	0.18-0.40 nmol/s/L
Bilirubin (total)	5.1-17.1 µmol/L

Normal values may vary depending on the laboratory performing the measurement. Within-subject variation occurs as a result of age and variations in the pretest standardization procedures.

TABLE 13-6

Common Tests of Multisystem Function and their Normal Values: Tests of Immunologic Function

	DIFFERENTIAL WHITE BLOOD CELL COUNT	
	ABSOLUTE VALUE (N/µL)	*RELATIVE VALUE (BY %)*
Neutrophils	3000-7000	60-70
Lymphocytes	1000-4000	20-40
Monocytes	100-600	2-6
Eosinophils	50-400	1-4
Basophils	25-100	0.5-1

Normal values may vary depending on the laboratory performing the measurement. Within subject variation occurs from age and variations in the pretest standardization procedures.

Liver Function

Liver function is especially important in that dysfunction of this organ can be life-threatening. The liver has a primary role in carbohydrate and protein metabolism; it produces bile and is responsible for detoxification of the blood. Its function is assessed by tests of liver enzymes such as amylase and alkaline phosphatase.

Some common tests of hepatic function are summarized in Table 13-5, along with their normal values.

Immunologic Function

Immunologic function is dependent on the adequacy of the function of several tissues and organs, namely, bone marrow, the thymus gland, the lymph nodes, and the vessels of the lymphatic system, spleen, tonsils, and intestinal lymphoid tissue. Immunologic function can break down if insufficient protective immune factors are produced, or if the system is overwhelmed by an invading organism for which the body has inappropriate or insufficient resistance.

Some common tests of immunological function are summarized in Table 13-6, along with their normal values. Specific detailed accounts of immmunodiagnostic studies and tests for autoimmune deficiencies are beyond the scope of this chapter but can be reviewed in Fischbach (2004) and Le Fever Kee (2000).

SUMMARY

This chapter describes the rationale for multisystem assessment in the patient being managed for cardiopulmonary dysfunction and discusses some common tests of multisystem function. The cardiopulmonary system affects and is affected by virtually every organ system in the body. Thus primary cardiopulmonary dysfunction can lead to complications in many organ systems and vice versa; dysfunction of other organ systems can have cardiopulmonary manifestations. In addition, the signs and symptoms of systemic conditions can mimic other conditions treated by physical therapists. Therefore, the physical therapist must be able to differentiate among these presentations so as to determine whether a pathology will respond to management by physical therapy, what treatments are not indicated, and what treatments may be contraindicated. Multisystem monitoring provides the fundamental information needed to refine and progress the treatment prescription. These abilities are essential in this era of increased professional responsibility and with the advent of direct patient access.

Review Questions

1. Describe the common tests for blood composition and the clinical implications of abnormally high and low values.
2. Describe pulmonary function tests.
3. Describe tests of heart function.
4. Describe tests of peripheral vascular function.
5. Describe tests of renal function.
6. Describe tests of endocrine function.
7. Describe tests of liver function.
8. Describe tests of immune function.

REFERENCES

Bauer, J.D. (1982). Clinical laboratory methods, ed 9. St. Louis: CV Mosby.

Dean, E. (1987). Assessment of the peripheral circulation: an update for practitioners. The Australian Journal of Physiotherapy 33:164-1671.

Dean, E. (1999). Preferred practice patterns in cardiopulmonary physical therapy: a guide to physiologic measures. Cardiopulmonary Physical Therapy Journal 10:124-134.

Fischbach, F. (2004). A manual of laboratory diagnostic tests, ed 7. Philadelphia: Lippincott Williams & Wilkins.

Guyton, A.C., & Hall, J.E. (2000). Textbook of medical physiology, ed 10. Philadelphia: Elsevier.

Jacobs, D.S., Kasten, B.L., & Demott, W.R. (2001). Laboratory test handbook, ed 5. Cleveland, Ohio: Lexi-Comp.

Le Fever Kee, J. (2000). Handbook of laboratory and diagnostic tests with nursing implications, ed 4. Paramus, NJ: Prentice Hall.

Pagana, K.D., & Pagana, T.J. (2002). Mosby's diagnostic and laboratory test reference, ed 6. Philadelphia: Elsevier.

Siest, G., Henny, J., Schiele, F., & Yonge, D.S. (1985). Interpretation of clinical laboratory tests. Foster City, Calif.: Biomedical Publications.

Wallach, J. (2000). Interpretation of diagnostic tests: a synopsis of laboratory medicine, ed 7. Philadelphia: Lippincott Williams & Wilkins.

CHAPTER 14

Special Tests

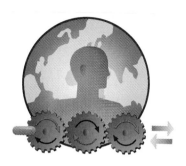

Gail M. Huber

KEY TERMS

Computed tomography
Echocardiography
Ejection fraction
Hibernating myocardium
Magnetic resonance imaging

Myocardial viability
Radionuclide angiography
Radionuclide imaging
Stunned myocardium
Ventilation-perfusion scan

The medical workup of a patient with cardiac or pulmonary disease uses many tools. The patient interview, physical examination, chest radiograph, and electrocardiogram (ECG) can provide adequate information to make a diagnosis. However, when the diagnosis remains unclear, more complex technology is required. Nuclear medicine offers a variety of noninvasive tests for evaluation of cardiac and pulmonary function. Echocardiography is another noninvasive method that provides information about the cardiovascular system, including valve function, ventricular performance, and estimation of filling pressures. It is particularly useful in children. Unlike tests of the cardiovascular system, special tests of the respiratory system are less commonly used in the initial diagnosis and treatment of disease. This is the result of the generally high-quality information obtained from standard radiograph examination when combined with the patient's respiratory symptoms and the results of the physical examination (Lillington, 1987).

However, the circumstances of some patients require the use of invasive tests. Pulmonary and cardiac angiography is not without risk; however, for evaluating blood flow in the heart and lungs, as well as for determining cardiac anatomy and direct volume and pressure measures, it is without equal. Transesophageal echocardiography is another invasive test.

Following the initial assessment of the problem, these same special tests may be used to assist in the determination of appropriate therapy and to evaluate prognosis and response to treatment. The noninvasive tests are most important in determining ongoing surgical, interventional, or medical therapy. Physical therapists should understand these invasive and noninvasive tests for several reasons. It is useful to understand how the information is used to make a differential diagnosis and determine treatment. These tests have helped to clarify our understanding of the physiology and pathophysiology of the system. Therapists need to understand the pathophysiologic basis for a patient's movement dysfunctions to select the most appropriate treatment strategies. Many special tests can be and are being used in research to evaluate treatment interventions. For example, radiolabeled aerosols are used to evaluate mucociliary clearance, providing a method to evaluate the effectiveness of pulmonary hygiene techniques (Miller & O'Doherty, 1992). Clinically, physical therapists need to use information from the tests to develop a framework for predicting how the patient may respond to a physical therapy intervention. For example, nuclear imaging can provide information about left ventricular ejection fraction. This information helps the physical therapist determine whether the patient should be stratified into a high-risk or a low-risk category. The monitoring of an exercise session may depend on the risk level, and the interpretation of the patient's response to treatment may be affected.

This chapter reviews some of the technology used to examine the cardiac and pulmonary systems. First, the general method used to acquire data is described. Second, the type of data available from the technology is defined and specific applications to the cardiac and pulmonary systems are discussed.

NUCLEAR IMAGING SYSTEMS
Physics of Nuclear Imaging

A general view of how nuclear imaging systems work should help the physical therapist understand some of the differences among the wide variety of tests used today. This area of medicine continues to experience rapid growth and change as technology changes the equipment used to perform the tests, the radiopharmaceuticals available, and the speed at which data can be acquired and analyzed.

Radionuclide imaging allows for the noninvasive acquisition of images of a variety of body tissues. An imaging system requires three basic parts. The first requirement is a radiopharmaceutical that emits gamma radiation and is taken up by the body tissue of interest. Next, a radiation detector or camera is needed. Finally, computers are required to collect and analyze the data. Thus, an image is formed based on the brightness of the tissue, which is proportional to the radiation the tissue has absorbed (Maass-Moreno, 2003).

Radionuclides are elements that are unstable; they gain stability by emitting particles or photons. This is called radioactive decay, and gamma radiation is released. Radionuclides are either cyclotron- or generator-produced. The cyclotron accelerates alpha particles, deuterons, and protons to energies suitable for the production of the required radionuclide (Murphy, 2003). A radionuclide generator is a system of parent and daughter radionuclides in equilibrium. The system is constructed so that the daughter can be removed from time to time for patient use (Kim, 1987). A generator system produces short-lived radionuclides (Murphy, 2003).

These elements are often attached to other substrates for transport in the body to the particular tissue of interest. The elements have differing characteristics, such as energy output and half-life. Because of their varied distribution in the body tissues, they provide different information.

Detection of the radioactive energy emitted by a specific radiopharmaceutical requires a camera. When certain materials are struck by ionizing radiation, light is emitted. A scintillation detector detects this light (Figure 14-1). A gamma camera is a scintillation detector able to detect photons exiting the body. It uses a large, collimated crystal monitored by an array of photomultiplier tubes (Beller, 1995). A collimator is a device that allows only those photons traveling in an appropriate direction to reach the crystal. There are several types of collimators: parallel-hole collimators, pinhole collimators, and converging and diverging collimators. The photomultiplier tube records the amount of light from the crystal and converts

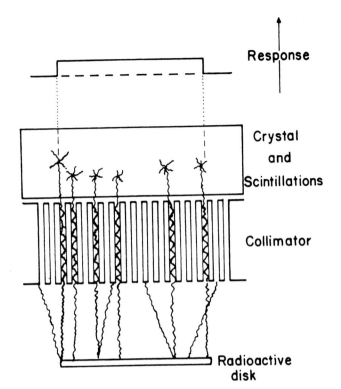

FIGURE 14-1 Diagrammatic illustration of a multi-hole collimator where gamma-rays admitted in line with the collimator holes are transmitted to the crystal, whereas gamma-rays emitted obliquely are absorbed by the collimator septa. *(From Hendee, W.R., & Ritenour, R., [Eds] [1992]. Medical imaging physics, ed 3. St. Louis: CV Mosby.)*

it into a voltage that is proportional to the intensity of the light (Beller, 1995).

The camera system is connected to a computer that stores the light images. The computer is able to derive two-dimensional images from the data. The computer can also quantify the data and perform a variety of data analyses (Beller, 1995).

Planar Imaging

A single-crystal camera (Anger) produces a two-dimensional, or planar, image. Multicrystal cameras (Blau and Blender) also produce planar images but are able to perform fast dynamic imaging used in first-pass and gated studies. Planar images are unable to reflect the depth of an image (Maass-Moreno, 2003). Planar imaging may be the only option available to obese patients who do not "fit" the single photon emission computed tomography (SPECT) camera or cannot remain immobile (Watson, 2003).

SPECT Imaging

If a gamma camera is rotated around the patient and multiple projections are obtained, a three-dimensional distribution of tracer is acquired. This image is a tomograph (i.e., a cross-sectional slice of the body). This is the basis for SPECT (Liao, 2001). The same gamma-emitting pharmaceuticals are used.

Regular gamma cameras or specially designed systems can be used (Iskandrian, 1987). SPECT imaging produces higher spatial resolution (Schwaiger, 1994) and greater sensitivity to coronary artery disease (CAD) than do planar images (Beller, 1994). SPECT images also allow for quantitation of radio-activity (Maass-Moreno, 2003). However, attenuation artifacts (absorption of the radioactive energy by other body tissues such that the camera does not detect it) are greater than in planar images, particularly those images involving the inferior wall of the heart in men and the anterior wall in women, and may produce false-positive scans (Schwaiger, 1994). The quality of the images is dependent on the use of stringent quality-control measures and on the experience of the staff. Image quality is also patient-dependent. Patients must be able to lie perfectly still for 15 to 20 minutes, with their hands over their heads, while data are collected.

Physical therapists can identify patients who would have difficulty with arm movements or with remaining still. For these patients, other imaging modalities such as echocardiography may be appropriate.

Positron Emission Tomography

Positron emission tomography (PET) uses positron-emitting radionuclides. The images obtained by PET can provide information regarding metabolism in lung tissue and cardiac muscle, myocardial perfusion, and myocardial receptor density (Maddahi, 1994). PET is valuable in delineating myocardial areas with reversible and irreversible injury and in assessing the feasibility of surgical revascularization, coronary angioplasty, or thrombolysis with respect to potentially salvageable tissue (Niemeyer, 1992). Many of the radionuclides used in PET scans require a cyclotron for generation and a specialized detection system. PET images offer superior resolution compared with SPECT images (Schwaiger, 1994). PET also allows greater correction for attenuation artifact (Schwaiger, 1994). PET imaging is a newer technology that offers improvement in sensitivity and specificity when compared with SPECT (Mullani, 1992). PET studies use short scanning times (5 to 20 minutes). Due to the short half-life of PET tracers, scans can be repeated relatively soon (Schelbert, 2003). The studies can be done at rest or with a pharmacologic stress agent (Schwaiger, 1994). Cost and location near a cyclotron to generate nuclides continues to limit the widespread use of this technology.

NUCLEAR TESTS OF THE CARDIOVASCULAR SYSTEM
First-Pass and Gated Equilibrium Scans

In a first-pass study, data are collected on a radiolabeled bolus of blood as it passes through the cardiac chambers, which is one method of radionuclide angiography. A first-pass scan allows for clear identification of the four cardiac chambers. During first-pass studies, data are collected over several cardiac cycles. Gated equilibrium studies or multiple-uptake gated acquisition (MUGA) scans average several hundred cardiac cycles. Each R wave of the ECG triggers the

acquisition of data, thus the average cycle observed is the compilation of many cycles (Williams, 2003). The quality of the image is best when the patient has a stable sinus rhythm. Patients with irregular heart rates such as atrial fibrillation produce images of poorer quality.

Exercise Stress Studies

Many of the tests performed using radionuclides are coupled with an exercise test. A treadmill exercise test is performed, and at the peak of exercise, a tracer is injected. Shortly afterwards (the timing depends on the tracer), images are acquired. Exercise imaging enhances the identification of ischemic areas. These tests are then often compared with rest studies. Rest/stress or stress/rest protocols can be used.

Pharmacologic Stress Studies

Some patients are unable to exercise to an intensity sufficient to produce stress on the cardiovascular system. When patients are unable to exercise, pharmacologic agents can be used to dilate the coronary arteries or increase the metabolic demand of the heart. Dipryridimole (Persantine), adenosine, and dobutamine are often used (Liao, 2001). Pharmacologic stress tests can be coupled with SPECT and PET nuclear imaging techniques or with echocardiography to determine regions of ischemic myocardium suggesting functionally significant blockage in the coronary artery supplying that territory.

Nuclear-Derived Measurements

Data derived from radionuclide images provide information about perfusion and function. Radionuclides taken up by the myocardium provide a picture of the heart that includes wall thickness and an outline of the chamber. In radionuclide angiography, which includes first-pass and gated studies, the blood is highlighted as it passes through the chambers. Qualitative and quantitative measurements can be taken. The most important of these measurements, the ejection fraction (right and left ventricle), is a measure of myocardial function. It is derived from quantitative counts of the ventricular area during diastole and systole (Williams, 2003):

$$\frac{(\text{end-diastolic counts} - \text{end-systolic counts}) \times 100}{\text{end-diastolic counts}}$$

End-Diastolic Counts

Left ventricular ejection fraction (LVEF) has been shown in several studies (Coronary Artery Surgery Study, Multi-center Postinfarction Research Group Database) to be highly predictive of 1-year survival (Maddahi, 1994; Port, 1994). LVEF values normally range between 55% and 75%, whereas an LVEF below 40% indicates moderate to severe congestive heart failure (Dyer, 2003; Jessup, 2003). Right ventricular ejection fraction (RVEF) has been found to have a wide range of normal values (35% to 75%) (Kinch, 1994) but is not clearly predictive of function without data about wall motion abnormalities. The strongest radionuclide predictor of outcome is the exercise LVEF. When predicting outcome, multivariate analysis of clinical data, catheterization, and radionuclide measurements has shown that the radionuclide results (exercise LVEF, resting end-diastolic volume, and change in heart rate [HR]) have the same prognostic power as the catheterization data (Port, 1994).

Another important measurement is wall motion. Quantitative and qualitative evaluation of the movement of the myocardium can be made. Wall thickness and wall movement are compared during systole and diastole. Assessments are made of akinesia, the absence of wall motion; global or regional hypokinesia, the reduction of wall motion; and dyskinesia, the outward bulging of the wall during systole (Otto, 2000). Global left ventricular function is a strong predictor of survival. It can help clinicians differentiate a weak heart from one that is stiff, allowing the appropriate treatment. Regional wall function, when correlated with knowledge of coronary artery anatomy, allows for the identification of potential blockages or areas of infarct. Assessing wall thickness can provide information about hypertrophy or aneurysm but that is done more reliably by echocardiography.

Anatomic measurements can be made of chamber size. From these data, chamber volume can be calculated, as well as stroke volume and cardiac output (Table 14-1).

Tests to Evaluate Myocardial Perfusion

Perfusion of the myocardium is a vital factor in the viability and function of the heart. Information about myocardial perfusion is used for diagnostic decisions, treatment decisions, and prognosis. Perfusion of the myocardium under rest and exercise conditions is important in the diagnosis of CAD. The efficacy of reperfusion strategies, such as angioplasty and thrombolytic therapy, must be evaluated. Identifying tissue that is viable but still at risk is one of the newer applications of myocardial perfusion tests. Information gained from combined perfusion and metabolic studies has helped to increase the understanding of ischemic myocardium. Two types of contractile dysfunction have been delineated. Hibernating myocardium is the result of prolonged ischemia. The contractility of the muscle fiber is affected so that there may appear to be regional wall motion abnormalities. The tissue is alive but not contracting. It is theorized that this is a measure to reduce energy expenditure and ensure myocyte survival. The second condition, myocardial stunning, occurs under conditions of acute ischemia. In this case, there is contractile dysfunction during the acute ischemic episode that persists for some time after perfusion has returned to normal. Both conditions are reversible. Patients demonstrating hibernating myocardium may benefit from revascularization procedures. Patients with stunned myocardium may require only supportive care until contractile function returns (Schelbert, 1994).

Thallium 201

Thallium 201 is the radioactive isotope most often used in myocardial perfusion studies (Wacker, 1994). It is a cyclotron-produced isotope that emits low-energy radiation (69 to 83 kiloelectron volt [keV]). Administered intravenously, its distribution throughout the body depends on blood flow. Thallium concentrations in the myocardium depend on four processes. First, there is a linear relationship between thallium concentration and coronary blood flow. Second, extraction-transport across the cell membrane depends on active and passive transport mechanisms. Thallium is thought to be transported across the cell membrane through the sodium-potassium ATPase pump (Maddahi, 1994). The third process is washout, also called redistribution. Thallium enters the cell initially and then is redistributed until an equilibrium is attained based on a net balance between thallium 201 input through recirculation and intrinsic thallium washout (Beller, 1994). Finally, concentrations are decay-related, dictated by the half-life of the isotope (Brown, 1994; Iskandrian, 1987).

Thallium 201 images can be qualitatively and quantitatively evaluated. Normally perfused myocardium demonstrates uniform uptake of the tracer. Uniform uptake can occur as long as blockages are less than 50% of the artery. Ischemic but viable myocardium initially appears as areas of decreased uptake, these areas fill in over time, a function of redistribution. Because blood flow is decreased, clearance of thallium 201 from the defect region is slower (Maddahi, 1994). In infarcted areas, these defects remain unchanged over time. Qualitative evaluation requires visual inspection of the images. Quantitative evaluation is performed by computer. The computer analyzes the amount of radioactivity taken up in a particular region of interest. It then quantifies this count so that regions can be compared with each other and with normalized data. In this way, unperfused or hypoperfused areas can be identified (Figure 14-2).

Thallium 201 is used to acquire planar and SPECT images for rest studies, exercise stress studies, and pharmacologic stress studies. The traditional thallium 201 stress study calls for injection of the tracer at the peak of exercise, with collection of the stress data shortly after. The redistribution study is completed 4 hours later. Newer study protocols include reinjection of thallium before the 4-hour redistribution study (Go, 1992) and use in dual-isotope studies (Berman, 1994). Reinjection of thallium and repeat imaging 24 hours after initial study can help identify severely ischemic (greater than 90% blockage) areas, which may take much longer to demonstrate redistribution.

Technetium 99m Sestamibi

Technetium (Tc) 99m sestamibi was developed because of the number of advantages it has over thallium imaging. Sestamibi provides improved SPECT image quality as a result of higher count rates and higher energy, in the 140 keV range. Tc 99m sestamibi is generator-produced. The isotope has a 6-hour half-life (Berman et al, 1994). Because of the short half-life, higher doses can be injected, and although the percentage of extraction is lower, sestamibi uptake in relation to flow is similar to that of thallium. These factors result in higher count rates, which thus allow the use of gated images

TABLE 14-1

Summary of Special Tests of the Cardiopulmonary System

SPECIAL TESTS	CLINICAL FINDINGS
Cardiac Tests	
Nuclear Imaging	
Planar, SPECT, first-pass, gated Thallium 201, technitium 99m sestamibi, technitium teboroxime	Evaluates myocardial perfusion; used in exercise stress studies and to assess reversibility of defects. Quantitatively can be used to determine: EF, SV, CO, regional function, ventricular volumes, intra-cardiac shunt, valvular regurgitation.
Positron emission tomography (PET) scans, FDG 18, acetate 11 C	Assesses myocardial viability by evaluating glucose metabolism (FDG) or oxidative metabolism (acetate 11 C). Can identify areas that improve with reperfusion.
Infarct avid scans, technetium 99m pyrophosphate, indium 111 antimyosin	Identifies areas of infarction by binding with elements released by the death of myocardial tissue.
Computed Tomography (CT)	
EBCT	Identifies calcium concentration in tissues, which is related to the amount of atherosclerotic plaque.
Magnetic Resonance Imaging (MRI)	
MRI with contrast (Gd-DTPA)	Identifies ventricular volumes, EF, CO. Contrast imaging can be used to identify perfusion defects, flow, areas of infarction.
Echocardiography	
M-mode, 2-D, transesophageal (TEE), Doppler, myocardial contrast echo (MCE)	Evaluates myocardial structure; 2-D used in exercise stress; quantitatively measures: chamber size, wall thickness, valve structure and function, pressure and flow through valve, valve area, EF studies; MCE can be used to examine perfusion.
Angiography	Quantitative measures of pressure, resistance, flow, O_2 consumption, arteriovenous oxygen difference EF, CO.
Pulmonary Tests	
Nuclear Imaging	
Perfusion scan, MAB	Identifies regions of decreased pulmonary perfusion; used to identify pulmonary embolism.
Ventilation scan, 99m Tc DTPA, gallium scan	Identifies regions of decreased ventilation; used in conjunction with 133-Xe perfusion scan to identify patients with pulmonary embolism; identifies neoplastic or inflammatory pulmonary lesions.
PET scan, FDG	Aids in differential diagnosis of solitary pulmonary nodules, inflammation, and malignant lesions.
Computed Tomography (CT)	
HRCT, spiral CT	HRCT used in the diagnosis of bronchiectasis; spiral CT can be used to diagnose PE.
Magnetic Resonance Imaging (MRI)	
MRI with contrast (Gd-DTPA)	MRI with contrast used for MR angiography; dynamic MRI used in workup of lung transplant to examine ventilation, pulmonary mechanics.
Angiography	For diagnosis of pulmonary embolism.

CO, Cardiac output; *EF*, ejection fraction; *SV*, stroke volume.

and first-pass acquisition studies. Higher count rates are preferred when evaluating obese patients. One of the greatest limitations of Tc 99m sestamibi is that it does not readily redistribute; therefore, the reversibility of defects cannot be ascertained as well as with thallium. This factor is one reason thallium is much more popular. Two-day protocols or dual isotope protocols can be used to overcome this limitation (Berman, 1994). Lack of redistribution has been exploited in evaluating the impact of thrombolytic therapy in acute

situations. A patient with an acute myocardial infarction (MI) can be injected with tracer, given thrombolytics, stabilized, and scanned 4 hours later. The scan results show myocardial perfusion at the time of injection, when the myocardium was ischemic. Later scans demonstrate the new perfusion situation.

Technetium 99m Teboroxime

Another isotope is technetium 99m teboroxime. It is not yet widely accepted because of its rapid washout and the

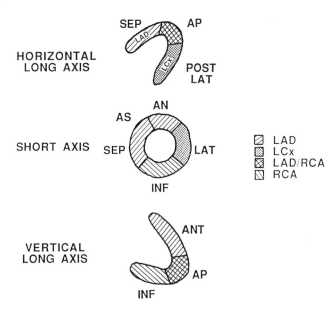

FIGURE 14-2 Illustration of the SPECT series. Representative midventricular slices of the three projections most frequently used for SPECT thallium display. *LAD*, left anterior descending; *LCx*, left circumflex; *RCA*, right coronary artery; *SEP*, septum; *AP*, apical; *LAT*, lateral; *POST LAT*, posterior lateral; *INF*, inferior. *(From Fisher, K.C. [1990]. Qualitative SPECT thallium imaging: technical considerations and clinical applications. In Guiberteau, M.J. [Ed]. Nuclear cardiovascular imaging. New York: Churchill Livingstone.)*

visualization problems related to hepatic uptake (Berman et al, 1991; Go, 1992). The half-life for teboroxime is 5 to 6 minutes (Johnson, 1994). It has a myocardial extraction fraction higher than either sestamibi or thallium (Johnson, 1994). Tc 99m teboroxime uptake parallels myocardial blood flow under both ischemic and nonischemic conditions (Johnson, 1994) and does not appear to rely on active cellular processes.

Because of the short half-life, rapid-acquisition imaging systems are required so that the images do not reflect washout. SPECT and first-pass studies can be performed, but Tc 99m teboroxime does not permit gated SPECT acquisition (Berman, 1991). Protocols using this isotope are designed to take advantage of the rapid uptake and washout. When used with pharmacologic stress studies, a rest-stress study can be completed within minutes (Johnson, 1994). This may have future application in studying reperfusion following balloon angioplasty or reperfusion therapy with thrombolytic agents (Johnson, 1994). PET tracers are also used to evaluate perfusion and will be discussed later. They include ammonia N 13, rubidium 82, and water O 15.

Tests to Evaluate Myocardial Viability

Identification of the size of an infarct has traditionally been helpful in determining prognosis. Infarct avid tracers were used. The tracers bind with elements released by necrotic myocardial tissue.

With the development of reperfusion strategies, angioplasty, bypass grafting, and thrombolytic therapy, it was noted that areas that appeared to be nonfunctional on perfusion scans regained function once the area regained adequate blood supply. Tests were developed that were able to distinguish these areas of stunned or hibernating myocardium. These tests of myocardial viability often look at metabolism.

According to Maddahi, four different PET approaches have been used for the assessment of myocardial viability: (1) perfusion-fluorodeoxyglucose (FDG) metabolism imaging; (2) determination of oxidative metabolism using acetate 11 C; (3) uptake and retention of rubidium 82; and (4) the water perfusable tissue index (Maddahi, 1994).

Fluorodeoxyglucose F 18

Fluorodeoxyglucose F 18 is a glucose analogue that crosses the capillary and sarcolemmal membrane at a rate proportional to that of glucose. It becomes trapped in the myocardium because it is not a useful substrate in metabolic pathways. FDG distribution is relative to uptake of unlabeled glucose (Maddahi, 1994).

Identification of areas with normal metabolism, altered metabolism, or no metabolism is based on the use of glucose as an energy substrate. Normally, perfused myocardial cells use fatty acids for ATP production when a person is in a fasting state, and they use glucose as the primary energy source in the postprandial state. Ischemic myocardium uses glucose in the fasting state and in the postprandial state. Infarcted areas show no metabolic activity. Therefore, increased uptake of FDG in the postprandial state occurs in both hibernating and normal myocardium, but in the fasting state, it occurs only in the hibernating myocardium. Clinical studies in infarct patients show that areas with persistent thallium 201 perfusion defects have evidence of remaining metabolic activity in 47% of regions when studied with a PET scan, indicating overestimation of irreversible injury. Use of reinjection and late-redistribution imaging has significantly lowered this number (Hendel, 1994). The implication derived from this finding is that in areas with perfusion defects, if glucose activity remains, the region is viable (mismatch pattern); conversely, if such activity is absent, the area is likely to be infarcted or necrotic (match pattern) (Niemeyer, 1992). Viewed in functional terms, mismatch simply implies the potential for improvement; match implies no potential for improvement in contractility after successful revascularization (Schelbert, 1994).

Acetate 11 C

Another way to evaluate myocardial viability is to use an isotope that is incorporated into the metabolic pathways related to myocardial oxygen consumption. Acetate 11 C, in its activated form, acetyl CoA, represents the entry point for all metabolic pathways into the tricarboxylic acid cycle, which is tightly coupled to oxidative metabolism. Its advantage over FDG F 18 is that it does not rely on substrate use (i.e., glucose vs. fat metabolism). It accurately reflects oxidative metabolism and can distinguish viable from nonviable myocardium in both acute and chronic ischemic conditions (Bergman, 1994).

Technetium 99m Pyrophosphate

Technetium 99m pyrophosphate (TcPyp) identifies areas of myocardial infarction by forming a complex with calcium, which is released when myocardial cells die. TcPyp scans have the best results when obtained 24 to 48 hours post-infarction. This time frame, obviously, occurs after reperfusion strategies would have been employed. The sensitivity of this scan is high, but its specificity is low, because a number of other processes can result in a positive scan (e.g., myocardial trauma, ventricular aneurysm, and uptake in skeletal structures) (Niemeyer, 1992).

Indium 111 Antimyosin

Indium 111 antimyosin is a radiolabeled monoclonal antibody that identifies infarcted myocardial tissue. It binds with myocardial myosin, which is released when a muscle cell dies. It can be used in conjunction with thallium 201 to distinguish infarcted tissue from perfused viable tissue. It is most reliable when performed 48 hours after infarction (Niemeyer, 1992).

NUCLEAR TESTS OF THE PULMONARY SYSTEM
Ventilation-Perfusion Lung Scan

The ventilation-perfusion lung scan is a combination of two separate imaging procedures. It is used primarily in the diagnosis of pulmonary embolism, and has limited use for other clinical problems (Lillington, 1987). The perfusion portion requires the injection of radioactive tracer. Technetium 99m macroaggregated albumin is (almost universally accepted as) the perfusion tracer of choice (Juni & Alavi, 1991). The ventilation scan requires the inhalation of radioactive gas, usually 133-XE gas or Tc 99m diethylene triamine pentaacetic acid (DTPA) aerosol. Other isotopes can be used for ventilation scanning (e.g., Kr-81M, Xenon-127), but they are more difficult to obtain (Figure 14-3).

A normal perfusion scan essentially rules out recent pulmonary embolus. If the perfusion scan is abnormal, it is compared with the ventilation scan for match or mismatch of defects. An interpretation scheme is used, such as Biello or Pioped, which classifies the probability of pulmonary embolism into normal, low, intermediate (indeterminate), or high (Juni, 1991; Miller & O'Doherty, 1992). Patients with high-probability scans should begin anticoagulation therapy (Juni, 1991). Patients with intermediate (indeterminate) scans may need to have a pulmonary angiogram before beginning treatment (Miller & O'Doherty, 1992).

Miller and O'Doherty (1992) note other applications of ventilation/perfusion scanning to include monitoring of response to radiotherapy and assessment of resectability of bullae. The scan is used to predict whether a patient can tolerate a pneumonectomy on the basis of percent flow to the opposite lung and extent of disease present.

Gallium Scintigraphy

Gallium 67 citrate concentrates in neoplastic and inflammatory lesions of the lung (Lillington, 1987). Gallium is more sensitive than normal chest radiographs in identifying infectious and noninfectious inflammatory processes. This is particularly important in identifying opportunistic infections in the immunocompromised patient. In patients with acquired immune deficiency syndrome (AIDS), the sensitivity of gallium in scanning for *Pneumocystis carinii* pneumonia approaches 94% to 96% (Kramer & Divgi, 1991). The radioisotope is injected but it is 48 to 72 hours before imaging can be performed (Miller & O'Doherty, 1992).

Gallium is commonly used in the evaluation of patients with interstitial lung disease; this includes sarcoidosis and amiodarone toxicity and is used after cytotoxic therapy using bleiomycin as well as many other entities (Miller & O'Doherty, 1992). In conjunction with neoplasms, the scan's use is limited to assessing tumor extent (Kramer & Divgi, 1991).

Positron Emission Tomography

PET scans utilizing FDG isotopes are being used to identify metabolically active tissue (glucose metabolism) in the lungs. It has found application in the differential diagnosis of pulmonary nodules, inflammation, and potential malignant lesions (Gould et al, 2001). PET with FDG is used as a diagnostic tool for pulmonary nodules and mass lesions (Gould et al, 2001). Solitary pulmonary nodules (SPN) are often found during screening tests. They are of significant concern due to the risk of malignancy. Gould and colleagues (2001) performed a metaanalysis and concluded that sensitivity is 96.8% and specificity is 77.8% for detecting malignancy in SPNs. PET-FDG is not recommended for nodules smaller than 1 cm (Tan et al, 2003). In addition to the difficulty in accessing PET scanners, cost may also limit their application, as PET-FDG can cost six times more than conventional CT scans of the chest, based on Medicare reimbursement (Tan et al, 2003).

ANGIOGRAPHY

Angiography is the radiographic examination of the arterial system using an opaque contrast dye that is injected into the arterial segment to characterize flow. Angiography requires an x-ray-generator tube and an image intensifier/cine camera (Reagan et al, 1994). The radiopaque dye is injected into the vascular supply of the region of interest. Radiographic images can then monitor the contrast material as it moves through the circulation. The development of coronary angiography via cardiac catheterization techniques allowed for the development of many of the catheter-based interventions used today (Ryan, 2002).

Cardiac

The gold standard with which many of the cardiac noninvasive tests are compared is that of cardiac catheterization. It is an

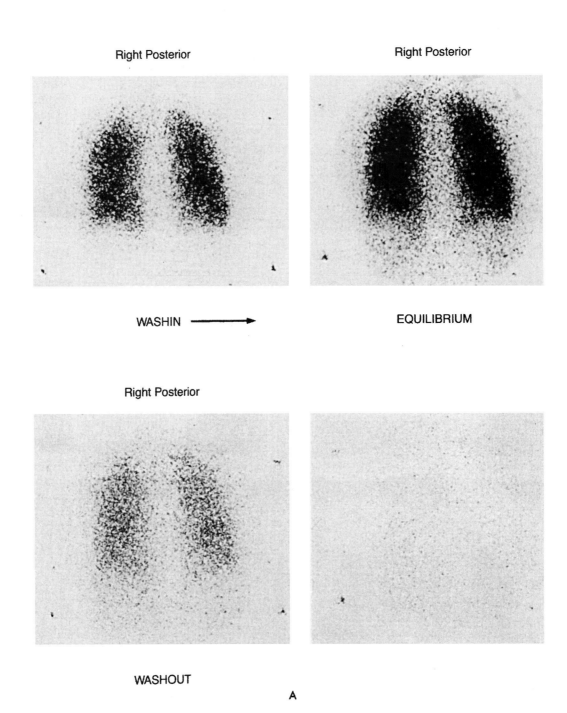

FIGURE 14-3 The value of ventilation/perfusion lung scans in the diagnosis of thromboembolism. A xenon inhalation lung scan (**A**) discloses normal ventilation parameters during the washin, equilibrium, and washout phases. *Continued*

Anterior

Posterior

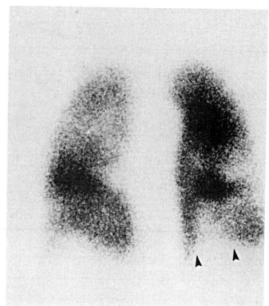

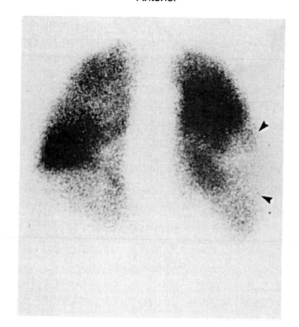

Right Posterior Oblique

Left Posterior Oblique

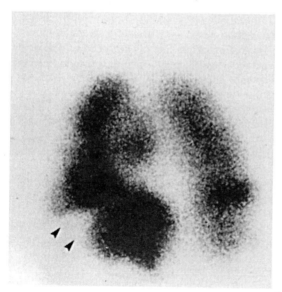

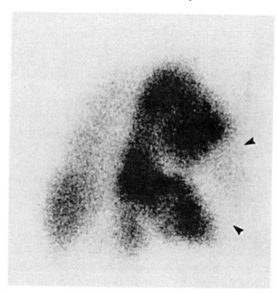

B

FIGURE 14-3 cont'd   Corresponding technetium 99m-labeled macroaggregated albumin perfusion lung scans (**B**) in anterior, posterior, and right and left posterior oblique projections identify multiple segmental filling defects throughout both lungs (*arrowheads*). These findings, in concert with the ventilation study are virtually diagnostic (high probability) of pulmonary thromboembolism. The patient was a 65-year-old man with acute dyspnea. (*From Fraser, R.S., Paré, P.D., Coman N., & Muller, N.L. [1999]. Diagnosis of diseases of the chest, ed 4. Philadelphia: WB Saunders.*)

invasive test with a small but serious risk to the patient. Complications include death, stroke, myocardial infarction (MI), bleeding, arterial trauma or thrombus, renal dysfunction, and arrhythmias (Reagan et al, 1994). The test is indicated in patients with a high risk of atherosclerotic heart disease whose stress perfusion scans are positive. Patients with diagnosed CAD with angina that is unresponsive to medical therapy may also require catheterization.

The procedure for cardiac catheterization of the left side of the heart requires the threading of a catheter, guided by fluoroscopy, through the femoral artery or brachial artery to the aorta. Direct measurements of chamber pressures, blood flow, and oxygen saturation can be obtained. When selective coronary arteriography is performed, radiopaque contrast material is injected from the catheter into the left main or right coronary artery. Cine recordings are made after the injection, and injections are repeated until the entire coronary tree is visualized. The location of an arterial obstruction can be identified as can the percentage of blockage (stenosis) (Figure 14-4).

More recently, it has been possible to obtain additional physiologic measures that provide flow and pressure data at the site of the lesion within the coronary artery (Kern, 2000). These measures have become particularly important for monitoring outcomes after the administration of reperfusion therapy (e.g., thrombolytics, angioplasty, stenting) (Gibson et al, 2002; Kern et al, 1996). Coronary artery flow grades (such as thrombolysis in myocardial infarction [TIMI] grades 0 to 3) are based on the visual analysis of the rate of opacification of the artery of interest, typically 90 minutes postintervention (Kern et al, 1996). TIMI myocardial perfusion grades (TMPG 0-3), or myocardial blush, grade the reperfusion of the myocardium by the contrast medium (Gibson et al, 2002). Higher TIMI and TMPG grades have been associated with reduced mortality over 2 years (Gibson et al, 2002).

Cardiac ventriculography is a procedure in which dye is injected into the ventricle, and the entire chamber becomes outlined. Several cardiac cycles are recorded on cine. It provides valuable information about global and segmental wall motion, valve motion, and the presence of abnormal anatomy (Grossman, 1986).

Pulmonary

The diagnosis of pulmonary embolism is the primary indication for pulmonary angiography. It is the gold standard against which ventilation-perfusion scans are compared (Juni, 1992). Contrast dye is injected into the pulmonary circulation through the pulmonary artery. Additional techniques such as balloon occlusion, segmental injections, or increased magnification improve the sensitivity of the test (Lillington, 1987). Interobserver reliability studies performed on the interpretation of pulmonary angiograms are 83% to 86% (Juni, 1992).

ECHOCARDIOGRAPHY

Another noninvasive method of evaluating the heart uses the physical properties of sound. Echocardiography provides information about the blood flow, structure, and function of the heart. Motion mode (M-mode) and two-dimensional (2-D) images are highly reliable methods of evaluation. Recent developments of technique and technology include color-flow Doppler echo, transesophageal echo, and intravascular echocardiography. These techniques, when used in combination, can provide much of the information previously available only by cardiac catheterization (Hartnell, 1994).

Physics of Echocardiography

Imaging systems that use ultrasound require a source for generation of the sound wave, a transducer, and a receiver to pick up the reflected sound waves. Sound is absorbed or reflected differentially by specific tissues. Therefore, the sound wave reflected from muscle differs from that reflected from vascular space or valvular structures. Returning signals are converted into electrical signals that generate an image. This is the basis for M-mode and 2-D echo. In M-mode echocardiography, the transducer transmits a single sound wave through the chest wall (transthoracic echocardiography, or TTE). A thin slice of the heart, an "ice-pick" view, directly under the sound wave, reflects the wave back to the transducer. M-mode, though useful, is rarely used; 2-D is the primary diagnostic mode. In 2-D echocardiography, the transducer is able to pick up a wedge section of the heart. In 2-D the transducer acts as the transmitter and receiver. A real-time 2-D picture of the heart is recorded on videotape. The heart can be viewed in motion, and wall motion can be evaluated (Figure 14-5).

Doppler Echocardiography

Doppler echocardiography relies on the Doppler effect to determine velocity. When a sound wave is aimed at moving objects such as red blood cells, the known frequency transmitted from the soundhead and the reflected frequency differ, a phenomenon known as a frequency shift. The greater the frequency shift, the greater the speed of the targeted object (Waggoner & Perez, 1990). *Velocity of flow* is the term used to express Doppler frequency shifts. Both continuous-wave and pulsed-wave Doppler formats are used.

Color-flow Doppler echocardiography was introduced in the mid-1980s. It is usually superimposed on a 2-D image in real time but can also be used with M-mode. It is a method that displays anatomic and spatial blood flow velocity estimates with indication of flow direction in real time (Waggoner, 1990). Color is matched on the basis of the direction of flow, and shading is indicative of intensity based on the mean velocity flow estimates (Waggoner & Perez, 1990). It is used primarily to assess the extent of regurgitant jets across "leaky valves," as well as to indicate areas of abnormal shunts such

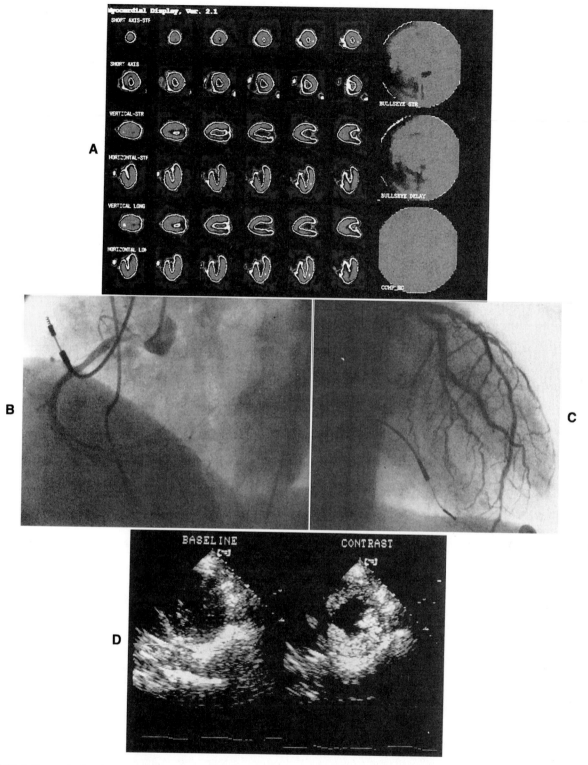

FIGURE 14-4 Stress single-photon emission computed tomography reoriented and polar plot images. **A,** Right coronary artery arteriogram; **B,** left anterior descending coronary artery arteriogram; **C,** circumflex coronary arteriogram; and the short-axis two-dimensional echocardiographic images (**D**) at baseline (*left*) and after contrast injection down the LAD coronary artery (*right*). Although this patient had a normal dobutamine thallium-201 SPECT with no discernible perfusion defect after comparison to the normal databank (*COMPSC*) (**A**), the right coronary artery is noted to have a subtotal ostial stenosis (**B**). No collaterals are observed to the right coronary artery after left main contrast injection (**C**). However, on echocardiography (**D**), intense contrast enhancement is noted in the inferior wall after injection of sonicated microbubbles down the LAD, verifying the presence of coronary collaterals to the right coronary artery. Despite a severe right coronary artery stenosis, this patient did not develop a stress perfusion defect because of the well-developed collateral circulation, which was apparent on echocardiography but not arteriography. *(From Malunarian, J.J. [1999]. State of the art for CAD detection: thallium 201. In Zarit, B.L. & Beller, G.A. [Eds]. Nuclear cardiology, ed 2. St. Louis: CV Mosby.)*

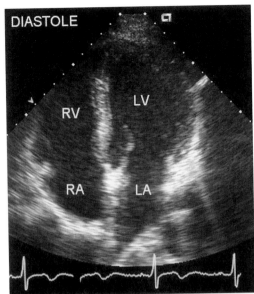

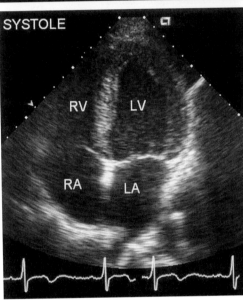

FIGURE 14-5 Normal 2-D echo images at end-diastole (*above*) and end-systole (*below*). (*From Otto, C.M. [2000]. Textbook of clinical echocardiography, ed 2. Philadelphia: WB Saunders.*)

as atrial septal defects. Turbulence created by narrowed valves creates wide color shading.

Measurements Derived from Echocardiography

Echocardiographic results can be viewed qualitatively and quantitatively. An experienced viewer can analyze the anatomic relationships and structure of the heart and the wall motion, valve movement and configuration, and chamber size.

Quantitative measures are calculated from the Doppler frequency shifts. Velocity measures can be used in other equations to estimate pressure and valve area. The modified Bernoulli equation is used to calculate pressure changes around the valve:

$$\Delta P \text{ (mm Hg)} = 4 \times V_{max}^2 \text{ (m/sec)},$$

where P is the pressure gradient across the valve and V is the velocity of blood flow through the valve.

These measurements allow the calculation of stenotic valve gradients and right-sided filling pressures, valve regurgitation, and ventricular septal defects (Waggoner & Perez, 1990). Valve regurgitation and shunt calculations are more complicated than the Bernoulli equation alone.

Another important quantitative measure is the estimated area of the valve. The continuity equation is used to estimate valve area. It is based on the principle of conservation of mass (i.e., in a normal heart, the volume of blood that enters the right atrium should be conserved as it passes through the other chambers). Flow volume at different sites is related to the flow velocity and the cross-sectional area of the site. Therefore,

$$A_1 \times V_1 = A_2 \times V_2,$$

where V_1 is the velocity of flow at one side of the valve, V_2 is the flow velocity at the other side of the valve, and A is the cross-sectional area (Waggoner & Perez, 1990; Wilson & Vacek, 1990).

Exercise Studies

Exercise echocardiography can be done with physiologic stress (treadmill or bicycle exercise) or with pharmacologic stress (dipyridamole, adenosine, or dobutamine). Pharmacologic stress offers the advantage of the patient's being in a stable position throughout the test. Under physiologic stress conditions, the bicycle test, in the upright or supine position, is preferred because imaging cannot be performed during a treadmill test (Armstrong & Griffin, 2000).

Transesophageal Echocardiography

Because of consistent technical difficulties with transthoracic echocardiography (TTE), the technique of transesophageal echo (TEE) was developed to improve spatial resolution. TEE can obtain M-mode, 2-D, and color-flow Doppler images by using a small probe mounted on the tip of a modified gastroscope. The probe can be advanced into the esophagus and even into the stomach and positioned so that multiple views of the heart are available (Kerber, 1988). Initially, the technique was performed intraoperatively on anesthetized patients and on intubated patients in the intensive care unit. It is now used on patients who are awake but mildly sedated (Schneider, 1993). TEE is commonly used for diagnosis of valve function and congenital heart disease and for the determination of thromboembolic risk. It has become an important monitoring tool during cardiac catheterization procedures and surgery (Peterson et al, 2003).

TEE is used to assess cardiac valve function as well as to monitor treatment. It is able to visualize the mitral and tricuspid valves more clearly than TTE. It is used to monitor prosthetic valve function, as well as to diagnose and monitor infective endocarditis, particularly the status of valve vegetation. TEE provides superior visualization (compared with TTE) of the left atrium and left atrial appendage, which is often the source of thrombi causing transient ischemic attack (TIA) or stroke. TEE Doppler studies can examine left atrial flow velocities, which also indicate increased stroke risk. They have been used successfully to decrease morbidity in patients with atrial fibrillation undergoing cardioversion by reducing hemorrhagic events (Klein et al, 2001).

Myocardial Contrast Echocardiography

The ability of echocardiography to evaluate myocardial perfusion was historically based on observation of wall-motion abnormalities. The development of a contrast agent that can be used with echo techniques has ushered in noninvasive techniques that do not rely on radioactive agents (see Figure 14-3). Microbubbles of air encapsulated in a thin shell are introduced by intravenous infusion or bolus injection into the venous system as the contrast agent (Rocchi et al, 2003). These small bubbles (< 6 to 10 μm) oscillate when exposed to ultrasound energy and produce harmonic signals (a multiple of the ultrasound frequency) that are then used to produce the images (Mulvagh, 2000).

COMPUTED TOMOGRAPHY

Computed tomography (CT) was first developed in the 1970s; it allows the visualization of cross-sectional views of body organs as compared to the planar views of standard radiographs (Fraser, 1999). Technologic developments allowing such rapid scan times that a CT of the respiratory system can be completed in a single breath-hold have resulted in scans of improved spatial resolution and diagnostic utility (Bakal, 2003). Electron beam CT has found application in the examination of the cardiac system and is currently used as part of risk stratification tests in asymptomatic patients (O'Rourke, 2003).

Physics of Computed Tomography

A computed tomographic scan (CT scan) acquires images of a fixed thickness, a cross-sectional slice, that allows examination of a specific part of the body. CT scanners utilize an x-ray source, collimators, x-ray detectors, and computers to reconstruct the cross-sectional images from the acquired data (Fraser, 1999). The x-ray source rotates around the patient; its speed dictates how long it takes to acquire a single slice— about 1 second. The slice thickness and the space between slices determine the quality of the spatial resolution of the images. The spatial resolution required is determined by the type of tissue being examined and the suspected diagnosis. Imaging can be done with a single-detector or a newer multiple-detector row scanner (4, 8, or 16 rows) (Nikolaou, 2003). Multidetector CT scanners (MDCT) allow for faster acquisition of images. Spiral CT scanners simultaneously rotate the source and move the table and patient for continuous data acquisition and improved resolution (Dawn, 2001). The most rapid scanning times are achieved by electron beam computed tomography (EBCT), also called ultrafast CT. EBCT uses an electron gun to generate x-rays to a fixed tungsten "target" (O'Rourke, 2000). The electron beam is electronically moved rather than mechanically rotated; that results in images that can be made in milliseconds. Their cost and a limited number of available EBCT scanners limit their routine use (Nikolaou, 2003).

Cardiac

EBCT is currently utilized to identify calcium in atherosclerotic plaques within the coronary arteries, primarily as a screening test in asymptomatic individuals and as a diagnostic test in symptomatic individuals (O'Rourke, 2000). A scoring system developed to quantify the amount of calcium in the coronary arteries is used to identify the future risk of cardiac events (O'Rourke, 2000). Scores are based on Housenfeld units, which are based on the tissue attenuation factor. In general, the greater the amount of calcium detected, the greater the amount of atherosclerotic plaque in the coronary arteries. A limitation of EBCT is that it cannot localize the plaque anatomically. Sensitivity and specificity for EBCT for CAD are 91% and 49%, respectively (O'Rourke, 2000). Research is currently being carried out to determine whether EBCT tests add valuable data to cardiac risk assessment (Kondos, 2003). In a sample of nearly 9000 asymptomatic low- to intermediate-risk middle-aged adults, the relative risk of a cardiac event significantly increased at higher quartiles of calcium scores (Kondos, 2003).

Pulmonary

Compared with the standard radiographs, CT is not commonly used in the initial diagnosis of pulmonary disease. The CT scan has been found to be a useful first-line diagnostic tool in the evaluation of mediastinal disease, including mediastinal masses, staging of mediastinal cancers, and identification of cysts (Lillington, 1987).

High-resolution computed tomography (HRCT) has improved the documentation of morphologic changes associated with chronic airflow obstruction. Webb's (1994) review of the application of this new technology identified the utility of this test in various obstructive diseases. HRCT is sensitive in the diagnosis of early emphysema, although it is rarely used clinically. In cystic disease, such as histiocytosis X and lymphangiomyomatosis, HRCT is able to reveal cysts less than 10 mm in diameter as well as indicate wall thickness.

In the diagnosis of bronchiectasis, HRCT demonstrates a high specificity (Figure 14-6). It is the procedure of choice after plain chest radiographs. HRCT can discriminate among the three different types of abnormal bronchi seen in bronchiectasis (cylindrical, varicose, and cystic) but again, there is little clinical significance (Webb, 1994). It can be used to differentiate lymphangitic spread of cancer versus heart

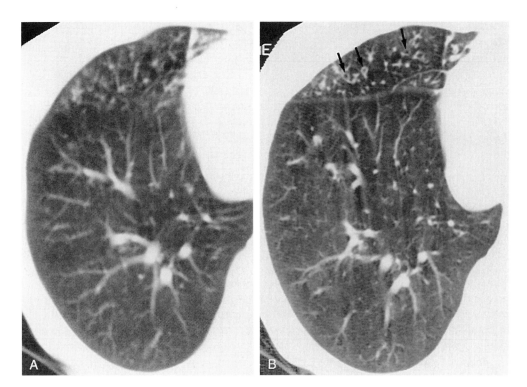

FIGURE 14-6 HRCT versus conventional CT for bronchiectasis. A conventional 10-mm-collimation CT scan (**A**) in a 65-year-old woman demonstrates small focal areas of ground-glass attenuation and consolidation in the right middle lobe. An HRCT scan (1.5 mm collimation) (**B**) performed immediately after the conventional CT scan demonstrates right middle lobe bronchiectasis (*arrows*). *(From Fraser, R.S., Paré, P.D., Coman, N., & Muller, N.L. [1999]. Diagnosis of diseases of the chest, ed 4. Philadelphia: WB Saunders.)*

failure when the distinction is unclear clinically. HRCT also can be used to evaluate the clearing of persistent pneumonias. Overall, HRCT has helped to clarify disease morphology, but the clinical significance for diagnosis and for a patient's pulmonary function is less clear.

Spiral CT with and without a contrast agent has been found beneficial in the diagnosis of acute pulmonary embolism (Powell, 2003). With a sensitivity and specificity of 90% it may rival the more widely used ventilation-perfusion scan to identify pulmonary embolism. In combination with a V/Q scan, a pulmonary embolism can more reliably be ruled out (Powell, 2003).

MAGNETIC RESONANCE IMAGING

Technically, the technology of magnetic resonance imaging (MRI), adopted clinically in the 1970s, uses nuclear magnetic resonance to build tissue images (i.e., nuclei are made to resonate in a magnetic field) (Forder & Pohost, 2003). However, because MRI is a technique that does not use radiopharmaceuticals or ionizing radiation, it was thought to be less confusing if the word *nuclear* were left out of the name. In addition to being noninvasive, no exposure to radiation is involved. With the development of ultrafast imaging, MRI has found use in the examination of the cardiovascular and pulmonary systems.

Physics of Magnetic Resonance Imaging

MRI relies on the creation of a stable, powerful magnetic field that causes hydrogen (also carbon-13, fluorine-19, and sodium-23) nuclei to align with the field. A radio frequency pulse specific to the hydrogen (or other) nuclei causes the nuclei to resonate (Forder & Pohost, 2003; Gould, 2004). Additional magnets that apply magnetic fields of differing gradients are used to locate the image. When the radio frequency is turned off, the nuclei release the stored energy. This energy is analyzed via Fourier transformation, which results in the image. The images are highly dependent on the timing and magnitude of the radiofrequency (Mayo, 1994). Data acquisition can take 20 to 90 minutes, during which time the patient must remain immobile. The application of MRI to the cardiac and pulmonary system was initially limited by the continuous movement of the heart and lungs, but the development of ultrafast imaging has overcome some of these problems (Gast et al, 2003). Contrast materials such as gadolinium diethylenetriamine pentaacetic acid (Gd-DTPA) can be used to enhance signal intensity.

Cardiac

MRI is a useful technique in evaluating cardiac structures. It can identify cardiac masses and is the modality of choice for evaluating the pericardium. MRI is secondary to CT in evaluating the mediastinum, especially constrictive pericarditis (Mayo, 1994). Analysis of cardiac images also allows the measurement of right and left ventricular volumes, ejection fraction, and cardiac output (Forder & Pohost, 2003).

Tests to Evaluate Myocardial Perfusion

Contrast agents such as Gd-DPTA can be used in stress MRI studies to examine perfusion defects in the myocardium (Nikolaou, 2003). Cardiac MRI is able to characterize blood flow as well as uptake and washout of the contrast agent. Different from other modalities, cardiac MRI can distinguish tissue layers, enabling identification of areas of subendocardial or transmural defects (Nikolaou, 2003).

Tests to Evaluate Myocardial Viability

The viability of cardiac tissue can be examined with MRI, using delayed-contrast enhancement Gd-DTPA as the contrast agent (Forder & Pohost, 2003). Images are taken 10 minutes after the intravenous administration of the agent. An inversion time pulse sequence allows the normal myocardial tissue to fade and the infarcted or scar tissue to be enhanced.

Pulmonary

Evaluation of the lung parenchyma presents unique problems because of respiratory movement, low proton density, and the air-tissue interface (Gast et al, 2003). The development of ultrafast imaging pulse sequences called dynamic MRI has improved the utility of this noninvasive test for evaluation of the pulmonary system. Contrast agents such as Gd-DTPA are used to perform MR angiography to diagnose pulmonary emboli (Meaney et al, 1997). The utilization of MRI to provide noninvasive evaluation of pulmonary emboli has application in special cases in which typical tests are inconclusive (Meaney et al, 1997). Without contrast, dynamic MRI is being used to study the biomechanical function of the diaphragm and chest wall in patients with and without pulmonary disease. These studies are important for patients undergoing lung volume reduction surgery (Suga et al, 2000).

The use of gaseous contrast agents such as hyperpolarized helium-3 (HHe-3), with dynamic MRI and lung motion correction, is a promising new development that allows examination of gas distribution in the lungs (Gast et al, 2003; Samee et al, 2003). These studies have shown that dynamic MRI with HHe-3 contrast can discriminate healthy lung grafts from native diseased lung in transplant patients (Gast et al, 2003) and can identify ventilation defects that correlate with decreased FEV_1 in patients with asthma (Samee et al, 2003).

BRONCHOSCOPY

Bronchoscopy is often used both as a diagnostic tool and as a therapeutic treatment modality (Mars & Ciesla, 1993). It allows direct visualization of the trachea and its major subdivisions.

Fiberoptic bronchoscopy has virtually replaced bronchography (Lillington, 1987). In fiberoptic bronchoscopy, a flexible tube is inserted into the trachea of mildly sedated patients. This tube is able to enter small brochial subdivisions. Secretions can be removed for evaluation or as a treatment. It is also possible to obtain biopsy samples by using tiny forceps or cell brushings. Bronchoscopy is particularly important in the diagnosis of bronchogenic carcinoma (Price & Wilson, 1986).

SUMMARY

Many tests are available to identify cardiopulmonary dysfunction. The attending physician determines which tests are appropriate for the patient's particular medical condition. When the tests are completed, results are given, and an evaluation of the results is documented. Physical therapists should understand the results of the tests and how they will apply to a patient's function and response to exercise. This understanding applies to the selection of exercises and workloads the physical therapist prescribes for the patient. Until a physical therapist reaches a certain maturity level, as well as a level of understanding and application of the test results to patient treatment, it is highly encouraged that the physical therapist discuss the tests and their results with the patient's physician. These discussions are excellent opportunities for learning, both for the physical therapist and for the physician, who can gain a better appreciation of what physical therapy has to offer a patient with cardiopulmonary dysfunction.

Review Questions

1. Why is the ejection fraction an important measure of myocardial function?
2. What is the difference between stunned myocardium and hibernating myocardium?
3. How does EBCT identify CAD risk?
4. Which tests can be used to evaluate myocardial viability?
5. Which test provides the best anatomic information?

REFERENCES

Armstrong, G.P., Griffin, B.P. (2000). Exercise echocardiographic assessment in severe mitral regurgitation. Coronary Artery Disease 11:23-30.
Bakal, C.W. (2003). Advances in imaging technology and the growth of vascular and interventional radiology: a brief history. Journal of Vascular and Interventional Radiology 14:855-860.
Beller, G. (1994). Myocardial perfusion imaging with thallium-201. Journal of Nuclear Medicine 35:674-680.
Beller, G. (1995). Clinical nuclear cardiology. Philadelphia: WB Saunders.
Bergman, S. (1994). Use and limitations of metabolic tracers labeled with positron-emitting radionuclides in the identification of viable myocardium. Journal of Nuclear Medicine 35(Suppl 4): 15S-22S.

Berman, D., Hosen, S., Van Train, K., Germano, G., Maddahi, J., & Friedman, J. (1994). Myocardial perfusion imaging with technitium-99M-sestamibi: comparative analysis of available imaging protocols. Journal of Nuclear Medicine 35:681-688.

Berman, D., Kiat, H., Van Train, K., Garcia, E., Friedman, J., & Maddahi, J. (1991). Technetium 99m sestamibi in the assessment of chronic coronary artery disease. Seminars in Nuclear Medicine 21:190-212.

Brown, K. (1994). The role of stress redistribution thallium-201 myocardial perfusion imaging in evaluating coronary artery disease and perioperative risk. Journal of Nuclear Medicine 35:703-706.

Dawn, S.K., Gotway, M.B., & Webb, W.R. (2001). Multidetector-row spiral computed tomography in the diagnosis of thoracic diseases. Respiratory Care 46:912-921.

Dyer, G.S.M., & Tifer, M.A. (2003). Heart Failure. In Lilly, L.S. (Ed). Pathophysiology of heart disease, ed 3. Philadelphia: Lippincott Williams & Wilkins.

Forder, J.R., & Pohost, G.M. (2003). Cardiovascular nuclear magnetic resonance: basic and clinical applications. Journal of Clinical Investigation 111:1630-1639.

Fraser, R.S., Paré, P.D., Coman N., & Muller, N.L. (1999) Diagnosis of diseases of the chest, ed 4. Philadelphia: WB Saunders.

Gast, K.K., Puderbach, M.U., Rodriguez, I., Eberle, B., Markstaller, K., Knitz, F., Schmiedeskamp, J., Weiler, N., Schreiber, W.G., Mayer, E., Thelen, M., & Kauczor, H.U. (2003). Distribution of ventilation in lung transplant recipients: evaluation by dynamic ^{3}He-MRI with lung motion correction. Investigative Radiology 38:341-348.

Gibson, C.M., Cannon, C.P., Murphy, S.A., Marble, S.J., Barron, H.V., & Braunwald, E., TIMI Study Group. (2002). Relationship of the TIMI myocardial perfusion grades, flow grades, frame count, and percutaneous coronary intervention to long-term outcomes after thrombolytic administration in acute myocardial infarction. Circulation 105:1909-1913.

Go, R.T., MacIntyre, W.J., Cook, S.A., & Neumann, D.R. (1992). Myocardial perfusion imaging in the diagnosis of coronary artery disease. Current Opinion in Radiology 4:23-33.

Gould, M.K., Maclean, C.C., Kuschner W.G., Rydzak, C.E., & Owens, D.K. (2001). Accuracy of positron emission tomography for diagnosis of pulmonary nodules and mass lesions. Journal of the American Medical Association 285:914-924.

Gould, T.A. How MRI works. www.howstuffworks.com; retrieved August 19, 2004.

Grossman, W. (1986). Cardiac catheterization and angiography, ed 3. Philadelphia: Lea & Febiger.

Hartnell, G. (1994). Developments in echocardiography. Radiologic Clinics of North America 32:461-475.

Hendel, R. (1994). Single-photon imaging for the assessment of myocardial viability. Journal of Nuclear Medicine 35(Suppl 4): 23S-31S.

Iskandrian, A.S. (1987). Nuclear cardiac imaging: principles and applications. Philadelphia: FA Davis.

Jessup, M., Brozena, S. (2003). Heart failure. New England Journal of Medicine 348:2007-2018.

Johnson, L. (1994.) Myocardial perfusion imaging with technetium-99m-teboroxime. Journal of Nuclear Medicine 35:689-692.

Juni, J., & Alavi, A. (1991). Lung scanning in the diagnosis of pulmonary embolism: the emperor redressed. Seminars in Nuclear Medicine 21:281-296.

Kerber, R. (Ed). (1988). Echocardiography in coronary artery disease. Mount Kisco, NY: Futura Publishing.

Kern, M.J. (2000). Coronary physiology revisited: practical insights from the cardiac catheterization laboratory. Circulation 101:1344-1351.

Kim, E. (1987). Nuclear diagnostic imaging: practical clinical applications. New York: Macmillan.

Kinch, J., & Ryan, T. (1994). Right ventricular infarction. New England Journal of Medicine 330:1211-1215.

Klein, A.L., Grimm, R.A., Murray, R.D., Apperson-Hansen, C., Asinger, R.W., Black, I.W., Davidoff, R., Erbel, R., Halperin, J.L., Orsinelli, D.A., Porter, T.R., Stoddard, M.F., & Assessment of Cardioversion Using Transesophageal Echocardiography Investigators. (2001). Use of transesophageal echocardiography to guide cardioversion in patients with atrial fibrillation. New England Journal of Medicine 344:1411-1420.

Kondos, G.T., Hoff, J.A., Serukov, A., Daviglus, M.L., Garside, D.B., Devries, S.S., Chomka, E.V., & Erbel, R. (2003). Electron-beam tomography coronary artery calcium and cardiac events. Circulation 107:2571-2576.

Kramer, E., & Divgi, C. (1991). Pulmonary applications of nuclear medicine. Clinics in Chest Medicine 12:55-75.

Liao, T., & Park, K.W. (2001). Noninvasive tests of myocardial perfusion: stress tests and their values. International Anesthesiology Clinic 39:1-10.

Lillington, G. (1987). A diagnostic approach to chest disease. Baltimore: Williams and Wilkins.

Maass-Moreno, R., & Bachrach, S.L. (2003). Imaging instrumentation. In Iskandrian, A.E., & Verani, M.S., (Eds). Nuclear cardiac imaging, ed 3. Oxford, UK: Oxford University Press.

Maddahi, J., Schelbert, H., Brunken, R., & DiCarli, M. (1994). Role of thallium-201 and PET imaging in evaluation of myocardial viability and management of patients with coronary artery disease and left ventricular dysfunction. Journal of Nuclear Medicine 35:707-715.

Mars, M., & Ciesla, N. (1993). Chest physical therapy may have prevented bronchoscopy and exploratory laparatomy: a case report. Cardiopulmonary Physical Therapy Journal 4:4-6.

Mayo, J. (1994). Magnetic resonance imaging of the chest. Advances in Chest Radiology 32:795-809.

Meaney, J.F., Weg, J.G., Chenevert, T.L., Stafford-Johnson, D., Hamiliton, B.H., & Prince, M.R. (1997). Diagnosis of pulmonary embolism with magnetic resonance angiography. New England Journal of Medicine 336:1422-1427.

Miller, R.F., & O'Doherty, M.J. (1992). Pulmonary nuclear medicine. European Journal of Nuclear Medicine 19:355-368.

Mullani, N.A., & Volkow, N.D. (1992). Positron emission tomography instrumentation: a review and update. American Journal of Physiologic Imaging 3/4:121-135.

Mulvagh, S.L. (2000). Myocardial perfusion by contrast echo-cardiography: diagnosis of coronary artery disease using contrast-enhanced stress echocardiography and assessment of coronary anatomy and flow reserve. Coronary Artery Disease 11:243-251.

Murphy, P.H. (2003). Radiation physics and radiation safety. In Iskandrian, A.E., & Verani, M.S. (Eds). Nuclear cardiac imaging, ed 3. Oxford, UK: Oxford University Press.

Nikolaou, K., Poon, M., Sirol, M., Becker, C.R., & Fayad, Z.A. (2003). Complementary results of computed tomography and magnetic resonance imaging of the heart and coronary arteries: a review and future outlook. Cardiology Clinics 21:639-655.

Niemeyer, M.G., Van der Wall, E.E., Pauwels, E.K.J., van Dijkman, P.R.M., Blokland, J.A.K., deRoos, A., & Bruschke, A.V.G. (1992). Assessment of acute myocardial infarction by nuclear imaging techniques. Angiology 43:720-733.

O'Rourke, R.A., Brundage, B.H., Froelicher, V.F., Greenland, P., Grundy, S.M., Hachamovitch, R., Pohost, G.M., Shaw, L.J., Weintraub, W.S., Winters, W.L., Jr., Forrester, J.S., Douglas, P.S., Faxon, D.P., Fisher, J.D., Gregoratos, G., Hochman, J.S., Hutter, A.M. Jr., Kaul, S., & Wolk, M.J. (2000). American College of Cardiology/American Heart Association expert consensus document on electron-beam computed tomography for the diagnosis and prognosis of coronary artery disease. Journal of the American College of Cardiology 36:326-340.

Otto, C.M. (2000). Textbook of clinical echocardiography. Philadelphia: WB Saunders.

Peterson, G.E., Brickner E., & Reimold S.C. (2003). Transesophageal echocardiography. Circulation 107:2398-2402.

Port, S. (1994). The role of radionuclide ventriculography in the assessment of prognosis in patients with CAD. Journal of Nuclear Medicine 35:721-725.

Powell, T., & Muller, N.L. (2003). Imaging of acute pulmonary thromboembolism: should spiral computed tomography replace the ventilation-perfusion scan? Clinical in Chest Medicine 24:29-38.

Price, S., & Wilson, L. (1986). Pathophysiology: clinical concepts of disease processes. New York: McGraw-Hill.

Reagan, K., Boxt, L., & Katz, J. (1994). Introduction to coronary arteriography. Radiologic Clinics of North America 32:419-433.

Rocchi G., Fallani, F., Bracchetti, G., Rapezzi, C., Ferlito, M., & Levorato, M. (2003). Noninvasive detection of coronary artery stenosis: a comparison among power-Doppler contrast echo, ^{99}Tc-Sestamibi SPECT and echo wall-motion analysis. Coronary Artery Disease 14:239-245.

Ryan, T.J. (2002). The coronary angiogram and its seminal contributions to cardiovascular medicine over five decades. Circulation 106:752-756.

Samee, S., Altes, T., Powers P., de Lange, E.E., Knight-Scott, J., Rakes, G., Mugler, J.P. 3rd, Ciambotti, J.M., Alford, B.A., Rookeman, J.R., & Platts-Mills, T.A. (2003). Imaging the lungs in asthmatic patients by using hyperpolarized helium-3 magnetic resonance: assessment of response to methacholine and exercise challenge. Journal of Allergy and Clinical Immunology 111:1205-1211.

Schelbert, H. (1994). Metabolic imaging to assess myocardial viability. Journal of Nuclear Medicine 35(Suppl 4):8S-14S.

Schneider, A., Hsu, T., Schwartz, S., & Pandian, N. (1993). Single, biplane, multiplane, and three-dimensional transesophageal echocardiography. Cardiology Clinics 11:361-387.

Schwaiger, M. (1994). Myocardial perfusion imaging with PET. Journal of Nuclear Medicine 35:693-698.

Suga, K., Tsukuda T., Awaya, H., Matsunaga, N., Sugi, K., & Esato, K. (2000). Interactions of regional respiratory mechanics and pulmonary ventilatory impairment in pulmonary emphysema: assessment with dynamic MRI and xenon-133 single-photon emission CT. Chest 117:1646-1655.

Tan, B.B., Flaherty, K.R., Kazerooni, E.A., Iannettoni, M.D. (2003). The solitary pulmonary nodule. Chest 123:89S-96S.

Wackers, F.J.T. (1994). Radionuclide evaluation of coronary artery disease in the 1990's. Cardiology Clinics 12:385-389.

Waggoner, A.D., & Perez, J. (1990). Principles and physics of Doppler. Cardiology Clinics 12:385-389.

Watson, D.D. (2003). Acquisition, processing, and quantification of nuclear cardiac images. In Iskandrian, A.E., & Verani, M.S. (Eds). Nuclear cardiac imaging, ed 3. Oxford, UK: Oxford University Press.

Williams, K.A., Borer, J.S., & Supino, D. (2003). Radio nuclide angiography. In Iskandrian, A.E., & Verani, M.S. (Eds). Nuclear cardiac imaging, ed 3. Oxford, UK: Oxford University Press.

Webb, W.R. (1994). High-resolution computed tomography of obstructive lung disease. Radiologic Clinics of North America 32:745-757.

Wilson, D., & Vacek, J. (1990). Echocardiography. Postgraduate Medicine 87:191-202.

CHAPTER 15

Clinical Assessment of the Cardiopulmonary System

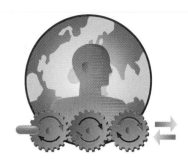

Susan M. Butler McNamara

KEY TERMS

Barrel chest
Bronchophony
Crackles
Cyanosis
Dyspnea
Egophony
Fremitus

Hyperresonant
Resonant
Rhonchi
Tachypnea
Wheeze
Whispered pectoriloquy

The background needed to perform a thorough assessment of a patient with a cardiopulmonary diagnosis is provided by the first element of the patient management model in *The Guide to Physical Therapist Practice: Examination*. The components of examination that are to be covered are history, system review (emphasis on cardiopulmonary), and the tests and measures used in the evaluation of this patient population.

This information allows the physical therapist to have a baseline against which to compare subsequent reassessments, which may occur daily. Any progress or deterioration in status can be easily identified and appropriate changes made in the treatment interventions.

HISTORY: CHART REVIEW AND PATIENT INTERVIEW

The first component in the examination is getting a history. It can be done indirectly, through the medical chart, or directly, by interviewing the patient. In the inpatient setting, a chart review is the first point of contact, whereas in the outpatient population, the only information may be what is obtainable from the patient. Time management is an ever-present issue in today's era of cost containment and health care reform, so a

medical chart review should be conducted in an organized fashion. Most physical therapists develop their own methods.

One strategy for reviewing charts is to use the following sequence:

1. Read the history and the physical and admission medical notes (i.e., the preadmission symptoms).
2. Read the last medical note.
3. *Scan* the remainder of the chart.
4. Read any reports from medical specialists and consultants, such as pulmonologists, neurologists, or oncologists.
5. Review any pertinent lab tests, such as chest radiograph, arterial blood gases (ABGs), complete blood count (CBC).
6. Review medications, in particular, pulmonary and cardiac drugs.
7. Review any procedures performed (e.g., surgery, intubation).
8. Review the psychosocial information (e.g., family, architectural barriers).

The last step is crucial in this time of shortened hospital stays. Any detail of the patient's background that would affect discharge planning is crucial to know, even on the first day of treatment. Additional information that may be helpful to

211

review and that falls into the category of "as time allows" is any documentation recorded by other health professionals, such as nurses, occupational therapists, or speech pathologists. Finally, when the initial chart review is finished, a mental picture of the patient should exist, even before the physical therapist steps into the patient's hospital room.

Details regarding the patient interview have been covered in Chapter 7. However, there are questions that should be posed to any patient, regardless of whether his or her primary condition is cardiopulmonary. The patient whose referring problem is musculoskeletal or neurologic still must have operational cardiac and respiratory systems. The questions asked could include the following: What is the smoking history? Does the patient have a family history of premature coronary artery disease (i.e., a parent or sibling who had a myocardial infarction)? Can the symptoms presented also be signs of a cardiovascular or pulmonary illness? Does the patient have an active versus a sedentary lifestyle? What activities precipitate symptoms? Do these symptoms include breathlessness?

Every patient should be seen as a human being with multiple organ systems. The patient's problem, whether orthopedic or cardiopulmonary, should not be viewed in isolation. An example is the outpatient with a physical therapy diagnosis of low back pain. When questioned about limiting symptoms, the patient might describe cramping leg pain, which is suggestive of peripheral vascular disease (PVD).

SYSTEM REVIEW AND TESTS AND MEASURES: PHYSICAL EXAMINATION OF THE CHEST

The traditional components of a chest assessment incorporate the other two elements of examination: system review, visual inspection and vital signs, and the tests and measures of auscultation, mediate, percussion, and palpation. When the information provided by each of these techniques is integrated with the patient's history and chart contents, the physical therapist can then piece together the puzzle and complete the other components of evaluation, diagnosis, and prognosis. For instance, to auscultate breath sounds without judging the symmetry of the chest wall would fail to provide needed clues to the total patient picture; thereby, the development of an appropriate plan of care for the patient is made more difficult.

Before each individual aspect of the assessment is discussed, a review of the pertinent anatomic landmarks and topographic lines is to be discussed. Knowledge of the superficial anatomy and its relationship to the underlying heart and lungs aids the therapist in decision making. The topographical lines allow for more accurate description of the physical findings.

TOPOGRAPHIC ANATOMIC LANDMARKS

Key anatomic structures include the following.

- Sternum
- Clavicles

> **BOX 15-1**
>
> ### Anatomic Structures
>
> *Suprasternal notch*: A depression palpable at the top of the sternum
> *Sternomanubrial angle*: A bony bump where the manubrium meets the body of the sternum; about 5 cm distal to suprasternal notch; also known as the angle of Louis; palpating lateral to this junction, the second ribs are found; they are reference points for identifying intercostal spaces and successive ribs; also, a superficial marking for where the underlying trachea divides into right and left mainstem bronchi.
> *Costal angle*: The angle formed by the joining of the costal margins with the sternum; normally, no greater than 90 degrees.
> *Vertebra prominens*: The spinous process of the seventh cervical vertebra (C7); allows numbering of thoracic vertebra.

- Suprasternal notch
- Sternomanubrial angle (angle of Louis)
- Costal angle
- Vertebra prominens

See Box 15-1 and Figures 15-1 and 15-2 for specific definitions and anterior and lateral views of the thorax. Imaginary topographic lines are used to more clearly describe any physical findings (e.g., location of surgical incisions, abnormal breath sounds, etc.) (Figure 15-3).

The anterior view of the thorax has three vertical lines.

- Midsternal line (MSL)—a vertical line bisecting the sternum
- Midclavicular lines (MCLs)—they lie parallel to the MSL, bisecting each clavicle; the lower lung borders cross the sixth ribs at the MCLs

Laterally, there are also three vertical lines, originating in their respective axillary folds.

- Anterior axillary line (AAL)
- Midaxillary line (MAL)
- Posterior axillary line (PAL)—like the MCLs, these lines are also bilateral

The posterior chest has the following three lines.

- Vertebral or midspinal line—runs through the spinous processes of the vertebrae
- Midscapular lines (MSLs)—they lie parallel to the midspinal line, bisecting the inferior angles of the scapulae

VISUAL INSPECTION

Inspection is the foremost element of a systematic review of the chest. Not only should the features of the patient be observed, but also the equipment and any aspect of the patient's surroundings that would contribute to delineating the

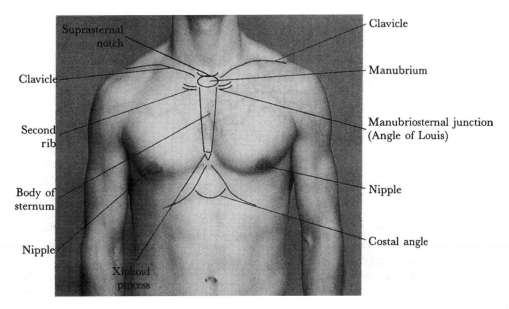

FIGURE 15-1 Topographic landmarks of the chest. *(From Seidel, H.M. [2003]. Mosby's guide to physical examination, ed 5. Philadelphia: Mosby.)*

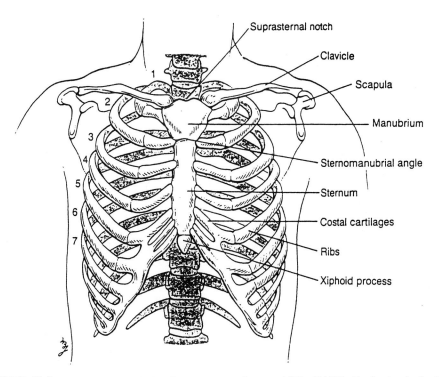

FIGURE 15-2 Anterior view of the thorax. *(From Swartz, M.H. [2002]. Textbook of physical diagnoses—history and examination, ed 4. Philadelphia: WB Saunders.)*

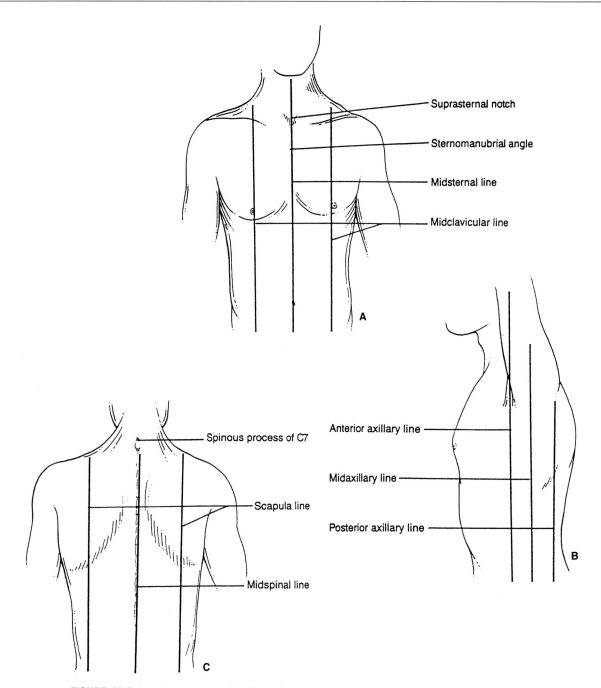

FIGURE 15-3 Imaginary topographic lines. **A,** Anterior view. **B,** Lateral view. **C,** Posterior view. *(Adapted with permission from Swartz, M.H. [2002]. Textbook of physical diagnoses—history and examination, ed 4. Philadelphia: WB Saunders.)*

true picture of that patient. Remember, the physical therapist has already gathered a preliminary picture of the patient based on review of the chart. Now, the ultimate test: how realistic was that initial impression? What are the outward clinical signs that the therapist should look for? Here it will be broken down into categories for clarity.

General Appearance

Does the patient appear comfortable? Is there any facial grimacing? Is the patient awake and alert or disoriented? Is there any nasal flaring or pursed-lip breathing? These are signs of respiratory distress. Nasal flaring can be defined as the outward movement of the nares with inspiration (Swartz,

2002). Are the accessory muscles of respiration (i.e., sternocleidomastoid and trapezius) hypertrophied? How is the patient positioned? Is the patient resting comfortably or leaning forward over the bedside table and struggling for breath? What is the patient's build—stocky, thin, or cachectic? Is the patient's mobility limited? Can the patient sit unsupported? Should the assessment be performed in stages, allowing the patient to be supine and then to lie on each side? Is there any extra equipment in the patient's surroundings? Is the patient using supplemental oxygen? Is the oxygen delivered through a nasal cannula or a mask? What is the fraction of inspired oxygen (FiO_2)? Are there any monitoring lines, and where are they located? For instance, if an arterial line is present, is it placed in the radial or the femoral artery? Are there electrocardiogram (ECG) leads? Is it a hard line (directly connected to a monitor) or a telemetry line (communicating through radio transmitter)? Are there intravenous (IV) sites? Are they peripheral (antecubital) or central (subclavian or jugular)? Is there a urinary catheter?

Skin

Does the skin have a pink, healthy color or a pallor? Is cyanosis present? Cyanosis is a bluish tinge that can be seen centrally or peripherally. Central cyanosis is a result of insufficient gas exchange within the lungs and is not usually seen unless oxygen saturation is less than 80%. A bluish tint may be seen at the mucous membranes (e.g., tongue and lips). Peripheral cyanosis, on the other hand, occurs when oxygen extraction at the periphery is excessive. This type is more closely associated with states of low cardiac output. Areas to observe for peripheral cyanosis include fingertips, toes, nose, and nail beds. A differentiating feature between central and peripheral cyanosis is that peripheral cyanosis normally occurs in the cooler body parts such as nail beds and usually vanishes when the part is warmed. In contrast, central cyanosis does not disappear when the area is warmed.

Are any scars, bruises, or ecchymoses observed? Are there reddened areas suggestive of prolonged pressure? Do the bony landmarks appear more prominent than usual? Are there any signs of trauma to the thorax or any other body parts? Does the skin appear edematous? Does this edema appear to limit joint motion? Are there any surgical incisions, new or old? Do these incisions appear to be healed or seem reddened and swollen? Is there evidence of clubbing of the digits? Digital clubbing can be defined as the loss of angle between the nail bed and the distal interphalangeal joint (Figure 15-4). The cause of clubbing is explained by a variety of theories, including increased perfusion. Its association with arterial oxygen desaturation has been noted, but this is not an exclusive phenomenon; clubbing has also been observed in nonpulmonary diseases such as hepatic fibrosis and Crohn disease. (George et al, 1990; Seidel et al, 2003; Swartz, 2002).

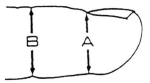

FIGURE 15-4 A, Clubbing of the fingers is best assessed by determining the ratio of the diameter at the base of the nail, **B,** to the diameter at the distal interphalangeal joint. This ratio is normally less than 1. *(From George, R.B. [1990]. Chest medicine, ed 2. Baltimore: Williams and Wilkins.)*

Neck

Are the accessory muscles of respirations being recruited for a resting breathing pattern? Do the sternocleidomastoid or trapezius muscles appear prominent? This is an early sign of obstructive lung disease (Swartz, 2002).

Jugular Venous Distention

The jugular veins empty into the superior vena cava and reflect right-sided heart function. Right atrial pressure (RAP) is evident based on the extent to which the jugular venous pulse (JVP) can be visualized. The more superficial external jugular veins may be seen superior to the clavicles; the internal jugular veins, though larger, lie deep beneath the sternocleidomastoids and are less visible. Jugular venous distention (JVD) can be best seen when the patient lies with the head and neck at an angle of 45 degrees (Figure 15-5). The presence or absence of symmetry of JVD should be noted. The veins are distended bilaterally if there is a cardiac cause such as congestive heart failure (CHF). A unilateral distention is an indication of a localized problem. (Seidel et al, 2003).

CHEST WALL CONFIGURATION

The normal thoracic cage is elliptically shaped when free of disease. The anteroposterior (AP)-to-lateral diameter is 1:2 or 5:7. The angle of the ribs is less than 90 degrees. The ribs articulate with the vertebra posteriorly, at a 45-degree angle. The thorax should be observed both anteriorly and posteriorly. With chronic obstructive pulmonary disease (COPD), the ribs become more horizontal and the AP diameter increases; thus the term *barrel chest* is used. In infants, the chest is round, with the anteroposterior and transverse or lateral diameters of about equal dimensions. As a child grows to adulthood, the chest becomes more elliptical. With the aging process, the chest returns to a more rounded appearance. The increased anteroposterior diameter in this population is a result of the multiple factors of decreasing lung compliance, decreased strength of the thoracic and diaphragmatic muscles, and skeletal changes in the thoracic spine. The symmetry or absence thereof of the thoracic cage should also be noted. Asymmetry can be the result of structural defects or an underlying intrathoracic pathology. Again, any asymmetry should be observed from both anterior and posterior views.

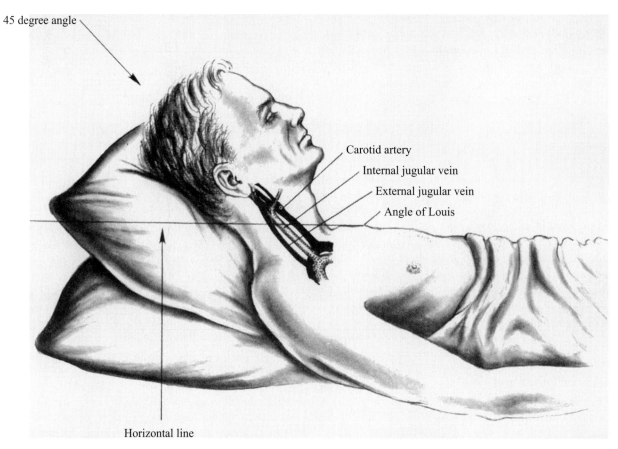

45 degree angle

Carotid artery
Internal jugular vein
External jugular vein
Angle of Louis

Horizontal line

FIGURE 15-5 Proper positioning to observe jugular venous distention. *(From Seidel, H.M.. [2003]. Mosby's guide to physical examination, ed 5. Philadelphia: Mosby.)*

Structural defects of the anterior chest may include the following: pectus excavatum, or funnel chest—a depressed lower sternum that usually causes restriction only when it is severe; pectus carinatum, or pigeon chest—a prominent upper sternum that does not restrict chest wall movement; and flail chest—the chest wall moves inward with inspiration, such as with multiple rib fractures.

Other structural defects are spinal deformities. These are best viewed posteriorly. Kyphoscoliosis is one example of how a posterior and lateral spinal deviation can limit chest wall and lung expansion. Another example is a patient with COPD, who usually has a forwardly tilted head and thoracic kyphosis (Figure 15-6).

BREATHING PATTERN

Respiratory rates normally range between 14 and 20 breaths per minute in adults (ages 15 and older). In children, the following ranges are used: newborn, 30-60 breaths per minute; early childhood, 20-40 breaths per minute; late childhood, 15 to 25 breaths per minute (Bickley & Szilagyi, 2003).

Eupnea is a normal breathing cycle. Apnea is a temporary halt in breathing. Tachypnea is a rapid, shallow breathing pattern; this is an indicator of respiratory distress. Bradypnea exists when respiration is slowed to less than 12 breaths per minute. Causes could be neurologic or metabolic. Kussmaul breathing is an increased rate and depth of respirations and is associated with metabolic acidosis.

Dyspnea describes the sensation of breathlessness or shortness of breath and is seen in cardiopulmonary disorders. The level of dyspnea worsens as the severity of the disease increases. An easy method for documenting the level of dyspnea is to count the numbers of words that the patient is able to speak per breath. For instance, six-word dyspnea is not as significant as one-word dyspnea. The type of activities that elicit shortness of breath should also be ascertained. For example, is breathlessness precipitated by stair climbing, taking a shower, and so forth? The normal ratio of inspiratory time to expiratory time is 1:2. As the respiratory rate increases, this ratio decreases to 1:1. This is seen in respiratory distress; as the patient struggles to breathe in, the expiratory phase is shortened, and a vicious circle continues. With pursed-lip

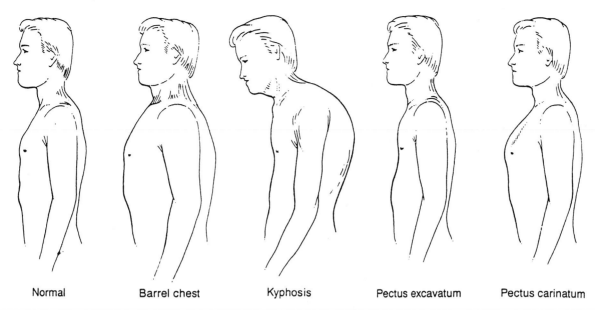

Normal   Barrel chest   Kyphosis   Pectus excavatum   Pectus carinatum

FIGURE 15-6 Chest wall configurations. *(From Swartz, M.H. [2002]. Textbook of physical diagnoses: history and examination, ed 4. Philadelphia: WB Saunders.)*

breathing, the idea is to prolong the expiratory phase and slow the breathing pattern.

AUSCULTATION

Auscultation is the art of listening to sounds produced by the body. Lung and heart sounds are the focus of this chapter. Skill in auscultation is dependent on the following four factors.

1. A functional stethoscope
2. Proper technique
3. Knowledge of the different categories of lung sounds: normal, abnormal, adventitious breath sounds, and voice sounds
4. Knowledge of the various categories of heart sounds and murmurs

Stethoscope

A stethoscope need not be fancy to be effective. A physical therapist skilled in auscultation can use any basic stethoscope and be able to identify lung sounds. The stethoscope functions more as a filter to the extraneous noises than as an amplifier. A basic stethoscope consists of ear pieces, tubing, and a chest piece. The bell portion of the chest piece assesses low-pitched sounds (i.e., heart sounds). The diaphragm portion discerns high-pitched sounds (Figure 15-7). The tubing should not be so long that sound transmission is dampened. The length of the tubing should be between about 30 cm (12 inches) and 55 cm (21 to 22 inches). The earpieces should fit the physical therapist's ears comfortably and allow the tuning out of external sounds. Another consideration is to position the ear pieces anteriorly, or forward toward the ear canals. Finally, an

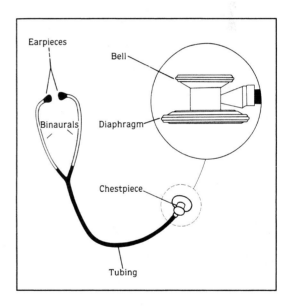

FIGURE 15-7 Stethoscope. *(From Wilkins, R.L., Hodgkin, J.E., & Lopez, B. [2004]. Fundamentals of lung and heart sounds, ed 3. St. Louis: Mosby.)*

aside gained from the author's clinical experience: warming the diaphragm with the hands before placing it on the patient's skin is a first step in developing good patient rapport.

Technique

Environment is another element in the correct performance of auscultation. The room or cubicle should be as quiet as possible. Television and radio should be turned down or off.

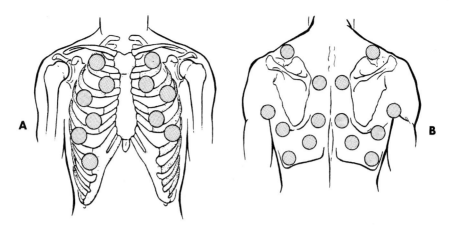

FIGURE 15-8 Stethoscope placement for auscultation of breath sounds. **A,** The chest. **B,** The back. *(From Buckingham, E.B. [1979]. A primer of clinical diagnosis, ed 2. New York: Harper & Row.)*

Any extraneous noises should be minimized or eliminated. This is especially important when auscultation is a new technique for the therapist. The patient should be in a sitting position, if possible, for lung sounds. The anterior, lateral, and posterior aspects of the chest should be auscultated both craniocaudally (apices to bases) and side to side (Figure 15-8). The physical therapist places the diaphragm on the patient's skin so that it lies flat. The patient is instructed to breath in and out through the mouth. A slightly deeper breath than tidal breathing is suggested. A minimum of one breath per bronchopulmonary segment allows for a comparison of the intensity, pitch, and quality of the breath sounds. Movement of the diaphragm from one side to the other side while, at the same time, moving it craniocaudally, enables the therapist to compare the right side of the chest to the left side of the chest. Clothing should be removed or draped so that it does not interfere in the assessment of the breath sounds.

Chest Sounds

Chest sounds may be divided into the following categories.

1. Breath sounds—normal, abnormal, adventitious
2. Voice sounds—egophony, bronchophony, whispered pectoriloquy
3. Extrapulmonary sounds—pleural or friction rubs
4. Heart sounds

Breath Sounds

The terminology of breath sounds given in this chapter is a compilation of multiple resources and clinical experience. Recognition of normal breath sounds is the key to the identification of abnormal and adventitious sounds because it offers the listener a point of reference. Normal breath sounds can be broken down into bronchial, bronchovesicular, and vesicular. The American Thoracic Society (ATS) and the

BRONCHIAL
loud, high pitched; hollow quality; heard over manubrium; louder on expiration; distinct pause between inspiration (I) and expiration (E)

BRONCHOVESICULAR
mixture of bronchial and vesicular; I: E is 1:1; heard over main-stem bronchi anteriorly, ICS #1 and #2; posteriorly, between scapulae

VESICULAR
soft, low pitched; heard over peripheral lung tissue; no pause between I and E; ratio is 3:1

FIGURE 15-9 Normal breath sounds.

American College of Chest Physicians (ACCP) have attempted to provide standardization of the nomenclature and continues to conduct surveys of health care professionals for use of this terminology in clinical practice.

Bronchial sounds can be described as high-pitched and are heard in both the inspiratory and the expiratory phase. A distinguishing feature is the pause that exists between the inspiratory and expiratory phases (Figure 15-9). This sound is also described as tracheal because its normal location is over the trachea. Bronchovesicular sounds are similar in that they are also high-pitched and have equal inspiratory and expiratory cycles. However, a differentiating feature is the lack of a pause (see Figure 15-9). Bronchovesicular sounds are heard best wherever the bronchi, or central lung tissue, are close to the surface. These areas are supraclavicular and suprascapular (the apices) and parasternal and interscapular (the bronchi). The ATS and ACCP, in their 1977 recommendations for pulmonary nomenclature, used the term *bronchial* to include both bronchial and bronchovesicular sounds. The finite difference is minor (the pause between the inspiratory and expiratory phases). This recommendation is meant to provide uniformity to lung-sound terminology. Vesicular breath sounds are heard over the remaining peripheral lung fields. These sounds have primarily an inspiratory component, with only the initial one third of the expiratory phase audible. Their intensity is also softer because of the dampening effect of the spongy lung tissue and the cumulative effect of the air entry from numerous terminal bronchioles. The idea that vesicular sounds reflect air entry in the alveoli has been disproved. Thus, as the therapist auscultates from top to bottom, the breath sounds are quieter at the bases than at the apices. Infants and small children have louder, harsher breath sounds. This is as result of the thinness of the chest wall and the airways' being closer to its surface.

Abnormal Breath Sounds

Abnormal breath sounds can be described as changes in the sound transmission as a result of an underlying pathologic process. Sound is filtered by the lung tissues because these organs are air-filled; thus sound transmission is dampened over the bases more than over the apices. On the other hand, sound transmission is enhanced when a liquid or solid is the medium. Certain lung pathologies produce abnormal lung sounds. Abnormal sounds can be divided into three types: bronchial, decreased, and absent. Bronchial sounds occur in peripheral lung tissue when it becomes airless—either partially or completely. In a consolidating type of pneumonia, the lung tissue is "airless" because of the complete obstruction of segmental or lobar bronchi by secretions. Sound from the adjacent bronchi is enhanced and becomes higher pitched, and the expiratory component is louder and more pronounced. Compression of lung tissue from an extrapulmonary source also produces bronchial sounds. Examples include compression secondary to increased pleural fluid (pleural effusion) or tumor. *Tubular breath sounds* is a term used synonymously to describe abnormal bronchial breath sounds.

Decreased or absent breath sounds occur when sound transmission is diminished or abolished. Decreased breath sounds occur when the normal vesicular sounds are further diminished. The term *absent sounds* means that no sounds are audible. Decreased or absent sounds can be caused by an internal pulmonary pathology or can be secondary to an initially nonpulmonary condition. Hyperinflation caused by emphysema causes decreased sound transmission as a result of the destruction of the acinar units and causes increased air as a result of the loss of normal lung structure. The loss of lung compliance resulting from pulmonary fibrosis also may produce decreased or absent breath sounds. Extrapulmonary causes include tumors, neuromuscular weakness (i.e, muscular dystrophy), and musculoskeletal deformities (i.e., kyphoscoliosis). Pain is a common cause for decreased or absent breath sounds. When the patient attempts to take a

deep breath, the volume is limited because of the onset of pain. The causes of the pain can be varied—from incisional (i.e., midsternotomy) to traumatic (fractured ribs). If no underlying pathologies are present, decreased breath sounds may be a reflection of the depth of respiration or the thickness of the chest wall (e.g., in obesity or with the presence of bandages). The skill of auscultation lies in the differentiation between normal and abnormal breath sounds.

Adventitious Breath Sounds

Adventitious breath sounds are the extraneous noises produced over the bronchopulmonary tree and are an indication of an abnormal process or condition. These sounds may be more easily identifiable than abnormal sounds. Adventitious sounds are classified as crackles (rales), rhonchi, and wheezes. Crackles (rales) are described as discontinuous, low-pitched sounds. They occur predominantly during inspiration. The sound of rubbing hair between the fingers or of Velcro popping simulates crackles. Crackles usually indicate a peripheral airway process. Rhonchi are low-pitched but continuous sounds. These occur in both inspiration and expiration. Snoring is a term used to describe its quality. Rhonchi are attributed to an obstructive process in the larger, more central airways. Wheezes are continuous but high-pitched. A hissing or whistling quality is present. Wheezes occur predominantly during expiration and are an indication of bronchospasm (i.e., asthma). However, wheezes can also be caused by the movement of air through secretions; thus, inspiratory wheezes can be described.

Extrapulmonary Sounds

An adventitious sound that is nonpulmonary is the friction rub. It can be described as a rubbing or leathery sound and it occurs during both inspiration and expiration. The sound is produced when the visceral (inner) pleural lining rubs against the parietal (outer) pleura and is a sign of a primary pleural process such as inflammation or neoplasm. Pain is usually associated with a friction rub.

Voice Sounds

Voice sounds are vibrations heard through a stethoscope and produced by the speaking voice as it travels down the tracheobronchial tree and through the lung parenchyma. These sounds, over the normal lung, are low-pitched and have a muffled or mumbled quality. The transmission of these vocal vibrations can be increased or decreased in the presence of an underlying pulmonary pathologic process. Bronchophony describes the phenomenon of increased vocal transmission. Words or letters are louder and clearer. It is caused by conditions in which there is increased lung density, as in consolidation due to pneumonia. The patient is usually asked to repeat "blue moon" or "one, two, three." Egophony, too, is described when there is increased transmission of the vocal vibrations. In this

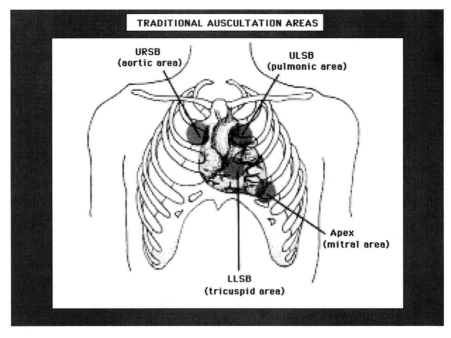

FIGURE 15-10 Cardiac auscultation. *(From http://www.kumc.edu/kumcpeds/cardiology/tofmsllecture/ auscultaitonareas.gif; retrieved.)*

case, the patient is asked to say "eeee." The underlying process distorts the *e* sound so that an "aaa" sound is heard over the peripheral area by the examiner. Egophony coexists with bronchophony.

Whispered voice sounds also produce low-pitched vibrations over the chest that are muffled by normal lung parenchyma. In whispered pectoriloquy, these whispered voice sounds become distinct and clear; "one, two, three" or "ninety-nine" are used to evaluate this sound. Whispered pectoriloquy can be present when bronchophony and egophony are absent. This sign is helpful in identifying smaller or patchy areas of lung consolidation.

Voice sounds are a method of confirming abnormal breath sounds. If a patient with significant atelectasis secondary to compression of lung tissue presents with bronchial breath sounds, then egophony and bronchophony are also audible.

Web sites are available where the beginner in auscultation can actually hear lung sounds. The two Web sites included in this chapter's references have links to these auditory sites. Also, going to Google and searching the key word *auscultation* may reveal others.

HEART SOUNDS

As with lung sounds, superficial topographic landmarks assist the therapist in auscultation of heart sounds and murmurs. The left ventricular apex is normally located at the MCL in the fifth intercostal space (ICS). The cardiac apex is also known as the point of maximum impulse (PMI). There are four reference areas for cardiac auscultation; they do not correspond directly to the underlying cardiac anatomy. On the other hand, these areas do relate to the events arising at the individual cardiac valves. These four areas are defined as the following.

- Aortic: second ICS, at right sternal border (RSB)
- Pulmonic: second ICS, at left sternal border (LSB)
- Tricuspid: fourth and fifth ICS, LSB
- Mitral: cardiac apex, fifth ICS, MCL

Technique

An environment that is as quiet as possible is recommended. Positions used for cardiac auscultation include the following: supine—used for all areas; left lateral decubitus (sidelying)—listening to cardiac apex or mitral area, bell usually used; and sitting—used for all areas.

Heart Sounds

The first heart sound (S_1) signifies the closing of the atrioventricular valves. Its duration is 0.10 seconds; it is heard the loudest at the cardiac apex. The two components of S_1 are tricuspid and mitral. Both the diaphragm and the bell of the stethoscope can be used to hear S_1. Its loudness is enhanced by any condition in which the heart is closer to the chest wall (i.e., thin chest wall) or in which there is an increased force to the ventricular contraction (e.g., tachycardia resulting from exercise) (Figure 15-10).

The second heart sound (S_2) represents the closing of the semilunar valves and the end of ventricular systole. Its components are aortic and pulmonic. During expiration, these two components are not distinct because the time difference in the closure of the valves is less than 30 milliseconds. However, during inspiration, a splitting of S_2 is audible. This physiologic split results from the increased venous return to the right heart secondary to the decreased intrathoracic pressure that occurs during inspiration. The pulmonic valve closure is delayed as the right ventricular systolic time is lengthened. A split S_2 is heard normally in children and young adults. The diaphragm of the stethoscope should be used to hear the split. The pulmonic component is the softer sound and is best heard at the LSB, in the second to fourth ICS. The two components may be heard best in the aortic and pulmonic areas, respectively. When the split is heard in both phases of respiration, an underlying cardiac abnormality is suspected. Causes may include right bundle branch block and pulmonary hypertension. (Swartz, 2002; Tilkian & Conover, 1993).

Gallops

The third heart sound (S_3) is a faint, low frequency sound and reflects the early (diastolic) ventricular filling that occurs after the atrioventricular valves open. S_3 is normal in children and young adults; however, it is usually abnormal in individuals over age 40. An extra effort must be made to auscultate S_3; the bell of the stethoscope should be used. The ideal position to hear S_3 would be left sidelying; the bell would be placed over the cardiac apex. Causes of a pathological S_3 may include ventricular failure, tachycardia, or mitral regurgitation. "Ken-TUCK-y" is one sound that has been used to approximate the sound sequencing of S_3 in the cardiac cycle (S_1, S_2, S_3).

The fourth heart sound (S_4) signifies the rapid ventricular filling that occurs after atrial contraction. When present, it is heard before S_1. S_4 may be heard in the "normal" individual with left ventricular hypertrophy. The location of S_4 is similar to that of S_3. Its sound can be described as dull because of the sudden motion of stiff ventricles in response to increased atrial contraction. Pathologies eliciting an S_4 may include systemic hypertension, cardiomyopathies, and coarctation of the aorta. "TENN-es-see" is a sound that approximates the sound sequencing when S_4 is present (S_4, S_1, S_2).

Murmurs

Cardiac murmurs are the vibrations resulting from turbulent blood flow. They may be described based on position in cardiac cycle (systole, diastole), duration, and loudness. Systolic murmurs occur between S_1 and S_2; diastolic murmurs occur between S_2 and S_1. A continuous murmur starts in S_1 and lasts through S_2 for a portion or all of diastole. The loudness of a murmur is a factor of the velocity of blood flow and the turbulence created as it flows through a specific opening such as a valve. Grades I to VI are described as follows.

- I: faint—requires concentrated effort to hear
- II: faint—audible immediately
- III: louder than II—intermediate intensity
- IV: loud—intermediate intensity; associated with palpable vibration (thrill)
- V: very loud—thrill present
- VI: audible without stethoscope

Murmurs that are grade III or higher are usually associated with cardiovascular pathology.

MEDIATE PERCUSSION

Mediate, or indirect, percussion allows the therapist to assess the density of the underlying organs. Striking the chest wall produces vibrations in the underlying structures which, in turn, give rise to sound waves or percussion tones. The quality of that tone depends on the density of the tissue or organ (i.e., it becomes louder over air-filled structures). These tones are described by the following terms.

- Resonant: loud or high amplitude, low pitch, longer duration; heard over air-filled organs such as the lungs
- Dull: low amplitude, medium to high pitch, short duration; heard over solid organs such as the liver
- Flat: high-pitch, short duration; heard over muscle mass such as the thigh
- Tympanic: high-pitch, medium duration; heard over hollow structures such as the stomach
- Hyperresonant: very low-pitch, prolonged duration; heard over tissue with decreased density (increased air to tissue ratio); abnormal in adults; heard over lungs with emphysema

Technique

The middle finger of the nondominant hand is placed firmly on the chest wall in an intercostal space and parallel to the ribs. The top of the middle finger of the dominant hand strikes the distal phalanx of the stationary hand with a quick, sharp motion. The impetus of the blow comes from the wrist rather than the elbow and has been likened to that of a paddle ball player (Swartz, 2002) (Figure 15-11). As with auscultation, the therapist must follow the sequence of apices to bases and side to side so that comparisons can be made. This technique is not usually used in infants because percussion is too easily transmitted by a small chest.

Diaphragmatic Excursion

Assessment of diaphragmatic movement can be made with mediate percussion. The patient is asked to breathe deeply and hold that breath. The lowest level of the diaphragm on maximal inspiration coincides with the lowest point where a resonant tone is heard. The patient is then asked to exhale, and mediate percussion is repeated. The lowest area of resonance now moves higher, as the diaphragm ascends with relaxation.

The distance between these two points is described as the diaphragmatic excursion; the normal range is 3 to 5 cm (Figure 15-12). Diaphragmatic movement is decreased in patients with COPD.

PALPATION

Physical therapists use palpation in all areas of practice. Touch is an integral part of physical therapy. As part of the chest examination, palpation is used to assess areas of tenderness, abnormalities, chest wall excursion, edema, tactile fremitus, and tracheal deviation.

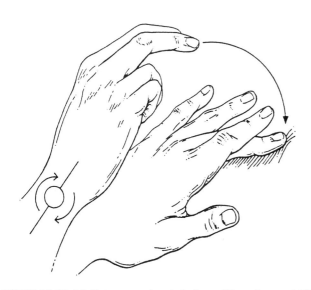

FIGURE 15-11 Mediate percussion technique. *(From Swartz, M.H. [2002]. Textbook of physical diagnoses—history and examination, ed 4. Philadelphia: WB Saunders.)*

Tenderness

Specific superficial or deep landmarks are identified by means of palpation. Determination of gross spinal alignment can be performed by tracing the spinous processes in a cephalocaudal direction. Certain structures can be identified, such as the T-4 vertebra or the sternal angle; this only augments the physical therapist's evaluation. Areas of tenderness can be assessed for degree of discomfort and reproducibility. Differentiation of chest wall discomfort of an organic nature, such as in angina, from that of a musculoskeletal condition may be made through palpation. In a patient complaining of chest pain, angina may be ruled out if the physical therapist can reproduce or increase the discomfort by increasing tactile pressure. However, one must also determine that corroborating symptoms (e.g., diaphoresis, tachycardia) are not present. Angina or chest pain secondary to myocardial ischemia usually results from exertion and may be relieved by rest. Crepitus is a crunchy sound often associated with articular structures. However, when bubbles of air occur within subcutaneous tissue, a crackling sensation can be palpated. An air leak from a chest-tube site is one circumstance in which when crepitus is palpated over the chest wall. Crepitus can also be secondary to a pleural or friction rub.

Edema

Palpation allows the physical therapist to assess peripheral edema. Dependency of body parts can cause swelling due to cardiac and noncardiac conditions. Assessment of edema is performed by pressing two fingers into the particular areas for 2 to 3 seconds. If an impression is left once the fingers are removed, then pitting or dependent edema is present. The degree of edema is based on the length of time that the indentation lasts. 1+ is the least; 4+ is the worst.

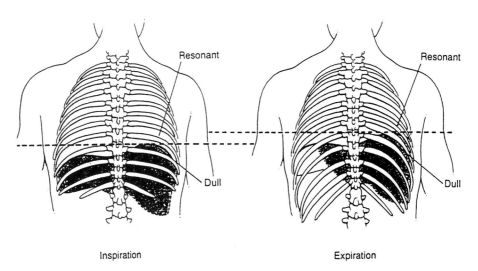

Inspiration

Expiration

FIGURE 15-12 Diaphragmatic excursion. *(From Swartz, M.H. [2002]. Textbook of physical diagnoses—history and examination, ed 4. Philadelphia: WB Saunders.)*

Chest Wall Excursion

Evaluation of thoracic expansion allows the therapist to observe a baseline level by which to measure progress or decline in a patient's condition. Chest wall movement can be restricted unilaterally as a result of lobar pneumonia or a surgical incision. A symmetrical decrease in chest wall motion occurs in the patient with COPD.

The hyperinflation associated with COPD produces an increase in the anteroposterior diameter with a progressive loss of diaphragmatic excursion. Normal chest wall excursion is about 3.25 inches (8.5 cm) in a young adult between 20 and 30 years of age. One method is to use a tape measure at the level of the xiphoid. However, the most common method involves direct hand contact. This technique is performed in all planes and from top to bottom. Symmetry and extent of movement are noted. The procedures for this method follow.

- Apical or upper lobe motion (Figure 15-13)

  1. The physical therapist faces the patient. The area to be examined is exposed and draped as needed.
  2. The physical therapist's hands are placed over the anterior chest. The heel of the hand is about the level of the fourth rib and the fingertips reach toward the upper trapezii.
  3. The thumbs lie horizontal at about the level of the sternal angle and meet at the midline, slightly stretching the skin.
  4. The patient is asked to inhale.
  5. The hands should be relaxed to allow for movement beneath.
  6. The symmetry and extent of movement are assessed.

- Anterolateral or middle lobe/lingula motion (Figure 15-14)

  1. See above.
  2. The physical therapist's hands are placed with the palms distal to the nipple line, and the thumbs meeting in the midline. The fingers lie in the posterior axillary fold.
  3. See steps 4 to 6 above.

- Posterior excursion/lower lobe motion (Figure 15-15)

  1. The physical therapist stands behind the patient.
  2. The area to be examined is exposed with draping used as appropriate.
  3. The physical therapist's hands are placed flat on the posterior chest wall at the level of the tenth rib. The thumbs meet at the midline; fingers reaching toward the anterior axillary fold.
  4. See steps 4 to 6 above.

Tactile Fremitus

Spoken word produces vibration over the chest wall. Voice sounds have been previously discussed under auscultation. When the physical therapist's hands are placed on the chest wall, the vibrations of spoken words can be felt; they are described as tactile fremitus. The presence or absence of tactile fremitus provides information about the density of the underlying lungs and thoracic cavity (Swartz, 2002).

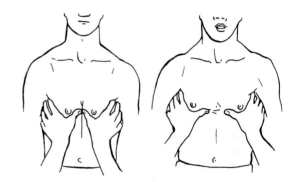

FIGURE 15-14 Evaluation of middle lobe and lingula motion (anterolateral excursion). *(From Cherniak, R.M. [1983]. Respiration in health and disease, ed 3. Philadelphia: WB Saunders.)*

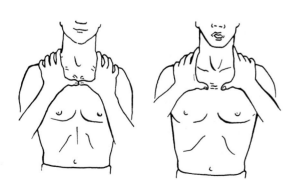

FIGURE 15-13 Evaluation of upper lobe motion. *(From Cherniak, R.M. [1983]. Respiration in health and disease, ed 3. Philadelphia: WB Saunders.)*

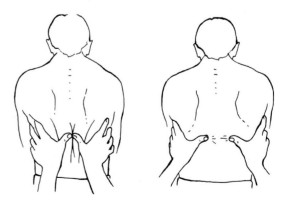

FIGURE 15-15 Evaluation of lower lobe motion (posterior excursion). *(From Cherniak, R.M., [1983].Respiration in health and disease, ed 3. Philadelphia: WB Saunders.)*

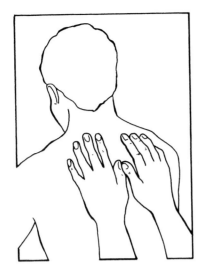

FIGURE 15-16 Technique for evaluating fremitus, method one.

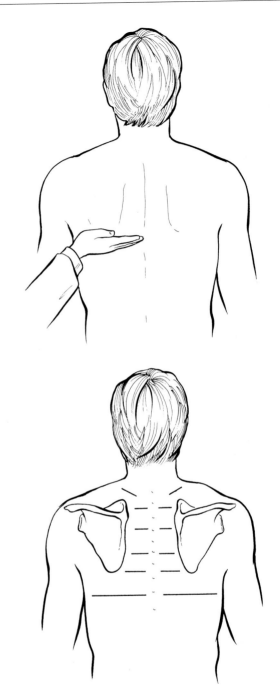

FIGURE 15-17 Technique for evaluating tactile fremitus, method two. *(From Swartz, M.H. [2002]. Textbook of physical diagnoses— history and examination, ed 4. Philadelphia: WB Saunders.)*

Technique

Two methods can be used (Figures 15-16 and 15-17). The first technique is one in which the therapist uses the palmar surface of one or both hands. The second method involves the use of the ulnar border of one hand. With both techniques, the sequence is, again, cephalocaudal and side to side. In either method, the next step is to ask that the patient speak a predetermined phrase. The two most commonly used are "ninety-nine" or "one, two, three." A light but firm touch is recommended.

Tracheal Deviation

The trachea's midline position can be examined anteriorly (Figure 15-18). The physical therapist places an index finger in the medial aspect of the suprasternal notch. This is repeated on the opposite side. An equal distance between the clavicle and the trachea should exist bilaterally. Tracheal deviation may be caused by a pneumothorax, atelectasis, or a tumor, among possible conditions. Whether the deviation is ipsilateral or contralateral depends on the underlying cause. A right pneumothorax or pleural effusion deviates the trachea away (toward the left); a left lower lobe atelectasis, however, deviates the trachea toward the affected side (i.e., the left).

CASE STUDIES

Case Study 1

A 30-year-old man with cystic fibrosis presents with a 1-week history of increased sputum production, loss of appetite, fatigue, and a 3-pound (6.6 kg) weight loss. With a system review of the chest (visual inspection) and the tests and measures of auscultation, mediate percussion, and palpation, the following findings are shown.

- Visual inspection: Forward head, kyphotic posture, and increased anteroposterior diameter are present; the patient appears thin and fatigued; no dyspnea is observed; the patient has an effective and wet cough

- Visual inspection: Tachypnea; respiratory rate of 44; ratio of inspiration to expiration ratio = 1:1; weak, shallow cough
- Auscultation: Bronchial over right midanterior chest; egophany also present
- Mediate percussion: Dull over affected area
- Palpation: Trachea midline, markedly decreased CWE on right side

Anticipated outcomes may include the following.

1. The patient will demonstrate an effective cough
2. The patient will demonstrate decreased work of breathing

Treatment interventions may include manual chest percussion, vibration/shaking, postural drainage to right middle lobe area and instruction in huff coughing. Games that may be incorporated to facilitate the huffing as well as increasing the I:E ratio include blowing bubbles, windmills, kazoos. Hand-held airway clearance devices such as the Flutter, Thera PEP, or A Cappella may also be used.

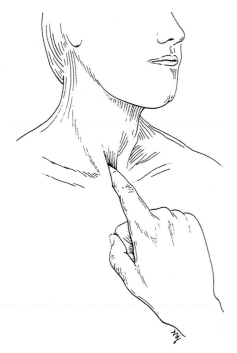

FIGURE 15-18 Technique for determining the position of the trachea. *(From Swartz, M.H. [2002]. Textbook of physical diagnoses—history and examination, ed 4. Philadelphia: WB Saunders.)*

- Auscultation: Decreased breath sounds with scattered crackles throughout all lung fields, especially over right posterior upper lobe and right middle lobe
- Palpation: Limited chest wall excursion (CWE), especially laterally
- Mediate percussion: Dull over right middle and lower chest, especially laterally

The evaluation component utilizes the above findings to identify the appropriate outcomes and treatment interventions. Based on the acuity of the examination, acute exacerbation of cystic fibrosis may be the the diagnosis. The focus may be on secretion clearance and identification of the most appropriate airway clearance techniques. Would the high-frequency chest oscillations (ThAIRapy Vest) or manual techniques of chest percussion, vibration/shaking, and specific postural drainage positions be the choice for this patient? Scheduling airway clearance techniques by means of respiratory therapy and inhaled medications is indicated as well. Ongoing daily reexamination will determine whether the treatment interventions need to be modified or continued as is.

Case Study 2

An 8-year-old female admitted to the pediatric inpatient unit presents on chart review (history) with a 4-day history of recurrent fevers, shortness of breath, and lethargy. A chest radiogram shows a right middle lobe infiltrate.

Case Study 3

A 72-year-old woman presents with symptoms of persistent fevers, left chest wall discomfort, and history of a fall 1 week ago. A CT scan shows a loculated pleural effusion on the left. A left chest tube has been inserted for drainage. The working medical diagnosis is empyema. The patient is a nonsmoker. The following information is learned during the examination component of the patient management model.

- Visual inspection: RR 30; I:E ratio = 1:2; epidural catheter for pain control; effective dry cough
- Auscultation: Absent breath sounds halfway up left lower lateral chest wall
- Mediate percussion: Flat over left lower lateral chest wall
- Palpation: Trachea deviated to right; decreased CWE on left; range of motion of left shoulder joint limited in flexion and abduction at about 90 degrees maximum; no preadmission shoulder limitations

Outcomes and treatment interventions must expand beyond the pulmonary diagnosis of empyema because the surgical insertion of a chest tube as well as the fall have impacted the musculoskeletal system as well. With a dry and effective cough, secretion clearance is not an issue, but atelectasis is.

An anticipated outcome would be for the patient to demonstrate no abnormal lung sounds as a result of increased lung volumes. Interventions would include breathing strategies (i.e., diaphragmatic breathing). The breathing strategies could be incorporated into range-of-motion exercises for the shoulder. Incentive spirometry may also facilitate increased lung volumes. Finally, as the patient's condition becomes less acute, one may ascertain whether a balance impairment was the cause of the initial fall.

TABLE 15-1

Differentiation of Common Pulmonary Conditions

	INSPECTION	PALPATION	PERCUSSION	AUSCULTATION
Emphysema	Increased anteroposterior diameter; use of accessory muscles; thin individual	Decreased tactile fremitus	Increased resonance; decreased excursion of diaphragm	Decreased lung sounds; decreased vocal fremitus
Chronic bronchitis	Possible cyanosis; short, stocky individual	Often normal	Often normal	Early crackles
Pneumonia	Possible cyanosis	Increased tactile fremitus; splinting on affected side	Dull	Late crackles; bronchal breath sounds
Pulmonary embolism	Sudden onset of dyspnea; chest pain	Usually normal	Usually normal	Usually normal
Pneumothorax	Rapid onset	Absent fremitus; trachea may be shifted to other side; may have decreased chest wall excursion on affected side	Hyperresonant	Absent breath sounds
Pleural effusion	May be no outward clinical sign	Decreased fremitus; trachea shifted to other side; decreased chest wall excursion on affected side	Dullness	Absent breath sounds
Atelectasis	Often no outward clinical sign	Decreased fremitus; trachea shifted to same side; decreased chest wall excursion on affected side	Dullness	Absent breath sounds

Adapted with permission from Swartz, MH: Textbook of physical diagnoses—history and examination, ed 2, Philadelphia, 1994, WB Saunders.

See Table 15-1 for a differentiation of diagnoses by the elements of a chest physical examination.

SUMMARY

As demonstrated in the case studies, each of the examination skills discussed contributes to the physical therapist's ability to solve the puzzle of the individual patient. This initial component of the patient management model makes it possible to perform the remaining components of evaluation, diagnosis, and prognosis.

Review Questions

1. Describe the sequence used to auscultate lung sounds.
2. State the difference between peripheral and central cyanosis.

3. How are normal bronchial breath sounds different from abnormal bronchial breath sounds?
4. Name two causes for a pathologic S_3.
5. Name two causes for decreased breath sounds.
6. Formulate a plan for the evaluation of a patient with an acute right lower lobe pneumonia.
7. Which components of the chest physical examination might a physical therapist include in the initial assessment of a geriatric patient with a recent left total hip replacement and a history of COPD?

REFERENCES

Bickley, L.S., Szilagyi, P.G. (2003). Bates' guide to physical examination and history taking, ed 8. Philadelphia: Lippincott Williams & Wilkins.
Buckingham, E.B. (1979). A primer of physical diagnosis, ed 2. New York: Harper and Row.

Cherniak, R.M., & Cherniak, L. (1983). Respiration in health and disease, ed 3. Philadelphia: WB Saunders.

Fraser, R.S., Muller, N.L., Colman N., & Pare, P.D. (1999). Fraser and Pare's diagnosis of diseases of the chest, ed 4. Philadelphia: WB Saunders.

George, R.B., Light, R.W., Matthay, M.A., & Matthay, R.A. (1990). Chest medicine, ed 2. Baltimore: Williams and Wilkins.

Lehrer, S. (1993). Understanding lung sounds, ed 2. Philadelphia: WB Saunders.

Mikami,R., Murao, M., Cugell, D.W., Chretien, J., Cole, P., Meier-Sydow, J., Murphy, R.L., & Loudon, R.G. (1987). International symposium on lung sounds. Chest 92:342-345.

Seidel, H.M., Ball, J.W., Dains, J.E., & Benedict, G.W. (2003). Mosby's guide to physical examination, ed 5. Philadelphia: Mosby.

Swartz, M.H. (2002). Textbook of physical diagnoses—history and examination, ed 4. Philadelphia: WB Saunders.

(2001). The guide to physical therapist practice, ed 2.

Tilkian, A.G., & Conover, M.D. (1993). Understanding heart sounds and murmurs, ed 3. Philadelphia: WB Saunders.

A practical guide to clinical medicine. University of California, San Diego. www.medicine.ucsd.edu/clinicalmed; retrieved .

Kansas University, KA. http://www.kumc.edu/kumcpeds/cardiology/tofmsllecture/auscultationareas.gif; retrieved

Wilkins, R.I., Hodgkin, J.E., & Lopez, B. (2004). Fundamentals of heart and lung sounds, ed 3. St. Louis: Mosby.

Wilkins, Dexter, J.R., Murphy, R.L. Jr., & DelBono, E.A. (1990). Lung sound nomenclature survey. Chest 98:886-889.

Willerson, J.T., & Cohn, J.N. (1995). Cardiovascular medicine. New York: Churchill Livingstone.

C H A P T E R   1 6

Monitoring Systems in the Intensive Care Unit

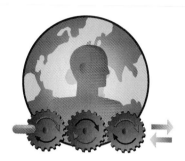

Elizabeth Dean and Christiane Perme

KEY TERMS

Acid-base balance
Critical illness polyneuropathies
ECG monitoring
Fluid and electrolyte status
Hemodynamic status

Intraaortic balloon counter pulsation
Intracardiac pressures
Intracranial pressure monitoring
Neuropyschological status

The primary goal of the intensive care unit (ICU) team is to achieve hemodynamic stability and optimal oxygen transport for each patient with a view to eventual return to maximal functional participation in life and activity. This chapter presents an introduction to monitoring systems used in the evaluation of cardiopulmonary status in patients in the ICU and describes some related elements of cardiopulmonary regulation and control that are relevant to the assessment of risk and oxygen transport status, and to physical therapy intervention.

ICUs have become highly specialized. Medical advances now preserve lives that would have been lost in the past. Patients admitted to the ICU, therefore, require intense and often invasive yet life-preserving medical management. ICUs can be categorized as either general or specific. In major hospital centers, units are often designed and staffed for the exclusive management of specific types of conditions, such as medical, surgical, trauma, burns, coronary, or neonatal care. Although monitoring priorities may differ among specialized ICUs, the principles are similar and relate either directly or indirectly to the foremost goal of preserving life by optimizing oxygen transport and minimizing threat to it and by preventing the risks associated with recumbency and restricted mobility.

The cardiopulmonary status of the patient in the ICU is often jeopardized by fluid and electrolyte disturbances and acid-base imbalance. This chapter describes the regulation of these systems and the clinical implications of imbalance, with special reference to the patient in the ICU. The principal monitoring systems used in assessing cardiopulmonary sufficiency in the ICU are highlighted, including the electro-cardiogram (ECG) monitor, arterial and venous lines, intra-cardiac monitoring, and the intracranial pressure (ICP) monitor. Ventricular-assist devices, including the intraaortic counter pulsation technique used to augment myocardial efficiency, are also described.

Familiarity with the extensive monitoring facilities in the ICU allays some of the apprehensions the physical therapist may have about practicing in intensive care. On introduction to the unit, the physical therapist is immediately struck by the high-tech environment. Quality care in this setting depends on harnessing the potential of high-tech monitoring equipment to optimize assessment, treatment selection, and effectiveness, as well as to reduce untoward risk for the patient.

Figure 16-1 illustrates a general view of a typical ICU. A closer view of a patient in the ICU shows life-support equipment and the various lines and catheters that are in place (Figure 16-2, *A, B*). A closer view of the patient demonstrates

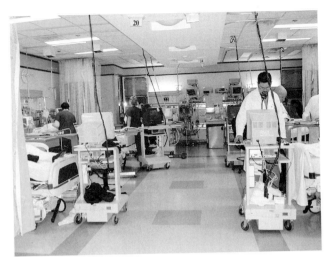

FIGURE 16-1 General view of an intensive care unit.

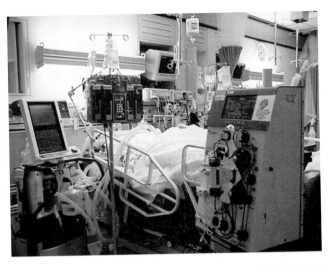

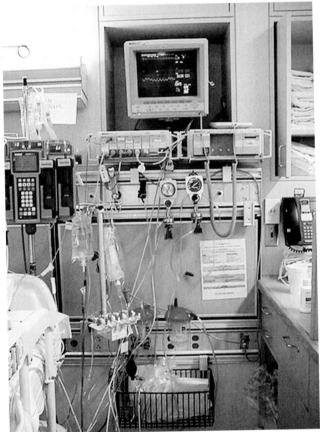

FIGURE 16-2 A, Closer bedside view of a patient in the intensive care unit. Note that with all the equipment, the patient is almost lost. **B**, Bedside monitoring equipment.

precisely where the various lines and catheters are positioned and identifies where caution must be observed. Treatments are modified according to the types and positions of the lines and catheters for each patient (Figure 16-3, *A*, *B*, and *C*).

INTRAVENOUS LINES

Intravenous (IV) lines are routinely established in the superficial veins of patients, such as those on the back of the hand, often before admission to the ICU if the patient is admitted through the emergency room or transferred from the ward. These lines provide an immediate route for fluids, electrolytes, nutrition, and medications. The specific lines used depend on the patient's needs, based on the history, laboratory tests, physical examination, and on-going evaluation.

FLUID AND ELECTROLYTE BALANCE

When the normal regulation of fluid intake, utilization, and excretion are disrupted, fluid, electrolyte, and acid-base imbalances result. Essentially, all medical and surgical conditions threaten these life-dependent mechanisms to some degree. Minor imbalances may be corrected by modification of the patient's nutrition and fluid intake. More major imbalances can be life-threatening, necessitating immediate, highly invasive medical intervention.

Imbalances are reflected as excesses, deficits, or as an abnormal distribution of fluids within the body (Phipps et al, 2000). Excesses result from increased intake and decreased loss of fluid and electrolytes. Deficits result from abnormal shifts of fluid and electrolytes among the intravascular and extravascular fluid compartments of the body. Excesses occur with kidney dysfunction promoting fluid retention and with respiratory dysfunction, which promotes carbon dioxide retention. Deficits are commonly associated with reduced intake of fluids and nutrition. Diaphoresis and wounds can also contribute to significant fluid loss. Diarrhea and vomiting

drain the gastrointestinal tract of fluid stores. Hemorrhage is always responsible for fluid and electrolyte loss. Deficits may be secondary to fluid entrapment and localized edema within the body (third-spacing), making this source of fluid unavailable for regulation of homeostasis.

Moderate to severe fluid imbalance can be reflected in the systemic blood pressure and central (jugular) venous pressure

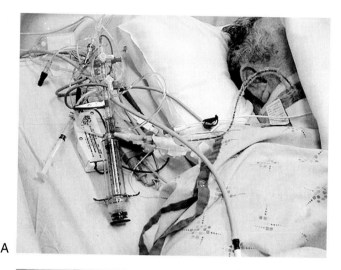

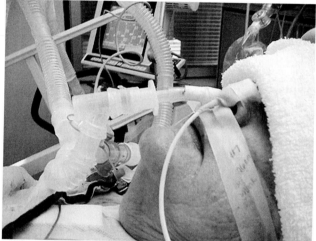

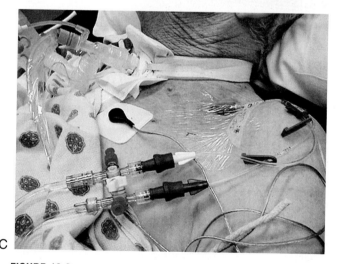

FIGURE 16-3 A, Note the Swan-Ganz catheter on the right jugular vein. **B,** The patient is on a ventilator with a nasoendotracheal tube in place. **C,** Tracheostomy and left subclavian central venous catheter.

(CVP). Elevated blood pressure can be indicative of fluid overload, but an intravascular fluid deficit of 15% to 25% must develop before blood pressure drops significantly. The jugular vein becomes distended with fluid overload. Normally, the jugular pulse is not visible 2 cm above the sternal angle when the individual rests at a 45-degree angle. If the jugular pulse is noted, this can be a sign of fluid overload.

Fluid replacement is based on a detailed assessment of the patient's needs. Whole blood is preferred for replacing blood loss. Plasma, albumin, and plasma volume expanders such as Dextran can be used to substitute for blood loss and to help reestablish blood volume. Albumin and substances such as Dextran increase plasma volume by increasing the osmotic pressure of the blood, hence the reabsorption of fluid from the interstitial space. Low-molecular-weight Dextran has the added advantage of augmenting capillary blood flow by decreasing blood viscosity and is therefore particularly useful in treating shock.

Clinical Picture

Excesses and deficits of fluids and electrolytes can be determined on the basis of laboratory determinations of serum levels of the specific electrolytes. Electrolyte levels and hematocrit are decreased with fluid excess (hemodilution) and are increased with fluid loss (hemoconcentration).

Excess fluid can be managed by controlled fluid intake, normal diuresis, and diuretic medications. Replacement of fluid and electrolyte losses can be achieved by oral intake, tube feeding, IV infusion, and parenteral hyperalimentation.

Assessment of fluid and electrolyte balance is based on both subjective and objective findings (Table 16-1). At the bedside, the physical therapist must be alert to complaints of headache, thirst, and nausea, as well as changes in dyspnea, skin turgor, and muscle strength. More objective assessment is based on fluid intake, output, and body weight. Fluid balance is so critical to physical well-being and cardiopulmonary sufficiency that fluid input and output records are routinely maintained at bedside. These records also include fluid volume lost in urine and feces, wound drainage, and fluids aspirated from any body cavity (e.g., abdomen and pleural space).

A patient's weight may increase by several kilograms before edema is apparent. The dependent areas of the body manifest the first signs of fluid excess. Patients on bed rest show sacral swelling; patients who can sit on the edge of the bed or in a chair for prolonged periods tend to show swelling of the feet and hands.

Decreased skin turgor can indicate fluid deficit. Tenting of the skin over the anterior chest in response to pinching may suggest fluid depletion. Wrinkled, toneless skin is more common in younger patients.

Weight loss may be deceptive in the patient on IV fluids, who can be expected to lose half a kilogram a day (approximately 1 pound). This sign, therefore, should not necessarily be interpreted as underhydration. In contemporary ICU care, supplemental nutrition is a priority to maintain fluid and

TABLE 16-1

Assessment of Fluid and Electrolyte Imbalance

AREA	FLUID EXCESS/ELECTROLYTE IMBALANCE	FLUID LOSS/ELECTROLYTE IMBALANCE
Head and neck	Distended neck veins, facial edema	Thirst, dry mucous membranes
Extremities	Dependent edema "pitting," discomfort from weight of bed covers	Muscle weakness, tingling, tetany
Skin	Warm, moist, taut, cool feeling when edematous	Dry, decreased turgor
Respiration	Dyspnea, orthopnea, productive cough, moist breath sounds	Changes in rate and depth of breathing
Circulation	Hypertension, jugular pulse visible at 45-degree sitting angle, atrial dysrhythmias	Pulse rate irregularities, dysrhythmia, postural hypotension, sinus tachycardia
Abdomen	Increased girth, fluid wave	Abdominal cramps

Modified from Phipps, W.J. Long, B.C. Woods, N.F. (Eds), (1991). Medical-surgical nursing: concepts in clinical practice, ed 4. St. Louis, Mosby.

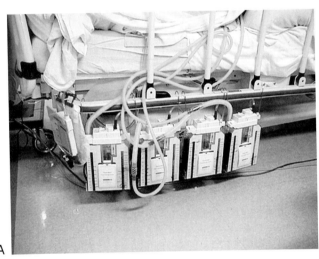
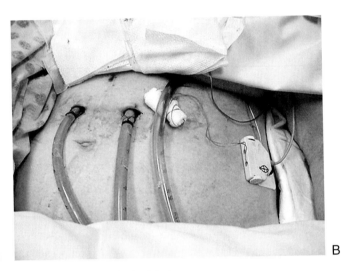

FIGURE 16-4 A, Chest tube drainage. **B,** Anterior view; mediastinal drains.

electrolyte balance, minimize weight loss, preserve strength and stamina, and support healing and recovery. Prescribing nutritional supplements for the patient in the ICU is a specialty in the field of nutrition and can take various forms, depending on the patient's specific needs.

The cardiopulmonary assessment can reveal changes in fluid balance. Lung sounds are valuable in identifying fluid overload. Vesicular sounds may become more bronchovesicular in quality. Crackles may increase in coarseness. In the presence of fluid retention involving the pleurae, breath sounds diminish to the bases. Dyspnea and orthopnea may also be symptomatic of fluid excess.

An early sign of congestive heart failure (CHF) with underlying fluid overload is an S_3 gallop (Ken-TUCK-y) caused by rapid ventricular filling.

Vigilance by the physical therapist with respect to fluid and electrolyte balance is essential in all areas of practice, not only in the ICU. Fluid imbalance is common in older people and in young children, so it needs to be watched for on the ward, in the home, and in the community.

CHEST TUBE DRAINAGE AND FLUID COLLECTION SYSTEMS

Chest tubes are large catheters placed in the pleural cavity to evacuate fluid and air and to drain into a graduated collection reservoir at bedside (Phipps et al, 2000). A typical chest tube drainage and collection system is shown in Figure 16-4, *A*. The removal of thick fluids such as blood and organized exudates by chest tubes is often indicated to prevent entrapment and loculation. Chest tubes are commonly inserted in the sixth intercostal space in the mid or posterior axillary line. Chest tubes inserted into the pleural space are used to evacuate air or exudate. Chest tubes can also be inserted into the mediastinum to evacuate blood such as after open heart surgery (Figure 16-4, *B*).

Any collection system is designed to seal the drainage site from the atmosphere and offer minimal resistance to the drainage of fluid and gas. This is accomplished by immersing the end of the collection tube in water. This is referred to as an underwater seal system. Additional reservoirs are included to decrease the resistance to fluid leaving the chest. This resistance is greater in a single-reservoir system in which the reservoir serves as both the collection receptacle and the underwater seal. A third reservoir can be added to the system; it is attached to the suction and serves as a pressure regulator. The more elaborate drainage systems are used for precise measurement of fluid loss in patients after thoracic and cardiovascular surgery.

The amount of exudate collected in the reservoir is measured every several hours or more often if the patient is losing considerable amounts of fluid or less than the amount predicted. This information is incorporated into the overall fluid-balance assessment. In addition, changes in the quantity and quality of exudates should be noted by the physical therapist before, during, and after changes in position and therapeutic interventions.

ACID-BASE BALANCE

Control of acid-base balance in the body is achieved by regulation of the hydrogen ion concentration in the body fluids (Guyton & Hall, 2000; Shapiro et al, 1994). The pH of the body is normally maintained within a narrow range of 7.35 to 7.45, or slightly alkaline. When pH of the blood drops below 7.35, a state of acidosis exists; above 7.45, a state of alkalosis exists. Regulation of pH is vital because even slight deviations from the normal range cause marked changes in the rate of cellular chemical reactions. A pH below 6.8 or above 8 is incompatible with life.

Acid-base balance is controlled by several regulatory buffer systems, primarily the carbonic acid-bicarbonate, phosphate, and protein buffer systems. These systems act very quickly to prevent moment-to-moment changes in pH. In compensation, pH is returned to normal primarily by altering the component not primarily affected (i.e., if the primary cause is respiratory, the compensating mechanism is metabolic). If the primary cause is metabolic, the compensating mechanism is respiratory. The lungs compensate for metabolic problems over hours, whereas the kidneys compensate for respiratory problems over days (Chapter 10).

Clinical Picture

A guide to the clinical presentation of acid-base imbalances is shown in Table 16-2. Along with the major distinguishing characteristics of acid-base imbalance described in this chapter and elsewhere in this volume, potassium excess (hyperkalemia) is associated with both respiratory and metabolic acidosis, and neuromuscular hyperexcitability is associated with both respiratory and metabolic alkalosis.

BLOOD GASES

Analysis of the composition of arterial and mixed venous blood provides vital information about respiratory, cardiac, and metabolic function (Ganong, 2003; West, 2004; see Chapter 10). For this reason, blood gases are usually analyzed

TABLE 16-2
Signs and Symptoms of Common Acid-Base Disturbances

Respiratory Acidosis	**Metabolic Acidosis**
Hypercapnia	Bicarbonate deficit
Hypoventilation	Hyperventilation
Headache	Headache
Visual disturbances	Mental dullness
Confusion	Deep respirations
Drowsiness	Stupor
Coma	Coma
Depressed tendon reflexes	Hyperkalemia
Hyperkalemia	Cardia dysrhythmias (secondary to hyperkalemia)
Ventricular fibrillation (secondary to hyperkalemia)	
Respiratory Alkalosis	**Metabolic Alkalosis**
Hypocapnia	Bicarbonate excess
Lightheadedness	Depressed respirations
Numbness/tingling of digits	Mental confusion
Tetany	Dizziness
Convulsions	Numbness/tingling of digits
Hypokalemia	Muscle twitching
Cardiac dysrhythmias (secondary to hypokalemia)	Tetany
	Convulsions
	Hypokalemia
	Cardia dysrhythmias (secondary to hypokalemia)

daily in the ICU. In cases where the patient's condition is changing for better or worse over a short period of time or when a specific treatment response is of interest, blood gases may be analyzed several times daily. With an arterial line in place, frequent blood gas analysis is feasible and not traumatic for the patient. Should the patient be anemic, however, blood loss associated with repeated arterial blood sampling may mean that it is contraindicated. Thus, requests for arterial blood gas analysis need to be particularly stringent in patients who are anemic.

Arterial saturation (SaO_2), the proportion of hemoglobin combined with oxygen, can be readily monitored noninvasively by a pulse oximeter (SpO_2). The earlobe or a finger is initially warmed by rubbing before attaching the oximeter sensor. Within seconds, the SpO_2 can be read directly from the monitor. Pulse oximetry is a useful adjunct for routine evaluation of the effectiveness of mechanical ventilation, the effect of anesthesia, and the treatment response. Continuous estimation of SaO_2 is particularly useful before, during, and after mobilization and exercise, position changes, and other therapeutic interventions. The SaO_2 may appear to be reduced in patients who are anemic or jaundiced or have reduced cardiac output. The SpO_2 is less valid in patients with poor peripheral perfusion, who have cold extremities, or who have pigmented skin. The oxygenation of patients in the ICU varies considerably over time and even moment-to-moment, irrespective of sedation, high post end-expiratory pressure, or inverse ventilation (Tsai et al, 1999).

Mixed venous oxygen saturation ($S\bar{v}O_2$) provides a useful index of oxygen delivery and utilization at the tissue level (Copel & Stolarik, 1991). $S\bar{v}O_2$ is highly correlated to tissue oxygen extraction, and thus is a good index of the adequacy of oxygen delivery. The $S\bar{v}O_2$ is particularly useful as a significant warning sign, a guide to myocardial function, and has been used as a tool to titrate positive end-expiratory pressure support. The normal value of $S\bar{v}O_2$ is 75%. $S\bar{v}O_2$ values of less than 60% or a drop of 10% for several minutes is a cause for concern. Excessive $S\bar{v}O_2$ values above 80% are also cause for concern. High $S\bar{v}O_2$ values may occur in patients with left-to-right shunts in the heart, hyperoxia, hypothermia, cyanide toxicity, sepsis, anesthesia, and drug-induced paralysis. Despite its general clinical usefulness, $S\bar{v}O_2$ is a nonspecific indicator of the adequacy of oxygen transport (i.e., of the balance between oxygen supply and demand). Abnormal $S\bar{v}O_2$ values do not indicate precisely where the problem lies; so other hemodynamic variables need to be considered. Further, $S\bar{v}O_2$ has been reported to fluctuate as much as ± 6% in patients in the ICU in response to routine activity and treatment (Noll et al, 1992). Maintaining normal $S\bar{v}O_2$ in patients with multiple trauma improves survival rates over those in whom oxygen transport values are maintained at above normal levels (Kremzar et al, 1997). Enhancing cardiac output and hemoglobin as well as $S\bar{v}O_2$ is essential to increase oxygen delivery (DO_2) above its critical level and avoid tissue oxygen debt (Vallet et al, 2000). Impaired extraction at the tissue level has been attributed to heterogeneity of oxygen delivery (Walley, 1996).

Hypoxemia

In health, age and body position are factors that reduce arterial oxygen tension (Oakes, 2000). Arterial oxygen levels diminish with age as a result of reduced alveolar surface area, pulmonary capillary blood volume, and diffusing capacity. Normal PaO_2 levels in older people should exceed 110-0.5 (age). In a young adult, PaO_2 ranges from 90 to 100 mm Hg in the upright seated position. In the supine position, this range is reduced to 85 to 95 mm Hg and in sleeping, to 70 to 85 mm Hg. These values are clinically significant in that in older people, smokers, and people with pathology, these positional effects are accentuated. Despite sedation in patients who are critically ill, spontaneous variability of PaO_2 is considerable, and factors unduly influencing it must be controlled when using PaO_2 as an outcome (Tsai et al, 1999).

Hypoxemia refers to reduced oxygen tension in the blood. Some common signs and symptoms of various degrees of hypoxemia in adults appear in Table 16-3. Although the brain is protected by autoregulatory mechanisms, an arterial oxygen tension of 60 mm Hg produces signs of marked depression of the central nervous system, reflecting the extreme sensitivity of cerebral tissue to hypoxia.

TABLE 16-3

Signs and Symptoms of Hypoxemia

PaO_2	SIGNS AND SYMPTOMS
80-100 mm Hg	Normal
60-80 mm Hg	Moderate tachycardia, possible onset of respiratory distress
50-60 mm Hg	Malaise
	Lightheadedness
	Nausea
	Vertigo
	Impaired judgment
	Incoordination
	Restless
	Increased minute ventilation
35-50 mm Hg	Marked confusion
	Cardiac dysrhythmias
	Labored respiration
25-35 mm Hg	Cardiac arrest
	Decreased renal blood flow
	Decreased urine output
	Lactic acidosis
	Poor oxygenation
	Lethargy
	Maximal minute ventilation
	Loss of consciousness
<25 mm Hg	Decreased minute ventilation (secondary to depression of respiratory center)

Hypoxemia is compensated primarily by increased cardiac output, improved perfusion of vital organs and, in the long term, polycythemia. Secondary mechanisms of compensation include improved unloading of oxygen at the tissue level as a result of tissue acidosis and anaerobic metabolism, which is achieved through a rightward shift of the oxyhemoglobin dissociation curve.

The progressive physiological deterioration observed at decreasing arterial oxygen levels will occur at higher oxygen levels if any one of the major compensating mechanisms for hypoxemia is defective. Even a mild drop in PaO_2, for example, is poorly tolerated by a patient with reduced hemoglobin and impaired cardiac output. Alternatively, the signs and symptoms of hypoxemia may appear at lower arterial oxygen levels (e.g., in patients with chronic airflow limitation who have adapted to reduced PaO_2 levels).

Monitoring oxygen kinetics is essential to understanding oxygen transport status in patients who are critically ill and to intervening early (Walley, 1996; Wiedemann et al, 1984). DO_2 and $\dot{V}O_2$ and their constituents can be measured directly or indirectly with calorimetry. Patients who survive heart failure have different oxygen kinetic profiles from those who do not (Inoue et al, 1993). In response to improved cardiac index and DO_2 in survivors, $\dot{V}O_2$ did not change, whereas the oxygen extraction ratio (OER) decreased. In nonsurvivors, $\dot{V}O_2$ increased and the OER did not change. Such profiles can be of assistance in establishing baseline information, in detecting changes early, and in modifying physical therapy interventions.

Hyperoxia

Mean tissue oxygen tensions rise less than 10 mm Hg when pure oxygen is administered to a healthy subject under normal conditions. Therefore, the function of nonpulmonary tissues is little altered. In the lung, high concentrations of oxygen replace nitrogen in poorly ventilated regions. This results in collapse of areas with reduced ventilation-perfusion matching (denitrogen atelectasis). Lung compliance is diminished.

High concentrations of oxygen (inspired oxygen fractions greater than 50%) directly injure bronchial and parenchymal lung tissue. The toxic effect of oxygen is both time- and concentration-dependent. Very high concentrations of oxygen may be tolerated for up to 48 hours. However, high concentrations of oxygen in combination with positive pressure breathing can predispose the patient to oxygen toxicity and lung parenchymal injury. At concentrations of inspired oxygen less than 50%, clinically detectable oxygen toxicity is unusual, regardless of the duration of oxygen therapy.

Hypocapnia

Acute reductions in arterial carbon dioxide levels (hypocapnia) results in alkalosis and diminished cerebral blood flow secondary to cerebral vasoconstriction. The major consequences of abrupt lowering of $PaCO_2$ are altered peripheral and central nerve function. Mechanical ventilation may initially cause an abrupt decrease in arterial PCO_2 and lead to a life-threatening situation. In addition to blood gas analysis, end tidal CO_2 measurement is useful in that it provides an index of $PaCO_2$.

Hypercapnia

CO_2, the principal end product of metabolism, is a relatively benign gas. CO_2 has a key role in ventilation and in regulating changes in cerebral blood flow, pH, and sympathetic tone. Acute increases in CO_2 (hypercapnia) depress the level of consciousness secondary to the effect of acidosis on the nervous system. Similar but slowly developing increases in CO_2, however, are relatively well tolerated. A high $PaCO_2$ is suggestive of alveolar hypoventilation, which causes a reduction in alveolar and arterial PO_2. Some patients with severe chronic airflow obstruction have been reported to be able to lead relatively normal lives with $PaCO_2$ in excess of 90 mm Hg if hypoxemia is countered with supplemental oxygen. Acute administration of oxygen to patients with chronic obstructive lung disease, however, may be hazardous, because it interferes with their hypoxic drive to breathe, on which they are reliant.

Acute hypercapnia enhances sympathetic stimulation, causing an increase in cardiac output and in peripheral vascular resistance. These effects offset the effect of excess hydrogen ions on the cardiovascular system, allowing better tolerance of low pH than with metabolic acidosis of a similar degree. At extreme levels of hypercapnia, muscle twitching and seizures may be observed. Trends in $PaCO_2$ can be monitored indirectly using end tidal CO_2 measurements.

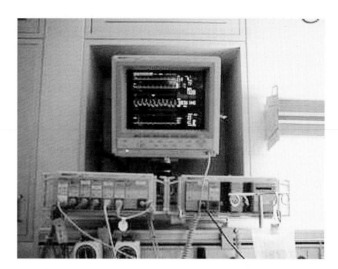

FIGURE 16-5 ECG monitor.

ECG MONITORING

A single-channel ECG monitor with an oscilloscope, strip recorder, and digital heart rate display is typically located above the patient at bedside in the ICU (Figure 16-5). The ECG can often be observed both at bedside and at a central monitoring console, where the ECGs of all patients in the ICU may be observed simultaneously.

The ECG monitor allows for continuous surveillance of the patient, regardless of activity. Low and high heart rates are determined; rates below and above those rates will trigger an alarm. For routine monitoring in the coronary care unit, a modified chest lead is often used. Three electrodes are positioned on the chest to provide optimal information regarding changes in rhythm and heart rate and thereby ensure close patient monitoring. The positive electrode is positioned at the fourth intercostal space at the right sternal border. The negative electrode is positioned at the first intercostal space in the left midclavicular line. The ground electrode, used to dissipate electrical interference, is often positioned at the first intercostal space in the right midclavicular line, although the ground electrode may be positioned wherever convenient. Other electrode placements may be required, for example, in patients with pacemakers or in patients with chest burns. The electrode wires are usually secured to the patient's gown.

Problems with the monitor usually result from faulty technique, electrical interference, or movement artifact. A thickened baseline can be caused by 60-cycle electrical interference. An erratic signal often results from coughing and movement. The cause of any irregularity must be explained and untoward changes in electrical activity of the myocardium ruled out. It is a dangerous practice for the physical therapist to turn off the ECG alarm system during treatment.

Cardiac dysrhythmias can be broadly categorized into tachdysrhythmias and bradydysrhythmias. Tachydysrhythmias are subdivided into supraventricular and subjunctional tachycardias. Bradydysrhythmias are subdivided into sinus

---

TABLE 16-4

Clinical Picture of Common Dysrhythmias

DYSRHYTHMIA	IN HEALTHY INDIVIDUALS WITH NO UNDERLYING CARDIOVASCULAR DISEASE	IN INDIVIDUALS WITH UNDERLYING CARDIOVASCULAR DISEASE
I. Tachycardias		
A. Supraventricular tachycardia	No symptoms Abrupt-onset palpitations, lightheadedness nausea, fatigue	May precipitate congestive heart failure, acute coronary insufficiency, myocardial infarction, pulmonary edema
1. Sinus tachycardia	Awareness of the heart on exertion or with anxiety	Secondary to some precipitating factor, e.g., fever, electrolyte imbalance, anemia, blood and fluid loss, infection, persistent hypoxemia in COPD, acute MI, congestive heart failure, thyrotoxicosis
2. Paroxysmal atrial tachycardia (PAT)	Prevalent, sudden onset, precipitated by coffee, smoking, and exhaustion	Common supraventricular tachycardia Spontaneous onset of regular palpitations that can last for several hours May be obscured by myocardial insufficiency and CHF in older patients Increased anxiety and report of fatigue
3. Atrial flutter	Rare May be difficult to distinguish from PAT May be precipitated by alcohol, smoking, physical and emotional strain	Rapid regular-irregular rate Suggests block at AV node Atrial flutter waves in jugular venous pulse
4. Atrial fibrillation	Rare, occasionally with alcohol excess in the young	Usually secondary to a variety of cardiac disorders
5. Paroxysmal atrial tachycardia with block	Rare	Common arrhythmia seen with digitalis toxicity
B. Subjunctional	Rare	Usually related to MI, pulmonary embolus, severe CHF Often unconscious, cyanotic, ineffective pulse, blood pressure and respiration
1. Ventricular tachycardia	Rare	Predisposed to ventricular fibrillation
2. Ventricular fibrillation	Rare	Ineffective cardiac output, unconscious, dusky; cardiac arrest threatens
II. Bradycardias		
A. Sinus bradycardia	Physiologic in very fit young adults	In older patients may suggest sinus node and conduction system pathology; can produce syncope or CHF
B. Heart block	Rare	Hypotension, dizziness, light-headedness, syncope In chronic block with sustained bradycardia, CHF may be more frequent Most common dysrhythmia iatrogenically produced with digitalis excess Associated with numerous cardiac conditions; commonly in age-related degenerative disease in conducting system, inferior and occasionally anterior MIs

---

bradycardia and those related to heart block and conduction abnormalities. The subjunctional tachycardias and ventricular dysrhythmias are particularly life-threatening. Ventricular tachycardia and ventricular fibrillation are medical emergencies requiring immediate recognition and treatment.

The characteristic features of dysrhythmic ECG tracings are illustrated in Chapter 12. Physical therapists specializing in ICU management should be thoroughly familiar with ECG interpretation and the implications of the various dysrhythmias on patient management. For further elaboration of ECG

application and interpretation, refer to Kinney and Packa (1995) and Dubin (2000).

Clinical Picture

The clinical picture associated with cardiac dysrhythmias depends on the nature of the dysrhythmia, the age and condition of the patient, the medications and, specifically, the absence or presence of underlying heart disease. The distinguishing clinical features of common atrial and ventricular dysrhythmias are outlined in Table 16-4.

The subjunctional or ventricular dysrhythmias are typically associated with severe illness. Cyanosis and duskiness of the mucosal linings and periphery may be apparent. The patient is unresponsive, the pulse is ineffective, and spontaneous respirations are likely to be absent. In this case, defibrillation is initiated by the nursing and medical staff to restore an effective, more normal rhythm. The high incidence of myocardial conduction irregularities warrants a defibrillator being present at all times in the ICU for rapid implementation of this common cardioversion procedure by the medical and nursing staff. Ventricular dysrhythmias may be better tolerated if ventricular rate is low, thereby improving cardiac output. Even in this circumstance, however, these dysrhythmias present an emergency.

The ECG of a patient with a pacemaker reflects either an imposed fixed or intermittent rhythm and rate, depending on whether a fixed-rate or a demand pacemaker has been inserted. The electrical impulse from the pacemaker has a unique ECG wave form.

HEMODYNAMIC MONITORING

Hemodynamic status reflects the adequacy of blood volume and electromechanical coupling of the myocardium to effect adequate cardiac output and peripheral perfusion commensurate with changing metabolic demand. In individuals who are not critically ill, monitoring fluid input and output, and heart rate and blood pressure may suffice in providing a profile. To monitor a patient's hemodynamics more closely in the ICU, however, the insertion of various invasive lines may be indicated in addition to the lines and leads needed to monitor basic fluid and electrolyte balance and ECG. These require invasive arterial and venous lines.

Intraarterial Lines

An arterial line is established by direct arterial puncture. It is usually in the radial artery; however, it can also be seen in the femoral or brachial artery (Figure 16-6, *A, B*). Blood pressure can be measured directly from this line. A digital monitor displays systolic and diastolic blood pressures above the patient at bedside. High and low blood pressure levels are set, above and below which the alarm will sound. Blood gas analysis can be performed routinely with an intraarterial line in place without repeated the puncture of a blood vessel.

Pulmonary Artery Balloon Flotation Catheter (Swan-Ganz Catheter)

The pulmonary artery balloon floatation catheter (Swan-Ganz catheter) is designed to provide an accurate and convenient means of hemodynamic assessment in the ICU by monitoring intracardiac pressures (Buchbinder & Ganz, 1976; Swan, 1975) and, in combination with other measures, assessing cardiac reserve, an important determinant of outcome following critical illness (Timmins et al, 1992). The catheter is usually inserted into the internal jugular vein, the subclavian

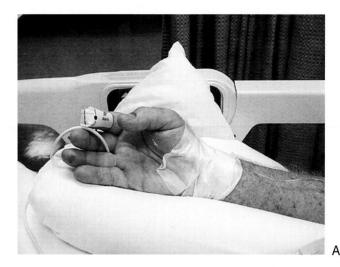

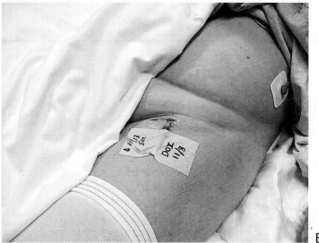

FIGURE 16-6 **A**, Radial arterial line. Also note the pulse oxymeter sensor on the finger. **B**, Femoral arterial line.

vein, or a large peripheral arm vein and is directed by the flow of blood into the right ventricle and pulmonary artery (see Figure 16-3, *A*). The catheter is securely taped to the patient's arm, which is splinted with an arm board to prevent dislodging. The procedure is associated with little risk and discomfort. Some of the complications that have been associated with pulmonary artery catheterization, however, include infection, venous thrombosis, myocardial irritation, air embolism, and pulmonary ischemia or infarct to segmental lung tissue (Puri et al, 1980).

Complex catheters are available for monitoring a variety of parameters. In a two-lumen catheter, the first lumen is used to measure pulmonary artery pressure (PAP) and obtain mixed venous blood samples. The second lumen terminates in a balloon with a volume of less than 1 ml, which is inflated and deflated to obtain pulmonary artery occlusion or wedge pressure (PAOP or PAWP). The normal range of the systolic PAP is 20 to 30 mm Hg, and it normally reflects right ventricular pressure

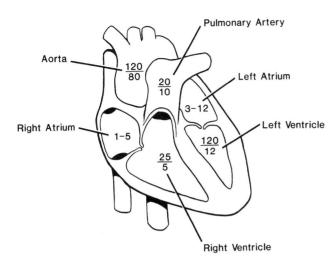

FIGURE 16-7 Normal cardiac pressures in each heart chamber.

(RVP). The diastolic PAP ranges from 7 to 12 mm Hg and reflects left ventricular pressure in the absence of pulmonary disease. The average range of PAWP is 8 to 12 mm Hg and gives an estimation of mean left atrial pressure (LAP) and the pressure in the left ventricle (LVP). More elaborate catheters have pacing wires, thermistors for cardiac output determination, and sensors for arterial saturation. Cardiac output has been reported to remain relatively stable in ventilated patients who are critically ill and receiving high positive end-expiratory pressures (15 cm H_2O) and inverse ratio ventilation (2:1) (Huang et al, 2000). Figure 16-7 shows the normal cardiac pressures in each heart chamber. Abnormal cardiopulmonary function and fluid disturbances may cause these readings to vary.

The PAP increases as a result of elevated pulmonary blood flow, increased pulmonary arteriolar resistance secondary to primary pulmonary hypertension or mitral stenosis, and left ventricular failure. Measurement of PAP and PAWP in particular allows for more prudent management of heart failure and cardiogenic shock.

The PAP, PAWP, and end diastolic LVP are directly related. Impaired left ventricular contractility that compromises normal emptying (e.g., left ventricular failure, mitral stenosis, or mitral insufficiency) results in an elevated end diastolic LVP which, in turn, elevates PAWP and PAP. An end diastolic, a PAP, or a PAWP greater than 12 mm Hg is considered abnormal.

The PAP and PAWP are low during hypotension secondary to hypovolemia. Infusion of normal saline, whole blood, or low-molecular-weight Dextran elevates the blood volume and blood pressure. Restoration of blood volume returns end diastolic PAP and PAWP to normal.

Elevation of the end diastolic PAP secondary to heart failure with pulmonary edema can typically be reduced with appropriate medication. The effectiveness of a drug and its prescription parameters can be assessed by the observed changes in the end diastolic PAP.

Deterioration of cardiovascular status and worsening of the clinical signs and symptoms of heart failure elevate end-diastolic PAP and PAWP, decrease cardiac output, decrease arterial and right atrial oxygen tension, and increase the oxygen difference between arterial and venous blood. As the heart pump continues to fail, arterial oxygen tension decreases, suggesting abnormal lung function and probably elevated LAP. Pulmonary dysfunction at this stage includes diffusion abnormalities, redistribution of pulmonary blood flow into the less well-ventilated upper lobes, and right-to-left shunting, which causes deoxygenated blood to bypass well-ventilated regions of the lungs. All patients with acute infarction or shock have reduced arterial oxygen tension. When the failing heart is unable to effectively eject blood through the aorta to the systemic circulation, fluid may back up into the lungs. Pulmonary congestion must be cleared before the patient can appropriately respond to oxygen administration.

Despite the enormous benefits of direct invasive hemo-dynamic monitoring to patient assessment and management, the benefits of basic hemodynamic assessment are a fundamental part of the cardiopulmonary assessment, regardless of whether the patient has an invasive line inserted (Kirby et al, 1990). Basic hemodynamic monitoring includes heart rate, ECG, blood pressure, and peripheral tissue perfusion. These are fundamental to the physical therapy assessment of all patients across settings. Even though ECG may not necessarily be monitored by the physical therapist directly in non-ICU settings, knowledge of its status is imperative in order to establish whether an individual is safe to treat and, if so, whether an individual should be premedicated before treatment, how treatment should be modified, and what precautions should be taken.

Measurement of Central Venous Pressure

CVP is monitored by means of a venous line or catheter inserted into the subclavian, basilic, jugular, or femoral vein (see Figure 16-3, *C*). The catheter is advanced to the right atrium by way of the inferior or superior vena cava, depending on the site of insertion. Minimal risk of phlebitis or infection is associated with this procedure.

CVP is the blood pressure measured in the vena cavae or right atrium. Normal CVP ranges from 0 to 5 cm H_2O or from 5 to 10 cm H_2O if measured at the sternal notch or midaxillary line, respectively. Essentially, the CVP provides information about the adequacy of right heart function, including effective circulating blood volume, effectiveness of the heart as a pump, vascular tone, and venous return. Measurement of CVP is particularly useful in assessing fluid volume and fluid replacement. If the patient has chronic airflow limitation, ventricular ischemia, or infarction, the CVP will reflect changes in pathology rather than fluid volume.

Specifically, CVP provides an index of right atrial pressure (RAP). The relationship between RAP and end diastolic LVP is unreliable; therefore, end diastolic PAP and PAWP are used

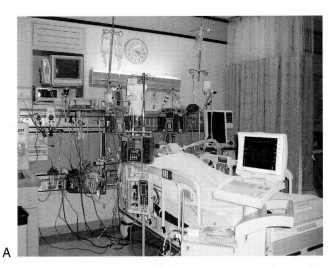

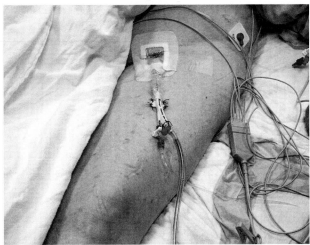

FIGURE 16-8 A, Patient on an intraaortic balloon pump (IABP) support. **B,** Closeup of the IABP insertion on the femoral artery.

as the principal indicators of cardiopulmonary sufficiency in patients in failure and shock.

INTRAAORTIC BALLOON COUNTER PULSATION DEVICE

Intraaortic balloon counter pulsation (Figure 16-8, *A*) provides mechanical circulatory assistance by using an intraaortic balloon. The balloon is inserted into the femoral artery (see Figure 16-8, *B*). To maintain proper placement and good circulation, the patient's leg must be extended. The presence of an intraaortic balloon must be taken into consideration whenever the patient is being treated and positioned. Inflation and deflation of the balloon with helium is correlated with the ECG. The intraaortic balloon is deflated during ventricular systole and assists the emptying of the aorta. Stroke volume is potentiated, afterload is reduced (hence, ventricular pressure), and myocardial oxygen delivery enhanced. The balloon is inflated during diastole, thereby restoring arterial pressure and coronary perfusion. Counterpulsation improves cardiac output, reduces evidence of myocardial ischemia, and reduces

ST-segment elevation. Intraaortic balloon counterpulsation is commonly used after open-heart surgery and for CHF, medically refractory myocardial ischemia, ventricular septal defects, and left main coronary stenosis in patients who are in shock. The intraaortic balloon pump provides protection for the myocardium in many instances until surgery can be performed. Limb ischemia, the most common complication, occurs in 10% to 15% of patients.

Left ventricular assist devices are used postoperatively in patients after open-heart surgery when they have developed cardiogenic shock and are unresponsive to conventional management. These devices take over the pumping action of the left ventricle and decrease myocardial workload and oxygen consumption. These types of assistive devices may have considerable potential in the management of refractory heart failure.

MEASUREMENT OF INTRACRANIAL PRESSURE

ICP results from many neurological insults, including head injury, hypoxic brain damage, aneurysm, hemorrhage, and cerebral tumor, and it may require surgery. In the adult, the cranial vault is rigid and noncompliant. Increases in the volume of the cranial contents result in an elevated ICP and decreased cerebral perfusion pressure.

Changes in consciousness are the earliest and most sensitive indicators of increased ICP (Borozny, 1987; Luce, 1985). Altered consciousness reflects herniation of the brainstem and compression of the midbrain. Compression of the oculomotor nerve and the pupilloconstrictor fibers results in abnormal pupillary reactions that are associated with brain damage.

The effects of ICP on blood pressure and pulse are variable. Blood pressure may be elevated secondary to elevated ICP and hypoxia of the vasomotor center. A reflex decrease in pulse occurs as blood pressure rises.

Compression of upper motor neuron pathways interrupts the transmission of impulses to lower motor neurons; progressive muscle weakness results. A contralateral weakened hand grasp, for example, may progress to hemiparesis or hemiplegia. The Babinski sign, hyperreflexia, and rigidity are additional motor signs that provide evidence of decreasing motor function as a result of upper motor neuron involvement.

Herniation can produce incoordinate respirations that are correlated with the level of brainstem compression. Cerebrate rigidity results from tentorial herniation of the upper brainstem. This results in the blocking of the motor inhibitory fibers and the familiar extended body posture. Seizures may be present. These neuromuscular changes may further compound existing cardiopulmonary complications in the patient in the ICU.

Clinically, increased ICP is best detected by altered consciousness, blood pressure, pulse, pupillary responses, movement, temperature, and respiration (Luce, 1985). The ICP monitor provides direct measurement of ICP. A hollow screw is positioned through the skull into the subarachnoid space. The screw is attached to a Luer-Lok, which is connected to a transducer and oscilloscope for continuous monitoring.

The prevention of further increase in ICP and a corresponding reduction in cerebral perfusion pressure is a treatment priority. High ICP and low cerebral perfusion pressure are highly correlated with brain injury. Measures to reduce venous volume are maintained until ICP has stabilized within normal range. Prudent body positioning is used to enhance venous drainage by elevating the bed 15 to 30 degrees and maintaining the head above heart level. Neck flexion is avoided by the placement of a neck support or sand bags. Fluid intake and output are carefully regulated and monitored; the patient may need to be fluid restricted. Stimulation of the Valsalva maneuver is avoided because intrathoracic pressure and ICP may increase correspondingly.

The normal range of the ICP is 0 to 10 mm Hg for adults and 0 to 5 mm Hg for patients under 6 years of age. The ICP may reach 50 mm Hg in the normal brain; typically, however, this pressure returns to baseline levels instantaneously. In patients with high levels of ICP and low cerebral compliance, extra care must be exercised during routine management and therapy. An ICP up to 30 mm Hg that is elicited by turning or suctioning may be acceptable, provided the pressure drops immediately following removal of the pressure-potentiating stimulus. Patients may be mechanically hyperventilated to keep arterial P_{CO_2} at low levels, because hypercapnia dilates cerebral vessels and hypocapnia constricts them.

To establish whether a patient will tolerate a treatment that requires movement or body positioning, an indication of cerebral compliance is needed. This can be obtained by observing changes in ICP during routine nursing procedures or by titrating small degrees of movement or position change and observing the rate at which the ICP returns to baseline following the challenge. Rapid return to baseline minimizes the risk of reduced cerebral perfusion pressure secondary to the increased ICP. A slow return to baseline or sustained elevation of ICP is consistent with poor cerebral compliance and indicates that treatment should be modified or possibly not performed at all, depending on the absolute level of the ICP. Physical therapy assessment only may be indicated until compliance improves.

ASSESSMENT OF BRAIN ACTIVITY

The Glasgow Coma Scale is a common tool for the clinical assessment and evaluation of the adequacy of basic brain function; it includes review of motor, sensory, pain, arousal, and cognitive status. An electroencephalogram, or EEG, provides useful information about gross cerebral functioning and changes in level of consciousness. A single-channel EEG monitor can be readily used in the ICU to reveal evidence of posttraumatic epilepsy when the clinical signs may be inhibited by muscle relaxants. An EEG assessment may be of benefit to the physical therapist in assessing arousal, prognosis, the capacity of the patient to cooperate with management, the response to treatment of cerebral function, and the planning and prescribing of treatment.

NEUROMUSCULAR ASSESSMENT

The neuromuscular assessment is a fundamental component of the assessment of the patient in the ICU. The patient may have been admitted for a primary neuromuscular problem. In addition, any patient in the ICU is at risk for critical illness polyneuropathy (CIP), which has been associated with the administration of steroids and neuromuscular blockade (Anzueto, 1999). The neuromuscular manifestations of CIP are difficult to assess in a valid manner. Despite this, their early identification is essential so as to avoid significant weakness, irreversible deterioration, delayed recovery, and prolonged dependence on mechanical ventilation (Hund et al, 1996). Other causes need to be ruled out. Prognosis is good if it is detected early and rehabilitation is instituted.

Because many patients in the ICU are administered sedatives and muscle relaxants, placing them at increased risk for CIP, the physical therapist needs to monitor arousal and sedation states. The use of agitation and sedation scales can be useful in monitoring arousal and the patient's capacity to cooperate with treatment (Detriche et al, 1999; Ely et al, 2003). The physical therapist has an important role in minimizing the need for pharmacologic sedation by optimizing pain control, relaxation, comfort, and the individual's perception of control.

Peripheral-nerve electrical stimulation (e.g., of the median nerve) is used to monitor potential neuropathies in a patient in a coma or under neuromuscular blockade. Such stimulation is sufficient to activate the pathways of the ascending reticular activating system associated with consciousness and to hasten awaking from coma (Cooper et al, 1999). In addition, patients score better on repeated assessment with the Glasgow Coma Scale initially and at 1 month after injury, and they have shorter ICU stays.

COGNITIVE ASSESSMENT

The ICU experience can contribute to cognitive impairment or worsen it in patients who are already impaired (Di Carlo et al, 2001; Pisani et al, 2003). These effects can extend for several months beyond the ICU stay (Jackson et al, 2003). Risk factors include functional dependence and low body mass, as well as previous cognitive impairment (Bo et al, 2003). Preexisting cognitive impairment must be identified and changes in cognition should be monitored so they can be detected early. Strategies can be implemented to avoid cognitive impairment, including frequent orientation of the patient to time and place, surrounding the individual with familiar objects and family and friends, using familiar tape recordings (voices or music), taking time to talk to the patient, and being reassuring. Further, strategies to reduce anxiety, stress, restlessness, and negative mood states can reduce the duration of hospitalization in patients in the ICU (Shi et al, 2003).

Acute distress disorder comparable to traumatic stress syndrome has been described recently in individuals after accidental injuries. In addition to the nature of the accident itself and the associated threat to life, factors contributing to an individual's overall stress include hospitalization, length of the ICU stay, the ICU experience, and pain management (Fuglsang et al, 2002; Rundshagen et al, 2002). Thus, optimizing the patient's perception of care is important in preventing and offsetting symptoms of acute distress.

With improvement in the management of acute respiratory distress syndrome (ARDS), long-term studies have examined the relationship between cognitive performance, employability, and return to work in survivors. These patients may exhibit long-term cognitive deficits and impaired health status, which contribute to disability and marked reduction in health-related quality of life (Rothenhausler et al, 2001). An understanding of these potential consequences will help their prevention and the comprehensive management of ARDS.

PAIN ASSESSMENT

Pain has been described as one of the vital signs. Assessing pain in the ICU is particularly challenging, given that patients cannot readily communicate their discomfort and pain. Physical therapists need to monitor discomfort and pain as part of the ongoing assessment to ensure that the patient is as comfortable as possible, that they do not contribute to compromised oxygen transport by increasing distress and $\dot{V}o_2$, that they do not interfere with sleep and recovery, and that noninvasive interventions are exploited as much as possible to reduce the necessity of pharmacologic agents that can compromise the patient's capacity to cooperate with treatment and may contribute to CIP. Optimal management can be achieved only with accurate assessment and ongoing evaluation as the basis of progressing treatment. Pain assessment tools include the McGill pain questionnaire, a pain analog scale, the "faces" scale, and others (Blenkharn, 2002). The format to which the patient can most readily respond to should be selected.

SUMMARY

The capacity of individuals in the ICU to participate in life and perform the requisite activities is severely compromised because of life-threatening illness or injury (i.e., involving the oxygen transport system). The immediate purpose of the ICU is to provide intense life-preserving, specialized care with the view of ultimately returning the individual to a healthy and productive life. Monitoring cardiopulmonary function and oxygen transport is an essential component of the management of the patient in the ICU. Regulation of homeostasis is disrupted in disease or following medical and surgical interventions. Physical therapists practicing in the unit must have a thorough understanding of homeostatic regulation and of the monitoring of fluid and electrolyte balance, acid-base balance, and blood gases. Physical therapy has an essential role in

restoring homeostasis in patients requiring intensive care by using conservative, noninvasive approaches, in addition to averting the musculoskeletal, neuromuscular, and multisystem complications associated with restricted mobility and recumbency. The selection of treatment and the assessment of treatment response are based upon quantitative evaluation of the parameters affecting oxygen transport and cardiopulmonary function as well as the patient's subjective sense of well-being. Meticulous monitoring contributes substantially to the rational management of the patient in the ICU whose status may change from one hour to the next (i.e., the optimization of physical therapy efficacy, in addition to minimizing deleterious treatment outcomes), and to vigilance in preventing deterioration or complications or in detecting them early. This information is critical in establishing the indications for physical therapy intervention, prescribing treatment parameters, and determining when to progress or discontinue treatment. The windows of opportunity for intervention are often narrow, so the physical therapist should be able to identify these expeditiously, on the basis of frequent serial assessment, and to intervene appropriately. Further, psychosocial assessment is fundamental to eliciting the most favorable outcomes and provides the basis for designing optimal programs for patient. Other important outcomes include reduced requirement for invasive care (i.e., drugs and surgery); reduced length of stay in the ICU and in hospital afterwards; patient education that is relevant to the patient's well-being in the short term and the long term; and reduced health care costs. Physical therapists have a major role in exploiting noninvasive, ethical interventions in the ICU and in helping to minimize the costs of this expensive, high-tech, labor-intense area of care. Databases and longitudinal studies of the profiles and long-term outcomes of patients following various critical illnesses after return to the community are needed. Such prognostic information would help to refine the assessment of patients by physical therapists and the short- and long-term management of patients in the ICU.

Review Questions

1. Explain how the International Classification of Function relates to physical therapy goals for patients in the ICU and how this classification can be applied in this setting with special reference to the role of monitoring.

2. Explain the determinants of fluid and electrolyte balance and factors that contribute to fluid excesses and deficits.

3. Describe the basis of acid and base balance.

4. Describe the physiological effects of hypoxia and hypercapnia.

5. Explain the physiological basis of ECG monitoring and common supraventricular and ventricular dysrhythmias.

6. Explain (a) the physiological basis of the pulmonary artery balloon floatation catheter, and

(b) what is represented by altered CVP, RAP (systolic and diastolic), PAP (systolic and diastolic), and the PAWP.

7. Describe the basis of the intraaortic balloon counter pulsation device with respect to improving myocardial function.

8. Describe intracranial pressure monitoring, its physiological basis, and the clinical implications of such monitoring.

9. What are neuropathies and myopathies; what is their clinical significance in the ICU; and what are the implications for the physical therapist?

10. Provide the rationale for cognitive assessment in the ICU.

11. What is the physical therapist's role in pain assessment in the ICU environment?

12. As primarily a noninvasive practitioner, what is the physical therapist's role in patient management in the high-tech ICU environment?

REFERENCES

Anzueto, A. (1999). Muscle dysfunction in the intensive care unit. Clinics in Chest Medicine 20:435-452.

Blenkharn, A., Faughnan, S., & Morgan, A. (2002). Developing a pain assessment tool for use by nurses in an adult intensive care unit. Intensive Critical Care Nursing 18:332-341.

Bo, M., Massaia, M., Raspo, S., Bosco, F., Cena, P., Molaschi, M., & Fabris, F. (2003). Predictive factors of in-hospital mortality in older patients admitted to a medical intensive care unit. Journal of the American Geriatric Society 51:529-533.

Borozny, M.L. (1987). Intracranial hypertension: implications for the physiotherapist. Physiotherapy Canada 39:360-366.

Buchbinder, N., & Ganz, W. (1976). Hemodynamic monitoring: invasive techniques. Anesthesiology 45:146-155.

Cooper, J.B., Jane, J.A., Alves, W.M., & Cooper, E.B. (1999). Right median nerve electrical stimulation to hasten awakening from coma. Brain Injury 13:261-267.

Copel, L.C., & Stolarik, A. (1991). Continuous Svo₂ monitoring: a research review. Dimensions of Critical Care Nursing 10:202-209.

Detriche, O., Berre, J., Massaut, J., & Vincent, J.L. (1999). The Brussels sedation scale: use of a simple clinical sedation scale can avoid excessive sedation in patients undergoing mechanical ventilation in the intensive care unit. British Journal of Anaesthesia 83:698-701.

Di Carlo, A., Perna, A.M., Pantoni, L., Basile, A.M., Bonacchi, M., Pracucci, G., Trefoloni, G., Bracco, L., Sangiovanni, V., Piccini, C., Palmarini, M.F., Carbonetto, F., Biondi, E., Sani, G., & Inzitari, DF. (2001). Clinically relevant cognitive impairment after cardiac surgery: 6-month follow-up study. Journal of Neurological Science 188:85-93.

Dubin, D. (2000). Rapid interpretation of EKGs: a programmed course, ed 6. Tampa, Fla: Cover Publishing.

Ely, E.W., Truman, B., Shintani, A., Thomason, J.W., Wheeler, A.P., Gordon, S., Francis, J., Speroff, T., Gautam, S., Margolin, R., Sessler, C.N., Dittus, R.S., & Bernard, G.R. (2003). Monitoring sedation status over time in ICU patients: reliability and validity of the Richmond Agitation-Sedation Scale (RASS). Journal of the American Medical Association 289:2983-2991.

Fuglsang, A.K., Moergeli, H., Hepp-Beg, S., & Schnyder, U. (2002). Who develops acute stress disorder after accidental injuries? Psychotherapy and Psychosomatics 71:214-222.

Ganong, W.F. (2003). Review of medical physiology, ed 21. New York: McGraw-Hill Professional Publishing.

Guyton, A.C., & Hall, J.E. (2000). Textbook of medical physiology, ed 10. Philadelphia: Elsevier.

Huang, C.C., Tsai, Y.H., Chen, N.H., Lin, M.C., Tsao, T.C., Lee, C.H., & Hsu, K.H. (2000). Spontaneous variability of cardiac output in ventilated critically ill patients. Critical Care Medicine 28:941-946.

Hund, E.F., Fogel, W., Krieger, D., DeGeorgia, M., & Hacke, W. (1996). Critical illness polyneuropathy: clinical findings and outcomes of a frequent cause of neuromuscular weaning failure. Critical Care Medicine 24:1328-1333.

Inoue, T., Morooka, S., Sakai, Y., Fujito, T., Hoshi, K., Ashai, S., & Takabatake, Y. (1993). Oxygen demand-supply relationship in peripheral tissues as a therapeutic indicator in acute myocardial infarction with advanced heart failure. Cardiology 82:30-35.

Jackson, J.C., Hart, R.P., Gordon, S.M., Shintani, A., Truman, B., May, L., & Ely, E.W. (2003). Six-month neuropsychological outcome of medical intensive care unit patients. Critical Care Medicine 31:1226-1234.

Kinney, M.R., & Packa, D.R. (1995). Andreoli's comprehensive cardiac care, ed 8. Philadelphia: Elsevier.

Kirby, R.R., Taylor, R.W., & Civetta, J.M. (1996). Critical care, ed 2. Philadelphia: Lippincott Williams & Wilkins.

Kremzar, B., Spec-Marn, A., Kompan, L., & Cerovic, O. (1997). Normal values of Svo₂ as a therapeutic goal in patients with multiple injuries. Intensive Care Medicine 23:65-70.

Luce, J.M. (1985). Neurologic monitoring. Respiratory Care 30:471-479.

Noll, M.L., Fountain, R.L., Duncan, C.A., Weaver, L., Osmanski, V.P., & Halfmann, S. (1992). Fluctuation in mixed venous oxygen saturation in critically ill medical patients: a pilot study. American Journal of Critical Care 1:102-106.

Oakes, D.F. (2000). Clinical practitioners pocket guide to respiratory care, ed 5. Orono: Health Education Publications.

Phipps, W.J., Long, B.C., & Woods, N.F. (Eds) (2000). Medical-surgical nursing: concepts and clinical practice, ed 7. Philadelphia: Elsevier.

Pisani, M.A., Inouye, S.K., McNicoll, L., & Redlich, C.A. (2003). Screening for preexisting cognitive impairment in older intensity care unit patients: use of proxy assessment. Journal of the American Geriatric Society 51:689-693.

Puri, V.K., Carlson, R.W., Bander, J.J., & Weil, M.H. (1980). Complications of vascular catheterization in the critically ill: a prospective study. Critical Care Medicine 8:495-499.

Rothenhausler, H.B., Ehrentraut, S., Stoll, C., Schelling, G., & Kapfhammer, H.P. (2001). The relationship between cognitive performance and employment and health status in long-term survivors of the acute respiratory distress syndrome: results of an exploratory study. General Hospital Psychiatry 23:90-96.

Rundshagen, I., Schnabel, K., Wegner, C., & Am Esch, S. (2002). Incidence of recall, nightmares, and hallucinations during analgosedation in intensive care. Intensive Care Medicine 28:38-43.

Shapiro, B.A., Peruzzi, W.T., & Kozelowski-Templin, R. (1994). Clinical application of blood gases, ed 5. St. Louis: Mosby.

Shi, S.F., Munjas, B.A., Wan, T.T., Cowling, W.R., 3rd, Grap, M.J., & Wang, B.B. (2003). The effects of preparatory sensory information on ICU patients. Journal of Medical Systems 27:191-204.

Swan, H.J. (1975). Second annual SCCM lecture. The role of hemodynamic monitoring in the management of the critically ill. Critical Care Medicine 3:83-89.

Timmins, A.C., Hayes, M., Yau, E., Watson, J.D., & Hinds, C.J. (1992). The relationship between cardiac reserve and survival in critically ill patients receiving treatment aimed at achieving supranormal oxygen delivery and consumption. Postgraduate Medical Journal 68(Suppl 2):S34-S40.

Tsai, Y.H., Lin, M.C., Hsieh, M.J., Chen, N.H., Tsao, T.C., Lee, C.H., & Huang, C.C. (1999). Spontaneous variability of arterial oxygenation in critically ill mechanically ventilated patients. Intensive Care Medicine 25:37-43.

Vallett, B., Tavernier, B., & Lund, N. (2000). Assessment of tissue oxygenation in the critically-ill. European Journal of Anaesthesiology 17:221-229.

Walley, K.R. (1996). Heterogeneity of oxygen delivery impairs oxygen extraction by peripheral tissues: theory. Journal of Applied Physiology 81:885-894.

West, J.B. (2004). Respiratory physiology—the essentials, ed 7. Baltimore: Williams & Wilkins.

Wiedemann, H.P., Matthay, M.A., & Matthay, R.A. (1984). Cardiovascular-pulmonary monitoring in the intensive care unit (Part 1). Chest 85:537-549.

Cardiovascular and Pulmonary Physical Therapy Interventions

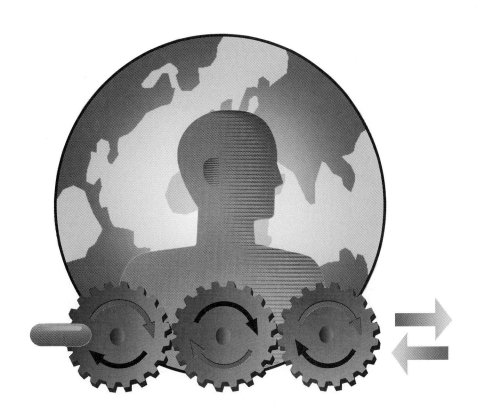

C H A P T E R 1 7

Optimizing Outcomes: Relating Interventions to an Individual's Needs

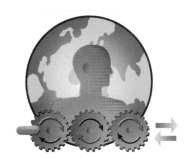

Elizabeth Dean

KEY TERMS

Activity (WHO, 2000)
Clinical decision making
Clinical judgment
Clinical reasoning
Diagnosis
Extrinsic factors
International Classification of Function
  (WHO, 2000)
Intrinsic factors

Oxygen transport limitations
Oxygen transport threats
Participation (WHO, 2000)
Pathophysiological factors
Problem definition
Restricted mobility and recumbency factors
Structure and function (WHO, 2000)
Treatment prescription

As direct access to patients becomes more global, the capacity of the physical therapist to diagnose problems that are amenable to, as well as not amenable to physical therapy is crucial for optimal, safe, and responsible care. After formulating the diagnoses in partnership with the patient as much as possible, the physical therapist prioritizes them to address those most injurious to the patient, which may not necessarily be the reason the individual initially came to see a physical therapist or was referred. This is the essence of evidence-based practice in the context of epidemiological indicators, or evidence-based planning (see Chapter 1).

This chapter provides a basis for clinical decision making and treatment prescription in physical therapy for patients ranging from the individual who is medically unstable and critically ill to the individual who is medically stable with cardiopulmonary dysfunction or risk and living in the community. In addition, physical therapists have an active role on wellness and its promotion in the form of structured programs as well as one-on-one. Thus, the individuals they counsel include those without primary or overt cardiovascular/cardiopulmonary pathology.

Clinical reasoning is the process of critically analyzing the patient's status (participation in life and activities, and anatomic structures or physiological function) with respect to the individual's psychosocial, cultural, and environmental contexts (see Chapter 1). What is the individual able to do (and not able to do); what is the status of the organ systems; and how do these two interrelate? The answers to these questions serve as the basis of the detailed diagnostic workup by the physical therapist. This process results in the diagnoses or problems that are then prioritized so the patient's major needs are addressed appropriately. Initial priorities include life-preserving interventions (including addressing threats) and the minimizing of physical and psychological distress. Facilitators and barriers to the patient's adhering to the treatment recommendations and lifestyle education are clearly identified, and education and treatments are adapted to meet the needs of the individual. With this database, the

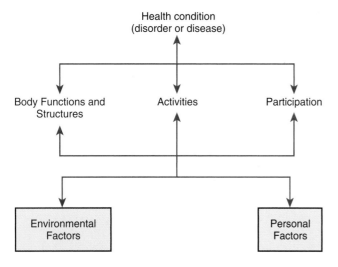

FIGURE 17-1 Model of ability. *(Adapted from the Model of Disablement, World Health Organization, 2000.)*

TABLE 17-1

Tools for Evaluating Domains of Quality of Life (Activity and Participation)

SCALE	DEVELOPERS
General Well-being Scales	
Medical Outcomes Study Short Form (SF-36)	Stewart et al, 1988
Sickness Impact Profile (SIP)	Gibson et al, 1975
Quality of Well-being Scale	Kaplan et al, 1984
Quality of Life Systemic Inventory	McGavin et al, 1977
Nottingham Health Profile	Hunt et al, 1980
Illness Effects Questionnaire	Greenberg et al, 1989
Dartmouth Primary Care Cooperative Information	Wasson et al, 1992
Duke Health Profile	Parkenson et al, 1981
Multidimensional Health Locus of Control Inventory	Wallston & Wallston, 1981
Symptom Questionnaire	Kellner, 1987
Cardiac-specific Scales	
Minnesota Living with Heart Failure Questionnaire	Rector et al, 1987
Outcomes Institute Angina Type Specification	Rogers et al, 1994
Quality of Life after Myocardial Infarction	Oldridge et al, 1991
Ferrans and Powers Quality of Life Index-Cardiac Version	Ferrans & Powers, 1992
Pulmonary-specific Scales	
Chronic Respiratory Disease Questionnaire	Guyatt et al, 1987
St. George's Respiratory Questionnaire	Jones et al, 1992
Pulmonary Functional Status Scale	Weaver & Narsavage, 1992
Pulmonary Functional Status and Dyspnea Questionnaire	Lareau et al, 1994
Living with Asthma Questionnaire	Hyland, 1991

physical therapist prescribes interventions so that their outcomes are maximized in the short term and the long term.

INTERNATIONAL CLASSIFICATION OF FUNCTION

Participation

Of most importance to people is their capacity to live a life consistent with their needs and wants, according to their sociocultural norms. Health has been defined by the World Health Organization as emotional, spiritual, intellectual, as well as physical well being, and not merely the absence of pathology (World Health Organization, 2000). Participation refers to the capacity of individuals to fulfill these needs in a social context and thereby fulfill the multiple roles in their lives—as parent, child, sibling, employee, employer, student, or homemaker, and in avocational pursuits (Figure 17-1). Participation in life is assessed by open-ended questions asked during the history and interview. In addition, an increasing number of scales are available for clinical use. Table 17-1 shows some common scales, categorized as generic or condition-specific, that can be used to assess quality of life, life satisfaction, sickness impact, and subjective sense of well-being. These can be useful outcome measures (technically, these scales provide scores that are indexes rather than actual measures of the constructs) for the physical therapist and the patient. Many of these scales have been shown to be reliable as well as valid. Validating these scales is conceptually and methodologically challenging, hence, their limitations must be appreciated.

Activity

Participation in life and fulfilling one's roles and obligations require being able to perform a range of activities specific to them to some level of proficiency (see Figure 17-1). The role

of a parent, for example, requires being able to identify the needs of children, plan and coordinate activities involved with their care (bathing, dressing, performing physical activities and playing with them, taking them to school, and so on). To fulfill the needs of being a truck driver, the individual needs to drive to work, be able to climb into the truck, be able to check the engine, go under the truck, be able to load and unload it, read a map, as well as drive a standard transmission. To be an elementary school teacher requires being able to move around the classroom, help children with physical tasks, anticipate their needs, anticipate danger, and be able to respond quickly. The assessment must identify the composite activities that are limited and that impact an individual's capacity to participate in fulfilling his or her roles.

Structure and Function

Limitations of anatomic structure and physiological function interfere with the performance of specific activities that are involved in fulfilling roles and obligations in life (i.e., participating in life) (see Figure 17-1). Some limitations may be specific to a particular role, and some may interfere across roles. The assessment identifies the limitations of structure and function and the degree to which they interfere with given activities and roles in life. Some limitations of structure and function related to oxygen transport do not necessarily limit activity or participation, yet they can be the most clinically important, life-threatening problems (e.g., high blood pressure, cardiac dysrhythmias, abnormal clotting factors, high blood sugar, and aerobic deconditioning). Given the prevalence of the diseases of civilization and their risk factors, each individual needs to be assessed for risk of heart disease, smoking-related conditions, hypertension and stroke, diabetes, and cancers (see Chapter 1). Knowledge of a patient's bone health and risk for osteoporosis and arthritis is also prudent.

Physical therapists have a primary role in assessing these risks for several reasons. First, these problems can be the most important clinically in terms of health and threat to life for the patient, either directly or indirectly. Second, identifying these problems enables the physical therapist to work collaboratively with the team in addressing and following them in a coordinated, integrated manner. If a patient was not referred and new problems are detected, the physician needs to be alerted. With direct-access practice, this is a primary responsibility of the contemporary physical therapist. If risks factors have been identified or have manifested clinically, the patient may be on medication or may be a candidate for surgery. The physical therapist has a primary role in avoiding or minimizing the need for invasive care (specifically, drugs and surgery), which constitutes a singularly important and often underestimated goal of the physical therapist, who is committed to noninvasive care. The physical therapist must monitor a patient's responses to invasive care (i.e., drugs and surgery) closely with the intention of reducing such intervention. Third, the physical therapist needs to institute relevant and targeted health education for lifelong behavior change (i.e., assess the patient's needs, including knowledge deficits, learning readiness, and learning style; tailor the education materials to the learner; and assess the outcome of the educational intervention as compared to other physical therapy interventions) (see Chapters 1 and 27). Fourth, the presence of risk factors may require a higher level of patient monitoring. Fifth, physical therapy interventions and their prescriptive parameters may need to be modified based on an individual's risk factors. Sixth, special attention to medications may be indicated, and they may need to be coordinated with physical therapy management. And seventh, the presence of risk factors for the *diseases of* civilization requires long-term management and follow-up.

Psychosocial and cultural factors are assessed to identify beliefs, attitudes, lifestyle behaviors, and expectations of care (see Chapter 1). A learning assessment (see Chapter 28) is conducted to identify knowledge deficits, the learning style of the patient, and readiness to participate in treatment. Identifying facilitators and barriers that will impact the outcome of the therapeutic relationship is central to ensuring maximal therapeutic outcomes, including an individual's subjective sense of well-being and empowerment.

Clinical decision making and treatment prescription are based on the answers to several questions related to oxygen transport status that underpins one's capacity for activity and participation and one's health threat. With respect to a given patient, the following must be considered:

1. What are the problem with respect to participation; activity; and structure and function (impairments); and what are their interrelationships? (Hint: their interrelationships will be individual-specific.)
2. What is the prognosis with and without intervention?
3. What is the relationship between the prognosis for each problem and the treatment objectives and prescription?
4. What are the treatments of choice, and why?
5. What are the treatment priorities, and why?
6. What are the prescriptive parameters for each, and why? How should they be sequenced, and why?
7. What is the course of treatment, and why? What are the requirements for follow-up in the short and long term, and why?

Considering that a patient can have oxygen transport limitations in the absence of participation and activity limitations and that, based on epidemiological evidence, many people do, oxygen transport limitations and risks need to be evaluated in each patient. Underlying risk, without overt manifestation clinically or in daily life, can constitute significant risk to the patient and the potential for significant impact on participation and activity. Furthermore, physical therapy by definition stresses patients physiologically, so knowledge of such threat is essential to ensure that the appropriate monitoring is instituted to maximize safety and that treatments are modified to maximize therapeutic outcome in the short and long term.

The principles involved in relating cardiopulmonary physical therapy interventions to the patient's needs depend on an analysis of what the patient's needs are with respect to participation in life and the composite activities. The degree to which limitations of anatomic structure and physiological function (with a focus on impairments of the steps in the oxygen transport pathway; see Chapter 2) impact activity and participation is assessed. The relationship of impairment to ability and participation cannot be assumed. Verification can be extracted from the history and overall assessment, including measures and indexes of the individual's capacity to perform activities and participate in life. These aspects of the assessment can be captured in standardized questionnaire tools that reveal the impact of health-related quality of life and sickness that can be used as outcome measures in conjunction with measures of anatomic structure and physiological function (see Table 17-1). Changes in structure and function with treatment may or may not have a corresponding effect on the impact of health-related quality of life or sickness. Such knowledge may help to identify those individuals whose quality of life and sickness impact will improve most, and where treatment needs to be targeted (Ferrucci et al, 2000).

A physiologically based treatment hierarchy is presented based on the premise that physiological function, including oxygen transport, is optimal when humans are upright and moving (see Chapters 18 and 19). Applying a systematic physiological approach to diagnosis and the analysis of the patient's problems, with respect to limitations in the oxygen transport pathway, leads directly to the most efficacious treatments. Such an approach provides a rational basis for modifying or discontinuing treatment based on the use of appropriate treatment outcome measures.

WHAT IS THE PROBLEM?

Consistent with the International Classification of Function, there are three primary levels of analysis, namely, structure and function (impairment); ability (limitations or disability); and participation in life (limitations or handicap); and they are affected by facilitating factors and barriers (WHO, 2000) (see Figure 17-1). Structure and function refer to the underlying anatomic and physiological limitations that may or may not contribute to the patient's symptoms but are clinically important and warrant remediation or being considered in management. Limitation of activities contributes to a compromised capacity to fulfill one's roles in life, such as those of occupation, profession, parent, and member of various groups that give one an identity. Usually, a patient presents clinically with complaints of being unable to complete tasks or fulfill roles because of pathophysiological, psychological, or environmental and physical barriers and limitations.

Measures and tools are standardized (concerning validity and reliability, see Chapter 7) for the assessment of each of these levels. With an increased focus on the quality of participation in life, numerous scales have emerged to quantify the subjective sense of well-being and health-related quality of life (see Table 17-1 for some examples).

Oxygen transport is determined by a multitude of factors that affect different steps in the oxygen transport pathway and thereby impact participation in life and related activities (see Figure 17-1; see Chapter 2). For treatment to be directed specifically to the underlying problems, the physical therapist needs to consider several levels of analysis of the deficits contributing to impaired or threatened oxygen transport. To be proficient in such analysis, the physical therapist must have a thorough knowledge of the multiple factors that contribute to abnormal gas exchange or contribute to such abnormality. This knowledge base includes a thorough understanding of the relevant anatomy and physiology; the multisystem and integrative pathophysiology; the impact of medical, surgical, and nursing procedures; the effects of various laboratory tests and procedures; and the impact of pharmacologic agents on cardiopulmonary function (Box 17-1). Assessment of oxygen transport reserve and reserve capacity is fundamental to the management of all patients (Weissman et al., 1994) and their risk factors (Goldhill et al, 1999), regardless of disease acuity. Routine procedures contribute to fluctuations in oxygen demands (Jerusum, 1997). Optimizing the ratio of oxygen

---

BOX 17-1

Fundamental Knowledge and Expertise to Diagnose Limitations in Oxygen Transport and Risk Factors

Oxygen transport deficits and how they impact or threaten participation and activity

Normal cardiopulmonary and cardiovascular anatomy and physiology

Knowledge about how the above are affected by normal conditions such as aging and lifestyle habits (e.g., smoking, stress, and the physical environment)

Physiological adaptation to hypoxia and cardiopulmonary impairment

Cardiopulmonary and cardiovascular pathophysiology and disease processes, and how they affect normal cardiopulmonary and cardiovascular function

Multisystem and integrative pathophysiology that can have a secondary effect on cardiopulmonary function and oxygen transport

Effects of medical, surgical, and nursing procedures on oxygen transport and gas exchange

Investigative laboratory procedures and tests and their effects on cardiopulmonary function

Pharmacologic effects on cardiopulmonary function of any medication

---

BOX 17-2

Steps in Diagnosing Limitations in Oxygen Transport (Structure and Function, WHO, 2000)

1. Determine what factors are specifically contributing to impaired oxygen transport and which steps in the pathway are affected
2. Determine those factors that threaten oxygen transport and the steps in the pathway that are involved
3. Determine the relative magnitude of the effect of each factor that is either impairing or threatening oxygen transport, and prioritize the importance of each
4. Distinguish those factors that are amenable to and those that are *not* amenable to physical therapy in that in the latter, treatment may have to be modified, and the type and level of monitoring may have to be reevaluated
5. Given the answers to 1 through 4, select, prioritize, and apply specific treatments prescriptively, to address each factor that contributes to cardiopulmonary dysfunction and is amenable to physical therapy

---

delivery to consumption improves clinical outcomes in patients who range from being medically stable to being unstable (Corriveau et al, 1989; Kelly, 1996; Lugo et al, 1993).

For a given patient, the cardiopulmonary physical therapist prescribes treatment by extracting the relevant information from the history, the laboratory tests and investigative procedures, and the assessment (Box 17-2; see Part II). Although physical therapists are primarily noninvasive practitioners, they use and request the results of invasive tests and investigations in their assessments and evaluations. Problems are prioritized on the basis of the relative magnitude of each one's threat or effect on oxygen transport limitation. Once the mechanisms of the cardiopulmonary and cardiovascular dysfunction have been identified, specific treatments are selected and prioritized, and then the prescriptive parameters of each treatment are defined. With respect to education, a learning assessment is an essential component of the overall assessment; it identified knowledge deficits and prescribes learning interventions consistent with the patient's needs (Chapter 28).

The diagnoses, or List of Problems

This diagnostic workup is designed to relate oxygen transport limitations and threats to an individual's participation in life and its composite activities. Analysis of oxygen transport limitations are described here.

Impaired Oxygen Transport

Two levels of problems must be identified, namely, functional and physiological limitations. Functional limitations are those that affect the patient's ability to perform activities of daily living (ADLs), such as reduced activity or exercise tolerance as a result of reduced peripheral oxygenation; reduced mobility related to deconditioning resulting from resting in bed; extremity or internal injury; anticoagulant therapy; drug-induced paralysis; impaired physical mobility related to muscle weakness and partial paralysis; paralysis; a depressed level of consciousness; or anemia.

Anatomic and physiological limitations are deficits in oxygen transport overall and specifically at the individual steps in the pathway. Examples of the limitations at each step in the pathway appear in Boxes 17-3 and 17-4.

Threatened Oxygen Transport

Although the complications of restricted mobility and static body positions are well understood, the precise prescription

---

BOX 17-3

Examples of Limitations in and Threats to the Steps in the Oxygen Transport Pathway

Central Control of Breathing

Altered central nervous system (CNS) afferent input and control of breathing
Impaired efferent pathways
Pharmacologic depression
Substance-abuse depression

Airways

Aspiration related to lack of gastrointestinal (GI) motility
Aspiration secondary to esophageal reflux
Obstruction secondary to airway edema, bronchospasm, or mucus
Inhaled foreign bodies

Lungs

Altered breathing pattern secondary to decreased lung compliance
Ineffective breathing pattern related to decreased diaphragmatic function and increased lung volumes, respiratory muscle weakness, respiratory muscle fatigue, CNS dysfunction, guarding, reflex, fatigue, and respiratory inflammatory process
Ineffective airway clearance related to restricted mobility, immobility, sedation, and pulmonary dysfunction secondary to long smoking history, impaired mucociliary transport, absent cilia, or dyskinesia of cilia, retained secretions, ineffective cough and mucociliary mechanisms, infection, inability to cough efficiently, artificial airway/intubation and endotracheal tube, drug-induced paralysis, and sedation
Large airway obstruction secondary to compliant oropharyngeal structures
Chest wall rigidity and decreased compliance
Loss of normal chest wall excursion movements (pump- and bucket-handle motions) and capacity to move appropriately in all three planes of motion
Chest wall and spinal deformity
Impaired lung fluid balance and acute lung injury

Blood

Bleeding abnormalities, altered body temperature (hypothermia, hyperthermia), fever, inflammation, hypermetabolism secondary to mediator systems
Altered body temperature related to integumentary disruption
Low hematocrit secondary to GI bleed (more prone to hypoxia)
Anemia
Thrombocytopenia
Disseminated intravascular coagulation
Abnormal clotting factors (i.e., balance between clotting and not clotting, sludging of blood)
Thromboemboli
Bleeding disorders with liver disease; abnormal clotting factors

Gas Exchange

Alveolar collapse, atelectasis, intrapulmonary shunting or pulmonary edema, shallow breathing and tenacious mucus, body position, consolidation and alveolar collapse, ventilation/perfusion mismatch, airway constriction, fluid volume excess, pleural effusions, breathing at low lung volumes, abdominal distension and guarding, ineffective airway clearance, pulmonary microvascular thrombi and altered capillary permeability secondary to circulating mediators, closure of small airways secondary to dynamic airway compression, decreased functional residual capacity, and intrapulmonary shunting, increased lung surface tension
Diffusion defects

Respiratory Muscles

Upper abdominal surgery, weakness, fatigue, neuromuscular disease, ileus related to gastric distension, mechanical dysfunction

Myocardial Perfusion

Coronary artery occlusion
Tachycardia

Box Continued

BOX 17-3

Examples of Limitations in and Threats to the Steps in the Oxygen Transport Pathway—cont'd

Potential for cardiac dysrhythmia related to reperfusion
Cardiac dysrhythmia related to myocardial hypoxia
Compression by edema or space-occupying lesions

Heart

Decreased venous return and cardiac output secondary to volume deficit, ascites, myocardial ischemia, hemorrhage, and coagulopathies
Conduction defects
Mechanical defects
Defects in electromechanical coupling
Abnormal distension characteristics and myocardial wall compliance
Abnormal afterload

Blood Pressure

Volume deficit/bleeding
Alteration in peripheral tissue perfusion related to acute myocardial infarction, myocardial depression, maldistribution of blood volume, and altered cellular metabolism
Volume excess

Tissue Perfusion

Impaired cardiac output
Impaired secondary to disseminated microvascular thrombi
Atherosclerosis and thromboembolic events, decreased circulating blood volume, decreased vascular integrity, and inflammatory process
Decreased cardiac output related to reduced venous return, impaired right ventricular function, dysrhythmias, increased afterload, and bradycardia

Low oxygen content in the blood
Thromboembolism, vasoconstriction secondary to toxins, sepsis, etc., blood flow alterations and hypermetabolism secondary to mediator systems

Fluid Volume Excess

Related to excessive intravenous administration
Related to impaired excretion
Apparent hypervolemia secondary to restricted mobility and recumbency (e.g., resulting from hemodynamic instability)
Renal failure
Water intoxication
Therapeutic volume expansion, acute myocardial infarction (MI) and acute renal failure related to renal retention of sodium and water and increased levels of aldosterone, renin, angiotensin II, and catecholamines

Fluid Volume Deficit

Fluid volume deficit related to volume losses during surgery and inadequate oral intake, blood loss, internal injuries (e.g., hematoma and third-spacing phenomenon; hormonal imbalance; increased intestinal motility; vomiting; diarrhea; fluid sequestration in tissues; nasogastric [NG] suction and diarrhea; hypovolemia; sepsis and shock; surface capillary leak and fluid loss as in burns and excoriated wounds; fluid shifts)

Tissue Oxygenation

Multisystem organ failure with altered peripheral tissue perfusion and gas exchange at the cellular level

BOX 17-4

Factors that can Contribute Indirectly to Oxygen Transport Limitations

Factors elated to Infection

Pulmonary and nonpulmonary infections increase the demands on the oxygen transport system

Cognitive Factors

Impaired neurological status and central cardiopulmonary control
Alteration in mental status secondary to inadequate cerebral perfusion with hypotension and cardiogenic shock
Sleep pattern disturbance; altered blood gases, and fatigue
Anxiety and agitation related to powerlessness and lack of knowledge, breathlessness, pharmacologic paralysis, impaired verbal community secondary to intubation, paralysis, etc.

Psychosocial Factors

Anxiety related to the condition, shortness of breath, hospitalization, etc.
Social isolation secondary to impaired communication
Fear and hopelessness
Pain response

Nutritional Factors

Altered nutritional needs secondary to greater need than resting state (i.e., increased caloric need and nutrients associated with illness, inability to ingest food, inability to absorb food)
Restricted ingestion of food and water
High caloric needs secondary to infectious process and protein catabolism

parameters for mobilization and body positioning to avoid these complications have not been defined in detail (Chapters 18 and 19). With respect to cardiopulmonary complications, a one- or two-hourly turning regimen is commonly accepted. For the patient who is flaccid or comatose, range-of-motion (ROM) exercises every several hours facilitates blood flow through dependent areas and enhances alveolar ventilation as well as mobilizing joints and muscles. Antiembolic stockings and pneumatic compression devices are routinely used to minimize circulatory stasis in the legs and thereby the potential for thrombi formation.

The physical therapist has a major role in preventing infection of all types but particularly cardiopulmonary infections. Cardiopulmonary assessment and treatment involve handling and close physical contact with patients. Thus the risk of nosocomial infection is high in patients who are hospitalized. Some standard means of preventing infection include meticulous hand washing before and after visiting each patient, avoiding contact with open wounds, and attending to the care of invasive lines and catheters. The physical therapist moves and repositions patients often, so it is essential that the positions of lines, leads, and catheters be continuously monitored. The physical therapist must consider when it is appropriate to don gown, mask, and gloves so as to protect and be protected from the patient adequately.

Factors that Contribute to or Threaten Oxygen Transport

The factors that can impair oxygen transport directly or can threaten it fall into four primary categories (Box 17-5): the underlying cardiopulmonary pathophysiology, restricted mobility (loss of physical exercise stress), recumbency (loss of vertical gravitational stress), extrinsic factors (i.e., those related to the patient's care), and intrinsic factors (i.e., those related to the patient).

Restricted Mobility and Recumbency: Special Examples of Extrinsic Factors

Although bed rest can be considered an extrinsic factor (i.e., a therapeutic intervention that contributes to cardiopulmonary dysfunction), the negative sequelae of this intervention are often not appreciated clinically because of the widespread use of rest in bed. Therefore, to draw the clinician's attention to the fact that the effects of this intervention need to be considered in each patient, the effects of restricted mobility and recumbency are analyzed separately (see Chapters 18 and 19).

Treatment Goals

Once the deficits and threats to oxygen transport have been determined, the goals of treatment fall into three categories: short-term, long-term, and preventive.

Short-term treatment goals are:

1. To empower the patient to manage symptoms and learn strategies to reduce health risk through effective education for life-long health.
2. To correct or reverse cardiopulmonary dysfunction that underlies the threat to or limitations on participation in life and its composite activities.
3. To reduce the rate of deterioration.
4. To avoid worsening the patient's condition.
5. To avoid, reduce, or postpone the need for drugs (including supplemental oxygen) and surgery.

Long-term treatment goals are:

1. To empower the patient through health education that promotes life-long health and well-being, and to minimize the likelihood of the recurrence of problems.
2. To enhance the efficiency of the steps in the oxygen transport pathway overall.
3. To enhance the efficiency of those specific steps in the oxygen transport pathway that compensate for impaired steps that may or may not be reversibly affected.
4. To maximize oxygen transport capacity so as to sustain and optimize healing and allow for maximal functional activity.
5. To avoid, reduce, or postpone the need for drugs (including supplemental oxygen) and surgery.
6. To minimize the need for doctor- and hospital-based care.
7. To reduce the cost of invasive doctor- and hospital-based care and related health care costs.

Preventive treatment goals are:

1. To promote life-long health (full participation in life and its activities) and subjective well-being through patient empowerment and self-responsibility—health and participation for all.

BOX 17-5

Factors that can Limit Oxygen Transport

1. Cardiopulmonary pathophysiology (see Chapter 5)
   - Primary (acute, chronic, acute on chronic)
   - Secondary (chronic, acute on chronic)

   Noncardiopulmonary pathophysiology (abnormalities in other systems that can impair oxygen transport [see Chapter 6])
   - Central nervous system
   - Musculoskeletal
   - Gastrointestinal
   - Endocrine (diabetes)
   - Renal
   - Liver abnormalities
   - Nutritional deficits and obesity
2. Restricted mobility
   - Loss of physical-exercise stress (see Chapter 18)
   - Recumbency
   - Loss of vertical-gravitational stress (see Chapter 19)
3. Extrinsic factors
   - Those related to the patient's care (see Chapter 2)
4. Intrinsic factors
   - Those related to the patient (see Chapter 2)

2. To maximize oxygen transport and aerobic conditioning and to prevent cardiopulmonary dysfunction.
3. To prevent multisystem organ complications and all-cause infection that will lead to restricted movement, recumbency, and potential deterioration.
4. To provide supportive palliative care for patients at the end of life.
5. To reduce the impact and burden of the diseases of civilization on individuals, their families, their communities, society as a whole, and the health of the world's population.

PRACTICE PATTERNS

The American Physical Therapy Association's *Guide to Physical Therapist Practice* (2001) has evolved over the past decade, and it reflects a broad scope of practice. The guide describes examination (history, systems review, and tests and measures), evaluation, diagnosis, prognosis (including plan of care), and intervention (with anticipated goals and expected outcomes). Each pattern addresses reexamination, global outcomes, and criteria for termination of physical therapy services. The evaluation consists of a review of health rather than having a primary focus on illness. The iterative cycle of clinical decision making based on outcomes and the modification of treatment interventions are designed to achieve the expected outcomes within a prescribed time frame (Figure 17-2). Based on the consensus of hundreds of clinicians in the United States, several primary practice patterns have been defined for each specialty. Based on the evaluation, a patient's profile may best be described by one or more practice patterns, within one or more specialty areas of practice. There are eight practice patterns in the cardiovascular and pulmonary area (Box 17-6). These patterns and the Guide (2001) provide a frame of reference for practice rather than serving as a basis for practice. Patients are increasingly complex, given increasing life expectancy and concomitant comorbidities, coupled with lifestyle factors and their impact on the patient's presenting complaint or underlying risk factors. Therefore, categorizing a patient in one or more practice patterns may be insufficient to address the patient's complaints. These patterns serve as a guide only. They are not diagnoses, nor do they replace good clinical reasoning and judgment.

WHAT IS THE TREATMENT AND WHY?

Clinical Decision Making

The basis for clinical decision making in the management of the patient with cardiopulmonary dysfunction or its risk is to pair the most efficacious treatments specifically with impaired or threatened steps in the oxygen transport pathway. Considerable time may pass between treatments, so optimal therapeutic effect is dependent on the efficacy of between-treatment treatments (i.e., teaching the patient to carry out prescriptive treatment whenever possible and eliciting the

assistance of the patient's family or nursing staff in supporting the patient in doing so).

When confined to a hospital, many patients spend an inappropriate amount of time recumbent and in restricted body positions; they turn and move less frequently and are upright and moving a smaller proportion of the time. Depending on the particular oxygen transport deficits of a patient, the body positions the patient assumes can have a positive, negative, or neutral effect on oxygen transport. Thus, the positions the patient assumes and his or her reduced activity level must be monitored and any potential ill effects anticipated, countered or, preferably, prevented.

Examples of some common treatment goals in managing the patient with cardiopulmonary dysfunction are shown in Box 17-7. Specific treatments are identified to address these goals and for each deficit or threat to oxygen transport. Treatment goals and specific treatments are prioritized according to the relative significance of the impact of each on oxygen transport.

A physiologically based treatment hierarchy is shown in Box 17-8. The treatment hierarchy is based on the premise that physiological function, including oxygen transport, is optimal when the human organism is upright and moving. Thus, the purpose of the hierarchy is to exploit the treatments that are most physical first: active mobilization and exercise in the upright position. The hierarchy ranges from those to the interventions that are the least physical: conventional chest physical therapy techniques such as ROM, postural drainage and percussion, and suctioning. The latter may simulate some of the physiological effects of being upright and moving, but their effects are more limited and less scientifically well-substantiated, and they affect fewer steps in the oxygen transport pathway. They do not substitute for the more active physical interventions that are higher in the treatment hierarchy. All interventions features in the hierarchy have some role in the management of cardiopulmonary dysfunction or its risks but are used in descending order to ensure that the most efficacious interventions are exploited first.

Treatment Plan

The treatment plan consists of interventions that will most expediently and efficiently remediate the problems that have been identified. These interventions are prioritized according to the greatest effect they are predicted to have on remediating the oxygen transport deficit or minimizing any threat to oxygen transport and on maximizing their benefit-to-risk ratio. Depending on the specific treatment goals and the adequacy of balance between oxygen supply and demand, the coordination of physical therapy treatments with other care (e.g., nursing care and certain tests and procedures) is commonly indicated.

Treatment Prescription

Once the specific pathophysiological problems underlying deficits or threats to oxygen transport have been identified,

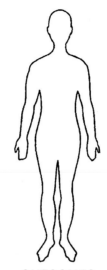

DIAGNOSIS
Both the process and the end result of evaluating examination data, which the physucal therapist organizes into defined clusters, syndromes, or categories to help determine the prognosis (including the plan of care) and the most appropriate intervention strategies.

**PROGNOSIS
(Including Plan of Care)**
Determination of the level of optimal improvement that may be attained through intervention and the amount of time required to reach that level. The plan of care specifies the interventions to be used and their timing and frequency.

EVALUATION
A dynamic process in which the physical therapist makes clinical judgments based on data gathered during the examination. This process also may identify possible problems that require consultation with or referral to another provider.

INTERVENTION
Purposeful and skilled interaction of the physical therapist with the patient/client and, if appropriate, with other individuals involved in care of the patient/client, using various physical therapy methods and techniques to produce changes in the condition that are consistent with the diagnosis and prognosis. The physical therapist conducts a reexamination to determine changes in patient/client status and to modify or redirect intervention. The decision to reexamine may be based on new clinical findings or on lack of patient/client progress. The process of reexamination also may identify the need for consultation with or referral to another provider.

EXAMINATION
The process of obtaining a history, performing a systems review, and selecting and administering tests and measures to gather data about the patient/client. The initial examination is a comprehensive screening and specific testing process that leads to a diagnostic classification. The examination process also may identify possible problems that require consultation with or referral to another provider.

OUTCOMES
Results of patient/client management, which include the impact of physical therapy interventions in the following domains: pathology/pathophysiology (disease, disorder, or condition); impairments, functional limitations, and disabilities; risk reduction/prevention; health, wellness, and fitness; societal resources; and patient/client satisfaction.

FIGURE 17-2 Iterative process of clinical reasoning and decision making. *(From The Guide to Physical Therapist Practice. APTA 2001).*

BOX 17-6

Cardiovascular and Pulmonary Preferred Practice Patterns Based on Oxygen Transport Limitations and Risks

Pattern A: Primary Prevention/Risk Reduction for Cardiovascular/Pulmonary Disorders
Pattern B: Impaired Aerobic Capacity/Endurance Associated With Deconditioning
Pattern C: Impaired Ventilation, Respiration/Gas Exchange, and Aerobic Capacity/Endurance Associated With Airway Clearance Dysfunction
Pattern D: Impaired Aerobic Capacity/Endurance Associated With Cardiovascular Pump Dysfunction or Failure
Pattern E: Impaired Ventilation and Respiration/Gas Exchange Associated With Ventilatory Pump Dysfunction or Failure

Pattern F: Impaired Ventilation and Respiration/Gas Exchange Associated With Respiratory Failure
Pattern G: Impaired Ventilation, Respiration/Gas Exchange, and Aerobic Capacity/Endurance Associated with Respiratory Failure in the Neonate
Pattern H: Impaired Circulation and Anthropometric Dimensions Associated With Lymphatic Systems Disorders

(From American Physical Therapy Association. [2001]. Guide to physical therapist practice, ed 2. Washington, DC: American Physical Therapy Association.)

BOX 17-7

Common Treatment Goals in the Management of a Patient with Cardiopulmonary Dysfunction or Its Risk

OVERALL GOAL: Directed at optimizing or preserving participation and activity by addressing structural and functional deficits in oxygen transport and gas exchange
  Direct treatment a specific steps involved
  ↑ Efficiency of all steps in the pathway
  Augment medical management
  Use medical management to augment physical therapy
  Coordinate with nursing management (e.g., in critical care)

SPECIFIC GOALS: Directed at specific steps in the oxygen transport pathway
  ↑ Air entry and alveolar ventilation (minimize airflow resistance)
  ↑ Air distribution (optimize lung compliance and chest wall compliance and reduce airway resistance)
  ↑ Ventilation and perfusion matching

↑ Diffusion
↑ Oxyhemoglobin saturation
↓ Work of breathing (from increased resistance, reduced or excessive compliance)
↓ Work of the heart (from increased preload, contraction, increased afterload)
↑ Efficiency of heart mechanics
Minimize ECG irregularities (identify factors that contribute to irregularities; anticipate problems)
Optimize blood flow distribution
Optimize oxygen extraction ratio
↓ Excessive or unnecessary energy expenditure
Optimize CO_2 removal
Optimize blood volume and distribution to maintain hemodynamic status
Optimize hydration

BOX 17-8

Physiological Treatment Hierarchy for Management of Limited Oxygen Transport to Optimize Participation and Activity

PREMISE: The position of optimal physiological function is being upright and moving

I. Mobilization and Exercise

Goal: To elicit an exercise stimulus that addresses one of the three effects on the various steps in the oxygen transport pathway, or some combination thereof
A. Acute effects
B. Long-term effect
C. Preventive effects

II. Body Positioning

Goal: To elicit a gravitational stimulus that simulates being upright and moving as much as possible: active, active-assisted, or passive
A. Hemodynamic effects related to fluid shifts
B. Cardiopulmonary effects on ventilation and its distribution, perfusion, ventilation, and perfusion matching and gas exchange

III. Breathing control Maneuvers

Goal: To augment alveolar ventilation, to facilitate mucociliary transport, and to stimulate coughing
A. Coordinated breathing with activity and exercise
B. Spontaneous eucapnic hyperventilation
C. Maximal tidal breaths and movement in three dimensions
D. Sustained maximal inspiration
E. Pursed-lip breathing to end-tidal expiration
F. Incentive spirometry

IV. Coughing Maneuvers

Goal: To facilitate mucociliary clearance with the least effect on dynamic airway compression and the fewest adverse cardiovascular effects
A. Active and spontaneous cough with closed glottis
B. Active-assisted (self-supported or supported by other)
C. Modified coughing interventions with open glottis (e.g., forced expiratory technique, huff)

V. Relaxation and Energy-Conservation Interventions

Goal: To minimize the work of breathing and of the heart and to minimize undue oxygen demand
A. Relaxation procedures at rest and during activity
B. Energy conservation, (i.e., balance of activity and rest, performing activities in an energy-efficient manner, improved movement economy during activity)
C. Pain-control interventions

VI. ROM Exercises (Cardiopulmonary Indications)

Goal: To stimulate alveolar ventilation and alter its distribution
A. Active
B. Assisted-active
C. Passive

VII. Postural Drainage Positioning

Goal: To facilitate airway clearance using gravitational effects
A. Bronchopulmonary segmental drainage positions

VIII. Manual Techniques

Goal: To facilitate airway clearance in conjunction with specific body positioning
A. Autogenic drainage
B. Manual percussion
C. Shaking and vibration
D. Deep breathing and coughing

IX. Suctioning

Goal: To facilitate the removal of airway secretions collected centrally
A. Open suction system
B. Closed suction system
C. Tracheal tickle
D. Instillation with saline
E. Use of manual hyperinflation bag (bagging)

BOX 17-9

Parameters of the Treatment Prescription in the Management of a Patient with Cardiopulmonary Dysfunction or its Risk

Determine whether to treat or not to treat at this time

Define measures and outcomes on which treatment progression and determination of whether goals have been met are based

Define parameters of treatment based on history, laboratory investigations, tests, and assessment

Treatment types

Intensity of each treatment (if applicable)

Duration of each treatment

Frequency of each treatment

Instruct patient in the between-treatment treatment and, if applicable, also instruct the nurse, a family member, or both

Reassess every treatment

Modify as necessary within each treatment

Modify and progress treatments as indicated

Determine when treatment is to be discontinued

Request additional supportive information, tests, and investigations as indicated throughout the course of treatment

Predict time course for optimal effects and course of treatment to determine treatment efficacy; modify as necessary

Schedule and coordinate treatments in conjunction with other interventions: medical, surgical, nursing, respiratory therapy (weaning), oxygen supplementation, symphathomimetic drugs, ADLs; and balance with sleep and rest periods, food intake and feeds, peak energy times, peak of drug potency and effects, e.g., pain, reduced sedation, reduced neuromuscular blockade

---

BOX 17-10

Use of Modalities and Aids

Goal: To incorporate the use of the modalities and aids that enhance the prescribed interventions over the short and the long term

Modalities

Treadmill, ergometer, rowing machine
Weights
Pulleys
Nebulizers and aerosols
Flutter valve
BIPAP* and CPAP†
Incentive spirometer
Orthoses, braces, and supports

Pharmacologic Agents

Oxygen
Bronchodilators
Vasodilators
Antihypertensives
Antiinflammatories
Mucolytics
Surfactant
Analgesics

*Bilevel positive airway pressure
†Continuous positive airway pressure.

WHAT IS THE COURSE OF TREATMENT?

Once a treatment has been prescribed, the prescription must be reviewed at each treatment session and modified accordingly (i.e., the prescription parameters change as the patient's condition changes). In addition, the parameters may be modified within a treatment on the basis of the patient's response. The physical therapist also decides when to discontinue a given treatment as well as which overall methods of cardiopulmonary physical therapy to employ; these decisions too are based on the patient's responses to the treatment and on the outcome. Some change in treatment should be effected with one or two treatment sessions so as to ensure that improvement is being maximized. If no improvement is noted, an explanation is found and the intervention is changed to elicit improvement. When no improvement is demonstrated, particularly in patients who are seriously ill, physical therapy may have a role in preventing deterioration, so it should not be withdrawn. However, a rationale should always be proposed for continued treatment in the event of no demonstrated change. Continued intervention may be indicated, for example, in a patient in an induced coma. Hemodynamic and oxygen transport status must be maintained in anticipation of the induced coma's being removed. In most other situations, however, some improvement toward the eventual goal of maximizing activity and participation status should be expected from every treatment.

Measures to assess treatment response and outcome are selected so that they reflect (1) activity and participation

they are differentiated into (1) those that can be addressed by physical therapy (i.e., noninvasive physical interventions); (2) those that are not amenable to physical therapy but need to be considered during treatment so as to determine whether treatment is contraindicated or needs to be modified and whether specific outcome and treatment-response measures are indicated; and (3) those that are best managed invasively, which may necessitate referral to a physician.

Problems amenable to physical therapy are prioritized. Optimal treatments are identified for each problem, and their parameters are prescribed. The treatment goals are identified: to reverse pathophysiological mechanisms contributing to impaired oxygen transport: to compensate for irreversible pathophysiological deficits (improve efficiency of other steps in the oxygen transport pathway); to decelerate deterioration; to avoid making the patient worse; to provide palliative care, support, and comfort; and to prevent the occurrence of problems in the future (see section on Treatment Goals). Based on the goals of treatment, the parameters of the treatment are defined. Treatment parameters in the management of a patient with cardiopulmonary problems are shown in Box 17-9. To achieve these goals, a range of modalities and aids may be needed in the short term and in the long term (Box 17-10).

BOX 17-11

Measures and Outcomes to Assess Limitations in the Steps in the Oxygen Transport Pathway

Central Control of Breathing

Central drive to breathe test
Arterial blood gases
Cerebral perfusion and pressure

Ambient Air

Partial pressures of O_2, N_2 and CO_2
Air pollution and quality
Humidity

Airways

Clinical assessment including auscultation
Pulmonary function tests
Arterial blood gases
Chest radiograph
Histamine challenge exercise tests

Lungs

Clinical assessment, including inspection, percussion, palpation, and auscultation
Pulmonary function tests
Ventilation and perfusion scans
Diffusion capacity test
Arterial blood gases
Chest radiograph
Immunological status
Respiratory muscle assessment
Assessment of the structure and integrity of chest wall
Lung water studies

Blood

Circulating blood volume and cardiac output
Arterial oxygen content
Venous oxygen content
Plasma volume
Red and white blood cell counts
Protein constituents
Platelets
Hemoglobin
Coagulability
Viscosity
Stasis
Hydration
Immunological status

Pulmonary Circulation

Perfusion scan
Pulmonary artery balloon floatation catheter to assess central venous pressure, pulmonary artery pressures, wedge pressure

Heart

Clinical assessment, including percussion, palpation, and auscultation
Inspection and clinical observation tests, including jugular venous distension test
Heart rate, systolic and diastolic blood pressures, and rate pressure product
ECG
Hemodynamic studies to assess cardiac output, stroke volume, cardiac distensibility, and ejection fraction
Ultrasound procedures to examine mechanical integrity
Scans
Coordination of electromechanical behavior of heart
Coronary artery perfusion studies
Stress test
Hemodynamic monitoring including central venous pressure, pulmonary artery pressures, and wedge pressure
Angiography
Chest radiograph

Peripheral Circulation

Clinical assessment findings
Segmental blood pressures of the extremities
Ultrasound studies
Arterial and venous lab studies and investigations
Adequacy and efficiency of lymphatic drainage system of the heart and lungs, and peripheral circulation
Stress test

Tissue

Enzyme studies
Tissue biopsies
Vascularization of tissue
Adequacy and efficiency of arterial and venous tissue
Blood flow
Tissue fluid balance; hydrostatic pressure, oncotic pressure, and lymphatic pressure
Blood work including serum lactates and $S\dot{V}O_2$
Tissue oxygenation and pH
Nuritional and hydration status

---

status, (2) the status of oxygen transport overall, and (3) the integrity of the step or steps in the oxygen transport pathway that were identified as being the primary problems contributing to cardiopulmonary or cardiovascular dysfunction in the original assessment (Box 17-11; see Part II). Cardiopulmonary dysfunction is determined on the basis of the history, assessment, and laboratory investigations, such as pulmonary function testing, breathing pattern, cardiac function testing, fluid balance and renal function, arterial blood gases, arterial saturation, vital signs, and hemodynamic variables, including heart rate

and ECG, blood pressure, and rate pressure product. Subjective reports are also clinically relevant, such as subjective ratings of perceived exertion, breathlessness, angina, and fatigue. These same measures are used to detect improved oxygen transport and gas exchange.

Considering that clinical decision making is based largely on the results of tests and measures, it is essential that these measures have certain characteristics. Measurements must be objective and their procedures standardized to maximize test validity and reliability. Although physical therapists specialize in noninvasive assessment procedures as well as treatments, noninvasive measures are prone to imprecision, hence to measurement error and unreliability. It is therefore essential that assessment measurements be performed in a systematic manner and according to measurement guidelines so as to maximize their quality and usefulness in guiding and directing treatment (Chapter 7). Invasive interventions, including blood work, scans, and radiographs, are also fundamental to the physical therapist's assessment and on-going evaluation. Assessment measurements always precede treatment to ensure that treatment and its prescriptive parameters are appropriate. Measurements during treatment provide information about the patient's responses, both beneficial and detrimental. This feedback determines the parameters of treatment, and whether the treatment should be modified in some way or possibly discontinued. The overall treatment response is established by further monitoring and assessment at the termination of treatment and often at periodic intervals posttreatment so that delayed effects can be monitored. Frequent and periodic measurements over time are referred to as serial measurements and provide useful trend data. The pre- and posttreatment responses and any noteworthy responses during treatment are charted along with sufficient information about the procedures that were used (i.e., assessment as well as treatment procedures).

Physical therapists often require the results of invasive tests such as blood work or invasive hemodynamic monitoring to establish treatment response and outcome; thus, these need to be requested as required.

Assessment and reevaluation data provide feedback to the physical therapist about her or his clinical decision making and therapeutic outcomes, as well as about the effectiveness of the prescribed interventions in the management of a given patient. Further, patient or client satisfaction with his or her physical therapist and with management, elicited by means of a formal evaluation by the patient, are critical for evaluating service and the overall outcome of physical therapy for each individual.

SUMMARY

This chapter provides a framework for clinical reasoning and decision making based on oxygen transport characteristics that underlie a limitation in activity and participation in life, as defined by the model of ability advocated by the World Health Organization. Carried out in partnership with the patient as much as possible, the process includes diagnoses and treatment prescriptions in the management of patients with cardiopulmonary dysfunction, who range from the individual who is medically unstable and critically ill to the individual who is medically stable with cardiopulmonary dysfunction or its risk and living in the community. The purpose of a systematic approach to clinical decision making is to maximize treatment efficacy and cost effectiveness. This is done by focusing on physiological and evidence-based practice within the context of evidence-based planning

(epidemiology), and monitoring to gauge improvement after every treatment so as to ensure that the patient is progressing. The clinical decision-making process involves diagnosis (i.e., specific analysis of the patient's problems—limitations in activity and participation) in relation to the physiology and underling pathophysiology, the contribution of restricted mobility and recumbency, and extrinsic (related to the patient's care) and intrinsic (related to the patient's characteristics) factors. Based on this analysis, treatment interventions and their parameters are prescribed so that they have the greatest physiological and scientific justification for being likely to return an individual to health and participation in life. Treatments and their prescription parameters should have a clear and justifiable rationale. Specific monitoring of the steps in the oxygen transport pathway that are impaired is essential to establishing and confirming the diagnoses, determining the most efficacious treatment, evaluating the treatment response, refining and progressing the treatment, and determining when to discontinue a given treatment and physical therapy overall. The specific components of the treatment prescription include the treatment, its intensity (if applicable), duration, and frequency, as well as its course and progression. A problem-solving approach to patient care has become essential in all health care professions, given the prohibitive cost of such care and the need for all health care to be physiological, evidence-based, cost effective, and ethically justifiable. As noninvasive practitioners, physical therapists need to evaluate their effectiveness in avoiding, reducing, or postponing the need for invasive care, such as drugs and surgery. These singularly important outcomes are crucial, yet all too often underestimated in practice.

Review Questions

1. Describe the three levels of assessment, based on the World Health Organization's model of ability and participation.
2. Describe the use of the oxygen transport pathway as a conceptual model of cardiopulmonary practice and as the basis for defining problems related to cardiopulmonary dysfunction and risk (structure and function level).
3. Distinguish among the short-term goals, long-term goals, and preventive goals of cardiopulmonary physical therapy management. Relate to participation, activity, and structure and function.
4. Discuss the significance of the reduction of invasive care (avoidance, reduction, and postponement of drugs and surgery) as a primary outcome for patients under the care of physical therapists who specialize largely in noninvasive management.
5. Distinguish the four categories of factors that contribute to cardiopulmonary dysfunction or threat (i.e., pathophysiology, restricted mobility and recumbency, extrinsic factors, and intrinsic factors).

6. Describe the factors that must be considered in treatment prescription.

7. Describe the factors that must be considered in determining the course of treatment.

8. Describe the process of modifying, progressing, or discontinuing treatment with respect to the iterative process of evaluation and modifying treatment prescription.

9. What is the role of prognosis in treatment planning in the short- and long-term?

10. Describe why physical therapists prescribe interventions rather than administer standardized treatments for given limitations of oxygen transport.

REFERENCES

American Physical Therapy Association. (2001). Guide to physical therapist practice, ed 2. Washington, DC: American Physical Therapy Association.

Corriveau, M.L., Rosen, B.J., & Dolan, G.F. (1989). Oxygen transport and oxygen consumption during supplemental oxygen administration in patients with chronic obstructive pulmonary disease. American Journal of Medicine 87:633-637.

Cutler, P. (1998). Problem solving in clinical medicine, ed 3. Baltimore: Williams and Wilkins.

Dantzker, D.R. (1997). Cardiopulmonary critical care, ed 3. Philadelphia: Elsevier.

Dean, E. (1994). Oxygen transport: a physiologically based conceptual framework for the practice of cardiopulmonary physiotherapy. Physiotherapy 80:347-355.

Dean, E. (1999). Preferred practice patterns in cardiopulmonary physical therapy: a guide to physiologic measures. Cardiopulmonary Physical Therapy Journal 10:124-134.

Epstein, C.D., & Henning, R.J. (1993). Oxygen transport variables in the identification and treatment of tissue hypoxia. Heart & Lung 22:328-348.

Ferrans, C., & Powers, M. (1992). Psychometric assessment of the Quality of Life Index. Research in Nursing & Health 15:29-38.

Ferrucci, L., Baldasseroni, S., Bandinelli, S., de Alfieri, W., Cartei, A., Calvani, D., Baldini, A., Masotti, G., & Marchionni, N. (2000). Disease severity and health-related quality of life across different chronic conditions. Journal of the American Geriatric Society 48:1490-1495.

Gibson, B., Gibson, J., & Bergner, M. (1975). The sickness impact profile: development of an outcome measure of health care. Annals of Internal Medicine 65:1304-1310.

Goldhill, D.R., Worthington, L., Mulcahy, A., Tarling, M., & Summer, A. (1999). The patient-at-risk team: identifying and managing seriously ill ward patients. Anaesthesia 54:853-860.

Goldring, R.M. (1984). Specific defects in cardiopulmonary gas exchange. American Review of Respiratory Diseases 129:S57-S59.

Greenberg, G., Peterson, R., & Heilbronner, R. (1989). Illness effects questionnaire. Philadelphia: Children's Rehabilitation Hospital, Thomas Jefferson University Hospital, unpublished.

Guyatt, G., Berman, L., Townsend, M., Pugsley, S.O., & Chambers, L.W. (1987). A measure of quality of life for clinical trials in chronic lung disease. Thorax 42:773-778.

Hayes, S.C., Barlow, D.H., & Nelson-Gray, R.O. (1999). The scientist practitioner: research and accountability in clinical and educational settings, ed 2. Boston: Allyn & Bacon.

Hillegass, E.A., & Sadowsky, H.S. (2001). Essentials of cardiopulmonary physical therapy, ed 2. Philadelphia: WB Saunders.

Hunt, S., McEwen, J., & McKenna, S. (1980). A quantitative approach to perceived health. Journal of Epidemiology and Community Health 34:281-295.

Hyland, M. (1991). The living with asthma questionnaire. Respiratory Medicine 85:13-16.

Irwin, S., & Tecklin, J.S. (2004). Cardiopulmonary physical therapy, ed 4. Philadelphia: Elsevier.

Jerusum, J. (1997). Tissue oxygenation and routine nursing procedures in critically ill patients. Journal of Cardiovascular Nursing 11:12-30.

Jones, P., Quirk, F., Baveystock, C., & Littlejohns, P. (1992). A self-complete measure of health status for chronic airflow limitation. American Review of Respiratory Disease 145:1321-1327.

Kaplan, R., Atkins, C., & Timms, R. (1984). Validity of a quality-of-well-being scale as an outcome measure in chronic obstructive pulmonary disease. Journal of Chronic Diseases 37:85-95.

Kellner, R. (1987). Manual of the symptom questionnaire. Albuquerque, NM: Department of Psychiatry, School of Medicine, University of New Mexico, unpublished.

Kelly, K.M. (1996). Does increasing oxygen delivery improve outcome? Yes. Critical Care Clinics 12:635-644.

Lareau, S., Carrieri-Kohlman, V., Janson-Bjerklie, S., & Roos, P.J. (1994). Development and testing of the Pulmonary Functional Status and Dyspnea Questionnaire. Heart Lung 23:242-250.

Lugo, G., Arizpe, D., Dominguez, G., Ramirez, M., & Tamariz, O. (1993). Relationship between oxygen consumption and oxygen delivery during anesthesia in high-risk surgical patients. Critical Care Medicine 21:64-69.

McGavin, C., Gupta, S., Lloyd, E., & McHardy, G.J. (1977). Physical rehabilitation for the chronic bronchitic: results of a controlled trial of exercises in the home. Thorax 32:307-311.

Oldridge, N., Guyatt, G., Jones, N., Crowe, J., Singer, J. Feeny, D., McKelvie, R., Runions, J., Streiner, D., & Torrance, G. (1991). Effects on quality of life with comprehensive rehabilitation after acute myocardial infarction. American Journal of Cardiology 67:1084-1089.

Parkerson, G., Gehlbach, S., Wagner, E., James, S.A., Clapp, N.E., & Muhlbaier, L.H. (1981). The Duke-UNC Health Profile: an adult health status measure for primary care. Medical Care 10:806-828.

Patrick, D.F. (1992). Clinical decision making. In Zadai, C. (Ed). Clinics in physical therapy. Pulmonary management in physical therapy. New York: Churchill Livingstone.

Rector, T., Kubo, S., & Cohn, J. (1987). Patients' self-assessment of their congestive heart failure. Heart Failure October/November: 198-209.

Riegelman, R.K. (1991). Minimizing medical mistakes. Boston: Little, Brown.

Rogers, W., Johnstone, D., Yusuf, S., Weiner, D.H., Gallagher, P., Bittner, V.A., Ahn, S., Schron, E., Shumaker, S.A., & Sheffield, L.T. (1994). Quality of life among 5,025 patients with left ventricular dysfunction randomized between placebo and enalapril: the study of left ventricular dysfunction. Journal of the American College of Cardiology 23:393-400.

Schon, D.A. (1983). The reflective practitioner. New York: Basic Books.

Stewart, A., Hays, R., & Ware, J.J. (1988). The MOS short-form general health survey: reliability and validity in a patient population. Medical Care 26:724-735.

Wallston, K.A., & Wallston, B.S. (1981). Health locus of control scales. In Lefcourt, H.M. (Ed). Research with the locus of control construct. New York: Academic Press.

Wasserman, K., Hansen, J.E., Sue, D.Y., Stringer, W.W., & Whipp, B.J. (2004). Principles of exercise testing and interpretation: including pathophysiology and clinical applications, ed 4. Philadelphia: Lippincott Williams & Wilkins.

Wasson, J., Keller, A., Rubenstein, L., Hays, R., Nelson, E., & Johnson, D. (1992). Benefits and obstacles of health status assessment in ambulatory settings: the clinician's points of view. The Dartmouth Primary Care COOP Project. Medical Care 30:42-49.

Weaver, T., & Narsavage, G. (1992). Physiological and psychological variables related to functional status in chronic obstructive pulmonary disease. Nursing Research 41:286-291.

Weissman, C., Kemper, M, & Harding, J. (1994). Response of critically ill patients to increased oxygen demand: hemodynamic subsets. Critical Care Medicine 22:1809-1816.

World Health Organization. (2000). International Classification of Functioning, Disability and Health. www.sustainable-design.ie/arch/ICIDH-2PFDec-2000.pdf; retrieved December 2004.

World Health Organization. (2000). Definition of health. www.who.int/about/definition; retrieved December 2004.

C H A P T E R   1 8

Mobilization and Exercise

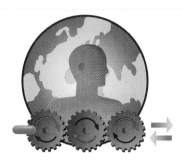

Elizabeth Dean

KEY TERMS   Exercise
Metabolic demand
Mobilization
Oxygen transport

Prescription
Recumbency
Restricted mobility

As clinical exercise physiologists, the physical therapist's primary "drugs" include mobilization and exercise. These drugs are used to prevent, remediate, or delay limitations in participation and activity by addressing limitations in structure and function. First, the terms *mobilization* and *exercise* are defined. Then the basis for prescribing mobilization and exercise as primary physical therapy treatment interventions, with the primary intent to optimize oxygen transport, is reviewed. The prime purpose of this chapter is to differentiate the routine application of mobilization and exercise from their prescriptive application. The three distinct objectives of prescribing mobilization and exercise for the purpose of maximizing oxygen transport are differentiated. These include the exploitation of their preventive, acute, and long-term effects. Mobilization and exercise can be prescribed specifically to elicit whichever of these distinct effects is indicated. Exercise to exploit each of these effects can be prescribed to address limitations in specific organ systems. Mobilization and exercise are prescribed on the basis of their specific indications, contra-indications, and potential side effects for a given individual.

DEFINITIONS

Mobilization is defined as the therapeutic and prescriptive application of low-intensity exercise in the management of

cardiovascular and pulmonary dysfunction, usually in patients who are acutely ill. Primarily, the goal of mobilization is to exploit the acute effects of exercise so as to optimize oxygen transport. Even a relatively low dose of mobilization stimulus can impose considerable metabolic demand on a patient with cardiovascular or pulmonary compromise. Whenever possible, mobilization is performed in the upright position, the physiological position (Chapter 19) to optimize gravitational stress on fluid shifts and thereby central and peripheral hemodynamics. Thus, mobilization is prescribed to elicit both a gravitational stimulus and an exercise stimulus.

Exercise refers to its prescription in the management of subacute and chronic cardiovascular or pulmonary dysfunction. Primarily, the goal of exercise is to exploit the cumulative effects of and adaptation to long-term exercise (i.e., over time) and in this way optimize the function of all steps in the oxygen transport pathway.

Both mobilization and exercise can be prescribed for their preventive effects. In this case, the parameters of the prescription focus on exploiting their multisystemic effects, including their cardiovascular and pulmonary effects, in addition to other effects such as neurological, musculoskeletal, and integumentary (skin).

Oxygen consumption, denoted $\dot{V}O_2$, refers to the amount of oxygen that an individual requires, and that is determined by fluctuating metabolic requirements. Oxygen demand is least at rest, increases to intermediate levels during submaximal activity, and reaches a peak at the maximal level of exercise an individual can volitionally tolerate. Metabolic cost increases with illness and injury as a result of healing and repair, as discussed later. In the descriptions of the literature, the reader will encounter two terms: $\dot{V}O_2$max and $\dot{V}O_2$peak. Although often used interchangeably, these terms are technically distinct. In the update of the literature in this and other chapters, whatever term used by the cited investigators in describing their work is used. Literature published in recent years tends to adopt the more precise terminology, $\dot{V}O_2$peak, when describing the $\dot{V}O_2$ achieved by an individual when performing a maximal effort during a specified exercise testing condition.

The physiological distinction between the terms is as follows. $\dot{V}O_2$max is a more theoretical value, and $\dot{V}O_2$peak is a practical value. A true maximal value would reflect the oxygen consumption of all muscles working maximally. However, exercise tests are selective and tend to work the legs or the arms; or the legs in different ways, for example, cycling a lower-extremity ergometer as opposed to walking on a treadmill. The more muscle groups that work simultaneously, the closer $\dot{V}O_2$peak approximates the true $\dot{V}O_2$max. Maximal effort resulting from leg work generates a greater $\dot{V}O_2$peak than maximal effort resulting from arm work; and further, maximal effort resulting from treadmill walking or running generates a greater $\dot{V}O_2$peak than maximal leg work on a cycle ergometer, about 10% more. This greater $\dot{V}O_2$peak may be explained by the larger muscle mass of the legs than the arms in the first situation, and the arm work and requirement for increased postural stabilization in the second situation. Whether $\dot{V}O_2$max can be achieved is an academic question. Maximal effort exerted during Nordik skiing approximates theoretical $\dot{V}O_2$max most closely in that this activity requires strenuous arm and leg work coupled with the need for marked postural stabilization.

BASES FOR THE PRESCRIPTION OF EXERCISE STRESS

The prescription of exercise is fundamental in the management of primary and secondary cardiovascular and pulmonary dysfunction. Exercise science has advanced exponentially over the past 50 years and has been the primary basis for physical therapy for almost 100 years. Guidelines have been developed for prescribing exercise to maximize functional work capacity or aerobic capacity for healthy persons and individuals with chronic heart and lung disease (American College of Sports Medicine, 2000; Astrand et al, 2003; Belman & Wasserman, 1981; Blair et al, 1988; Froelicher & Myers, 2000; Hasson, 1994; Irwin & Tecklin, 2004; Wasserman & Whipp, 1975; Woods, 2004). Physical therapists as clinical exercise specialists exploit the effects of exercise in most patients and adapt the prescription based on the patient's clinical presentation and needs. Exercise training is based on the findings of a maximum graded exercise test. Submaximal

exercise testing is often indicated for patients with severely impaired functional work capacity because of the inherent risks associated with maximal testing and the potential for invalid test results (Compton et al, 1989; Noonan & Dean, 2000). Guidelines for submaximal exercise testing, test interpretation, and prescription of exercise based on the submaximal exercise test are less well defined (Dean & Ross, 1992a; 1993; Shephard et al, 1968).

The prescription of mobilization and exercise to optimize oxygen transport in the patient with acute cardiopulmonary dysfunction has been a relatively neglected area of research compared with exercise prescription in the management of chronic cardiopulmonary dysfunction. This is surprising given that early mobilization is a key component of cardiopulmonary physical therapy in the management of patients who are acutely ill. Orlava (1959) was the first to report the beneficial application of mobilization in the management of acute cardiopulmonary compromise, specifically, bronchopulmonary pneumonia. The physiological literature supports an unequivocal role for therapeutic mobilization to maximize oxygen transport in patients with acute cardiopulmonary dysfunction (Dean & Ross, 1992b). Despite this conclusive body of knowledge, Orlava's work has not been extended significantly in the literature since her work was published more than 45 years ago. Even for patients who are critically ill, the goal is to evaluate their oxygen transport reserve capacity and use it as a basis for estimating the limits of a patient's physiological tolerance for mobilization, with a view to returning the patient to living within the community (Weissman et al, 1994). The more critically ill the patient, the greater the need to assess the relationship between the patient's $\dot{V}O_2$ and oxygen delivery (DO_2) (see Chapter 2) (Weissman & Kemper, 1991), so that the patient's capacity for oxygen transport is not exceeded.

Unlike exercise prescription for the patient with chronic cardiovascular and pulmonary dysfunction, the patient with acute dysfunction cannot be exercise-tested in the conventional manner because of the risks of an untoward exercise response. Given the profound and direct effects of mobilization and exercise on cardiopulmonary and cardiovascular function, it is essential that the physical therapist be able to identify the specific effects of exercise required and define the optimal therapeutic stimulus (i.e., the stimulus that yields the maximal benefit to oxygen transport with the least risk).

Acute and chronic cardiovascular and pulmonary pathology have the additional challenges of compromising functional capacity in two important ways. First, in acute illness, the patient tends to be recumbent in bed a great proportion of the time and, second, in both acute and chronic illnesses, the physical activity of the patient is reduced. Recumbency and restricted mobility have physiologically distinct effects on oxygen transport and are the primary determinants of bed-rest deconditioning (Chase et al, 1966; Convertino et al, 1982; Winslow, 1985). The impact of these factors is exaggerated in smokers, young people, older adults, obese individuals, and patients who are mechanically ventilated.

The goals of mobilization and exercise are directed at correcting impairments and enhancing the patient's capacity for activity and participation (see overview of the International Classification of Function in Chapters 1 and 17). Outcomes related to improving abilities and participation include self-care, home management, return to work, and resumption of avocational activities. Return to work warrants special mention. Return to work is often related to oxygen transport capacity in terms of aerobic and muscle power. However, there are economic, psychosocial, and environmental factors that need to be considered. So these factors, too, should be part of the overall assessment and incorporated into the overall goal setting.

OXYGEN TRANSPORT AND METABOLIC DEMAND OF PATIENTS

In health, when individuals have optimal physiological reserve, both the acute and the long-term responses to an exercise stimulus can be predicted. Specifically, minute ventilation ($\dot{V}_E$) and cardiac output (CO), hence DO_2, increase commensurate with work rate and oxygen demand.

In patients whose oxygen transport capacity is reduced or threatened, mobilization and exercise constitute a metabolic load that is superimposed on other factors and can increase metabolic cost (Box 18-1). Hospitalized patients tend to be hypermetabolic. In addition to their basal metabolic demands, their energy demands are increased secondary to such factors as increased body temperature, healing and repair processes, increased work of breathing and of the heart, pain, and anxiety and in response to routine interventions and procedures, including cardiovascular and pulmonary physical therapy. The goal, therefore, in prescribing mobilization and exercise, is to ensure a safety margin wherein the patient's demand for oxygen does not exceed the available supply or delivery. This is usually indicated clinically by worsening of the patient's oxygen transport, objectively and subjectively.

Of the physical therapy interventions, mobilization, exercise, body positioning, arousal, breathing control maneuvers, coughing, postural drainage, manual techniques, bagging, suctioning and range-of-motion (ROM) exercises can increase $\dot{V}_O_2$ and overall metabolic demand (Dean et al, 1995; Weissman et al, 1984). Therefore, the capacity of the oxygen transport system to meet the patient's metabolic demands must be established during the physical therapy assessment. Can the oxygen transport system support the patient's metabolic demands? If so, what reserve capacity is available to support a mobilization or exercise stimulus? The exercise stimulus is designed to exploit the potential of the reserve capacity. Establishing reserve capacity is essential to optimize the efficacy of the therapeutic exercise stimulus (i.e., neither subthreshold or suprathreshold).

Metabolic demand and $\dot{V}_O_2$ are determined by multiple factors. In patients, the effect of arousal, anxiety, pain, and noxious stimulation, in addition to the hypermetabolic demands of recovery, contribute to energy cost and demand on the

---

Factors That Contribute to Increased Metabolic Demand and Oxygen Consumption in Patient Populations

Pathophysiological Factors

Fever (e.g., secondary to an infectious agent or inflammation, surgery, multiple trauma, severe illness)
Thermoregulatory challenges (i.e., too hot or too cold, altered ambient temperature and humidity)
Healing and repairing (i.e., secondary to illness, trauma, surgery)
Combating infection

Intervention-related Factors

Alerting, noxious, and painful responses to routine nursing, medical, and physical therapy interventions, including injections, insertion of lines, procedures, and neurological checks)
Feeding; enterally or parenterally
Being handled physically (e.g., by health care workers)
Body position
Changing body position (i.e., passive, active assist, or active changes)
Range of motion exercises (i.e., passive, active assist, or active)
Mobilization and exercise
Pharmacologic agents

Psychosocial Factors

Social contact (e.g., health care workers, family)
Anxiety
Discomfort
Pain

Miscellaneous

Noise
Disrupted circadian rhythms when ill, hospitalized, or away from daylight

---

oxygen transport system. Thus, relaxing and calming patients is a central component of physical therapy because these interventions minimize undue oxygen demand, as do physical therapy interventions for pain management. Although relaxation, often coupled with sedation or analgesia, is central to physical therapy management in other settings, relaxation procedures should be applied in the management of patients with cardiovascular and pulmonary dysfunction in situations in which agitation, anxiety, and pain contribute to increased oxygen demand. This is especially true in intensive care, where oxygen transport is compromised or threatened in most patients (see Chapters 34 and 35).

CELLULAR ENERGETICS IN RESPONSE TO MOBILIZATION AND EXERCISE

The cardiopulmonary unit supports oxygen transport and cellular respiration (Weber et al, 1983). Oxygen is continuously being used by every cell in the body for oxidative phosphoryl-ation and the synthesis of adenosine triphosphate (ATP). The splitting of a phosphate bond from ATP to form adenosine diphosphate yields a considerable amount of energy for metabolism. The energy for this process comes from the reduction of hydrogen in the formation of water and carbon dioxide, which are the end products of the Krebs cycle and the electron transfer chain (i.e., cellular respiration). These metabolic processes, which make up oxidative phosphorylation, take place in the mitochondria of the cells (see Chapter 2).

The balance between $\dot{V}o_2$ and Do_2 is precisely regulated to ensure that there is not only an adequate supply of oxygen but also that, under normal resting conditions, approximately four times as much oxygen is delivered to the tissues as is used. This safety margin permits the immediate availability of oxygen when the system is perturbed by physical, gravitational, or psychological challenges (see Chapter 2).

Anaerobic metabolism is prevalent during all-out, short, sprint-type activities, such as hockey, soccer, and volleyball. Although physical therapists tend to focus on aerobic rather than anaerobic training, in conditions in which Do_2 is comp-romised, patients may rely on anaerobic metabolism to sustain ATP production and breakdown to provide energy. Although the term anaerobic implies that the exercise is performed in the absence of oxygen, anaerobic metabolism provides a short-term means of supporting phosphorylation, using substrates other than oxygen to generate and split ATP. If insufficient oxygen is available, the amount of ATP that can be generated anaerobically is limited. Thus this process can be sustained for only a short period. Lactic acid accumulates in the blood during anaerobic metabolism. In healthy, untrained individuals, lactic acid increases exponentially at an exercise intensity of about 55% of maximal aerobic capacity (McArdle et al, 2000). Anaerobic capacity and specifically the anaerobic threshold can increase with training; however, anaerobic training effects are less than the training effects achieved with aerobic training.

Anaerobic metabolism is thought to be triggered by tissue hypoxia. The term *anaerobic* is somewhat of a misnomer in that oxygen is needed to pay the oxygen debt that it creates. Thus, in health, the need for oxygen is delayed rather than eliminated. In disease states, anaerobic metabolism occurs when a patient's oxygen transport system cannot meet the metabolic demand required, as in patients with sepsis and multisystem organ dysfunction. Serum lactate levels are elevated in these patients, resulting in metabolic acidosis, which is unfavorable to the maintenance of homeostasis.

During exercise, the cellular Po_2 is lower than the surrounding interstitial fluid Po_2. Oxygen diffuses rapidly through cell membranes. At the onset of physical exercise, the increased metabolic demand of the muscle and supporting tissues increases the oxygen diffusion gradient. Feedback mechanisms are triggered to increase Do_2, which depends primarily on arterial oxygen content and CO. The first line of defense is the response to an increase in pericellular pH. The concentration of carbon dioxide is increased and this, as a result of the decrease in pH, facilitates the dissociation of oxygen from hemoglobin (i.e., it shifts the oxyhemoglobin dissociation curve to the right). CO, the product of stroke volume and heart rate (SV × HR), increases commensurate with metabolic demand. The immediate response to oxygen utilization and lowered tissue oxygen is an increase in CO to increase Do_2. This averts arterial desaturation that is not normally observed in health, even with extreme exertion. With progressive exercise intensity, SV increases disproportionately at lower intensities to increase CO, with HR contributing to a greater extent at moderate and high exercise intensities. However, older individuals exercising at high intensity in upright positions rely more on the Frank-Starling effect than on HR (Rodeheffer, 1986). In health, exercise-induced cardiac fatigue has been proposed as a limiter to prolonged exercise (Dawson et al, 2003); however, the mechanisms of the associated reduced left ventricular systolic and diastolic function are unclear.

The increase in systemic CO results in increased venous return and pulmonary CO. The SV plateaus at 40% of $\dot{V}o_2$max, and thereafter CO is augmented by increases in HR. One exception in health is in elite athletes, whose SV may continue to increase commensurate with exercise intensity (Zhou et al, 2001). To oxygenate a greater volume of blood in the lungs, an increased volume of air must be inspired. To increase minute alveolar ventilation ($\dot{V}_E$), tidal volume (V_T) and respiratory rate (RR) increase. At low intensities of exercise, V_T increases disproportionately to RR, whereas at moderate to high intensities, V_T plateaus and further increases in $\dot{V}_E$ are effected by an increase in RR (Jones & Fletcher, 1997). Exercise is associated with a small increase in airway diameter and length of pulmonary structures, hence, a reduction in airway resistance. Zone 2, the zone of greatest alveolar ventilation to perfusion ($\dot{V}_A$/Q) matching in the lungs, is increased as a result of pulmonary capillary dilation and recruitment. Diaphragmatic excursion is enhanced and the distributions of ventilation and perfusion are more uniform throughout the lung, which minimizes airway closure and atelectasis. Exercise increases the excursion, which leads to inflation of the lungs in three planes (anteroposterior, transverse, and cephalocaudal, particularly in the upright position).

Rhythmic inflation and deflation of the lungs associated with physical activity has several clinically important effects. First, this action increases alveolar ventilation ($\dot{V}_A$) by a primary increase in V_T. Second, exercise-induced lung motion facilitates lymphatic flow and drainage. Optimal lymphatic drainage is essential for lung water balance with the increased volume of blood being processed through the pulmonary circulation and lung parenchyma. This action may explain, in part, the beneficial effect of mobilization on the distribution and function of pulmonary immune factors (Pyne, 1994). The increased movement of the lungs during exercise has a primary effect on mucociliary transport and mucus clearance (Wolff et al, 1977). Physical activity may also minimize bacterial colonization in the airways, hence, reduce the risk of pulmonary infection (Skerrett et al, 1989). Finally, lung movement stimulates surfactant production and its distribution over parenchymal tissue. Surfactant is essential for reducing surface tension in the alveoli, maintaining alveolar stability, and maintaining lung compliance, thereby minimizing airway closure and areas of lung collapse.

The heart and peripheral circulation are primed and respond to the increased demands of acute exercise. Hemodynamic adjustments occur immediately with the onset of exercise stress and in fact may precede it due to anticipation. To maximize the CO available, blood shifts from the venous capacitance reservoirs such as the venous compartments of the gut and extremities, particularly the legs and working muscles. At rest, most of the circulation (70%) is contained within the highly compliant venous circulation. The Starling law of the heart regulates the forward movement of blood commensurate with the volume of blood that is received. The heart chambers are normally distensible; they adjust to changing volumes of blood returning to the heart and pump more forcefully when stretched than at rest to eject it through the pulmonary and peripheral circulations. Muscle enzymes that extract oxygen at the cellular level are also primed and are synthesized commensurate with chronic metabolic demand.

EFFECTS OF MOBILIZATION AND EXERCISE ON OXYGEN TRANSPORT

In health, optimal function of oxygen transport depends on the integrity of each step in the oxygen transport pathway and on the interdependent function of all the steps. Cardiovascular and pulmonary dysfunction can lead to dysfunction in one or more steps in the oxygen transport pathway. Because of the interdependence of the steps in the pathway and the ability of functional steps to compensate for dysfunctional steps, gross measures of the efficacy of gas exchange and oxygenation can be normal. The number of steps in the pathway that are affected by disease and the severity of the disease determine the degree of impairment of oxygen transport overall and the degree to which this impairment is reflected in gross measures of oxygen transport.

To optimize the capacity of the various steps in the oxygen transport pathway, the oxygen transport system has to be exposed to two principal stressors: (1) gravitational stress and (2) exercise stress. These stressors are tantamount to life in that they enhance the biochemical, physical, and mechanical efficiency of the various steps in the oxygen transport pathway and the patient's capacity to respond rapidly to changes in the physical environment.

The absence of gravitational stress and exercise stress are the two primary factors contributing to bed-rest deconditioning. Thus the exploitation of both gravitational and exercise stress in preventing cardiovascular and pulmonary dysfunction is indicated. Further, mobilization and exercise are the two most vital physiological interventions available to the physical therapist for remediating cardiovascular and pulmonary dysfunction. Body position has marked effects on pulmonary and cardiovascular function, hence, exercise performance. The more acutely ill the patient is, the more body position needs to be coupled with mobilization to increase aerobic capacity and tolerance to exercise stress (Cotsamire et al, 1987).

PRESCRIPTION OF MOBILIZATION AND EXERCISE: PREVENTIVE EFFECTS

Humans are designed to be upright and moving. The deconditioning associated with restricted activity in patients is comparable to detraining in athletes (Mujika & Padilla, 2000a, 2000b) yet is distinct from bed-rest deconditioning, which is associated with recumbency as well as restricted mobility. Adaptation to gravitational stress and exercise stress demonstrates the remarkable plasticity of the oxygen transport system.

Deconditioning secondary to restricted activity leads to resting tachycardia and to reduced CO and $\dot{V}O_2$ at peak exercise. Blood volume is reduced. Oxygen extraction at the peripheral level is also limited. Commensurate changes take place in muscle. Type I and type II fibers are altered, and metabolic enzyme activity is down-regulated to adapt to the inactive state; muscle adapts by atrophying accordingly. Endocrine changes take place commensurate with the level of deconditioning, including reduced growth hormone production. The cell membranes become less sensitive to insulin, thus chronic inactivity can be associated with glucose intolerance.

When people are both recumbent and inactive, both gravitational stress (the vertical gravitational gradient) and exercise stress are removed. Bed rest is one of the most commonly used yet unquestioned therapeutic practices. Despite its widespread acceptance, the body positions it promotes, namely, being supine and immobile, are nonphysiological (Chapter 19). The harmful sequelae of this posture have been well documented (see overview Dean & Ross, 1992b), yet the more severely ill the patient is the more confined that individual is to the bed, and the greater the risk of multisystem complications (Box 18-2).

The immediate effects of restricted mobility are those associated with recumbency; these are followed within 24 to 48 hours by cardiopulmonary and musculoskeletal changes. Within 24 hours, marked fluid shifts occur and blood volume is reduced by 10% to 15%. Within days, these effects can impair oxygen transport. These systemic effects are more profound in premature infants, young and older people, smokers, and obese and deconditioned individuals. These effects are further compounded when a patient has either primary or secondary cardiovascular and pulmonary compromise. The less aerobically fit an individual, the less physiological reserve capacity is available in the cardiovascular and pulmonary systems. In the event of a medical or surgical insult, such a patient will have an increased risk for morbidity and mortality than a fitter counterpart. Thus the importance of aerobic fitness cannot be overemphasized for patients anticipating procedures as well as in health.

BOX 18-2

Physiological Consequences of Bed Rest

I Fluid volume redistribution

↓ Plasma and blood volume
↓ Total heart and left ventricular volumes
↑ Hematocrit
Diuresis and natriuresis
Venous stasis

II Muscular inactivity

↑ Insulin resistance
↓ Muscle mass
↓ Muscle strength
↓ Muscle endurance

III Altered distribution of body weight and pressure

Urine stasis, retention, tendency toward calculus formation
Hypercalciuria
Bone demineralization
Local skin changes

IV Aerobic deconditioning

↑ HR at rest and at all levels of activity
↓ Resting and maximum stroke volume

↓ Maximum cardiac output
↑ Risk of venous thrombosis and thromboembolism
↓ Orthostatic tolerance
↓ Aerobic conditioning
↓ $\dot{V}O_2$max
↑ Venous compliance

V Other

Catabolism
Anorexia
Paralytic ileus
Constipation
↑ Sensitivity to thermal stimuli; increased sweating and hyperemia
↑ Anxiety, hostility, depression, psychosis
↑ Auditory threshold
↑ Focal point, decreased near point of visual acuity
Alteration in clearance of some drugs

Adapted from Woods, S.L. (2004). Cardiac nursing, ed 5. Philadelphia: JB Lippincott, Williams & Wilkins.

As previously described, a primary effect of mobilization and exercise on the cardiopulmonary system is enhanced mucociliary transport and airway clearance (Wolff et al, 1977). Frequent changes in body position augment airway clearance and minimize the pooling and stagnation of bronchial secretions, hence, airway obstruction and airflow resistance (Chapter 19).

The primary effects of bed rest on the cardiopulmonary system result from recumbency and a down-regulation of oxygen transport (Ferretti et al, 1998). Pulmonary sequelae of recumbency include reduced lung volumes and capacities, particularly functional residual capacity (FRC), residual volumes (RV), and forced expiratory volumes (Blair & Hickman, 1995; Craig et al, 1971; Hsu & Hickey, 1976; Powers, 1944; Risser, 1980; Svanberg, 1957). A reduction in FRC in the supine position compared with the sitting position has been attributed to both a decrease in thoracic volume and an increase in thoracic blood volume, hence pulmonary venous engorgement (Sjostrand, 1951). Thus alveolar-arterial oxygen difference and arterial oxygen tension are reduced during periods of bed rest (Cardus, 1967; Clauss et al, 1968; Ray et al, 1974). Closing volumes are increased, precipitating arterial desaturation in recumbent positions and subsequent complications.

The cardiovascular sequelae of prolonged recumbency include an increase in resting and submaximal HR (Deitrick et al, 1948), a decrease in $\dot{V}O_2$max (Saltin et al, 1968), and a decrease in total blood volume and plasma volume, and an increase in hematocrit (Deitrick et al, 1948; Saltin et al, 1968;

Friman, 1979). Down-regulation of oxygen transport with bed rest reflects reduced CO and arterial oxygen content due to reduced hemoglobin (Ferretti et al, 1998). The combination of an increase in blood viscosity and a decrease in venous blood flow results in an increased risk of thromboemboli (Lentz, 1981; Wenger, 1982).

With bed rest and recumbency, orthostatic intolerance in combination with resting tachycardia and reduced exercise capacity occur, reflecting diminished reflex activity of the sympathetic nervous system. Baroreceptor-mediated activity is blunted and appears to involve abnormal processing in the central nervous system at the level of the ventrolateral medulla (Hasser & Moffitt, 2001). The net effect is abnormal vascular tone that contributes to changes in vascular and cardiac function and in hypovolemia, resulting in orthostatic intolerance. The lower peripheral vascular resistance that occurs when in the supine position compared with being upright suggests there is the potential for greater vasoconstriction; however, it is not evoked to maintain blood pressure (BP). This observation supports the theory that the arterial baroreceptor reflex is reset to a lower operating pressure; this has been suggested to explain the hemodynamic effects of exercise (Raine et al, 2001).

Bed-rest-induced diuresis increases renal load. Patients with renal insufficiency are particularly seriously affected by this effect and other sequelae of bed rest (Krasnoff & Painter, 1999). As a result, they may exhibit dysrhythmias, muscle wasting, weakness, neuropathy, glucose intolerance, and reduced bone density.

Musculoskeletal changes that occur with deconditioning due to bed rest include loss of muscle mass and strength as well as muscle and ligament shortening, joint contractures, skin lesions, and decubitus ulcers (Kasper et al, 2002; Rubin, 1988). At the cellular level disuse atrophy begins within 4 hours of bed rest. Compared with type IIa muscle fibers in vastus lateralis, type I fibers have been reported to be more seriously affected by bed rest, and they respond less favorably to muscle-resistance training (Trappe et al, 2004). Differences in fiber type may explain why muscles in the lower limbs are differentially affected; for example, the plantar flexors are particularly affected (Akima et al, 1997). Also, gender differences in muscle strength loss with bed rest have been reported (Yamamoto et al, 1997). Skeletal muscle protein synthesis is compromised by bed rest, aging, nutritional deficit, uncontrolled diabetes mellitus, and sepsis (Farrell, 2001). Disuse osteoporosis results from reduction of the mechanical stress caused by gravity and from lack of active muscle contraction across joints. Prevention is a primary goal because recovery of mineral loss in bone is prolonged and its loss is potentially irreversible (Takata & Yasui, 2001). Bone mass is restored later than muscle mass and function after a period of restricted mobility, and that contributes to fracture risk (Bloomfield, 1997).

CNS changes include slowed electrical activity of the brain, emotional and behavioral changes, slowed reaction times, sleep disturbances, and impaired psychomotor performance (Rubin, 1988; Ryback et al, 1971; Zubeck & MacNeil, 1966). Diminished sympathetic activity is the primary factor responsible for orthostatic intolerance, along with hypovolemia, and the result is bed-rest deconditioning (Kamiya et al, 2003).

Metabolic changes that occur during periods of bed rest and the relative absence of muscle contraction include reduced insulin sensitivity and glucose intolerance (Mikines et al, 1991); increased calcium excretion due to bone loss; and increased nitrogen excretion secondary to protein loss from atrophying muscle (Deitrick et al, 1948; Donaldson et al, 1969; Hulley et al, 1971). In sedentary people, plasma lipids are elevated and skeletal muscle becomes insulin resistant (Stannard & Johnson, 2003). Insulin sensitivity and triglyceride levels are highly responsive to change in diet, activity level, and thermogenic state. Fit people are highly insulin sensitive, whereas unfit sedentary people tend to be insulin insensitive. Reversal and the normalizing of insulin sensitivity are dependent on increasing muscle contraction.

Bed rest has been associated with a reduction in cytokine function and antibody counts, hence in reduced immunity and an increased risk of infection (Ahlinder et al, 1970; Sonnenfeld, 1999). Lymph flow is reduced with bed rest, and that may predispose patients to further risk of infection (Havas et al, 1997).

Of clinical importance is the fact that deterioration of cardiovascular and pulmonary function occurs at a faster rate than musculoskeletal deterioration, and that the rate of recovery from the negative effects of bed rest is generally slower than the rate of impairment (Kottke, 1966; Sandler et al,

1988). These effects of bed rest are accentuated in older adults (Harper & Lyles, 1988) and are likely to further compound the oxygen transport and other deficits of patients with pathology.

The preventive effects of exercise are evident in prehabilitation. Examples include conditioning a patient prior to a surgical intervention or hospital admission (Topp et al, 2002). Individuals are prescribed exercise programs commensurate with their age, functional status, and anticipated procedure or surgery. The purpose is to reduce complications, speed recovery, minimize the time until discharge, and promote a complete return to daily living as soon as possible.

Finally, disuse deconditioning has been implicated in aging. Half of the physical decline associated with aging has been attributed to this factor (Landin et al, 1985). With regular physical activity and prescribed aerobic and strengthening programs, these changes may be substantially offset. As a result, functional capacity is optimized and, in the event of illness, the individual has better physiological reserve to deal with the pathophysiological insult. Irrespective of age, however, exercise-induced physiological and health advantages are lost following cessation of exercise (Lennon et al, 2004). Restricted mobility in the elderly is associated with clinical depression (Lampinen & Heikkinen, 2003).

Cardiorespiratory fitness is related to the volume of regular physical activity; however, its relationship to health measures is less strong (Oja, 2001). Physical inactivity has been causally implicated in the diseases of civilization, but the precise dose of activity or exercise needed to provide protection against illness and disease is not precisely known. One exception is in ischemic heart disease, in which a threshold intensity of 6 metabolic equivalents (METs) in conjunction with a minimal volume of regular physical activity is recommended for optimal cardiovascular health (Shephard, 2001). The precise dose for prevention of hypertension and stroke is less clear (Kohl et al, 2001). Moderate as opposed to heavy exercise has been recommended (Shephard, 2001). The choice of relative or absolute intensity of effort depends on the desired preventive outcomes.

Hazards of Bed Rest

The negative multisystem sequelae of bed rest have been unequivocal for 60 years (Allen et al, 1999; Bassey & Fentem, 1974; Chobanian et al, 1974; Dean & Ross, 1992b; Dock, 1944; Harrison, 1944; Ross & Dean, 1989). The classic study by Saltin et al (1968) demonstrated marked multisystem deterioration with three weeks of bed rest in five healthy young men and the restoration of aerobic capacity with strenuous training afterwards. In a follow-up of the same subjects 30 years later (McGuire et al, 2001a), all were found to have an age-related decrement in aerobic power. When their exercise responses were compared over that timeframe, bed rest had had a more profound impact on physical work capacity than thirty years of aging. Thus, the use of bed rest as a primary medical intervention requires justification. The recumbent, immobile positions associated with bed rest adversely affect most organ systems by means of an apparent down-regulation of the oxygen transport system (Ferretti et al, 1998). This is clinically important because in conventional patient management, there is a direct relationship between how sick the patient is and the amount of time she or he is confined to bed. In addition, the musculoskeletal, neurological, gastrointestinal, and genitourinary systems are adversely affected. Deconditioning associated with bed rest reduces $\dot{V}O_2$max and the oxygen transport reserve to perform physical work (Convertino et al, 1997).

The cardiovascular deconditioning resulting from bed rest include the loss of fluid-volume and pressure regulating mechanisms, the loss of plasma volume, and diuresis (Grenon et al, 2004a, 2004b; Hirayanagi et al, 2004a, 2004b). In turn, the hematocrit is increased, and the risk of developing deep vein thromboses and thromboemboli is increased. This is exacerbated by increases in blood viscosity, platelet count, platelet stickiness, plasma fibrinogen (Wang et al, 1995), and stasis of venous blood flow.

Venous thromboembolic disease is preventable with conservative management, including prophylactic anticoagulation in some instances (Jacobs, 2003). In addition to restricted mobility, other risk factors include being elderly, undergoing venous catheterization, and hormone replacement therapy. Conditions that are associated with risk include previous thromboembolus, myocardial infarction, heart failure, severe lung disease, cancer, obesity, and paralytic conditions such as stroke. After acute stroke, patients are particularly at risk due to paresis, recumbency, restricted mobility, and circulatory stasis (Harvey, 2003). The work of the heart is increased in a patient who is immobile and recumbent, as is the work of breathing. The work of the heart is greater as a result of the increased filling pressures and heart rate associated with chronic recumbency and the increased blood viscosity. The work of breathing is increased due to reduced lung volumes secondary to visceral encroachment on the underside of the diaphragm, increased intrathoracic blood volume, and restricted chest wall motion.

With bed rest, the blood vessels of the muscles and splanchnic circulation dilate. With prolonged bed rest, they may lose their ability to constrict. The ability of these vessels to constrict is essential for preventing the pooling of blood and maintaining circulating blood volume when the patient assumes the upright position. Following bed rest, a patient may feel lightheaded or dizzy and may faint. Individual differences in terms of orthostatic intolerance have been reported and need to be assessed (Grenon et al, 2004a, 2004b). Individuals with greater venous compliance in the legs recruit mechanisms to compensate, such as activation of the renin-angiotensin-aldosterone system, activation of the sympathetic nervous system, and inhibition of the parasympathetic nervous system, so they tolerate orthostatic challenges better.

With only a few days of bed rest, muscle atrophy is initiated, leading to weakness, discoordination, and balance difficulty (Lentz, 1981; Saltin et al, 1968). With severe weakness, excessive strain may be placed on ligaments and joints. Muscles and their inert structures are differentially affected. In the knee extensors, for example, tendon stiffness is reduced and their hysteresis characteristics become exaggerated, whereas this does not occur in the plantar flexors (Kubo et al, 2004). Muscle imbalance may result from poor postural alignment. The limited positioning alternatives in bed may contribute to poor postural alignment, stiffness, and soreness. Bed rest allocates weight bearing to various body parts not adapted for weight bearing. Skin breakdown most commonly occurs over bony prominences, such as the sacrum, trochanters, elbows, scapulae, and heels. Risk factors for pressure ulcers include age, prolonged hospitalization, restricted mobility and general debility, low body weight, low diastolic BP, and surgical intervention (Lindgren et al, 2004). Immobile patients are at risk for bone demineralization. Of particular importance in older populations, in patients with disabilities, in postmenopausal women, and in patients on steroids is calcium loss. Prevention of disuse osteoporosis is the primary aim because remineralization of bone, even with aggressive exercise, body positioning, electrical stimulation, and possible pharmacological agents, is unlikely (Takata & Yasui, 2001). In patients who are critically ill, cytokines have been implicated in inactivity-related inflammation and muscle injury and atrophy. Activity has been proposed as a countermeasure (Winkelman, 2004).

Bed rest also affects psychological status. Patients may become depressed or sensorily deprived or may develop a psychoneurosis (Ishizaki et al, 2000).

The evidence supports the following:

1. Evidence supporting bed rest as an efficacious intervention is lacking.
2. The use of bed rest remains nonspecific and excessive.
3. Bed rest has multisystemic negative effects, so must be prescribed as specifically and judiciously as medication.
4. Methods other than bed rest to manage very ill patients such as those in the intensive care unit (ICU) must be developed.

Alternatives to the Nonspecific Use of Bed Rest

Physical therapists need to become active in designing furniture and devices that are better suited to patients' normal physiological functioning and to the needs of those patients' course of recovery. Such appliances would include the presence in ICUs of a greater number of stretcher chairs that enable easy transfer of patients from bed to chair and upright positioning and a greater availability of patient-lifting devices. Chairs that can be used to change the patient's body position and facilitate mobilizing need to be designed and used routinely.

Kinetic and rotating beds are electromechanical beds that turn the patient through an arc of about 30 degrees to both sides from the supine position over several minutes (Powers & Daniels, 2004; Schimmel et al, 1977). These beds are used for heavy-care patients who are critically ill and are unable to turn or are difficult to turn. Even though studies have shown these beds can enhance oxygenation in severely compromised patients such as those with acute respiratory distress syndrome (Nelson & Anderson, 1989; Summer et al, 1989; Yarnel et al, 1986), they should be used selectively to avoid reliance on passive positioning by the bed rather than more active and active-assisted patient positioning. These constitute the initial stages of mobilization and ambulation.

The use of tilt tables to promote mobilization can be hazardous because the muscle pumping action when the legs are dependent is minimal. Passive standing on a tilt table constitutes a greater hemodynamic stress than active standing. Upright sitting postures with the legs dependent may elicit greater physiological benefit than passive standing and with less risk due to their increased hemodynamic stress. Leg movement elicited by stepping in place, however, can counter the marked fluid shifs associated with the upright position.

Indications for Bed Rest

Despite the universal acceptance of bed rest as a medically therapeutic intervention, indications for its therapeutic use have not been documented, and its efficacy continues to be questioned (Allen et al, 1999). Furthermore, much more is known about the adverse and potentially life-threatening hazards of bed rest than about its benefits. Bed rest should clearly be used as selectively as other medical interventions to ensure that specific benefits are being derived and that the multisystemic negative sequelae are minimized. Many procedures such as surgery are associated with considerable pain, so being relatively immobile and recumbent in bed is believed to minimize postsurgical discomfort. Minimizing the effects of gravity and the need to bear weight is commonly indicated in patients after orthopedic surgery. The bed enables a patient with multiple wounds and fractures to be immobilized and supported in a fixed position that is believed to promote healing. Conditions that are associated with edema require minimizing the effect of gravity on the affected limbs. Whether edema can be controlled by localized elevation rather than bed rest must be established. Some conditions, particularly in their acute stages, so as to reduce the work of the heart, as in cases of myocardial infarction, may require some activity restriction. However, 50 years ago, restriction to a chair was reported to be more beneficial than restriction to bed in patients with heart disease (Levine & Lown, 1954). Despite this finding, many patients continue to recline in beds rather than sit upright in chairs and initiate ambulation. Mobilizing patients and permitting bathroom privileges has also been reported to be less stressful than having to use a bedpan (Kinney et al, 1995).

Prescription of an Adequate Exercise Stimulus to Elicit its Preventive Effects

Although much is known about the protective benefits of cardiopulmonary fitness and conditioning and about the negative effects of bed rest and restrictive mobility, little has been documented about prescribing exercise to counter orthostatic intolerance in a given patient (Convertino et al, 1997). Further, the characteristics of deconditioning, or detraining, in a given individual are determined by age, gender, conditioning status prior to bed rest, underlying pathophysiology, fluid and electrolyte balance, medications, and the duration of bed rest (Mujika & Padilla, 2000a). The preventive effects of an exercise stimulus can be defined as that exercise dose that will maintain the patient's conditioning level and prevent deterioration. At present, the prescription of preventive mobilization and exercise is nonspecific. Aerobic exercise and resistance muscle training have differential effects in countering the effects of restricted mobility (Alkner & Tesch, 2004; Shackelford et al, 2004). Although the upright position is the primary means of countering orthostatic changes associated with recumbency, exercise may have a limited role (Greenleaf, 1997). Even though high-intensity, short-duration, isotonic cycle ergometry training (ITE) and intermittent resistive isokinetic training (IKE) have no effect on orthostatic intolerance associated with recumbency in healthy people, ITE maintains plasma volume, red blood cells, and positive fluid balance, and IKE has no effect on plasma loss but mitigates red blood cell loss.

These differential training effects are of considerable clinical interest; however, their effects resulted from high-intensity training, and further recumbent exercise should not be considered a substitute for the gravitational stress associated with the upright position. Although patients who are severely ill are not usually capable of performing intense exercise, it is important to note that the responses to upright exercise by healthy people after 5 days of bed rest are maintained with a daily bout of 30 minutes of intense interval upright exercise training (Lee et al, 1997). Further, moderately intense exercise performed against lower body negative pressure to simulate an upright 1-g environment, fails to counter orthostatic intolerance after 15 days of bed rest (Schneider et al, 2002b). Also, aerobic pedaling exercise in the supine position during bed rest may be inadequate to maintain hemodynamic function and $\dot{V}O_2$max (Suzuki et al, 1994). Finally, with respect to the parameters of prescriptions for mobilization, the intensity of the training appears to be singularly important in attenuating the deconditioning effects of bed rest. In terms of importance, intensity is followed by frequency (Mujika & Padilla, 2000b).

Resistance training fails to counter the cardiovascular deconditioning associated with bed rest (Belin De Chantemele et al, 2004). Some evidence suggests that isometric exercise during bed rest can attenuate the decrement in $\dot{V}O_2$peak and maintain muscle integrity better than isotonic exercise (Greenleaf et al, 1985). Markers of lactic dehydrogenase, hence anaerobic threshold, increase with both types of exercise. Over time, however, reduced hydrostatic stress contributes to reduced lactic dehydrogenase in both types of training. Research is needed to refine exercise prescription for the preventive effects of exercise in recumbent patients whose mobility is restricted. For example, the following questions need to be answered:

- What preventive mobilization/exercise is best for which individuals and under what conditions (i.e., what are the principles of prescription)?
- How do different types of exercise compare with respect to preventive effects when all else is constant (i.e., patient's age and demographic profile, smoking history, general health, presenting illness and severity, body weight, nutritional status, aerobic condition, stress levels, cognitive status, and medication schedule)?
- Does exercising in some body positions elicit better preventive effects than exercise in other body positions?
- What principles establish the mobilization/exercise intensity, duration, and frequency that are optimal for a given individual whose mobility is restricted?
- What types of exercise are best suited for cross-transfer of their effects between the ipsilateral and contralateral limbs, to limit deconditioning during unilateral immobilization?

The question that arises is, what constitutes an adequate stimulus to maximize the preventive effects of exercise for a given patient, particularly a patient who is critically ill? Although the preventive effects of exercise are accepted, this important question has not been adequately researched. Some general practices, however, have become accepted clinically for patients who are acutely ill. These practices include turning patients. The turning frequency that is widely accepted is every 2 hours. There is no literature, however, to support evidence of greater preventive effects when a patient is turned every 2 hours rather than hourly or every 4 hours. Sitting up and ambulating are two other practices that are used. The timing of these interventions, however, is often based on convenience, on what else may be happening with the patient, or on a once- or twice-a-day regimen, rather than on a prescriptive basis. Patients who sit or walk for preventive reasons may assume suboptimal and even deleterious slumped or asymmetric positions. Patients and their caregivers need to be reminded about the importance of proper body position at all times, and patients should be provided with appropriately supported chairs, firm bolsters, and adjustable beds that maintain optimal body positions. The benefits can be augmented by scheduling such interventions when the patient is rested, or coordinating with medications.

Like exercise prescribed for its beneficial acute and long-term effects, exercise to elicit its optimal preventive effects should be prescribed on the basis of the individual's age; premorbid functional work capacity; type, distribution, and severity of disease; and capabilities. Such preventive mobilization or exercise must be prescribed in such a way as to avoid having any deleterious effects on the patient's overall condition. Even after highly invasive investigative procedures such as heart catheterization, patients can benefit from safe early ambulation (Rosenstein et al, 2004).

BOX 18-3

Acute Pathophysiological Conditions That Benefit From the Acute Effects of Mobilization and Exercise

Atelectasis
Pulmonary consolidation
Pulmonary infiltrates
Bronchopulmonary and lobar pneumonias
Bronchiolitis
Alveolitis
Pleural effusions
Acute lung injury and pulmonary edema
Hemothorax
Pneumothorax
Cardiopulmonary insufficiency
Cardiopulmonary sequelae of surgery
Cardiopulmonary sequelae of restricted mobility

PRESCRIPTION OF MOBILIZATION AND EXERCISE: ACUTE RESPONSES

The clinical decision-making process involved in defining the optimal mobilization and exercise stimulus for a given patient is multifactorial. On the basis of the patient's history, the history of the current illness, the assessment, and the results of the lab tests and procedures, the integrity of each step in the oxygen transport pathway is determined, as is the integrity of this system overall to preserve arterial oxygenation and pH. Box 18-3 shows some common conditions associated with acute cardiopulmonary dysfunction for which there is a rational basis for exploiting the *acute* effects of mobilization as a primary treatment intervention.

There are three primary components in assessing acute exercise responses: establishing a stable baseline founded on standardizing the preexercise conditions; and determining the appropriateness of the quantitative and qualitative changes in the objective and subjective responses during the onset of activity, the steady-state phase of activity, cool-down, and recovery. Recovery is an important part of the exercise response assessment. Postexercise hypotension in a healthy person, for example, is greater and longer after intense exercise (Forjaz et al, 2004). After the cessation of intense exercise, CO is initially maintained by increased SV; it is maintained by the HR after low-intensity exercise.

The physiological benefits of acute exercise are shown in Box 18-4. The principal outcomes include increased $\dot{V}_E$ secondary to increased V_T, RR, or both; improved airflow rates; and improved mucus transport. CO is increased secondary to increased SV, HR, or both, and to increased tissue oxygen extraction. The particular benefits of acute mobilization and exercise that are the goals are directed at each patient's specific pathophysiological deficits. Once the specific effects of acute mobilization or exercise that are needed are identified and matched to the patient's underlying pathophysiology, then the mobilization or exercise stimulus can be prescribed (Box 18-5).

BOX 18-4

Acute Physiological Effects of Mobilization and Exercise

Pulmonary System

↑ Regional ventilation
↑ Regional perfusion
↑ Regional diffusion
↑ Zone 2 (i.e., area of ventilation perfusion matching)
↑ Tidal volume
Alter breathing frequency
↑ Minute ventilation
↑ Efficiency of respiratory mechanics
↓ Airflow resistance
↑ Flow rates
↑ Strength and quality of a cough
↑ Mucociliary transport and airway clearance
↑ Distribution and function of pulmonary immune factors

Cardiovascular System

Hemodynamic effects

↑ Venous return
↑ Stroke volume
↑ Heart rate
↑ Myocardial contractility
↑ Stroke volume, heart rate, and cardiac output
↑ Coronary perfusion
↑ Circulating blood volume
↑ Chest tube drainage

Peripheral circulatory effects

↓ Peripheral vascular resistance
↑ Peripheral blood flow
↑ Peripheral tissue oxygen extraction

Lymphatic System

↑ Pulmonary lymphatic flow
↑ Pulmonary lymphatic drainage

Hematological System

↑ Circulatory transit times
↓ Circulatory stasis

Neurological System

↑ Arousal
↑ Cerebral electrical activity
↑ Stimulus to breathe
↑ Sympathetic stimulation
↑ Postural reflexes

Neuromuscular System

↑ Regional blood flow
↑ Oxygen extraction

Endocrine System

↑ Release, distribution, and degradation of catecholamines

Genitourinary System

↑ Glomerular filtration
↑ Urinary output
↓ Renal stasis

Gastrointestinal System

↑ Gut motility
↓ Constipation

Integumentary System

↑ Cutaneous circulation for thermoregulation

Multisystemic Effects

↓ Effects of anesthesia and sedation
↓ Deleterious cardiopulmonary effects of surgery
↓ Risk of loss of gravitational stimulus in conjunction with the upright position

---

The study of a patient's capacity to respond to maximal or submaximal exercise is fundamental to the physical therapy assessment of most patients. $\dot{V}O_2$max reflects the sum of the conductances of an integrated system of oxygen transport from the inspired air to the mitochondria. CO is in part passively regulated by the elastic characteristics of the peripheral circulation (Sheriff & Mendoza, 2004), so its anatomic and physiological integrity is essential to Do_2. The diffusive conductance of muscle is a particularly important component, and it has become a focus of the research related to impaired exercise capacity in patients with heart failure, chronic lung disease, and chronic renal disease (Wagner, 1996). This may explain why the correction of central cardiovascular defects in oxygen transport fails to restore exercise capacity in these patients.

The increased metabolic demand of acute exercise results in a slight increase in airway diameter and in increased $\dot{V}_E$, $\dot{V}_A$, V_T, RR, air flow rates, CO, SV, HR, BP, and rate pressure product (RPP; the product of heart rate and systolic BP). In healthy people and those with heart disease, RPP is highly correlated with myocardial $\dot{V}O_2$ and, therefore, with myocardial work (Gobel et al, 2003), $\dot{V}O_2$, and carbon dioxide production ($\dot{V}CO_2$). Generally, SV increases disproportionately more than HR at low intensities of exercise to affect CO. With increasing intensity, SV contributes proportionately less to HR, which continues to increase until the maximum HR is achieved with incremental exercise. In moderately active young women, however, SV plateaus through moderate to heavy exercise intensity and then undergoes a secondary increase at very heavy work loads (Ferguson et al, 2001). With endurance training, SV is increased, largely reflecting increased diastolic filling and emptying rates and an increase in blood volume. Older people may not increase their maximal CO and SV in response to training, in favor of peripheral adaptation (Spina et al, 2000). The area of greatest ventilation-to-perfusion matching in the midzones of the lungs, zone 2, is increased secondary to increased dilation and recruitment of pulmonary capillaries (West, 1995).

BOX 18-5

Acute Mobilization and Exercise: Clinical Decision Making and Prescription

Step 1

Identify *all* factors contributing to deficits in oxygen transport (Chapter 2):

1. The underlying pathophysiology of the disease or condition
2. Restricted mobility and recumbency
3. Extrinsic factors related to the patient's care
4. Intrinsic factors related to the individual patient

Identify the parameters that need monitoring before, during, and after each session

Step 2

Determine whether mobilization and exercise are indicated and, if so, which form of either will specifically address the oxygen transport deficits identified in step 1.

Step 3

Match the appropriate mobilization or exercise stimulus to patient's oxygen transport capacity.

   Examples: activities of daily living, walking unassisted, standing erect with assist and taking a few steps, transferring from bed to chair,* seated dangling position over bed side, moving in bed†

Step 4

Set the intensity within therapeutic and safe limits of the patient's oxygen transport capacity.

Step 5

Combine the various body positions, especially the erect position, with the following maneuvers:

1. Thoracic mobility exercises (flexion, extension, side flexion, and rotation)
2. Active, active assist, or passive range of motion exercises
3. Breathing control exercises, especially when coordinated with body movements
4. Coughing, spontaneous and voluntary, supported by self or others

Step 6

Set the duration of the mobilization sessions according to the patient's responses such as changes in the measures and indexes of oxygen transport rather than according to time.

Step 7

Repeat the mobilization sessions as often as possible according to their beneficial effects and their being safely tolerated by the patient.

Step 8

Increase the intensity of the mobilization stimulus, the duration of the session, or both, commensurate with the patient's capacity to maintain optimal oxygen transport when confronted with an increased mobilization stressor, and in the absence of distress; monitored variables should remain within the predetermined threshold range.

Step 9

Progression continues until:

1. the patient's functional status provides a base for resuming activities and full participation in life, with or without further physical therapy, and
2. the threat to the oxygen transport system is minimized.

---

*All sitting positions require upright erect sitting; propped up, semirecumbent, slouched, or slumped positions, although approximating the upright position, are not physiologically comparable.
†No amount of movement or activity is too small to derive acute or long-term benefits.

The hemodynamic benefits of exercise are maximized in the upright position as opposed to recumbent positions because exercise alone fails to counter the loss of volume-regulating mechanisms associated with recumbency (Sandler, 1986). Most important is the role of gravitational stress on maintaining BP control and reducing orthostatic intolerance. (See Chapter 19 for the effects of position changes on hemodynamics.) During exercise, end-diastolic volume and SV have been reported to be greater in the upright position than the supine position in endurance athletes, which supports greater reliance on the Frank-Starling law (Warburton et al, 2002). Thus, body position determines the relative contributions of HR, myocardial contractility, and the Frank-Starling mechanism to CO during exercise. Patients with impaired venous return and myocardial contractility may benefit from moderate-intensity recumbent cycling in which central circulation and local vasodilation are favored (Leyk et al, 1994). Plasma volume increases with acute intense exercise, and this has been shown to be position dependent (Nagashima

et al, 1999). Plasma albumen content increases in upright compared with supine positions, and this is thought to be responsible for the increase in plasma volume. By coupling upright positioning with exercise, physical therapy may directly help to normalize fluid balance and hemodynamics in patients whose fluid homeostasis is threatened.

The effect of acute exercise on blood coagulation and platelet aggregability is of particular interest in individuals with existing risk factors for clotting. The risk of stroke, for example, is of clinical importance in people with atrial fibrillation. Moderate levels of activity are associated with minimal procoagulatory effects, compared with high-intensity exercise, which increases platelet activity (Goette et al, 2004). Whether this increased platelet activity constitutes a risk factor clinically has yet to be determined.

The role of exercise in preventing deep vein thrombosis is well established. Although controversy has existed regarding its role in the management of deep vein thrombosis, aggressive approaches, including walking based on judicious assessment, have been proposed (Aldrich & Hunt, 2004). Recent evidence has shown that leg compression coupled with walking is superior to bed rest for the management of outpatients with acute deep vein thrombosis (Blattler & Partsch, 2003). Further, a systematic review and metaanalysis have corroborated that mobilization does not increase the rate of pulmonary embolism or complications above that found with bed rest (Trujilio-Santos et al, 2004).

Mobilization and exercise stimulate the endocrine system. Catecholamines, released to support the cardiovascular system, sustain a given exercise work rate. Increased sympathetic activity secondary to mobilization can help reduce the patient's need for sympathomimetic pharmacologic agents (Bydgeman & Wahren, 1974), and that is an important physical therapy outcome. Sympathetic nerve stimulation is increased, resulting in sympathetic neurotransmitters being processed more efficiently (i.e., synthesized and biodegraded). This is a significant effect that can be used as a goal for the prescription of mobilization. When exogenous catecholamines are used to augment Do_2 (optimally to $600\,ml/min/m^2$) in patients in surgical ICUs, the survival rate is improved and there are no increases in the number of cardiac events over those in control patients (Yu et al, 1995). Whether this effect, which is probably mediated by improved cardiac reserve, could be achieved by exercise-induced sympathetic stimulation warrants study. An additional benefit of sympathetic arousal in patients who are critically ill is the proposed anti-inflammatory effects associated with increased catecholamines (Uusaro & Russell, 2000).

Muscle training in patients who are critically ill has been shown to have general as well as local benefits in terms of acute and long-term effects as well as its preventive effects. Peripheral and respiratory muscles are important targets of exercise prescription in this patient population, and such training may have implications for avoiding mechanical ventilation or, if mechanical ventilation is indicated, facilitating weaning (Cirio et al, 2003). Resistance exercise is an effective countermeasure to muscle atrophy when a patient is recumbent (Alkner & Tesch, 2004; Reeves et al, 2002).

Central nervous system (CNS) responses to mobilization include arousal via activation of the reticular activating system and priming of the various organ systems involved (Browse, 1965). With respect to autonomic function, para-sympathetic inhibition occurs at the start of exercise, followed by sympathetic activation to augment the force and rate of myocardial contraction. Substrate utilization and transfer to working tissue as well as the capacity for oxygen to be supplied to muscle are precisely regulated through coordinated control of body temperature, breathing, cardiac function, and vasoactivity, both systemically and locally; and at the tissue level, they are regulated by the control of local metabolism and the production of vasoactive and chemoactive substances.

The metabolic effects of acute exercise, in particular, on glucose metabolism and growth hormone synthesis are of considerable clinical relevance in that these functions are fundamental to health and recovery. Restricted physical activity causes hyperinsulinemia and hyperglycemia and reduces growth hormone synthesis (Smorawinski et al, 1998). Thus, the acute effects of exercise are instrumental in offsetting these changes.

Acute exercise has profound effects the immune system. A single bout of moderate exercise has a positive effect on immunity (Nieman, 2003). Whether there is a dose-dependent effect is not known. Whether there is a cumulative effect of short periods of less intense exercise, such as for the patient who is acutely ill or who has a low functional capacity, is also not known.

The prescription of mobilization and exercise to stimulate their acute benefits parallels that of the prescription of exercise for its long-term, central and peripheral aerobic effects. The exercise parameters for achieving long-term adaptations in healthy people have been defined by the American College of Sports Medicine (2000) (Table 18-1) and are generally well accepted: the individual engages in aerobic exercise at a heart rate intensity of 70% to 85% of a maximum heart rate, for 20 to 40 minutes, three to five times a week. Aerobic training effects are usually observed within 2 months. In severely deconditioned individuals and in some patient populations, however, such a prescription would not be realistic, ethical, or indicated. Thus, exercise is prescribed that is sufficient to elicit progressive oxygen transport adaptation within defined limits of certain objective and subjective responses, such as perceived exertion, shortness of breath, angina, discomfort/pain, and general fatigue. Considerable research, however, is needed to refine the prescription of mobilization and exercise for their acute effects in patients with acute cardiopulmonary and cardiovascular dysfunction. Furthermore, specifications for the low-level exercise needed to effect long-term aerobic adaptation have not been elucidated in detail. However, based on physiological understanding of acute exercise responses and of cardiopulmonary pathophysiology, principles for prescribing mobilization to exploit its acute effects related to oxygen transport can be formulated.

TABLE 18-1

Exercise Prescription Parameters to Elicit Long-Term Aerobic Benefits in Healthy People

PARAMETER	SPECIFICATION
Exercise type	Rhythmic activity involving the large muscle groups—legs, arms, or both
Intensity	70% to 85% of the age-predicted HRmax or observed HRmax
Duration	20 to 40 minutes
Frequency	3 to 5 times a week
Course	6 to 8 weeks

Adapted from the American College of Sports Medicine. (2000). Guidelines for exercise testing and prescription, ed 6. Philadelphia: Lippincott, Williams & Wilkins.

After an acute stroke, patients undergo threat to oxygen transport in addition to the risks of restricted mobility during the acute period. A recent review of patients during this period reported low activity levels (Bernhardt et al, 2004). Early mobilization not only reduces the risk of restricted mobility, it initiates the rehabilitation process along its continuum toward return to daily function.

Gender differences in acute aerobic exercise responses exist between men and women; one example is in people with hypertension (Reybrouck & Fagard, 1999). The lower $\dot{V}O_2$max in women has been attributed to both central and peripheral factors. The higher $S\bar{v}O_2$ observed in women contributes to their reduced arteriovenous oxygen difference. These findings can be explained by women's smaller muscle mass, capillary density, and oxidative capacity. Older women show depressed cardiac function in comparison with younger women, whereas this difference is not observed between older and younger men (Yoshioka et al, 2003). Specifically, the percent increase in ejection fraction and the decrease in vascular resistance are depressed. This may be explained by endothelial dysfunction in postmenopausal women, which impairs peripheral vascular function during exercise.

Acute aerobic exercise responses to resistance muscle training have become more interesting clinically because the aerobic responses may have to be used as a guide to the muscle training prescription, particularly in individuals with cardiovascular risk factors and in those who are severely ill. One study examined the metabolic and cardiorespiratory responses of healthy people to maximal intermittent knee isokinetic exercise at 60 degrees per second and 180 degrees per second (Marzorati et al, 2000). In the last 2 minutes of exercise, $\dot{V}O_2$, $\dot{V}_E$, HR, and BP were comparable, consistent with a steady rate. The slope for the increase in $\dot{V}O_2$ was steeper in the 60 degrees per second protocol than in the 180 degrees per second, whereas HR was unaffected by angular velocity. Neither systolic nor diastolic BP was related to exercise intensity or angular velocity of exercise. Although the metabolic and cardiorespiratory responses to intermittent isokinetic exercise of the knee mimic dynamic exercise, qualitative differences likely reflect an isometric component associated with postural stabilization. Thus, the cardiorespiratory capacity of patients must be screened to ensure that they can safely meet this demand or, conversely, so that the resistance training program can secondarily augment cardiovascular conditioning.

The acute hemodynamic responses to resistance muscle training are seldom considered when muscle training is prescribed for clinical populations such as people with low back pain. The patients have weak muscle strength and commonly have poor physical conditioning. Repetitive McKenzie exercises are commonly used in management; they include forward flexion while standing and lying down and back extension while standing and lying down. The hemodynamic responses to these exercises have been reported to be distinct (Al-Obaidi et al, 2001). HR and BP are maximal in back extension lying down and are progressively lower in

---

BOX 18-6

Examples of Activities Used to Exploit the Acute Effects of Mobilization

Mobilization Stimuli

Ambulation—independently, with one or more assisting
Cycle ergometry—lower and upper extremities
Activities of daily living—independently, with one or more assisting
Standing—independently, with one or more assisting
Transferring—independently, with one or more assisting
Dangling—independently, with one or more assisting
Cycle ergometry in bed (lower extremity)
Turning in bed
Bed exercises

Mobilization Aids

For the patient:

Walking aids (crutches, cane, IV pole for support, wheelchair, orthoses)
Weights
Pulleys
Monkey bar
Grab bars
Grab rope
Portable oxygen
Portable ventilator

For the physical therapist:

Transfer belts
Mechanical lifts for patients

---

forward flexion lying down and forward flexion standing, and least for back extension standing. Thus, the aerobic and isometric hemodynamic consequences of resistance muscle training must be considered, irrespective of the purpose of that training, whether it is for management of back pain or for heart disease.

Mobilization Testing

Evaluating a patient's response to a mobilization stimulus can be assessed in two ways. First, the patient can be exposed to a mobilization challenge test. The patient is monitored before, during, and after mobilization activities comparable to monitoring for a graded exercise test (Box 18-6). Relatively low-intensity activities, such as bed exercises, moving in bed, changing body position, sitting up, dangling over the bed's side, transferring to a chair, doing chair exercises, and taking short walks with assistance, constitute a sufficient stimulus to elicit the acute effects of exercise as well as gravitational stimulus. The degree of assistance required to perform the activity should be noted because it demonstrates the patient's individual effort. Also, if a patient's status is unstable and oxygen transport is jeopardized, monitoring that patient during usual care, such as turning the patient and performing daily activities and nursing and medical procedures, can provide an indication of the patient's physiological responses to mobilization and the capacity of the oxygen transport system to meet metabolic demand. Any movement that is sufficient to perturb the oxygen transport system, no matter how minimal, is sufficient to elicit short- and long-term gains.

For mobilization testing and for training, patients who are acutely ill may benefit from recumbent exercise if upright is not tolerated. Body position affects exercise parameters as well as resting parameters. End-diastolic and end-systolic left ventricular volumes and SVs are larger in the supine position than in a 70-degree upright tilt, at rest, or during exercise (Cotsamire et al, 1987). CO was comparable, given an increase in HR in the semirecumbent position. When subjects were tested maximally, the left ventricular ejection fraction was greater in the semirecumbent position than in the supine position. Overall, exercise capacity was greater in the supine and full upright positions than in the semirecumbent position. Thus, body position affects exercise responses directly by its effect on hemodynamics and cardiac function.

Differences between genders exist in response to bed rest; for example, the types of muscle-function changes that occur differ. Mechanical efficiency when cycling decreases in both healthy men and women after 20 days of horizontal bed rest (Suzuki et al, 1997). Delta efficiency (work/energy liberation), however, is significantly greater for men in upright exercise than in supine exercise. There is no change for women. This is thought to reflect a selective decrement in slow-twitch muscle fibers associated with a decrease in leg-muscle mass in men during bed rest.

Gait speed has been proposed as a means of predicting discharge for individuals with acute stroke. Within the first 5 weeks following stroke, the 5-meter walk test at a comfortable pace, as opposed to the 10-meter walk test, the timed up-and-go test, and other common functional assessment indexes, is the measure of choice for detecting change in walking ability (Salbach et al, 2001).

Monitoring

Patients for whom mobilization is prescribed require monitoring. Because of the stress to the oxygen transport system that mobilization elicits, the following variables, in addition to oxygen transport variables, are most useful: HR, systolic and diastolic BP, RPP, RR, SaO_2, arterial blood gases, and ECG. The RPP is an index of myocardial $\dot{V}O_2$ during exercise and an indicator of the work of the heart (Steele et al, 1978). In individuals with ischemic heart disease, the anginal threshold often can be defined by the RPP. After bed rest, healthy individuals have blunted sympathetic responses to isometric exercise in the antigravity muscles (Kamiya et al, 2004). Thus, patients who have had periods of recumbency and restricted activity may show similar abnormal responses to exercise. Subjective responses, including discomfort and pain, fatigue, exertion, and breathlessness, can be recorded as needed. Visual analog scales are commonly used, as are modified Borg scales (0, or nothing at all, to 10, maximal symptoms). Subjective responses are more inherently variable

and unreliable, therefore potentially less valid (Whaley et al, 1997). Nonetheless, intrasubject reliability may be acceptable if measures are conducted in a standardized manner.

Mobilization Prescription

Prescribing a mobilization stimulus for its acute effects parallels the prescription of exercise for its long-term effects but with some important differences. In patients with acute disease, a mobilization or stimulus often results in a greater response gain than is found with such a stimulus in patients with subacute or chronic illness. In addition to the rapid favorable response an acutely ill patient may have to acute exercise, the patient may exhibit a negative response just as quickly. Thus, judicious monitoring of treatment responses in these patients is essential; the prescription is response driven. Finally, patients for whom mobilization is indicated have had variable periods of recumbency that can alter their hemodynamics and autonomic function as well as their capacity to respond normally to mobilization (Kacin et al, 2002). Hemodynamic responses even to static exercise can be blunted, and this may vary from day to day. Further, such responses can vary from hour to hour in acutely ill patients, and day to day in patients with chronic dysfunction.

The scheduling of and preparation for a mobilization session is crucial to the response that can be expected. The following conditions should be adhered to as closely as possible, and their details should be recorded so that any factor that influences the response to treatment can be identified. The patient should be rested, should not have eaten heavily in the previous couple of hours, should be as attentive and aroused as possible, and should be experiencing minimal pain, discomfort, or other distress. Review of a patient's medication schedule will ensure that treatments are well timed with respect to analgesia and medications that interfere with a good treatment response, such as narcotics. The patient's clothing should not be restrictive, and any lines, leads, and catheters should not be taut. Any equipment, monitors, or arterial and intravenous lines should be appropriately positioned to avoid disconnections or mishaps. Mobilizing a patient in intensive care requires the positioning of the mechanical ventilator and other supports before moving the patient. Portable ventilators facilitate mobilizing and ambulating patients (McCluskey et al, 2001). The physical therapist must prepare assistants before moving a patient, particularly if one or more assistants is required. Despite the number of persons assisting, the goal is usually to have the patient perform as much of the mobilization activity as possible. Even small degrees of physical movement can provide sufficient stress to the cardiopulmonary system to be beneficial.

The basic components of a mobilization session should approximate the components of an exercise session described by the American College of Sports Medicine for long-term training effects (2000) (Figure 18-1). Wherever possible, the session should include warm-up, steady-rate, cool-down, and recovery. These components are less distinct when a patient

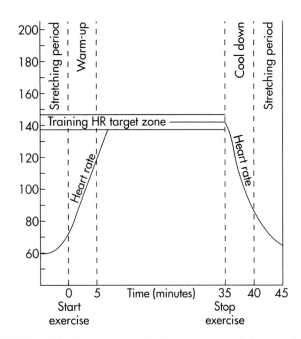

FIGURE 18-1 Components of the exercise training session: stretching, warm-up, training zone, cool-down, and stretching. *(From American College of Sports Medicine. [2000]. Guidelines for exercise testing and prescription, ed 6. Philadelphia: Lippincott, Williams & Wilkins.)*

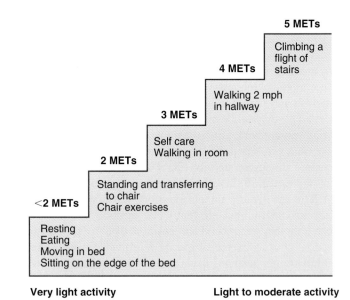

FIGURE 18-2 Progression of mobilization in patients with acute medical and surgical conditions based on a consideration of METs. *(Adapted from Woods, S.L. [2004]. Cardiac nursing, ed 5. Philadelphia: Lippincott, Williams & Wilkins.)*

has minimal functional capacity or is being mobilized to remediate acute cardiopulmonary dysfunction. The rhythmic movement of large muscle groups is still ideal. Prolonged static maneuvers are usually avoided, particularly if the patient is severely ill, because of their disproportionate hemodynamic response. The movements that are usually considered when mobilizing a patient include turning, sitting up, shifting, transferring, standing, and taking some steps. The progression of the levels of mobilization and exercise for medical and surgical patients, based on a consideration of metabolic cost (up to light to moderate activity), is illustrated in Figure 18-2. This schema represents the low end of the incremental staircase of activities based on the MET level shown in Figure 18-3 for a broader range of physical activities (up to very heavy activity).

Patients progress from one level to the next on the basis of their objective and subjective responses. Mobilization can be metabolically demanding for patients with acute cardiopulmonary dysfunction. Thus, pacing the mobilization session allows the patient to rest between stages. The patient is reassured and encouraged to relax and coordinate deep breathing and coughing with the activity. Throughout the session, attention is given to the patient's biomechanical alignment, postural erectness, and stability. Back extension or body positioning minimizes the slumping of the chest wall and compromised ventilation. In this way, chest wall expansion is maximized in three dimensions. The erect position is efficient and requires the least amount of energy to maintain. Less demand is placed on the accessory muscles of respiration

in erect sitting, and this effect is enhanced further by leaning forward and supporting the arms.

This chapter emphasizes the principles of mobilization and progression for the patient who is acutely-ill but medically stable. Patients who are medically unstable, including those in the ICU, have special considerations, which are addressed in Chapters 33, 34, 35, and 36. Regardless of setting, however, the rate at which progression occurs is always dependent on the patient's response.

Mobilization Training

The optimal therapeutic dose of the acute mobilization stimulus is based on the patient's presentation and history; the specific parameters are determined by the goals of the treatment and the acute effects of exercise that are indicated. The intensity of mobilization for many patients, for example, is that intensity that elicits optimal V_Ts and $\dot{V}_A$, increased RR and air-flow rates, enhanced mucociliary transport, and cough stimulation, without arterial desaturation, hemodynamic instability, or respiratory distress.

Over time, exposure to an acute exercise stimulus of an appropriate intensity, for an appropriate duration, and at an appropriate frequency will stimulate long-term aerobic adaptation to that stimulus. Underprescribing the exercise stimulus results in less potent effects, and overprescribing results in excessive, deleterious effects. Although the latter may be tolerated in the short run, the patient's well-being may be jeopardized by suboptimal treatment responses, overtraining signs and symptoms, and risk.

The duration of each mobilization session and the frequency of sessions are response dependent rather than time

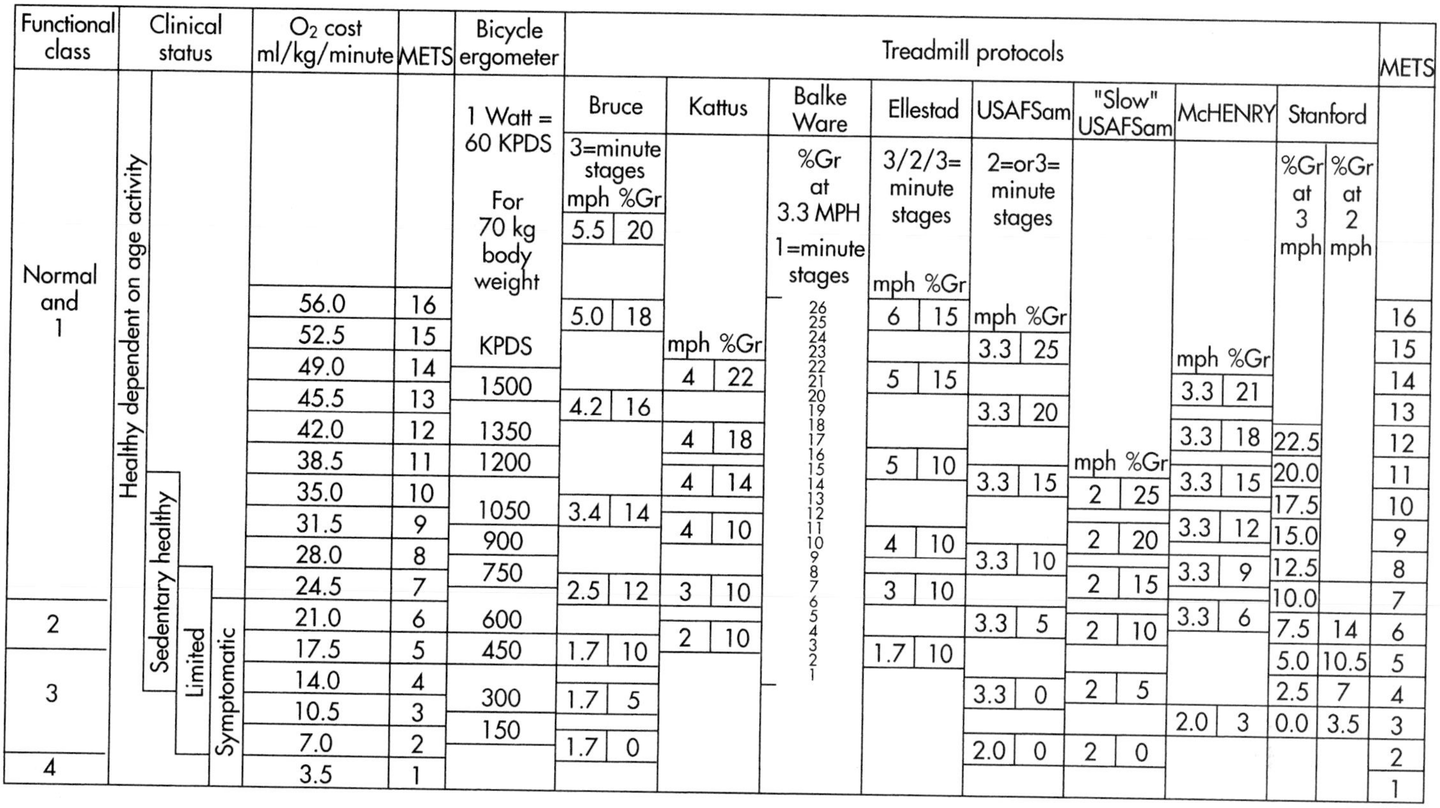

Oxygen cost of work stages of some commonly used exercise test protocols:

Functional class	Clinical status	O₂ cost ml/kg/minute	METS	Bicycle ergometer (1 Watt = 60 KPDS; For 70 kg body weight)	Bruce mph	Bruce %Gr	Kattus mph	Kattus %Gr	Balke Ware %Gr at 3.3 MPH	Ellestad mph	Ellestad %Gr	USAFSam mph	USAFSam %Gr	"Slow" USAFSam mph	"Slow" USAFSam %Gr	McHENRY mph	McHENRY %Gr	Stanford %Gr at 3 mph	Stanford %Gr at 2 mph	METS
Normal and 1	Healthy dependent on age activity				5.5	20														
		56.0	16		5.0	18				6	15									16
		52.5	15	KPDS					26			3.3	25							15
		49.0	14	1500			4	22	25 24 23	5	15					3.3	21			14
	Sedentary healthy	45.5	13		4.2	16			22 21 20			3.3	20							13
		42.0	12	1350			4	18	19 18 17							3.3	18	22.5		12
		38.5	11	1200					16 15 14	5	10			2	25	3.3	15	20.0		11
		35.0	10				4	14	13 12 11			3.3	15			3.3	12	17.5		10
	Limited	31.5	9	1050	3.4	14	4	10	10 9	4	10			2	20	3.3	9	15.0		9
		28.0	8	900					8 7			3.3	10	2	15			12.5		8
		24.5	7	750	2.5	12	3	10	6 5 4	3	10							10.0		7
2	Symptomatic	21.0	6	600					3 2 1			3.3	5	2	10	3.3	6	7.5	14	6
		17.5	5	450	1.7	10	2	10		1.7	10							5.0	10.5	5
3		14.0	4									3.3	0	2	5			2.5	7	4
		10.5	3	300	1.7	5										2.0	3	0.0	3.5	3
		7.0	2	150	1.7	0														2
4		3.5	1									2.0	0	2	0					1

FIGURE 18-3 Oxygen cost of work stages of some commonly used exercise test protocols. *(From Froehlicher V.F., & Myers, J.N. [2000]. Exercise and the heart, ed 4. Philadelphia: Elsevier.)*

dependent. The optimal mobilization threshold, in which physiological variables increase but not in excess of predetermined acceptable and safe limits, should be maintained for as long as possible within the patient's fatigue and comfort levels and in the absence of adverse responses. The mobilization sessions should be repeated as often as the patient can tolerate them (i.e., as often as the patient exhibits beneficial responses or no deterioration and adequately recovers between treatments). Treatment sessions for acute cardiopulmonary dysfunction are usually shorter and more common than for patients with chronic cardiopulmonary dysfunction. The patient's condition changes rapidly, with respect to both improvement and deterioration. Progression of mobilization for its immediate acute effects is usually rapid. Progression of exercise for its long-term effects may occur every several weeks, whereas progression of mobilization for its acute effects may occur as frequently as every treatment to every few days. Over time, exposure to a progressive mobilization stimulus leads to long-term physiological adaptations throughout the oxygen transport pathway. The goal is to achieve the oxygen transport status that is consistent with being able to discharge the patient from care to home, or to the next lowest level of care (e.g., from critical care to the ward).

In patients who are severely and acutely ill, passive rather than active exercise may be the only feasible option. Little research has been done to examine the acute and chronic effects of such exercise. When passive cycling is compared with active cycling (10% of $\dot{V}O_2$max) in healthy people, however, $\dot{V}O_2$, HR, exertion, and electromyogram (EMG) activity are predictably lower (Krzeminski et al, 2000). The shortening of the duration of the preejection period, and this period in relation to ejection time, however, are similar. Plasma catecholamines remain at resting levels for both types of exercise, but blood lactates increase in both, with higher levels occurring in active cycling. Thus, the inotropic response to exercise probably depends on both skeletal muscle mechanoreceptors and the Frank-Starling mechanism (preload and shortening in the preejection period).

Monitoring

The more acute the patient's condition, the more physiological variables need to be recorded as outlined previously. The capacity to measure multiple objective measures is available in special care and intensive care units, and often these are continuously monitored. Subjective responses are also vital to refine the adequacy of the mobilization stimulus (not too much and not too little); however, severely ill patients are often unable to respond effectively. Compared with the condition of chronic patients, the condition of acute patients tends to vary more within and between sessions and afterwards, which necessitates greater monitoring.

Monitoring should be performed continuously or at least frequently in patients for whom acute mobilization has been prescribed. First, a baseline of the patient's resting metabolic state must be established. Second, the metabolic responses to stimuli that perturb oxygen transport and the lability of these responses must be established. Obtaining such a profile provides some indication of the upper limit for the target intensity range of mobilization. The target intensity range can be defined in terms of an upper and a lower level of various physiological variables. The most commonly used are HR, ECG, BP, RPP, RR, and perceived exertion or breathlessness. Monitoring during nursing procedures and other types of routine care provides an indication of the patient's functional capacity without having to conduct a modified exercise test. Similarly, detailed monitoring is conducted during a mobilization or exercise challenge. The patient's response is compared with resting baseline measures. The quality as well as the immediacy of the response is documented. The characteristics of the quality of response are also recorded. Is the response commensurate with the intensity of the exercise stimulus? With cessation of exercise, do the responses revert to baseline? If so, how fast? Do the variables return to baseline or remain above baseline? In addition, qualitative assessment is made based on the physical therapist's subjective impressions. The patient's self-reports are also important.

The variables to be measured depend on the patient (see Chapters 2 and 17). Most commonly, HR, ECG, BP, RPP, RR, and subjective symptoms are considered basic measures and indexes of exercise response that require no invasive procedures. At the other end of the spectrum is the critically ill patient who has various invasive lines and monitoring equipment, including hemodynamic monitoring and intracranial pressure monitoring. This patient requires more specific and frequent measures of oxygen transport. Several measures in high dependency care areas can be monitored continuously, such as cardiac rhythm, HR, and BP.

The use of transcutaneous oxygen and carbon dioxide tensions as indexes of gas exchange has been considered limited in exercise testing, yet their use would overcome the need for arterial cannulation (Carter & Banham, 2000). The use of these measures as estimates of gas exchange has been shown to be reliable, provided the electrodes are heated and the workload changes are gradually increased to allow for latency in response time.

Adaptation to an Acute Mobilization Stimulus

When an individual is exposed to repeated exercise stress of a specific threshold intensity and for a response-dependent duration and frequency, there is a cumulative adaptive response to that repeated stimulation, or a long-term, training response. In deconditioned individuals and in those whose oxygen transport system has been compromised by disease, the exercise intensity associated with relatively low-intensity mobilizing activities (such as bed exercises, moving in bed,

sitting up, dangling over bedside, transferring to chair, chair exercises, and short walks with assistance) constitute sufficient, progressive gravitational and exercise stimuli to initiate adaptation to being upright and moving. However, it is important to stress that optimal adaptation occurs only if these activities are prescribed at the requisite intensity, duration, and frequency, and the exercise prescription progresses commensurate with the individual's adaptation. Mechanical ventilation is not a contraindication to mobilization. In fact, new generations of mechanical ventilators are portable and perform comparably to conventional ventilation. They are associated with minimal adverse effects on hemodynamic variables and oxygen transport (McCluskey et al, 2001), and can facilitate mobilization and ambulation.

Mobilization activities prescribed to enhance oxygen transport can be coupled with resistive muscle work to increase muscle strength and endurance (e.g., weights, use of a monkey bar for moving in bed and sitting up, manual resistive exercise, the use of wrist or ankle weights, ergometry, and walking). Coordinating postural changes, thoracic mobility, and upper-extremity exercises with inspiratory and expiratory efforts can be effective in stimulating increased V_T and improving ventilation-perfusion matching. Chapters 22 and 23 illustrate how such movement and breathing patterns can be coupled so as to maximize oxygen transport in patients with neurological conditions. Such coordinated exercise, however, can also be used in patients with acute cardiopulmonary conditions. Isometric exercises, postures that require increased muscle work for stabilization, and activities that elicit the Valsalva maneuver produce disproportionate hemodynamic responses, which could be detrimental. The capacity of the patient to respond appropriately to these loads must be established beforehand to avoid undue risk.

In the management of acute cardiopulmonary dysfunction, the parameters of mobilization stimuli include a relatively low intensity (although it is often perceived as intense by the patient), short duration, and high frequency of sessions. If the patient is severely compromised as in end-stage heart or lung disease, interrupted or interval training is indicated. This type of training is characterized by either on-off exercise, which allows for rest in between bouts of exercise, or high-low intensities of activity. The volume of work that can be achieved in an interrupted protocol by a severely compromised patient is greater than that achievable during continuous activity. With physiological adaptation over time, the exercise period can be increased and the rest period decreased and possibly eliminated. When high- and low-intensity exercises are alternated, the workload can be progressed by increasing the respective loads in each phase or by increasing the duration of the higher load period. If the patient has a low functional work capacity but sufficient physiological reserve, adaptation can be rapid, necessitating small, frequent progressions. As the patient's aerobic capacity increases, the response gains are correspondingly smaller. If the patient has both poor functional capacity and poor physiological reserve capacity, progress would be correspondingly slower.

TABLE 18-2

Relationships Among Mobilization and Exercise Prescription Parameters

	SESSION DURATION	SESSION FREQUENCY
Incremental activity		
Mobilization activities	Short (e.g., 5 min)	1 time per 1 to 2 hours
(e.g., self-care, moving in bed, bed exercises, sitting up in bed, sitting on the edge of the bed, standing, transferring to chair, walking)	Long (e.g., 20 min)	4 to 6 times per day
Interval continuous aerobic exercise	Short (e.g., 5 min)	1 time per 1 to 2 hours
	Long (e.g., 20 min)	4 to 6 times per day
Continuous aerobic exercise (light)	Short (e.g., 5 min)	1 time per 1 to 2 hours
	Long (e.g., 20 min)	4 to 6 times per day
Continuous aerobic exercise (moderate)	Short (e.g., 10 min)	2 to 3 times per day
	Long (e.g., 30 min)	1 time a day or two days
Continuous aerobic exercise (heavy)	Short (e.g., 20 min)	Daily
	Long (e.g., 30 to 45 min)	3 to 5 times per week

Intensity is set to the needs of the individual (i.e., oxygen transport and aerobic capacity are being stressed sufficiently to meet the treatment goals, with risk being minimized). The duration and frequency of treatments are based on the individual's responses and tolerance, with these being maintained within an optimal margin of safety and of recovery profiles.

When mobilization is prescribed to remediate acute cardiopulmonary dysfunction, particularly in patients in the ICU, extensive and often invasive monitoring is required. This permits detailed assessment and ongoing metabolic assessment of the patient's treatment responses and recovery. With these supports, mobilization and exercise can be prescribed effectively for these patients. Judicious monitoring minimizes inherent risks of either under- or overprescribing the intensity of the exercise stimulus (see Part II). Monitoring leads, lines, and catheters may restrict body positions and activities. Such encumbrances, however, do not preclude most activities, including ambulation. Moving relatively immobile patients who are confined to their beds with lines and leads is crucial, because it is these patients who benefit significantly from exercise stress but succumb most severely to its removal.

The goal is to adapt the patient to multiple short mobilization sessions per day, as frequently as once per hour as indicated and as tolerated, and progressively increase the intensity of these sessions, reduce the duration and correspondingly reduce the frequency of sessions. Table 18-2 illustrates the inverse relationship between mobilization and exercise intensity, with the duration and frequency of the sessions.

PRESCRIPTION OF MOBILIZATION AND EXERCISE: LONG-TERM RESPONSES

In health, the long-term effects of exercise occur in response to a specific and sufficient exercise stimulus to which the individual is exposed for a finite period. With respect to aerobic training or adaptation, the essential training parameters appear in Table 18-1. As central and peripheral adaptation to the exercise stimulus occurs, each step in the oxygen transport system becomes more efficient in facilitating Do_2, $\dot{V}o_2max$, and extraction at the cellular level (Astrand et al, 2003; Froelicher & Myers, 2000; McArdle et al, 2000). The long-

term effects of aerobic exercise are summarized in Box 18-7. In addition to an increase in $\dot{V}o_2max$, training results in exercise-induced bradycardia and increased SV at rest and in reduction in the physiological demands of submaximal work rates. Specifically, ventilation and hemodynamic responses to submaximal exercise are decreased. Endurance training increases parasympathetic activity and decreases sympathetic activity at rest (Carter, 2003). Arterial stiffness is decreased (Gates et al, 2003), and microcirculatory function and tissue perfusion are improved (Franzoni et al, 2004). The subjective experience of exercise stress is also reduced. These training effects are commensurate with increases in the efficiency of oxygen transport at each step in the pathway. Unlike the effects in patients with low functional work capacity, however, exercise does not improve ventilatory performance, as is evidenced by the relationship between ventilation and the production of carbon dioxide:

$$\dot{V}_E - \dot{V}co_2 \text{ slope}$$

and

$$\dot{V}_E/\dot{V}co_2$$

(Clark et al, 1994). Because of the marked ventilatory reserve in health, it is normally CO, rather than ventilation that limits exercise. However, there is some evidence that the respiratory system can limit endurance in healthy sedentary people (Boutellier & Piwko, 1992).

Although change in $\dot{V}o_2peak$ is the gold standard for aerobic conditioning, theoretically, submaximal $\dot{V}o_2$ values for given work rates do not change with training (Williams & Williams, 1983) unless improvement in movement efficiency and economy has occurred. With training, an individual reduces the physiological responses to each exercise load on an incremental exercise test, so is able to achieve a higher work load, thus higher $\dot{V}o_2peak$ with training.

BOX 18-7

Long-Term Physiological Effects of Mobilization and Exercise

Cardiopulmonary System

↓ Submaximal minute ventilation
↑ Respiratory muscle strength and endurance
↑ Collateral ventilation
↑ Pulmonary vascularization

Cardiovascular System

↑ Myocardial muscle mass
↑ Myocardial efficiency
Exercise-induced bradycardia
↓ Stroke volume at rest and submaximal work rates
↓ Resting heart rate and blood pressure
↓ Submaximal heart rate, blood pressure, and rate pressure product
↓ Submaximal perceived exertion and breathlessness
↑ Efficiency of thermoregulation
↓ Orthostatic intolerance when performed in the upright position

Hematological System

↑ Circulating blood volume
↑ Number of red blood cells
Optimize hematocrit
Optimize cholesterol
↓ Blood lipids

Central Nervous System

↑ Sense of well-being
↑ Concentration

Neuromuscular System

Enhance neuromotor control
↑ Efficiency of postural reflexes associated with type of exercise
↑ Efficiency of reflex control
↑ Movement efficiency and economy

Musculoskeletal System

↑ Muscle vascularization
↑ Myoglobin
↑ Muscle metabolic enzymes
↑ Glycogen storage capacity
↑ Biomechanical efficiency
↑ Movement economy
Muscle hypertrophy
↑ Muscle strength and endurance
↑ Ligament tensile strength
Maintain bone density

Endocrine System

↑ Efficiency of hormone production and degradation to support exercise

Immunological System

↑ Resistance to infection

Integumentary System

↑ Efficiency of skin as a heat exchanger
↑ Sweating efficiency
↓ Skin abrasions and breakdown
↑ Healing

That maximum HR (HRmax) is genetically determined and does not change with training has been challenged (Zavorsky, 2000). Factors that down-regulate HR have been implicated in resetting maximum heart rate. Such factors include the baroreceptors, autonomic function, the electrophysiology of the sinoatrial node, and a reduction in the number and density of beta-adrenergic receptors.

The rheology of blood plays an important role in cardiovascular disease. Platelet adhesiveness and aggregation are reduced with regular aerobic exercise (Wang et al, 1995). Optimal platelet adhesiveness along with blood volume maintain optimal blood viscosity, which is important for blood flow through the heart and blood vessels and for perfusion of peripheral tissue. Increased plasma viscosity and hematocrit have been attributed to exercise-induced hemoconcentration due to the shift of fluid from the blood to the interstitium (El-Sayed, 1998). With long-term endurance training, the plasma volume expands, which may reduce the resistance of blood flow to working muscle.

Exercise is a powerful controller of normal BP and an effective intervention to control high BP in patients with hypertension. The antihypertensive effects of long-term aerobic exercise are mediated through a reduction in total peripheral resistance and altered blood rheology. In addition, exercise may lead to weight loss, which contributes to lower BP. Individuals who are normotensive experience no changes in BP with an aerobic exercise program, even though peripheral resistance is reduced (Wijnen et al, 1994).

Aerobic exercise improves the hemodynamic responses and lipid profiles of individuals with cardiac disease. (see Chapter 24). Walking, cycling, and running are common types of aerobic exercise. However, patients from other cultures and those who do not enjoy these types of exercise may prefer t'ai chi, which also has been shown to have beneficial effects on BP, lipid profiles, and relaxation (Jones et al, 2005; Tsai et al, 2003).

Hemoglobin concentration and the number of circulating red blood cells are essential to effecting optimal oxygen transport (see Chapters 2 and 13). A single bout of exercise as well as long-term exercise can influence the erythropoietin processes in bone marrow (Szygula, 1990). In the extreme, exercise can interfere with these processes and result in "sports anemia." This condition can reflect postexercise plasma expansion, increased hemolysis with intense exercise, iron deficiency, bleeding into the digestive and urinary systems, and abnormal erythropoiesis.

The responses of the CNS to training include autonomic nervous system conditioning that is associated with BP control and thermoregulation (Kreider, 1991). Training is associated with a more sensitive vascular response to stress, which may reflect greater alpha-adrenergic sensitivity (Boutcher et al, 2001). The capacity to sweat is primed in response to exercise, which ensures that the muscle and internal organs remain at a temperature that is metabolically and energetically optimal for a given workload.

As the body adapts to the exercise training stimulus (overload principle), the intensity should be increased to elicit further training benefit. This is the basis for the physiological adaptation to a training stimulus. Depending on the goals of the exercise prescription, a decision is made after several weeks about whether the exercise intensity should be increased to further increase aerobic capacity or whether a maintenance program is indicated. The training program is progressed by establishing a new exercise intensity that usually is based on 70% to 85% of the HRmax achieved in a repeat of the initial exercise test.

Changes in cardiac structure and function after prolonged exercise by healthy people have been of interest to researchers in their attempt to understand changes during ill health. Questions such as "Does the heart muscle show signs of fatigue and impaired function with such exercise?" have been posed. One study of highly trained male athletes showed some cardiac damage along with reduced diastolic filling and contractility of the left ventricle after completion of a half-ironman triathlon (Shave et al, 2004).

The effect of exercise on glucose kinetics is important clinically for several reasons. First, illness creates metabolic stress on glucose metabolism; second, bed rest reduces insulin sensitivity; third, sedentary lifestyle and high-glycemic diets contribute to hyperglycemia and insulin insensitivity; and fourth, physical therapy's primary drug, exercise, places stress on energy substrates, including glucose metabolism, commensurate with the type, intensity, and duration of exercise. The time course of changes in glucose metabolism is important to the physical therapist because the patient must be protected from hypoglycemia and the effects of training on the muscles' sensitivity to insulin must be optimized. Even though these changes are well known to occur with multiple weeks of aerobic training, serial measures over the training period show that after 10 days there are benefits to glucose kinetics (Mendenhall et al, 1994).

Resistance muscle training has been a mainstay of physical therapy for motor recovery and conditioning effects in patient populations. There has been an increasing interest in the hemodynamic effects of resistance training and their interactions. After a resistance training program, healthy older adults show improved aerobic exercise responses. Cardio-vascular responses to exertion are reduced, peak responses are delayed, and recovery from maximum exertion is faster (Vincent et al, 2003). Training effect is determined by a dose-dependent relationship between intensity of resistance training and aerobic exercise responses, in addition to the individual's pre training status (Izquierdo et al, 2003). These effects are of benefit to patients with primary cardiovascular

and pulmonary dysfunction; thus, modified resistance training has become an integral component of traditional cardiac and pulmonary rehabilitation programs (see Chapter 24). Resistance muscle training, however, is associated with increased arterial wall stiffness, hence reduced compliance and increased pulse pressure (Dart & Kingwell, 2001). Increased pulse pressure is a risk factor for ischemic heart disease, which suggests the need for caution in prescribing exercise that has a selective effect on pulse pressure.

Caution should be taken with high-resistance exercise, which is defined relative to the individual's strength and endurance status. Sit-ups, for example, require relatively strong abdominal contraction and can elicit a heavy resistance contraction or strong isometric effort in weak individuals. In turn, intrathoracic pressure increases, SV decreases, and vascular injury may be precipitated. There have been reports of catastrophic neurological consequences (stroke and spinal epidural hematoma) in two healthy young men (Uber-zak & Venkatesh, 2002). Thus, prior to prescribing abdominal exercise, patients should be screened for risk factors. Breathing control should be incorporated to reduce intrathoracic and intrabdominal pressure. The physical therapist needs to be vigilant about detecting neurological signs and symptoms early.

Aggressive mobilization/exercise has been reported to have significant functional impact in the management of patients in the ICU. Prolonged intensive physical training, for example, has been reported to result in the regeneration of skeletal muscle after prolonged catabolism and weight loss (Bulow et al, 1993).

Respiratory muscle fitness may affect exercise performance in healthy individuals. Isolated respiratory muscle training increases respiratory muscle endurance and endurance time in response to whole-body exercise (Boutellier, 1998; Inbar et al, 2000; Markov et al, 2001). Although $\dot{V}O_2$max is unaffected, $\dot{V}_E$ and blood lactate decrease after training. In addition, respiratory muscle training can attenuate breathlessness in healthy people during exercise. However, improvements in respiratory muscle strength and endurance with specific training have been reported not to transfer to $\dot{V}O_2$max in athletes (Williams et al, 2002). Although optimizing respiratory muscle fitness through whole-body functional exercise is the goal in patient care, these findings have some clinical implications.

Upper-body and lower-body work have distinct physiological characteristics (Schneider et al, 2002a). These responses may have to be avoided (as in the hemodynamic stress of upper-body work in an individual with myocardial dysfunction) or exploited (as in an individual with lower-body paralysis). Oxygen kinetics differ for the two types of work, as do their hemodynamic responses. $\dot{V}O_2$ kinetics are prolonged in arm cranking compared with leg cycling. This change is consistent with increased type II fiber recruitment. Type II fibers are metabolically inefficient compared with fast, glycolytic, type I fibers.

Aerobic power declines with age. The capacity to train, however, is not age-limited, as training effects have been reported in octogenarians (Ehsani et al, 2003). Often older people show greater gains in response to training because of their reduced levels of baseline conditioning. Oxygen kinetics may be slowed with aging. Training responses reflect an increasing contribution to aerobic training by peripheral as opposed to central adaptations (McGuire et al, 2001b). Furthermore, based on a 30-year follow-up study, age-related decline in aerobic power over the course of 30 years was reversable with aerobic training (McGuire et al, 2001b). Tasks and exercises that involve various physiological systems are differentially affected by aging as well as by training. Training profiles of young and middle-aged adults show an age-related performance decline in cardiorespiratory endurance but not in muscle endurance (Knapik et al, 1996). This finding has implications for norms of fitness and prognosis for recovery. Finally, lack of exercise has been implicated in the incidence of cognitive impairment in the elderly (Ho et al, 2001). Physiological changes associated with aging, particularly those related to exercise capacity, are often confounded by deconditioning and related physical deterioration in older people rather than being an immutable consequence of aging (Zeleznik, 2003).

Circadian rhythms refer to physiological changes that occur in response to the fluctuating synthesis and secretion of hormones and other endocrine regulators over time (usually over 24 hours). These have a profound effect on physiological function. Circadian rhythms can be exploited in optimizing functional performance. Younger people may want to exercise later in the day, whereas older people might optimize their activity and exercise in the morning (Atkinson & Reilly, 1996). These differences are important to the physical therapist concerned with optimizing performance in patient populations whose response to activity and functional capacities may be dependent on time of day. Growth hormone production is determined by circadian fluctuations, sleep, and exercise (Godfrey et al, 2003). Growth hormone is implicated in metabolism and physical performance throughout life. Thus, exercise-induced growth hormone is an important effect of exercise that can optimize levels of growth hormone for general health, well-being, and successful aging. Circadian rhythms can be desynchronized during illness and, in particular, during hospitalization. That is why normal day and night cycles should be maintained, even in critical care units, so as to augment patients' recovery.

Exercise induces white blood cell production, so it is important for optimizing natural immunity (McKenzie et al, 1999). Generally, moderate levels of regular aerobic exercise are associated with improved immune function (MacKinnon, 2000a). Within the first 10 minutes of intense exercise, leucocytosis increases as do the thrombocytes responsible for increasing platelet production. These changes are not associated with exercise-related hypovolemia or hyperthermia. Whether leukocytosis and exercise are dose-dependent or there is a critical exercise intensity that has to be achieved to stimulate leucocytosis has yet to be established. Prolonged exhaustive exercise has been associated with compromised immunity, which may be avoided with optimal rest and recovery along with good nutrition and possibly vitamin C supplements (MacKinnon, 2000b). After prolonged heavy exercise in athletes, an "open window" of susceptibility to infection lasting 3 to 72 hours after exercise has been described (Nieman, 2000). The risk for infection may be exacerbated by travel, lack of rest and sleep, inappropriate diet, weight loss, and mental strain, and it may be prevented or reversed by better rest and diet and more exercise (Mascitelli & Pezzetta, 2003). Training strategies recommended for athletes so they can optimize their immunocompetence have relevance for clinical populations. Exercise sessions are monitored for individuals' susceptibility to infection, their general health, and the intensity and duration of the exercise session as well as recovery, rest, optimal diet, and stress management (Gleeson, 2000; Pyne et al, 2000).

After decades of research in exercise science based on men and college-aged students in particular, an increasing number of studies have identified gender differences in exercise responses. Higher $\dot{V}O_2$ peak and muscle strength are found in men, even when adjusted for body weight. These are explained primarily by hormonal differences, specifically estrogen and progesterone in women and testosterone and androgen in men. Differences in autonomic function contribute to the reduced risk by women for heart disease and to their increased longevity (Carter et al, 2003). Women have greater parasympathetic control of the heart and less sympathetic activity.

To evaluate an apparently healthy individual who is beginning an exercise program, the Physical Activity Readiness Questionnaire (PAR-Q) is an established screening device (Figure 18-4). The answers help establish whether a progressive exercise program is indicated or whether there are contraindications to the individual's undertaking a progressive exercise program. The person may require a medical workup if cardiopulmonary risk factors or musculoskeletal limitations exist. Underlying conditions may have to be addressed beforehand or concurrently.

EXERCISE TESTING AND TRAINING IN PATIENT POPULATIONS

Numerous conditions, including nonprimary cardiopulmonary conditions, have been shown to benefit from the long-term effects of aerobic exercise (Box 18-8; see Chapters 24 and 25). Thus, for each patient with these conditions, the exercise prescription differs. Comparable with prescribing mobilization in acute conditions, prescribing exercise for long-term adaptations is based on the patient's presentation, history, premorbid status and conditioning level, lab and investigative reports related to physiological reserve capacity, the exercise test, and the goals of the exercise prescription. To promote health, as few as 30 minutes of moderately intense exercise a day on most days of the week is required (Varo Cenarruzabeitia et al, 2003). However, based on the American College of Sports Medicine (2000) guidelines, optimal aerobic exercise

Physical Activity Readiness
Questionnaire - PAR-Q
(revised 2002)

PAR-Q & YOU

(A Questionnaire for People Aged 15 to 69)

Regular physical activity is fun and healthy, and increasingly more people are starting to become more active every day. Being more active is very safe for most people. However, some people should check with their doctor before they start becoming much more physically active.

If you are planning to become much more physically active than you are now, start by answering the seven questions in the box below. If you are between the ages of 15 and 69, the PAR-Q will tell you if you should check with your doctor before you start. If you are over 69 year of age, and you are not used to being very active, check with your doctor.

Common sense is your best guide when you answer these questions. Please read the questions carefully and answer each one honestly: check YES or NO.

YES	NO	
☐	☐	1. Has your doctor ever said that you have a heart condition <u>and</u> that you should only do physical activity recommended by a doctor?
☐	☐	2. Do you feel pain in your chest when you do physical activity?
☐	☐	3. In the past month, have you had chest pain when you were not doing physical activity?
☐	☐	4. Do you lose your balance because of dizziness or do you ever lose consciousness?
☐	☐	5. Do you have a bone or joint problem (for example, back, knee or hip) that could be made worse by a change in your physical activity?
☐	☐	6. Is your doctor currently prescribing drugs (for example, water pills) for your blood pressure or heart condition?
☐	☐	7. Do you know of <u>any other reason</u> why you should not do physical activity?

If you answered

YES to one or more questions

Talk with your doctor by phone or in person BEFORE you start becoming much more physically active or BEFORE you have a fitness appraisal. Tell your doctor about the PAR-Q and which questions you answered YES.

- You may be able to do any activity you want — as long as you start slowly and build up gradually. Or, you may need to restrict your activities to those which are safe for you. Talk with your doctor about the kinds of activities you wish to participate in and follow his/her advice.
- Find out which community programs are safe and helpful for you.

NO to all questions

If you answered NO honestly to <u>all</u> PAR-Q questions, you can be reasonably sure that you can:
- start becoming much more physically active – begin slowly and build up gradually. This is the safest and easiest way to go.
- take part in a fitness appraisal – this is an excellent way to determine your basic fitness so that you can plan the best way for you to live actively. It is also highly recommended that you have your blood pressure evaluated. If your reading is over 144/94, talk with your doctor before you start becoming much more physically active.

DELAY BECOMING MUCH MORE ACTIVE:
- if you are not feeling well because of a temporary illness such as a cold or a fever – wait until you feel better; or
- if you are or may be pregnant – talk to your doctor before you start becoming more active.

PLEASE NOTE: if your health changes so that you then answer YES to any of the above questions, tell your fitness or health professional. Ask whether you should change your physical activity plan.

<u>Informed Use of the PAR-Q</u>: The Canadian Society for Exercise Physiology, Health Canada, and their agents assume no liability for persons who undertake physical activity, and if in doubt after completing this questionnaire, consult your doctor prior to physical activity.

No changes permitted. You are encouraged to photocopy the PAR-Q but only if you use the entire form.

NOTE: if the PAR-Q is being given to a person before he or she participates in a physical activity program or a fitness appraisal, this section may be used for legal or administrative purposes.

"I have read, understood and completed this questionnaire. Any questions I had were answerd to my full satisfaction."

NAME _____

SIGNATURE _____ DATE _____

SIGNATURE OF PARENT _____ WITNESS _____
or GUARDIAN (for participants under the age of majority)

Note: This physical activity clearance is valid for a miximum of 12 months from the date it is completed and becomes invalid if your condition changes so that you would answer YES to any of the seven questions.

 © Canadian Society for Execise Physiology   Supported by: Health Canada Santé Canada   continued on other side...

FIGURE 18-4 The Physical Activity Readiness Questionnaire (PAR-Q). *(From Health Canada. [2005]. Canadian Society for Exercise Physiology. www.csep.ca.)*

BOX 18-8

Chronic Conditions That Benefit From the Long-Term Effects of Mobilization and Exercise

Cardiovascular Conditions

Congenital heart disease
Acquired heart disease
Postsurgical heart conditions
Angina
Hypertension
Hyperlipidemia
Hypercholesterolemia
Chronic heart failure
Heart transplantation
Peripheral vascular disease

Cardiopulmonary Conditions

Chronic obstructive pulmonary disease
Chronic ventilatory insufficiency and failure
Interstitial lung disease
Asthma
Cystic fibrosis
Postthoracotomy conditions
Lung transplantation

Neurological Conditions

Stroke
Parkinson syndrome
Quadriplegia
Paraplegia
Cerebral palsy
Down syndrome
Multiple sclerosis
Poliomyelitis and post polio syndrome

Endocrine Conditions

Thyroid dysfunction
Diabetes mellitus

Neoplastic Conditions

General conditioning
Prevention in some cases

Musculoskeletal Conditions

Osteoarthritis
Rheumatoid arthritis
Ankylosing spondylitis
Osteopenia and osteoporosis

Connective Tissue Conditions

Systemic lupus erythematosus
Scleroderma

Nutritional Disorders

Insulin resistance associated with physical inactivity
Obesity
Anorexia

Conditions Requiring Organ Transplantation

Pre- and postsurgical stages

Other Systemic Conditions

Chronic fatigue syndrome
Chronic depression
Renal disease
Liver disease
Alcoholism
Nonalcoholic and alcoholic cirrhosis of the liver

Other

Pregnancy

---

adaptation requires an exercise stimulus of 70% to 85% of HRmax for 20 to 40 minutes, 3 to 5 times a week for at least 6 to 8 weeks. However, the effect of exercise intensity on $\dot{V}O_2$max and on CO continues to be studied (Lepretre et al, 2004). Improvement in $\dot{V}O_2$max does not appear to be achieved by the same central and peripheral adaptations across a range of exercise intensities. Some individuals have high $\dot{V}O_2$max, CO, and SV without a history of training (Martino et al, 2002). This may reflect a genetically determined greater blood volume.

Exercise Testing

Exercise testing can pose a risk to the patient, so exercise testing must have clear indications, and any contraindications must be ruled out. On the other hand, earlier guidelines for exercise testing in patients, particularly those with cardiac disease, were too conservative (Fletcher et al, 1993). Patients can be exercised aggressively provided that the indications are based upon a comprehensive assessment and a judiciously selected exercise test and protocol and provided that the patient is appropriately monitored throughout testing.

The indications for exercise testing are numerous (Box 18-9). They range from quantifying maximum functional, aerobic, or oxygen transport capacities to assessing endurance during low-level activities of daily living (ADLs). The capacity of the oxygen transport system is the most important determinant of maximum oxygen uptake in healthy people. Metabolic studies including $\dot{V}O_2$ provide a link between impairment and functional capacity (Singh, 2001) and can distinguish cardiac versus pulmonary contribution to exercise intolerance (Myers & Madhavan, 2001). $\dot{V}O_2$ studies require the use of a nose clip or face mask, which may contribute to perceived exertion in addition to the increased dead space that is created by the inspiratory circuit. In a study comparing the two devices in patients with congestive heart failure, no difference in gas-exchange measurements was observed (Baran et al, 2001). Perceived exertion, however, was not reported. This is an important finding given that $\dot{V}O_2$peak is a strong predictor of survival (see Chapter 24).

BOX 18-9

Common Indications for Exercise Testing in Patient Populations

Diagnosis of Limitations of Structure and Function

Primary cardiovascular and pulmonary dysfunction
Secondary cardiovascular and pulmonary dysfunction

Diagnosis of Factors Contributing to Limitations of Activity and Participation

Assessment

Maximal functional work capacity
Submaximal functional work capacity
Endurance
Dyspnea
Chest pain
Ability to work
Employment options
Cardiopulmonary and cardiovascular conditioning
Limitations due to noncardiopulmonary factors
Movement economy
Effect of medication (supplemental oxygen, blood pressure medication, antianginal medication, oral hypoglycemic agents and insulin, analgesics, bronchodilators)
Adequacy of diabetes management
Adequacy of orthotics, walking aids, and prostheses

Prescription

Exercise program
Medications (effects and regulation)

BOX 18-10

Relative and Absolute Contraindications to Exercise Testing

Absolute Contraindications

Congestive heart failure
Acute electrocardiogram changes in myocardial ischemia
Unstable angina
Ventricular or dissecting aneurysm
Ventricular tachycardia
Multifocal ectopic beats
Repetitive ventricular ectopic activity
Untreated or refractory tachycardia
Supraventricular dysrhythmia
Recent thromboembolic event (pulmonary or other)
Uncontrolled asthma
Uncontrolled heart failure
Pulmonary edema
Uncontrolled hypertension (>250 mm Hg systolic, >120 mm Hg diastolic)
Acute infections

Relative Contraindications

Recent myocardial infarction (less than 4 weeks earlier)
Aortic valve disease
Severe cardiomegaly
Pulmonary hypertension
Resting tachycardia
Resting electrocardiogram abnormalities
Poorly controlled diabetes
Severe electrolyte disturbance
Severe systemic hypertension
Significant conduction disturbance
Complete atrioventricular block
Fixed-rate pacemakers
Acute cerebrovascular disease
Respiratory failure
Left ventricular failure
Epilepsy

Adapted from Jones, N.L., & Fletcher, J. (1997). Clinical exercise testing, ed 4. Philadelphia: WB Saunders.

$\dot{V}O_2$ studies have become a primary component of the workup of patients with abnormal exercise tolerance for diagnostic and assessment purposes and for exercise prescription. Metabolic measurement carts are used to conduct these studies. To ensure valid and reliable data, the gases used by the cart must be calibrated and testing procedures tightly standardized before the test as well as during it. A practice session is recommended to reduce learning effects and sympathetic arousal (Dean et al, 1989). Prior to the commencement of the test, a couple of minutes of baseline measures are taken against which the acute exercise responses and the recovery responses can be compared. The metabolic measurement cart can be programmed to display a variety of exercise variables and graphs of interest. The exercise test results are interpreted according to an evaluation of the resting baseline values, the responses of the exercise variables to changes in the exercise test protocol (qualitatively and quantitatively appropriate), the interrelationship of these changes, and whether they achieve some peak value, such as HR or perceived exertion. Beforehand, a decision is made with respect to whether the test is sign- or symptom-limited. Any unusual responses or events during the test are documented. The full impact of the test may not be manifested for several hours or even the next day, so the patient is followed so these changes or effects can be evaluated as well. In some patients, lactate measures that require invasive blood work or, minimally, a finger prick, may be indicated.

Contraindications to exercise testing and, in particular, maximal testing are classified as relative or absolute (Box 18-10). Absolute contraindications prohibit the safe conduct of an exercise test, whereas the presence of relative contraindications requires that the test, protocol, physiological variables monitored, or end point of the test be modified. Both the indications for the test and any contraindications must be clearly established before performing an exercise test.

The guidelines used to test and train healthy people with no disease are not directly generalizable to patients with chronic illness who are medically stable. Because of functional impairments in these patients (secondary to cardiopulmonary, cardiovascular, neuromuscular, or musculoskeletal dysfunction), exercise testing and training must be modified. Moreover, patients who are physically challenged experience more

TABLE 18-3

Subjective Scales of Exercise Responses

	PERCEIVED EXERTION	BREATHLESSNESS	DISCOMFORT/PAIN	FATIGUE
0	Nothing at all	Nothing at all	Nothing at all	Nothing at all
0.5	Very very weak	Very very light	Very very light	Very very light
1	Very weak	Very light	Very weak	Very light
2	Weak	Light	Weak	Light
3	Moderate	Moderate	Moderate	Moderate
4	Somewhat strong	Somewhat hard	Somewhat strong	Somewhat hard
5	Strong	Hard	Strong	Hard
6				
7	Very strong	Very heavy	Very strong	Very heavy
8				
9				
10	Very very strong	Very very hard	Very very strong	Very very hard
	Maximal	Maximal	Maximal	Maximal

Based on the Borg rating of perceived exertion scale.

subjective symptoms in response to exercise than do healthy people, so monitoring the subjective responses to exercise is essential. The Borg scale of rating perceived exertion can be modified for clinical use to score breathlessness, discomfort, pain, and fatigue (Table 18-3) (Borg, 1970, 1982). If the end points of the scale have been well described and are understood by the patient, the ratings can be used to compare the patient's subjective exercise responses over repeated tests. The patient's subjective reports can be correlated with the exercise response and so can provide a basis for exercise prescription as well as avoiding adverse responses.

The functional impairments and capacities of the patient determine the nature of the exercise test; it can be one of various types, depending on the objective of testing and potential training. If exercise training is an objective of the exercise test, the activity used in the test should be comparable to that to be used in training. Physiological responses and adaptation to exercise are specific to the training stimulus (the specificity-of-exercise principle). Thus, if walking is to be the training activity, the test should be a walking test, not a cycling test.

There are numerous variants of standard exercise tests (Table 18-4). They are categorized as continuous tests or interrupted tests. Continuous tests include maximal and submaximal incremental tests and steady-rate tests; interrupted tests include maximal interval and submaximal interval tests. Interrupted tests are designed for patients with low functional work capacity who cannot sustain prolonged periods of aerobic exercise. These patients can perform more work over time when the workload is intermittent. Specifically, the test allows for alternating fixed periods of work and rest or of high and low intensities of exercise. The proportions of work to rest or high to low exercise intensity is set according to the patient's level of impairment. One patient, for example, may be able to tolerate 3 to 5 minutes of relatively high-intensity

TABLE 18-4

Exercise Tests That Can Be Applied to Patient Populations

TEST TYPE	INDICATIONS
Continuous Tests	
Maximal	Generally medically stable patient
	No significant musculoskeletal abnormalities
	Test maximal functional capacity
	Basis for aerobic exercise program
Incremental	Incremental work rates, usually 2 to 5 minutes in duration
Steady rate	Endurance test at a given work rate, usually a comfortable walking or cycling speed
Submaximal	For patients in whom maximal testing is contraindicated
Incremental	Approximate maximal exercise testing
	Test of near-maximal functional capacity or some significant proportion of maximum
Steady rate	Establish baseline of response to steady-rate exercise, usually at 60% to 75% of predicted HRmax
	Establishes an index of endurance, cardiopulmonary conditioning and may give an index of movement economy
Interrupted Tests	
Maximal or submaximal	Establish level of functional capacity in patients with extremely low functional work capacity
	On-off protocol or high-low intensity protocol, such as 5 min on to 1 min off, alternate high- and low-intensity exercise in cycles, such as 1 minute high to 15 seconds low

BOX 18-11

Preexercise Test Conditions

Establish the indications for an exercise test.
Determine absolute and relative contraindications to conducting an exercise test.
Ensure that patient is free of any acute illnesses, including influenza and colds for 48 hours.
Ensure that patient understands the purpose of the test and provides signed consent.
Ensure that patient has not eaten heavily, has avoided caffeinated beverages, and has refrained from smoking for at least 3 hours before testing.
Ensure that patient is rested and has not exercised or been excessively exerted for at least 24 hours before testing.
Standardize time of day and the influence of circadian rhythm.
Ensure that patient is appropriately dressed: shorts, nonbinding clothes, short-sleeve shirt, socks, running or walking shoes that have proper support, and secured laces or fastenings.

Orthoses should be worn unless the test is evaluating changes in functional capacity with and without an orthosis.
Ensure that patient understands the subjective rating scales and is able to read them when they are held at an appropriate distance.
Select the type of exercise test, the protocol, and the exercise test termination criteria beforehand.
Ensure that the patient is familiar with and has practiced performing the test or test activity, preferably before the test day, so as to reduce arousal, improve movement efficiency, and maximize test validity.
Based on the purpose of the test, determine beforehand the premedication status of the patient. If medicated (e.g., bronchodilators or analgesics), ensure that they are at peak effect during test.
Room temperature (standardized and recorded).

work alternated with bouts of 1 to 2 minutes of low-intensity work, whereas another patient may be able to tolerate only 1 minute of low-intensity work alternated with 10 to 20 seconds of rest.

For maximal standardization and the capacity to perform comprehensive monitoring, stationary exercise modalities such as the treadmill, ergometer, or step are recommended. However, there may be indications to perform an exercise test without a modality, such as the 12-minute walk test or some variant like 6 or 3 minutes (McGavin et al, 1976). Standardization of such tests, however, is more challenging. Practice has a significant effect on the results of the 12-minute walk test, so this test must be repeated to achieve a valid test. Also, the instructions for this test are less well standardized clinically than are those for the treadmill or ergometer; this jeopardizes stringent test control and thus must be tightly standardized (Dean & Ross, 1992a).

Like other diagnostic and testing procedures, the validity and reliability of the exercise test depend on standardization of the procedures. Test validity and reliability can easily be compromised in the absence of repeated testing and controls (Kraemer et al, 1989; Noonan & Dean, 2000). Early ergometer training responses in resting along with submaximal heart rates and reduction in EMG activity in the arms and legs can reflect familiarization (Ziemba et al, 2003). Repeated exercise tests reflect the marked effects of practice. Practice reduces energy output, improves practice-related coordination, and reduces muscle activation (Lay et al, 2002). However, with good quality control, a test's validity and reliability can be maximized, even in patients with severe disease such as chronic heart failure (Meyer et al, 1997). The preexercise test conditions and the preparation and testing procedures must be standardized (Boxes 18-11 and 18-12).

The test is terminated as soon as the sign or symptom criteria for terminating the test are reached, or the criteria for prematurely terminating the test are reached (Box 18-13).

Recording the test conditions and procedures in detail is essential. An example of an exercise test data sheet that can be modified to any testing protocol that includes an exercise modality is shown in Box 18-14, *A*. Many patients are unable to be exercise tested using a modality; these patients can walk on a marked circuit, and the results are recorded on an exercise test data sheet like the one shown in Box 18-14, *B*. Systematic and detailed record keeping will maximize the test's validity and its interpretation and will ensure that the same procedures are used in follow-up tests, thereby maximizing the comparability of the results of repeated tests. It is imperative that retests be comparable in every respect to the original test in terms of the preparation of the patient and the procedures.

One application of exercise testing in patient populations that has been of interest is to predict $\dot{V}O_2peak$ (Noonan & Dean, 2000). Prediction of $\dot{V}O_2peak$ involves a large margin of error in healthy populations, and that margin could be expected to be greater in patients who are likely to be more deconditioned, have comorbidities, and be prone to greater variations in their exercise responses. The Astrand-Ryhming Cycle Ergometer Test continues to be one of the most frequently used submaximal tests for exercise prescription as well as for prediction of $\dot{V}O_2peak$ (Astrand, 1954). Prediction of $\dot{V}O_2peak$ is obtained from a nomogram in which the $\dot{V}O_2peak$ is estimated from the submaximal HR. To improve its accuracy, an age-correction factor is used to adjust for the age-dependent decrement in HRpeak (Astrand, 1960). This ergometer test has the clinical advantage of being applicable to less ambulatory people.

Three equations have been compared to predict $\dot{V}O_2peak$ in patients with hypertension and fibromyalgia (Dominick et al, 1999): one equation is from the American College of Sports Medicine (ACSM); one equation is from the Fitness and Arthritis in Seniors Trial (FAST); and the third equation was developed by Foster and colleagues (FOSTER). Predicted

BOX 18-12

Preparation and General Procedures for an Exercise Test

Preparation

Patient changes into exercise clothes and shoes (not new); ensure that laces are secure.

If the ergometer is used, the seat-to-pedal distance must be established before the test, and the seat should be adjusted to allow for 15 degrees of knee extension when the foot is lowermost in the pedal in the revolution cycle; the knee must not extend fully.

Patient sits quietly in a supported chair to establish a resting baseline.

Monitors are attached (e.g., heart rate, electrocardiogram, blood pressure cuff, pulse oximeter), and the subjective rating scales are explained.

Testing procedures are explained and demonstrated; the patient has an opportunity to ask questions.

General Procedures

Unnecessary conversation and interaction with the patient are kept to a minimum throughout all stages of the test, including postexercise recovery, so as to optimize the validity of the measurements and the test results overall.

Resting baseline measures are taken over 5 minutes or until they have reached a plateau.

Patient stands on treadmill or sits erect on cycle ergometer with feet securely strapped into place on the pedals; the metatarsal heads should be positioned comfortably over the pedals.

Patient uses two fingers for balance on one side, if, possible, when walking on the treadmill, rather than a hand grip; if on the ergometer, does not excessively grasp the handlebar.

Additional baseline measures are recorded in this position for 2 to 3 minutes or until the baseline is stable.

The test timer is started.

The warm-up portion of the protocol begins.

The selected protocol is carried out.

Patient is monitored objectively and subjectively at least every couple of minutes throughout all stages of the test, including postexercise recovery.

The test is terminated when the preset exercise test termination criteria or any of the criteria for prematurely terminating an exercise test are reached.

The cool-down begins.

When the cool-down portion of the protocol is complete, the patient moves to the supported chair for the postexercise recovery phase, with legs slightly elevated and uncrossed.

Postexercise recovery continues until resting baseline measures have been reached or are within 5% to 10%.

Obtain a report from patient about how patient feels.

Disconnect the monitoring equipment.

Continue to observe patient for any untoward postexercise signs or symptoms.

BOX 18-13

Criteria for Prematurely Terminating an Exercise Test

Miscellaneous

Wish of individual for any reason
Failure of monitoring equipment

General Signs and Symptoms

Fatigue
Lightheadedness, confusion, ataxia, pallor, cyanosis, dyspnea, nausea, or peripheral vascular insufficiency
Onset of angina

Electrocardiogram Signs

Symptomatic supraventricular tachycardia
Sinus tachycardia displacement (3 mm) horizontal or downsloping from rest
Ventricular tachycardia

Exercise-induced left bundle branch block
Onset of second- or third-degree atrioventricular block
R wave on T wave premature ventricular contractions (one)
Frequent multifocal premature ventricular contractions (frequent runs of three or more)
Atrial fibrillation when absent at rest
Appearance of a Q wave

Other Cardiovascular Signs

Any fall in blood pressure below the resting level
Exercise hypotension (> 20 mm Hg drop in systolic blood pressure)
Excessive blood pressure increase (systolic $\geq$ 220 or diastolic $\geq$ 110 mm Hg)
Inappropriate bradycardia (drop in heart rate greater than 10 beats/min with increase or no change in work load)

Adapted from the American College of Sports Medicine. (2000). Guidelines for exercise testing and prescription, ed 6. Philadelphia: Williams and Wilkins; and Jones, N.L., & Fletcher, J. (1997). Clinical exercise testing, ed 4. Philadelphia: WB Saunders.

$\dot{V}o_2$peak for all equations was different from the actual measured values. However, the FAST and FOSTER equations predicted values within 1 MET for both patient groups; the ACSM equation predicted values that were different by more than 2 METs.

The distance walked in the 6-minute walk test can provide valid information regarding the functional capacity of elderly patients with chronic heart failure (Peeters & Mets, 1996). The results are highly correlated with $\dot{V}o_2$max and can differentiate between classes III and IV of the New York Hospital Association classification of functional capacity.

Nutrition and preexercise meals as they relate to exercise testing and training of individuals with pathology have been given little attention in the literature compared with the

BOX 18-14

PANEL A: Exercise Test Data Sheet for Treadmill or Ergometer

Patient name:

Patient number:

Date:

Weight (kg):   Height (cm):   Body mass index:

Reason for test:

Type of test:

Resting HR: Resting BP:

FEV_1:   FVC: FEV_1/FVC: SpO_2:

Medications and timing in relation to test: _____

Review of preexercise checklist ☐

Level of handrail support: N/A ☐   Yes ☐

     Level _____

Use of orthotics and types: N/A ☐   Yes ☐

     Type _____

Minute or stage	Speed or tension	Grade or RPM	Heart rate and/or ECG changes	Blood pressure	Rate pressure product	SpO_2	Rating of perceived exertion or breath-lessness	Discomfort/pain (not anginal)	Comments

What was the reason for test? _____

     How often does the patient experience the level of exertion reached on the test in daily life?

     (e.g. 1×/wk   1×/month   3×/day   never

     other) _____

BOX 18-14

PANEL B: Exercise Test Data Sheet for a Walk or Circuit Test

Patient name:

Patient number:

Date:

Weight (kg):   Height (cm):   Body mass index:

Reason for test:

Type of test:

Resting HR: Resting BP:

FEV_1:   FVC: FEV_1/FVC: SpO_2:

Medications and timing in relation to test: _____

Review of preexercise checklist ☐

Use of orthotics and types N/A ☐   Yes ☐

   Type _____

Use of walking aids during the test N/A ☐   Yes ☐

   Type _____

Minute	Runway or circuit distance	Heart rate and/or ECG changes	Blood pressure	Rate pressure product	SpO_2	Rating of perceived exertion or breathlessness	Discomfort/pain (not anginal)	Comments
0 or Baseline	0							

What was the reason for test termination? _____

How often does the patient experience the level of exertion reached on the test in daily life?

(e.g.,   1×/wk   1×/month   3×/day   never

other) _____

attention given to the nutrition of healthy people and athletes. Nutritional preparation in respect to macro- and micronutrients and the timing of meals with respect to activity and exercise could have a major impact on the functional capacity of an individual with oxygen transport impairments and low functional capacity. The performance by healthy people in a bout of moderate- to high-intensity exercise for 35 to 40 minutes is improved if they consume a meal moderately high in carbohydrates and low in fat and protein 3 hours before exercise, rather than 6 hours before (Maffucci & McMurray, 2000). Missing or delaying meals could alter performance on a test or the outcome of training. Because it has been relatively overlooked in patient populations, nutrition as well as hydration should be a focus of the physical therapy assessment and standardized for the pretest and posttest and training sessions.

Exercise testing is considered resource-intense because of the need for highly qualified individuals to perform tests that are safe, valid, and reliable. In addition, pretest conditions must be met, and the patient has to devote a significant amount of time to taking one or more repeated tests. As a means of streamlining such testing, one study, using two different protocols, compared arterial blood gases and respiratory and metabolic measures in patients who reported shortness of breath (Zeballos et al, 1998). One protocol was an incremental exercise test and the other a constant-work protocol. The data generated by both protocols were comparable; however, $PaCO_2$ was somewhat higher during the incremental test, as were exercise stress indexes when compared above the anaerobic threshold. No differences were observed below this threshold.

Exercise Tests and Protocols

Exercise tests are used for diagnosis, assessment and evaluation, prognosis, and exercise prescription. The purpose is one major consideration in selecting the specific test and its protocol. The exercise test can be a continuous maximal, a submaximal incremental or steady-rate, or an interrupted maximal or submaximal test. The protocol for the test and the end points to be used in terminating the test are determined beforehand on the basis of the indications for the test and the objectives. Some commonly used protocols are shown in Figure 18-3 along with a comparison of the energy expenditure required by the various work stages in their protocols.

The 12-minute walk test and its variants, 6-minute and 3-minute walk tests, were designed to test patients with lung disease (McGavin et al, 1976). These tests have been favored clinically, because they are functional and do not require exercise equipment. However, these tests are often used for patients who have extremely impaired exercise capacity and are unable to tolerate being tested on an exercise modality. A major disadvantage, therefore, is that the patient cannot be as comprehensively monitored. Thus, patients who are to undergo a 12-minute walk test or one of its variants must be selected with care.

When the 6-minute walk test is applied to healthy older adults, it has been shown to be reliable; two familiarization tests are needed to minimize arousal and the learning effect (Kervio et al, 2003). In the same trial, the subjects walked, on average, at 80% of $\dot{V}O_2$max. Based on a comparison with the performance of patients with COPD to an "encouraged" 6-minute walk test and a standard incremental cycling test, the prognostic value of the walk test was reported to be high (Troosters et al, 2002). Patients achieved a high steady-rate $\dot{V}O_2$ in the walk test. No differences were reported in $\dot{V}O_2$, HR, and arterial blood gases between the two tests at peak. However, $\dot{V}_E$ and $\dot{V}CO_2$ were lower in the walk test. When performance was "encouraged," the 6-minute walk test was reported to have good prognostic value.

The 6-minute walk test has been favored as an expedient and inexpensive means of evaluating the functional capacity of older adults with multiple comorbidities. A short distance walked by this cohort is associated with having a low level of education; being non-Caucasian; having a reduced capacity to perform activities of daily living; self-reporting poor health; having a history of heart disease, stroke, or diabetes; and showing abnormal levels of C-reactive protein, fibrinogen, and white blood cell count (Enright et al, 2003).

The 6-minute walk test can provide a useful measure of the distance an individual can walk. Because it fails to account for body weight, a determinant of exercise capacity, the validity of the 6-minute walk test has been questioned. To enhance its usefulness, Carter and colleagues (2003) proposed the use of the product of the distance of the 6-minute walk and the body weight, to yield the work involved in the 6-minute walk. This measure provides a more valid measure of exercise performance and, in addition, can be converted to provide an index of calorie expenditure, hence, a standardized basis of comparison across exercise modalities.

The shuttle test has been another commonly used exercise test for patients with disabilities. When performance on this test is compared with the 6-minute walk distance in patients with COPD, the two tests appear to assess different pathophysiological processes (Onorati et al, 2003). The shuttle test is considered a more accurate predictor of maximal exercise capacity than the 6-minute walk test.

Reproducibility of exercise test results is a particular concern in patient populations whose status may change from day to day. When tested weekly for 4 weeks, patients with stable COPD have been reported to have reproducible submaximal physiological exercise responses and ratings of perceived exertion in response to a constant work rate (Covey et al, 1999). Exercise performance at a constant work rate is a functional indicator of endurance. On serial exercise testing of patients with chronic heart failure, the mechanical efficiency of walking markedly improves, which gives rise to an apparent placebo effect, and this effect has been reported to be independent of motivation and changes in conditioning (Russell et al, 1998). This factor can invalidate the findings of a single test. Highly trained individuals show a more marked neuroendocrine (sympathoadrenal and hypothalamopituitary

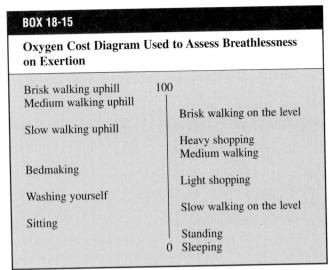

From McGavin, C.R., Artivini, M., Naoe, H., & McHardy, .G.J.R. (1978). Dyspnea, disability, and distance walked: comparison of estimates of exercise performance in respiratory disease. British Medical Journal, 22:241-243.

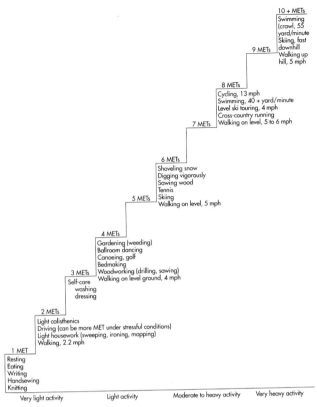

FIGURE 18-5 Energy cost in METSs of activity and exercise. *(From Woods, S.L. [2004]. Cardiac nursing, ed 5. Philadelphia: JB Lippincott, Williams & Wilkins.)*

adrenal) response in a second bout than in the first bout of exercise performed on the same day (Ronsen et al, 2001). There is a need to study the implications of neuroendocrine changes with repeated exercise tests in patient populations.

Knowledge of the patient's functional ability based on verbal report is useful and serves as a guideline for selecting the type of exercise test, its parameters, and the test termination criteria. Although these verbal reports do not replace an exercise test, they can be used as an adjunct. The diagram of oxygen cost is shown in Box 18-15. This visual analog scale is constructed of a 100-mm line with physical activities hierarchially sequenced based on oxygen cost; the high end of the scale represents strenuous activity (walking briskly uphill) and the low end of the scale represents no activity, or sleep. The patient crosses the line at the point where breathlessness does not allow continuation at the patient's best. Figure 18-5 shows an incremental staircase of workloads associated with step increments in metabolic cost, that is, multiples of resting or near resting metabolic rate (resting metabolic rate = 1 MET, or 3.5 ml O_2/min/kg of body weight). Metabolic costs of activities range from very light to very heavy activities. One limitation of such charts in indicating the metabolic costs of various activities and exercises is that they can be used only as a general guide in patients with cardiopulmonary compromise, as they do not take into consideration the increased work of breathing and the work of the heart that observed in patients with cardiopulmonary dysfunction, or the increased energy cost associated with abnormal biomechanics as observed in patients with neuromuscular and musculoskeletal conditions.

With respect to exercise capacity in patient populations, aerobic performance has been of primary interest for diagnosis, assessment, evaluation, and prognosis. $\dot{V}O_2$ studies provide a range of exercise performance data including anaerobic capacity, which is often ignored. Recently, however, the anaerobic threshold has been considered an important marker of cardiovascular insufficiency and exercise performance that has importance in evaluating the performance of individuals with low functional work capacity, such as the elderly and patients with left ventricular dysfunction, and in prescribing exercise for them (Nappi et al, 1997; Wasserman 2002). In addition, examining the anaerobic threshold may have particular relevance to individuals in these groups, who may be ill-advised to undergo maximal stress tests.

The oxygen uptake efficiency slope (OUES), which is based on a submaximal test, has been proposed as a valid and reliable index of exercise performance in patients with congestive heart failure (Hollenberg & Tager, 2000). This method was tested on older healthy individuals and on patients on the basis of the rationale that maximal testing is not always valid, feasible, or safe. The OUES involves plotting $\dot{V}O_2$ against the logarithm of total ventilation at submaximal work rates. On repeated tests, the OUES is less variable than endurance or $\dot{V}O_2$peak. Thus, the OUES is an objective and reproducible measure of cardiorespiratory reserve based on submaximal effort. The measure reflects ventilatory-circulatory-metabolic coupling and is influenced primarily by pulmonary dead-space ventilation and exercise-induced lactic acidosis.

Exercise testing and training can be challenging in individuals with marked physical disability such as those with severe stroke. Because of this limitation, many patients are denied the potential benefits of diagnostic exercise testing and exercise training. The use of external body supports is one means of providing support during standardized exercise testing on a treadmill. One study examined the metabolic effects of a 15% body-weight support in individuals without impairments (MacKay-Lyons, 2001). End expiratory gas variables were not affected, except for maximal V_T, which was lower with the body support; however, time to achieve peak values was increased. The responses of patient populations who would require variable levels of body support have yet to be determined.

Exercise testing has a role in preoperative assessment. In combination with other tests and examination, exercise testing in patients as a component of the workup for abdominal aortic aneurysm repair with measurement of $P\bar{v}O_2$ can identify patients at risk for perioperative complications (Nugent et al, 1998). Exercise testing has been used to define a gas-exchange threshold for patients with COPD who are being considered for thoracic surgery (Torchio et al, 1998). A $\dot{V}O_2$peak of less than 20 ml O_2/kg/min has been recommended as the threshold for predicting perioperative complications. Routine preoperative exercise testing has been advocated. Exercise testing has also been recommended to assist in determining the operability of a patient with lung cancer (Gilbreth & Weisman, 1994; Walsh et al, 1994). Patients may be excluded from lung resection surgery based on conventional medical criteria, yet included based on their $\dot{V}O_2$peak. These patients have shown survival benefit.

Monitoring

Common variables measured during an exercise test include HR, ECG, systolic and diastolic BP, RPP, RR, SpO_2, and subjective responses such as perceived exertion, breathlessness, discomfort, pain, and fatigue. Assessment of dyspnea is central to monitoring individuals with breathing and exertional impairments. The Borg scale and the visual analog scale are applicable to individuals with dyspnea and, if assessed in a systematic manner, they can provide valid and reliable measures when used in the patient groups for which they were designed, so they should be used routinely (Cullen & Rodak, 2002). Measures are taken every few minutes after the patient has been exercising at a given intensity for a few minutes when a response to steady-rate exercise is being assessed. This allows for relative stabilization of oxygen kinetics during dynamic exercise. Subjective responses to exercise and daily activities are often the most important to the patient as these are typically what interferes with their social participation and its composite activities.

The short- and long-term recovery responses, both quantitative and qualitative, in patient populations are important components of the exercise testing profile. A thorough understanding of normal physiological recovery responses is needed by the physical therapist to benchmark abnormal responses. Sustained elevated BP after cessation of exercise, for example, has been reported to be more sensitive than ECG for detecting myocardial insufficiency. Further, systolic BP after exercise is a strong predictor of hypertension, coronary artery disease, and cardiovascular mortality. An increase in systolic BP and the percent maximum systolic BP 2 minutes post exercise is directly and independently related to risk for stroke (Kurl et al, 2001).

Exercise Training Prescription

One of the most common indications for exercise testing is to establish whether a training program is indicated and, if so, what the training parameters should be. The components of exercise training for patients is the same as those for healthy people, specifically, selection of the type of exercise; its intensity, duration, and frequency; and the course of training and its progression. New advances in athletic training that may have application to clinical populations include titrating training day by day in response to a detailed analysis of the responses to and recovery from the previous exercise session. This method is based on modeling the effects of training, detraining, and overtraining (Banister, 1992; Morton, 1997). This method does not assume that the interval between exercise sessions is the same across individuals or the same for a given individual from one day to the next. The proponents of the model believe that training is optimized by the avoidance of under- or overtraining, and that the training effect is better if it is accumulated over time, rather than according to the conventional methods that subscribe to a rigid exercise intensity, duration, and frequency over some interval (e.g., 6 to 8 weeks). Other areas of study necessary for population patients include the use of adjuncts to maximize endurance.

Individualizing an exercise prescription rather than administering a standardized program is essential to maximizing outcomes in the same way a that physician must individualize a drug prescription (Vallet et al, 1997). The word *prescription* implies individualization to a person's needs and goals with respect to social participation and its composite activities. Thus, comparable to the athlete, the selection of the type of exercise for training and that used in the exercise test is based on the objectives of the training. Hemodynamic responses are dependent on the type of exercise and the degree of static exercise and postural stabilization involved and on the muscle mass involved. Depending on the patient's status and diagnoses, hemodynamic responses have to be considered. The HR response to ergometer rowing using the arms and legs, for example, is lower than running for the same relative workload (Yoshiga & Higuchi, 2002). This reflects increased venous return. $\dot{V}O_2$max and O_2 pulse are also greater in rowing.

Water exercise, including chair exercise in the water and running, are undergoing a revival in physical therapy for the management of chronic conditions. Water provides buoyancy, prevents injury, reduces spinal loading and lower extremity loading, minimizes muscle soreness, and optimizes temperature control to facilitate exercise performance. Long-term effects of water exercise such as deep-water running include increased blood volume, increased stroke volume, and increased cardiac output (Reilly et al, 2003). Water exercise for strength or cardiovascular endurance has benefits for training and for recovery from injury. Aquatic exercise programs have the advantage of being offered to groups as a way of improving fitness in healthy individuals and in people with pathologies such as stroke (Chu et al, 2004).

The intensity is usually set at some proportion of the HR response or some other response, to a maximum or near-maximum work rate that was safely tolerated during the exercise test. The training intensity for an individual who is able to tolerate several incremental work stages on a graded exercise test may be optimal between 70% to 85% of the HRpeak, or 60% to 80% of the $\dot{V}O_2$ achieved in the test. Alternatively, in health, a training zone can be estimated based on a predicted HRmax such as 220 − age. This predicted maximum is associated with significant error ± 10 beats (i.e., deviation from the actual HRmax achieved in a maximal test), thus the HR at which training is eventually conducted is refined on the basis of other indexes, such as the talk test and general responses. The ratio of HRmax (actual or predicted) and resting HR (the Heart Rate Ratio Method) provides a good estimate of $\dot{V}O_2$max in healthy men and may have some application in some patient populations (Uth et al, 2004).

A patient who is unable to tolerate a couple of increases in work stage is more likely to benefit from an exercise intensity range of 60% to 75% of the HRpeak achieved. In some patients, HR is an invalid indicator of exercise intensity because of the pathology or medications (Dean, 1993; Dean & Ross, 1992b). Thus, other responses, such as BP, arterial saturation, or subjective parameters such as rating of perceived exertion or breathlessness, can be used. The duration and frequency of the exercise program are established based on the patient's functional capacity, physiological reserve capacity, and exercise responses (Table 18-2, for general guidelines). Patients with low functional capacities but with adequate physiological reserve capacity respond to a training stimulus quickly (short training course), so should be progressed accordingly. Patients with low functional capacities, however, and with limited physiological reserve capacity adapt more slowly (long training course). The shorter the training course, the sooner a retest is indicated to progress and reset the training parameters. To ensure that the patient continues to be trained safely and optimally, the training parameters should be progressed based on an exercise retest.

Developing exercise programs for the masses of sedentary people in the community constitutes one of the greatest challenges to the physical therapist. Motivating people to be physically active in their daily lives and undertake a formal program of exercise is a skill in itself (see physical activity pyramid in Chapter 1). Intermittent bouts of exercise accumulated throughout the day are showing acceptance by the public and are producing favorable results. The 10,000-steps-per-day program encourages individuals to wear a pedometer and become conscious of how closely they approximate this guideline, which has been associated with an "active" lifestyle (Tudor-Locke & Barnett, 2004). With this objective information, people may be more inclined to increase the number of their daily steps so as to improve their health by elevating the range of their daily steps from the inactive to the active lifestyle. Another creative public health initiative is a stair-climbing program in the community. Such a program has been directed to sedentary young women (Boreham et al, 2000). The 7-week program of stair climbing involves progressing from one flight to several flights daily using a public-access stairway of 199 steps. This short-term exercise program resulted in aerobic conditioning as evidence by reduced $\dot{V}O_2$, HR, and lactate during stair climbing and by improved cholesterol levels. Such innovative approaches have enormous potential for improving public health.

The prescription of the parameters for optimal physiological recovery has not been described in detail. However, the practice of progressive, decremental exercise intensity in the form of a warm-up is supported. Such activity facilitates venous return and the return of HR and other exercise parameters to baseline values (Takahashi & Miyamoto, 1998). In addition, light activity after exercise promotes the degradation of circulating catecholamines. Priming exercise in athletes improves performance (Jones et al, 2003), and this result can be expected in nonathletes as well. However, the parameters (i.e., exercise type, intensity, and duration) of an optimal warm-up have yet to be defined, and they may depend on the individual, general health and fitness, weight, age, and morbidity.

Cross-training principles analogous to those used in athletes apply to patients (Mujika & Padilla, 2000a, 2000b). Based on the assessment of oxygen transport deficits and threats and goals for the individual (e.g., function, health, fitness, prevention, or a combination), a decision is made regarding the prescription of a single mode or a dissimilar mode of training. Because of the specificity of exercise principles, the generalization of a single-mode exercise can not be assumed; thus, other types of exercise, including task-specific exercise, may have to be included. Also, consideration should be given to the cross-transfer effects of exercising one side of the body. Cross-transfer between ipsilateral and contralateral limbs should be considered when focusing attention on one side of the body or to limit detraining during periods of unilateral immobilization.

An overtraining phenomenon has been described in healthy people. Athletes whose performance has dropped off may improve performance outcomes with several weeks of rest (Koutedakis et al, 1990). The role of overtraining in people with underlying pathology, whether induced by the pathology or resulting from an excessive therapeutic exercise prescription, is not well understood. The extent to which some severely compromised patients are, in fact, overtrained as a mere consequence of their activities of daily living is not known. It is possible that the syndrome of inability to maintain work performance, persistent fatigue, frequent illness (in particular upper respiratory tract infections), disturbed sleep, and altered mood states may reflect overwork in patients that is analogous to overtraining in athletes (MacKinnon et al, 2000). With respect to immunity, reduced neutrophil function may be implicated in both situations. In athletes, this overtraining syndrome due to excessive physical exertion and inadequate recovery has been related to autonomic dysfunction and increased cytokine production. Because regular intense exercise can suppress mucosal immunity and because saliva is the most commonly used secretion for assessing mucosal immunity, monitoring the saliva of athletes during critical training periods provides an index of risk status. The usefulness of mucosal assessment in clinical populations warrants investigation. Relaxation has been shown to offset the exercise-induced suppression of secretory immunoglobulin associated with upper respiratory tract infection in healthy people (Reid et al, 2001). The role of relaxation and its immune protection warrants exploitation in clinical populations. Immunity may be optimized with an appropriate balance of exercise, rest, and recovery. Achieving an optimal balance of exercise and rest or recovery warrants study in patient populations when focused on optomizing social participation.

Prescriptive rest, including optimal sleep in patient populations, comparable to that of athletes should be considered as closely as the prescriptive parameters of exercise itself to produce optimal physical performance.

BOX 18-16

Patient's Checklist Before Exercise Testing or Training Session

☐ Feeling well over the past 48 hours
☐ No infections (e.g., upper respiratory tract infection) or influenza
☐ No temperature
☐ No unaccustomed muscle or joint discomfort or pain
☐ No chest tightness or pain
☐ No unaccustomed breathing difficulty or fatigue
☐ Adequate night's sleep
☐ Has not eaten heavily within past 3 hours
☐ Best time of day
☐ Wearing or using orthoses, walking aids, and devices
☐ Clothing appropriate for exercise conditions (indoors or outdoors)
☐ Appropriate socks and footwear that is comfortable, well-fitting, and has secured laces (double-knotted)
☐ Has water within reach
☐ Taken preexercise medications at specified time
☐ Has nitroglycerine within reach (patients with cardiac dysfunction)
☐ Has inhaler within reach (patients with pulmonary dysfunction)
☐ Has sugar supply within reach (patients with diabetes)
☐ Standardize and record the use of orthotics and walking aids

---

Exercise Training
General procedures

Before an exercise session, the patient needs to review a checklist to ensure that exercise is not contraindicated on that day. This is particularly important for patients whose conditions change rapidly or whose disease course tends to fluctuate, as in multiple sclerosis, cystic fibrosis, chronic fatigue syndrome, and congestive heart failure. Box 18-16 provides a checklist to be used in preparation for exercise testing and training sessions. Such a checklist, however, must be tailored to each patient. Aids and devices for older patients must provide assistance that is optimal and safe and promotes the most independence. Inappropriate aids are associated with poor patient outcomes in this population, and their use requires more surveillance by carers (Taylor & Hoenig, 2004).

Active exercise is always selected to elicit optimal oxygen transport stress for improving aerobic and muscle power. Passive exercise, however, may have a limited role in some patients. Compared with active exercise, little is known about the physiological responses to passive exercise. When low-intensity active and passive cycling are compared in healthy people, inotropic changes are elicited primarily with active exercise, thus are dependent on mechanoreflexes stimulated by the metabolic products of skeletal muscle (Krzeminski et al, 2000). Cardiac output is increased by an increase in HR during active cycling and by an increase in stroke volume during passive cycling. It is interesting to note that, blood lactate increases in both active and passive cycling, but is higher during active cycling. These findings are of some physiological interest and may have potential therapeutic application; however, active exercise is the therapeutic priority, no matter how minimal the absolute intensity, duration, and frequency may be initially. The degree to which passive exercise could be exploited in individuals unable to cooperate with an exercise program, or whether passive exercise could augment active exercise, warrants further study.

Specific procedures

In a supervised setting, the general procedures used in exercise training are comparable to those used for testing. Specifically, the patient prepares for the training session in a standardized manner and is monitored according to his or her condition. The components of the session are the same with respect to warm-up, cool-down, and recovery. The main part of the exercise program, however, will usually be steady-rate or interrupted exercise. Varying work rates may be indicated for some patients.

In the majority of situations, the goal is to transfer the responsibility of surveillance and monitoring from the physical therapist to the patient. Depending on the patient's pathology and ability to learn how to monitor exercise responses accurately, this process takes varying amounts of time.

Planning of transition to home and the community is considered from the beginning. The patient's daily needs at home serve as the basis for the exercise program; his or her skills need to be transferred from the physical therapist and clinic to the home environment.

Monitoring

For safety reasons and to ensure that the patient is within the target training range of the variables selected to set exercise intensity, the patient must be closely monitored. This is particularly true if the patient has any risk of untoward or adverse reactions to exercise. If a patient is considered to be at any risk, exercise training should take place only in a supervised setting. A stable patient may begin an exercise program in a supervised setting, but with training and education can usually be transferred to an unsupervised setting. Education includes self-monitoring of exercise responses, maintaining exercise intensity within the appropriate limits, and keeping a record of the details of their exercise sessions. When the patient is safely carrying out the exercise program independently in the community, some mechanism is needed to follow up on the patient's progress. If the objective is continued conditioning, the patient should be rescheduled for a retest. If the patient is on a maintenance program, the physical therapist is responsible for reminders about exercise and injury precautions and about notifying the physical therapist or physician if significant adverse effects are observed.

HR, BP, RR, and other measure are taken according to standardized procedures. Electronic equipment and mechanical devices must be calibrated. A break point in the double product (HR × systolic BP) and work-rate relationship can provide a good estimate of the anaerobic threshold in patients with exercise intolerance as well as in healthy persons (Riley et al, 1997).

Patients on sympathomimetic drugs or with various pathologies will have abnormal exercise responses. Thus, knowledge of these factors is essential to determine whether a measure is valid.

The World Health Organization recommends repeated BP measurements be performed in the sitting or supine position followed by standing (WHO, 1999), and that the cuff be positioned at the level of the right atrium, irrespective of body position. One concern about this recommendation is that systolic and diastolic BP is lower in a sitting than in a supine position, so the two readings are not equivalent (Netea et al, 2002). Blood pressure may be under- or overestimated if the level of the cuff is not at the level of the right atrium, regardless of body position. Further, this effect may be amplified in patients with autonomic dysfunction such as that found in patients with diabetes.

Nutritional status and rest/sleep status must be assessed in patient populations by physical therapists to maximize exercise capacity and function comparable to competitive athletes. Mobilization and exercise must be prescribed to maximize these effects during acute and chronic long-term exercise.

SUMMARY

Physical therapists are clinical exercise physiologists whose primary "drugs" include mobilization and exercise to address limitations in participation and activity irrespective of whether these limitations result from primary or secondary cardiovascular/pulmonary dysfunction. This chapter describes three distinct goals associated with the prescription of mobilization and exercise in the management of impaired oxygen transport: to exploit the preventive effects, acute effects, and long-term effects of exercise so as to maximize an individual's capacity for activity and participation in life when that person is limited by impairment of oxygen transport at the structural and functional levels.

The physical therapist must have a comprehensive and detailed understanding of how mobilization and exercise have potent and direct effects on oxygen transport preventively, acutely, and in the long term. The specific mobilization or exercise prescription is based on a comprehensive multisystem assessment, an analysis of oxygen transport dysfunction or failure, and the treatment goals for a given patient.

If the preventive effects of mobilization or exercise on oxygen transport are required, the prescription focuses on maximizing these benefits for a given patient by prescribing exercise that is of sufficient intensity, duration, and frequency to preserve adequate aerobic capacity and endurance for that patient. Mobilization or exercise may be prescribed for its preventive effects in conjunction with its acute or long-term effects. Although the principles of prescribing mobilization and exercise for their optimal preventive effects have not been elucidated scientifically, exercise in some form is indicated commensurate with levels of recumbency and restricted activity.

If the acute effects of mobilization or exercise are indicated to remediate oxygen transport limitations, the prescription specifies the parameters of an appropriate mobilization or exercise stimulus, usually of relatively low intensity, short duration, and high frequency. The treatment effects are often immediate. Because treatment responses can be dramatic, the prescription is progressed relatively quickly, depending on the patient's responses to the treatment. Prescribing mobilization to remediate acute cardiopulmonary dysfunction requires the same precision and specificity as prescribing exercise for chronic cardiopulmonary dysfunction.

If the long-term effects of exercise are indicated, the exercise stimulus is defined in an appropriate prescription, generally involving higher intensity, longer duration, and less frequency, compared with the prescription for the acute effects, and is designed to be followed for several weeks or more before demonstrable physiological adaptation can be observed and progression of the stimulus indicated.

These three levels of prescription of mobilization and exercise are physiologically distinct and should be prescribed specifically by the physical therapist for a given patient, giving consideration to their indications, contraindications, and side effects for that individual.

Finally, the physical therapist needs to be proficient in the assessment of nutritional status and sleep/rest status in every patient. These are important variables in facilitating and inhibiting response to exercise comparable to that in athletic training.

Review Questions

1. Describe how the physical therapy exploitation of the effects of mobilization and exercise are congruent with the levels of the Model of Ability, that is, structure and function, activity, and participation.

2. Distinguish between mobilization and exercise.

3. Distinguish among the prescription of mobilization/exercise for their preventive effects, their acute effects, and their chronic effects.

4. Describe the negative sequelae of restricted mobility and bed rest.

5. Describe the distinction between "prescriptive" mobilization or exercise and its "routine" clinical use to prevent the sequelae of recumbency and restricted activity.

6. Explain the effects of mobilization on enhancing the efficiency of oxygen transport.

7. Explain the effects of exercise on enhancing the efficiency of oxygen transport.

8. Describe the differences in the mobilization/exercise prescription parameters (i.e., type of exercise stimulus, intensity, duration, frequency, and course) when prescribing mobilization/exercise for its (a) preventive effects, (b) acute effects, and (c) chronic effects.

9. Describe the factors that can invalidate exercise test results and jeopardize test realiability and thus must be tightly controlled by the physical therapist.

10. Describe how the physical therapy assessment of nutrition and sleep/rest can be used to augment clinical outcomes.

REFERENCES

Ahlinder, S., Birke, G., Norberg, R., Plantin, L.O., & Reizenstein, P. (1970). Metabolism and distribution of IgG in patients confined to prolonged strict bed rest. Acta Medica Scandinavica 187:267-270.

Akima, H., Kuno, S., Suzuki, Y., Gunji, A., & Fukunaga, T. (1997). Effects of 20 days of bed rest on physiological cross-sectional area of human thigh and leg muscles evaluated by magnetic resonance imaging. Journal of Gravitational Physiology 4:S15-S21.

Aldrich, D., & Hunt, D.P. (2004). When can the patient with deep vein thrombosis begin to ambulate? Physical Therapy 84:268-273.

Alkner, B.A., & Tesch, P.A. (2004). Efficacy of a gravity-independent resistance exercise device as a countermeasure to muscle atrophy during 29-day bed rest. Acta Physiologica Scandinavica 181:345-357.

Allen, C., Glasziou, P., & Del Mar, C. (1999). Bed rest: a potentially harmful treatment needing more careful evaluation. Lancet 354:1229-1233.

Al-Obaidi, S., Anthony, J., Dean, E., & Al-Shuwai, N. (2001). Cardiovascular responses to repetitive McKenzie lumbar spine exercise. Physical Therapy 81:1524-1533.

American College of Sports Medicine. (2000). Guidelines for exercise testing and prescription, ed 6. Philadelphia: Lippincott Williams & Wilkins.

Astrand, I. (1960). Aerobic capacity in men and women with special reference to age. Acta Physiologica Scandinavica 49(Suppl) 169:2-92.

Astrand, P.-O., Rodahl, K., Dahl, H., & Stromme, S. (2003). Textbook of work physiology: physiological bases of exercise, ed 4. Philadelphia: Human Kinetics.

Astrand, P.-O., & Ryhming, I. (1954). A nomogram for calculation of aerobic capacity from pulse rate during submaximal work. Journal of Applied Physiology 7:218-221.

Atkinson, G., & Reilly, T. (1996). Circadian variation in sports performance. Sports Medicine 21:292-312.

Banister, E.W. (1992). Dose/response effects of exercise modeled from training: physical and biochemical measures. Annals of Physiology and Anthropology 11:345-356.

Baran, D.A., Rosenwinkel, E., Spierer, D.K., Lisker, J., Whelan, J., Rosa, M., & Goldsmith, R.L. (2001). Validating facemask use for gas exchange analysis in patients with congestive heart failure. Journal of Cardiopulmonary Rehabilitation 21:94-100.

Bassey, E.J., & Fentem, P.H. (1974). Extent of deterioration in physical condition during postoperative bed rest and its reversal by rehabilitation. British Medical Journal 4:194-196.

Belin De Chantemele, E., Blanc, S., Pellet, N., Duvareille, M., Ferretti, G., Gauquelin-Koch, G., Gharib, C., & Custaud, M.A. (2004). Does resistance exercise prevent body fluid changes after a 90-day bed rest? European Journal of Applied Physiology 29:555-564.

Belman, M.J., & Wasserman, K. (1981). Exercise training and testing in patients with chronic obstructive lung disease. Basics of Respiratory Disease 10:1-6.

Bernhardt, J., Dewey, H., Thrift, A., & Donnan, G. (2004). Inactive and alone: physical activity within the first 14 days of acute stroke unit care. Stroke 35:1005-1009.

Blair, E., & Hickman, J.B. (1995). The effect of change in body position on lung volumes and intrapulmonary gas mixing in normal subjects. Journal of Clinical Investigation 34:383-389.

Blair, S.N., Painter, P., Pate, R.R., Smith, L.K., & Taylor, C.B. (Eds). (1988). Resource manual for guidelines for exercise testing and training. Philadelphia: Lea & Febiger.

Blattner, W., & Partsch, H. Leg compression and ambulation is better than bed rest for the treatment of acute deep vein thrombosis. International Angiology 22:393-400.

Bloomfield, S.A. (1997). Changes in musculoskeletal structure and function with prolonged bed rest. Medicine and Science in Sports and Exercise 29:197-206.

Boreham, C.A., Wallace, W.F., & Nevill, A. (2000). Training effects of accumulated daily stair-climbing exercise in previously sedentary young women. Preventive Medicine 30:277-281.

Borg, G. (1982). Psychophysical basis of perceived exertion. Medical Science in Sports and Exercise 14:377-381.

Borg, G.A.V. (1970). Psychophysiological bases of perceived exertion. Scandinavian Journal of Rehabilitation Medicine 2:92-98.

Boutcher, S.H., Nurhayati, Y., & McLaren, P.F. (2001). Cardiovascular response of trained and untrained old men to mental challenge. Medicine and Science in Sports and Exercise 33:659-664.

Boutellier, U. (1998). Respiratory muscle fitness and exercise endurance in healthy humans. Medicine and Science in Sport and Exercise 30:1169-1172.

Boutellier, U., & Piwko, P. (1992). The respiratory system as an exercise limiting factor in normal sedentary subjects. European Journal of Applied Physiology and Occupational Physiology 64:145-152.

Browse, N.L. (1965). The physiology and pathology of bed rest. Springfield, Ill.: Charles C. Thomas.

Bulow, H.H., Kanstrup, L., Henriksen, O., Ingemann-Jensen, L., & Qvist, J. (1993). CT and magnetic resonance imaging and spectroscopy for noninvasive study of regeneration of skeletal musculature after intensive therapy. Ugeskrift for Laeger 19:2273-2276, English abstract..

Bydgeman, S., & Wahren, J. (1974). Influence of body position on the anginal threshold during leg exercise. European Journal of Clinical Investigation 4:201-206.

Cardus, D. (1967). O$_2$ alveolar-arterial tension differences after 10 days' recumbency in man. Journal of Applied Physiology 23:934-937.

Carter, J.B. (2003). Effect of endurance exercise on autonomic control of heart rate. Sports Medicine 33:33-46.

Carter, R., & Banham, S.W. (2000). Use of transcutaneous oxygen and carbon dioxide tensions for assessing indices of gas exchange during exercise testing. Respiratory Medicine 94:350-355.

Carter, R., Holiday, D.B., Nwasuruba, C., Stocks, J., Grothues, C, & Tiep, B. (2003). Six-minute walk work for assessment of functional capacity in patients with COPD. Chest 123:1408-1415.

Chase, G.A., Grave, C., & Rowell, L.B. (1966). Independence of changes in functional and performance capacities attending prolonged bed rest. Aerospace Medicine 17:1232-1237.

Chobanian, A.V., Lille, R.D., Tercyak, A., & Blevins, P. (1974). The metabolic and hemodynamic effects of prolonged bed rest in normal subjects. Circulation 49:551-559.

Chu, K.S., Eng, J.J., Dawson, A.S., Harris, J.E., Ozkaplan, A., & Gylfaddotir, S. (2004). Water-based exercise for cardiovascular fitness in people with chronic stroke: a randomized controlled trial. Archives of Physical Medicine and Rehabilitation 85:870-874.

Cirio, S., Piaggi, G.C., De Mattia, E., & Nava, S. (2003). Muscle retraining in ICU patients. Monaldi Archives of Chest Diseases 59:300-303.

Clark, A.L., Skypala, I., & Coats, A.J. (1994). Ventilatory efficiency is unchanged after physical training in healthy persons despite an increase exercise tolerance. Journal of Cardiovascular Risk 1:347-351.

Clauss, R.H., Scalabrini, B.Y., Ray, J.F., & Reed, G.E. (1968). Effects of changing body positions upon improved ventilation-perfusion relationships. Circulation 37(Suppl 4):214-217.

Compton, D.M., Eisenman, P.A., & Henderson, H.L. (1989). Exercise and fitness for persons with disabilities. Sports Medicine 7:150-162.

Convertino, V.A. (1997). Cardiovascular consequences of bed rest: effect on maximal oxygen uptake. Medicine and Science in Sport and Exercise 2:191-196.

Convertino, V.A., Bloomfield, S.A., & Greenleaf, J.E. (2003). An overview of the issues: physiological effects of bed rest and restricted physical activity. Medicine and Science and Sports and Exercise 29:187-190.

Convertino, V.A., Hung, J., Goldwater, D., & DeBusk, R.F. (1982). Cardiovascular responses to exercise in middle-aged men after 10 days of bed rest. Circulation 65:134-140.

Cotsamire, D.L., Sullivan, M.J., Bashore, T.M., & Leier, C.V. (1987). Position as a variable for cardiovascular responses during exercise. Clinics in Cardiology 10:137-142.

Covey, M.K., Larson, J.L., & Wirtz, S. (1999). Reliability of submaximal exercise tests in patients with COPD. Chronic obstructive lung disease. Medicine and Science in Sports and Exercise 31:1257-1264.

Craig, D.B., Wahba, W.M., Don, H., Couture, J.G., & Becklake, M.R. (1971). "Closing volume" and its relationship to gas exchange in the seated and supine positions. Journal of Applied Physiology 31:717-721.

Cullen, D.L., & Rodak, B. (2002). Clinical utility of measures of breathlessness. Respiratory Care 47: 986-993.

Dart, A.M., & Kingwell, B.A. (2001). Pulse pressure: a review of mechanisms and clinical relevance. Journal of the American College of Cardiology 37:975-984.

Dawson, E., George, K., Shave, R., Whyte, G., & Ball, D. (2003). Does the human heart fatigue subsequent to prolonged exercise? Sports Medicine 33:365-380.

Dean, E., Ross, J., Bartz, J., & Purves, S. (1989). Improving the validity of clinical exercise testing: the relationship between practice and performance. Archives of Physical Medicine and Rehabilitation 70:599-604.

Dean, E. (1993). Advances in rehabilitation for older persons with cardiopulmonary dysfunction. In Katz, P.R., Kane, R.L., & Mezey, M.D. (Eds). Advances in long-term care. New York: Springer.

Dean, E., Murphy, S., Parrent, L., & Rousseau, M. (1995). Metabolic consequences of physical therapy in critically-ill patients. Proceedings of the World Confederation of Physical Therapy Congress, Washington, D.C.

Dean, E., & Ross, J. (1992a). Mobilization and exercise conditioning. In Zadai, C. (Ed). Clinics in physical therapy. Pulmonary management in physical therapy. New York: Churchill Livingstone.

Dean, E., & Ross, J. (1992b). Discordance between cardiopulmonary physiology and physical therapy. Toward a rational basis for practice. Chest 101:1694-1698.

Dean, E., & Ross, J. (1993). Movement energetics of individuals with a history of poliomyelitis. Archives of Physical Medicine and Rehabilitation 74:478-483.

Deitrick, J.E., Whedon, G.D., & Shorr, E. (1948). Effects of immobilization upon various metabolic and physiologic functions of normal man. American Journal of Medicine 4:3-36.

Dock, W. (1944). The evil sequelae of complete bed rest. Journal of the American Medical Association 125:1083-1085.

Dominick, K.L., Gullette, E.C., Babyak, M.A., Mallow, K.L., Sherwood, A., Waugh, R., Chilikuri, M., Keefe, F.J., & Blumenthal, J.A. (1999). Predicting peak oxygen uptake among older patients with chronic illness. Journal of Cardiopulmonary Rehabilitation 19:81-89.

Donaldson, C.L., Hulley, S.B., & McMillan, A.V. (1969). The effect of prolonged simulated non-gravitational environment on mineral balance in the adult male. NASA Contact CR-108314. Moffett Field, Cal.: NASA.

Ehsani, A.A., Spina, R.J., Peterson, L.R., Rinder, M.R., Glover, K.L., Villareal, D.T., Binder, E.F., & Holloszy, J.O. (2003). Attenuation of cardiovascular adaptations to exercise in frail octogenarians. Journal of Applied Physiology 95:1781-1788.

El-Sayed, M.S. (1998). Effects of exercise and training on blood rheology. Sports Medicine 26:281-292.

Enright, P.L., McBurnie, M.A., Bittner, V., Tracy, R.P., McNamara, R., Arnold, A., & Newman, A.B. The 6-min walk test: a quick measure of functional status in elderly adults. Chest 123: 387-398.

Farrell, P.A. (2001). Protein metabolism and age: influence of insulin and resistance exercise. International Journal of Sport, Nutrition and Exercise Metabolism 11(Suppl):S150-S163.

Ferguson, S., Gledhill, N., Jamnik, V.K., Wiebe, C., & Payne, N. (2001). Cardiac performance in endurance-trained and moderately active young women. Medicine and Science in Sports and Exercise 33:1114-1119.

Ferretti, G., Girardis, M., Moia, C., & Antonutto, G. (1998). Effects of prolonged bed rest on cardiovascular oxygen transport during submaximal exercise in humans. European Journal of Applied Physiology and Occupational Physiology 78:398-402.

Fletcher, B.J., Dunbar, S., Coleman, J., Jann, B., & Fletcher, G.F. (1993). Cardiac precautions for non-acute inpatient settings. American Journal of Physical Medicine and Rehabilitation 72:140-143.

Forjaz, C.L., Cardosa, C.G., Jr., Rezk, C.C., Santaella, D.F., & Tinucci, T. (2004). Postexercise hypotension and hemodynamics: the role of exercise intensity. Journal of Sports Medicine and Physical Fitness 44:54-62.

Franzoni, F., Galetta, F., Morizzo, C., Lubrano, V., Palombo, C., Santoro, G., Ferrannini, E., & Quinones Galvan, A. (2004). Effects of age and physical fitness on microcirculatory function. Clinical Science (London) 106:329-335.

Friman, G. (1979). Effect of clinical bed rest for seven days on physical performance. Acta Medica Scandinavica 205:389-393.

Froelicher, V.F., & Myers, J.N. (2000). Exercise and the heart, ed 3. Philadelphia: Elsevier.

Gates, P.E., Tanaka, H., Graves, J., & Seals, D.R. (2003). Left ventricular structure and diastolic function with human aging: relation to habitual exercise and arterial stiffness. European Heart Journal 24:2213-2220.

Gilbreth, E.M., & Weisman, I.M. (1994). Role of exercise stress testing in preoperative evaluation of patients for lung resection. Clinics in Chest Medicine 15:389-403.

Gleeson, M. (2000). The scientific basis of practical strategies to maintain immunocompetence in elite athletes. Exercise Immunology Review 6:75-101.

Gobel, F.L., Norstrom, L.A., Nelson, R.R., Jorgensen, C.R., & Wang, Y. (1978). The rate-pressure product as an index of myocardial oxygen consumption during exercise in patients with angina pectoris. Circulation 57:549-556.

Godfrey, R.J., Madgwick, Z., & Whyte, G.P. (2003). The exercise-induced growth hormone response in athletes. Sports Medicine 33:599-613.

Goette, A., Weber, M., Lendeckel, U., Welte, T., Lutze, G., & Klein, H.U. (2004). Effect of physical exercise on platelet activity and the von-Willebrand factor in patients with persistent lone atrial fibrillation. Journal of Interventionistic Cardiology and Electrophysiology 10:39-46.

Greenleaf, J.E. (1997). Intensive exercise training during bed rest attenuates deconditioning. Medicine and Science in Sports and Exercise 29:207-215.

Greenleaf, J.E., Juhos, L.T., & Young, H.L. (1985). Plasma lactic dehydrogenase activities in men during bed rest with exercise training. Aviation and Space Environmental Medicine 56:193-198.

Grenon, S.M., Hurwitz, S., Sheynberg, N., Xiao, X., Ramsdell, C.D., Mai, C.L., Kim, C., Cohen, R.J., & Williams, G.H. (2004a). Role of individual predisposition in orthostatic intolerance before and after simulated microgravity. Journal of Applied Physiology 96:1714-1722.

Grenon, S.M., Sheynberg, N., Hurwitz, S., Xiao, X., Ramsdell, C.D., Ehrman, M.D., Mai, C.L., Kristjansson, S.R., Sundby, G.H., Cohen, R.J., & Williams, G.H. (2004b). Renal, endocrine, and cardiovascular responses to bed rest in male subjects on a constant diet. Journal of Investigative Medicine 52:117-128.

Gylfadottir, S. (2003). The six-minute walk test: a methodologic perspective and with special reference to individuals with poliomyelitis. University of British Columbia, Canada, thesis.

Harper, C.M., & Lyles, Y.M. (1988). Physiology and complications of bed rest. Journal of the American Geriatrics Society 36:1047-1054.

Harrison, T.R. (1944). The abuse of rest as a therapeutic measure for patients with cardiovascular disease. Journal of the American Medical Association 125;1075-1077.

Harvey, R.L. (2003). Prevention of venous thromboembolism after stroke. Topics in Stroke Rehabilitation 10:61-69.

Hasser, E.M., & Moffitt, J.A. (2001). Regulation of sympathetic nervous system function after cardiovascular deconditioning. Annals of the New York Academy of Science 940:454-468.

Hasson, S.M. (Ed). (1994). Clinical exercise physiology. St. Louis: Mosby.

Havas, E., Komulainen, J., & Vihko, V. (1997). Exercise-induced increase in serum creatine kinase is modified by subsequent bed rest. International Journal of Sports Medicine 18:578-582.

Health Canada. (2005). Canadian Society for Exercise Physiology, www.csep.ca; retrieved January 2005.

Hirayanagi, K., Iwase, S., Kamiya, A., Sasaki, T., Mano, T., & Yajima, K. (2004). Functional changes in autonomic nervous system and baroreceptor reflex induced by 14 days of 6 degrees head-down bed rest. European Journal of Applied Physiology 92:160-167.

Hirayanagi, K., Kamiya, A., Iwase, S., Mano, T., Sasaki, T., Oinuma, M., & Yajima, K. (2004). Autonomic cardiovascular changes during and after 14 days of head-down bed rest. Autonomic Neuroscience 27:110, 121-128.

Ho, S.C., Woo, J., Sham, A., Chan, S.G., & Yu, A.L. (2001). A 3-year follow-up study of social, lifestyle and health predictors of cognitive impairment in a Chinese older cohort. International Journal of Epidemiology 30:1389-1396.

Hollenberg, M., & Tager, I.B. (2000). Oxygen update efficiency slope: an index of exercise performance and cardiopulmonary reserve requiring only submaximal exercise. Journal of the American College of Cardiology 36:194-201.

Hsu, H.O., & Hickey, R.F. (1976). Effect of posture on functional residual capacity postoperatively. Anesthesiology 44:520-521.

Hulley, S.B., Vogel, J.M., Donaldson, C.L., Bayers, J.M., Friedman, R.J., & Rosen, S.N. (1971). The effect of supplemental oral phosphate on the bone mineral changes during prolonged bed rest. Journal of Clinical Investigation 50:2506-2518.

Inbar, O., Weinter, P., Azgad, Y., Rotstein, A., & Weinstein, Y. (2000). Specific inspiratory muscle training in well-trained endurance athletes. Medicine and Science in Sport and Exercise 32:1233-1237.

Irwin, S., & Tecklin, J.S. (Eds). (2004). Cardiopulmonary physical therapy, ed 4. Philadelphia: Elsevier.

Ishizaki, Y., Fukuoka, H., Ishizaki, T., Katsura, T., Kim, C.S., Maekawa, Y., & Fujita, M. (2000). Evaluation of psychological effects due to bed rest. Journal of Gravitational Physiology 7:183-184.

Izquierdo, M., Hakkinen, K., Ibanez, J., Anton, A., Garrues, M., Ruesta, M., & Gorostiaga, E.M. (2003). Effects of strength training on submaximal and maximal endurance performance capacity in middle-aged and older men. Journal of Strength Conditioning Research 17:129-139.

Jacobs, L.G. (2003). Prophylactic anticoagulation for venous thromboembolic disease in geriatric patients. Journal of the American Gerontological Society 51:1472-1478.

Jones, N.L., & Fletcher, I. (1997). Clinical exercise testing, ed 4. Philadelphia: Elsevier.

Jones, A.Y.M., Dean, E., & Scudds, R. (2005). Effectiveness of a community-based t'ai chi program and implications for public health initiatives. Archives of Physical Medicine and Rehabilitation 86:619-625.

Jones, A.M., Koppo, K., & Burnley, M. (2003). Effects of prior exercise on metabolic and gas exchange responses to exercise. Sports Medicine 33:949-971.

Kacin, A., Mekjavic, I.B., Rodman, S., Kolegard, R., & Eiken, O. (2002). Influence of active recovery followed prolonged bed rest on static exercise pressure response. Journal of Gravitational Physiology 9:91-92.

Kamiya, A., Michikami, D., Fu, Q., Iwase, S., Hayano, J., Kawada, T., Mano, T., & Sunagawa, K. (2003). Pathophysiology or orthostatic hypotension after bed rest: paradoxical sympathetic withdrawal. American Journal of Physiology. Heart and Circulatory Physiology 285:H1158-H1167.

Kamiya, A., Michikami, D., Shiozawa, T., Iwase, S., Hayano, J., Kawada, T., Sunagawa, K., & Mano, T. (2004). Bed rest attenuates sympathetic and pressor responses to isometric exercise in anti-gravity leg muscles in humans. American Journal of Physiology, Regulation, Integration and Comparative Physiology 286: R844-R850.

Kasper, C.E., Talbot, L.A., & Gaines, J.M. (2002). Skeletal muscle damage and recovery. AACN Clinical Issues 13:237-247.

Kervio, G., Carre, F., & Ville, N.S. (2003). Reliability and intensity of the six-minute walk test in healthy elderly subjects. Medicine & Science in Sports and Exercise 35:169-174.

Kinney, M.R., & Packa, D.R. (1995). Andreoli's comprehensive cardiac care, ed 7. Philadelphia: Elsevier.

Knapik, J.J., Banderet, L.E., Vogel, J.A., Bahrke, M.S., & O'Conner, J.S. (1996). Influence of age and physical training on measures of cardiorespiratory and muscle endurance. European Journal of Applied Physiology and Occupational Physiology 72:490-495.

Kohl, H.W. 3rd. (2001). Physical activity and cardiovascular disease: evidence for a dose response. Medicine & Science in Sports & Exercise 33(6 Suppl):S472-S483.

Kottke, F.J. (1966). The effects of limitation of activity upon the human body. Journal of the American Medical Association 196:825-830.

Koutedakis, Y., Budgett, R., & Faulmann, L. (1990). Rest in under-performing elite competitors. British Journal of Sports Medicine 24:248-252.

Kraemer, M.D., Sullivan, M., Atwood, J.E., Forbes, S., Meyers, J., & Froelicher, V. (1989). Reproducibility of treadmill exercise data in patients with atrial fibrillation. Cardiology 76:234-242.

Krasnoff, J., & Painter, P. (1999). The physiologic consequences of bed rest and inactivity. Advances in Renal Replacement Therapy 6:124-132.

Kreider, R.B. (1991). Physiologic consideration of ultraendurance performance. International Journal of Sports and Nutrition 1:3-27.

Krzeminski, K., Kruk, B., Nazar, K., Ziemba, A.W., Cybulski, G., & Niewiadomski, W. (2000). Cardiovascular, metabolic and plasma catecholamine responses to passive and active exercise. Journal of Physiology and Pharmacology 51:267-278.

Kubo, K., Akima, H., Ushiyama, J., Tabata, I., Fukuoka, H., Kanehisa, H., & Fukunaga, T. (2004). Effects of 20 days of bed rest on the viscoelastic properties of tendon structures in lower limb muscles. British Journal of Sports Medicine 38:324-330.

Kurl, S., Laukkanen, J.A., Rauramaa, R., Lakka, T.A., Sivenius, J., & Salonen, J.T. (2001). Systolic blood pressure response to exercise stress test and risk of stroke. Stroke 32:2036-2041.

Lampinen, P., & Heikkinen, E. (2003). Reduced mobility and physical activity as predictors of depressive symptoms among community-dwelling older adults: an eight-year follow-up study. Aging Clinical and Experimental Research 15:205-211.

Landis, R.J., Linnemeier, T.J., Rothbaum, D.A., Chappelear, J., & Nobel, R.J. (1985). Exercise testing and training of the elderly patient. Cardiovascular Clinics 15:201-218.

Lay, B.S., Sparrow, W.A., Hughes, K.M., & O'Dwyer, N.J. (2002). Practice effects on coordination and control, metabolic energy expenditure, and muscle activation. Human Movement Science 21:807-830.

Lee, S.M., Bennett, B.S., Hargens, A.R., Watenpaugh, D.E., Ballard, R.E., Murthy, G., Ford, S.R., & Fortney, S.M. (1997). Upright exercise or supine lower body negative pressure exercise maintains exercise responses after bed rest. Medicine and Science in Sport and Exercise 29:892-900.

Lennon, S., Quindry, J.C., Hamilton, K.L., French, J., Staib, J., Mehta, J.L., & Powers, S.K. (2004). Loss of exercise-induced cardioprotection following cessation of exercise. Journal of Applied Physiology 96:1299-1305.

Lentz, M. (1981). Selected aspects of deconditioning secondary to immobilization. Nursing Clinics of North America 16:729-737.

Lepretre, P.M., Koralsztein, J.P., & Billat, V.L. (2004). Effect of exercise intensity on relationship between VO_2max and cardiac output. Medicine and Science in Sports and Exercise 36: 1357-1363.

Levin, S.A., & Lown, B. (1952). Armchair treatment of acute coronary thrombosis. Journal of the American Medical Association 148:1365-1369.

Leyk, D., Essfeld, D., Hoffmann, U., Wunderlich, H.G., Baum, K., & Stegemann, I. (1994). Postural effect on cardiac output, oxygen uptake and lactate during cycle exercise of varying intensity. European Journal of Applied Physiology and Occupational Physiology 68:30-35.

Lindgren, M., Unosson, M., Fredrikson, M., & Ek, A.C. (2004). Immobility—a major risk factor for development of pressure ulcers among adult hospitalized patients: a prospective study. Scandinavian Journal of Caring Science 18:57-64.

MacKay-Lyons, M., Makrides, L., & Speth, S. (2001). Effect of a 15% body weight support on exercise capacity of adults without impairments. Physical Therapy 81:1790-1800.

MacKinnon, L.T. (2000a). Special features for the Olympics: effects of exercise on the immune system: overtraining effects on immunity and performance in athletes. Immunology and Cell Biology 78:502-509.

MacKinnon, L.T. (2000b). Chronic exercise training: effects on immune function. Medicine and Science in Sport and Exercise 32:S369-S376.

Maffucci, D.M., & McMurray, R.G. (2000). Towards optimizing the timing of the pre-exercise meal. International Journal of Sport Nutrition and Exercise Metabolism 10:103-113.

Markov, G., Spengler, C.M., Knopfli-Lenzin, C., Stuessi, C., & Boutellier, U. (2001). Respiratory muscle training increases cycling endurance without affecting cardiovascular responses to exercise. European Journal of Applied Physiology 85:233-239.

Marzorati, M., Perini, R., Milesi, S., & Veiesteinas, A. (2000). Metabolic and cardiorespiratory responses to maximal intermittent knee and isokinetic exercise in young health humans. European Journal of Applied Physiology 81:275-280.

Martino, M., Gledhill, N., & Jamnik, V. (2002). High VO_2max with no history of training is primarily due to high blood volume. Medicine and Science in Sports and Exercise 34:966-971.

Mascitelli, L., & Pezzetta, F. (2003). Anti-inflammatory effects of physical exercise. Archives of Internal Medicine 163:1682-1688.

McArdle, W.D., Katch, F.I., & Katch, V.L. (2000). Essentials of exercise physiology, ed 2. Philadelphia: Lippincott Williams & Wilkins.

McCluskey, A., Gwinnutt, C.L., Hardy, L., Haslett, R., Bowles, B., & Kishen, R. (2001). Evaluation of the Pneupac Ventipac portable ventilator in critically ill patients. Anaesthesia 56:1073-1081.

McGavin, C.R., Artvinli, M., Naoe, H., & McHardy, G.J.R. (1978). Dyspnea, disability, and distance walked: comparison of estimates of exercise performance in respiratory disease. British Medical Journal 2:241-243.

McGavin, C.R., Artivini, M., Naoe, H., & McHardy, G.J.R. (1978). Dyspnea, disability, and distance walked: comparison of estimates of exercise performance in respiratory disease. British Medical Journal 1:822-823.

McGavin, C.R., Gupta, S.P., & McHardy, G.J.R. (1976). Twelve-minute walking test for assessing disability in chronic bronchitis. British Medical Journal 1:822-823.

McGuire, D.K., Levine, B.D., Williamson, J.W., Snell, P.G., Blomqvist, C.G., Saltin, B., & Mitchell, J.H. (2001a). A 30-year follow-up of the Dallas Bedrest and Training Study: I. Effect of age on the cardiovascular response to exercise. Circulation 104:1350-1357.

McGuire, D.K., Levine, B.D., Williamson, J.W., Snell, P.G., Blomqvist, C.G., Saltin, B., & Mitchell, J.H. (2001b). A 30-year follow-up of the Dallas Bedrest and Training Study: II. Effect of age on cardiovascular adaptation to exercise training. Circulation 104:1358-1366.

McKenzie, M.A., Greenleaf, J.E., Looft-Wilson, R., & Barnes, P.R. (1999). Leucocytosis, thrombocytosis, and plasma osmolality during rest and exercise: an hypothesis. Journal of Physiology and Pharmacology 50:259-273.

Mendenhall, L.A., Swanson, S.C., Habash, D.L., & Coggan, A.R. (1994). Ten days of exercise training reduces glucose production and utilization during moderate-intensity exercise. American Journal of Physiology 266:E136-E143.

Meyer, K., Westbrook, S., Schwaibold, M., Hajric, R., Peters, K., & Roskamm, H. (1997). Short-term reproducibility of cardio-pulmonary measurements during exercise testing in patients with severe chronic heart failure. American Heart Journal 134:20-26.

Mikines, K.J., Richter, E.A., Dela, F., & Galbo, H. (1991). Seven days of bed rest decrease insulin action on glucose uptake in leg and whole body. Journal of Applied Physiology 70:1245-1254.

Morton, R.H. (1997). Modeling training and overtraining. Journal of Sports Science 15:335-340.

Mujika, I., & Padilla, S. (2000a). Detraining: loss of training-induced physiological and performance adaptations. I: Short-term insufficient training stimulus. Sports Medicine 30:79-87.

Mujika, I., & Padilla, S. (2000b). Detraining: loss of training-induced physiological and performance adaptations. II: Long-term insufficient training stimulus. Sports Medicine 30:145-154.

Myers, J., & Madhavan, R. (2001). Exercise testing with gas exchange analysis. Cardiology Clinics 19:433-445.

Nagashima, K., Mack, G.W., Haskell, A., Nishiyasu, T., & Nadel, E.R. (1999). Mechanism for the posture-specific plasma volume increase after a single intense exercise protocol. Journal of Applied Physiology 86:867-873.

Nappi, A., Cuocolo, A., Imbriaco, M., Nicolai, E., Varrone, A., Morisco, C., Romano, M., Trimarco, B., & Salvatore, M. (1997). Ambulatory monitoring of left ventricular function: walk and bicycle exercise in congestive heart failure. Journal of Nuclear Medicine 38:948-953.

Nelson, L.D., & Anderson, H.B. (1989). Physiologic effects of steep positioning in the surgical intensive care unit. Archives of Surgery 124:352-355.

Netea, R.T., Elving, L.D., Lutterman, J.A., & Thien, T. (2002). Body position and blood pressure measurement in patients with diabetes mellitus. Journal of Internal Medicine 25:393-399.

Nieman, D.C. (2000). Special feature for the Olympics: effects of exercise on the immune system: exercise effects on systemic immunity. Immunology and Cell Biology 78:496-501.

Nieman, D.C. (2003). Current perspective on exercise immunology. Current Sports Medicine Review 2:239-242.

Noonan, V., & Dean, E. (2000). Submaximal exercise testing: clinical application and interpretation. Physical Therapy 80:782-807.

Nugent, A.M., Riley, M., Megarry, J., O'Reilly, M.J., MacMahon, J., & Lowry, R. (1998). Cardiopulmonary exercise testing in the pre-operative assessment of patients for repair of abdominal aortic aneurysm. Irish Journal of Medical Science 167:238-241.

Oja, P. (2001). Dose response between total volume of physical activity and health and fitness. Medicine and Science in Sports and Exercise 33(6 Suppl):S428-S437.

Onorati, P., Antonucci, R., Valli, G., Berton, E., De Marco, F., Serra, P., & Palange, P. (2003). Non-invasive evaluation of gas exchange during a shuttle walk test vs. a 6-min walking test to assess exercise tolerance in COPD patients. European Journal of Applied Physiology 89:331-336.

Orlava, O.E. (1959). Therapeutic physical culture in the complex treatment of pneumonia. Physical Therapy Review 39:153-160.

Peeters, P., & Mets, T. (1996). The 6-minute walk as an appropriate exercise test in elderly patients with chronic heart failure. Journal of Gerontology. A. Biological Sciences and Medical Sciences 51:147-151.

Powers, J.H. (1944). The abuse of rest as a therapeutic measure in surgery. Journal of the American Medical Association 125:1079-1083.

Powers, J., & Daniels, D. (2004). Turning points: implementing kinetic therapy in the ICU. Nursing Management 35(Suppl): 1-7.

Pyne, D.B. (1994). Regulation of neutrophil function during exercise. Sports Medicine 17:245-258.

Pyne, D.B., Gleeson, M., McDonald, W.A., Clancy, R.L., Perry, C., Jr., & Fricker, P.A. (2000). Training strategies to maintain immuno-competence in athletes. International Journal of Sports Medicine 21(Suppl 1):S51-S60.

Raine, N.M., Cable, N.T., George, K.P., & Campbell, I.G. (2001). The influence of recovery posture on post-exercise hypotension in normotensive men. Medicine and Science in Sports and Exercise 33:404-412.

Ray, J.F., Yost, L., Moallem, S., Sanoudos, G.M., Villamena, P., Paredes, R.M., & Clauss, R.H. (1974). Immobility, hypoxemia, and pulmonary arteriovenous shunting. Archives of Surgery 109:537-541.

Reeves, N.J., Maganaris, C.N., Rerretti, G., & Narici, M.V. (2002). Influence of simulated microgravity on human skeletal muscle architecture and function. Journal of Gravitational Physiology 9:P153-P154.

Reid, M.R., Drummond, P.D., & MacKinnon, L.T. (2001). The effect of moderate aerobic exercise and relaxation on secretory immunoglobulin A. International Journal of Sports Medicine 22:132-137.

Reilly, T., Dowzer, C.N., & Cable, N.T. (2003). The physiology of deep-water running. Journal of Sports Science 21:959-972.

Reybrouck, T., & Fagard, R. (1999). Gender differences in the oxygen transport system during maximal exercise in hypertensive subjects. Chest 115:788-792.

Riley, M., Maehara, K., Porszasz, J., Engelen, M.P., Barstow, T.T., Tanaka, H., & Wasserman, K. (1997). Association between the anaerobic threshold and the break-point in the double product-work rate relationship. European Journal of Applied Physiology and Occupational Physiology 75:14-21.

Risser, N.L. (1980). Preoperative and postoperative care to prevent pulmonary complications. Heart and Lung 9:57-67.

Rodeheffer, R.J., Gerstenblith, G., Beard, E., Fleg, J.L., Becker, L.C., Weisfeldt, M.L., & Lakatta, E.G. (1986). Postural changes in cardiac volumes in men in relation to adult age. Experimental Gerontology 21:367-378.

Ronsen, O., Haug, E., Pedersen, B.K., & Bahr, R. (2001). Increased neuroendocrine response to a repeated bout of endurance exercise. Medicine and Science in Sport and Exercise 33:568-575.

Rosenstein, G., Cafri, C., Weinstein, J.M., Yeroslavtsev, S., Abuful, A., Ilia, R., & Fuchs, S. (2004). Simple clinical risk stratification and the safety of ambulation two hours after 6 French diagnostic heart catheterization. Journal of Invasive Cardiology 16:126-128.

Ross, J., & Dean, E. (1989). Integrating physiological principles into the comprehensive management of cardiopulmonary dysfunction. Physical Therapy 69:255-259.

Rubin, M. (1988). The physiology of bed rest. American Journal of Nursing 88:50-56.

Russell, S.D., McNeer, F.R., Beere, P.A., Logan, L.J., & Higginbotham, M.B. (1998). Improvement in the mechanical efficiency of walking: an explanation for the "placebo effect" seen during repeated exercise testing of patients with heart failure. Duke University Clinical Cardiology Studies (DUCCS) Exercise Group. American Heart Journal 135:107-114.

Ryback, R.S., Lewis, O.F., & Lessard, C.S. (1971). Psychobiologic effects of prolonged bed rest (weightless) in young healthy volunteers. Study II. Aerospace Medicine 42:529-535.

Salbach, N.M., Mayo, N.E., Higgins, J., Ahmed, S., Finch, L.E., & Richards, C.L. (2001). Responsiveness and predictability of gait speed and other disability measures in acute stroke. Archives of Physical Medicine and Rehabilitation 82:1204-1212.

Saltin, B., Blomqvist, G., Mitchell, J.H., Johnson, B.L., Wildenthal, K., & Chapman, C.B. (1968). Response to exercise after bed rest and after training. Circulation 38(VII):S1-S78.

Sandler, H. (1986). Cardiovascular effects of inactivity. In Sandler, H., & Vernikos, J. (Eds). Inactivity physiological effects. New York: Academic Press.

Sandler, H., Popp, R.L., & Harrison, D.C. (1988). The hemodynamic effects of repeated bed rest exposure. Aerospace Medicine 59:1047-1053.

Schimmel, L., Civetta, J.M., & Kirby, R.R. (1977). A new mechanical method to influence pulmonary perfusion in critically ill patients. Critical Care Medicine 5:277-279.

Schneider, D.A., Wing, A.N., & Morris, N.R. (2002a). Oxygen uptake and heart rate kinetics during heavy exercise comparison between arm cranking and leg cycling. European Journal of Applied Physiology 88:100-106.

Schneider, S.M., Watenpaugh, D.E., Lee, S.M., Ertl, A.C., Williams, W.J., Ballard, R.E., & Hargens, A.R. (2002b). Lower-body negative pressure exercise and bed-rest-mediated orthostatic intolerance. Medicine and Science in Sport and Exercise 34:1446-1453.

Shackelford, L.C., LeBlanc, A.D., Driscoll, T.B., Evans, H.J., Rianon, N.J., Smith, S.M., Spector, E., Feeback, D.L., & Lai, D. (2004). Resistance exercise as a countermeasure to disuse-induced bone loss. Journal of Applied Physiology 97:119-129.

Shave, R., Dawson, E., Whyte, G., George, K., Gaze, D., & Collinson, P. (2004). Altered cardiac function and minimal cardiac damage during prolonged exercise. Medicine and Science in Sports and Exercise 36:1098-1103.

Shepherd, R.J. (2001). Absolute versus relative intensity of physical activity in a dose response context. Medicine and Science in Sports and Exercise 33(6 Suppl):S400-S418.

Shepherd, R.J., Allen, C., Benade, A.J., Davies, C.T., Di Prampero, P.E., Hedman, R., Merriman, J.E., Myhre, K., & Simmons, R. (1968). Standardization of submaximal exercise test. Bulletin of the World Health Organization 38:765-775.

Sheriff, D.D., & Mendoza, J.R. (2004). Passive regulation of cardiac output during exercise by the elastic characteristics of the peripheral circulation. Exercise and Sports Science Review 32:31-35.

Singh, V.N. (2001). The role of gas exchange analysis with exercise testing. Primary Care 28:159-179.

Sjostrand, T. (1951). Determination of changes in the intrathoracic blood volume in man. Acta Physiologica Scandinavica 22:116-128.

Skerrett, S.J., Niederman, M.S., & Fein, A.M. (1989). Respiratory infections and acute lung injury in systemic illness. Clinics in Chest Medicine 10:469-502.

Smorawinski, J., Kaciuba-Uscilko, H., Nazar, K., Kaminska, Korszun, P., & Greenleaf, J.E. (1998). Comparison of changes in glucose tolerance and insulin secretion induced by three-day bed rest in sedentary subjects and endurance or strength trained athletes. Journal of Gravitational Physiology 5:P103-P104.

Sonnfeld, G. (1999). Space flight, microgravity, stress, and immune responses. Advances in Space Research 23:1945-1953.

Spina, R.J., Rashid, S., Davila-Roman, V.G., & Ehsani, A.A. (2000). Adaptations in beta-adrenergic cardiovascular responses to training in older women. Journal of Applied Physiology 89:2300-2305.

Stannard, S.R., & Johnson, N.A. (2004). Insulin resistance and elevated triglyceride in muscle: more important for survival than 'thrifty' genes? Journal of Physiology 554:595-607.

Steele, P.P., Maddoux, G., Kirch, D.L., & Vogel, R.A. (1978). Effects of propranolol and nitroglycerin on left ventricular performance in patients with coronary arterial disease. Chest 73:19-23.

Summer, W.R., Curry, P., Haponik, E.F., Nelson, S., & Elston, R. (1989). Continuous mechanical turning of intensive care unit patients shortens length of stay in some diagnostic-related groups. Journal of Critical Care 4:45-53.

Suzuki, Y., Iwamoto, S., Haruna, Y., Kuriyama, K., Kawakubo, K., & Gunji, A. (1997). Effects of 20 days horizontal bed rest on mechanical efficiency during steady-state exercise at mild-moderate work intensities in young subjects. Journal of Gravitational Physiology 4:S46-S52.

Suzuki, Y., Kashihara, H., Takenaka, K., Kawakubo, K., Makita, Y., Goto, S., Ikawa, S., & Gunji, A. (1994). Effects of daily mild supine exercise on physical performance after 20 days of bed rest in young persons. Acta Astraunaut 33:101-111.

Svanberg, L. (1957). Influence of position on the lung volumes, ventilation and circulation in normals. Scandinavian Journal of Clinical and Laboratory Investigations 25:1-195.

Szygula, Z. (1990). Erythrocytic system under the influence of physical exercise and training. Sports Medicine 10:181-197.

Takahashi, T., & Miyamoto, Y. (1998). Influence of light physical activity on cardiac responses during recovery from exercise in humans. European Journal of Physiology and Occupational Physiology 77:305-311.

Takata, S., & Yasui, N. (2001). Disuse osteoporosis. Journal of Medical Investigation 48:147-156.

Taylor, D.H., & Hoenig, H. (2004). The effect of equipment usage and residual task difficulty on use of personal assistance, days in bed, and nursing home placement. Journal of the American Gerontological Society 52:72-79.

Topp, R., Ditmyer, M., King, K., Doherty, K., & Hornyack, J. 3rd. (2002). The effect of bed rest and potential of prehabilitation on patient in the intensive care unit. AACN Clinical Issues 13:263-276.

Torchio, R., Gulotta, C., Parvis, M., Pozzi, R., Giardino, R., Borasio, P., & Greco Lucchina, P. (1998). Gas exchange threshold as a predictor of severe postoperative complications after lung resection in mild-to-moderate chronic obstructive lung disease. Monaldi Archives of Chest Diseases 53:127-133.

Trappe, S., Trappe, T., Gallagher, P., Harber, M., Alkner, B., & Tesch, P. (2004). Human single muscle fibre function with 84 day bed-rest and resistance exercise. Journal of Physiology 557: 501-513.

Troosters, T., Vilaro, J., Rabinovich, R., Casas, A., Barbera, J.A., Rodriguez-Roisin, R., & Roca, J. (2002). Physiological responses to the 6-min walk test in patients with chronic obstructive lung disease. European Respiratory Journal 20:564-569.

Trujilio-Santos, A.J., Martos-Perez, F., & Perea-Milla, E. Bed rest or early mobilization as treatment of deep vein thrombosis: a systematic review and meta-analysis. Medical Clinics (Barcelona) 122:641-647, English abstract.

Tsai, J.C., Wang, W.H., Chan, P., Lin, L.J., Wang, C.H., Tomlinson, B., Hsieh, M.H., Yang, H.Y., & Liu, J.C. (2003). The beneficial effects of Tai Chi Chuan on blood pressure and lipid profile and anxiety states in a randomized controlled clinical trial. Journal of Alternative and Complementary Medicine 9:747-754.

Tudor-Locke, C., & Bassett, D.R., Jr. (2004). How many steps/day are enough? Preliminary pedometer indices for public health. Sports Medicine 34:1-8.

Uber-zak, L.D., & Venkatesh, Y.S. (2002). Neurologic complications of sit-ups associated with the Valsalva maneuver: 2 case reports. Archives of Physical Medicine and Rehabilitation 83:278-282.

Uth, N., Sorensen, H., Overgaard, K., & Pedersen, P.K. (2004). Estimation of Vo$_2$max from the ratio between HRmax and HRrest: the Heart Rate Ratio Method. European Journal of Applied Physiology 91:111-115.

Uusaro, A., & Russell, J. A. (2000). Could anti-inflammatory actions of catecholamines explain the possible beneficial effects of supranormal oxygen delivery in critically-ill surgical patients? Intensive Care Medicine 26:299-304.

Vallet, G., Ahmaidi, S., Serres, I., Fabre, C., Bourgouin, D., Desplan, J., Varray, A., & Prefaut, C. (1997). Comparison of two training programmes in chronic airway limitation patients: standardized versus individualized protocols. European Respiratory Journal 10:114-122.

Varo Cenarruzabeitia, J.J., Martinez Hernandez, J.A., & Martinez-Gonzalez, M.A. (2003). Benefits of physical activity and harms of inactivity. Medical Clinics (Barcelona) 121:665-672.

Vincent, K.R., Vincent, H.K., Braith, R.W., Bhatnagar, V., & Lowenthal, D.T. (2003). Strength training and hemodynamic responses to exercise. American Journal of Geriatric Cardiology 12:97-106.

Wagner, P.D. (1996). Determinants of maximal oxygen transport and utilization. Annual Review of Physiology 58:21-50.

Walsh, G.L., Morice, R.C., Putman, J.B., Jr., Nesbitt, J.C., McMurtrey, M.J., Ryan, M.B., Reising, J.M., Willis, K.M., Morton, J.D., & Roth, J.A. (1994). Resection of lung cancer is justified in high-risk patients selected by exercise oxygen consumption. Annals of Thoracic Surgery 58:704-710.

Wang, J.S., Jen, C.J., & Chen, H.I. (1995). Effects of exercise training and deconditioning on platelet function in men. Arteriosclerosis and Thrombosis 15:1668-1674.

Warburton, D.E., Haykowsky, M.J., Quinney, H.A., Blackmore, D., Teo, K.K., & Humen, D.P. (2002). Myocardial responses to incremental exercise in endurance-trained athletes: influence of heart rate, contractility and the Frank-Starling effect. Experimental Physiology 87:613-622.

Wasserman, K. (2002). Anaerobic threshold and cardiovascular function. Monaldi Archives of Chest Diseases 58:1-5.

Wasserman, K.L., & Whipp, B.J. (1975). Exercise physiology in health and disease. American Review of Respiratory Diseases 112:219-249.

Weber, K.T., Janicko, J.S., Shroff, S.G., & Likoff, M.J. (1983). The cardiopulmonary unit: the body's gas transport system. Clinics in Chest Medicine 4:101-110.

Weissman, C., & Kemper, M. (1991). The oxygen uptake-oxygen delivery relationship during ICU interventions. Chest 99: 430-435.

Weissman, C., Kemper, M., Damask, M.C., Askanazi, J., Hyman, A.I., & Kinney, J.M. (1984). Effect of routine intensive care interactions on metabolic rate. Chest 86:815-818.

Weisssman, C., Kemper, M., & Harding, J. (1994). Response of critically-ill patients to increased oxygen demand: hemodynamic subsets. Critical Care Medicine 22:1809-1816.

Wenger, N.K. (1982). Early ambulation: the physiologic basis revisited. Advances in Cardiology 31:138-141.

West, J.B. (2004). Respiratory physiology—the essentials, ed 7. Baltimore: Williams & Wilkins.

Whaley, M.H., Brubaker, P.H., Kaminsky, L.A., & Miller, C.R. (1997). Validity of rating of perceived exertion during graded exercise testing in apparently healthy adults and cardiac patients. Journal of Cardiopulmonary Rehabilitation 17:261-267.

Wijnen, J.A., Kool, M.J., van Baak, M.A., Kuipers, H., de Haan, C.H., Verstappen, F.T., Struijker Boudier, H.A., & Van Bortel, L.M. (1994). Effect of exercise training on ambulatory blood pressure. International Journal of Sports Medicine 15:10-15.

Winkelman, C. (2004). Inactivity and inflammation: selected cytokines as biologic mediators in muscle dysfunction during critical illness. AACN Clinical Issues 15:74-82.

Winslow, E.H. (1985). Cardiovascular consequences of bed rest. Heart Lung 14:236-246.

Williams, D.H., & Williams, C. (1983). Cardiovascular and metabolic responses of trained and untrained middle-aged men to a graded treadmill walking test. British Journal of Sports Medicine 17:110-116.

Williams, J.S., Wongsathikun, J., Boon, S.M., & Acevedo, E.O. (2002). Inspiratory muscle training fails to improve endurance capacity in athletes. Medicine and Science in Sport and Exercise 34:1194-1198.

Wolff, R.K., Dolovich, M.B., Obminski, G., & Newhouse, M.T. (1977). Effects of exercise and eucapnic hyperventilation on bronchial clearance in man. Journal of Applied Physiology 43:46-50.

Woods, S.L. (2004). Cardiac nursing, ed 5. Philadelphia: Lippincott, Williams & Wilkins.

World Health Organization (1999). Bulletin of the World Health Organization, 77; and International Society of Hypertension (1999). Guidelines for the management of hypertension. Hypertension 17:183-293.

Yarnel, J.R. Helbock, M., & Schwiter, E.J. (1986). Rotorest kinetic treatment table (Rotobed) in patients with acute respiratory failure. In Green, B.A., & Summer, W.R. (Eds). Continuous oscillating therapy: research and practical applications. Miami: University of Miami Press.

Yamamoto, T., Sekiya, N., Miyashita, S., Asada, H., Yano, Y., Morishima, K., Okamoto, Y., Goto, S., Suzuki, Y, & Gunji, A. (1997). Gender differences in effects of 20 days horizontal bed rest on muscle strength in young subjects. Journal of Gravitational Physiology 4:S31-S36.

Yoshioka, J., Node, K., Hasegawa, S., Paul, A.K., Mu, X., Maruyama, K., Nakatani, D., Kitakaze, M., Hori, M., & Nishimura, T. (2003). Impaired cardiac response to exercise in post-menopausal women: relationship with peripheral vascular function. Nuclear Medicine Communication 24:383-389.

Yu, M., Takanishi, D., Myers, S.A., Takiguchi, S.A., Severino, R., Hasaniya, N., Levy, M.M., & McNamara, J.J. (1995). Frequency of mortality and myocardial infarction during maximizing oxygen delivery: a prospective, randomized trial. Critical Care Medicine 23:1025-1032.

Zavorsky, G.S. (2000). Evidence and possible mechanisms of altered maximum heart rate with endurance training and tapering. Sports Medicine 29:13-26.

Zeballos, R.J., Weisman, I.M., & Connery, S.M. (1998). Comparison of pulmonary gas exchange measurements between incremental and constant work exercise above the anaerobic threshold. Chest 113:602-611.

Zeleznik, J. (2003). Normative aging of the respiratory system. Clinics in Geriatric Medicine 19:1-18.

Zhou, B., Conlee, R.K., Jensen, R., Fellingham, G.W., George, J.D., & Fisher, A.G. (2001). Stroke volume does not plateau during graded exercise in elite male distance runners. Medicine and Science in Sport and Exercise 33:1849-1854.

Ziemba, A.W., Chwalbinska,-Moneta, J., Kaciuba-Uscilko, H., Kruk, B., Krzeminska, K., Cybulski, G., & Nazar, K. (2003). Early effects of short-term aerobic exercise training: physiological responses to graded exercise. Journal of Sports Medicine and Physical Fitness 43:57-63.

Zubeck, J.P., & MacNeil, M. (1966). Effects of immobilization: behavioural and EEG changes. Canadian Journal of Psychology 20:316-336.

CHAPTER 19

Body Positioning

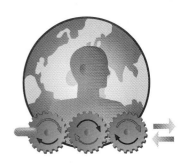

Elizabeth Dean

KEY TERMS   Body position changes   Prescriptive body positioning
                 Cardiopulmonary function   Routine body positioning
                 Gravitational gradients   Static body positioning
                 Oxygen transport

The purpose of this chapter is threefold. First, therapeutic body positioning prescribed by physical therapists to optimize cardiopulmonary function and oxygen transport is differentiated from routine body positioning. Second, the physiological effects of static body positions as opposed to dynamic body position changes on cardiovascular and pulmonary function and oxygen transport are described. Third, the principles for prescribing therapeutic versus routine body positioning are presented.

Body positions that simulate the normal physiological effects of gravity and position change on oxygen transport are the clinical priority; being "upright and moving" is the physiological body position. When, because of disease or injury, patients are unable to be upright and moving consistent with the demands of normal living, the physical therapist simulates the patient's being upright and moving by means of specific body positions. Whether body positions are assumed actively by the patient or the patient is positioned passively by the physical therapist depends on the patient's status and needs.

Specific indications for body positioning and the decision-making process are highlighted. The chapter does not provide treatment prescriptions for given conditions because no specific patient is being considered. Understanding the physiological effects of body position on oxygen transport and how pathophysiology disrupts these normal processes is fundamental to prescribing body positioning for a given patient. An optimal body position can be prescribed only on the basis of consideration of all factors that impact on oxygen transport: the effects of the patient's pathophysiology and its specific presentation in that individual, the effect of restricted mobility and recumbency, the effect of extrinsic factors related to the patient's care, and the effect of intrinsic factors related to the patient (Chapter 17). It is only with an integrated analysis of these factors overall that (1) the most beneficial body positions can be predicted; (2) the least beneficial body positions can be identified and used minimally; and (3) the appropriate outcome measures can be selected.

GRAVITY AND NORMAL PHYSIOLOGICAL FUNCTION: IMPLICATIONS FOR CARDIOPULMONARY PHYSICAL THERAPY

The human is an orthograde organism. From moment to moment, gravity exerts its influence on the human body and particularly affects oxygen transport. The combined effects of gravity on the lungs, heart, and peripheral circulation are central to their interdependent function and to establishing normal oxygen transport. Knowledge of the effects of gravity on cardiopulmonary function in health and the deleterious effects of pathophysiological states on cardiopulmonary

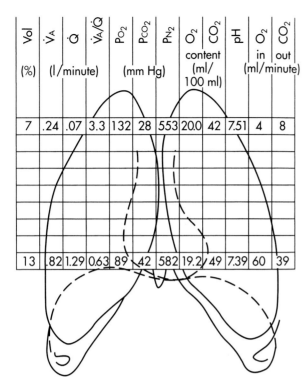

Vol (%)	$\dot{V}_A$ (l/minute)	$\dot{Q}$	$\dot{V}_A/\dot{Q}$	P_{O_2} (mm Hg)	P_{CO_2}	P_{N_2}	O_2 content (ml/ 100 ml)	CO_2	pH	O_2 in (ml/minute)	CO_2 out
7	.24	.07	3.3	132	28	553	20.0	42	7.51	4	8
13	.82	1.29	0.63	89	42	582	19.2	49	7.39	60	39

FIGURE 19-1 Regional physiological differences down the upright lung. V_A, Alveolar ventilation; Q, perfusion; V_A/Q, ventilation perfusion ratio. *(From West, J.B. [2004]. Respiratory physiology—the essentials, ed 7, Baltimore: Williams & Wilkins.)*

function (both primary pathology of the cardiopulmonary system and pathology of this system secondary to pathology in one or more other systems, as described in Chapter 6) provides a foundation for therapeutic body positioning as a primary intervention to optimize oxygen transport. Because of its potent and direct effect on oxygen transport, therapeutic body positioning can maintain or augment arterial oxygenation so that invasive, mechanical, and pharmacologic forms of respiratory support can be postponed, reduced, or avoided—a primary objective of cardiopulmonary physical therapy.

In health, normal oxygen transport is maintained by being upright and moving—the physiological body position. A patient who may have prolonged periods of recumbency is also exposed to gravity continuously, but not to the same extent as in the upright position. Each body position the patient assumes differentially affects the steps of the oxygen transport pathway due to alterations in gravitational stress. Oxygen transport can be improved, maintained, or worsened with changes in body position. Despite being essential to normal cardiopulmonary function, gravity is the principal contributor to inhomogeneity of physiological function down the lungs (West, 2004). Figure 19-1 illustrates the effect of this gradient with respect to alveolar ventilation ($\dot{V}_A$), perfusion (Q), ventilation and perfusion ratio ($\dot{V}_A/Q$), Pao_2, Pco_2, Pn_2, oxygen content, carbon dioxide (CO_2) content, pH, and the flow of oxygen and CO_2 in and out of the lungs.

Thus the lungs should not be likened to balloons, either physiologically or anatomically.

Based on a detailed analysis of all factors contributing to impaired oxygen transport and gas exchange (Chapter 17), the body positions that will have an optimal effect on oxygenation and those that may be deleterious must be distinguished from each other. In this way, a greater proportion of time can be spent by the patient in beneficial positions and less time in deleterious positions. Body positions themselves are associated with energetic stress, particularly in positions with greater gravitational stress, so the upright position can be more energetically demanding than supine positions, which are more demanding than lateral positions (Jones et al, 2004). Compression forces also impact the heart and cardiac output. Lying on the left side, for example, can compromise cardiac output, particularly within 12 hours after surgery in patients whose cardiac index is less than 2.3 L/min/m² (Doering & Dracup, 1988).

In health, gravitational effects and movement continually perturb the distributions of ventilation ($\dot{V}_A$) and perfusion (Q), and optimize $\dot{V}_A/Q$ matching commensurate with physiological demand. When body positions that are initially beneficial to the patient are assumed for too long, hydrostatic, gravitational, and compression forces acting on the heart, blood volume, lymphatic system, lungs, and chest wall, including the diaphragm, eventually compromise oxygen transport, offsetting any benefit. Therefore, close monitoring is essential to ensure that the patient is turned to another position before the effects become detrimental. Frequent changes in body position and avoidance of prolonged periods in any single position minimize this risk.

The length of time a body position is maintained is response-dependent rather than time-dependent (Bliss, 2004), and it reflects individual differences, including pathology, severity, age, and body mass. Knowledge of the deleterious effects of prolonged periods in a single position supports the prescription of both frequent body position changes and extreme sequential body positions. These perturbations simulate the normal perturbations that the cardiovascular and pulmonary systems experience in health during normal mobility and body position changes in daily life. The ability to weigh the relative beneficial and deleterious effects of each possible body position (through 360 degrees in the horizontal plane and 180 degrees in the vertical plane, ranging from approximately 20 degrees head down to 20 degrees leaning forward) on a given patient's gas exchange is critical in prescribing body positioning.

PRESCRIPTIVE VERSUS ROUTINE BODY POSITIONING

The literature supports the benefits of frequent body position changes, particularly for a patient who is relatively immobile, unalert, severely debilitated, obtunded, breathing at low lung volumes, obese, aged or very young or has lost the sigh mechanism. The practice of routinely turning patients every 2 hours continues to be an accepted standard of care. Even

BOX 19-1

Indications for Body Positioning to Optimize Oxygen Transport

Cardiopulmonary Indications

↓ Regional alveolar volume
↓ Regional ventilation
↓ Regional perfusion
↓ Regional diffusion
Compromised ventilation to perfusion matching
Pulmonary shunting
↓Lung volumes and capacities, particularly functional residual capacity, vital capacity, and tidal volume
Closure of dependent airways
Abnormal breathing frequency
Abnormal minute ventilation
Monotonous pattern of tidal ventilation
Suboptimal position of the hemidiaphragms
↓ Respiratory muscle efficiency
Airway resistance
Suboptimal lung compliance
Suboptimal flow rates
Weak ineffective cough
Poor biomechanical efficiency of cough's strength and productivity
↑ Work of breathing
Abnormal arterial blood gases, gas exchange, and oxygenation
Impaired mucociliary transport and mucus clearance
Untoward gravitational, mechanical and compression forces on the lungs, chest wall, diaphragm, and the gut
Impaired viscerodiaphragmatic breathing
Suboptimal pattern of breathing

Cardiovascular and Lymphatic Indications

Suboptimal preload and afterload
↑ Work of the heart
Impaired systolic ejection fraction to pulmonary and systemic circulations
Suboptimal venous return
Untoward gravitational, mechanical, and compression forces on the myocardium, great vessels, mediastinal structures, and lymphatic system
Suboptimal fluid shift from central to dependent areas (extremities) and vice versa to maintain fluid volume regulating mechanisms

Other Systemic Indications

↓ Patient arousal
Undue energy expenditure
Discomfort
Pain
Posturally increased muscle tone
↑ Intrathoracic pressure
↑ Intraabdominal pressure
↑ Intracranial pressure
Biomechanically suboptimal body positions
↓ Chest tube drainage
↓ Urinary drainage
Impaired peripheral perfusion

---

though the efficacy of this practice has not been firmly established, intensive care units (ICUs) fall short of this minimal guideline (Krishnagopalan et al, 2002). The practice is based on the belief that the deleterious consequences associated with assuming a static position for a prolonged period will be prevented. More frequent turning, however, may have greater physiological benefits in patients who are critically ill, and this suggests that patients who are less severely ill may also benefit from being gravitationally challenged systematically. The preventive effects of a routine turning regimen are distinct from the acute effects of body positioning on oxygen transport, which is the primary focus of this chapter.

PHYSIOLOGICAL EFFECTS OF VARIOUS BODY POSITIONS

Body positioning has potent and direct effects on most steps of the oxygen transport pathway, thus can be prescribed to elicit these effects preferentially. Because humans function optimally when upright and moving, therapeutic interventions that elicit or simulate being upright and moving (i.e., elicit both gravitational and exercise stress) are most justified physiologically (see Chapter 17). The recumbent supine position, a common position assumed by patients who are hospitalized, is nonphysiological and is deleterious to oxygen transport. The side-lying positions have an effect that is intermediate between that of upright and supine. The prone position, which

is underutilized clinically, can have such a significant powerful effect on oxygen transport that a good rationale must be made for *not* incorporating this position into the treatment prescription.

The indications for therapeutic body positioning and the indications for frequent body position changes to optimize oxygen transport are shown in Boxes 19-1 and 19-2. For each of the indications listed, an optimal therapeutic body position can be selected for a given patient. A description of the physiological effects of several primary body positions follow, namely, the upright supine, side-lying, head-down, and prone positions. However, this information cannot be applied out of context. The specific positions prescribed for a given patient are based on consideration of the multiple factors that impair oxygen transport (Chapter 17) in conjunction with a physiological analysis of the most justifiable positions.

Because of the potent and direct effects of body positioning on the steps in the oxygen transport pathway in health and in disease, it is unknown whether the beneficial effects reported with the use of postural drainage are attributable to enhanced mucociliary transport; or to the direct effect of positioning the good lung down on improving the gas exchange of that lung by increasing alveolar volume of the affected, nondependent lung; or to both. Typically, studies evaluating conventional chest physical therapy, including postural drainage, have failed to control for the direct effect of body positioning on oxygen

Indications for Frequent Changing of Body Position

Cardiopulmonary Indications

Alter chest wall configuration
Shift distribution of alveolar volume
Shift distribution of ventilation
Shift distribution of perfusion
Shift distribution of diffusion
Shift distribution of ventilation to perfusion matching
Shift mechanical physical compression of the heart on adjacent alveoli
Shift position of the heart, thereby altering chamber end diastolic filling pressures, preload, afterload, and work of the heart
Shift distribution of mucus transport and accumulation
Stimulate effective and productive cough
Facilitate pumping action needed for optimal lymphatic drainage
Perturb pattern of monotonous tidal ventilation
Perturb breathing pattern
Shift gravitational, mechanical, and compression forces on the lungs, chest wall, diaphragm, and gut
Simulate normal inflation-deflation sigh cycles
Shift intraabdominal pressure

Cardiovascular Indications

Shift gravitational, mechanical, and compression forces on the myocardium, great vessels, mediastinal structures, and lymphatic system
Stimulate fluid volume shifts particularly to the dependent limbs

Other Systemic Indications

Alter arousal state
Promote relaxation
Promote comfort
Control pain
Prevent skin breakdown, risk of infection, and resulting positioning limitations
Shift abnormal postural tone patterns
Optimize chest tube drainage
Promote urinary drainage

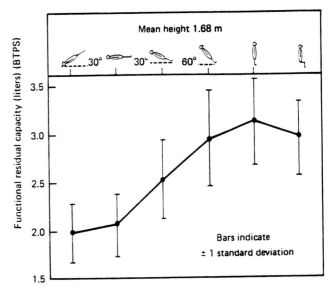

FIGURE 19-2 Changes in functional residual capacity in various body positions. *(From Lumb, A., & Nunn, J.F. [1999]. Nunn's applied respiratory physiology, ed 5. London: Elsevier.)*

transport, or for the direct effects of increased arousal and mobilization that occur when a patient's body position is changed (Dean, 1994a; Ross & Dean, 1989). This is a serious methodological problem that pervades the literature evaluating conventional practices, so-called chest physical therapy, and one that has to be considered when interpreting the results of studies of these procedures. Unless these potent confounding variables are controlled, the degree to which conventional chest physical therapy has a beneficial effect over and above the effects of positioning, as well as of mobilization and increased arousal, cannot be established (Dean, 1994b).

Upright Positions

Although the upright position is common to both the physiological and anatomical positions, movement in the upright constitutes the true physiological position in that the upright position coupled with movement (e.g., walking, cycling, or movement in sitting) is consistent with the requirements of daily activities. To meet the energetic demands of these activities, oxygen transport is optimized to the greatest degree, in that ventilation and perfusion are more uniform than they would be without the additional exercise stimulus. The upright standing position maximizes lung volumes and capacities, with the exception of closing volume, which is decreased (Svanberg, 1957). Functional residual capacity (FRC), the volume of air remaining in the lungs at the end of end tidal expiration, is greater in standing than in sitting and exceeds that in the supine position by as much as 50% (Figure 19-2). Maximizing FRC is associated with reduced airway closure and maximal arterial oxygenation (Hsu & Hickey, 1976; Ray et al, 1974). Figure 19-3 illustrates the relationship of FRC and closing capacity as a function of age. Because of age-related pulmonary changes, the closing capacity of the dependent airways increases with age; this effect is further accentuated with recumbency. Airway closure is evident in the supine position in the healthy 45-year-old person and in the upright seated position in the healthy 65-year-old person (Leblanc et al, 1970). Compression atelectasis results from cardiac weight, abdominal pressure, and pleural effusions, the effects of which are determined by the specific position of the patient (Rouby et al, 2003). These positional effects are further accentuated in patient populations with cardiopulmonary, thoracic, and abdominal pathologies, so the upright position is favored, and the supine position should be minimized so as to prevent airway closure and impaired gas exchange.

With respect to pulmonary function testing, the upright sitting position with legs dependent is the standard reference position (American Thoracic Society, 1987). When upright,

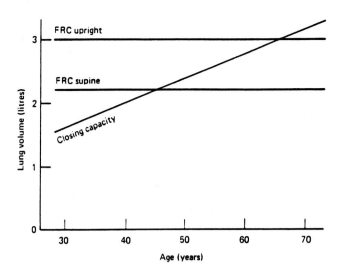

FIGURE 19-3 Functional residual capacity (FRC) and closing capacity as a function of age. *(From Lumb, A., & Nunn, J.F. [1999]. Nunn's applied respiratory physiology, ed 5. London: Elsevier.)*

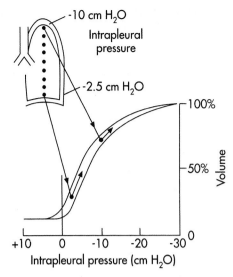

FIGURE 19-5 Schematic of the regional differences in ventilation down the upright lung. *(From West, J.B. [1985]. Ventilation/bloodflow and gas exchange, ed 4. Oxford: Blackwell Scientific.)*

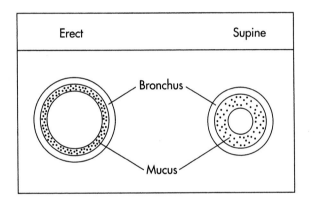

FIGURE 19-4 Effect of body position on bronchiolar diameter. *(From Browse, N.L. [1965]. The physiology and pathology of bed rest. Springfield, Ill.: Charles C. Thomas.)*

the diameter of the main airways increases slightly. If the airways are obstructed, even small degrees of airway narrowing induced by recumbency can increase airway resistance (Figure 19-4). When a person is upright, the vertical gravitational gradient is maximal, the anteroposterior dimension of the chest wall is the greatest, and compression of the heart and lungs is minimized (Weber et al, 1983). The shortened position of the diaphragmatic fibers is countered by an increase in the neural drive to breathe when a person is in the upright position (Druz & Sharp, 1982). Maximal expiratory pressure is augmented with progressively upright positions in patients with chronic obstructive lung disease as well as in those in health; standing results in the highest values and head-down positions the lowest (Badr et al, 2002). Thus, coughing and other forced expiratory maneuvers should be encouraged when the individual is in the optimal erect, upright position.

The distribution of ventilation is determined primarily by the effect of gravity, which changes down the lung due to the

anatomic position and the suspension of the lungs within the chest. At FRC in the upright position, the intrapleural pressure at the apex is -10 cm H_2O and at the base -2.5 cm H_2O (Figure 19-5). The intrapleural pressure is less negative in the base because of the suspended mass of the lungs. Because of the greater negative intrapleural pressure in the apices, thus low compliance, these lung units have a larger initial volume, hence smaller volume changes occur during respiration. Because the lung units at the base have a smaller initial volume, thus high compliance, larger volume changes occur during respiration. Therefore, depending on their relative position with respect to gravity, different regions of the lung are at different points on the pressure volume curve.

A common clinical concern is patients' breathing at low lung volumes (e.g., patients in pain, patients who have undergone thoracic or abdominal incisions, older and younger patients, obese patients, pregnant patients, patients with gastrointestinal dysfunction, such as paralytic ileus and ascites, organomegaly, or intrathoracic or intraabdominal masses, patients who are malnourished, and patients who are mechanically ventilated or have spinal cord injuries). Breathing at low lung volumes reverses the normal intrapleural pressure gradient such that in the upright lung the apices have a negative intrapleural pressure compared with the bases, which have a positive intrapleural pressure (i.e., exceeding airway pressure) (Figure 19-6). This results in the apices' being more compliant, thus better ventilated than the bases. The bases are prone to airway closure in individuals breathing at low lung volumes.

Another factor that reverses the normal intrapleural pressure gradient is mechanical ventilation. Despite its necessity in the management of patients in respiratory failure, mechanical ventilation can contribute to hypoxemia in several ways. First, it reverses the normal intrapleural pressure gradient

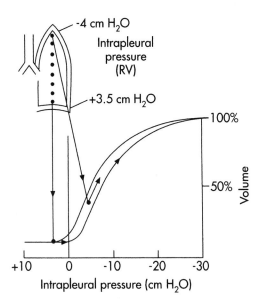

FIGURE 19-6 Schematic of the regional differences in ventilation at low lung volumes. *(From West, J.B. [1985]. Ventilation/bloodflow and gas exchange, ed 4. Oxford: Blackwell Scientific.)*

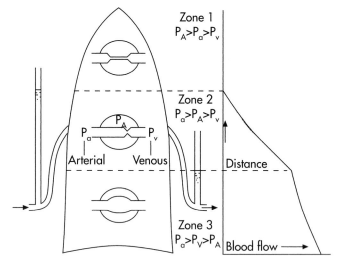

FIGURE 19-7 Schematic of pressures affecting the pulmonary capillaries and blood flow. *(From West, J.B. [1985]. Ventilation/bloodflow and gas exchange, ed 4. Oxford: Blackwell Scientific.)*

so that the uppermost lung fields are preferentially ventilated. Because the dependent lung fields are preferentially perfused, $\dot{V}_A/Q$ mismatch is promoted. Positive pressure ventilation has the additional complication of increasing intrathoracic pressure and reducing venous return and cardiac output. These factors, in addition to the negative pressure required to open the inspiratory valve, can increase the work of breathing associated with mechanical ventilation (Cane et al, 1990; Rivara et al, 1984).

Although gravity is the primary determinant of interregional differences in the distribution of ventilation in the healthy lung, intraregional differences, secondary to differences in compliance and resistance of contiguous lung units, also contribute (Ross et al, 1992). These effects are exaggerated in patient populations (Bates, 1989).

The distribution of perfusion down the upright lung is also primarily gravity dependent (Figure 19-7). The pressures affecting blood flow through the pulmonary capillaries and resulting in the typical uneven distribution (inhomogeneity) of blood flow are alveolar pressure and the arterial and venous pressures. In zone 1, at the apex, alveolar pressure predominates over arterial and venous pressures, so there is little or no blood flow. Zone 2, in the middle zone, reflects the blood flow from the recruitment of pulmonary vessels. Arterial pressure exceeds alveolar pressure and blood flow. Zone 3, in the lower area of the lung, reflects the blood flow from the distension of pulmonary vessels; arterial and venous pressures exceed alveolar pressure. And zone 4 (not illustrated), in the most dependent portion of the lung, has little or no pulmonary blood flow because of the interstitial pressure acting on the pulmonary blood vessels and creating a compression force (West, 2004).

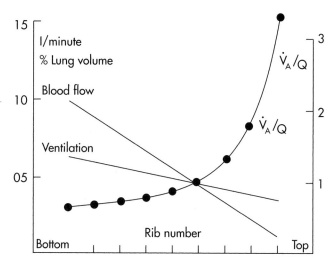

FIGURE 19-8 Distributions of ventilation and blood flow down the upright lung and the distribution of ventilation perfusion matching down the upright lung. *(From West, J.B. [1985]. Ventilation/bloodflow and gas exchange, ed 4. Oxford: Blackwell Scientific.)*

The matching of $\dot{V}_A$ and Q reflects the interfacing of the distributions of $\dot{V}_A$ and Q down the upright lung. Both $\dot{V}_A$ and Q increase down the upright lung; however, $\dot{V}_A$ increases disproportionately more than Q (Figure 19-8). As a result, the optimal area for $\dot{V}_A/Q$ matching is in the mid zone, where the ratio is about 1.0 (West, 1985).

The upright position is associated with significant hemodynamic effects. These effects reflect primarily the central blood volume, which is shifted from the thoracic compartment to the dependent venous compartments when a person assumes the upright position from the supine (Blomqvist & Stone, 1963; Gauer & Thron, 1965; Sandler, 1986). End-diastolic

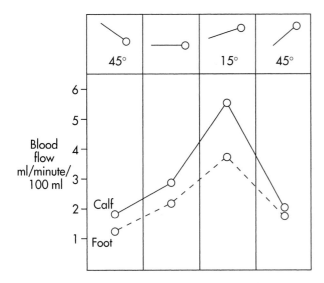

FIGURE 19-9 Effect of body position on peripheral blood flow. *(From Browse, N.L. [1965]. The physiology and pathology of bed rest. Springfield, Ill.: Charles C. Thomas.)*

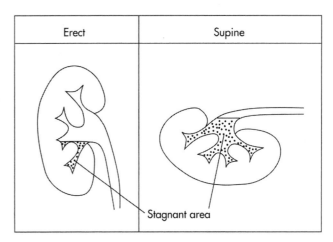

FIGURE 19-10 Effect of body position on drainage from the pelvis of the kidney. *(From Browse, N.L. [1965]. The physiology and pathology of bed rest. Springfield, Ill.: Charles C. Thomas.)*

volume and stroke volume are decreased, which results in a compensatory increase in heart rate (Thandani & Parker, 1978). Cardiac output is correspondingly decreased. The net effect of these physiological changes is a reduction in myocardial work (Langou et al, 1977). This finding is corroborated by the observation that the anginal threshold is increased in patients with cardiac conditions when they are upright (Prakash et al, 1973). Further, intermittent gravitational stress following myocardial infarction or bypass surgery maintains orthostatic tolerance and thereby prevents bed-rest deconditioning (Convertino, 2003).

Peripheral vascular resistance increases and blood flow decreases with the assumption of an upright position greater than 45 degrees to offset dependent fluid shifts and potential blood pressure drop (Figure 19-9). An upright angle of at least 60 degrees is needed to optimize cardiac output and sympathetic tone (Zaidi et al, 2000). Another important effect of body position on fluid volume is the promotion of urinary drainage from the renal pelvi to the bladder when in the upright position, as a result of the reduced area for urinary stasis when in this position as opposed to the supine position (Figure 19-10). Optimal renal function is essential to preserving normal hemodynamic status.

Older individuals who are relatively immobile tend to sit for prolonged periods. Without frequent exposure to standing upright, however, the phenomenon of seated postural hypotension may result (Cohen et al, 2003). In addition, dependent circulatory stasis and other consequences of restricted mobility such as deconditioning are promoted in this position.

Supine Position

The indiscriminant use and overwhelming acceptance of bed rest evolved historically over the past 150 years. In the mid-

1800s, the use of immobilization to heal bones and injuries was extended to the management of other conditions in the belief that internal organs could be rested as a therapeutic intervention as well. The injudicious application and overuse of bed rest to address medical problems has been challenged over several decades (Dock, 1944; Harrison, 1944; Moreno & Lyons, 1961; Powers, 1944; Winslow, 1985). Although there has been a marked decrease in the use of prolonged periods of bed rest based on innumerable studies over the past several decades of its negative sequelae (Dean & Ross, 1992b), the merits of bed rest as a therapeutic modality and the parameters for its prescription (i.e., indications and specifications to achieving healing and recovery without deterioration) have not been scientifically established.

The supine position inherent in bed rest alters the configuration of the chest wall, the anteroposterior position of the hemidiaphragms, the intrathoracic pressure, the intra-abdominal pressure secondary to the shifting of the abdominal viscera in this position, and the mechanics of cardiac function (Behrakis et al, 1983; Craig et al, 1971; Don et al, 1971; Druz & Sharp, 1981; Klingstedt et al, 1990a; Roussos et al, 1976; Sasaki et al, 1977). The normal anteroposterior configuration becomes more transverse. The hemidiaphragms are displaced cephalad, which reduces FRC in this position (Hsu & Hickey, 1976). Prefaut and Engel (1981) observed that hypoxic vaso-constriction secondary to closure of the dependent airways in the supine position contributed to preferential perfusion of the nondependent lung zones. Finally, in the supine position, excess pulmonary secretions tend to pool on the dependent sides of the airways. The upper side may dry out, exposing the patient to infection and obstruction (Figure 19-11).

An increase in intrathoracic blood volume in the supine position also contributes to a reduction in FRC and lung compliance and to increased airway resistance (Lumb & Nunn, 1999; Sjostrand, 1951). Collectively, these effects predispose the patient to airway closure and an increase in the work of

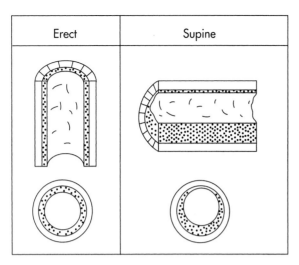

FIGURE 19-11 Effect of body position on the distribution of mucus within the bronchi. *(From Browse, N.L. [1965]. The physiology and pathology of bed rest. Springfield, Ill.: Charles C. Thomas.)*

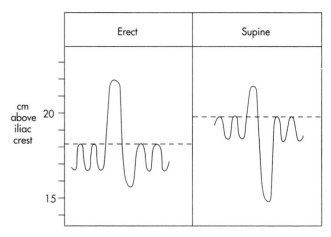

FIGURE 19-12 Effect of body position on the level and movements of the diaphragm during respiration. *(From Browse, N.L. [1965]. The physiology and pathology of bed rest. Springfield, Ill.: Charles C. Thomas.)*

breathing. Although a healthy person can accommodate to these physiological changes, a healthy person does not assume this position for prolonged periods without unconsciously shifting. A hospitalized patient, however, is less likely to adapt to these immediate changes and their long-term effects. They may be less responsive to the need to shift position or unable to respond to afferent stimuli prompting a need to change position. These effects are accentuated in older people whose arterial oxygen tensions progressively diminish with age (Lumb & Nunn, 1999; Ward et al, 1966), and are lower in the supine position compared with the reference sitting position (Hardie et al, 2002).

Several cardiovascular changes occur on assuming the supine position (e.g., hemodynamic or intolerance to position change). A central shift of blood volume from the extremities to the central circulation initiates orthostatism (Matzen et al, 1991; Sandler, 1986). This fluid shift increases both the preload and the afterload of the right side of the heart. This increased volume tends to distort the interventricular septum and reduce left ventricular volume and preload. The relatively increased central blood volume inhibits the release of antidiuretic hormone and atrial natriuretic peptide from the right side of the heart (Perko et al, 1994) and diuresis is stimulated (Norsk, 2000). Between 10% and 15% of fluid is lost within 24 hours (Sandler, 1986), which can manifest clinically as cardiac underfilling, orthostatic intolerance, and negative fluid balance (Dean & Ross, 1992a). Altered autonomic nervous system function also has been implicated in the etiology of bed rest deconditioning (Hasser & Moffit, 2001; Hughson et al, 1994). Individuals with impaired autonomic control (those with high spinal cord lesions) exhibit greater reductions in mean arterial pressure and stroke volume compared with able-bodied individuals (Houtman et al, 2000). Because of local vascular regulation, cerebral circulation can be maintained. Finally, when individuals are confined to bed rest abruptly, they show more dehydration than do individuals confined to bed rest for a longer term, and

it occurs faster, possibly because of less opportunity to compensate (Zorbas et al, 2003). Although the prescriptive parameters regarding the optimal gravitational stress required to offset the hemodynamic changes that occur with the supine position have yet to be elucidated (degree of upright angle, duration, and frequency) (Zhang et al, 2000), there are other effects of the upright position that support its frequent use in patients whose mobility is restricted. Anatomic regions adapt to the relative microgravity effects of the supine position differently according to the redistribution of transmural pressures and flows within the various vascular beds (Zhang, 2001). Knowledge of these physiological adaptations is essential for refining therapeutic countermeasures.

Although lower body negative pressure (LBNP) may have a role in space exploration for maintaining orthostatic stability and has been shown to offset change with bed rest such that exercise capacity is maintained (Watenpaugh et al, 2000), LBNP will not likely be a feasible or practical modality in acute management. Despite its reported benefit in countering the adverse fluid shifts associated with recumbency, LBNP does not address other negative effects of bed rest.

Because of a reduction in the vertical gravitational gradient, and therefore in the intrapleural pressure gradient of the lung, in the supine position, the distribution of $\dot{V}_A/Q$ matching appears more uniform and evenly matched in this position (Bates, 1989). These changes, however, must be considered in conjunction with other changes associated with the supine position, namely reduced FRC, reduced vital capacity, reduced flow rates, increased area of dependent lung, and increased closure of the dependent airways as well as its associated hemodynamic consequences. These deleterious factors offset any theoretical benefit of the supine position on V/Q matching (Ross & Dean, 1992). However, in a patient who is unresponsive, hemodynamically unstable, and clining to life, a recumbent position may be the only alternative (see end of life issues in Chapter 33).

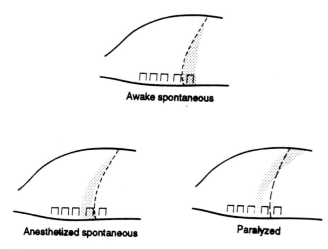

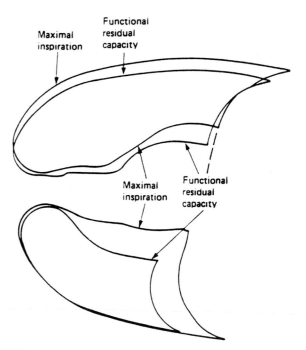

FIGURE 19-13 Position of the diaphragm in an awake, spontaneously breathing subject and in anesthetized subjects with and without paralysis. The broken line is the end-expiratory position of the diaphragm in the awake state in the supine position. The shaded area shows the excursion of the diaphragm during inspiration and expiration. *(From Froese, A.B., & Bryan, A.C. [1974]. Effects of anesthesia and paralysis on diaphragmatic mechanics in man. Anesthesiology 41:242-255.)*

FIGURE 19-14 Outlines of the lungs at two lung volumes in a conscious, spontaneously breathing subject in the right side-lying position. *(From Lumb, A., & Nunn, J.F. [1999]. Nunn's applied respiratory physiology, ed 5. London: Elsevier.)*

The position of the diaphragm and its function are dependent on body position. Figure 19-12 illustrates the effect of body position on the level and movement of the diaphragm consistent with compromised lung function recorded in recumbent positions. In the supine position, the resting level of the diaphragm is influenced differentially by anesthesia and neuromuscular blockade (Froese & Bryan, 1974). Figure 19-13 illustrates these effects. In the spontaneously breathing subject, the excursion of the diaphragm is greater posteriorly because of the dependent viscera beneath the posterior portion of the diaphragm. During anesthesia with or without paralysis, the diaphragm ascends 2 cm into the chest. When paralysis is induced, the loss of diaphragmatic tone results in greater excursion of the nondependent rather than the dependent part of the diaphragm.

A study of hemodynamic postural effects in healthy subjects supports that the horizontal position maximizes central blood volume (Harms et al, 2003). This position, however, cannot be considered clinically optimal because of such effects as intrathoracic and intrabdominal compression.

Side-Lying Positions

Side-lying may be theoretically less deleterious compared with the supine position (Hurewitz et al, 1985; Ibanez et al, 1981; Ross & Dean, 1992; Roussos et al, 1977). The side-lying position accentuates anteroposterior expansion at the expense of transverse excursion of the dependent chest wall. In this position, the dependent hemidiaphragm is displaced cephalad because of the compression of the viscera beneath it. This results in a greater excursion during respiration and to

greater contribution to the ventilation of that lung and to gas exchange as a whole. The FRC in side-lying falls between that in the upright and supine positions. Compared with supine, in side-lying compliance is increased, resistance is reduced, and the work of breathing is reduced, whereas these measures are reversed when side-lying is compared to the upright position. Figure 19-14 illustrates the difference in lung volumes between maximal inspiration and FRC in a spontaneously breathing subject in right side-lying. Although ventilation is enhanced to the dependent lung, inspiratory lung volume and FRC are reduced. Compared with the reference sitting position, FEV_1 and FVC are reduced similarly in left and right side-lying with no differential effects of side-lying on diffusing capacity and closing volume (Manning et al, 1999). These lung-function effects in side-lying may reflect altered lung geometry with position change and a reduction in the vertical diameter of each lung in side-lying compared with that which occurs in the supine position (Klingstedt et al, 1990b).

Side-lying increases end diastolic ventricular pressure on the dependent side secondary to compression of the viscera beneath the diaphragm and to reduced lung compliance on that side (Lange et al, 1988). Although such changes can be readily accommodated in health, they may further impair gas exchange in individuals with oxygen transport deficits.

Optimal $\dot{V}_A/Q$ matching occurs in the upper one third of each lung in the side-lying position (Kaneko et al, 1966). The total area for optimal $\dot{V}_A/Q$ matching, therefore, is likely greater than that in the upright position, which contributes theoretically to an improved $\dot{V}_A/Q$ matching. These apparent improvements, however, are offset by reduced lung volumes and airflow rates in this position.

In both healthy people and patients, arterial oxygen tension is greater in side-lying than in supine (Clauss et al, 1968). This is true for patients receiving supplemental oxygen as well as for those who are not. Thus side-lying can be used to enhance the efficiency of gas exchange and thereby minimize or avoid the use of supplemental oxygen. Arterial blood gases have been reported to be improved in patients with unilateral lung disease (Remolina et al, 1981; Sonnenblick et al, 1983) when they are positioned with the good lung down and worsened when the affected lung is down. When lung pathology is bilateral, arterial blood gases are better when patients lie on the right side than when they lie on the left. This can be explained by the greater size of the right lung and the reduced compression of the heart on the lung in this position compared with left side-lying (Dean, 1985; Zach et al, 1974). The practice of "down with the good lung," however, has been questioned in patients with unilateral lung collapse secondary to central airway lesions (Chang et al, 1993). Not all patients respond favorably when the good lung is down. Research is necessary to distinguish the characteristics of responders and nonresponders to refine the prescription of body positions.

The side-lying rather than the supine position is often a preferred position for patients who are hospitalized, yet its physiological consequences are not well understood. The pulmonary effects of side-lying have been reported for healthy older people (Manning et al, 1999). FEV_1 and FVC are reduced comparably for right and left side-lying compared with a reference sitting position. Although diffusing capacity and homogeneity of ventilation appear to be unchanged, they may be adversely affected in patient populations with single and combined pathologies that impact oxygen transport.

Patients who are hemodynamically unstable require special consideration with respect to body positioning. These patients may be less able to benefit from active mobilization and are more reliant on positional perturbation than on movement to promote optimal gas exchange. In one study of patients with severe respiratory failure and receiving inotropic support, the extreme left lateral position contributed to a hyperdynamic state, and the right lateral position predisposed the patients to hypotension likely due to impaired right ventricular preload (Bein et al, 1996). Spirometric evidence from patients who were intubated supports decreased dynamic lung compliance in the lateral and prone positions compared with supine (Tanskanen et al, 1997). Body positioning warrants judicious prescription, with particular attention to the angle of the lateral position and the duration and to monitoring to observe the effect.

Prolonged side-lying has been shown to mobilize lung water in patients with pulmonary edema, and to a lesser extend in patients with pulmonary inflammation (Zimmerman et al, 1982). Physical therapy interventions that entail gravitational challenges, therefore, can have a direct effect on lung water distribution and possibly compartmentalization that,

in turn, may affect pulmonary compliance and gas exchange. Similarly, pleural effusions respond to the effect of gravity. In patients with unilateral effusions, when the effusion is positioned lowermost in side-lying, oxygenation is lower than when the effusion is positioned uppermost (Duan et al, 1997). This may be explained by the effusion impairing $\dot{V}_A/Q$ matching and gas exchange in the lowermost lung.

Head-Down Position

The head-down position augments oxygen transport in some patients by improving pulmonary mechanics. Patients with chronic airflow limitation, for example, tend to have hyperinflated chests and flattened diaphragms in which the contraction of the diaphragm is inefficient because of the position of its muscle fibers on the length tension curve. The head-down position causes the viscera to be displaced cephalad beneath the diaphragm. The diaphragm is positioned more normally and rests at a higher and more mechanically efficient position in the chest (Barach & Beck, 1954; De Troyer, 1983). In this position, patients may experience relief from dyspnea, reduced accessory muscle use, reduced upper chest breathing patterns, and reduced minute ventilation. Patients with pathology in the lung bases may also benefit from the head-down position in that this position favors gas exchange in the more functional upper lung fields and promotes alveolar distension of bases, which are uppermost in the head-down position. Other patients, however, such as those with respiratory muscle fatigue, may have increased respiratory distress in this position due to the added resistive loading of the diaphragm because of the weight of the viscera beneath. These observations support the need to prescribe body positioning on an individual basis with consideration of the multiple factors that may impair oxygenation as well as enhance it.

Prone Position

There is mounting physiological and scientific justification for use of the prone position to enhance arterial oxygenation and reduce the work of breathing in patients with cardiopulmonary dysfunction who may or may not be mechanically ventilated. The prone position shifts the mobile structures of the thoracic and abdominal cavities (Ball et al, 1980). The heart and great vessels are displaced anteriorly. The liver, spleen, and kidney shift anteriorly and caudally.

The prone position increases arterial oxygen tension, tidal volume, and dynamic lung compliance (Albert et al, 1987; Valter et al, 2003; Wagaman et al, 1979). The pleural pressure gradient is homogenized, hence the distribution of $\dot{V}_A$ and alveolar inflation are augmented. In addition, this position reduces stroke volume, increases sympathetic activity, and augments urine output (Pump et al, 2002). There has been increasing interest in exploiting these benefits in patients who are critically ill where mobilizing options are more limited (see Chapters 34 and 35). The prone position has some role in avoiding mechanical ventilation in patients who are conscious and alert, thereby reducing the risk of ventilator-associated complications (Valter et al, 2003). Most of the studies of prone positioning have been conducted in patients with acute respiratory distress syndrome (Ball et al, 2001; Langer et al, 1988; see Chapter 36). Prone is associated with improving oxygenation in 70% to 80% of cases (Pelosi et al, 2002). The effect of prolonged duration in the prone position has been studied, and the benefits appear to be dose-dependent (McAuley et al, 2002). The physiological outcomes of prone positioning in the management of acute lung injury are thought to reflect primarily its pathoetiology.

Complications associated with prolonged periods in the prone position, including skin breakdown, are common, so close monitoring is essential. To prevent or manage these complications, intermittent prone positioning has been advocated. Intermittent prone positioning of patients with acute respiratory distress syndrome and best positive end-expiratory pressure (PEEP) therapy can reduce FIO_2 levels to be reduced to less than 0.50, the critical level for oxygen toxicity (Michaels et al, 2002).

In a study using a canine model of acute lung injury, the prone position was observed to augment oxygenation in conjunction with low PEEP, and to offset the negative hemodynamic effects of high PEEP (Lim et al, 1999). This finding is consistent with clinical outcome studies. The two common variants of the prone position are prone abdomen-restricted and prone abdomen-free. Prone abdomen-restricted refers to lying prone with the abdomen in contact with the bed, whereas in the prone abdomen-free position the patient's hips and chest are elevated so that the abdomen is free. Both prone positions augment gas exchange, but the prone abdomen-free position, comparable to the hands-and-knees position (Mellins, 1974), enhances lung compliance, tidal volume, FRC, and diaphragmatic excursion to a greater degree and minimizes compression of the heart and abdominal viscera on the lungs (Rouby et al, 2003). In one study, supplemental oxygen was reduced in four of five patients who were mechanically ventilated and whose positioning regimen included the prone abdomen-free position (Dougles et al, 1977). Although patients in respiratory failure have been shown to benefit from the prone position, certain precautions must be observed. The patient is positioned so that all pressure points, particularly on the head and face, and stress on the tubing and circuitry of the mechanical ventilator tubing are minimized. The patient should be monitored continuously. A semiprone position can provide many of the physiological benefits of a full prone position and can minimize the risks, particularly in patients who are mechanically ventilated and those with cervical spine pathology. In addition, the semiprone position simulates the prone abdomen-free position. The semiprone position may be more conservative, more comfortable, and safer for the patient who is severely ill, potentially hemodynamically unstable, older, or has a protruding abdomen.

For patients unable to be mobilized, use of some variant of the prone position is even more important. Excessive recumbency, particularly in patients who are being positioned through a restricted arc (e.g., supine and one-quarter turns to either side), should be offset by some variant of the prone position, and this position should be incorporated often. Inevitably, patients exposed to a restricted arc of positioning may readily develop atelectasis in the dependent lung fields. Patients who are mechanically ventilated and have monotonous patterns of tidal ventilation are at particular risk. The only means of preventing and countering compression and hydrostatically induced atelectasis is by positioning dependent areas uppermost and repositioning the patient frequently.

The time course for the development of such hydrostatic complications is dependent on the patient's status, which may change from hour to hour in an individual who is critically ill. Although it is essential to monitor objective measures of oxygen transport and the adequacy of the steps in the oxygen transport pathway, subclinical changes will precede clinically measurable changes. By the time changes manifest in clinical measures, significant pathology may be present. Prevention, anticipation, and early detection are key.

PHYSIOLOGICAL EFFECTS OF FREQUENT CHANGES IN BODY POSITION

Box 19-2 lists some of the physiological effects of frequent changes in body position that are mediated primarily through their effects on respiratory mechanics, cardiac mechanics, airway closure, mucociliary transport, lymphatic drainage, and altered neural activation of the diaphragm. These effects, resulting from a change in position, are distinct from the benefits derived from a particular static body position. The benefits of changing position can be enhanced by moving to an extreme position (i.e., moving from supine to prone, rather than moving from supine to side-lying). Extreme body position changes simulate, but do not replace, the physiological stir-up and perturbations that occur with normal mobility and being upright. When the stir-up regimen was originally proposed, Dripps and Waters (1941) did not appreciate fully the physiological implications of regular upright standing (Convertino, 1992). The net effect of changing body position is stirring-up of the constituent distributions of $\dot{V}_A$, Q, and $\dot{V}_A$/Q matching and shifting of internal organs and their compression on the structures of the cardiopulmonary unit. Areas of dependent atelectasis, physiological dead space and shunting, and mucus distribution are dramatically shifted. The stir-up stimulates lymphatic drainage, surfactant production and distribution through stretching of the lung parenchyma, and the distribution and function of pulmonary immune factors (Pyne, 1994). Frequent physical perturbations also may inhibit bacterial colonization (Skerrett et al, 1989). In addition, frequent body position changes shift and redistribute compression forces acting on the diaphragm, myocardium, and mediastinal structures and the compression of the lungs by the myocardium and mediastinal structures.

Frequent body position changes are used by physical therapists to stimulate the patient and increase arousal to a more alert and wakeful state (Figure 19-15). The more upright the patient, the greater the neurological arousal and the greater the stimulus to breathe; this effect is augmented by encouraging the patient to be self-supporting. Commensurate with an increase in arousal, the patient is stimulated to take deeper breaths and, hence, to increase $\dot{V}_A$. When body positioning is coupled with mobilization, vasodilation and recruitment of the pulmonary capillaries are stimulated, and this, in turn, improves the homogeneity of the distributions of $\dot{V}_A$ and Q, hence augmenting $\dot{V}_A$/Q matching.

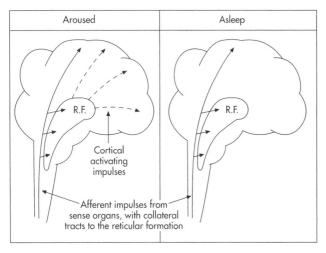

FIGURE 19-15 Effect of arousal on cerebral activity. *(From Browse, N.L. [1965]. The physiology and pathology of bed rest. Springfield, Ill.: Charles C. Thomas.)*

PRESCRIPTION OF THERAPEUTIC BODY POSITIONS AND BODY POSITION CHANGES

Prescription of body positioning is based on an analysis of the factors that contribute to impaired oxygen transport for each patient (Doering, 1993). Specific positions are selected to simulate as closely as possible the physiological function of the normal, healthy, upright cardiopulmonary unit and oxygen transport, and the perturbations and stirring-up that occurs hemodynamically during normal mobility and being upright (Convertino, 1992). A hierarchy of body positioning alternatives based on the physiological justification of the various positions appears in Box 19-3. These positions range from the most to the least physiological. The hierarchy is based on the premise that oxygen transport is optimal when upright and moving. Mobilization in the upright position increases tidal volume and respiratory rate, hence minute ventilation, flow rates, and mucociliary transport and clearance and enhances the efficiency and effectiveness of airway clearance and coughing. Thus, incorporating active movement into the body position change is optimal.

Despite the well-documented benefits of the judicious application of therapeutic body positioning to enhance oxygen transport, it does not replace the more physiological intervention of mobilization and exercise to maximize oxygen transport. Rather, once the effects of mobilization/exercise have been maximally exploited, body positioning is the next best physiological approximation to a mobilized upright state. However, even the mobilized patient benefits from therapeutic body positioning between mobilization sessions and during the night and rest periods. The progressive sequence of body

---

Physiological Hierarchy of Body Positions

Most Physiological Body Position

Upright and moving in a 1 *g* gravitational field and exposed to a range of body positions and body-position changes over time
Relaxed erect standing (not too prolonged)
Erect sitting (self-supported or with assist) with feet moving (e.g., active, active assisted, or passive cycling motion)
Erect sitting (self-supported or with assist) with feet dependent
Lean-forward sitting, with arms supported and feet dependent
≥ 45-degree sitting with legs dependent
Erect long sitting (legs nondependent)
< 45-degree sitting (legs nondependent)
Prone and semiprone/side-lying
Supine

Least Physiological Body Position

Provisos

The upright erect sitting position implies that the back, head, and neck are vertical and aligned, with flexion only at the hips; the patient is not slumped or recumbent.

The less able the patient is to assist in positioning, the greater the need for more extreme positions and greater turning frequency.
If the patient is totally unable to move (i.e., in a coma or paralyzed), extreme body positions are indicated if they are not contraindicated because of hemodynamic instability or increased intracerebral pressure. The upright position is used as much as possible, provided the patient is physically supported for safety and monitored in terms of treatment response. Passive standing on a tilt table is hemodynamically questionable; it is preferable that patients be placed in a high Fowler position, with legs positioned dependently, using the knee breaks in the bed.
Regimens of 360-degree horizontal turning and 180-degree vertical turning (ranging from 20 degrees head-down to 20 degrees lean-forward) are used unless contraindicated. Positioning through a maximal arc simulates as closely as possible the three-dimensional movement of the chest wall during normal respiration.

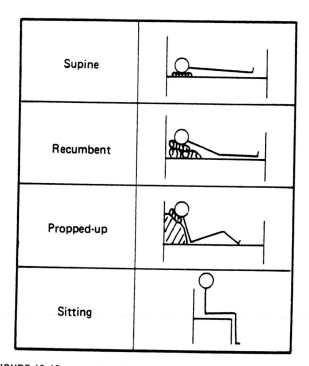

Supine	
Recumbent	
Propped-up	
Sitting	

FIGURE 19-16 Approximations of the upright position from supine. The recumbent and propped-up positions are not comparable physiologically to the upright sitting position. *(From Browse, N.L. [1965]. The physiology and pathology of bed rest. Springfield, Ill.: Charles C. Thomas.)*

positioning with movement is considered from the outset in planning for fully functional recovery and return to daily life.

Body position should first be exploited when coupled with movement followed by the erect sitting positions with legs dependent. Figure 19-16 illustrates several variants of the sitting position. Each of these positions has distinct effects on oxygen transport, so the specific upright position has to be prescribed specifically, as the supported and propped-up positions in bed do not substitute for upright, erect sitting. These variants have a role only when the patient deteriorates while being positioned upright or when in that position. Sitting with the feet down and supported is preferable to the long sit because of the gravitationally induced hemodynamic benefits associated with this position. Sitting up in bed fails to position the patient in a perfectly vertical upright position. The head-up position in bed can be maximized and the use of knee breaks in the bed provides a gravitational stimulus to the circulating blood volume.

One challenge when positioning patients in bed is the tendency to lose the position, usually from the compliance of the mattress and supporting pillows. Patients lose optimal positions in bed very quickly, so they should be monitored to ensure that the specific positions are maintained. An uncorrected slumped position can compromise pulmonary function and gas exchange. Pillows should not be used to maintain a body position because they are easily compressed

and shifted. Blankets and sheets tightly rolled and secured with tape and rigid bolsters are more effective in maintaining a patient's body position.

Although there is a role for modified positions such as half side-lying, these positions are often overused at the expense of full turns to each side or prone or semiprone positions. Patients can be positioned safely, with appropriate supervision and monitoring, and comfortably in these full positions by observing the normal precautions of passive positioning.

A common practice is to progressively turn patients in one-quarter turns, such as supine to side-lying and back to supine and so forth. However, the use of extreme positions and extreme position changes may yield greater physiological benefit with respect to the degree of perturbation and stir-up elicited (Piehl & Brown, 1977). Extreme position changes result in significant alterations in the distributions of $\dot{V}_A$, Q, and $\dot{V}_A$/Q matching. Mucociliary transport is stimulated, and secretion accumulation and stagnation is minimized. In addition, the more extreme the body position, the greater the degree of arousal stimulated, particularly in the upright positions, and arousal is essential in patients who are critically ill.

Another important consideration is the time course of changes in oxygen transport with positions and position changes. There are three plausible outcomes: a favorable response, no response, or an unfavorable response. With the passage of time, all three outcomes will deteriorate. The specific time depends on the multitude of factors contributing to impaired oxygen transport. With judicious monitoring, the duration of a position can be maintained as long as the patient responds favorably, and it is modified before or at the first sign of deteriorating gas exchange.

Because of the marked changes that can be expected with body positioning and body positioning changes, the physical therapist has a narrow window of opportunity to assess and treat the patient before, during, and after position changes (immediate and delayed effects).

Mechanical Body Positioning

Mechanical turning beds can benefit oxygen transport in patients who are severely ill (Brackett & Condon, 1984; Fink et al, 1990; Gentillelo et al, 1988; Gonzalez-Arias et al, 1983; Kelley et al, 1987; Meinig et al, 1986; Summer et al, 1989). These beds are indicated for patients who are moderately hemodynamically unstable and on neuromuscular blockers, and thus tolerate manual turns poorly. Such turning frames are contraindicated, however, for patients who are less ill. Even for patients who require multiple assistants and extra caution and time to turn and position effectively, these issues should never deny a patient a much needed treatment with proven efficacy.

The benefit of these beds on oxygen transport in patients who are critically ill has implications for the management of patients who are less severely ill. Continuous mechanical rotation can be simulated by increasing the frequency and arc of positions when manually positioning patients.

PRACTICAL CONSIDERATIONS IN POSITIONING PATIENTS

Prescriptive body positioning can require a significant amount of the physical therapist's time as well as other team members' time. Such prescriptive positioning is based on clear indications and well-defined parameters; it is not to be confused with "routine" positioning. For any hospitalized patient who is recumbent and inactive rather than being out of hospital, body positioning is a 24-hour concern, both during treatment and between treatments. Such patients are at risk of impaired oxygen transport. The team as a whole has a responsibility to ensure that complications related to static positioning and restricted mobility are prevented (Markey & Brown, 2002).

Despite the time and labor involved in turning a patient to the prone position, particularly if mechanically ventilated, the benefits of this position outweigh the time and effort required to place a patient in the prone position, even for short periods. Given the benefits that can be derived from the prone position, justification has to be made for *not* doing so. Frequently, therapeutic body positioning can be effectively coordinated with nursing interventions and other procedures. With all body positions, but especially the prone position in patients who are severely ill, potential inclusion and exclusion criteria should be reviewed, along with pre-turn considerations, the turning technique, assistants, monitoring the effectiveness of the prone position, passive movements, and limb positioning (Ball et al, 2001). Finally, any problems or adverse responses to the prone, as to other positions, are documented.

Extreme body positions and body position changes are the interventions of choice after mobilization has been fully exploited or in the event that the role of mobilization is limited for a given patient. When extreme positions are less feasible, modified positions may be used. Even though the greatest benefits will be derived from extreme changes as they simulate the normal range of changes the human body is exposed to in health, small changes can be effective in altering intrapleural gradients slightly so that previously closed alveoli will be opened even though previously opened ones may be prone to closure. Although modified positions and small degrees of position change should not be relied upon, their potential benefits should not be minimized in patients for whom extreme positions are contraindicated. Before and after each position change are prime opportunities to assess the patient, and to encourage deep breathing and coughing or to suction the patient, as indicated.

MONITORING RESPONSES TO A BODY POSITION OR POSITION CHANGES

The prescriptive parameters of body positioning and body position changes include the positions selected, the duration in each position, the sequence of position changes, the cycle of all positions, and position changes overall. Because a patient necessarily assumes a body position at all times (can never be free of gravitational forces), positioning patients between treatments can contribute as much to the overall treatment response as the treatment itself because the patient spends more time in the between-treatment positions than in the within-treatment positions.

The duration and frequency of the positions and the frequency of body position changes are response dependent rather than time dependent. Monitoring is the basis for defining and modifying the body positioning prescription. The physiological variables to be monitored depend on the patient's specific presentation and on cardiopulmonary dysfunction and its severity and distribution. Monitoring the patient who is not critically ill includes subjective and objective evaluation of indexes of the adequacy of oxygen transport (Part II). Among the most important are oxygen delivery, oxygen consumption, oxygen extraction, and gas exchange indicators such as the A/AO_2 difference and the PAO_2/PaO_2. Subjectively, the patient's facial expression, respiratory distress, dyspnea, anxiety, peripheral edema, and discomfort and pain are assessed. Objectively, heart rate, blood pressure, respiratory rate, SaO_2, flow rates, and bedside spirometry can be readily assessed. The appropriate standardization and procedures need to be used to ensure that the measures are both valid and reliable (see Chapter 7). Because physiological variables change from moment to moment, serial measures over a period of time should be taken to establish an average value rather than using peak or discrete measures which may misrepresent a treatment effect.

To interpret and compare various measures, the FIO_2 and any change in FIO_2 must be recorded. The use of the ratio $PaO_2:FIO_2$ enables comparison of gas exchange within and between patients when FIO_2 levels differ or change (Dean & Ross, 1992c). Similarly, for patients who are mechanically ventilated, any changes in the ventilatory parameters must also be noted, in addition to other interventions that have a direct effect on oxygen transport. Only in this way will the clinician be able to reasonably conclude that the position or position change was instrumental in enhancing oxygen transport.

Measures and outcomes are recorded before (pretreatment baseline), during, and at periodic intervals following the treatment. A valid stable pretreatment baseline is essential to determine the therapeutic effect of a given position on oxygen transport. Variables monitored during the treatment are focused on ensuring that the treatment is having a beneficial effect, in addition to its not having any deleterious effect on the patient subjectively or with respect to any parameter of oxygen transport. As long as beneficial effects are being recorded, a position can usually be safely maintained in the absence of other contraindications; however, diminishing returns can be expected as the period becomes prolonged. Patients maintained in static positions for more than 1 to 2 hours need to be monitored closely. A position change is physiologically defensible after this duration, rather than risking diminishing returns and potentially worsening the patient's condition.

Although sicker than a noncritically ill counterpart, the patient who is critically ill has the advantage of having more monitoring devices and lines in place. These give access to several measures and indexes of oxygen transport, and certain hemodynamic and pulmonary variables are available continuously to ensure that the outcome is therapeutic and the patient is safe.

SUMMARY

The premise underlying body positioning is that the physiological body position consistent with social participation and activity is "upright and moving." The specific purpose of this chapter is to differentiate therapeutic body positioning prescribed by the physical therapist to optimize oxygen transport, from "routine" body positioning, which has the primary objective of maintaining gas exchange and preventing complications. The physiological effects on cardiopulmonary and cardiovascular function and oxygen transport of different body positions and of changing body positions are described. The primary goal is to strive toward the physiological position for optimizing oxygen transport (i.e., upright and preferably moving). Issues related to optimizing the prescription of therapeutic body positioning and monitoring treatment outcome are presented.

This chapter focuses on the physiological effects of body positioning, an intervention that has well-documented, direct, and potent effects on oxygen transport. Establishing a clear rationale for prescribing a specific body position or body position changes is essential. The rationale, however, is based on multiple factors in addition to the physiological considerations presented. This chapter highlights the principles that must be considered in the decision-making process for prescribing therapeutic body positioning.

Review Questions

1. Relate the physiological body position of being upright and moving to the categories of participation and activity in the International Classification of Function.
2. Describe the effects of gravity on cardiopulmonary function and oxygen transport.
3. Distinguish *prescriptive* from *routine* body positioning.
4. In reference to the seated upright position, describe the effects of the following body positions (i.e., supine, side-lying, head down, and prone) on cardiopulmonary function and oxygen transport in health.
5. In reference to the seated upright position, describe the effects of the following body positions (i.e., supine, side lying, head down, and prone) on cardiopulmonary function and oxygen transport in disease.
6. Explain how a physiologically ideal body position with respect to oxygen transport can be deleterious over time.
7. Distinguish between the prescription of therapeutic body positions and the frequency of body position changes.
8. Describe the principles of monitoring oxygen transport variables before, during, and after positioning a patient.
9. Explain why body positioning protocols cannot be defined for the management of specific pathological conditions, although this is often the way in which it is studied scientifically.

REFERENCES

Albert, R.K., Leasa, D., Sanderson, M., Robertson, H.T., & Hlastala, P. (1987). The prone position improves arterial oxygenation and reduces shunt in oleic-acid induced acute lung injury. American Review of Respiratory Diseases 135:628-633.

American Thoracic Society. Standardization of spirometry. (1987). Update. American Review of Respiratory Diseases 136:1285-1298.

Badr, C., Elkins, M.R., & Ellis, E.R. (2002). The effect of body position on maximal expiratory pressure and flow. Australia Journal of Physiotherapy 48:95-102.

Ball, C., Adams, J., Boyce, S., & Robinson, P. (2001). Clinical guidelines for the use of the prone position in acute respiratory distress syndrome. Intensive Critical Care Nursing 17:94-104.

Ball, W.S., Wicks, J.D., & Mettler, F.A., Jr. (1980). Prone-supine change in organ position: CT demonstration. American Journal of Roentgenology 135:815-820.

Barach, A.L., & Beck, G.J. (1954). Ventilatory effects of head-down position in pulmonary emphysema. American Journal of Medicine 16:55-60.

Bates, D.V. (1989). Respiratory function in disease, ed 3. Philadelphia: WB Saunders.

Behrakis, P.K., Baydur, A., Jaeger, M.J., & Milic-Emili, J. (1983). Lung mechanics in sitting and horizontal body positions. Chest 83:643-646.

Bein, T., Metz, C., Keyl, C., Pfeifer, M., & Taeger, K. (1996). Effects of extreme lateral posture on hemodynamics and plasma atrial natriuretic peptide levels in critically ill patients. Intensive Care Medicine 22:651-655.

Bliss, M.R. (2004). The rationale for sitting elderly patients in hospital out of bed for long periods is medically unsubstantiated and detrimental to their recovery. Medical Hypotheses 62: 471-478.

Blomqvist, C.G., & Stone, H.L. (1963). Cardiovascular adjustments to gravitational stress. In Shepherd, J.T., & Abboud, F.M. (Eds). Handbook of physiology, section 2: circulation, vol 2. Bethesda, Md.: American Physiological Society.

Brackett, T.O., & Condon, N. (1984). Comparison of the wedge turning frame and kinetic treatment table in the acute care of spinal cord injury patients. Surgical Neurology 22:53-56.

Browse, N.L. (1965). The physiology and pathology of bed rest. Springfield, IL: C.C. Thomas.

Cane, R.D., Davison, R., & Shapiro, B.A. (1990). Case studies in critical care medicine, ed 2. Philadelphia: Elsevier.

Chang, S.C., Chang, H.I., Shiao, G.M., & Perng, R.P. (1993). Effect of body position on gas exchange in patients with unilateral central airway lesions: down with the good lung? Chest 103:787-791.

Clauss, R.H., Scalabrini, B.Y., Ray, J.F., & Reed, G.E. (1968). Effects of changing body position upon improved ventilation-perfusion relationships. Circulation 37(Suppl 2):214-217.

Cohen, N., Gorelik, O., Fishlev, G., Almoznino-Sarafian, D., Alon, I., Shteinshnaider, M., & Modai, D. (2003). Seated postural hypotension is common among older inpatients. Clinical Autonomic Research 13:447-449.

Convertino, V.A. (1992). Effects of exercise and inactivity on intra-vascular volume and cardiovascular control mechanisms. Acta Astronaut 27:123-129.

Convertino, V.A. (2003). Value of orthostatic stress in maintaining function status soon after myocardial infarction or cardiac artery bypass grafting. Journal of Cardiovascular Nursing 18:124-130.

Craig, D.B., Wahba, W.M., Don, H.F., Couture, J.G., & Becklake, M.R. (1971). Closing volume and its relationship to gas exchange in seated and supine positions. Journal of Applied Physiology 31:717-721.

Dean, E. (1985). Effect of body position on pulmonary function. Physical Therapy 65:613-618.

Dean, E. (1994a). Invited commentary to "Are incentive spirometry, intermittent positive pressure breathing, and deep breathing exercises effective in the prevention of postoperative pulmonary complications after upper abdominal surgery? A systematic overview and meta-analysis." Physical Therapy 74:10-15.

Dean, E. (1994b). Tightening up physical therapy practice: the confounding variable—friend or foe? Physiotherapy Canada 46:77-78, editorial.

Dean, E., & Ross, J. (1992a). Mobilization and exercise conditioning. In Zadai, C.C. (Ed). Clinics in physical therapy. Pulmonary management in physical therapy. New York: Churchill Livingstone.

Dean, E., & Ross, J. (1992b). Discordance between cardiopulmonary physiology and physical therapy: toward a rational basis for practice. Chest 101:1694-1698.

Dean, E., & Ross, J. (1992c). Oxygen transport: the basis for contemporary cardiopulmonary physical therapy and its optimization with body positioning and mobilization. Physical Therapy Practice 1:34-44.

De Troyer, A. (1983). Mechanical role of the abdominal muscles in relation to posture. Respiratory Physiology 53:341-353.

Dock, W. (1944). The evil sequelae of complete bed rest. Journal of the American Medical Association 125:1083-1085.

Doering, L.V. (1993). The effect of positioning on hemodynamics and gas exchange in the critically ill: a review. American Journal of Critical Care 2:208-216.

Doering, L., & Dracup, K. (1988). Comparisons of cardiac output in supine and lateral positions. Nursing Research 37:114-118.

Don H.F., Craig, D.B., Wahba, W.M., & Couture, J.G. (1971). The measurement of gas trapped in the lungs at functional residual capacity and the effect of posture. Anesthesiology 35:582-590.

Douglas, W.W., Rehder, K., Beynen, F.M., Sessler, A.D., & Marsh, H.M. (1977). Improved oxygenation in patients with acute respiratory failure: the prone position. American Review of Respiratory Diseases 115:559-566.

Dripps, R.D., & Waters, R.M. (1941). Nursing care of surgical patients. I. The 'stir-up.' American Journal of Nursing 41:530-534.

Druz, W.S., & Sharp, J.T. (1981). Activity of respiratory muscles in upright and recumbent humans. Journal of Applied Physiology 51:1552-1561.

Druz, W.S. & Sharp, J.T. (1982). Electrical and mechanical activity of the diaphragm accompanying body position in severe chronic obstructive pulmonary disease. American Review of Respiratory Diseases 125:275-280.

Duan, L.F., Lu, S.Y., & Ling, A.Z. (1997). Effect of position change on the PaO_2 in patients with unilateral tuberculous pleural effusion. Zhonghua Hu Li Za Zhi 32:190-191, English abstract.

Fink, M.P., Helsmoortel, C.M., Stein, K.L., Lee, P.C., & Cohn, S.M. (1990). The efficacy of an oscillating bed in the prevention of lower respiratory tract infection in critically ill victims of blunt trauma: a prospective study. Chest 97:132-137.

Froese, A.B., & Bryan, A.C. (1974). Effects of anesthesia and paralysis on diaphragmatic mechanics in man. Anesthesiology 41:242-255.

Gauer, O.H., & Thron, H.L. (1965). Postural changes in the circulation. In Hamilton, W.F. (Ed). Handbook of Physiology. Washington: American Physiological Society.

Gentillelo, L., Thompson, D.A., & Tonnesen, A.S. (1988). Effect of a rotating bed on the incidence of pulmonary complications in critically ill patients. Critical Care Medicine 16:783-786.

Gonzalez-Arias, S.M., Goldberg, M.L., Baumgartner, R., Hoopes, D., & Rubin, B. (1983). Analysis of the effect of kinetic therapy on intracranial pressure in comatose neurosurgical patients. Neurosurgery 13:654-656.

Hardie, J.A., Morkve, O., & Ellingsen, I. (2002). Effect of body position on arterial oxygen tension in the elderly. Respiration 69:123-128.

Harms, M.P., van Lieshout, J.J., Jenstrup, M., Pott, F., & Secher, N.H. (2003). Postural effects on cardiac output and mixed venous oxygen saturation in humans. Experimental Physiology 88:611-616.

Harrison, T.R. (1944). The abuse of rest as a therapeutic measure for patients with cardiovascular disease. Journal of the American Medical Association 125:1075-1077.

Hasser, E.M., & Moffitt, J.A. (2001). Regulation of sympathetic nervous system function after cardiovascular deconditioning. Annals of the New York Academy of Science 940:454-468.

Houtman, S., Colier, W.N., Oeseburg, B., & Hopman, M.T. (2000). Systemic circulation and cerebral oxygenation during head-up tilt in spinal cord injured individuals. Spinal Cord 38:158-163.

Hsu, H.O., & Hickey, R.F. (1976). Effect of posture on functional residual capacity postoperatively. Anesthesiology 44:520-521.

Hughson, R.L., Yamamoto, Y., Maillet, A., Fortrat, J.O., Pavy-Le Traon, A., Butler, G.C., Guell, A., & Gharib, C. (1994). Altered autonomic regulation of cardiac function during head-up tilt after 28-day head-down bed-rest with counter-measures. Clinical Physiology 14:291-304.

Hurewitz, A.N., Susskind, H., & Harold, W.H. (1985). Obesity alters regional variation in lateral decubitus position. Journal of Applied Physiology 59:774-783.

Ibanez, J., Raurich, J.M., Abizanda, R., Claramonte, R., Ibanez, P., & Bergada, J. (1981). The effect of lateral position on gas exchange in patients with unilateral lung disease during mechanical ventilation. Intensive Care Medicine 7:231-234.

Jones, A.Y.M., & Dean, E. (2004). Body position change and its effect on hemodynamic and metabolic stress. Heart and Lung 33:281-290.

Kaneko, K., Milic-Emili, J., Dolovich, M.B., Dawson, A., & Bates, D.V. (1966). Regional distribution of ventilation and perfusion as a function of body position. Journal of Applied Physiology 21:767-777.

Kelley, R.E., Vibulsrest, S., Bell, L., & Duncan, R.C. (1987). Evaluation of kinetic therapy in the prevention of complications of prolonged bed rest secondary to stroke. Stroke 18:638-642.

Klingstedt, C., Hedenstierna, G., Baehrendtz, S., Lundqvist, H., Strandberg, A., & Tokics, L. (1990a). Ventilation-perfusion relationships and atelectasis formation in the supine and lateral positions during conventional mechanical and differential ventilation. Acta Anaesthesiologica Scandinavica 34:421-429.

Klingstedt, C., Hedenstierna, G., Lundqvist, H., Strandberg, A., Tokies, L., & Brismar, B. (1990b). The influence of body position and differential ventilation on lung dimensions and atelectasis formation in anaesthetized man. Acta Anaethesiologica Scandinavica 34:315-322.

Krishnagopalan, S., Johnson, E.W., Low, L.L., & Kaufman, L.J. (2002). Body positioning of intensive care patients: clinical practice versus standards. Critical Care Medicine 30:2588-2592.

Lange, R.A., Katz, J., McBride, W., Moore, D.M., & Hillis, L.D. (1988). Effects of supine and lateral positions on cardiac output and intracardiac pressures. American Journal of Cardiology 62:330-333.

Langer, M., Mascheroni, D., Marcolin, R., & Gattinoni, L. (1988). The prone position in ARDS patients. Chest 94:103-107.

Langou, R.A., Wolfson, S., Olson, E.G., & Cohen, L.S. (1977). Effect of orthostatic postural changes on myocardial oxygen demands. American Journal of Cardiology 39:418-421.

Leblanc, P., Ruff, F., & Milic-Emili, J. (1970). Effects of age and body position on airway closure in man. Journal of Applied Physiology 28:448-451.

Lim, C.M., Koh, Y., Chin, J.Y., Lee, J.S., Lee, S.D., Kim, W.S., Kim, D.S., & Kim, W.D. (1999). Respiratory and haemodynamic effects of the prone position at two different levels of PEEP in a canine lung injury model. European Respiratory Journal 13: 163-168.

Lumb, A., & Nunn, J.F. (1999). Nunn's applied respiratory physiology, ed 5. San Diego: Elsevier.

Manning, F., Dean, E., Ross, J., & Abboud, R.A.T. (1999). Effects of side lying on lung function in older individuals. Physical Therapy 79:456-466.

Markey, D.W., & Brown, R.J. (2002). An interdisciplinary approach to addressing patient activity and mobility in the medical-surgical patient. Journal of Nursing Care Quality 16:1-12.

Matzen, S., Perko, G., Groth, S., Friedman, D.B., & Secher, N.H. (1991). Blood volume distribution during head-up tilt induced central hypovolaemia in man. Clinical Physiology 11:411-422.

McAuley, D.F., Giles, S., Fichter, H., Perkins, G.D., & Gao, F. (2002). What is the optimal duration of ventilation in the prone position in acute lung injury and acute respiratory distress syndrome? Intensive Care Medicine 28:414-418.

Meinig, R.P., Leininger, P.A., & Heckman, J.D. (1986). Forces in patients treated in conventional and oscillating hospital beds. Clinical Orthopedics and Related Research 210:166-172.

Mellins, R.B. (1974). Pulmonary physiotherapy in the pediatric age group. American Review of Respiratory Diseases 110(Suppl 1): 37-142.

Michaels, A.J., Wanek, S.M., Dreifuss, B.A., Gish, D.M., Otero, D., Payne, R., Jensen, D.H., Webber, C.C., & Long, W.B. (2002). A protocolized approach to pulmonary failure and the role of intermittent prone positioning. Journal of Trauma 52:1037-1047.

Moreno, F., & Lyons, H.A. (1961). Effect of body posture on lung volumes. Journal of Applied Physiology 16:27-29.

Norsk, P. (2000). Renal adjustment to microgravity. Pflugers Archives 441(Suppl):R62-R65.

Pelosi, P., Brazzi, L., & Gattinoni, L. (2002). Prone position in acute respiratory distress syndrome. European Respiratory Journal 20:1017-1028.

Perko, G., Payne, G., Linkis, P., Jorgensen, L.G., Landow, L., Warberg, J., & Secher, N.H. (1994). Thoracic impedance and pulmonary atrial natriuretic peptide during head-up tilt induced hypovolemic shock in humans. Acta Physiologica Scandinavica 150:449-454.

Piehl, M.A., & Brown, R.S. (1977). Use of extreme position changes in acute respiratory failure. Critical Care Medicine 4:13-14.

Powers, J.H. (1944). The abuse of rest as the therapeutic measure in surgery. Journal of the American Medical Association 125: 1079-1083.

Prakash, R., Parmely, W.W., Dikshit, K., Forrester, J., Swan, H.J. (1973). Hemodynamic effects of postural changes in patients with acute myocardial infarction. Chest 64:7-9.

Prefaut, C.H., & Engel, L.A. (1981). Vertical distribution of perfusion and inspired gas in supine man. Respiratory Physiology 43: 209-219.

Pump, B., Talleruphuus, U., Christensen, N.J., Warberg, J., & Norsk, P. (2002). Effects of supine, prone, and lateral positions on cardiovascular and renal variables in humans. American Journal of Physiology. Regulatory, Integrative and Comparative Physiology 283:R174-R180.

Pyne, D.B. (1994). Regulation of neutrophil function during exercise. Sports Medicine 17:245-258.

Ray, J.F., 3rd, Yost, L., Moallem, S., Sanoudos, G.M., Villamena, P., Paredes, R.M., & Clauss, R.H. (1974). Immobility, hypoxemia, and pulmonary arteriovenous shunting. Archives of Surgery 109:537-541.

Remolina, C., Khan, A.U., Santiago, T.V., & Edelman, N.H. (1981). Positional hypoxemia in unilateral lung disease. New England Journal of Medicine 304:523-526.

Rivara, D., Artucio, H., Arcos, J., & Hiriart, C. (1984). Positional hypoxemia during artificial ventilation. Critical Care Medicine 12:436-438.

Ross, J., & Dean, E. (1989). Integrating physiologic principles into the comprehensive management of cardiopulmonary dysfunction. Physical Therapy 69:255-259.

Ross, J., & Dean, E. (1992). Body positioning. In Zadai, C.C. (Ed). Clinics in physical therapy, pulmonary management in physical therapy. New York: Churchill Livingstone.

Ross, J., Dean, E., & Abboud, R.T. (1992). The effect of postural drainage positioning on ventilation homogeneity in healthy subjects. Physical Therapy 72:794-799.

Rouby, J.J., Puybasset, L., Nieszkowska, A., & Lu, Q. (2003). Acute respiratory distress syndrome: lessons from computed tomography of the whole lung. Critical Care Medicine 31(Suppl):S285-S295.

Roussos, C.H., Fukuchi, Y., Macklem, P.T., & Engel, L.A. (1976). Influence on diaphragmatic contraction on ventilation distribution in horizontal man. Journal of Applied Physiology 40:417-424.

Roussos, C.H., Martin, R.R., & Engel, L.A. (1977). Diaphragmatic contraction and the gradient of alveolar expansion in the lateral posture. Journal of Applied Physiology 43:32-38.

Sandler, H. (1986). Cardiovascular effects of inactivity. In Sandler, H., & Vernikos, J. (Eds). Inactivity: physiological effects. Orlando: Academic Press.

Sasaki, H., Hida, W., & Takishima, T. (1977). Influence of body position on dynamic compliance in young subjects. Journal of Applied Physiology 42:706-710.

Sjostrand, T. (1951). Determination of changes in the intrathoracic blood volume in man. Acta Physiologica Scandinavica 22: 116-128.

Skerrett, S.J., Niederman, M.S., & Fein, A.M. (1989). Respiratory infections and acute lung injury in systemic illness. Clinics in Chest Medicine 10:469-502.

Sonneblick, M., Meltzer, E., & Rosin, A.J. (1983). Body positional effect on gas exchange in unilaeral pleural effusion. Chest 83:784-786.

Summer, W.R., Curry, P., Haponik, E.F., Nelson, S., & Elston, R. (1989). Continuous mechanical turning of intensive care patients shortens length of stay in some diagnostic-related groups. Journal of Critical Care 4:45-53.

Svanberg, L. (1957). Influence of posture on lung volumes, ventilation and circulation of normals. Scandinavian Journal of Clinical Laboratory Investigations 25:1-195.

Tanskanen, P., Kytta, J., & Randell, T. (1997). The effect of patient positioning on dynamic lung compliance. Acta Anaesthesiologica Scandinavica 41:602-606.

Thandani, U., & Parker, J.O. (1978). Hemodynamics at rest and during supine and sitting bicycle exercise in normal subjects. American Journal of Cardiology 41:52-58.

Valter, C., Christensen, A.M., Tollund, C., & Schonemann, N.K. (2003). Response to the prone position in spontaneously breathing patients with hypoxemic respiratory failure. Acta Anaesthesiologica Scandinavica 47:416-418.

Wagaman, M.J., Shutaack, J.G., Moomjiam, A.S., Schwartz, J.G., Shaffer, T.H., & Fox, W.W. (1979). Improved oxygenation and lung compliance with prone positioning of neonates. Journal of Pediatrics 94:787-791.

Ward, R.J., Tolas, A.G., Benveniste, R.J., Hansen, J.M., & Bonica, J.J. (1966). Effect of posture on normal arterial blood gas tensions in the aged. Geriatrics 21:139-143.

Watenpaugh, D.E., Ballard, R.E., Schneider, S.M., Lee., S.M., Ertl, A.C., William, J.M., Boda, W.L., Hutchinson, K.J., & Hargens, A.R. (2000). Supine lower body negative pressure exercise during bed rest maintains upright exercise capacity. Journal of Applied Physiology 89:218-227.

Weber, K.T., Janicki, J.S., Shroff, S.G., & Likoff, M.J. (1983). The cardiopulmonary unit: the body's gas exchange system. Clinics in Chest Medicine 4:101-110.

West, J.B. (1985). Ventilation/blood flow and gas exchange, ed 4. Oxford: Blackwell Scientific Publications.

West, J.B. (2004). Respiratory physiology—the essentials, ed 7. Baltimore: Williams & Wilkins.

Winslow, E.H. (1985). Cardiovascular consequences of bed rest. Heart Lung 14:236-246.

Zach, M.B., Pontoppidan, H., & Kazemi, H. (1974). The effect of lateral positions on gas exchange in pulmonary disease. American Review of Respiratory Diseases 110:49-53.

Zaidi, A., Benitez, D., Gaydecki, P.A., Vohra, A., & Fitzpatrick, A.P. (2000). Haemodynamic effects of increasing angle of head up tilt. Heart 83:181-184.

Zhang, L.F. (2001). Vascular adaptation to microgravity: what have we learned? Journal of Applied Physiology 91:2415-2430.

Zhang, L.N., Gao, F., Ma, J., & Zhang, L.F. (2000). Daily head-up tilt, standing or centrifugation can prevent vasoreactivity changes in arteries of simulated weightless rats. Journal of Gravitational Physiology 7:P143-P144.

Zimmerman, J.E., Goodman, L.R., St. Andre, A.C., & Wyman, A.C. (1982). Radiographic detection of mobilizable lung water: the gravitational shift test. American Journal of Roentgenology 138:59-64.

Zorbas, Y.G., Yarullin, V.L., Denogratov, S.D., & Deogenov, V.A. (2003). Fluid volume measurements in normal subjects to disclose body hydration during acute bed rest. International Urology and Nephrology 35:457-465.

C H A P T E R   2 0

Physiological Basis for
Airway Clearance Techniques

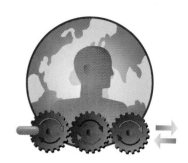

Anne Mejia Downs

KEY TERMS

Active cycle of breathing technique
Airway clearance techniques
Autogenic drainage
Flutter
Forced expiratory technique
High frequency chest wall oscillation
Intrapulmonary percussive ventilation

Manual hyperventilation
Percussion
Positive expiratory pressure
Postural drainage
Shaking
Trendelenberg
Vibration

Techniques for assisting the mobilization of secretions from the airways have long been advocated for use in the patient with an impairment in mucociliary clearance or an ineffective cough mechanism. The goals of this therapy are to reduce airway obstruction, improve mucociliary clearance and ventilation, and optimize gas exchange.

Airway clearance techniques (ACTs) have been referred to in the literature in a variety of ways, including chest physiotherapy, chest physical therapy (CPT), bronchial drainage, postural drainage therapy, and bronchial hygiene.

Research that studies the results of airway clearance is often difficult to evaluate because the components of a given treatment have not been standardized. The availability of equipment and education about a technique as well as cultural differences in its application confound the results. Differences in the outcome measures for a given technique also occur— some studies use wet or dry (dehydrated) sputum volume or radioaerosol clearance, whereas other studies use pulmonary function tests, radiographic evidence, or arterial blood gases to asses the effectiveness of an airway clearance technique. Even though a treatment has been shown to be effective in one cross section of patients, care must be taken not to generalize

the effectiveness of the treatment across all patients with pulmonary disease. The majority of secretion clearance research has been focused on patients with cystic fibrosis, as the need for ongoing secretion removal is apparent in this population.

Recently, the gold standard of airway clearance— specifically, a combination of postural drainage, percussion, and vibration with cough—has been challenged (Lapin, 1994). The indications for routine airway clearance with certain diagnoses have been questioned, and the conditions leading to effective application have been examined. Postural drainage and percussion have been shown to be ineffective in some cases and, in fact, to be detrimental to pulmonary status in others. Caregivers have also been shown to suffer from the performance of percussion; repetitive-motion injuries of the wrists have been documented as a result of regular performance of percussion (Ford et al, 1991; MMWR, 1989).

Alternative techniques have arisen out of the need to find effective methods for those patients not responsive to traditional methods. A desire to increase adherence with airway clearance, especially in patients approaching adolescence and adulthood, has led to an investigation of more independent techniques (Currie, 1986). Many of these techniques have been practiced for years in European countries, and they are now being introduced to practitioners in the United States.

It is important to remember, however, that secretion clearance is but one step toward realizing effective gas exchange in the complex oxygen transport pathway (Dean, 1992). Airway clearance, when indicated, should be integrated into a total approach, including positioning and mobilization, to optimize oxygen transport.

INDICATIONS FOR AIRWAY CLEARANCE

Oxygen transport is the primary purpose of the cardiopulmonary system (see Chapter 2). Ventilation of the alveoli is an important step in the oxygen transport chain; it allows optimal delivery of oxygen to the tissues. Several medical and surgical conditions may interfere with this process. Retained secretions or mucus plugs in the airways may interfere with the exchange of oxygen. The secretions must be mobilized from the peripheral, or smaller, airways to the larger, more central airways, where they may be removed by coughing or suction.

The following conditions are indications for airway clearance:

1. Cystic fibrosis—In this multisystem genetic disease, copious (often purulent), thick secretions and mucus plugs block the peripheral and central airways. Even infants diagnosed with cystic fibrosis, whether symptomatic or not, show evidence of small airway obstruction in the form of bronchial mucus casts (Wood, 1989). Recurrent bacterial infections combined with this mucus hypersecretion in the lungs leads to destruction of the bronchial walls, or bronchiectasis. Airway clearance continues to be an important therapy in the treatment of cystic fibrosis. This practice is supported by evidence of deteriorating lung function when regular treatments of postural drainage and percussion have been stopped (Desmond, 1983; Reisman, 1988).

2. Bronchiectasis—This condition results in a breakdown of the elastic tissue in the bronchial walls, causing severe dilation. Inflamed mucosa and copious purulent secretions are present in this condition. Airway clearance has been shown to benefit patients with bronchiectasis in the mobilization of sputum (Gallon, 1991; Mazzocco, 1985).

3. Atelectasis—This condition is caused by the collapse of alveolar segments, often by retained secretions. It has been documented in patients who have undergone surgery under general anesthesia, especially in cases of thoracic or abdominal surgery. ACTs are indicated in cases of atelectasis thought to be caused by mucus plugging (Hammon, 1981; Marini, 1979).

4. Respiratory muscle weakness—Many patients with neurological or metastatic diseases or general debilitation tend to hypoventilate or have increased work of breathing.

They are unable to maintain adequate control of respiratory secretions and often have weak, ineffective coughing (Massery, 1987). This is especially true in patients with diminished diaphragm innervation resulting from spinal cord injuries (Wetzel, 1990).

5. Mechanical ventilation—Patients on ventilatory support for any reason, including obtunded or comatose patients, are at risk for atelectasis and are unable to manage their secretions independently (Dickman, 1987).

6. Neonatal respiratory distress syndrome—These infants are born lacking surfactant in the lungs, which results in atelectasis. ACTs may be useful in clearing secretions and preventing atelectasis, but there should be a clear indication for this procedure and it must be monitored carefully in this population (Crane, 1995; Finer, 1978).

7. Asthma—This condition is characterized by the presence of hyperreactive airways and mucus plugging. ACTs may be beneficial to assist in the mobilization of mucus plugs but are not helpful in treating uncomplicated acute exacerbations (Eid, 1991).

There are several conditions that do not appear to benefit from ACTs. Patients with pneumonia or chronic bronchitis without large amounts of secretion production do not appear to benefit from airway clearance. No differences in outcome were found when these populations were treated with postural drainage and percussion (Britton, 1985; Rochester, 1980; Sutton, 1982; Wollmer, 1985). Viral bronchiolitis is an asthma-like lung disease occurring in infants less than 2 years of age. These patients do not appear to benefit from ACTs (Webb, 1985). Also of little benefit, and possibly harmful, is the inclusion of chest physical therapy in the routine care of postoperative patients without extensive secretions (Eid, 1991). Even in patients with a history of lung disease, the use of ACTs has failed to affect the incidence of atelectasis as a postoperative complication (Torrington, 1984).

Postural Drainage

Postural drainage (PD), also known as bronchial drainage, is a passive technique in which the patient is placed in positions that allow gravity to assist with the drainage of secretions from the bronchopulmonary tree (Figure 20-1). Positioning the patient to assist the flow of bronchial secretions from the airways has been a standard treatment for some time in patients with retained secretions (Zadai, 1981).

Knowledge of the anatomy of the tracheobronchial tree is vital to effective treatment. Each lobe to be drained must be aligned so that gravity can mobilize the secretions from the periphery to the larger, more central airways. The mechanism of postural drainage is considered to be a direct effect of gravity on bronchial secretions, although observations made by Lannefors (1992) that gravity influences regional lung ventilation and volume suggest that these mechanisms are also involved.

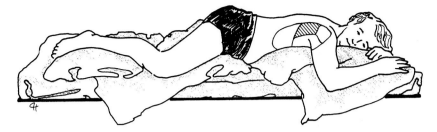

FIGURE 20-1 Postural drainage position for the right upper lobe—posterior segment (anterior view—patient positioned three quarters prone).

PD has been shown to be effective in mobilizing secretions in patients with cystic fibrosis (Lorin, 1071; Wong, 1977), bronchiectasis (Mazzacco, 1985), and other pulmonary diseases (Bateman, 1981; Zausmer, 1968). Other treatments, such as percussion, vibration, and the active cycle of breathing technique (ACBT), may be used while the patient is in postural drainage positions.

There are, however, many contraindications to optimal positioning for PD, especially the head-down or Trendelenberg positions required for the lower lobes (see Chapter 21).

Percussion

Percussion, sometimes referred to as chest clapping, is a traditional approach to secretion mobilization. A rhythmic force is applied with cupped hands to the patient's thorax over the involved lung segments, with the aim of dislodging or loosening bronchial secretions. This technique is performed with the patient in postural drainage positions and requires that a caregiver administer it. In the United States, percussion in conjunction with postural drainage continues to be a mainstay of the treatment of individuals with pulmonary disease, especially neonates and patients who are unresponsive.

The proposed mechanism of action of percussion is the transmission of a wave of energy through the chest wall into the lung. The resulting motion loosens secretions from the bronchial wall and moves them proximally, where ciliary motion and cough (or suction) can remove them. The combination of postural drainage and percussion has been shown to be effective in secretion removal (Denton, 1962; May, 1979; Radford, 1982).

A handheld mechanical percussor may be used by a caregiver to minimize fatigue or may be used by the patient to self-administer percussion. The effectiveness of mechanical as opposed to manual percussion has been studied. Maxwell and Redmond (1979) found mechanical percussion equivalent to manual percussion in effecting removal of secretions. Although there was a significant increase in pulmonary function with manual techniques, Pryor and colleagues (1979, 1981) supported the use of mechanical percussion in patients, using the forced expiration technique. A study by Rossman and colleagues (1982) was in disagreement, finding that mechanical percussion did not enhance postural drainage in secretion removal.

There are many contraindications to percussion. If the patient's pulmonary status is of greater concern than the relative contraindications, a decision may be made to administer the treatment, with appropriate modifications (see Chapter 21).

Vibration

Vibration is a sustained co-contraction of the upper extremities of a caregiver to produce a vibratory force that is transmitted to the thorax over the involved lung segment. Vibration is applied throughout exhalation, concurrent with mild compression to the chest wall. Vibration is often applied in postural drainage positions following percussion to the area. The patient or a caregiver may use a mechanical vibrator in place of manual vibration.

It is proposed that vibration enhances mucociliary transport from the periphery of the lung fields to the larger airways. Because it is often used in conjunction with PD and percussion, many studies do not separate the effects of vibration from those of the other components. In fact, many studies describe the techniques of PD, percussion, and vibration as a single entity and refer to the treatment as chest physical therapy, pulmonary therapy, or postural drainage therapy.

Pavia (1976) demonstrated a higher, though not statistically significant, rate of secretion clearance and sputum production with vibration. However, this study was conducted while subjects were in the upright position only, which does not replicate the use of vibration clinically.

Mackenzie and colleagues (1980) demonstrated significant improvement in total lung/thorax compliance after treatment with postural drainage, percussion, and vibration in mechanically ventilated patients. Feldman and colleagues (1979) demonstrated improved ventilatory function by showing a significant improvement in expiratory flow rates in patients receiving postural drainage, percussion, vibration, and directed coughing.

Shaking

Shaking consists of a bouncing maneuver, sometimes referred to as "rib springing," against the thoracic wall in a rhythmic fashion throughout exhalation. A concurrent pressure is given to the chest wall, compressing the thorax. Shaking is similar in application to vibration, with shaking being on one end of the spectrum in application of force and vibration being on the opposite end, supplying a gentler pressure. Many variations exist throughout the continuum between these techniques. Shaking may be used in postural drainage positions and requires the assistance of a caregiver. It may also be used in place of percussion or intermittently with percussion and vibration.

Shaking is assumed to work in the same manner as vibration, mobilizing secretions to the central, larger airways from the lung periphery. Because the compressive force to the thorax is greater, producing increased chest wall displacement, the stretch of the respiratory muscles may produce an increased inspiratory effort and lung volume (Levenson, 1992).

The same relative contraindications for percussion should be observed for shaking, because it involves the application of force to the thorax (see Chapter 21).

Manual Hyperinflation

This technique is used in patients with an endotracheal or tracheostomy tube that can be attached to a manual ventilation bag. One caregiver uses the bag to hyperinflate the lungs with a slow, deep inspiration and, after a short inspiratory pause, provides a quick release to allow rapid exhalation. A second caregiver applies shaking or vibration starting at the beginning of exhalation so as to mobilize secretions. The timing of this sequence is important if the desired effect is to be achieved (Webber, 1988). It has been likened to simulating a cough—deep inspiration, pause, and forceful exhalation. Manual hyperventilation requires two competent caregivers and is performed while the patient is in a postural drainage position.

The inspiration provided by the manual ventilation bag, which is deeper than an inspiration the patient could generate, promotes aeration of the alveoli. The compression of the thorax augments the high expiratory flow rate from the bag, accelerating the movement of the secretions from the smaller airways to the larger bronchi (Clement, 1968).

Clement (1968) reports that this method of airway clearance enables patients to be maintained on ventilators for long periods while retaining normal lung function. It has been demonstrated that treatment of atelectasis by hyperinflation and suction is enhanced by the addition of positioning and vibrations (Stiller, 1990).

Contraindications to manual hyperinflation are discussed in Chapter 21. Conditions requiring mechanical ventilation present additional challenges.

Active Cycle of Breathing

In New Zealand, Thompson (1973) described clearing bronchial secretions in patients with asthma by using a technique of forced expirations and diaphragmatic breathing. British physiotherapists modified the technique and further described it in the literature, first as the forced expiration technique (FET; Pryor, 1979) and later as the active cycle of breathing technique (ACBT; Webber & Pryor, 1993).

As described by Webber and Pryor (1993), the ACBT consists of repeated cycles of three ventilatory phases: breathing control, thoracic expansion exercises, and the FET. Breathing control is described as gentle tidal volume breathing with relaxation of the upper chest and shoulders. The thoracic expansion phase consists of deep inspiration and may be accompanied by percussion or vibration performed by a caregiver or the patient. This phase helps to loosen secretions. The forced expiration technique involves one or two huffs (forced expirations). Webber and Pryor (1993) report that huffing from a mid lung volume (a medium-sized inspiration) down to a low lung volume moves secretions from the peripheral to the upper airways. Upper airway secretions may be cleared by a huff from high lung volume (a deeper inspiration). The ACBT may be performed in the sitting position but has been shown to be more effective in gravity-assisted (postural drainage) positions (Steven, 1992).

The period of breathing control between the other phases is essential so as to prevent bronchospasm (Lapin, 1990). The period of thoracic expansion, which increases lung volume and promotes collateral ventilation, allows air to get behind secretions and assist in their mobilization (Prasad, 1993). Mead and colleagues (1967) described the physiological theory of equal pressure point (EPP), which is the basis for the FET. The EPP is the point in the airways where the pressure is equal to the pleural pressure. The forced expiratory maneuver produces compression of the airway peripherally to the EPP. A huff from high lung volume causes compression within the trachea and bronchi, which moves secretions from these larger airways. A huff continued to low lung volume shifts the EPP more peripherally, which moves more peripheral secretions (Webber, 1988).

A patient may perform ACBT independent of a caregiver. FET performed by patients independently has been shown to clear more sputum in a shorter amount of time than PD with self-percussion combined with percussion and shaking by a physical therapist (Pryor, 1979). Improvements in pulmonary function (Webber, 1986) and sputum clearance (Sutton, 1983) have been demonstrated in patients with cystic fibrosis who incorporated the FET into their postural drainage treatments.

Because huffing has been shown to stabilize collapsible bronchial walls, it increases the expiratory flow in patients with obstruction without causing airway collapse (Hietpas, 1979). Another benefit of this technique lies in its ability to maintain oxygen saturation. The decrease in oxygen saturation that has been demonstrated with postural drainage and percussion has been prevented by the use of the ACBT (Pryor, 1990). Hassani and colleagues (1994) showed that unproductive cough and FET resulted in the movement of secretions proximally from all regions of the lung in patients with mild hyposecretion. This suggests that FET might help to avoid prolonged retention of secretions, even in patients who produce little sputum.

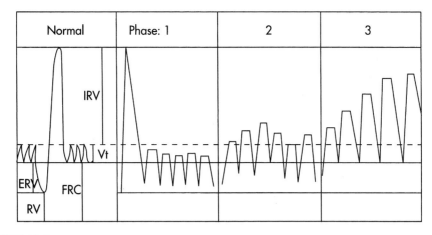

FIGURE 20-2 Phases of autogenic drainage shown on a spirogram of a normal person. Phase 1: unstick; phase 2: collect; phase 3: evacuate. (*VT*, Tidal volume; *ERV*, expiratory reserve volume; *RV*, reserve volume; *FRC*, functional residual capacity; *IRV*, inspiratory reserve volume; *IRV* + *VT* + *ERV*, vital capacity). *(From Schoni, M.H. [1989]. Autogenic drainage: a modern approach to physiotherapy in cystic fibrosis. Journal of the Royal Society of Medicine 82(Suppl 16):32-37.)*

Autogenic Drainage

In Belgium in 1976, Chevaillier introduced autogenic drainage (AD), or self-drainage, for the treatment of asthmatic patients. He observed that during sleep, as well as while playing and laughing during the day, mucus was mobilized better than it was during PD and clapping. AD is an antidyspnea technique based on quiet expirations in a relaxed state and without use of postural drainage positions (Chevaillier, 1992).

AD uses diaphragmatic breathing to mobilize secretions by varying expiratory airflow. It consists of three phases: (1) breathing at low lung volumes to "unstick" the peripheral secretions; (2) breathing at low to middle lung volumes (tidal volume) to collect the mucus in the middle airways; and (3) breathing at middle to high lung volumes to evacuate the mucus from the central airways (Chevaillier, 1984). The patient is seated in a relaxed position and exhales actively, with the mouth and glottis open, listening for the movement of mucus while avoiding a wheeze. The phases of the AD technique are depicted in Figure 20-2.

Schoni (1989) eloquently explained the physiology of AD's three phases. The first phase starts with a normal inspiration and is followed by a breath hold to ensure equal filling of lung segments by collateral filling; then a deep exhalation is made into the expiratory reserve volume range. By lowering the middle tidal volume below the functional residual capacity level, secretions from peripheral lung regions are mobilized by the compression of peripheral alveolar ducts. Midexpiratory tidal volume is lowered in the range of normal expiratory reserve volume. The second phase of AD consists of tidal volume breathing so that breathing is changed gradually from the expiratory reserve volume into the inspiratory reserve volume range, which mobilizes secretions from the apical parts of the lungs. The velocity of the airflow

must be adjusted at each level of inspiration so that the maximal expiratory airflow is reached without being high enough to cause collapse of the airways. Flow volume curves show that higher flows of longer duration can be achieved with AD (Dab, 1979), demonstrating that mucus can be moved farther and at a faster rate. The third phase consists of deeper inspiration into the inspiratory reserve volume, with huffing often used to help in evacuating the mobilized secretions. Control of airflow during this final phase is essential to the avoidance of uncontrolled, unproductive coughing.

The Belgian method has been modified by German practioners to use a combination of diaphragmatic and costosternal breathing in a treatment that is not separated into phases (David, 1991). The patient varies his or her midtidal volume in a passive exhalation followed by an active exhalation through pursed lips or through the nose. The German method of airway clearance includes other maneuvers in conjunction with AD, including inhalation therapy, FET, chest wall exercises, and physical activity.

AD has been compared to positive expiratory pressure (PEP) breathing and PD with percussion and vibration. More sputum was produced with AD in patients with hyperreactive airways (Davidson, 1988). In a 2-year crossover trial, AD was found to be as effective as conventional CPT among patients with cystic fibrosis for improving pulmonary function (Davidson, 1992). However, patients exhibited a strong preference for AD than for CPT, and that increases the likelihood of adherence. Miller (1993) showed greater clearance of inhaled radioisotopes with AD than with the ACBT, with no significant differences in sputum weight, spirometry, or transcutaneous oxygen saturation. Giles (1993) also studied oxygen (O_2) saturation in AD and found greater O_2 saturation with AD than with PD with percussion; there was greater sputum recovery with AD.

The technique of AD requires attention to airflow and volume and to cough suppression until secretions are mobilized; this is a key factor to success (Downs, 2004). Learning AD requires tactile and auditory feedback and continued modification of the patient's technique, at least initially, to achieve a good result. AD takes considerable time to learn and requires a great deal of cooperation by the patient. Therefore, it is not suitable for the very young or distractible patient.

Positive Expiratory Pressure

The development and utilization of PEP breathing came about in the 1980s in Denmark and is now widely used in the United States. High- or low-pressure PEP may be prescribed, although only low-pressure PEP is used in the United States.

Several devices deliver PEP; two of the most commonly used are the Acapella and TheraPEP (DHD Healthcare, Wampsville, NY). The application of PEP involves a mask or mouthpiece connected to a device that includes a one-way breathing valve and an adjustable level of expiratory resistance. This results in positive pressure in the airways during exhalation. A manometer in the circuit determines and monitors the pressure generated by the patient. A patient uses PEP breathing in a cycle of about 10 breaths at tidal volume, with slightly active expiration followed by huffing or coughing to expectorate secretions (Falk & Kelstrup, 1993).

In low-pressure PEP breathing, the resistance is regulated to achieve 10 to 20 cm of water pressure during expiration. The pressure should be sustainable during only slightly active expiration. High-pressure PEP breathing requires the patient to perform forced vital capacity maneuvers through expiratory resistance with a mask connected to a spirometer. The appropriate resistor is one that produces a flow volume curve demonstrating a maximal forced vital capacity, good plateau, and no curvilinearity (Prasad, 1993). In general, the range of pressure generated with high-pressure PEP breathing is 50 to 120 cm of water pressure. Low-pressure PEP breathing is used more often, as it offers equal effectiveness at a lower presumed risk of pneumothorax.

It is theorized that PEP breathing reinflates collapsed alveoli by allowing air to be redistributed through collateral channels—the pores of Kohn and the Lambert canals. Pressure is built up distal to an obstruction, promoting the movement of secretions toward the larger airways (Anderson, 1979; Groth, 1985). Airway stability is maintained with PEP breathing, which results in improved ventilation and gas exchange as well as in airway clearance (Hardy, 1994). In addition, supplemental oxygen and nebulized medication can be effectively delivered during treatment with PEP (Anderson, 1982).

PEP breathing has been shown to benefit patients at risk for postoperative atelectasis but has gained wider practice in the area of airway clearance, especially in patients with cystic fibrosis (Malhmeister, 1991). Numerous studies have demonstrated the effectiveness of PEP breathing. Tyrrell (1986) has shown the PEP mask to be as effective as conventional physiotherapy over a 1-month period, with no difference in pulmonary function. Falk (1984, 1993) demonstrated increased sputum production and clearance with the use of PEP over FET alone. However, Hofmeyer (1986) found FET produced a greater quantity of sputum without the addition of PEP. Oberwaldner (1986) evaluated lung function during 10 months of regular treatments with high-pressure PEP and found reduced pulmonary hyperinflation and airway instability and higher flow rates with PEP than with conventional CPT. These improvements in lung function deteriorated only 2 months after a return to conventional CPT. A study by Plfeger and colleagues (1992) compared PEP to AD and found that PEP cleared higher amounts of sputum and demonstrated increased lung function. Finally, decreased duration of hospitalization has been cited as a benefit of using PEP breathing for airway clearance (Simonova, 1992).

A form of PEP breathing in combination with high-frequency oscillation is available through a device developed in Switzerland. The Flutter VRP1 (VarioRaw, Aubonne, Switzerland) is a handheld device that interrupts the expiratory flow and decreases the collapsibility of the airways. The pipelike device consists of a steel ball, a plastic cone, a perforated cover, and a mouthpiece. The patient completes about 10 to 15 deep breaths, keeping the cheeks flat while the Flutter is tilted to achieve the maximum effects of the vibration in the chest. Following this, huffing is used to eliminate the airway secretions.

Exhalation through the Flutter device causes airway vibrations and oscillating endobronchial pressures (Althaus, 1993) to ease the expectoration of mucus. The PEP maintained by the Flutter (5 to 35 cm of water pressure) prevents dynamic airway compression and improves airflow acceleration. The improvement in expectoration is based on the increase in airway diameter and the improvement in airflow acceleration (Schibler, 1992).

Konstan and colleagues (1994) compared the amount of sputum expectorated with use of the Flutter to vigorous voluntary cough and to PD, percussion, and vibration. Subjects with cystic fibrosis produced more than three times the amount of sputum when using the Flutter than when using the other two methods, and no adverse effects were reported. Ambrosino (1991) reported success in the treatment of patients with chronic obstructive pulmonary disease by using the device. When compared with AD, the Flutter was found to produce equal amounts of expectorated mucus (Lindemann, 1992). When compared with the PEP mask, the Flutter produced slightly increased measures of spirometry, but the two techniques were otherwise comparable (Anonymous, 1989).

The advantages of the Flutter device lie in its portability and the ease with which its use can be learned. Increased independence and better compliance have also been cited as advantages of this technique. However, frequent assessment of patient technique and appropriate level of resistance is recommended (Lapin, 1990). Young children can be taught to use the device effectively, and because of its small size it can easily be used for multiple treatments throughout the day.

A newer device that provides PEP with oscillations is the Quake (Thayer Medical, Tucson, AZ). This device uses a crank to interrupt airflow and produce the oscillation, and the speed at which the crank is turned dictates the frequency of the vibration. This allows the user to vary the expiratory pressure, which is constant with the Flutter device. The mouthpiece can be replaced with a facemask, which is not possible with the Flutter.

High-Frequency Chest Wall Oscillation

Efforts aimed at mucus clearance by creating a differential airflow rate (i.e., greater expiratory than inspiratory flow rate) led to the development of a high-frequency chest wall oscillation (HFCWO) system. Hansen and Warwick (1990) designed a large-volume, variable-frequency air-pulse delivery system that can be used by patients with obstructive lung disease to promote mucus clearance.

The ThAIRapy Vest (Hill ROM, St. Paul, MN) system consists of an inflatable fitted vest connected to an air-pulse generator by flexible tubing. This device provides oscillation of the entire thoracic cavity at varying frequencies (5 to 25 Hz) and is used while sitting upright. The lung volume expired tends to increase with lower frequencies (less than 10 to 12 Hz), whereas the flow rates tend to increase with higher frequencies (12 to 20 Hz). A widely adopted protocol consists of three frequencies that vary the volume flow rate; each frequency is used for about 10 minutes. Continuous aerosolized medication or saline administered concurrently may assist with secretion mobilization (Warwick, 1992).

Two probable mechanisms of action have been offered to explain the significant increase in sputum mobilization that occurs with HFCWO (Klous, 1994). The first mechanism proposes that oscillatory airflow leads to changes in the consistency of mucus, which results in increased mobilization of secretions. Significant decreases in mucus viscoelasticity were observed during administration of oscillatory airflow (Tomkiewicz et al, 1994). The second mechanism proposes that the difference between the expiratory and inspiratory velocities produces shear forces strong enough to move mucus. Chang and colleagues (1988) demonstrated that nonsymmetrical airflow (peak expiratory flow rates greater than inspiratory flow rates) could be a significant factor leading to enhanced mucus clearance during the administration of HFCWO. Each chest compression produces a transient flow pulse similar to that observed during coughing, and by using the flows with the greatest rates and volumes, sufficient force is obtained to move mucus in the airway (Warwick, 1991).

HFCWO has been shown to increase mucus clearance rates in dogs, with the most pronounced effect in the 11- to 15-Hz frequency range (King, 1983). Radford and colleagues (1982) used bronchoscopy to demonstrate a marked increase in the speed and flow of mucus produced by oscillations at even higher frequencies than those attainable by manual percussion. Results of short-term use of the ThAIRapy vest have been mixed, but they show HFCWO to be at least as effective as conventional CPT. Robinson (1992) showed no significant improvement or deterioration of lung function with its use. In two different studies, Kluft (1992) and Faverio (1994) demonstrated increased wet and dry sputum weights using HFCWO as opposed to manual CPT, and Arens (1993) showed similar dry sputum weight but an increase in wet sputum weight and a significant improvement in pulmonary function with HFCWO as opposed to conventional CPT. One 2-year study showed improved lung function and greater sputum production in subjects with cystic fibrosis with the use of HFCWO rather than manual CPT (Warwick, 1991). No adverse effects were observed with long-term use of the ThAIRapy vest.

Hospitalized patients with acute exacerbation of lung disease have been shown to tolerate HFCWO well (Burnett, 1993), and the safety and tolerance of this method have been demonstrated in long-term mechanically ventilated patients (Whitman, 1993).

The fit of the vest requires attention because nausea, abdominal and chest wall discomfort, and complaints of urinary urgency may occur with an ill-fitting vest (Downs, 2004). The expense of the ThAIRapy vest and a similar apparatus, the MedPulse Respiratory Vest System (Electromed, New Prague, NM), may be a significant deterrent to its use; it is much more costly than other mechanical aids to airway clearance. However, in a study of HFCWO users insured by Blue Cross and Blue Shield, a 49% reduction in health care costs was shown in the year following initial use of the vest as compared with the year prior to HFCWO use (Ohnsorg, 1994). The impact of the use of the HFCWO device in a hospital department demonstrated a substantial savings resulting from therapy self-administration by patients (Klous, 1993).

Intrapulmonary Percussive Ventilation

The intrapulmonary percussive ventilation (IPV) device (Percussionaire, Sandpoint, ID) works in a manner similar to that of the HFCWO. However, the oscillation is delivered internally through a mouthpiece. IPV provides percussion at 6 to 14 Hz, with a positive expiratory pressure of 10 to 20 cm of water pressure and simultaneous delivery of an aerosol. IPV provides a safe and effective form of airway clearance (Marks, 1999).

It is theorized that changes in the frequency and pressure of the airflow delivered through the IPV device assist in stabilizing the airways and decrease the viscosity of the secretions. This results in increased sputum mobilization (Downs, 2004).

IPV has been found to be as effective as postural drainage and percussion in improving pulmonary function and sputum expectoration (Natale, 1994). Marks (2001) found no difference between IPV and Flutter in number of hospital or antibiotic days required and reported good acceptance of the method of airway clearance by patients. IPV may be beneficial for patients with asthma and neuromuscular disease as well as cystic fibrosis (Hardy, 1996; Homnick, 1995).

Two types of IPV are available: a hospital unit powered by 50 psi of gas and a home unit powered by a compressor. Use of the hospital unit must be supervised by a respiratory care practitioner, whereas the patient and caregivers receive training to use the home unit.

Exercise

In addition to its many effects on health and well-being, exercise has been shown to assist in secretion clearance. It has been suggested that exercise can replace all or part of a conventional chest physiotherapy routine in some patients or at some stages of lung disease (Andreasson, 1987; Cerny, 1989; Zach, 1982).

Exercise increases mucociliary transport in patients with chronic bronchitis (Oldenberg, 1979). Higher transpulmonary pressure with aerobic exercise may open closed bronchi as well as increase collateral ventilation to allow mucus to be moved (Andreasson, 1987). It has also been shown that exercise-induced hyperventilation is more effective than eucapnic hyperventilation in mobilizing bronchial secretions (Wolff, 1977). The contribution of expiratory airflow and exercise-induced coughing are other factors in effective secretion removal.

Some studies conclude that exercise alone is not sufficient and recommend its use as a complement to other forms of airway clearance. Airway clearance using PD and FET was shown to be more effective than exercise with a cycle ergometer in inducing sputum expectoration (Salh et al, 1989). Results from Bilton and colleagues (1992) demonstrated that any modality that included the ACBT in PD positions alone or in combination with exercise is better than exercise alone at clearing sputum.

Other studies have suggested that some forms of exercise may serve as a replacement for chest physiotherapy, citing a lack of decrease in lung function following the cessation of CPT but the continuation of an exercise program (Andreasson, 1987; Zach, 1984). In hospitalized patients with cystic fibrosis, no significant change in pulmonary function was reported when exercise was substituted for two of three daily treatments of PD, percussion, and vibration, and the weight of the sputum produced was equivalent (Cerny, 1989).

When mucus clearance was studied, no significant differences were found among exercise on a cycle ergometer, postural drainage, and PEP mask breathing (Lannefors, 1992). Increases in sputum expectoration on exercise days as opposed to nonexercise days have been reported (Baldwin, 1994; Zach, 1981). For patients with cystic fibrosis who demonstrate adherence to an exercise program alone or in addition to another form of secretion mobilization, there is evidence of positive prognostic value (Nixon, 1992).

It is difficult to compare these studies across the board, however, because the mode and length of exercise differ, as does the measurement of effectiveness of airway clearance. Exercise as an airway clearance technique is not suitable for the very young (less than 4 to 5 years of age), for patients with neuromuscular limitations, or for patients with severely limited exercise tolerance. Moreover, the potential need for supplemental oxygen during exercise should be monitored. Nonetheless, evidence suggests that an exercise program in addition to clearing secretions may decrease morbidity and mortality by improving exercise capacity (Lapin, 1993).

Contraindications and Precautions Concerning Airway Clearance

General Precautions and Contraindications to Postural Drainage Positioning

It is essential that the therapist and the health care team discuss treatment priorities. A decision to use postural drainage might be made despite a contraindication if the benefits were thought to outweigh the risks in a particular case.

For example, it is known that use of the Trendelenberg (head-down) position increases intracranial pressure in patients after neurosurgery (Humberstone, 1990). However, if the patient develops atelectasis, the stress of respiratory embarrassment may also increase intracranial pressure. In this instance, the decision may be made to position the patient to clear the atelectasis and subsequently return to a modified conservative regimen (Frownfelter, 1987).

A fall in arterial O_2 saturation has been reported with the use of postural drainage in chest physiotherapy, although the effects of PD were not separated from additional techniques (Huseby, 1976; Selsby, 1990). Therefore, O_2 saturation levels should be monitored during treatment, especially in patients with known low PaO_2 values.

Caution must also be used in treating a patient with end-stage lung disease in postural drainage positions because of the risk of hemoptysis (Hammon, 1979; Stern, 1978). Decreased cardiac output (Barrell, 1978; Laws, 1969) has been associated with chest physiotherapy treatment; however, the effects of postural drainage were not separated from those of percussion and vibration.

Many physical therapists working with the pediatric population do not use the head-down position in treating infants but rather a modified routine that excludes the Trendelenberg position. The head-down position has been shown to increase the incidence of gastroesophageal reflux in neonates (Crane, 1995). Button and colleagues (2004) found that the head-down position is associated with gastroesophageal reflux, distressed behavior, and lower oxygen saturation in infants with cystic fibrosis. A modified routine that eliminates head-down positioning is associated with fewer respiratory complications (Button, 2003). Box 20-1 summarizes the precautions and contraindications concering postural drainage.

General Contraindications and Precautions Concerning External Manipulation of the Thorax

In patients who are very young, who have limited ability to cooperate, or who are not adherent to other ACTs, percussion, shaking, and vibration offer methods for dislodging retained

---

BOX 20-1

Contraindications for Postural Drainage

All Positions Are Contraindicated for the Following

Intracranial pressure (ICP) > 20 mm Hg
Head and neck injury until stabilized
Active hemorrhage with hemodynamic instability
Recent spinal surgery (e.g., laminectomy) or acute spinal injury
Active hemoptysis
Empyema
Bronchopleural fistula
Pulmonary edema associated with heart failure (HF)
Large pleural effusions
Pulmonary embolism
Aged, confused, or anxious patients
Rib fracture, with or without flail chest
Surgical wound or healing tissue

Trendelenberg Position is Contraindicated for the Following

Patients in whom increased ICP is to be avoided
Uncontrolled hypertension
Distended abdomen
Esophageal surgery
Recent gross hemoptysis related to recent lung carcinoma
Uncontrolled airway at risk for aspiration

Trendelenberg Position is Contraindicated for the Following Cases in Neonates

Untreated tension pneumothorax
Recent tracheoesophageal fistula repair
Recent eye or intracranial surgery
Intraventricular hemorrhage (grades III and IV)
Acute heart failure or cor pulmonale

From AARC Clinical Practice Guideline. (1991); Postural drainage therapy. Respiratory Care 36:1418–1426; Crane, L. (1995). Physical therapy for the neonate with respiratory disease. In Irwin, S., & Tecklin, J.S. (Eds). Cardiopulmonary physical therapy. St. Louis: Mosby.

BOX 20-2

Contraindications to External Manipulation of the Thorax in Addition to Contraindications for Postural Drainage

Subcutaneous emphysema
Recent epidural spinal infusion or spinal anesthesia
Recent skin grafts, or flaps, on the thorax
Burns, open wounds, and skin infections of the thorax
Recently placed pacemaker
Suspected pulmonary tuberculosis
Lung contusion
Bronchospasm
Osteomyelitis of the ribs
Osteoporosis
Coagulopathy
Complaint of chest-wall pain

Additional Contraindications for Percussion of a Neonate

Intolerance to treatment as indicated by low oxygen saturation values
Rib fracture
Hemoptysis

From AARC Clinical Practice Guideline. (1991); Postural drainage therapy. Respiratory Care 36:1418–1426; Crane, L. (1995).Physical therapy for the neonate with respiratory disease. In Irwin, S., and Tecklin, J.S. (Eds). Cardiopulmonary physical therapy. Mosby: St. Louis.

---

secretions. However, because of the force transmitted to the thoracic cage with these techniques, there are many precautions and contraindications to consider. The therapist should not make this decision alone but should seek direction from the medical team. Chest physiotherapy is not a completely benign procedure and should not be performed in the absence of good indications (McDonnell, 1986).

Percussion has been shown to contribute to a fall in PaO_2 in acutely ill patients (Connors, 1980), especially in patients with cardiovascular instability (Gormenzano, 1972) and in neonates (Fox, 1978). The factor that seems most closely associated with or predictive of the effect is the patient's baseline PaO_2 (McDonnell, 1986). Cardiac dysrhythmias have been associated with chest percussion for bronchial drainage (Hammon, 1981). Huseby (1976) hypothesizes that hypoxemia may be the underlying mechanism of CPT-caused cardiac arrhythmias.

Patients with hyperreactive airways (e.g., asthma) show intolerance for percussion as part of chest physiotherapy.

Campbell and colleagues (1975) demonstrated a fall in FEV_1 associated with percussion; it was not evident when percussion was omitted. Administration of a bronchodilator before treatment with percussion abolished the fall in FEV_1. Wheezing has also been associated with percussion and vibration in patients with cystic fibrosis and COPD (Feldman, 1979; Tecklin, 1975).

Box 20-2 summarizes the precautions and contraindications for external manipulation of the thorax associated with percussion, shaking, and high-frequency chest compression. Vibration involves less force to the thorax and may be better tolerated than the aforementioned techniques. A nebulized bronchodilator may be administered during a treatment of high-frequency chest compression to avoid the consequences of hyperreactive airways.

Other Precautions

Manual hyperinflation has been shown to cause significant depression of cardiac output in patients who are unable to compensate hemodynamically and have little cardiac reserve (Clement, 1968; Laws, 1969). Significant and deleterious increases in ICP have also been demonstrated (Garradd, 1986). Webber (1988) offers these additional contraindications to manual hyperinflation: severe hypoxemia with few bronchial secretions, as in ARDS; acute pulmonary edema; air leak (e.g., pneumothorax); severe bronchospasm, as in acute asthma; and hemoptysis.

The use of PEP for airway clearance carries an increased risk of pneumothorax (Oberwaldner, 1986). Bronchodilator premedication should be considered when applying PEP in patients who show clinical or physiological signs of airway hyperreactivity (Pfleger, 1992).

The increased airflow produced by the huff cough, as in the ACBT, may aggravate bronchospasm (Hietpas, 1979). Additionally, Hietpas cautions that the movement of secretions into the larger airways by the huff cough may precipitate spontaneous explosive coughing.

Several precautions must be observed when using exercise as a form of airway clearance. Desaturation has been shown to occur with exercise in individuals with pulmonary disease (Henke, 1984; Lane, 1987), and therefore it becomes prudent to monitor oxygen saturation, providing supplemental oxygen for the exercise period when indicated. Exercise-induced bronchospasm must also be considered when pulmonary compromise is seen with exercise, especially with higher intensity exercise (Godfrey, 1975). When indicated, it is recommended to provide an inhaled bronchodilator 20 to 30 minutes before exercise to alleviate this symptom (Orenstein, 1985). Andreasson (1987) reports a risk of pneumothorax associated with exercise in patients with extensive bullae.

Factors Affecting Selection of Airway Clearance Techniques

Among patients with pulmonary disorders, poor adherence to the performance of airway clearance on a regular basis has been well documented (Currie, 1986; Litt, 1980; Muszynski-Kwan, 1988; Passero, 1981). The problem is increased among adolescents. Litt (1980) has also shown that the complexity and increased duration of a prescribed treatment has a negative influence on patient adherence. It has been suggested that enhanced adherence might be achieved if the treatment were specifically tailored to the individual patient's needs with regard to clinical status, family functioning, and family concerns. Negotiation between the patient and the caregiver to agree on follow-through with the prescribed treatment regimen is also effective (Shultz, 1980). For this reason, it is imperative to consider multiple factors in the recommendation of a specific technique of airway clearance, especially in a patient with a chronic disease (Box 20-3).

The age of the patient affects the usefulness of a particular technique. Infants and very young children are limited to conventional physical therapy (postural drainage, percussion, and vibration), because they are not able to cooperate with other methods of airway clearance. After the age of 3 or 4, a youngster may be taught huffing and breathing control and can be assisted with the ACBT. A vest for use with HFCWO is now available for children as young as 2 or 3 years of age. PEP, oscillating PEP, and exercise are also suitable for this age group, depending on the child's attention span and cooperation. Children 12 years of age and older are capable of using any of the ACTs, including AD, which requires more concentration than a younger child is typically able to exhibit consistently.

BOX 20-3

Factors to Be Considered When Selecting an Airway Clearance Technique

Motivation
Patient's goals
Physician/caregiver's goals
Effectiveness (of considered technique)
Patient's age
Patient's ability to learn
Skill of therapists/teachers
Fatigue or work required
Need for assistants or equipment
Limitations of technique based on disease type and severity
Costs (direct and indirect)
Desirability of combining methods

From Hardy, K.A. (1994). A review of airway clearance: new techniques, indications, and recommendations. Respiratory Care 39;440-452.

The lack of an assistant to provide airway clearance is a factor that prompts many patients to seek methods other than postural drainage and percussion. HFCWO, PEP, oscillating PEP, ACBT, exercise, and AD are techniques that provide independence from a caregiver. These methods have been chosen by adults living on their own, students away at school, and adolescents eager for independence. For optimal results, a health care team member skilled in the subject of airway clearance must regularly reevaluate each technique's effectiveness after it has been agreed that a patient exhibits independence in a given technique.

The clinical status of a patient during each hospital admission must be evaluated to determine the appropriateness of a particular ACT. For example, PD and percussion might worsen airway hyperreactivity, and care must also be taken when using ACBT in such a case. HFCWO, oscillating PEP, and exercise should be preceded by an inhaled bronchodilator in this case, and PEP and IPV can be performed concurrently with bronchodilator administration. AD lends itself well to use by patients with airway hyperreactivity.

Gastroesophageal reflux prohibits patients from performing airway clearance in conventional PD positions. In this instance, AD, PEP, and oscillating PEP, HFCWO, IPV, and exercise, or ACBT in upright positions, are the preferred treatments. In infants or neurologically impaired patients in whom PD and percussion are the treatments of choice, modified PD positions are used, with exclusion of the Trendelenberg position, and sufficient time is allowed between a feeding and a treatment with PD.

The severity of a patient's lung disease will affect the choice of ACT. Specifically, a patient with end-stage lung disease or an acute exacerbation might not have the required energy to effectively carry out an active ACT such as AD or PEP. A more passive technique would be appropriate, at least temporarily. Also, a marked decrease in pulmonary function limits the airflow control necessary for AD, PEP, or oscillating PEP.

Accessibility of equipment or trained personnel limits the use of some ACTs. A number of these techniques are new to many health care centers, especially in the United States, because they were pioneered in Europe. Proper instruction and review of a patient's technique is imperative to achieving optimal results, and in the case of PEP, the reassessment of resistance is recommended. For IPV, the equipment and trained personnel must be available in the hospital; if a home unit is to be used, proper training of the patient and caregiver must be included. In the case of AD, the method is limited by the number of instructors available to teach the technique to patients, and a great deal of time must be spent by the health care team member to learn it. The patient must possess motivation, have time to learn the technique, and be willing to fine-tune the technique with the therapist periodically.

In this era of cost containment, the financial requirements of a technique must also be taken into consideration, especially in the case of a chronic condition. The insurance coverage or additional financial resources of the patient could determine the availability of any given method. If several methods prove to be equally effective, it would be prudent to select the method requiring the least expense. Although one of the most common forms of airway clearance in the United States continues to be postural drainage and percussion by a caregiver, this often proves to be quite expensive if a family member is not available for ongoing home treatments. The equipment needed for ACTs varies. The generator required for HFCWO is much more expensive to purchase or rent on a monthly basis than is an IPV unit. Mechanical percussors or vibrators are moderately priced, and PEP and oscillating PEP devices are the least expensive of the techniques requiring equipment. A patient independently using ACBT or AD consumes the fewest financial resources.

Ultimately, the regular use of a particular ACT by a patient is governed by personal belief in the effectiveness of the method for his or her own disease process, the manner in which the method affects the family's life habits, and the patient's willingness to use the technique on a daily basis. Adherence is ultimately the best measure of any ACT's effectiveness.

Clinical outcome measures to assess the effectiveness of an ACT can be followed during clinical appointments or periods of hospitalization. Radiographic changes, breath sounds, and pulmonary function tests may demonstrate adequate airway clearance or the need to reassess the appropriateness of the technique and its application. Hemodynamic values such as heart rate, blood pressure, O_2 saturation, and arterial blood gas values may also be monitored to assess the response of a patient to a particular treatment. Though it is difficult to quantify, many patients subjectively rely on amount of sputum production to guide their choice of secretion clearance method. Other changes to monitor in sputum quality are color and viscosity. This measure provides immediate feedback to the patient without a visit to the hospital or clinic. Of course, the ultimate outcome measure is treatment adherence, as it will have long-lasting effects on the success of any airway clearance method.

SUMMARY

The goals of airway clearance are to decrease airway obstruction, improve secretion clearance, and improve ventilation and gas exchange. Routine application of ACTs in many conditions has not been shown to be effective in achieving these goals. ACTs are not without side effects or complications; routine use of these methods is not recommended without clear indications.

Indications for ACTs have been divided into those for acute illness and those for chronic disease states. In acute illness, traditional CPT (i.e., PD, percussion, and vibration) has been shown to be beneficial in patients with copious secretions and in the treatment of atelectasis (Kiriloff, 1985). For patients with cystic fibrosis, treatment with PEP and exercise in conjunction with PD, percussion, and vibration were also shown to be effective in an acute exacerbation (Boyd, 1994). Acute asthma, bronchitis, pneumonia without copious secretions, bronchiolitis, and routine postoperative conditions were not shown to benefit from PD, percussion, and vibration (Eid, 1991; Sutton, 1982).

In chronic disease states, patients with cystic fibrosis and bronchiectasis have been found to benefit from PD, percussion, and vibration (Kiriloff, 1985). PEP, autogenic drainage, ACBT, IPV, and exercise are effective in the ongoing management of patients with cystic fibrosis (Boyd, 1994; Downs, 2004).

In patients for whom traditional CPT is contraindicated or not effective, the caregiver must consider many factors in recommending an alternative form of airway clearance. The age of the patient is a primary factor in the appropriateness of a selected technique. For infants, PD, percussion, and vibration remain the mainstay of secretion clearance. In older children, the active cycle of breathing may be initiated, PEP may be taught, and high-frequency chest compression is available for children after 2 years of age. Exercise should be included in treatment as well. Adults and children who are 12 years of age or older have the complete range of ACTs at their disposal, including IPV and autogenic drainage.

Treatments aimed at secretion clearance require an individualized approach to tailor the treatment to the patient's condition and lifestyle, to continuously reevaluate the patient's status, and to monitor the response to treatment. Acceptance of the specific treatment technique by the patient and family is paramount; adherence is the key to achieving effective treatment, especially in chronic lung disease.

Further research in the area of airway clearance is certainly needed. Studies with consistent application of techniques, similar outcome measures, and consistent study design will assist practitioners in evaluating and recommending a given technique of airway clearance for a particular patient population.

Review Questions

1. Which ACTs would be the easiest (for the therapist and the patient) to incorporate into an established routine of conventional PD and percussion?
2. What possible factors could be considered a contra-indication to chest percussion with PD in a patient admitted to the hospital due to trauma or surgery?
3. What considerations are necessary when applying airway clearance methods to an infant or neonate?
4. What factors might make it difficult for a patient to accept a new method of airway clearance?
5. Which ACTs would be most appropriate during an acute exacerbation of a pulmonary disease?

REFERENCES

AARC Clinical Practice Guideline. (1991). Postural drainage therapy. Respiratory Care 36:1418-1426.

Althaus, P. (1989). The bronchial hygiene assisted by the Flutter VRP1 (module regulator of a positive pressure oscillation expiration). European Respiratory Journal 2(Suppl 8):693.

Althaus, P. (1993). Oscillating PEP. In Bronchial hypersecretion: current chest physiotherapy in cystic fibrosis (CF). International Committee for CF (IPC/CF).

Ambrosino, N. (1991). Clinical evaluation of a new device for home chest physiotherapy in nonhypersecretive COPD patients. American Review of Respiratory Diseases 4:260.

Andersen, J.B., Qvist, J., & Kann, T. (1979). Recruiting collapsed lung through collateral channels with positive end-expiratory pressure. Scandanavian Journal of Respiratory Diseases 4: 260-266.

Andersen, J.B., & Klausen, N.O. (1982). A new mode of administration of nebulized bronchodilator in severe bronchospasm. European Respiratory Journal 119(Suppl 6):97-100.

Andreasson, B., Jonson, B., Kornfalt, R., Nordmark, E., & Sandstrom, S. (1987). Long-term effects of physical exercise on working capacity and pulmonary function in cystic fibrosis. Acta Pediatrics of Scandanavia 76:70-75.

Arens, R., Gozal, D., Omlin, K.J., Vega, J., Boyd, K.P., Woo, M.S., & Keens, T.G. (1993). Comparative efficacy of high frequency chest compression and conventional chest physiotherapy in hospitalized patients with cystic fibrosis. Pediatric Pulmonology suppl. 9:239.

Baldwin, D.R. (1994). Effect of addition of exercise to chest physiotherapy on sputum expectoration and lung function in adults with cystic fibrosis. Respiratory Medicine 88:49-53.

Barrell, S.E., Abbas, H.M. (1978). Monitoring during physiotherapy after open heart surgery. Physiotherapy 64:272-273.

Bateman, J., Newman, S.P., Daunt, K.M., Sheahan, N.F., Pavia, D., & Clarke, S.W. (1981). Is cough as effective as chest physio-therapy in the removal of excessive tracheobronchial secretions? Thorax 36:683-687.

Bilton, D., Dodd, M.E., Abbot, J.V., & Webb, A.K. (1992). The benefits of exercise combined with physiotherapy in the treatment of adults with cystic fibrosis. Respiratory Medicine 86:507-511.

Boyd, S., Brooks, D., Agnew-Coughlin, J., & Ashwell, J. (1994). Evaluation of the literature on the effectiveness of physical therapy modalities in the management of children with cystic fibrosis. Pediatric Physical Therapy :70-74.

Britton, S., Bejstedt, M., & Vedin, L. (1985). Chest physiotherapy in primary pneumonia. British Medical Journal 290:1703-1704.

Button, B.M., Heine, R.G., Catto-Smith, A.G., Olinsky, A., Phelan, P.D., Ditchfield, M.R., & Story, I. (2003). Chest physiotherapy in infants with cystic fibrosis: to tip or not? A five-year study. Pediatric Pulmonology 35:208-213.

Button, B.M., Heine, R.G., Catto-Smith, A.G., Phelan, P.D., & Olinsky, P.D. (2004). Chest physiotherapy, gastro-oesophageal reflux, and arousal in infants with cystic fibrosis. Archives of Disease in Childhood 89:435-439.

Burnett, M. (1993). Comparative efficacy of manual chest physiotherapy and a high-frequency chest compression vest in treatment of cystic fibrosis [abstract]. American Review of Respiratory Disease 147(Suppl):A30.

Campbell, A.H., O'Connell, J.M., & Wilson, F. (1975). The effect of chest physiotherapy upon the FEV_1 in chronic bronchitis. Medical Journal of Australia 1:33-35.

Cerny, F.J. (1989). Relative effects of bronchial drainage and exercise for in-hospital care of patients with cystic fibrosis. Physical Therapy 69:633-639.

Crane, L. (1995).Physical therapy for the neonate with respiratory disease. In Irwin, S. & Tecklin, J.S. (Eds). Cardiopulmonary physical therapy, ed 3. St. Louis: Mosby.

Chang, H.K., Weber, M.E., & King, M. (1988). Mucus transport by high-frequency nonsymmetrical oscillatory airflow. Journal of Applied Physiology 65:1203-1209.

Chevaillier, J. (1992). Airway clearance techniques. Dallas: Sixth Annual North American Cystic Fibrosis Conference (course).

Clement, A.J., & Hubsch, S.K. (1968). Chest physiotherapy by the 'bag squeezing' method: a guide to technique. Physiotherapy 54:355-359.

Connors, A.F. Jr., Hammon, W.E., Martin, R.J., & Rogers, R.M. (1980). Chest physical therapy: the immediate effect on oxygenation in acutely ill patients. Chest 78:559-564.

Crane, L. (1995). Physical therapy for the neonate with respiratory disease. In Irwin, S., & Tecklin, J.S. (Eds). Cardiopulmonary physical therapy, ed 3. St. Louis: Mosby.

Currie, D.C. (1986). Practice, problems and compliance with postural drainage: a survey of chronic sputum producers. British Journal of Diseases of the Chest 80:249-253.

Dab, I., & Alexander, F. (1979). The mechanism of autogenic drainage studied with flow volume curves. Monographs of Paediatrics 10:50-53.

David, A. (1991). Autogenic drainage: the German approach. In Pryor, J. (Ed). Respiratory care. Edinburgh: Churchill Livingstone.

Davidson, N.G.T. (1988). Physiotherapy in cystic fibrosis: a comparative trial of PEP, AD, and conventional percussion and drainage techniques [abstract]. Pediatric Pulmonology 2(Suppl):132.

Davidson, A.G.F., Wong, L.T.K., Piric, G.E., & McIlwaine, P.M. (1992). Long-term comparative trial of conventional percussion and drainage physiotherapy versus AD in cystic fibrosis [abstract]. Pediatric Pulmonology 8(Suppl):235.

Dean, E., & Ross, J. (1992). Discordance between cardiopulmonary physiology and physical therapy. Chest 101:1694-1698.

Denton, R. (1962). Bronchial secretions in cystic fibrosis. American Review of Respiratory Disease 86:41-46.

Desmond, K., Schwenk, W.F., Thomas, E., Beaudry, P.H., & Coates, A.L. (1983). Immediate and long-term effects of chest physical therapy in patients with cystic fibrosis. Journal of Pediatrics 103:538-542.

Dickman, C., & Wilchynski, J.A. (1987). Respiratory failure. In Frownfelter, D. (Ed). Chest physical therapy and pulmonary rehabilitation, ed 2. Chicago: Year Book Medical.

Downs, A.M., & Lindsay, K.L.B. (2004). Physical therapy associated with airway clearance dysfunction. In Deturk, W.E. & Cahalin, L.P. (Eds). Cardiovascular and pulmonary physical therapy. New York: McGraw-Hill.

Eid, N., Buchheit, M.D., Neuling, M., & Phelps, H. (1991). Chest physiotherapy in review. Respiratory Care 36:270-282.

Falk, M., Kelstrup, M., Andersen, J.B., Kinoshita, T. , Falk, P., Stovring, S., & Gothgen, I. (1984). Improving the ketchup bottle method with PEP, PEP in cystic fibrosis. European Journal of Respiratory Disease 65:423-432.

Falk, M., Mortensen, J., Kelstrup., M., Lanng, S., Larsen, L., & Ulrik, C.S. (1993). Short-term effects of PEP and the FET on mucus clearance and lung function in cystic fibrosis [abstract]. Pediatric Pulmonology 9(Suppl):241.

Falk, M., & Kelstrup, M. (1995). PEP. In Physiotherapy in the treatment of cystic fibrosis (CF). International Physiotherapy Group for Cystic Fibrosis (IPC/CF).

Faverio, L., Kluft, J., Fink, R., Chaney, H., Becker, L., & Castagnino, M. (1994). A comparison of bronchial drainage treatments in patients with cystic fibrosis [abstract]. American Journal of Respiratory and Critical Care Medicine 149:A669.

Feldman, J., Traver, G.A., & Taussig, L.M. (1979). Maximal expiratory flows after postural drainage. American Review of Respiratory Disease 119:239-245.

Finer, N., & Boyd, J. (1978). Chest physiotherapy in the neonate: a controlled study. Pediatrics 61:282-285.

Ford, R.M., Godreau, K.M., & Burns, D.M. (1991). Carpal tunnel syndrome as a manifestation of cumulative trauma disorder in respiratory care practitioners [abstract]. Respiratory Care 36:137.

Frownfelter, D. (1987). Postural drainage. In Frownfelter, D. (Ed). Chest physical therapy and pulmonary rehabilitation, ed 2. Chicago: Year Book Medical.

Fox, W.W., Schwartz, J.G., & Shaffer, T.H. (1978). Pulmonary physiotherapy in neonates: physiologyogic changes and respiratory management. Journal of Pediatrics 92:977-981.

Gallon, A. (1991). Evaluation of chest percussion in the treatment of patients with copious sputum production. Respiratory Medicine 85:45-51

Garradd, J., & Bullock, M. (1986). The effect of respiratory therapy on intracranial pressure in ventilated neurosurgical patients. Australian Journal of Physiology 32:107-111.

Giles, D.R., Acurso, F.J., & Wagener, J.S. (1993). Acute effects of PD and clapping versus AD on oxygen saturation and sputum recovery in cystic fibrosis. Pediatric Pulmonology 9(Suppl):252.

Godfrey, S., Silverman, M., & Anderson, S. (1975). The use of the treadmill for assessing exercise-induced asthma and the effect of varying the severity and duration of exercise. Pediatrics 56(Suppl):893-898.

Gormenzano, J., & Branthwaite, M.A. (1972). Pulmonary physiotherapy with assisted ventilation. Anaesthesia 27:249-257.

Groth, S., Stafanger, G., Dirksen, H., Andersen, J.B., Falk, M., & Kelstrup, M. (1985). PEP (PEP-mask) physiotherapy improves ventilation and reduces volume of trapped gas in cystic fibrosis. Bulletin of European Physiopathology and Respiratory 21:339-343.

Hammon, W.E., & Martin, R.J. (1979). Fatal pulmonary hemorrhage associated with chest physical therapy. Physical Therapy 59:1247-1248.

Hammon, W.E., & Martin, R.J. (1981). Chest physical therapy for acute atelectasis. Physical Therapy 61:217-220.

Hansen, L.G., & Warwick, W.J. (1990). High-frequency chest compression system to aid in clearance of mucus from the lung. Biomedical Instrumentation and Technology 24:289-294.

Hardy, K.A. (1994). A review of airway clearance: new techniques, indications, and recommendations. Respiratory Care 39:440-452.

Hardy, K.A., & Anderson, B.D. (1996). Noninvasive clearance of airway secretions. Respiratory Care Clinics of North America 2:323-345.

Hasani, A., Pavia, D., Agnew, J., & Clarke, S.W. (1994). Regional mucus transport following unproductive cough and FET in patients with airways obstruction. Chest 105:1420-1425.

Hietpas, B.G., Roth, R.D., & Jensen, W.M. (1979). Huff coughing and airway patency. European Journal of Respiratory of Disease 24:710-713.

Henke, K.G., & Orenstein, D.M. (1984). Oxygen saturation during exercise in cystic fibrosis. American Review of Respirator Diseases 129:708-711.

Hofmeyer, J.L., Webber, B.A., & Hodson, M.E. (1986). Evaluation of PEP as an adjunct to chest physiotherapy in the treatment of cystic fibrosis. Thorax 41:951-954.

Homnick, D.N., White, F., & de Castro, C. (1995). Comparison of effects of an IPV to standard aerosol and chest physiotherapy treatment in cystic fibrosis. Pediatric Pulmonology 20:50-55.

Humberstone, N. (1990). Respiratory assessment and treatment. In Irwin, S., Tecklin, J.S. (Eds). Cardiopulmonary physical therapy, ed 2. St. Louis: Mosby.

Huseby, J., Hudson, L., Stark, K., & Tyler, M. (1976). Oxygenation during chest physiotherapy [abstract]. Chest 70:430.

King, M., Phillips, D.M., Gross, D., Vartian, V., Chang, H.K., & Zidulka, A. (1983). Enhanced tracheal mucus clearance with high-frequency chest wall compression. American Review of Respiratory Disease 128:511-515.

Kirifoff, L.H., Owens, G.R., Rogers, R.M., & Mazzocco, M.C. (1985). Does chest physical therapy work? Chest 88:436-444.

Klous, D., Boyle, M., Hazelwood, A., & McComb, R.C. (1993). Chest vest and cystic fibrosis: better care for patients. Advanced Respiratory Care Management 3:44-50.

Klous, D.R. (1994). High-frequency chest wall oscillation: principles and applications. St. Paul, Minn: American Biosystems.

Kluft, J., Becker, L., Castagnino, M., Gaiser, J., Chaney, H., & Fink, R. (1996). Comparison of bronchial drainage treatments in cystic fibrosis. Pediatric Pulmonology 22:271-274.

Konstan, M.W., Stern, R.C., & Doershuk, C.F. (1994). Efficacy of the Flutter device for airway mucus clearance in patients with cystic fibrosis. Journal of Pediatrics 124:689-693.

Lane, R., Cockroft, A., Adams, L., & Guz, A. (1987). Arterial oxygen saturation and breath issues in patients with cardiovascular disease. Clinical Science 72:693-698.

Lannefors, L., & Wollmer, P. (1992). Mucus clearance with three chest physiotherapy regimes in cystic fibrosis: a comparison between postural drainage, PEP, and physical exercise. European Respiratory Journal 5:748-753.

Lapin, A. (1990). Physical therapy in cystic fibrosis: a review. Cardiopulmonary Physical Therapy 1:11-12.

Lapin, C.D. (1993). Is exercise a substitute for airway clearance techniques? Dallas: Seventh Annual North American Cystic Fibrosis Conference (symposium).

Lapin, C.D. (1994). Conventional postural drainage and percussion: is this still the gold standard?—against. Pediatric Pulmonology 10(Suppl):87-88.

Laws, A.K., & McIntyre, R.W. (1969). Chest physiotherapy: a physiological assessment during intermittent positive pressure ventilation in respiratory failure. Canadian Anaesthetists' Society Journal 16:487-493.

Levenson, C.R. (1992). Breathing exercises. In Zadai, C.C. (Ed). Pulmonary management in physical therapy. New York: Churchill Livingstone.

Lindemann, H. (1992). Evaluation of VRP1 physiotherapy. Pneumology 46:626-630.

Litt, I.F., & Cushey, W.R. (1980). Compliance with medical regimens during adolescence. Pediatric Clinics of North America 27:3-15.

Lorin, M.I., & Denning, C.R. (1971). Evaluation of postural drainage by measurement of sputum volume and consistency. American Journal of Physical Medicine 50:215-219.

MacKenzie, C.F., Shin, B., Hadi, F., & Imle, P.C. (1980). Changes in total lung/thorax compliance following chest physiotherapy. Anesthesia and Analgesia, 59:207-210.

Mahlmeister, M.J., Fink, J.B., Hoffman, G.L., & Fifer, L.F. (1991). Positive-expiratory-pressure mask therapy: Theoretical and practical considerations and a review of the literature. Respiratory Care 36:1218-1229.

Marks, J.H., & Homnick, D.N. (1999). Safety and effectiveness of IPV compared to standard chest physiotherapy. Pediatric Pulmonology 19(Suppl):290.

Marks, J.H., Homnick, D.N., Hare, K., & Cucos, D. (2001). The Percussivetech HF compared to the Flutter device in cystic fibrosis patients: a six-month pilot study. Pediatric Pulmonology 22(Suppl):309.

Marini, J.J., Pierson, D.J., & Hudson, L.D. (1979). Acute lobar atelectasis: a prospective comparison of fiberoptic bronchoscopy and respiratory therapy. American Review of Respiratory Diseases 119:971-978.

Massery, M. (1987). Respiratory rehabilitation secondary to neurological deficits: understanding the deficits. In Frownfelter, D. (Ed). Chest physical therapy and pulmonary rehabilitation, ed 2. Chicago: Year Book Medical.

Maxwell, M., & Redmond, A. (1979). Comparative trial of manual and mechanical percussion technique with gravity-assisted bronchial drainage in patients with cystic fibrosis. Archives of Diseases of the Childhood 54:542-544.

May, D.B., & Munt, P.W. (1979). Physiologic effects of chest percussion and postural drainage in patients with stable chronic bronchitis. Chest 75:29-32.

Mazzocco, M.C., Owens, G.R., Kiriloff, L.H., & Rogers, R.M. (1985). Chest percussion and postural drainage in patients with bronchiectasis. Chest 88:360-363.

McDonnell, T., McNicholas, W.T., & Fitzgerald, M.X. (1986). Hypoxaemia during chest physiotherapy in patients with cystic fibrosis. Irish Journal of Medical Sciences 155:345-348.

Mead, J., Turner, J.M., Macklem, P.T., & Little, J.B. (1967). Significance of the relationship between lung recoil and maximum expiratory flow. Journal of Applied Physiology 22:95-108.

Miller, S., Hall, D., Clayton, C.B., & Nelson, R. (1993). Chest physiotherapy in cystic fibrosis (CF): a comparative study of autogenic drainage (AD) and active cycle of breathing technique (ACBT)(formerly FET). Pediatric Pulmonology 9(Suppl):240.

MMWR Publication from the Centers for Disease Control. (1989). Occupational disease surveillance: carpal tunnel syndrome. Journal of the American Medical Association 282:886-889.

Muszynski-Kwan, A.T., Perlman, R., & Rivington-Law, B.A. (1988). Compliance with and effectiveness of chest physiotherapy in cystic fibrosis: a review. Physiotherapy of Canada 40:28-32.

Natale JE., Pfeifle, J., & Homnick, D.M..(1994). Comparison of intrapulmonary percussive ventilation and chest physiotherapy: a pilot study in patients with cystic fibrosis. Chest 105: 1789-1793.

Nixon, P.A. (1992). The prognostic value of exercise testing in patients with cystic fibrosis. New England Journal of Medicine 327:1785-1788.

Oberwaldner, B., Evans, J.C., & Zach, M.S. (1986). Forced expirations against a variable resistance: a new chest physiotherapy method in cystic fibrosis. Pediatric Pulmonology 2:358-367.

Ohnsorg, F. (1994). A cost analysis of high-frequency chest wall oscillation in cystic fibrosis [abstract]. Boston: ALA/ATS International Conference.

Oldenberg, F.A. Jr., Dolovich, M.B., Montgomery, J.M., & Newhouse, M.T. (1979). Effects of postural drainage, exercise, and cough on mucus clearance in chronic bronchitis. American Review of Respiratory of Diseases 120:739-745.

Orenstein, D.M., Reed, M.E., Grogan, F.T. Jr., & Crawford, L.V. (1985). Exercise conditioning in children with asthma. Journal of Pediatrics 106:556-560.

Passero, M.A., Remor, B., & Salomon, J. (1981). Patient-reported compliance with cystic fibrosis therapy. Clinics of Pediatrics 20:265-268.

Pavia, D., Thomson, M.L., & Phillipakos, D. (1976). A preliminary study of the effect of a vibrating pad on bronchial clearance. American Review of RespiratoryDiseases 113:92-96.

Pfleger, A., Theissl, B., Oberwaldner, B., & Zach, M.S. (1992). Self-administered chest physiotherapy in cystic fibrosis: a comparative study of high-pressure PEP and autogenic drainage. Lung, 170:323-330.

Prasad, S.A. (1993). Current concepts in physiotherapy. Journal of the Royal Society of Medicine 86(Suppl 20):23-29.

Pryor, J.A., Webber, B.A., Hodson, M.E., & Batten, J.C. (1979). Evaluation of the forced expiration technique as an adjunct to postural drainage in treatment of cystic fibrosis. British Medical Journal 18:417-418.

Pryor, J.A., Parker, R.A., & Webber, B.A. (1981). A comparison of mechanical and manual percussion as adjuncts to postural drainage in the treatment of cystic fibrosis in adolescents and adults. Physiotherapy 67:140-141.

Pryor, J.A., Webber, B.A., & Hodson, M.E. (1990). Effect of chest physiotherapy on oxygen saturation in patients with cystic fibrosis 45:77.

Radford, R., Barutt, J., Billingsley, J.G., Hill, W., Lawson, W.H., & Willich, W. (1982). A rational basis for percussion-augmented mucociliary clearance. Respiratory Care 27:556-563.

Reisman, J., Rivington-Law, B., Corey, M., Marcotte, J., Wannamaker, E., Harcourt, D., & Levison, H. (1988). Role of conventional therapy in cystic fibrosis. Journal of Pediatrics 113:632-636.

Robinson, C., & Hernried, L. (1992). Evaluation of a high-frequency chest compression device in cystic fibrosis. Pediatric Pulmonology 8(Suppl):255.

Rochester, D.F., & Goldberg, S.K. (1980). Techniques of respiratory physical therapy. American Review of Respiratory Diseases 122:133-146.

Rossman, C.M., Waldes, R., Sampson, D., & Newhouse, M.T. (1982). Effect of chest physiotherapy on the removal of mucus in patients with cystic fibrosis. American Review of Respiratory Diseases 126:131-135.

Salh, W., Bilton, D., Dodd, M., & Webb, A.K. (1989). Effect of exercise and physiotherapy in aiding sputum expectoration in adults with cystic fibrosis. Thorax 44:1006-1008.

Schibler, A., Casaulta, C., & Kraemer, R. (1992). Rationale of oscillatory breathing as chest physiotherapy performed by the Flutter in patients with cystic fibrosis (CF) [abstract]. Pediatric Pulmonology 8(Suppl):244.

Selsby, D., & Jones, J.G. (1990). Some physiological and clinical aspects of chest physiotherapy. British Journal of Anaesthesia 64:621-631.

Schoni, M.H. (1989). Autogenic drainage: a modern approach to physiotherapy in cystic fibrosis. Journal of the Royal Society of Medicine 82(Suppl 16):32-37.

Shultz, K. (1980). Compliance with therapeutic regimens in pediatricics: a review of implications for social work practice. Social Work Health Care 5:267-278.

Simonova, O., Kapranov, N., Smirnova, E., & Stucalova, A. (1992). PEP-mask therapy in complex treatment of cystic fibrosis patients. Pediatric Pulmonology 8(Suppl):245.

Stern, R.C., Wood, R.E., Boat, T.F., Matthews, L.W., Tucker, A.S., & Doershuk, C.F. (1978). Treatment and prognosis of massive hemoptysis in cystic fibrosis. American Review of Respiratory Diseases 117:825-828.

Steven, M.H., Pryor, J.A., & Webber, B.A. (1992). Physiotherapy versus cough alone in the treatment of cystic fibrosis. New Zealand Journal of Physiotherapy 20:31-37.

Stiller, K., Geake, T., Taylor, J., Grant, R., & Hall, B. (1990). Acute lobar atelectasis: a comparison of two chest physiotherapy regimens. Chest 98:1336-1340.

Sutton, P.P., Pavia, D., Bateman, J.R., & Clarke, S.W. (1982). Chest physiotherapy: a review. European Journal of Respiratory Diseases 63:188-201.

Sutton, P.P., Parker, R.A., Webber, B.A., Newman, S.P., Garland, N., Lopez-Vidriero, M.T., Pavia, D., & Clarke, S.W. (1983). Assessment of the forced expiration technique, postural drainage and directed coughing in chest physiotherapy. European Journal of Respiratory Diseases 64:62-68.

Tecklin, J.S., & Holsclaw, D.S. (1975). Evaluation of bronchial drainage in patients with cystic fibrosis. Physical Therapy 55:1081-1084.

Thompson, B.J. (1973). The physiotherapist's role in the rehabilitation of the asthmatic. New Zealand Journal of Physiotherapy 4:11-16.

Tomkiewicz, R., Bivij, A., & King, M. (1994). Rheologic studies regarding high-frequency chest compression (HFCC) and improvements of mucus clearance in cystic fibrosis. Boston: ATS International Conference (abstract).

Torrington, K., Sorenson, D., & Sherwood, L. (1984). Postoperative chest percussion with postural drainage in obese patients following gastric stapling. Chest 86:891-895.

Tyrrell, J.C., Hill, E.J., & Martin, J. (1986). Face mask physiotherapy in cystic fibrosis. Archives of Diseases of Childhood 61:598-611.

Warwick, W.J., & Hansen, L.G. (1991). The long-term effect of high-frequency chest compression therapy on pulmonary complications of cystic fibrosis. Pediatric Pulmonology 11:265-271.

Warwick, W.J. (1992). Airway clearance by high frequency chest compression. Washington, D.C.: Sixth Annual North American Cystic Fibrosis Conference (symposium).

Webb, M.S.C., Martin, J.A., Cartlidge, P.H., Ng, Y.K., & Wright, N.A. (1985). Chest physiotherapy in acute bronchiolitis. Archives of Diseases of Childhood 60:1078-1079.

Webber, B.A., Hofmeyer, J.L., Morgan, M.D.L., & Hodson, M.E. (1986). Effect of postural drainage, incorporating the forced expiration technique, on pulmonary function in cystic fibrosis. British Journal of Diseases of the Chest 80:353-359.

Webber, B.A. (1988). Is postural drainage necessary? Sydney: Tenth International Cystic Fibrosis Conference.

Webber, B.A. (1988). Physiotherapy for patients receiving mechanical ventilation. In Webber, B.A. (Ed). The Brompton Hospital Guide to Chest Physiotherapy, ed 5. Oxford: Blackwell Scientific.

Webber, B., & Pryor, J. (Eds). (1993). Active cycle of breathing techniques. In Bronchial hypersecretion: current chest physiotherapy in cystic fibrosis (CF). International Physiotherapy Committee for Cystic Fibrosis (IPC/CF). p. 113-116.

Webber, B.A., & Pryor, J. A. (1993). Physiotherapy skills: techniques and adjuncts. In Physiotherapy for respiratory and cardiac problems. Edinburgh: Churchill Livingstone.

Wetzel. J.L., Lunsford, B.R., Peterson, M.J., & Alvarez, S.E. (1995). Respiratory rehabilitation of the patient with a spinal cord injury. In Irwin, S., & Tecklin, J.S. (Eds). Cardiopulmonary physical therapy, ed 3. St. Louis: Mosby.

Whitman, J., Van Beusekom, R., Olson, S., Worm, M., & Indihar, F. (1993). Preliminary evaluation of high-frequency chest compression for secretion clearance in mechanically ventilated patients. Respiratory Care 38:1081-1087.

Wolff, R.K., Dolovich, M.B., Obminski, G., & Newhouse, M.T. (1977). Effects of exercise and eucapnic hyperventilation on bronchial clearance in man. Journal of Applied Physiology: Respiratory Environment Exercise Physiology 43:46-50.

Wollmer, P., Ursing, K., Midgren, B., & Eriksson, L. (1985). Inefficiency of chest percussion in the physical therapy of chronic bronchitis. European Journal of Respiratory Disease 66:233-239.

Wong, J.W., Keens, T.G., Wannamaker, E.M., Crozier, D.N., Levison, H., & Aspin, N. (1977). Effects of gravity in tracheal transport rates in normal subjects and in patients with cystic fibrosis. Pediatrics 60:146-152.

Wood, R.E. (1989). Treatment of cystic fibrosis lung disease in the first two years. Pediatric Pulmonology 4:685-690.

Zach, M., Oberwaldner, B., & Hausler, F. (1982). Cystic fibrosis: physical exercise versus chest physiotherapy. Archives of Diseases of Childhood. 57:587-589.

Zadai, C.C. (1981). Physical therapy for the acutely ill medical patient. Physical Therapy 61:1746-1753.

Zausmer, E. (1968). Bronchial drainage: evidence supporting the procedures. Physical Therapy 48:586-591.

CHAPTER 21

Clinical Application of Airway Clearance Techniques

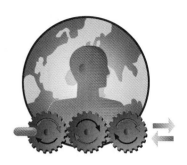

Anne Mejia Downs

Oxygen transport from the lungs to body tissues can be limited in patients that possess an ineffective cough or an impairment of normal mechanisms of mucociliary clearance. The caregiver must augment these mechanisms using the array of techniques available for airway clearance. Each technique has a physiological basis for improving the mobilization of secretions. When prescribing an optimal method of airway clearance, the caregiver must consider the pathophysiology and the symptoms of the disease, the availability of the technique to the patient, and the patient's acceptance of the technique.

The previous chapter addressed the physiological basis of each technique, the history of its use, and research to establish its effectiveness. This chapter provides an introduction to the application of these techniques to patients and addresses the benefits and burdens of each technique.

Airway clearance techniques differ with respect to equipment needs, the skill level required to perform them, and their usefulness with various clinical problems. Matching a patient with an appropriate method or combination of methods may increase effectiveness, reduce complications, and promote long-term adherence to the treatment. This will, in turn, help

with achieving the goals of airway clearance: reducing airway obstruction, improving ventilation, and optimizing gas exchange.

USE OF AIRWAY CLEARANCE TECHNIQUES

This chapter will address the application of airway clearance techniques (ACTs) with specific instructions for patient treatment. Contraindications and precautions for each ACT are addressed in Chapter 20. This section will speak to practical concerns regarding patient care.

Preparation for any secretion removal technique should include evaluation of the patient's pulmonary status (see Chapter 16) so that measures may be compared before and after a treatment is completed. A physical examination, including inspection, palpation, measurement of vital signs, and chest auscultation provides assessment of a treatment's effectiveness. Laboratory tests including chest x-ray, arterial blood gas measurements, and pulmonary function studies should be followed, because these may be used as outcome measures.

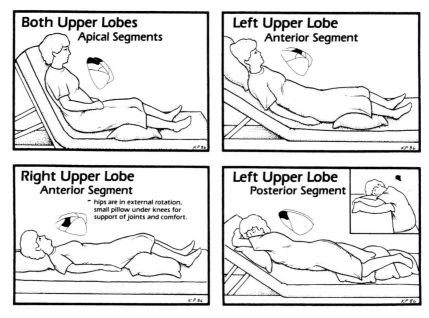

FIGURE 21-1 Upper lobes.

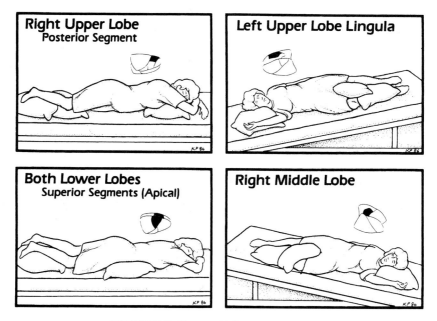

FIGURE 21-2 Upper, middle, and lower lobes.

Several factors must be taken into account when scheduling an optimal time for patient treatment. At least 1 half hour to 1 hour should be allowed for the completion of tube feedings or meals. The inhalation of bronchodilator medications should take place before airway clearance maneuvers to improve secretion removal by opening the airways. Inhaled antibiotics are best scheduled after airway clearance has taken place for optimal deposition of medication. Adequate pain control is necessary to receive a patient's best effort and cooperation with a treatment. It is also advisable to have all necessary equipment and personnel available at the start of the treatment.

POSTURAL DRAINAGE

Postural drainage (PD) is accomplished by positioning the patient so that the angle of the lung segment to be drained allows gravity to have its greatest effect (Figures 21-1 through 21-4). Modified positions should be used when there is a precaution or contraindication to the ideal position. For

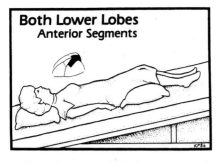

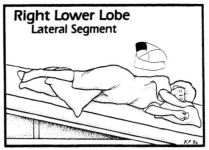

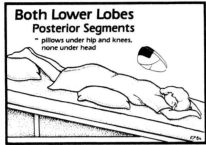

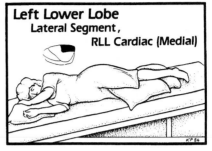

FIGURE 21-3 Lower lobes.

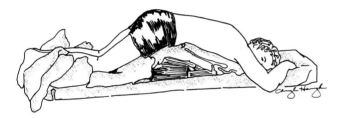

FIGURE 21-4 Both lower lobes—posterior segments (shown using telephone books or pillows for home use). A beanbag chair is also helpful for home treatments.

example, if an increase in intracranial pressure is a concern, the head of the bed should remain flat instead of being tipped into the Trendelenburg (head down) position.

Equipment Required For PD

1. For the hospitalized patient, there are a variety of beds that employ manual or electric devices to position the patient. Air therapy beds, most often used in the intensive care unit (ICU), are valuable aids for positioning, especially in patients who are large or unresponsive.
2. Make use of pillows or bedrolls to support body parts or relieve pressure areas.
3. For home treatment, aids in positioning might include pillows, a slant board (or ironing board if the patient is small), a foam wedge, sofa cushions, or a beanbag chair.

Preparation for PD

1. Nebulized bronchodilators before PD may facilitate the mobilization of sputum.

2. An adequate intake of fluids (as allowed) decreases the viscosity of the secretions, allowing easier mobilization.
3. Become familiar with the workings of the model of bed the patient is occupying, especially the movement of the bed into the Trendelenburg position.
4. In the ICU, it is imperative to be familiar with the multiple lines, tubes, and other devices attached to the patient. Allow enough slack from each device to position a patient for postural drainage.
5. Make sure there are enough personnel to position the patient with as little stress to both patient and staff as possible (Frownfelter, 1987).
6. Have suctioning equipment ready to remove secretions from an artificial airway or the patient's oral or nasal cavity after the treatment. Have tissues or a specimen cup available for the patient with an adequate cough to expectorate secretions.

Treatment with PD

1. After determining the lobe of the lung to be treated, position the patient in the appropriate position, using pillows or bedrolls as needed to support the patient comfortably in the position indicated. See Figures 21-1 through 21-4.
2. If postural drainage is used exclusively, each position should be maintained for 5 to 10 minutes, if tolerated, or longer when focusing on a specific lobe. Coordinating the positioning with nursing care for skin pressure relief may allow the time spent in a position to be extended. If postural drainage is used in conjunction with another technique, the time in each position may be decreased. For example, if percussion and vibration are performed while

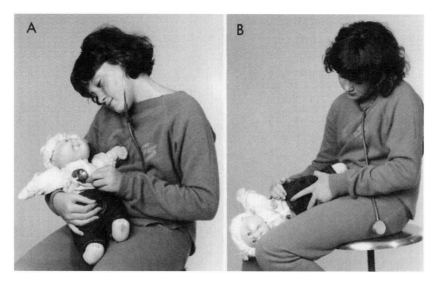

FIGURE 21-5 A and **B**, If children are able to role play the treatment, they will better understand what is expected and be more cooperative with therapy.

the patient is in each PD position, 3 to 5 minutes is sufficient.

3. A patient who requires close monitoring should not be left unattended in a Trendelenburg position, but this may be appropriate if a patient is alert and able to reposition herself.

4. It is not always necessary to treat each affected lung segment during every treatment; this may prove to be too fatiguing for the patient. The most affected lobes should be addressed with the first treatment of the day, with the other affected areas addressed during a subsequent treatment.

5. The patient should be encouraged to take deep breaths and cough after each position if possible, and again after the treatment is completed. Having the patient sit upright or lean forward optimizes this effort by allowing the use of the abdominals for a stronger cough (Frownfelter, 1987).

6. Secretions may not be mobilized immediately after the treatment but this may occur up to 1 hour later. The patient should be thus informed and reminded to clear secretions at a later time. A health care practitioner or family member should be included in this aspect of treatment, especially with patients who need encouragement (Frownfelter, 1987).

Advantages and Disadvantages of PD

PD is relatively easy to learn; the patient and/or caregiver must be familiar with the appropriate positioning for the affected lung fields. Treatment in the hospital may be coordinated with other patient activities such as positioning for skin pressure relief, bathing, or positioning for a test or procedure. Home treatment may be coordinated with activities such as reading or watching television.

For many patients, optimal PD positions will be contraindicated for a variety of reasons (see Chapter 20). Adherence

to PD may be reduced because of the length of the treatment, especially in the pediatric population, who will require considerable distractions to maintain a desired position for the appropriate length of time (Figure 21-5).

The cost of the equipment required for PD is minimal. Inexpensive items may be used for home treatment. The cost of a caregiver's time to provide the treatment, however, especially in the case of a chronic disease, may be substantial. A family member may be willing to learn the procedure, which would decrease the cost and provide flexibility in scheduling.

PERCUSSION

Percussion is performed with the aim of loosening retained secretions from the airways so they may be removed by suctioning or expectoration. The clapping of the caregiver's cupped hands against the thorax provides a rhythmical force over the affected lung segment, trapping air between the patient's thorax and the caregiver's hands (Figure 21-6). It is performed during both the inspiratory and expiratory phases of breathing. Percussion is used in postural drainage positions for increased effectiveness (Sutton, 1985; Bateman, 1979) and may also be used during the active cycle of breathing technique (ACBT).

Equipment Required for Percussion

1. The only equipment required for manual percussion is the caregiver's cupped hands to deliver the force to mobilize secretions.

2. For the adult and older pediatric population, electric or pneumatic percussors that mechanically simulate percussion are available. This enables a patient to apply self-percussion more effectively. Several models have variable frequencies of percussion, as well as different levels of intensity.

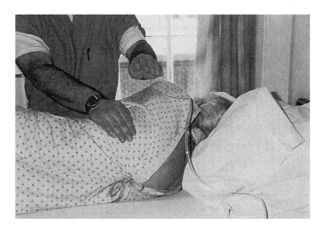

FIGURE 21-6 Chest percussion.

3. Several devices may be used to provide percussion to infants: padded rubber nipples, pediatric anesthesia masks, padded medicine cups, or the bell end of a stethoscope.

Preparation for Percussion

1. Placing the patient in appropriate PD positions (as the patient's condition allows) enhances the effect of percussion.
2. Place a thin towel or hospital gown over the patient's skin where the percussion is to be applied. The force of percussion over bare skin may be uncomfortable; however, padding that is too thick absorbs the force of the percussion without benefit to the patient.
3. Adjust the level of the bed so that the caregiver may use proper body mechanics during the treatment. The caregiver may become fatigued or injured as a result of lengthy or numerous treatments if proper body mechanics are ignored.

Treatment with Percussion

1. Position the hand in the shape of a cup with the fingers and thumb adducted. It is important to maintain this cupped position with the hands throughout the treatment, while letting the wrists, arms, and shoulders stay relaxed.
2. The sound of percussion should be a hollow as opposed to a slapping sound. If erythema occurs with percussion, it is usually a result of slapping or not trapping enough air between the hand and the chest wall (Imle, 1989).
3. The patient will better tolerate an even, steady rhythm. The rate of manual percussion delivered by caregivers can vary between 100 and 480 times per minute (Imle, 1989).
4. The force applied to the chest wall from each hand should be equal. If the nondominant hand is not able to keep up with the dominant hand, the rate should be slowed to match that of the slower hand. It might also be helpful to start with the nondominant hand and let the dominant hand match the nondominant hand (Frownfelter, 1987). The force does not have to be excessive to be effective; the amount of force should be adapted to the patient's comfort.

5. If the size of an infant does not allow use of a full hand, percussion may be done manually with four fingers cupped, three fingers with the middle finger "tented," or the thenar and hypothenar surfaces of the hand (Crane, 1990).
6. Hand position should be such that percussion does not occur over bony prominences of the patient. The spinous processes of the vertebrae, the spine of the scapula, and the clavicle should all be avoided. Percussion over the floating ribs should also be avoided because these ribs have only a single attachment.
7. Percussion should not be performed over breast tissue. This will produce discomfort and diminish the effectiveness of the treatment. In the case of very large breasts, it may be necessary to move the breast out of the way with one hand, (or ask the patient to do this) and percuss with the other hand.
8. A patient may be taught to perform one-handed self-percussion to those areas that can be reached comfortably, either manually or with a mechanical percussor. This does, however, virtually preclude the treatment of the posterior lung segments.

Advantages and Disadvantages of Percussion

The addition of percussion to a PD treatment may enhance secretion clearance and shorten the treatment. Patients, especially young children and infants, often find the rhythm soothing and are relaxed and sedated by percussion.

Patients with chronic lung disease who have used PD and percussion for many years and have found it effective may be reluctant to try an alternative method of airway clearance. Acceptance of this method is dependent on the consistent availability of a family member or other caregiver to provide the treatment. Mechanical percussors allow a patient more independence or decrease fatigue of a caregiver, and are especially useful in patients requiring ongoing treatment at home.

Percussion is not well tolerated by many patients postoperatively without adequate pain control. The force of percussion is also a threat to patients with osteoporosis or coagulopathy. Other contraindications are listed in Chapter 20. Percussion has been associated with a fall in oxygen saturation, which can be eliminated with concurrent thoracic expansion exercises and pauses for breathing control (Pryor, 1990).

Delivering percussion for extended periods on an ongoing basis can result in injury to the caregiver, whether a family member or a health care provider. Repetitive motion injuries of the upper extremities may occur in long-term delivery of percussion for airway clearance.

The expense of a mechanical device for percussion is minimal compared with the ongoing cost of a caregiver to provide percussion and PD, either in the hospital setting or at home. In the case of young children or unresponsive patients, there are few choices for airway clearance. For other populations, however, a more independent method can prove to be more cost-effective if adequate adherence is achieved.

VIBRATION/SHAKING

The techniques of vibration and shaking are on opposite ends of a spectrum. Vibration involves a gentle, high frequency force, whereas shaking is more vigorous in nature. Vibration and shaking are performed with the aim of moving secretions from the lung periphery to the larger airways where they may be suctioned or expectorated. Vibration is performed by co-contracting all the muscles in the caregiver's upper extremities to cause a vibration while applying pressure to the chest wall with the hands. Shaking is a stronger bouncing maneuver that also supplies a concurrent, compressive force to the chest wall.

Like percussion, vibration and shaking are used in conjunction with PD positioning. Unlike percussion, they are performed only during the expiratory phase of breathing, starting with peak inspiration and continuing until the end of expiration. The compressive forces follow the movement of the chest wall.

Equipment Required for Vibration/Shaking

1. For manual techniques, the only equipment required is the caregiver's hands.
2. Mechanical vibrators are available to administer the treatment and are useful for self-treatment by a patient or to reduce fatigue in the caregiver.
3. For infants, a padded electric toothbrush may be used (Crane, 1990).

Preparation for Vibration/Shaking

1. Place the patient in the appropriate PD position or modified position as the patient's status allows.
2. Place a thin towel or hospital gown over the patient's skin. The material should not be thick enough to absorb the effect of the vibration or shaking.
3. Proper body position of the caregiver is important to deliver an effective treatment and to decrease caregiver fatigue.

Treatment with Vibration/Shaking

1. Conventional chest physical therapy (CPT) is often referred to as a combination of PD and percussion followed by vibration or shaking.
2. For shaking, with the patient in the appropriate PD position, place your hands over the lobe of the lung to be treated and instruct the patient to take in a deep breath. At the peak of inspiration, apply a slow (approximately 2 times per second), rhythmic bouncing pressure to the chest wall until the end of expiration. The hands follow the movement of the chest as the air is exhaled. The frequency of shaking is 2 Hz (Gormenzano, 1972; Bateman, 1981).

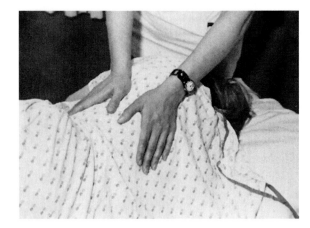

FIGURE 21-7 Vibration—hands positioned on both sides of the chest.

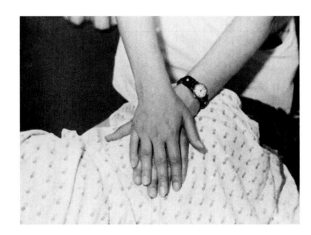

FIGURE 21-8 Vibration—hand placement one on top of the other.

3. For vibration, the hands may be placed side by side or on top of one another as shown in Figures 21-7 and 21-8. As with shaking, the patient is instructed to take in a deep breath while in a proper PD position. A gentle but steady co-contraction of the upper extremities is performed to vibrate the chest wall, beginning at the peak of inspiration and following the movement of chest deflation. The frequency of manual vibration is between 12 and 20 Hz (Gormenzano, 1972; Bateman, 1981).
4. If the patient is mechanically ventilated, the previously described techniques must be timed with ventilator-controlled exhalation.
5. If the patient has a rapid respiratory rate, either voluntary or ventilator-controlled, it may be necessary to apply vibration or shaking only during every other exhalation.
6. A mobile chest wall is necessary to apply a compressive force without causing discomfort. If a patient has limited chest wall movement, vibration will probably be better tolerated than shaking.

7. Mechanical vibrators may be used by patients themselves, although only limited attention can be paid to the posterior portions of the lungs.

Advantages and Disadvantages of Vibration/Shaking

The use of vibration or shaking with PD may enhance the mobilization of secretions. Shaking or vibration may be better tolerated than percussion, especially in the postsurgical patient.

Manual vibration and shaking allows the caregiver to assess the pattern and depth of respiration. The stretch on the muscles of respiration during expiration may encourage a deeper inspiration to follow. A mechanical vibrator, more commonly used with pediatric patients, may be preferable for delivery of long-term airway clearance.

The patient cannot apply these techniques herself, except in a limited manner with a mechanical vibrator, so adherence and regular administration of vibration depends on caregiver availability.

The same contraindications for percussion apply because shaking and vibration involve compression to the thorax. The technique of vibration is less constrained by these contraindications than is shaking.

MANUAL HYPERINFLATION

The technique of manual hyperinflation is used in patients with an artificial airway who are mechanically ventilated or who have a tracheostomy. This method of airway clearance promotes mobilization of secretions and reinflates collapsed areas of lung. Two caregivers are necessary to provide this treatment and the coordination between these two people is key to achieving satisfactory results. This technique is shown in Figure 21-9.

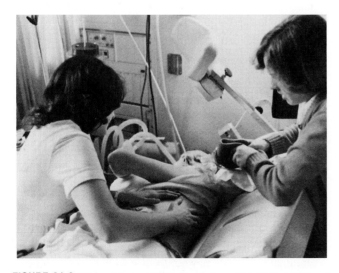

FIGURE 21-9 Manual hyperinflation using a self-inflating bag and chest compression with vibration.

Equipment Required for Manual Hyperinflation

1. A manual ventilation bag attached to an oxygen source is needed for lung inflation. A positive-end expiratory pressure (PEEP) valve may be attached. This is recommended when greater than 10 cm PEEP is being used for mechanical ventilation (Webber, 1993).
2. A second trained caregiver is necessary to provide shaking or vibration in an appropriate sequence with lung inflation.

Preparation for Manual Hyperinflation

1. It may be necessary to premedicate the patient with a sedative or analgesic so that airway clearance may be better tolerated.
2. The two caregivers providing the treatment should be positioned on opposite sides of the bed to allow greater freedom of movement and improved observation of the patient's response to treatment.
3. The positions for treatment will be primarily side lying with the head of the bed flat or slightly elevated to patient tolerance.

Treatment with Manual Hyperinflation

1. One caregiver squeezes the manual ventilation bag slowly to inflate the lungs. A pause is maintained momentarily at the peak of inflation to allow collateral ventilation to fill under-expanded areas of the lung. Release of the bag should be rapid and result in a high expiratory flow rate (Clement, 1968).
2. A second caregiver provides thoracic compression with shaking or vibration to assist with the mobilization of secretions. The compression phase should begin just before the inflation pressure has been released and continue until the end of the expiratory phase.
3. In a patient who is breathing spontaneously, "bag squeezing" with the manual ventilation bag should be timed to augment the patient's inspiratory effort, making vibration more effective (Imle, 1989).
4. After about six cycles of inspiration/expiration, the patient's airway is suctioned using sterile technique. The length of treatment is individualized and depends on the amount of secretions present in the airways and the areas of the lungs affected.
5. Manual hyperinflation may be performed with intubated infants or children using an appropriately sized ventilation bag. Care must be taken to apply slow inflation to avoid a high peak inspiratory pressure, which carries the risk of barotrauma (Webber, 1993).
6. When manual hyperinflation is contraindicated, shaking or vibration may be timed with the expiratory phase of the ventilator without additional inflation during inspiration (Webber, 1988).

BOX 21-1

Active Cycle of Breathing Technique

- Breathing control
Diaphragmatic breathing at normal tidal volume
- 3-4 Thoracic expansion exercises
Deep inhalation with relaxed exhalation at vital capacity, with or without chest percussion
- Breathing control
- 3-4 Thoracic expansion exercises
- Breathing control
- Forced expiratory technique
1-2 Huffs at mid to low lung volume
Abdominal muscle contraction to produce forced exhalation
- Breathing control

Adapted from Webber, B., Pryor, J. (1993). Physiotherapy skills: techniques and adjuncts. In Webber, B. Pryor, J. (Eds). Physiotherapy for respiratory and cardiac problems. Churchill Livingstone: Edinburgh.

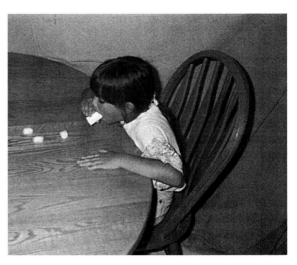

FIGURE 21-10 Using a peak flow meter mouthpiece for huffing.

Advantages and Disadvantages of Manual Hyperinflation

Manual hyperinflation may be helpful in managing airway secretions in those patients requiring long-term mechanical ventilation. In this patient population, the choice of airway clearance techniques is limited, especially when the patient is unresponsive. Manual hyperinflation simulates a cough by augmenting the inspiratory effort, momentarily maintaining a maximal inspiratory hold, and causing an increased expiratory flow.

Hyperinflation has the potential to cause significant barotrauma. There are a number of contraindications to this technique including unstable hemodynamics, pulmonary edema, air leak, and severe bronchospasm (Webber, 1988). In addition, it is not appropriate for infants with increased pulmonary resistance requiring high inflation pressures or in preterm infants at risk of pneumothorax (Webber, 1993). Other contraindications are discussed in Chapter 20. Manual hyperinflation requires two well-trained caregivers. This may be its biggest disadvantage.

ACTIVE CYCLE OF BREATHING TECHNIQUE

The active cycle of breathing technique (ACBT) involves three phases repeated in cycles: breathing control, thoracic expansion, and the forced expiratory technique (FET). This method encourages active participation of the patient and has been shown to be as effective when performed by the patient alone or with the aid of a caregiver (Pryor, 1979). PD positions may be used in conjunction with ACBT. This method of airway clearance may be used with some children as young as 3 or 4 years of age. The sequence of ACBT is shown in Box 21-1.

Equipment Required for ACBT

1. The only equipment required for this manual technique is the patient's or caregiver's hands to percuss or shake/vibrate the chest wall during the thoracic expansion phase.
2. Mechanical percussors or vibrators may be used during the thoracic expansion phase, either for self-percussion by the patient or for use by the caregiver.
3. If PD positions are used, equipment for positioning will be required.
4. To teach the huffing maneuver (part of the FET), it may be helpful to use a peak flow meter mouthpiece to keep the mouth and glottis open (Figure 21-10). Young children may be taught games of huffing at cotton balls or tissue to improve the technique (Webber, 1993). To help them focus on the expiratory maneuver, small children may also be taught to flap their arms to their lateral chest as they perform the huff, a technique referred to as the "chicken breath" (Mahlmeister, 1991).

Preparation for ACBT

1. Most patients tolerate treatment of two or three productive areas during one session.
2. The patient is positioned or positions herself in a PD position to stimulate drainage of a productive area of the lungs. The entire treatment may also be done in the upright sitting position.
3. A minimum of 10 minutes in any productive position may be necessary to clear a patient with a moderate amount of secretions. Patients after surgery or with minimal secretions may not require as much time, and very ill patients may fatigue before optimal treatment is given (Webber, 1993).

Treatment with ACBT

1. During the breathing control phase, the patient is instructed to breathe in a relaxed manner using normal tidal volume. The upper chest and shoulders should remain relaxed and the lower chest and abdomen should be active. The breathing control phase should last as long as is required for the patient to relax and prepare for the next phases, usually 5 to 10 seconds.
2. The emphasis during the thoracic expansion phase is on inspiration. The patient is instructed to take in a deep breath to the inspiratory reserve volume; expiration is passive and relaxed. The caregiver or the patient may place a hand over the area of the thorax being treated to facilitate increased chest wall movement.
3. Chest percussion, shaking, or vibration may be performed in combination with thoracic expansion as the patient exhales. For surgical patients or those with lung collapse, a breath hold or a sniff at the end of inspiration encourages collateral ventilation to redistribute air into collapsed segments and assist with reexpansion of the lung.
4. The FET phase consists of huffing interspersed with breathing control. A huff is a rapid, forced exhalation without maximal effort. This maneuver is comparable to fogging a pair of eyeglasses with warm breath so they may be cleaned. Unlike a cough in which the glottis is closed, a huff requires the glottis remain open. In an effective huff, the muscles of the abdomen should contract to provide greater expiratory force. Other characteristics of effective versus ineffective huffing are shown in Boxes 21-2 and 21-3.
5. Two different levels of huffing are characterized in the FET. To mobilize secretions from peripheral airways, a huff after a medium-sized breath in will be effective. This huff will be longer and quieter. To clear secretions that have reached the larger, proximal airways, a huff after a deep breath in will be effective. This huff will be shorter and louder.
6. The patient must pause for breathing control after one or two huffs. This will prevent any increase in airflow obstruction.

7. The ACBT should be adapted to the individual patient's needs. If secretions are tenacious, two cycles of the thoracic expansion phase may be necessary to loosen secretions before the FET can follow. In a patient with bronchospasm or unstable airways, the breathing control phase may be as long as 10 to 20 seconds (Webber, 1993). After surgery, the patient may be shown how to support the incision with her hands during the FET to achieve sufficient expiratory force.
8. When a huff from a medium-sized inspiration through complete expiration is nonproductive and dry sounding for two cycles in a row, the treatment may be concluded (Pryor, 1991).

Advantages and Disadvantages of ACBT

Incorporation of the ACBT into a treatment of PD and percussion allows the patient to participate actively in a secretion mobilization treatment and offers the prospect of independently managing airway clearance. The ACBT may be introduced at 3 or 4 years of age, with a child becoming independent in the technique at 8 to 10 years of age.

The technique may be adapted for patients with gastroesophageal reflux, bronchospasm, and an acute exacerbation of their pulmonary disease. A decrease in oxygen saturation caused by chest percussion may be avoided by using the ACBT (Pryor, 1990). When the technique is performed independently, the cost of using ACBT for the long term is minimal.

In young children and in extremely ill adults, it will be necessary for a caregiver to assist the patient with this technique. An assistant will also be required for the patient in whom percussion or shaking during the thoracic expansion phase increases the effectiveness of the treatment.

AUTOGENIC DRAINAGE

Autogenic drainage (AD) is a breathing technique that uses expiratory airflow to mobilize bronchial secretions. It is a self-drainage method that is performed independently by the patient in the upright sitting position. AD consists of three phases: (1) the "unsticking" phase, which loosens secretions in the peripheral airways, (2) the "collecting" phase, which moves the secretions to the larger, more central airways, and (3) the "evacuating" phase, which results in the removal of the secretions. This technique of airway clearance requires much patience and concentration to learn and is therefore not suitable for young children. It is ideal, however, for the adolescent or adult who prefers an independent method.

Equipment Required for AD

1. No equipment is needed for a patient to perform the technique of AD. The patient must possess good proprioceptive, tactile, and auditory perception of the mucus moving—this feedback makes it possible to adjust the technique of AD.
2. To teach this method to a patient, a caregiver needs keen tactile and auditory senses to coach a patient to move between the phases by listening to and feeling the location and the quality of the secretions.

Preparation for AD

1. The patient should be seated upright in a chair with a back for support. The surroundings should be devoid of distractions, allowing the patient to concentrate on the breathing technique.
2. The upper airways (nose and throat) should be cleared of secretions by huffing or blowing the nose.
3. The caregiver should be seated to the side and slightly behind the patient, close enough to hear the patient's breathing. One hand should be placed to feel the work of the abdominal muscles and the other hand placed on the upper chest (Figure 21-11).

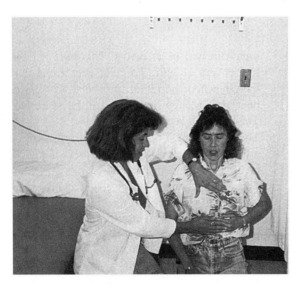

FIGURE 21-11 *Autogenic drainage.*

Treatment with Autogenic Drainage

1. In all phases inhalation should be done slowly, through the nose if possible, using the diaphragm or lower chest. A 2- to 3-second breath hold should follow, allowing collateral ventilation to get air behind the secretions.
2. Exhalation should occur through the mouth with the glottis open, causing the secretions to be heard. The vibrations of the mucus may also be felt with the hand placed on the upper chest. The frequency of these vibrations reveals their location. High frequencies mean that the secretions are located in the small airways; low frequencies mean that the secretions have moved to the large airways (Chevaillier, 1992).
3. The unsticking phase mobilizes mucus from the periphery of the lungs by lowering the mid-tidal volume below the functional residual capacity level (Schoni, 1989). In practice, inspiration is followed by a deep expiration into the expiratory reserve volume. The patient attempts to exhale as far into the expiratory reserve volume as possible, contracting the abdominal muscles to achieve this. This low lung volume breathing continues until the mucus is loosened and starts to move into the larger airways.
4. The collecting phase collects the mucus in the middle airways by increasing the lung volume over the unsticking phase. Tidal volume breathing is then changed gradually from expiratory reserve volume toward the inspiratory reserve volume range (Schoni, 1989) so that the lungs are expanded more with each inspiration. The patient increases both inspiration and expiration to move a greater volume of air. This low to middle lung volume breathing continues until the sound of the mucus decreases, signaling its movement into the central airways to be evacuated.
5. In the evacuating phase, the patient increases inspiration into the inspiratory reserve volume range. This middle-to-high lung volume breathing continues until the secretions are in the trachea and are ready to be expectorated. The collected mucus can be evacuated by a stronger expiration or a high-volume huff. Nonproductive coughing should be avoided, since it may result in collapse of airways. See Figure 21-12 for a diagram of the 3 phases of AD.
6. Compression of the airways should be avoided. If wheezing is heard, the expiratory flow rate must be decreased. Beginners may have to use pursed lips to avoid airway compression (Chevaillier, 1992). Instructing the patient to roll the tongue (if possible) may assist in controlling the expiratory flow rate.
7. A German modification of AD resulted from the observation that many patients had difficulty breathing in the expiratory reserve volume range. In the simplified procedure, the patient begins by varying the mid-tidal volume without excessive effort. After a passive but rapid expiration, an actively performed expiration follows, achieving exhalation to a low expiratory reserve volume (David, 1991). See Figure 21-13 for a description of German AD.

8. The duration of each phase of AD depends on the location of the secretions. The duration of a session depends on the amount and viscosity of the secretions. A patient who is experienced in AD will clear secretions in a shorter amount of time than a beginner. An average treatment will be 30 to 45 minutes in length.

Advantages and Disadvantages of AD

After instruction in the technique of AD has been completed, it may be performed independently by patients over 12 years of age and requires no additional equipment. Because it does not require the use of PD positions, it is appropriate for patients with gastroesophageal reflux. It is also recommended for use in patients with airway hyperreactivity (Pfleger, 1992).

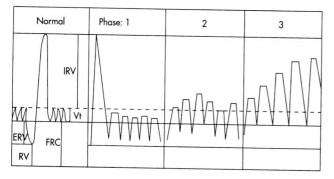

FIGURE 21-12 Phases of autogenic drainage shown on a spirogram of a normal person. Phase 1, unstick; phase 2, collect; phase 3, evacuate. *VT*, Tidal volume; *ERV*, expiratory reserve volume; *RV*, reserve volume; *FRC*, functional residual capacity; *IRV*, inspiratory reserve volume; *IRV + VT + ERV*, vital capacity. *(From Schoni, M.H. [1989]. Autogenic drainage: a modern approach to physiotherapy in cystic fibrosis. Journal of the Royal Society of Medicine 82[Suppl 16]:32-37.)*

Although it is widely used in Europe, the use of AD in the United States is limited by the lack of trained caregivers but is growing in popularity. To learn this technique, patients must demonstrate good self-discipline and possess the ability to concentrate. This method takes more practice than others. A patient must also be available for periodic reevaluation and refinement of the technique.

AD is not the treatment of choice for a patient who is unmotivated or uncooperative, and the study of flow volume curves suggests that AD would not be appropriate for small children even if they were cooperative (Dab, 1979).

The period of hospitalization for an acute pulmonary exacerbation is a difficult time for a patient to learn AD. In fact, patients who are skilled in the technique choose a more passive (less energy consuming) form of airway clearance at such a time until they return to their baseline pulmonary status.

POSITIVE EXPIRATORY PRESSURE

Positive expiratory pressure (PEP) creates a backpressure to stent the airways open during exhalation and promotes collateral ventilation, allowing pressure to build up distal to the obstruction. This method of airway clearance prevents collapse of the airways, which eases the mobilization of secretions from the periphery toward the central airways. A mask or mouthpiece apparatus provides a controlled resistance (10 to 20 cm water pressure) to exhalation and requires a slightly active expiration; tidal volume inspiration is unimpeded.

High-pressure PEP uses the same mask apparatus but at much higher levels of pressure (50 to 120 cm water pressure). Inspiration is performed to total lung capacity; this is followed by a forced expiratory maneuver against the PEP mask.

Intermittent or oscillatory PEP provides (1) positive expiratory pressure, (2) oscillation of the airways and (3)

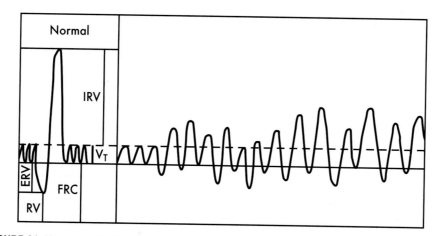

FIGURE 21-13 Autogenic drainage: German method. Autogenic drainage shown on a spirogram of a normal person. The method is not divided into separate phases. *Vt*, Tidal volume; *ERV*, expiratory reserve volume; *RV*, reserve volume; *FRC*, functional residual capacity; *IRV*, inspiratory reserve volume; *IRV + Vt + ERV*, vital capacity). *(From David, A. [1991]. Autogenic drainage—the German approach. In Pryor, J. (Ed). Respiratory care. Edinburgh: Churchill Livingstone.)*

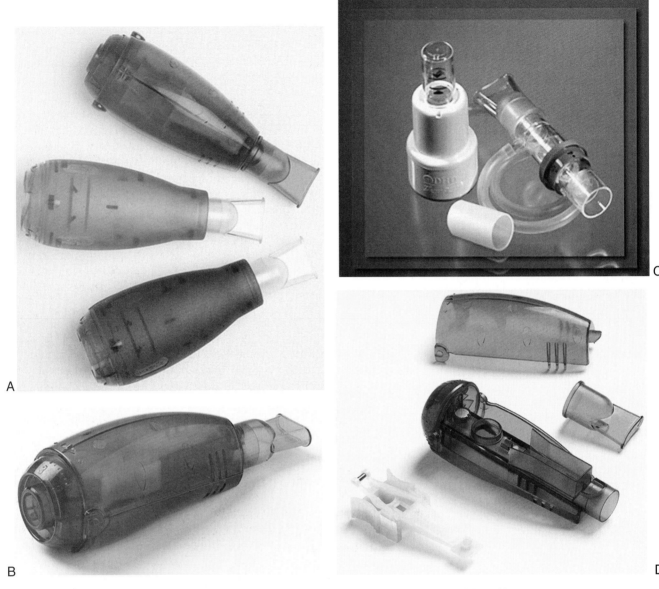

FIGURE 21-14 Positive expiratory pressure devices: TheraPEP and Acapella.

accelerated expiratory flow rates to loosen secretions and move them centrally.

PEP is performed in the upright position and can be used during acute episodes as well as chronic pulmonary conditions. Children over 4 years of age may be instructed in the technique, and PEP may provide an independent method of airway clearance in older children and adults.

Equipment Required For PEP

1. There are several different devices available to deliver positive expiratory pressure consisting of a mouthpiece attached to a valve with adjustable expiratory resistance. One of the more common devices used in the United States is TheraPEP (Figure 21-14). The TheraPEP device consists of a mouthpiece and an expiratory resistor that can

accommodate many levels of expiratory flow. It comes with a detachable pressure monitoring port and indicator to show 10 to 20 cm of water pressure. The TheraPEP can accommodate a mask of 3 different sizes and also allows the user to inhale through the device without removing it from the mouth.

2. Devices available for oscillatory or vibratory PEP are the Flutter valve, the Acapella, and the Quake. Scandipharm Pharmacy (Birmingham, AL) markets the Flutter VRP1 valve (VarioRaw, Switzerland), the first oscillatory PEP device available in the United States. It is a pipe-like mechanism consisting of a mouthpiece, a plastic cone, a steel ball, and a perforated plastic cover. Exhaled air causes the steel ball to roll up and down the cone causing airflow vibration. The Acapella has similar performance characteristics to the Flutter (Volsko, 2003). It comes

in two models: green for patients who can maintain an expiratory flow of 15 l/min or more and blue for patients whose expiratory flow rate is less than 15 l/min. (see Figure 21-14). The Acapella consists of a mouthpiece attached to the body of the unit that uses a counterweighted plug and magnet to create airflow oscillation and an expiratory resistance dial at the other end. The Quake (Thayer Medical, Tucson, AZ) consists of a mouthpiece integrated into the outer housing and a crank with a handle that allows the user to manually adjust the frequency and pressure intensity. The speed of the rotation of the crank varies the frequency of airflow vibrations. This allows the use of a wider range of oscillation frequencies than other devices.

3. For high-pressure PEP therapy, the Astra Meditec (Stroud, Gloucester) mask is used (not available in the United States). The equipment consists of a ventilation mask, a one-way valve and various resistors. Spirometry is used to determine the appropriate resistance for each patient individually, but generally, a 1½ mm resistor is used for infants, a resistor of up to 21½ to 3 mm for older children and adults, and 31½ mm for adults with COPD.

4. A mask can be used in place of the mouthpiece on most of the PEP and oscillatory PEP devices for both the adult and pediatric populations and is preferred by some practitioners. The rationale for using a mask is that the lung volumes should be increased during the entire phase of exhalation through the PEP device, which is more difficult to achieve when using a mouthpiece because the patient may open her mouth around the mouthpiece at the end of expiration causing a fall in lung volumes. (Button, 2002) The use of nose clips is recommended when using a mouthpiece.

5. A manometer may be placed proximal to the resistor in the initial stages of instruction in the use of PEP in most devices. First, the manometer helps to determine and monitor the appropriate level of resistance needed for the patient to achieve 10 to 20 cm of water pressure throughout exhalation. Second, the visual display of the manometer serves as feedback to assist the patient in mastering the technique (Mahlmeister, 1991).

6. Aerosol medication delivered by nebulizer or metered dose inhaler may be placed inline in many devices to be delivered simultaneously with PEP for airway clearance, improving the deposition of medication (Andersen, 1982; Frischnecht-Christensen, 1991). Supplemental oxygen may also be placed inline in many devices for patients who require this.

7. Bubble PEP is a variation of positive expiratory pressure that is particularly useful when treating children. Equipment needed includes: a length of tubing 15 to 18 inches long and a plastic container filled with a column of water 13 cm high (this will generate a positive expiratory pressure of around 20 cm of water pressure). A few drops of food coloring and/or 3 to 6 squirts of liquid detergent or bubble liquid may be added to make the treatment more entertaining. Place the tubing at the very bottom of the

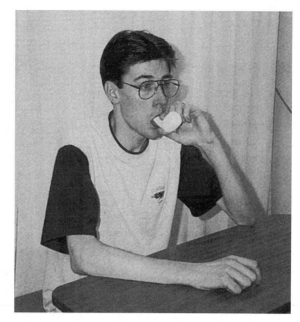

FIGURE 21-15 Use of Flutter valve.

container—it is important that the tube remain at the base of the column of water to generate the required expiratory pressure. If detergent or bubbles are included, place the container in a large bowl or on a towel to contain the overflow (Button, 2002).

8. All PEP devices should be cleaned regularly with hot, soapy water. In the hospital, the equipment should be sterilized according to infection control recommendations. A newer model of the Acapella, the Acapella Choice, disassembles more easily than the original models for cleaning.

Preparation for PEP

1. For PEP therapy, the patient should be seated upright with elbows resting on a table. Use of a mask may require securing the device with both hands for a tight seal. If needed, the patient may be in a reclining position for all PEP devices except the Flutter, which is position dependent. To use the Flutter valve, the patient should be seated upright (Figure 21-15).

2. If aerosolized medication is to be used simultaneously, the patient should be instructed in how to stop the flow of the aerosol when the mask or mouthpiece is removed during the PEP treatment session for coughing.

3. To determine the correct level of resistance for PEP, the patient inhales using tidal volume and exhales actively into the mask or mouthpiece. The resistor valve is adjusted while the level of PEP is monitored on the manometer. The resistance is gradually decreased until the PEP level supplying 10 to 20 cm of water pressure has been identified (Falk 1993). Mahlmeister (1991) reports most patients achieve this pressure range with flow resistors of 2.5 to

4.0 mm in diameter. Selection of the proper resistor produces the desired inspiratory to expiratory ratio of 1:3 or 1:4 (Mahlmeister, 1991). The use of too great a resistance will create an increased respiratory rate or too low a pressure, whereas too small of a resistor will create a slow respiratory rate or too high a pressure (McIlwaine, 1993).

4. For high-pressure PEP, appropriate resistance is determined by connecting the outlet of the PEP mask to a spirometer. Forced vital capacity maneuvers are performed through different expiratory resistors. The resistor producing the highest forced vital capacity through the PEP mask is selected for continued use (Oberwaldner, 1986).

Treatment with PEP

1. The patient should be instructed to breathe into the mask or mouthpiece to tidal volume using the lower chest and abdomen and pause with inspiratory hold for 2 to 3 seconds to equalize ventilation before exhaling (Button 2002). Exhalation into the mask or mouthpiece should be slightly active but not forced. The patient continues breathing into the mask or mouthpiece for 10 to 15 breaths, using a normal respiratory rate. After a series of 10 to 15 breaths, the mask or mouthpiece is removed from the face and the patient performs a series of huffs and/or coughing to expectorate any mucus that has been mobilized. It may be necessary to pause every 5 to 10 exhalations before resuming the session (Althaus, 1993)

2. The series of PEP breaths followed by huffs should be repeated about four to six times. The total treatment lasts about 15 to 20 minutes and should be performed twice during the day or as needed. The frequency and duration of the treatment must be individualized for each patient. During periods of pulmonary exacerbation, patients are encouraged to increase the frequency of PEP treatments rather than extend the length of individual sessions (Mahlmeister, 1991). Some patients have a tendency to hyperventilate and become dizzy; an inspiratory pause will prevent this (Button 2002).

3. Initially the patient and caregiver monitor the effort by means of the manometer, ensuring that a pressure of 10 to 20 cm of water pressure is achieved throughout exhalation (this is not possible with the Flutter). After the technique is mastered with the appropriate resistor, the manometer may be removed from the system. The appropriate resistance should be rechecked periodically during clinical visits or periods of hospitalization.

4. The recommended procedure for use of the Flutter is shown in Box 21-4. The full effects of the vibration induced by the Flutter (6 to 20 Hz) may be received by changing the angle of the device. Movement of the Flutter upward increases the pressure and frequency while movement of the device downward results in lower pressure and frequency (Althaus, 1993). The vibration of the chest may be palpated to provide feedback as to the optimal angle of the device.

BOX 21-4

Proper Patient Technique for Using Flutter

1. Gather supplies, relax, and assume proper posture and position.
   Begin stage 1, mucus loosening and mucus mobilization.
2. Slowly inhale beyond a normal breath, but do not fill lungs completely.
3. Hold breath for 2 to 3 seconds.
4. Place Flutter in mouth, adjust tilt, and keep cheeks stiff.
5. Exhale through Flutter at a reasonably fast but not too forceful speed.
6. Exhale beyond a normal breath, but do not empty lungs completely.
7. Attempt to suppress cough.
8. Repeat steps 2 through 7 for 5 to 10 breaths.
   Begin stage 2, mucus elimination
9. Slowly inhale, filling lungs completely.
10. Hold breath for 2 to 3 seconds.
11. Place Flutter in mouth, adjust tilt, and keep cheeks stiff.
12. Exhale forcefully through Flutter as completely as possible.
13. Repeat steps 9 through 12 for 1 to 2 breaths.
14. Initiate cough (or "huff" maneuver). Return to step 2 and repeat full sequence until lungs are clear or therapy is over.
15. Additional sessions may be added if necessary.
16. Clean Flutter and store in clean, dry location.

For more information about Flutter, contact Scandipharm, 22 Inverness Center Parkway, Birmingham, AL 35242; phone 800-950-8085; www.scandipharm.com.

5. When using the Quake, it is recommended to rotate the handle at a steady and comfortable rate of about 1 to 2 rotations per second during exhalation. At the end of exhalation, the user may either remove the Quake from the mouth to inhale or continue to rotate the handle and slowly begin to breathe in deeply, then repeat the exhalation cycle. Both the inhalation and exhalation rate and the speed of the handle rotation may be varied to produce the ideal level of vibration in the lungs (Thayer Medical).

6. The procedure for use of high-pressure PEP differs from that of low-pressure PEP. The expiratory pressure used in this method usually ranges between 50 and 120 cm of water pressure. The patient breathes in and out through the mask at tidal volume for 6 to 10 breaths, then inspiration is done to total lung capacity and a forced expiratory maneuver is performed against the PEP mask. This is repeated until all the mucus is mobilized (McIlwaine, 1993).

7. For Bubble PEP, the patient is instructed to blow through the tube with enough force to cause the bubbles to rise up to the top of the container. After a number of breaths, the patient is asked to do huffing or coughing before resuming the treatment. The therapist may prescribe the height of the column of water to alter the pressure, the number of breaths taken, and the huffs or coughs needed to tailor the treatment to each patient (Button 2002).

Advantages and Disadvantages of PEP

PEP therapy does not possess some of the limitations of conventional PD and percussion for secretion clearance and is therefore applicable to a wider patient population. It is relatively easy to learn in one or two sessions, and may be applied equally to the pediatric and adult populations. PEP is appropriate for use in hospitalized patients, as well as for long-term use at home.

The expense of the equipment is minimal, and once the patient is competent in the technique, it provides independence (except for small children). All of the PEP devices are quite portable, making airway clearance easier to perform during travel or when away from home during the day. PEP devices can be used in any position except the Flutter, which is position dependent.

Some musical instruments can provide a form of PEP therapy due to the manner in which they are played, with an inspiratory pause and resisted exhalation (Button 2002). These instruments include the clarinet, oboe, bassoon, French horn, trumpet, flute and voice.

A decision to use PEP should be carefully evaluated in cases of acute sinusitis, ear infection, epistaxis, and recent oral or facial surgery or injury (Mahlmeister, 1991). For PEP therapy to be effective, a patient should be able to cooperate and actively participate with the treatment. Although rare, pneumothorax has been reported with high-pressure PEP (Oberwaldner, 1986).

Low-pressure PEP is more commonly used in North America because it is felt to be as effective, easier, and safer to use and monitor than high-pressure PEP. In those patients in whom PEP is an appropriate airway clearance technique, a high degree of acceptance has been shown (Falk, 1984; Steen, 1991; Volsko, 2003). This may translate into better adherence in the long term.

HIGH FREQUENCY CHEST WALL OSCILLATION

High frequency chest wall oscillation (HFCWO), also referred to as high frequency chest compression, consists of an inflatable vest linked to an air-pulse generator. Although the sensation of the device is somewhat akin to mechanical percussion, it differs significantly in its mechanism of action. HFCWO works by differential airflow (i.e., the expiratory flow rate is higher than the inspiratory flow rate), allowing the mucus to be transported from the periphery to the central airways for expectoration. HFCWO has also been shown to decrease the viscosity of mucus, making it easier to mobilize. Figure 21-16 shows a patient using HFCWO.

Equipment Required for HFCWO

1. Two devices of HFCWO are available, the Vest Airway Clearance System (Hill-Rom, St. Paul, MN) and the MedPulse Respiratory Vest System (Electromed, Inc., Huntsville, AL). The original, larger unit is best used in a

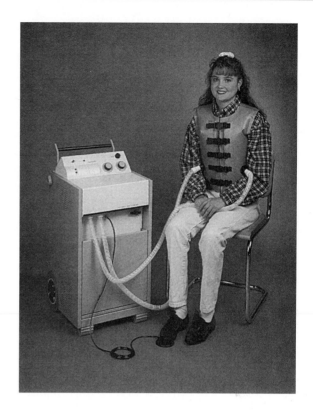

FIGURE 21-16 *Patient using the Vest Airway Clearance System for high frequency chest wall oscillation.*

clinical setting; it can be placed on a wheeled stand for easy mobility. Newer models of the air-pulse generator weigh as little as 17 lbs, providing more mobility than earlier models. These units will fit under an airplane seat and are easier to manage during travel.

2. The inflatable vest is constructed to fit over the entire thorax and should extend to the top of the thigh when the patient is sitting upright. Different sizes are available (from toddler to large adult). For the hospital setting, adjustable vests are available for use with multiple patients (following appropriate infection control guidelines for cleaning). For home use, each patient is fitted for her own vest. A shorter, chest vest is also available, which results in less pressure to the abdominal area, resulting in less gastric discomfort.

3. Simultaneous use of aerosolized medication is recommended for use throughout the treatment. This humidifies the air to counteract the drying effect of the increased airflow.

Preparation for HFCWO

1. The patient should be seated upright in a chair. The vest should fit properly, but breathing should not feel restricted while the vest is deflated. A single layer of clothing should be worn under the vest.

2. It is important that the tubing be securely connected to the air pulse generator.

3. Start the aerosol therapy before turning on the HFCWO system.
4. The pressure control setting should be adjusted according to patient comfort, opting for the highest pressure that is well tolerated.

Treatment with HFCWO

1. The treatment should progress through different frequencies, from low (7 to 10 Hz) to medium (10 to 14 Hz) and then to high (14 to 20 Hz), to achieve both higher flow rates and increased lung volume. Warwick (1991) reported that the frequencies associated with the highest flow rates were usually greater than 13 Hz, whereas those associated with the largest volume were usually less than 10 Hz.
2. The average length of time spent at each frequency is 10 minutes, but this will vary according to patient tolerance, amount and consistency of secretions, and the acuity of the patient's illness. After treatment at each frequency for the prescribed length of time, the patient should be instructed to huff or cough to clear loosened secretions.
3. HFCWO has also been used with patients requiring long-term mechanical ventilation. Whitman et al. (1993) found use of HFCWO to be safe and effective and that it resulted in time savings over conventional PD and percussion.
4. Patients requiring central intravenous (IV) access such as a Porta-cath or Hickman are able to use HFCWO with sufficient padding (such as a foam doughnut pillow) to relieve pressure around the access site.

Advantages and Disadvantages of HFCWO

This method of airway clearance allows independence and is easy to learn in a short period. HFCWO is now designed to accommodate children as young as 2 years of age, and a vest may be custom-made for very large or obese adults. HFCWO is appropriate for those patients in whom PD positions are contraindicated, and it has been used successfully in reclining patients who are unable to tolerate the upright sitting position.

Use of HFCWO may result in time savings at home as well as in a hospital or long-term care facility due to the fact that nebulized medications are administered concurrently with the airway clearance treatment and all lobes of the lungs are treated simultaneously. The amount of time for patient contact required for a hospital caregiver is much less with this method than with conventional PD and percussion. This efficiency would also benefit families in which there is more than one member requiring airway clearance (such as siblings with cystic fibrosis).

A disadvantage of HFCWO as a method of airway clearance is the cost of the equipment. A study by Ohnsorg (1994), however, demonstrated a decline in total health care costs for the year after HFCWO was put into use by 11 patients. A study of the impact of the device in a hospital setting (Klous, 1993) showed a substantial savings as a result of therapy self-administration. Replacement of the equipment should not be a factor, as a lifetime warranty is available for both devices. In those patients for whom it is appropriate (and reimbursable), HFCWO is an effective method of airway clearance. It provides independence for long-term use at home as well as for acute exacerbations in the hospital.

INTRAPULMONARY PERCUSSIVE VENTILATION

The intrapulmonary percussive ventilator (IPV) is an airway clearance device that simultaneously delivers intrathoracic percussion and aerosolized solution for bronchodilation (Homnick, 1994). An apparatus known as the phasitron is the functional component in the IPV. The phasitron provides high-frequency impulses during inspiration, while positive expiratory pressure is maintained throughout passive exhalation. The pressure generated with IPV is between 10 to 30 cm of water pressure.

IPV is similar to HFCWO except that a pneumatic device delivers the oscillation internally instead of externally. A mouthpiece delivers high flow rate mini-bursts of gases into the lungs at rates of 100 to 240 cycles per minute. Continuous pressure in the airways is maintained while pulsatile, percussive intra airway pressure rises and dilates the airways, enhancing intrabronchial secretion mobilization. The aerosol mist within the lungs reduces adhesive forces of retained secretions.

Equipment Required for IPV

1. One model of IPV meant for institutional use is the Percussionaire Model IPV-1 (Percussionaire Corp., Sandpoint, ID). Percussive rates or frequencies range from under 100 to greater than 225 cycles per minute. It has the capability to be used with an endotracheal tube, and can be installed on a stand for greater mobility.
2. The Percussionaire Impulsator is self-contained for home use, but may also be used in a clinical situation. It generates 40-psi source pressure, which provides for efficient delivery of impulses and aerosolized medication. Condensation is minimal compared to institutional models, so maintenance on the unit is low.

Treatment with IPV

1. Aerosolized medication in saline solution is delivered via the nebulizer component of the IPV unit.
2. Each percussive interval is programmed by the clinician or the patient at home. Treatment with IPV is titrated for patient comfort and visible thoracic movement. A thumb button is held for 5 to 10 second intervals to initiate the percussive impulses and released after an interval to allow exhalation. After each deep exhalation, the percussive interval starts again.
3. When the patient has the desire to cough or expectorate, the thumb button is released until coughing is completed or secretions are cleared.
4. An average treatment lasts about 20 minutes.

Advantages and Disadvantages of IPV

IPV is available for home use and can be continued during hospitalization. IPV allows for greater independence for adolescents and adults with long-term need for airway clearance. Homnick (1994) reported that three fourths of the patients using IPV in one study estimated increased sputum production, and satisfaction was high for comfort and independence.

IPV is neither appropriate for nor tolerated by young children. In other patients, a feeling of claustrophobia or chest fullness may hinder the decision to use IPV (Downs 2004). It is more expensive than a PEP device but less costly than a unit for HFCWO. The availability of IPV in the clinical setting is not as common as other airway clearance devices; therefore, respiratory care practitioners may not be as familiar or comfortable with its application. The use of IPV may increase as more research is done to demonstrate its benefit.

EXERCISE FOR AIRWAY CLEARANCE

A regular program of exercise has been shown to improve many outcomes in patients with lung disease. Peak oxygen consumption, maximal work capacity, respiratory muscle endurance, and exercise tolerance all improve with an exercise program (Orenstein, 1981, Andreasson, 1987). Secretion clearance is also improved with exercise (Zach, 1981; Oldenburg, 1979). Based on improvement in pulmonary function, exercise has been recommended as a replacement, partial or complete, for conventional chest physical therapy (PD and percussion) (Zach, 1982; Cerny, 1989; Andreasson, 1987). Exercise for secretion clearance has focused on aerobic or endurance exercise; however, any form of exercise must be adapted to the individual patient's status and abilities.

Equipment Required for Exercise

1. A walking program requires only a suitable pair of shoes and a safe location. Jogging, because of increased stress on the knees, requires shoes specifically for that purpose.
2. The following exercise equipment may be suitable for a patient who is beginning an exercise program: treadmill, bicycle ergometer, elliptical trainer, mini-trampoline, or arm ergometer.
3. For more accomplished exercisers or patients with a higher exercise tolerance, equipment may include a stair climber, cross-country ski machine, or rowing machine. Other activities that provide positive benefits are too numerous to mention; the patient's interests should be the primary factor for choosing.
4. Tools to monitor a patient's response to exercise include a sphygmomanometer, stethoscope, heart rate monitor, pulse oximeter, and a scale to measure patient's level of perceived exertion (Figure 21-17).
5. Supplemental oxygen and oxygen delivery supplies will be necessary for those patients who exhibit oxygen desaturation during exercise.

6	
7	Very, very light
8	
9	Very light
10	
11	Fairly light
12	
13	Somewhat hard
14	
15	Hard
16	
17	Very hard
18	
19	Very, very hard
20	

FIGURE 21-17 Original perceived exertion scale. *(From Borg, G. [1982]. Psychophysical basis of perceived exertion. Medicine and Science in Sports and Exercise 14:377.)*

Preparation for Exercise

1. Patients with hyperreactive airways should be premedicated with a prescribed bronchodilator before an exercise session.
2. Baseline vital signs should be recorded before beginning the activity. In a home setting, patients should be knowledgeable in self-monitoring exercise intensity. For those patients who require closer monitoring, a pulse oximeter may be rented from an oxygen supply company.

Treatment with Exercise

1. The principles of an exercise prescription addressing mode, intensity, duration, and frequency, as well as principles of warm up and cool down are addressed elsewhere in this text and should be followed when using exercise as a form of airway clearance. Individualizing an exercise program for each patient is important.
2. Patients in the hospital for an acute exacerbation may not be able to initially perform endurance exercise. They should be started slowly and progressed as tolerated. Monitoring of heart rate, blood pressure, oxygen saturation, respiratory rate, and level of perceived exertion before and during exercise, and during recovery, will allow titration of the workload for optimal performance.

3. The patient should be instructed in huffing or controlled coughing to expectorate secretions as they are loosened.
4. A regular, consistent program of exercise should be scheduled around the patient's daily activities to achieve adherence (e.g., walking the dog, sports at school, stopping by the health club after work).

Advantages and Disadvantages of Exercise for Airway Clearance

Exercise has the advantage of being the only airway clearance technique that is performed regularly by people without lung disease. This factor can make it appealing to those patients who do not want to call attention to their differences from their peers. Exercise may improve self-esteem, a sense of well being, and quality of life. The level of exercise tolerance in patients with cystic fibrosis has been demonstrated to be of prognostic value (Nixon, 1992).

Many patients do not tolerate the amount or frequency of exercise required to utilize it as the sole method of airway clearance. For this reason, it is recommended as an adjunct to other techniques. This is particularly true during an acute exacerbation when activity tolerance is limited, or in infants or patients with neurological or musculoskeletal limitations.

Care must be taken in prescribing exercise to patients with hyperreactive airways or a tendency toward oxygen desaturation. Use of bronchodilator medication and supplemental oxygen may be necessary to improve exercise tolerance, but these patients require closer monitoring as well.

Andreasson (1987) observed that regular contact with a caregiver seems to be necessary for successful exercise training, as does family support, especially in young children. Adherence will also be affected by a patient's preference for a particular activity, scheduling conflicts, and commitment by friends and family members.

SELECTION OF AIRWAY CLEARANCE TECHNIQUES

The process of prescribing an appropriate technique for secretion mobilization should be ongoing, with periodic reevaluation of the method and its effects on the patient. Because of the low adherence reported with conventional chest physical therapy (Passero, 1981), it is necessary for caregivers to address the many factors that may alter a patient's adherence to a particular method. These factors include the availability of the caregiver to teach the technique and the willingness of the patient to learn it; the patient's concurrent medical problems; the effectiveness of the technique (subjective and objective); support for the technique from family, friends, and health care personnel; age and lifestyle of the patient; and the cost of the treatment (Downs, 2004). Table 21-1 summarizes factors that influence the choice of an airway clearance technique.

AVAILABILITY

Many techniques of airway clearance that have been used in Europe for some time are new to health care providers in the United States. Use of a method may be limited by the lack of caregivers trained to instruct patients in a particular technique. This is especially true for AD, which takes longer for a caregiver to learn how to teach than does PEP or HFCWO. The ACBT is easily incorporated into conventional chest physical therapy by learning the FET and modifying the use of percussion or shaking. Manual hyperinflation, on the other hand, because of increased precautions for its use, requires more study and observation before implementation. Exercise for airway clearance may be out of the realm of a caregiver who is trained in respiratory care but not familiar with exercise principles.

The patient's availability must also be taken into consideration. A single outpatient clinic visit does not lend itself to instruction in AD, but instruction in PEP, ACBT, and HFCWO can be initiated and further training can be provided during return visits. On the other hand, if a patient is admitted for exacerbation of a pulmonary disease, the patient is a captive audience for instruction in a variety of techniques, including AD or a home exercise program once the acute stage has passed.

The key to success of airway clearance is the reevaluation of any technique used. The patient and caregiver must be available to demonstrate and review the technique periodically so that modifications can be made. A change in a patient's level of independence or motivation, a decline or marked improvement in pulmonary status, or a decrease in the effectiveness of a technique all necessitate reevaluation of the current method.

EFFECTIVENESS

Another consideration in selecting a technique is the effectiveness of the technique measured both subjectively and objectively. Objective measures include pulmonary function studies, chest x-rays, arterial blood gas values, changes in mechanical ventilator settings, changes in auscultation, and quantity of sputum produced. A patient's response to treatment can be evaluated by changes in heart rate, respiratory rate, oxygen saturation, and level of perceived exertion.

A patient's subjective response to the treatment has implications for adherence to any technique. The ease of sputum mobilization and the quantity of sputum expectorated are useful feedback for a patient. The effort that a treatment requires, or more importantly, the amount of energy remaining after completion of the treatment, will affect the patient's willingness to continue.

Complications that occur as a result of a technique or precautions associated with a particular method must guide a patient and caregiver to find an alternate technique in many instances. A patient hospitalized with an acute pulmonary exacerbation may need to be assisted with a more passive

TABLE 21-1

Considerations when Selecting an Airway Clearance Technique

TECHNIQUE	AGE OF PATIENT	ASSISTANT NEEDED	EQUIPMENT NEEDED	DURING ACUTE EXACERBATION	CONCURRENT NEBULIZER	PRECAUTIONS	COST
PD, percussion, vibration/shaking	Any age	Yes	Positioning aids; percussor/vibrator; devices for infants	Yes	Only in upright	See Chapter 20; may modify positions; repetitive motion injuries	Expensive if performed by caregiver long-term
Manual hyperinflation	Extra care with infants	Two assistants needed	Manual ventilation bag	Yes, with tracheostomy or mechanical ventilation	Not usually	Pulmonary edema, air leak, bronchospasm, unstable, risk of pneumothorax	Expensive due to caregivers, but usually used short-term
ACBT	Begin to teach at 3-4 years of age	Until 8-10 years of age	Positioning aids; percussor/vibrator	Yes	Only in upright	Only precautions for head-down positions (see Chapter 20)	Cost is low if done independently
AD	Age ≥12 years	No	None	Best to use an alternative	No	Takes time to learn	No cost
PEP	Begin to teach at 3-4 years of age	Until 8-10 years of age	Mouthpiece or mask; PEP device; manometer	Yes	Yes, except flutter	Sinusitis, epistaxis, ear infection, risk of pneumothorax	Minimal, but devices require replacement
IPV	Adolescents and adults	While in hospital	Home unit; unit for hospital setting	May not be well tolerated	Yes	Titrate for comfort and visible chest movement	Moderate expense
HFCWO	Age ≥2-3 years	For young children	Air pulse generator; appropriately sized vest	Yes	Yes	Chest tube, indwelling catheter, or other device in chest area	Very expensive
Exercise	Children, adolescents, and adults	For young children	Variable	No	Premedicate before exercise	Exercise-induced bronchospasm; oxygen desaturation; adjunct to ACT	Depends on type of exercise

method of secretion clearance until the patient's condition allows a return to a more independent technique. A patient with hyperreactive airways may find that bronchospasm renders percussion ineffective. The presence of gastroesophageal reflux may force the decision to use a technique that can be performed in an upright position. Sinus surgery may make use of a PEP mask intolerable. Placement of a chest tube may necessitate a temporary replacement for HFCWO.

SUPPORT

When airway clearance must take place on a daily basis, it becomes necessary to accommodate a patient's schedule. A patient may have a preference for the most effective treatment performed in the shortest amount of time. A patient may also be interested in performing another activity during the airway clearance treatment: AD or PEP may be performed while riding in a car (as a passenger); HFCWO can be conducted while studying for an examination or surfing the web; and a patient can be watching the news while running on a treadmill or during percussion by an assistant.

Many patients adopt a multifaceted approach to secretion clearance, becoming adept at several methods and using them as conditions dictate. Patients who use AD or exercise primarily will need to use an alternate form of airway clearance during an acute exacerbation of an illness. Use of HFCWO at home may necessitate use of a more portable technique when away from home during the day. Patients who rely on an assistant to perform percussion may need to learn a more independent method for occasions when the assistant is not available.

In a home where more than one family member requires ongoing airway clearance, as can be the case for parents of children with cystic fibrosis, spending the least amount of time for the greatest benefit becomes of primary importance. For an infant or young child, an adult must be responsible for performing secretion mobilization. As the child grows older and the choices of a technique increase, close supervision remains necessary. In the adolescent, even when physical assistance is no longer required, emotional support from family and friends is paramount to continued success with a technique. Finally, the support received from health care providers is vital to the patient's motivation to continue with a technique or to learn a new one.

COST

In this age of skyrocketing health care costs, especially for long-term care and chronic disease, the expense of a treatment must be considered. The initial cost of equipment, replacement costs, and the expense of assistance required all figure into the total cost of treatment.

The generator for HFCWO is the most costly piece of equipment presented here, but replacement should not be necessary. PEP devices are relatively inexpensive, with replacement of equipment expected to occur several times during a lifetime of use. AD and ACBT require no equipment.

Payment of a trained assistant for home use of PD and percussion when family support is not available is a great expense. Depending on the duration and frequency of treatment, this cost may outweigh that for other airway clearance techniques on a long-term basis.

Often the choice of an airway clearance technique is limited by the reimbursement available for equipment or assistance by a third party payer. Nonetheless, the caregiver must strike a balance between economic and clinical considerations in choosing a mode of therapy.

SUMMARY

Numerous airway clearance techniques have been shown to reduce obstruction, enhance mucociliary clearance, and improve ventilation, accomplishing the goal of improved oxygen transport. Their effectiveness has been demonstrated in multiple studies and evaluated with numerous outcome measures. Caregivers must incorporate this information into the real life situations presented by patients and choose a technique or combination of techniques that best suits each individual patient's needs.

An individualized approach to airway clearance requires consideration of a multitude of variables, physiological, psychological, and practical, that affects a patient's response to treatment. Health care providers are challenged to keep abreast of techniques and their modifications to best provide for the patient's needs. The role of the caregiver involves more than technical expertise. The caregiver is uniquely positioned to simplify medical language for patients and families and encourage adherence to airway clearance. Support of a treatment by a health care provider can increase the benefit derived from the treatment.

Further study is needed to compare and standardize techniques, follow long-term outcomes, and establish optimal treatment guidelines. This information will assist both patients and caregivers to maximize treatment with airway clearance techniques.

Review questions

1. Which ACTs can be performed without purchasing specialized equipment?
2. Are there any ACTs that are *not* suitable for patients in an intensive care unit?
3. What are the airway clearance methods most suited for instruction during a single outpatient clinic visit?
4. What outcome measures do you have at your disposal for evaluating the effectiveness of airway clearance?
5. How would you encourage adherence of a prescribed method of airway clearance in:
   - An independent adolescent with a spinal cord injury?
   - A 3-year-old newly diagnosed with cystic fibrosis?
   - An older adult with bronchiectasis?

REFERENCES

Althaus, P. (1993). Oscillating PEP. In Bronchial hypersecretion: current chest physiotherapy in cystic fibrosis (CF). International Committee for CF (IPC/CF).

Andersen, J.B., Klausen, N.O. (1982). A new mode of administration of nebulized bronchodilator in severe bronchospasm. European Journal of Respiratory Diseases 119(Suppl 63):97-100.

Andreasson, B., Jonson, B., Kornfalt, R., Nordmark, E. & Sandstrom, S. (1987). Long-term effects of physical exercise on working capacity and pulmonary function in cystic fibrosis. Acta Paediatr Scand 76:70-75.

Bateman, J., Newman, S.P., Daunt, K.M., Panà, D., & Clarke, S.W. (1979). Regional lung clearance of excessive bronchial secretions during chest physical therapy in patients with stable chronic airways obstruction. Lancet 1:294-297.

Bateman, J.R., Newman, S.P., Daunt, K.M., Sheahan, N.F., Pavia, D. & Clarke, S.W. (1981). Is cough as effective as chest physiotherapy in the removal of excessive tracheobronchial secretions? Thorax 36:683-687.

Button, B., McIlwaine M. (2002) Airway clearance techniques training class. Presented at the Sixteenth Annual North American Cystic Fibrosis Conference, New Orleans.

Cerny, F.J. (1989). Relative effects of bronchial drainage and exercise for in-hospital care of patients with cystic fibrosis. Physical Therapy 69:633-639.

Chevaillier, J. (1992). Airway clearance techniques. Presented at Sixth Annual North American Cystic Fibrosis Conference, Dallas.

Clement, A.J., Hubsch, S.K. (1968). Chest physiotherapy by the 'bag squeezing' method: a guide to technique. Physiotherapy 54:355-359.

Crane, L.D. (1990). Physical therapy for the neonate with respiratory disease. In Irwin, S., Tecklin, J.S. (Eds). Cardiopulmonary physical therapy. St. Louis: Mosby. p. 409-410.

Dab, I., Alexander, F. (1979). The mechanism of autogenic drainage studied with flow volume curves. Mon Paed 10:50-53.

David, A. (1991). Autogenic drainage-the German approach. In Pryor, J. (Ed). Respiratory care. Edinburgh: Churchill Livingstone.

Downs, A.M., Lindsay, K.L.B. (2004). Physical therapy associated with airway clearance dysfunction. In DeTurk, W.E., Cahalin, L.P., (Eds). Cardiovascular and pulmonary physical therapy: an evidence-based approach. New York: McGraw Hill. p. 463-490.

Falk, M., Kelstrup, M., Andersen, J.B., Kinoshita, T., Falk, P., Stovring, S., & Gothgen, L. (1984). Improving the ketchup bottle method with PEP, PEP in cystic fibrosis. European Journal of Respiratory Diseases 65:423-432.

Frownfelter, D. (1987). Postural drainage. In Frownfelter, D. (Ed). Chest physical therapy and pulmonary rehabilitation, ed 2. Chicago: Year Book Medical Publishers. p. 265-290.

Frischknecht-Christensen, E., Norregaard, O., Dahl, R. (1991). Treatment of bronchial asthma with terbutaline inhaled by conespacer combined with positive expiratory pressure mask. Chest 100:317-321.

Gormenzano, J., Branthwaite, M.A. (1972). Pulmonary physiotherapy with assisted ventilation. Anaesthesia 27:249-257.

Homnick, D., Spillers, C., White, F. (1994). The intrapulmonary percussive ventilator compared to standard aerosol therapy and chest physiotherapy in the treatment of patients with cystic fibrosis. Abstracted in Pediatric Pulmonology 10(Suppl):266.

Imle, P.C., (1989). Percussion and vibration. In Mackenzie, (Ed). Chest physical therapy in the intensive care unit, ed 2. Baltimore: Williams & Wilkins. p. 134-152.

Klous, D., Boyle, M., Hazelwood, A., & McComb, R.C. (1993). Chest vest and cystic fibrosis: better care for patients. Advanced Respiratory Care Management 3:44-50.

Klous, D.R. (1994). High-frequency chest wall oscillation: principles and applications. Published by American Biosystems, Inc., St. Paul. p. 626-630.

Mahlmeister, M.J., Fink, J.B., Hoffman, G.L., & Fifer, L.F. (1991). Positive-expiratory-pressure mask therapy: theoretical and practical considerations and a review of the literature. Respiratory Care 36:1218-1229.

McIlwaine, M. (1993). Airway clearance techniques (ACT) refresher class. Presented at Seventh Annual North American Cystic Fibrosis Conference, Dallas.

Natale, J.E., Pfeifle, J. & Homnick, D.N. (1994). Comparison of intrapulmonary percussive ventilation and chest physiotherapy: a pilot study in patients with cystic fibrosis. Chest 105:1789-1895.

Nixon, P.A. (1992). The prognostic value of exercise testing in patients with cystic fibrosis. New England Journal of Medicine 327:1785-1788.

Oberwaldner, B., Evans, J.C., Zach, M.S. (1986). Forced expirations against a variable resistance: a new chest physiotherapy method in cystic fibrosis. Pediatric Pulmonology 2:358-367.

Ohnsorg, F. (1994). A cost analysis of high-frequency chest wall oscillation in cystic fibrosis. Abstract presented at the ALA/ATS International Conference, Boston.

Oldenberg, F.A. Jr., Dolovich, M.B., Montgomery, J.M., & Newhouse, M.T. (1979). Effects of postural drainage, exercise, and cough on mucus clearance in chronic bronchitis. American Review of Respiratory Diseases 120:739-745.

Orenstein, D.M., Franklin, B.A., Doershuk, C.F., Hellerstein, H.K., Germann, K.J., Horowitz, J.G., & Stern, R.C. (1981). Exercise conditioning and cardiopulmonary fitness in cystic fibrosis. Chest 80:392-398.

Passero, M.A., Remor, B., Salomon, J. (1981). Patient-reported compliance with cystic fibrosis therapy. Clinical Pediatrics 20:265-268.

Pfleger, A., Theissl, B., Oberwaldner, B., & Zach, M.S. (1992). Self-administered chest physiotherapy in cystic fibrosis: a comparative study of high-pressure PEP and autogenic drainage. Lung 170:323-330.

Pryor, J.A., Webber, B.A., Hodson, M.E., & Batten, J.C. (1979). Evaluation of the forced expiration technique as an adjunct to postural drainage in treatment of cystic fibrosis. British Medical Journal 18:417-418.

Pryor, J.A., Webber B.A., Hodson, M.E. (1990). Effect of chest physiotherapy on oxygen saturation in patients with cystic fibrosis 45:77.

Pryor, J.A. (1991). The forced expiration technique. In Pryor, J.A. (Ed). Respiratory care. Edinburgh: Churchill Livingstone. p. 79-100.

Rodeberg, D.A., Maschinot, N.E., Housinger, T.A., & Warden, G.D. (1992). Decreased pulmonary barotrauma with the use of volumetric diffusive respiration in pediatric patients with burns: the 1992 Moyer Award. Journal of Burn Care Rehabilitation 13:506-511.

Samuelson, W., Woodward, F., Lowe, V. (1994). Utility of a dynamic air therapy bed vs. conventional chest physiotherapy in adult CF patients [abstract]. Pediatric Pulmonology 10(Suppl):266.

Schoni, M.H. (1989). Autogenic drainage: a modern approach to physiotherapy in cystic fibrosis. Journal of the Royal Society of Medicine 82(Suppl 16):32-37.

Steen, H.F., Redmond, A.O., O'Neill, D., & Beattie, F. (1991). Evaluation of the PEP mask in cystic fibrosis. Acta Paediatr Scand 80:51-56.

Sutton, P.P., Lopez-Vidriero, M.T., Panà, D., Newman, S.P., Clay, M.M., Webber, B., Parker, R.A., & Clarke, S.W. (1985). Assessment of percussion, vibratory-shaking and breathing exercise in chest physical therapy. European Journal of Respiratory Diseases 66:147-152.

Volsko, TA, DiFiore, J., & Chatburn, R.L. (2003). Performance comparison of two oscillating positive expiratory pressure devices: Acapella versus Flutter. Resp Care 48:124-130.

Warwick, W.J., Hansen, L.G. (1991). The long-term effect of high-frequency chest compression therapy on pulmonary complications of cystic fibrosis. Pediatric Pulmonology 11:265-271.

Webber, B.A. (1988). Physiotherapy for patients receiving mechanical ventilation. In Webber, B.A. (Ed). The Brompton hospital guide to chest physiotherapy, ed 5. Oxford: Blackwell Scientific Publications.

Webber, B., Pryor, J. (1993). Active cycle of breathing techniques. In Bronchial hypersecretion: current chest physiotherapy in cystic fibrosis (CF). Published by International Physiotherapy Committee for Cystic Fibrosis (IPC/CF).

Webber, B.A., Pryor, J.A. (1993). Physiotherapy skills: techniques and adjuncts. In Physiotherapy for respiratory and cardiac problems. Edinburgh: Churchill Livingstone.

Whitman, J., Van Beusekom, R., Olson, S., Worm, M., & Indihar, F. (1993). Preliminary evaluation of high-frequency chest compression for secretion clearance in mechanically ventilated patients. Respiratory Care 38:1081-1087.

Zach, M.S., Purrer, B., Oberwaldner B. (1981). Effect of swimming on forced expiration and sputum clearance in cystic fibrosis. Lancet 11:1201-1203.

Zach, M., Oberwaldner, B., Hausler, F. (1982). Cystic fibrosis: physical exercise versus chest physiotherapy. Archives of Diseases of the Child 57:587-589.

CHAPTER 22

Facilitating Airway Clearance with Coughing Techniques

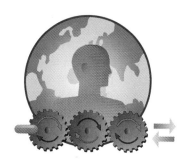

Donna Frownfelter and Mary Massery

KEY TERMS

Airway clearance deficits
Assisted cough
Complications with coughing
Cough
Cough Assist Machine
Cough pump

Cough stages
Mucous blanket
Reflex cough
Smoker's cough
Swallowing disturbance
Throat clearing

> Cough truly serves many purposes: a therapeutic technique, a diagnostic signpost, and a social necessity. If it didn't already exist, we would have to invent it.
>
> Glen A. Lillington, MD

Cough is one of the most frequently reported symptoms in patients with pulmonary impairments. It is important to get a good history and physical examination to determine the cause and course of the patient's cough. History should include sudden onset versus chronic; duration and type of cough—productive, nonproductive or wheezy; whether the cough disturbs sleep and function; and what relieves or aggravates it. Diagnostic testing may include chest imaging, pulmonary function tests, bronchoscopy, and evaluation for gastro-esophageal reflux (GER) (Kardos, 2000).

The cough is an interesting phenomenon. It can either be a reflex or a voluntary action. Generally, in healthy individuals, a cough is rarely heard unless a person has a cold, or an irritant is inhaled and a sneeze or a cough ensues to evacuate the foreign body. The mucociliary escalator functions to clear secretions and inhaled particulate matter. Unless the mucus is very thick, as in individuals with dehydration or abnormal secretions; or a foreign body is inhaled; or a bolus of food

"goes down the wrong hole," or into the trachea rather than the esophagus, a cough is not the usual mechanism to clear mucus. The mucus blanket and the cough mechanism are the two mechanisms for normal airway clearance.

Frequent coughing or throat clearing may signal that the airways are irritated, that mucus is not clearing normally, or that the person is in an uncomfortable situation. This is something to be aware of, especially when treating patients with cystic fibrosis or asthma, and patients with psychogenic issues. Depending on the reason for a cough, a variety of different approaches might be utilized. In most patients with primary pulmonary disease, the cough is related to the need for improved hydration and airway clearance. In patients with psychogenic coughs, psychotherapy, biofeedback, and relaxation techniques have proven to be effective (Riegel, 1995).

Many people are unaware of their coughing. For example, when asked if they cough, smokers with typical morning and ongoing smoker's coughs may deny coughing. Spouses will chime in, "He coughs and hacks all the time." An individual might constantly clear his or her throat and swallow mucus but will claim to be unproductive of mucus and free of a cough. It is important for therapists to be aware of both the reflex and the voluntary nature of their patients' coughs.

Frequent coughing or throat clearing may indicate other problems besides airway clearance deficits. For example, a patient may have postnasal drip from a sinus infection or allergy. When the mucus drips down into the back of the throat, it can cause a reflex cough to clear it. Other causes include bronchogenic carcinoma, nervousness, and smoking. In a pediatric patient, a foreign body or object inserted or inspired into the nose or airway should be ruled out. GER must be evaluated in children and adults with symptoms of cough (Williams, 2003; Chandra et al, 2004). A persistent cough or throat clearing might be indicative of asthma or other pulmonary diseases, but it may also be a result of GER and irritation to the upper airway. It is important to ask questions related to the patient's sleep. For example, does the person have heartburn or belching at least once a week after going to bed? Is there breathlessness at rest and nocturnal breathlessness? In a random group study in a large population of young adults, 4 % were found to have GER. People with asthma and GER (9% of asthmatics had GER) had more nocturnal cough and morning phlegm with sleep-related symptoms (Gislason, 2002). The authors concluded that there was a strong association between asthma and GER.

Cigarette smoking is known to stop mucociliary clearance. It has been noted that for every cigarette a person smokes, the cilia are paralyzed for approximately 20 minutes. Many individuals are chain smokers and consequently must cough to provide any airway clearance. They will often have significant amounts of phlegm raised first thing in the morning secondary to ciliary clearance while they slept.

Persistent cough has also been reported following pulmonary resection. The cause seems to be unclear but some studies focused on the population of patients who had had a lobectomy and mediastinal lymph node resection, some of whom also had had GER; they were at increased risk for continued cough, which was found to continue up to a year later. Of this group, 90% saw improvement in their coughing with medication (Sawabata, 2005).

If a patient demonstrates retained secretions on radiography, encourage hydration (drinking water), use airway clearance mobilization techniques, and carefully evaluate the cough. Instruct the patient in controlled coughing when mucus is felt in the throat or upper airways (see Chapter 21).

COUGH ASSOCIATED WITH EATING OR DRINKING

If a cough is associated with eating, drinking, or taking medications, the patient's swallowing mechanism should be examined and evaluated. A barium swallow (cookie swallow) is a fluoroscopic study in which the patient is given an opaque liquid, and a moving picture is observed to see if there is aspiration into the trachea. Populations commonly in need of evaluation of swallowing are patients with neurological disorders, such as those that occur with cerebrovascular accident (CVA), amyotrophic lateral sclerosis (ALS), cerebral palsy, Parkinson disease, and multiple sclerosis (MS). Patients who have trachestomy tubes may experience difficulty in swallowing

because the tube inhibits the normal movement of the larynx during swallowing. Elderly people with chronic cough should be carefully observed and monitored, as the chronic cough may be a defense mechanism to prevent aspiration (Teramoto, 2005). This is especially true if there are comorbities such as a previous stroke. This list is not inclusive; any patient who chokes when you offer fluids or who reports to you that food or water "Goes down the wrong way" should be referred for evaluation of the swallowing mechanism

Speech and language pathologists work with patients who have swallowing dysfunction (dysphagia) by helping them to learn techniques and procedures for safe swallowing. They work with the patients, spouses and parents to position patients for success, usually in a semi-Fowler sitting posture with head and neck flexion. In addition, the types and consistencies of food are evaluated. Many people have more difficulty with liquids than with puddings and other thicker consistencies. A thickening agent can be added to liquids to help patients to swallow safely. Food may be ground up if chewing is difficult. Every effort is made to help patients to eat and drink fluids successfully. However, if patients are unable to swallow safely, alternative means of nourishment, such as feeding tubes and gastric tubes, will have to be utilized. The method can be revisited later and feeding tried again when patients' conditions improve.

COUGH PUMP

The cough pump is intricate. Mucus must be transported upward against the gravitational force and propelled cephalad by the expiratory gas flow. Generally, cough is most effective because it has a large inspiration and high expiratory flow rates. Cough will clear to approximately the sixth or seventh generation of airway segments (segmental bronchi). If a patient has retained secretions, distal airway clearance techniques must move the secretions to an area where the cough can be effective. If the patient does not have the mechanical ability to cough (as in spinal cord injury), assistive cough techniques or mechanical methods, discussed later in this chapter, will have to be employed.

COMPLICATIONS OF COUGHING

Coughing can be hazardous to the patient. It should never be repeated routinely. The irritation, inflammation, and possible airway narrowing that can occur during forced exhalation may cause bronchospasm. If the cough is dry and unproductive, do not encourage frequent coughing. This is especially true for people with asthma and chronic obstructive pulmonary disease (COPD). If the patient demonstrates retained secretions, first employ an airway clearance device or treatment; then use an effective and controlled technique like the active cycles of breathing and forced expiratory technique (FET) to mobilize the secretions.

Tussive syncopy can occur when a patient goes into a series of coughs in which the intrathoracic pressure becomes so high

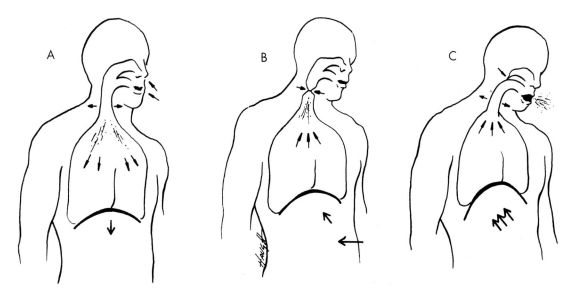

FIGURE 22-1 Cough mechanics. **A,** Stage 1: adequate inspiration. **B,** Stage 2: glottal closure; Stage 3: building up of intrathoracic and intraabdominal pressure. **C,** Stage 4: glottal opening and expulsion.

that venous return to the heart is impaired. The cardiac output falls and the patient becomes very dizzy, progressing to unconsciousness. Care must be exercised, especially in patients with primary and secondary cardiovascular and pulmonary disease. They must learn to control their coughing to prevent untoward side effects.

Stages of Cough

Four stages are involved in producing an effective cough (Linder, 1993). The first stage requires inspiring enough air to provide the volume necessary for a forceful cough. Generally, adequate inspiratory volumes for a cough are noted to be at least 60% of the predicted vital capacity for that individual. The second stage involves the closing of the glottis (vocal folds) to prepare for the abdominal and intercostal muscles to produce positive intrathoracic pressure distal to the glottis. The third stage is the active contraction of these muscles. The fourth and final stage involves opening of the glottis and the forceful expulsion of the air. The patient usually is able to cough three to six times per expiratory effort. A minimal threshold of FEV_1 (forced expiratory volume in 1 second) of at least 60% of the patient's actual vital capacity is a good indicator of adequate muscle strength necessary for effective expulsion (Figure 22-1). Bach and Saporito (1996) established a minimal peak cough flow rate (PCFR) of 160 L/min to effectively clear secretions and predict successful decannulition for patients with neuromuscular conditions. The use of a simple peak flow meter can help assess the cough. Drops in peak flow have been correlated in children, patients with spinal cord injury, and the elderly who have decreased ability to cough. This is a simple clinical test that could objectively measure the patients ability to provide the exhalation phase of the cough (Clough & Sly, 1995; Enright, 2001, Massery et al, 1999) During a cough, alveolar, pleural, and subglottal pressures

may rise as much as 200 cm H_2O (Bach, 1993; Jaeger et al, 1993; Linder, 1993).

COUGH EVALUATION

How do you assess whether a patient's cough is effective? The answer appears to be obvious: ask the patient to cough. However, the obvious answer often does not adequately analyze the functional performance of a cough, especially for a neurologically impaired patient. The clinician must first take time to prepare the patient for successful evaluation of cough. Guidelines for preparing the patient follow:

1. Do not ask the patient to cough while in whatever posture you happen to find him or her in. Ask, "What position do you like to cough in when you feel the need to cough?" Then ask the patient to assume that posture, or assist him or her in assuming a posture as close to the preferred posture as possible. Listen closely to his or her answers. A patient should spontaneously choose a posture that lends itself to trunk flexion, which is necessary for effective expulsion and airway protection. A red flag, or inappropriate choice, would be a preference for coughing while supine, which involves the opposite: trunk extension and poor mechanical alignment for airway protection.

2. Now the patient is ready to demonstrate coughing. Do not make the mistake of asking a patient to "show me a cough" or he or she may simply "show you" a cough. It may not be the way the patient coughs to clear secretions. Instead, continue to set the patient up for success by asking him or her to "show me how you would cough if you had secretions in your chest and you felt the need to cough them out." With these instructions you are asking the patient to show you something functional not theoretical.

BOX 22-1

Positioning and Instruction to Improve Cough Effectiveness

- Position the patient for success, especially in regard to trunk alignment.
- Maximize inspiratory phase through verbal cues, positioning, and active arm movement.
- Improve hold stage through verbal cues and positioning.
- Maximize intrathoracic and intraabdominal pressures with muscle contractions, physical assist, or trunk movement.
- Instruct the patient in appropriate timing and trunk movements for expulsion.
- Make the procedure physically active on the patient's part.

Cough effectiveness can now be assessed (Box 22-1). Guidelines for objective evaluation with pulmonary function tests have been indicated. This section focuses on analyzing the movement patterns during all four stages of a cough. An effective cough should maximize the function of each individual stage. Thus the clinician should see a deep inspiratory effort paired with trunk extension, a momentary hold, and then a strong cough or series of expiratory coughs on a single breath while the patient moves into trunk flexion.

Stage 1: Adequate Inspiration

Did the patient spontaneously inspire a deep breath before coughing or did he or she cough regardless of the inspiration or expiration cycle? Did the patient spontaneously use trunk extension, an upward eye gaze, or the arms to augment the inspiratory effort? Did the patient take enough time to fully inspire before coughing? If the patient inspires adequately, he or she should be able to sustain two to six coughs per expiratory effort for a cascade effect. Neurologically impaired patients who have inadequate inspiratory efforts usually present with only one or two coughs per breath and generally produce a quieter cough (Hoffman, 1987). If the patient cannot cough on demand (such as a young child or patient with cognitive impairment), ask the caretaker if he or she has time to "duck." If the patient inhales before the cough, the caretaker will learn unconsciously to listen for the inspiratory phase in order to move out of the way before the patient coughs.

Stage 2: Glottal Closure

Did the patient hold his or her breath at the peak of inspiration before the expulsion phase or did the patient go directly from inspiration to expiration? Did you hear a cough or a huff? A huff (or a complete absence of a hold between inspiration and expiration), when the patient intended to give you a cough, is an indication of insufficient glottal closure. This can result from a wide variety of situations, including glottal edema after prolonged intubation, partial or full paralysis of the vocal folds, hemiparesis of the vocal folds, or timing or sequencing

difficulty secondary to brain injuries, to name a few possibilities. A complete lack of glottal closure will not produce any cough sound because the vocal folds are not approximating (adducting). The huff technique may be encouraged when the patient tends to wheeze or after long-term intubation when there is vocal fold edema. But in the "normal" population, a good hold and cough are encouraged.

Stage 3: Building-up of Intrathoracic and Intraabdominal Pressure

Did you see active contraction of the intercostal and abdominal muscles? Did the patient spontaneously move into trunk flexion during this phase? Did the cough have a low, resonant sound? Inadequate force is usually heard as a higher pitched cough, often called a *throaty cough*. The sound is quieter overall and does not produce as many coughs per expiratory effort. It is sometimes associated with neck extension rather than flexion as the patient attempts to clear the upper airway only. The air appears to leak out rather than being propelled out of the larynx during the cough. Like inadequate lung volumes, inadequate pressure also prevents the patient from coughing more than once or twice on one expiratory effort.

Stage 4: Glottal Opening and Expulsion

The timing of the opening of the glottis and the forceful expulsion of the air is directly tied into the function of the third stage. During expulsion, does the patient appear to gag before successfully allowing the air to be expelled? Does the patient seem to get stuck holding his or her breath? Deficiencies in this area are often related to brain injuries and coordination difficulties. The opposite can also occur. Some patients get stuck at the end of expulsion, especially those with severe neurological impairments or bronchospasms, and may have difficulty initiating the next inspiratory effort.

If the patient is able to follow directions and has the muscular ability and cognition to learn cough techniques, patient instruction is the next step. If the person is unable secondary to neuromuscular weakness or frailty and cannot be independent in coughing, a decision must be made about the next step to be taken provide airway clearance of secretions. Assistive cough techniques, the Cough Assist Machine, and suctioning are considerations and are discussed later in this chapter.

PATIENT INSTRUCTION

When working with patients, especially those with primary pulmonary disease or primary disease superimposed on secondary disease (i.e., a patient with a CVA asthma), there are some helpful techniques that make secretion mobilization more effective.

Patients with asthma and emphysema tend to go into an expiratory wheeze when they force and prolong exhalation.

This can lead to bronchospasm and respiratory distress. Patients can be taught the pump cough, a variation on the huff technique. A huff is often used in patients to help them produce controlled, less stressful coughs. It may be used when patients have been intubated with an endotracheal tube for an extended time. The vocal folds are swollen and inflamed and will not close and form the tight seal necessary to build up the pressure for a cough. Patients are instructed to huff rather than cough. It is done with more open vocal folds, a low sound, and less effort, yet it is quite effective in mobilizing secretions, especially when combined with FET.

The pump cough extends the huff and, in this clinician's opinion, is more effective. The patient is instructed to take three mid-sized huffs followed by three short, easy coughs at low lung volume, not deep breaths or deep lung volumes. Three or four sequences are performed: huff, huff, huff; cough, cough, cough; huff, huff, huff; cough, cough, cough; huff, huff, huff; cough, cough, cough. Usually, if secretions are present, a spontaneous cough occurs, or the secretions will mobilize with the small coughs.

Patients with emphysema have over-distended lungs and difficulty in exhalation. Do not instruct the patient to take a deep breath and cough because this can cause more air trapping, which does not facilitate the expulsion of secretions. Patients will be more effective in trying to take controlled small or medium-sized breaths followed by huffs or a small series of coughs. The active cycles of breathing and forced expiratory pressure technique is also a good choice for these patients.

Several ideas are presented here because the therapist needs a "bag of tricks." Some techniques work well for some patients and not for others. Try several with each patient and let him or her determine what works best. Objective tests can also be used to determine the most effective intervention, such as a change in oxygen saturation, improved breath sounds via auscultation, improved expiratory flow rates, and a reduction in the patient's perceived work of breathing (dyspnea scale).

Another variation that decreases stress on the patient is to use a series of coughs starting with a small breath and a small cough, then a medium breath and a medium cough, then a large breath and a large cough. This is a good technique to use with postoperative patients, who become fatigued trying to cough maximally each time. It is an effort to get air distal to the secretions in various parts of the lungs, a form of autogenic drainage.

For patients with transient or permanent neuromuscular weakness or paralysis, further instructions may be necessary (Braun et al, 1984; Chatwin et al, 2003, Jaeger et al, 1993; Lahrmann, 2003; Sivasothy et al, 2001). These patients must use every physical trait to maximize the function of each stage of the cough (see Figure 22-1). Physically assisting these patients during the expulsion stage of the cough addresses only one aspect (Fishburn et al, 1990; Slack & Shucart, 1994). Care must be taken to look at all four stages to maximize the airway clearance potential of any assistive cough technique. First, the patient must be positioned for success. The beginning of any cough requires trunk extension or inspiratory movement to maximize inhalation, whereas the expulsion stage requires trunk flexion or expiratory movement to maximize exhalation (Massery, 1994). Thus for any given posture, the clinician must assess the following: (1) whether the posture allows for both trunk movements; (2) whether flexion and extension are possible, which movement is more important for that particular patient, and whether that posture facilitates its occurrence; (3) how gravity is affecting the patient's muscle strength and function in that posture; and (4) whether the patient can still protect the airway in this posture. When these questions have been answered satisfactorily, the clinician is ready to instruct the patient in the act of coughing.

An example may provide the best illustration of these instructions. A clinician may pick a modified sitting position for a patient with generalized weakness (e.g., incomplete spinal cord injury, developmental delay, or temporary weakness or exhaustion after a medical or surgical procedure). The patient looks slumped, so the clinician places a lumbar support (e.g., a lumbar roll, a towel, or a pillow) behind the lower back to increase trunk extension in that position. The patient is asked if he or she is comfortable and if he or she can swallow safely. Next, the clinician tries to maximize the first cough stage by asking the patient to take a deep breath. Observing that the patient did not appear to take in as deep a breath as the clinician thought possible, the clinician adds further instructions such as the following: (1) "Look upward while you inhale." (2) "Raise both of your arms up over your head as high as you can while you inhale." (3) "Squeeze your shoulders back while you inhale." (4) "Straighten or extend your back while you inhale." For those with more limited arm function, apply appropriate ventilatory strategies detailed in Chapter 23. Very subtle movements can then be requested, such as the following: (1) "Bring your arms up and out while you inhale." (2) "Rotate your arms outward while you inhale." (3) "Turn your forearm up while you inhale." Although less dramatic than the larger movements described previously, these subtle motions may significantly increase the patient's inspiratory effort and provide a more active means for the patient to participate in his or her own coughing program (Ishii & Matsuo, 2004).

Stage two involves closing the glottis. For some patients with weakness or timing problems, a sharp loud command to "hold it" at the peak of inspiration, may be sufficient to facilitate closure. Remember to allow enough time for the patient to take in a deep inspiratory effort before being asked to "hold." Some clinicians rush the first phase by saying, in quick succession, "Take a deep breath. Hold it," thus unintentionally limiting the time of the inspiratory effort. A more appropriate verbal cue would be: "Take a deep breath in … in … in … in … , and now hold it," allowing adequate time for the patient to inhale.

Stages three and four (building up pressure and expulsion) are discussed together because their timing is interdependent. The patient now needs to move into trunk flexion, with or without the clinician's assistance, to maximize expulsion.

Patients who can assist can be asked to do the opposite of stage one: (1) "Look down while you cough." (2) "Pull both of your arms down to your hips as you cough." (3) "Roll your shoulders forward while you cough." (4) "Bend your trunk forward while you cough." Likewise, patients with more limited arm function can be asked to do the following: (1) "Squeeze your arms to your chest while coughing." (2) "Roll your shoulders and arms inward while coughing." (3) "Turn your hands down (pronation) while coughing."

In this manner the clinician has used every conceivable resource to maximize a voluntary cough. Even the weakest cough can be made more effective by applying the following simple concepts: (1) position for success; (2) maximize inhalation first; (3) ask for a breath hold; (4) encourage maximal intrathoracic and intraabdominal pressures; (5) instruct the patient in appropriate timing and trunk movements for expulsion; and (6) make the procedure as active as possible for the patient. Objective and subjective assessments can confirm the improvement. However, even with excellent instructions, many patients with neurological disorders require a clinician's physical assistance to inhale more deeply or to exhale more forcefully because of muscle weakness or paralysis (MacLean et al, 1989).

ACTIVE ASSISTED COUGH TECHNIQUES

If after instruction and modification in the patient's cough as described previously, the patient still cannot produce an effective cough, then one of the following assistive cough techniques may be appropriate. However, a patient who needs some assistance to improve a cough is not excused from taking an active role in coughing. Keep the act of coughing as active as possible for each patient, whether that is accomplished by adding a few verbal cues to improve overall timing or posture while the patient independently performs the cough, or whether it is accomplished by adding eye gazes for a very weak patient who cannot move the upper extremities and breathes with the assistance of a ventilator. Encourage the patient to be responsible for his or her own care by teaching the concepts involved in producing an effective cough (Estenne & Detroyer, 1990). In that manner, you will help the patient develop the problem-solving skills necessary for modifications later. Modify and develop additional techniques based on the principles presented thus far. See Box 22-2 for techniques presented in this chapter.

Manually Assisted Techniques

Costophrenic Assist

The first assistive cough technique, the costophrenic assist, can be used in any posture. After assessing the most appropriate position for the patient (most often sitting or side-lying) and giving the patient instructions for maximizing all four coughing stages, the therapist places his or her hands on the costophrenic angles of the rib cage (Figure 22-2). At the end of the patient's next exhalation, the therapist applies a

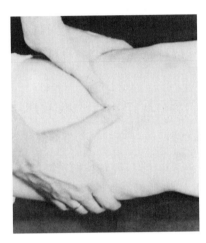

FIGURE 22-2 Assisted cough techniques in supine position; costophrenic assist.

quick manual stretch down and in toward the patient's navel to facilitate a stronger diaphragmatic and intercostal muscle contraction during the succeeding inhalation. The therapist can also apply a series of repeated contractions based on proprioceptive neuromuscular facilitation (the PNF approach; Sullivan & Markos, 1996) throughout inspiration to facilitate maximal inhalation. The patient may assist the maneuver by actively using his or her upper extremities, head and neck, eyes, trunk, or all of the above to maximize the inspiratory phase. The patient is then asked to "hold it." Just a moment before asking the patient to actively cough, the therapist applies strong pressure with his or her hands, again down and in toward the navel. In this manner the therapist is assisting both the buildup of intrathoracic pressure and the force of expiration. Of course, the patient would also actively participate by using his or her arms, trunk, or other body parts throughout the entire procedure (see Chapter 23).

This technique's obvious use would be for patients with weak or paralyzed intercostal or abdominal muscles. The therapist must remember to evaluate the effect of gravity and posture in each position for the appropriateness of this

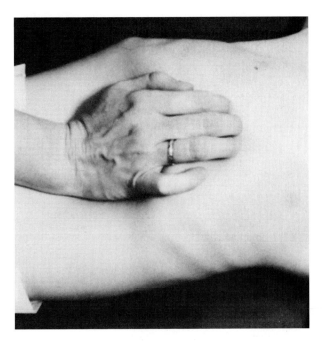

FIGURE 22-3 Hand position for Heimlich-type assist or abdominal thrust.

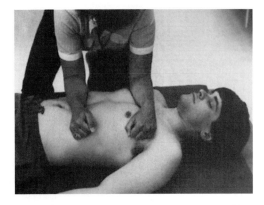

FIGURE 22-4 Assistive cough techniques in supine position; variation of the anterior chest compression assist.

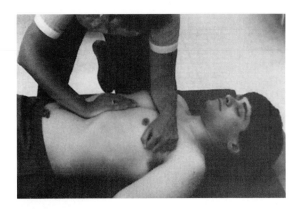

FIGURE 22-5 Assistive cough techniques in supine position; variation of the anterior chest compression assist.

technique (Massery, 1987). It is helpful for lower-airway clearance but does not directly assist in upper-chest clearance unless the patient is able to move his or her upper body independently while the therapist assists the lower chest. This technique is easy to learn and teach and can usually be used from the acute phase through the patient's rehabilitation phase, thus accounting for its popularity.

Heimlich-Type Assist, or Abdominal Thrust Assist

The second technique, the Heimlich-type assist, or abdominal thrust, requires the therapist to place the heel of his or her hand at about the level of the patient's navel, taking care to avoid direct placement on the lower ribs (Figure 22-3). After appropriate positioning, the patient is instructed to "take in a deep breath and hold it." Unfortunately, manual facilitation of inhalation is not feasible with this technique. As the patient is instructed to cough, the therapist quickly pushes up and in, under the diaphragm with the heel of his or her hand, as in a Heimlich maneuver. The patient is instructed to assist with appropriate trunk movements to the best of his or her ability. Technically, this procedure is very effective at forcefully expelling the air (Braun, 1984), as in a cough, but it can be extremely uncomfortable for the patient because of (1) its concentrated area of contact; (2) its abrupt nature, which may elicit an undesired high neuromuscular tone response or worse when combined with the sensory input that the therapist's manual contacts supply; (3) the force, which may cause gastrointestinal dysfunction such as GER. Because of its limited usefulness, the Heimlich-type assist, or abdominal thrust, should be used only when the patient does not respond to other techniques and the need to produce an effective cough is great.

The therapist can use both of the above techniques simultaneously when the patient is in the side-lying position. If the patient has a hemiplegic deficit or has a unilateral lung or thorax disease or trauma, emphasizing one side of the thorax over the other may be an appropriate focus during airway clearance treatments. One upper extremity is used to perform the Heimlich-type of assist while the other does a unilateral costophrenic assist. In this manner the therapist can compress simultaneously all three planes of ventilation in the lower chest. The possibilities of combining techniques and positions are almost endless once the therapist understands the principles on which they were developed.

Anterior Chest Compression Assist

The third assistive cough is called the *anterior chest compression assist* because it compresses both the upper and lower anterior chest during the coughing maneuver. This is the first single technique thus far to address the compression needs of the upper and lower chest in one maneuver. The therapist puts one arm across the patient's pectoralis region to compress the upper chest; the other arm is placed parallel on the lower chest (avoiding the xiphoid process) or the abdomen (Figure 22-4) or is placed as in the Heimlich-type maneuver (Figure 22-5). The commands are the same as in the other

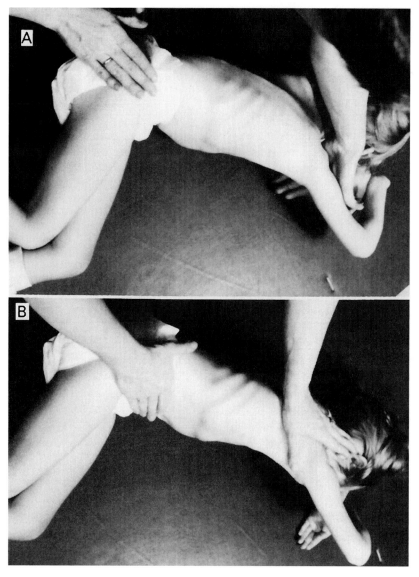

FIGURE 22-6   Counter-rotation assist. **A,** Hand placement during expulsion phase. **B,** Hand placement during inspiration phase.

techniques. Because of the direct manual contact on the chest, inspiration can be easily facilitated first, followed by a "hold." Thus the therapist can readily enhance the first two cough stages. The therapist then applies a quick force with both arms to simulate the force necessary during the expulsion phase. The directions of the force are (1) down and back on the upper chest, and (2) up and back on the lower chest or abdominal arm. When performed together, the compression force exerted by both arms makes the letter V.

The anterior chest compression technique is more effective than the costophrenic assist for patients with very weak chest wall muscles because of the added compression of the upper anterior chest wall. These authors have found the side-lying or $\frac{3}{4}$ supine position to be the most effective position for this technique. However, the anterior chest compression technique is not appropriate for a patient with a cavus condition of the

upper anterior chest because it promotes further collapsing of the anterior chest wall.

Counter-rotation Assist

The most effective assistive-cough technique for the widest cross-section of patients with neurological disorders, in these authors' clinical experience, is the fourth and final method described: the side-lying counter-rotation assist (Massery et al, 1999). The positioning and procedures required for the counter-rotation technique are described in detail in chapter 23 and apply for both the patient and the therapist (Figure 22-6). The therapist should recall that orthopedic precautions for the spine, rib cage, shoulder, and pelvis persist for this technique.

The therapist begins by following the patient's breathing cycle, with his or her hands positioned over the patient's shoulder and pelvis (see Figure 22-6). The therapist then gently assists the patient in inhalation and exhalation to promote better overall ventilation. This sequence is generally repeated for three to five cycles or until the patient appears to have achieved good ventilation to all lung segments.

At this point, the patient is ready to begin the coughing phase of the procedure. The patient is asked to take in as deep a breath as possible, with the therapist assisting the patient in chest expansion (see Figure 22-6, *B*). The patient is then instructed to "hold it" at the end of maximal inspiration. The patient is then commanded to cough out as hard as possible while the therapist quickly and forcefully compresses the chest with his or her hands in their flexion phase positions (see Figure 22-6, *A*).

The importance of following a true diagonal plane of facilitation during both the flexion and extension phases of this technique cannot be overemphasized. Failure to do so will result in the shifting of the air within the chest cavity rather than the desired forcing out of the air. This air shifting can occur to varying degrees when the upper and lower chest are not used together, as in all the other assistive cough techniques. When done properly, the counter-rotation assist is the only one to rapidly close off the chest cavity in all three planes of ventilation in all areas of the chest. Unless the patient voluntarily closes his or her glottis, it is impossible to prevent the air from being forcefully expelled. However, a common mistake made by the therapist is pulling the patient back into trunk extension during the expulsion phase rather than into trunk flexion. A good rule of thumb: if you can see your patient's face when you are applying the compression force, you have pulled him or her into extension. The head and neck should stay forward and flexed, so only a facial profile should be seen.

Other effects of counter-rotation make this procedure particularly beneficial for patients with low levels of cognitive functioning.

1. The rotation component is a natural inhibitor of high tone. Thus, this is the least likely of all techniques discussed so far to elicit an increase in abnormal tone during the coughing phase. In fact the opposite usually prevails. Gentle rotation before passive coughing in a patient who is comatose can reduce high tone and frequently reduces a high respiratory rate. Both of these reduce the possibility of the patient's keeping his or her glottis closed during the expulsion phase.
2. Counter-rotation is an excellent mobilizer for a tight chest, which in itself can facilitate spontaneous deeper breaths. Tidal volumes (TVs) can therefore be increased for many patients by mobilizing the chest walls.
3. Finally, rotation can be a vestibular stimulator and may assist in arousing the patient cognitively, allowing him or her to take a more active role in the procedure.

The true beauty of the technique is the fact that no active participation on the part of the patient is required for success. Incoherent or unresponsive patients, such as patients with low functioning following a head trauma, CVA, or cerebral palsy, will still demonstrate good secretion clearance with this technique. The mechanics of the procedure dictate that the air within the lungs be rapidly and forcefully expelled regardless of the patient's level of active participation. Obviously, patient participation is desirable to clear secretions even more effectively and to teach the patient eventually to clear his or her own secretions, but it is not critical.

Clinical experience has demonstrated that in patients who have extremely tenacious secretions, the use of vibration instead of quick chest compression during the cough itself may be more effective. This prolongs the cough phase and gives the secretions time to be moved along the bronchi for successful expulsion. These patients may also require a series of three or four cough cycles before clearing most of their secretions. In general, patients from all the diagnostic groups discussed thus far, with or without good cognitive functioning, are appropriate for this procedure. The majority of them find it to be the most comfortable and effective assistive means of expectorating secretions.

Self-Assisted Techniques

The coughing techniques discussed in this section are intended to be used as self-assisted procedures, so they are usually taught later in a patient's rehabilitation process. Five different techniques are presented in detail. Suggestions for variations are included. All self-assisted cough techniques can start out as physically assisted techniques; however, because they are more active and require greater gross motor movement, they lend themselves to self-assisted techniques.

Prone-on-Elbows, Head-Flexion Self-Assisted Cough

The prone position is not commonly used as a posture for coughing because the position itself inhibits full use of the diaphragm by preventing lower anterior chest and abdominal excursion following a neurological insult. This forces the patient to use an alternative breathing pattern that facilitates greater use of accessory muscles. Because this change in breathing patterns often occurs spontaneously, prone on elbows can be an effective posture for promoting spontaneous use of the accessory muscles in a more difficult activity (coughing). However, without the full recruitment of the diaphragm, the resultant cough will be weaker than it would be in other postures. Prone on elbows should not be the exclusive posture for a self-assisted cough. After mastering the timing of the procedure, most patients move back to another posture, usually sitting or side-lying, and to other techniques to capitalize on the functional increase in chest expansion and compression. For the population of patients who can assume a prone on elbows posture independently (i.e., some patients with tetraplegia), this technique may be used functionally. Here, they can assist their own coughs when the need arises, rather than wait for someone to assist them in a position change.

The head flexion assist requires good use of head and neck musculature, seen in patients sustaining a spinal level injury below C_4 (e.g., spinal cord injuries [SCIs], spina bifida). It can

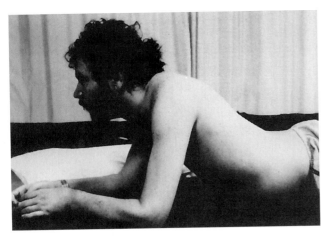

FIGURE 22-7 Head flexion assistive cough in prone on elbows; extension and inspiratory phase.

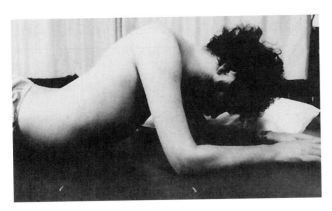

FIGURE 22-8 Head flexion assistive cough in prone on elbows; flexion and coughing phase.

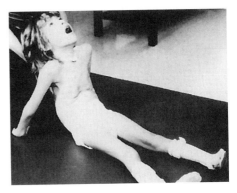

FIGURE 22-9 Tetraplegic–self-assisted cough in long-sitting; maximizing the inspiration phase.

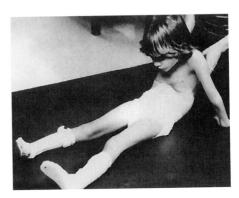

FIGURE 22-10 Tetraplegic–self-assisted cough in long-sitting; maximizing the expiration, or coughing, phase.

be used either as a self-assisted or a therapist-assisted procedure, using the principles of trunk extension to facilitate inspiration and trunk flexion to facilitate expiration. With the patient prone on elbows, the therapist instructs him or her to bring the head and neck up and back as far as possible, inhaling maximally (Figure 22-7). The patient is then instructed to cough out as hard as possible while throwing the head forward and down (Figure 22-8). This head-and-neck pattern can be assisted initially by the therapist to establish the desired movement pattern and gradually progressed to a resisted pattern to promote increased accessory muscle participation and to strengthen those muscle groups.

Long-Sitting Self-Assisted Cough

For the first procedure, tetraplegic–long-sitting self-assist, the patient is positioned on a mat in a long-sitting posture (legs straight out in front) and with upper extremity support. The therapist instructs the patient to extend his or her body backwards while inhaling maximally (Figure 22-9). The therapist then tells the patient to cough as the patient throws his or her upper body forward into a completely flexed posture, using shoulder internal rotation if possible (Figure

22-10). Once again, the extension aspect of the procedure is used to maximize inhalation, whereas the flexion aspect is used to maximize expiration. The self-directed chest compression occurs mainly on the superior-inferior plane of ventilation only.

The second procedure, the paraplegic–long-sit assist, uses the same principles as the techniques described for the tetraplegic–long-sit assist. These patients have active spinal extension musculature and can achieve greater trunk extension and flexion safely, thus achieving greater chest expansion before the cough and greater chest compression on a superior-inferior plane during the cough. The patient positions his or her upper extremities in a butterfly position or uses elbow retraction, depending on the level of injury (Figure 22-11). During the flexion phase, patients throw themselves onto their legs, thereby compressing both the upper and lower chest (Figure 22-12). This can be taught very successfully to patients with paraplegia, provided they have adequate trunk balance control. If the patient lacks hip flexion or is worried about bony contact or skin injury, place a pillow (or two as needed) on the legs. This will limit the hip flexion and minimize trauma from the quick thrust onto the legs.

Short-Sitting Self-Assisted Cough

The third assistive cough when sitting, the short-sitting self-assist, is typically performed in a wheelchair or over the

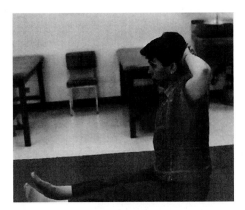

FIGURE 22-11 Paraplegic–self-assisted cough in long-sitting; inspiration.

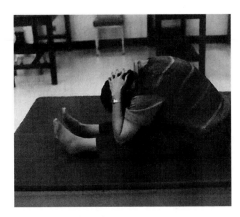

FIGURE 22-12 Paraplegic–self-assisted cough in long-sitting; expiration.

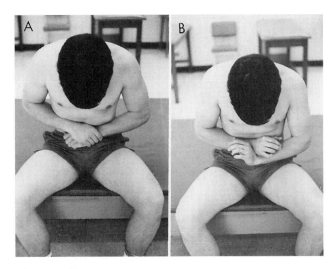

FIGURE 22-13 Assisted cough in short-sitting. **A,** Hand position for patient with good hand function. **B,** Hand position for patient with only wrist function.

edge of a bed. The patient is instructed to place one hand over the other at the wrist and place them in his or her lap. As in the previous technique, the patient is then asked to extend the trunk backwards while inhaling maximally, followed by a strong voluntary cough. During the cough, the patient pulls his or her hands up and under the diaphragm, resembling the motion of a Heimlich maneuver (Figure 22-13). The hands mimic the abdominal muscles, which would ordinarily contract to push the intestinal contents up and under the diaphragm to aid its recoil ability. This short-sitting technique uses the diaphragm more substantially than the long-sitting procedure and is therefore generally more effective as an assistive cough. It is an effective self-assisted method for patients who have weak diaphragms or abdominal musculature. Most patients with SCI or spina bifida at C_5 or below can learn this technique successfully. Patients with tetraplegia usually require trunk support from their wheelchairs to perform it independently and safely, whereas most patients with lower level lesions resulting in paraplegia can perform it from an unsupported short-sitting position. Patients who lack good upper-extremity coordination, such as many patients with Parkinson disease and MS, cannot perform the procedure

quickly or forcefully enough to make it effective and usually require assistance from another person.

Variations on all sitting techniques can be made readily. Clinicians are encouraged to use the concepts explained in the introduction to these cough techniques to develop techniques that work for their patients. For example, ask a patient in a wheelchair to lift his or her arms up while inhaling, hold, and then cough while throwing arms down toward feet or lap using maximum trunk flexion. (Use a seat belt for safety.) Another idea is to have the patient hook one arm on a push handle of the wheelchair and move the other arm up and back (as in a pattern of shoulder flexion, abduction, and external rotation [PNF D_2]) (Knott & Voss, 1956); make sure the patient's moving hand maximizes trunk rotation; have the patient inhale during the movement, hold, and cough as he or she throws trunk and arm down toward opposite knee. When devising the most appropriate self-assisted cough for your patient, remember to look for combination of trunk, arm, head, neck, and eye patterns that will maximize all four phases of the cough.

Hands-Knees, Rocking Self-Assisted Cough

The last assistive cough to be discussed is performed most commonly as a multipurpose activity to increase the patient's balance, strength, coordination, and functional use of breathing patterns (including quiet breathing and coughing) simultaneously. The patient assumes an all-fours position (hands-knees). He or she is then instructed to rock forward, looking up and breathing in as he or she moves to a fully extended posture (Figure 22-14). After this, the patient is told to cough out as he or she quickly rocks backwards to the heels with a flexed head and neck (Figure 22-15). Once again, the importance of the flexion and extension components of a cough are to be noted. The rocking can be done with or without a therapist's assistance. For patients with generalized

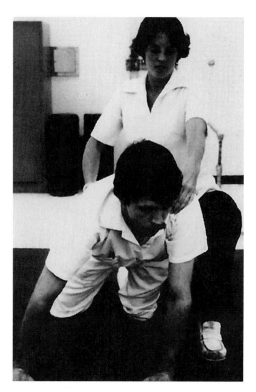

FIGURE 22-14 Assisted cough in hands-knees position; extension or inspiratory phase.

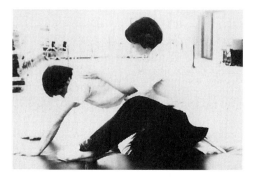

FIGURE 22-15 Assisted cough in hands-knees position; flexion or coughing phase.

or spotty weakness throughout (e.g., some patients with SCI, head trauma, Parkinson disease, MS, cerebral palsy, or spina bifida), this method is perfect for incorporating many functional goals into a single activity. It can help prepare them for more challenging respiratory activities that they will undoubtedly meet after their discharge from a rehabilitation center.

For patients with limited lower-extremity range of movement or skin concerns associated with a quick force, a pillow can be placed on the lower legs, thus restricting knee flexion and preventing direct contact of bony prominences.

Standing Self-Assisted Cough

Standing uses the same concepts and can be readily used for self-assisted coughs, provided the patient has adequate

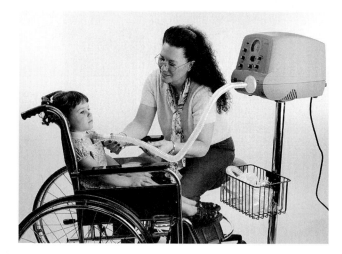

FIGURE 22-16 Cough Assist Machine.

standing balance and upper-extremity support. Use any technique previously described and modify for this posture. Combinations of trunk, head, and extremity movements during the cough maneuver are almost endless, so specific techniques are not itemized.

As mentioned previously in the chapter, if patients are unable to be independent and assist in coughing to remove secretions, other options will be necessary. At this point, suctioning has been the most commonly used aid in secretion removal. However, it is not always tolerated well by patients. Mouth suction for oral secretions is usually appreciated and easy to use, but patients with tracheostomies and endotracheal tubes have usually been suctioned more invasively into the trachea to remove secretions. There is a piece of equipment now readily available that many patients have found to be superior in comfort and in effectiveness in removing secretions, Cough Assist Machine, previously known as the cof-flator or the Mechanical In-Exsufflator.

MECHANICAL IN-EXSUFFLATOR

The Cough Assist Machine, previously known as the cof-flator or Mechanical In-Exsufflator (MI-E) is a noninvasive machine used for airway clearance. A positive-pressure phase (insufflation) is followed by a negative pressure phase (exsufflation) simulating a cough. This device can be used as a face mask or attached to a universal adaptor for a tracheostomy tube (Figure 22-16).

Adults and children with neuromuscular disease are susceptible to recurrent chest infections, which are a major cause of morbidity and mortality. The suggested mechanism of action of the Cough Assist Machine is to improve peak cough flow (Bach, 1993). In a study of 22 patients ages 10 to 56 (median age 21), spirometry and respiratory muscle strength were measured. Peak cough flows were measured with maximal coughs unassisted, then randomly with assistive coughs, non-invasive mechanical ventilation, Cough Assist Machine, and exsufflation alone. All the therapeutic techniques were well tolerated and showed similar patient acceptance. However, the Cough Assist Machine produced greater increases in cough pressures than the other cough-assist techniques (Chatwin et al, 2003). Considering the workload of caregivers and the ease of availability of the MI-E, many patients with neuromuscular weakness and artificial airways could well use this as an effective adjunct in the home as well as in other settings.

The Cough Assist Machine has been used primarily in adults but is being used more and more in children. In a study of 62 children (median age 11.3, ranging from 3 months to 28.6 years) with neuromuscular disease and impaired cough who were seen in a pediatric respiratory clinic, it was much preferred and was considered safe, well tolerated, and effective in 90% of this population for preventing pulmonary complications (Miske, 2004). In a similar study, patients with spinal cord injury also preferred the Cough Assist Machine and found it effective and more comfortable than other methods for removing secretions (Garstang, 2000). In a direct comparison of suctioning and the Cough Assist Machine for adult patients with neuromuscular impairments, this author and colleagues found no clinically significant difference between the two mechanical interventions; however, patients preferred the Cough Assist Machine 10 to 1 over suctioning (Massery et al, 2003).

SUMMARY

In all postures and in all techniques, for both assisted and self-assisted coughs, initial positioning and ventilatory strategies are of utmost importance to the success of the airway clearance technique. There is an effective idea waiting to be incorporated so all patients can improve their coughing, from the tiniest postural change to full-body movements and physical assists. Be creative in applying the concepts to all patient populations. Also consider the mechanical needs of patients who are not able to assist or be independent in the secretion removal that prevents pulmonary complications.

Review Questions

1. What is the purpose of a cough?
2. What are the two mechanisms of airway clearance?
3. Which patients would a therapist have to assist in their coughing?
4. How does the Cough Assist Machine work, and which patients would benefit from it?
5. What is a smoker's cough, and why does it occur?
6. What are the stages of a cough?
7. When should a therapist make a referral for a swallow study?
8. What effect does coughing have on the blood pressure and cardiac output?
9. What special techniques can be taught to patients with asthma to mobilize secretions?
10. What manual techniques are most effective in patients with spinal cord injury?

REFERENCES

Bach, J.R. (1993). Comparison of peak expiratory flows with manually assisted and unassisted coughing techniques. Chest 104:1553-1562.

Bach, J.R., & Saporito, L.R. (1996). Criteria for extubation and tracheostomy tube removal for patients with ventilatory failure. A different approach to weaning. Chest 110:1566-1571.

Braun, S.R., Giovannoni, R., & O'Connor, M. (1984). Improving cough in patients with spinal cord injury. American Journal of Physical Medicine 63:1-10.

Chandra, A., Moazzez, R., Bartlett, D., Anggiansah, A., & Owen, W.J. (2004). A review of the atypical manifestations of gastro-esophageal reflux disease. International Journal of Clinical Practice 58:41-48.

Chatwin, M., Ross, E., Hart, N., Nickol, A.H., Polkey, M.I., & Simonds, A.K. (2003) Cough augmentation with mechanical insufflation/exsufflation in patients with neuromuscular weakness. European Respiratory Journal 21:502-508.

Clough, J.B., & Sly, P.D. (1995). Association between lower respiratory tract symptoms and falls in peak expiratory flow in children. European Respiratory Journal 8:718-722.

Enright, P.L. (2001) Correlates of peak expiratory flow lability in elderly persons. Chest 120:1861-1868.

Estenne, M., & Detroyer, A. (1990). Cough in tetraplegic subjects: an active process. Annals of Internal Medicine 12:22–28.

Fishburn, M.J., Marino, R.J., & Dittuno, J.F. (1990). Atelectasis and pneumonia in acute spinal cord injury. Archives of Physical Medicine and Rehabilitation 71:197-200.

Gislason, T., Janson, C., Vermeire, P., Plaschke, P., Bjornsson, E., Gislason, D., & Boman, G.. (2002). Respiratory symptoms and nocturnal gastroesophageal reflux: a population-based study of young adults in three European countries. Chest 121:158-163.

Hoffman, L.A. (1987). Ineffective airway clearance related to neuromuscular dysfunction. Nursing Clinics of North America 22:151-166.

Ishii, M., Matsuo, Y., et al. (2004). Optimizing forced vital capacity with shoulder positioning in a mechanically-ventilated patient with amyotrophic lateral sclerosis. Cardiopulmonary Physical Therapy Journal 15:12-16.

Jaeger, R.J., Turba, R.M., Yarkony, G.M., & Roth, E.J. (1993). Cough in spinal cord injured patients: comparison of three methods to produce cough. Archives of Physical Medicine and Rehabilitation 74:1358-1361.

Kardos, P. (2000). Proposals for a rationale and for rational diagnosis of cough. Pneumologie 54:110-115.

Knott, M., & Voss, D.E. (1956). Proprioceptive neuromuscular facilitation: patterns and techniques. New York: Hoeber-Harper Books.

Lahrmann, H. (2003) Expiratory muscle weakness and assisted cough in ALS. Amyotrophic Lateral Sclerosis and Other Motor Neuron Disorders 4:49-51.

Linder, S.H. (1993). Functional electrical stimulation to enhance cough in quadriplegia. Chest 103:166-169.

MacLean, D., Drummond, C., & Macpherson, C., McLaren, G., & Prescott, R. (1989). Maximum expiratory airflow during chest physiotherapy on ventilated patients before and after the application of an abdominal binder. Intensive Care Medicine 5:396-399.

Massery, M.P. (1987). An innovative approach to assistive cough techniques. Topics in Acute Care Trauma Rehabilitation 3:73-85.

Massery, M.P. (1994). What's positioning got to do with it? Neurology Report 18:11-14.

Massery, M., Dreyer, H., et al. (1999). A pilot study investigating the effectiveness of assisted cough techniques and the clinical utility of a peak flow meter to measure peak cough expiratory flow in persons with spinal cord injury [abstract]. Proceedings for the World Congress for Physical Therapy 30.

Massery, M., Sammon, K., et al. (2003). Comparing airway clearance effectiveness using a suction machine and the Cough-Assist machine for patients in acute rehabilitation [abstract]. Cardiopulmonary Physical Therapy Journal 14:21.

Miske,L.J., Hickey, E.M., Kolb, S.M., Weiner, D.J., & Panitch, H.B. (2004). Use of the mechanical in-exsufflator in pediatric patients with neuromuscular disease and impaired cough. Chest 125:1406-1412.

Riegel, B., Warmoth, J.E., Middaugh, S.J., Kee, W.G., Nicholson, L.C., Melton, D.M., Parikh, D.K., & Rosenberg, J.C. (1995). Psychogenic cough treated with biofeedback and psychotherapy: a review and case report. American Journal of Physical and Medical Rehabilitation. 74:155-158.

Sawabata, N., Maeda, H., Takeda, S., Inoue, M., Koma, M., Tokunaga, T., & Matsuda, H. (2005). Persistent cough following pulmonary resection: observational and empiric study of possible causes. Annals of Thoracic Surgery 79:289-293.

Sivsaothy, P., Brown, L., Smith, I.E., & Shneerson, J.M. (2001). Effect of manually assisted cough and mechanical insufflation on cough flow of normal subjects, patients with chronic obstructive pulmonary disease (COPD) and patients with respiratory muscle weakness. Thorax 56:438-444.

Slack, R.S., & Shucart, W. (1994). Respiratory dysfunction with traumatic injury to the central nervous system. Clinics in Chest Medicine 15:739-749.

Sullivan, R.E., Markos, P.D., & Minor, A.D. (1982). An integrated approach to therapeutic exercise: theory and clinical application. Reston, Va.: Reston Publishing.

Sullivan, P.E., & Markos, P.D. (1996). Clinical procedures in therapeutic exercise. Stamford, Conn: Simon and Schuster Co.

Termoto, S., Ishii, T., Yamamoto, H., Yamaguchi, Y., Namba, R., Hanaoka, Y., Takizawa, M., Okada, T., Ishii, M., & Ouchi, Y. (2005). Significance of chronic cough as a defense mechanism or a symptom in elderly patients with aspiration and aspiration pneumonia. European Respiratory Journal 25:210-211.

Toder, D.S. (2000). Respiratory problems in the adolescent with development delay. Adolescent Medicine 11:617-631.

Williams, J.L. (2003). Gastroesophageal reflux disease: clinical manifestations. Gastroenterology Nursing 26:195-200.

C H A P T E R   2 3

Facilitating Ventilation Patterns and Breathing Strategies

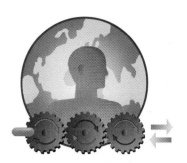

Donna Frownfelter and Mary Massery

KEY TERMS	Controlled breathing	Jacobsen's progressive relaxation
	Core stability	Ventilatory strategies
	Diaphragmatic breathing pattern	Work of breathing

Individuals with breathing impairments (whether primary or secondary in origin) require a variety of interventions to optimize ventilation and oxygen delivery. Some interventions are passive in nature, such as the positioning of the patient or the application of an abdominal binder for better diaphragmatic positioning. Some interventions require very active participation on the part of the therapist, patient, or both, such as in assisted-cough techniques, in glossopharyngeal breathing instruction, or in learning a more efficient breathing pattern. Other techniques are subtly incorporated into the patient's total physical rehabilitation program, such as the use of ventilation strategies pairing breathing with movement. All of these diverse aspects of treatment play an important role in the development of a successful rehabilitation program to meet the needs of patients with pulmonary impairments. No single intervention or approach is appropriate in all cases. Sound clinical judgment and experience must be exercised when applying these ideas in each person. The interventions identified in this chapter are not inclusive. They are meant to provide examples and guidelines and to stimulate the clinician's creative talents in order to incorporate the interventions into a comprehensive treatment program determined by individual needs that improves the outcomes of the patients (Box 23-1).

POSITIONING CONCERNS

All patients spend some portion of the day in a horizontal position for rest or sleep. Some who are acutely ill or medically compromised spent extended time in bed, and major emphasis must be placed on the mobilization of patients early and often so as to prevent immobility from exerting its negative effects on all body systems (see Chapter 18). However, the time spent in a horizontal position can be used as an opportunity to assist patients in passive drainage and preventing the retention of lung secretions. It can be a natural beginning in the development of a patient's long-term respiratory program (e.g., the prevention of respiratory complications in a patient with tetraplegia). Specific postural drainage positions are covered under airway clearance interventions (see Chapter 21). Using a combination of these positions and the patient's position in bed, in the hospital or at home, can help to achieve multiple goals. First, they can assist patients in passively clearing secretions that they may have difficulty clearing actively. Pneumonia is still the leading cause of death in patients with spinal cord injury who are tetraplegic (Beuret-Blanquart & Boucand, 2003). Second, these position changes provide for skin relief and better circulation. Finally, they assist in retarding the development

377

of joint contractures or other musculoskeletal abnormalities. A four-position rotation (i.e., supine, prone, and side-to-side) or a modified six-position rotation (supine, three quarter supine, side-lying, three quarter prone on each side) is usually an effective and reasonable means of incorporating these goals into a long-term prophylactic program.

Simple adaptations may make ventilation easier in each of these postures. For example, when the patient is in the supine position, placing the patient's arms up over his or her head facilitates greater anterior upper chest expansion (Iishii, 2004). Likewise, positioning the pelvis in a slight posterior tilt facilitates more diaphragmatic excursion. (Detailed explanations of positioning are discussed in Chapter 42.) Observation of all precautions and contraindications to passive positioning is still warranted and positions should be modified based on the individual need of each patient.

Just as passive positioning of the patient in bed helps to maintain bronchial hygiene and improve ventilation potential, optimal passive positioning of the patient's skeletal frame in an upright posture (sitting, standing) helps to maximize the mechanical advantages that facilitate breathing. For example, patients with spinal cord injuries (SCIs) resulting in tetraplegia will be unable to support their intestinal contents properly under the diaphragm to allow for maximal expansion of the chest in all three planes of ventilation (see Chapter 39). The use of an abdominal support from the iliac crest to the base of the xiphoid process provides positive-pressure support to restore intestinal positioning to an upright position (Figure 23-1). Research has documented well the significant improvements in vital capacity, inspiratory capacity, and tidal volume (TV) in sitting with the use of a strong abdominal support (Boaventura & Gastaldi, 2003). These binders have also been used in nursing care to provide for better circulation and the prevention of hypotension.

BOX 23-1

Categories of Therapeutic Interventions Presented in this Chapter to Optimize Ventilation Patterns

1. Positioning concerns
2. Ventilatory and movement strategies
3. Manual facilitation techniques
   - Facilitating controlled breathing patterns (diaphragmatic)
   - Mobilizing the thorax
   - Facilitating upper chest breathing patterns (accessory muscles)
   - Promoting symmetrical breathing patterns (unilateral dysfunction)
   - Reducing high respiratory rates
4. Glossopharyngeal breathing
5. Enhancing phonation skills

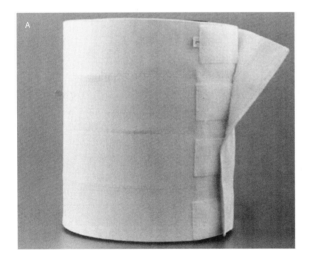

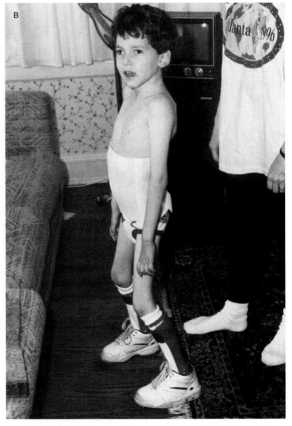

FIGURE 23-1 A, Abdominal binder, Velcro fastener. **B,** Placement of abdominal binder.

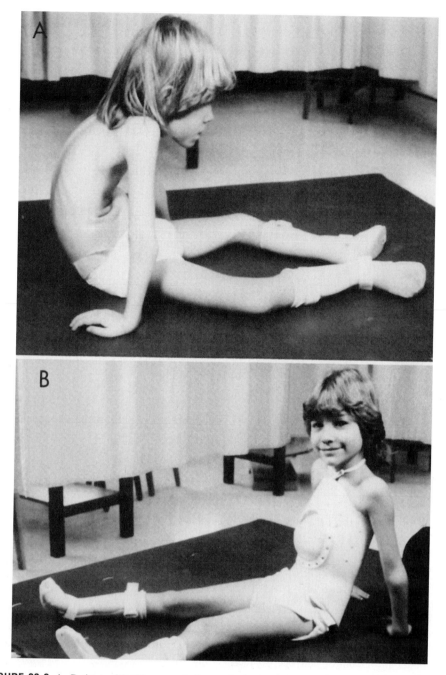

FIGURE 23-2 A, Patient with C5 congenital tetraplegia, independent long-sitting. **B,** Long-sitting with body jacket support. Note the changes in head position and eye contact, hip alignment, and shoulder rotation.

The abdominal binder's value in cosmesis may be under-rated. Many of the patients with neurological issues were once normal, healthy individuals with high self-esteem who took great pride in their appearances. They now present with protruding bellies (the anterior and inferior shift of the intestines resulting from flaccid abdominal muscles), which may be psychologically disturbing to them. Thus the use of a binder may greatly aid in the restoration of these patients' self-esteem, which should be a high-priority goal in any rehabilitation program.

A rigid type of abdominal support can be used when the vertebral column and the abdominal viscera need support. These are called body jackets or total contact thoracic lumbar sacral orthoses (TLSOs) (Figure 23-2). A TLSO is a rigid trunk support molded individually to the shape of the patient's entire trunk from the axilla down to the pubis. It is made up of two separate pieces, a front and a back, ideally with an anterior cutout in the abdomen to allow for normal diaphragmatic displacement of the viscera. In addition to these jackets, an elastic binder is applied across the cutout to

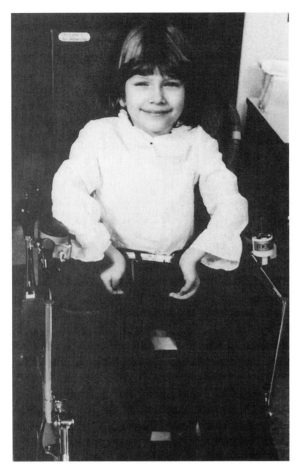

FIGURE 23-3 Wheelchair alignment considerations.

allow for diaphragmatic motion but to minimize excessive displacement of the abdominal contents. This is particularly appropriate for a growing child who needs more spinal stability and for the completely flaccid patient with tetraplegia, who may also require the same support. Because head and neck positioning are so dependent on trunk positioning, a body jacket may make the difference for these patients between being dependent or independent in an upright posture. It may result in significantly better head control and eye contact, longer phonation, and possibly better articulation. However, because it limits trunk movement, its usefulness for each patient must be assessed carefully.

The next consideration in passive respiratory techniques is proper wheelchair positioning. Optimal performance in ventilatory functioning, as well as many other areas of rehabilitation, depends on good alignment of the body against the force of gravity. Symmetry must be strived for through the use of a body jacket, lateral trunk supports in the wheelchair, abdominal binders, or some other means (Figure 23-3). This is especially important for patients with hemiplegia in whom habitual asymmetrical posturing leads to musculoskeletal problems later. Symmetrical breathing patterns and uniform aeration of all lung segments are augmented by careful upright positioning. Therefore, everything from the type of neck and

trunk support to the height and width of the arm rests to the length and type of the foot supports must be carefully analyzed for each patient.

VENTILATORY AND MOVEMENT STRATEGIES FOR IMPROVING FUNCTIONAL OUTCOMES

The patient is first positioned for successful ventilation. Then motor activities should be introduced. Interventions chosen will improve the patient's ventilatory support, or the therapist should capitalize on the patient's good ventilatory support to improve the motor activity. Using ventilatory strategies to improve motor performance or movement strategies to improve ventilation performance enables patients to achieve their functional goals sooner and have better health, including fewer respiratory complications. Generally, these simple concepts take no more than 1 to 2 additional minutes of therapy time, with no additional equipment costs other than a few extra pillows or towels. Therefore, time and money are not mitigating factors. However, these ideas do require the practitioner to look carefully at the patient before beginning any treatment intervention and to ask, "Have I positioned my patient for ventilatory success?"; "Am I simply treating the patient in whatever position I found her or him in?"; and "Have I carefully chosen my verbal cues to include a ventilatory response and a functional response?" The practitioner must actively include ventilation in every activity to help the patient understand that breathing transcends all activities. Breathing is the bridge to function. A summary of the most important ventilation-movement strategies is listed in Box 23-2.

Incorporating Simple Therapy Tasks
Inspiration

After the patient has been carefully positioned for respiratory success, as described previously, begin the patient's therapy or daily-living activities. From an anatomical perspective, the pattern of inspiration is naturally associated with the following: (1) trunk extension; (2) shoulder flexion, abduction, and external rotation movements; and (3) an upward eye gaze. Expiration is logically associated with the opposite: (1) trunk flexion; (2) shoulder extension, adduction, and internal rotation movements; and (3) a downward eye gaze. In a study looking at rhythmic pronation and supination wrist movements, inspiration and exhalation adapted and became coordinated with the arm movement (Gandevia, 2002; Temprado et al, 2002). Accordingly, then, the simple task of passive range of movement (ROM) can easily include the active goal of increasing ventilation by asking the patient to breathe in and look up when his or her arm is raised up into shoulder flexion. This encourages the patient to breathe in when his or her chest wall muscles are being stretched and the ribs are naturally opening up, causing both activities to be more successful. It also begins to teach the patient to use ventilatory strategies to optimize potential functional movement, such as in reaching up to a kitchen cabinet. Patients need to focus on avoiding breath holding and incorporating breathing during each activity.

Exhalation

Likewise, active or passive exhalation should be coordinated with the reverse upper-extremity ROM pattern (i.e., the arm returning from flexion back to the patient's side). This can be done using all types of exhalation patterns, including the following: (1) passive quiet exhalation; (2) forceful exhalation, as in blowing, coughing, or pursed-lips exhalation; or (3) vocalization patterns. Thus the therapist may ask the patient to slowly count out loud to 10 while the arm is being returned eccentrically to his or her side. The patient learns to correlate exhalation with shoulder extension while simultaneously learning a much more complex idea—that of controlling his or her rate and volume of expiration by including deliberate speech during exhalation maneuvers. Research is being done in the area of respiratory plasticity to evaluate changes with exercise and conditioning (Mitchell & Johnson, 2003; Morris et al, 2003). Clinical observation demonstrates that patients will incorporate new ventilation strategies and that they become less cognitive and more based in habit as they are repeated.

To improve exhalation potential, increase the patient's relative trunk flexion alignment. While still supine and performing upper-extremity ROM, this can be simply accomplished by asking the patient to lift his or her head and watch the hand as it returns to his or her side, which increases abdominal and intercostal activation, or by asking the patient to increase knee flexion, which increases posterior pelvic tilting and trunk flexion. Pairing trunk flexion with exhalation completes the trunk movement strategy for better ventilation.

Combining positioning with verbal cues for ventilation, as described in ROM activities, changes passive upper-extremity ROM exercises into dynamic upper-extremity ROM exercises. It encourages increased inspiratory and expiratory capacities, develops early functional motor planning strategies, and facilitates trunk mobility. In this manner the patient has the opportunity to learn from the beginning of his or her rehabilitation process that movement and breathing go hand in hand. Clinically, incorporating appropriate breathing patterns with movement early in the rehabilitation process discourages the development of Valsalva patterns or shallow breathing patterns when the motor activities become more difficult and

complex. Patients who are mechanically ventilated on an assist mode can accomplish this as well.

Dynamic Activities

Inhalation promotes trunk extension, exhalation promotes trunk flexion, and vice versa. This basic theme occurs naturally in all motor activities but may have ceased to become spontaneous after a neuromuscular or musculoskeletal insult. Valsalva, or breath holding, maneuvers during transitional movements, such as rolling or coming to a sitting or standing position, are often noted in these patients. By teaching them strategies that incorporate breathing into their motor plans for all motor activities, Valsalva patterns can be eliminated or minimized while simultaneously promoting better cardiac function.

The following activities are just a few of the common daily activities. They are typical gross motor activities, but the use of ventilatory strategies is a means of improving patients' abilities to perform them. Extrapolation of these concepts to all other motor activities should be carefully analyzed by each therapist for each individual patient, looking at the trunk patterns and type of muscle contraction that occurs in a given exercise or activity. At times there may be more than one effective ventilation strategy; there is no hard and fast rule. The important concept is that the patient breathe with the movement and not holding his or her breath.

Rolling

Ask patients to attempt to roll, and assess whether they tend to move with trunk extension or flexion to begin the roll. Those who roll in trunk extension patterns should be asked to breathe in while they roll and to look up. Those who roll with trunk flexion as their primary movement pattern should be instructed to roll while blowing out and tucking the chin. In doing so, patients work with, not against, natural whole patterns of movements that increase the likelihood of success.

Coming Up to Sitting

Pushing up to sitting from side-lying should be evaluated in much the same manner. If patients are more effective in coming to the upright position when using trunk extension, have them inhale as they push up to sitting. Asking them to look up as they move will reinforce the upper chest movements through the use of the symmetrical tonic neck reflex (STNR). If they have more success in pushing up with trunk flexion, have them blow out and tuck the chin while moving. It may be helpful to allow patients to try both strategies and see which is most effective. The important consideration is that they do not hold the breath while changing the position.

Dressing

Patients often express how short of breath they become with dressing. These activities, too, can benefit from the concepts discussed here. While putting on lower-extremity items such as pants, socks, and shoes in a long-sitting position, have the patient first take in a deep breath while extending his or her trunk. Then have the patient blow out, huff out, or cough while flexing the trunk to reach his or her toes. This combines the functional daily task of dressing with improving breath control, trunk control, and airway-clearance techniques.

Upper-extremity dressing and upper-extremity exercise can incorporate the same ideas. All movements should be coordinated with appropriate chest wall movements to maximize upper-extremity tasks. Thus, every time the arm is moving up above 90 degrees of shoulder flexion, the patient should be asked to breathe in, allowing for the normal shoulder/rib-cage rhythm to occur. Full shoulder flexion requires the opening of the intercostal spacing and the separation of the individual ribs. Many patients with neurological impairments have lost the intrinsic mobility of the chest wall and thus may have lost some functional shoulder ROM as well. Not pairing inspiration with shoulder flexion is likely to limit the patient's shoulder ROM to approximately 140 to 150 degrees. It may also encourage Valsalva maneuvers during the activity and may cause more shoulder pain.

Coming Up to Standing

Coming up to standing requires both trunk flexion and trunk extension. Patients often use a rhythmic initiation (rocking) to begin the sit-to-stand transfer. This is a good opportunity to begin teaching breath control. Patients breathe in and then as they rock forward, they exhale; rocking backwards, they inhale as the trunk extends. There can be several cycles of rocking and breathing prior to standing before control is attained. Thus, patients should initiate the forward trunk lean with exhalation and initiate the standing phase with inhalation and trunk and neck extension. Active neck extension during assumption of standing not only facilitates greater inhalation but, along with the influence of the tonic labyrinthine reflex (TLR), also facilitates more significant contractions of the trunk and hip extensors. Clinically, this often results in a more noticeably upright posture and may make the difference between an assisted standing pivot transfer and an independent one. Returning to sitting should be accompanied by slow, controlled exhalation, such as in pursed-lips blowing or counting out loud, so as to maximize the body's controlled descent into gravity's influence.

FACILITATING A CONTROLLED DIAPHRAGMATIC BREATHING PATTERN

Why would a therapist want to change a patient's breathing pattern? The answer is simple—when the pattern being used is ineffective. Ordinarily, people use the pattern of breathing that is the most efficient for them. However, when the work of breathing increases and there is musculoskeletal, neuromuscular, or pulmonary impairment, abnormal patterns that are not efficient may be adopted. The patient knows that it requires hard work to breathe but often does not know how to do it with greater ease, especially during stressful situations when

panic is present. The patient may spontaneously do pursed-lips breathing (PLB) but often in a forceful manner that may not relieve the dyspnea.

A healthy person uses approximately 5% of total oxygen consumption and 10% of vital capacity for the muscular work of breathing. Consequently, breathing at rest is generally perceived as effortless under normal conditions.

However, in the patients physical therapists evaluate and treat (often after surgery, respiratory disease, or dysfunction secondary to neurological insult or injury), the vital capacity may be significantly decreased and the oxygen consumption may be greatly increased because of the use of accessory muscles or the extra effort needed to breathe or cough. In a patient with tetraplegia, for example, the vital capacity may be reduced to 1000 to 1500 ml. If the normal TV (normal volume of breathing) is 500 ml, that means that with each breath the patient would use 33% to 50% of his or her vital capacity (maximal inspiration followed by maximal exhalation). This would greatly increase the work of breathing and oxygen consumption just for normal quiet breathing. The patient would have little pulmonary reserve. This can lead to respiratory muscle fatigue. During exercise or stress, the patient would have an increased subjective feeling of shortness of breath and feel an increase in the work of breathing. In addition, patients with spinal cord injury who are smokers experience excessive vital capacity losses (Linn et al, 2003). Commonly used terms to describe breathing patterns are listed in Box 23-3.

BOX 23-3

Breathing Pattern Terminology

Eupnea—Normal breathing, repeated rhythmic inspiratory-expiratory cycles

Hyperpnea—Increased breathing; usually refers to increased tidal volume with or without increased frequency

Polypnea, tachypnea—Increased frequency of breathing

Hyperventilation—Increased alveolar ventilation in relation to metabolic rate (an increase in alveolar ventilation); seen as a decrease in the arterial Pco_2

Hypoventilation—Decreased alveolar ventilation in relation to metabolic rate (a decrease in alveolar ventilation); seen as an increase in Pco_2

Apnea—Cessation of respiration in the resting expiratory position

Dyspnea—The patient's subjective feeling of shortness of breath

Apneusis—Cessation of respiration in the inspiratory position

Apneustic breathing—Apneusis interrupted periodically by exhalation

Cheyne-Stokes respiration—Cycles of gradually increasing tidal volume followed by gradually decreasing tidal volume (usually followed by an apneic period)

Biot respiration—Sequences of uniformly deep gasps and apnea, followed by deep gasps

Adapted from Comroe, J.H., Jr. (1974). Physiology of respiration, ed 2. St. Louis: Mosby.

BOX 23-4

Indications for Teaching Controlled-Breathing Techniques

Patients with any of the following:
- Pulmonary dysfunction, either primary or secondary causes
- Pain resulting from surgery, trauma, or disease
- Apprehension or nervousness
- Bronchospasm or impending bronchospasm in asthma
- Airway clearance dysfunction
- Restriction of inspiration resulting from musculoskeletal dysfunction, such as scoliosis, kyphoscoliosis, or pectus excavatum; obesity; pregnancy; pulmonary pathology such as fibrosis; scarring resulting from radiation therapy; neurologic weakness such as spinal cord injury, Parkinson disease, or myasthenia gravis
- Congestive heart failure, pulmonary edema, or pulmonary emboli
- Rib fractures
- Ventilated patients on assist control or intermittent mandatory ventilation
- Metabolic disturbances that have a compensatory respiratory response
- Debilitated or bedridden patients, who tend to have constant volume ventilation and retain secretions and are prone to pneumonia and atelectasis due to poor airway clearance

---

BOX 23-5

Goals of Teaching Controlled-Breathing Techniques

To decrease the work of breathing
To improve alveolar ventilation
To improve airway clearance by improving cough
To increase strength, coordination, and efficiency of respiratory muscles
To teach the patient how to respond to and control breathing
To assist in relaxation
To mobilize and maintain mobility of the thorax
To enable patients to feel self-control and confidence in managing disease or dysfunction

---

A listing of indications for teaching controlled-breathing techniques is given in Box 23-4.

It should be appreciated that breathing comfortably and in a controlled manner is associated with wellness and a sense of ease. Even normal individuals who are under stress and have increased work levels are more cognizant of the increase in work of breathing. For a patient who is struggling with every breath and wonders how it will be possible to get through the day, ventilatory strategies and breathing-control techniques can be the key to maximizing potential. A list of goals for teaching controlled-breathing techniques is found in Box 23-5.

Breathing control has long been used in yoga to focus and to promote meditation. This is a key to maximizing rehabilitation. Patients who cannot breathe cannot function! It is of primary importance to assess patients' breathing at rest and during exercise. People often hold their breath with exertion, especially during new activities, so it is vital to assess the cardiopulmonary and neuromuscular response to each new activity.

CONSIDERATIONS IN TEACHING BREATHING CONTROL TO PATIENTS WITH PRIMARY VERSUS SECONDARY PULMONARY DYSFUNCTION

Patients with primary lung disease, such as chronic obstructive pulmonary disease (COPD), asthma, bronchitis, or cystic fibrosis, present a picture very different from that of patients with secondary pulmonary deficits, SCI, Parkinson disease, myasthenia gravis, or Guillain-Barré syndrome.

In general, patients with primary lung disease tend to overuse their accessory muscles and greatly increase the work of breathing secondary to shortness of breath or coughing. They often complain that they have difficulty "getting the air out," which demonstrates the decreased expiratory flow rates noted on pulmonary function tests. This can lead to dynamic hyperinflation, in which patients continue to gasp and increase the respiratory rate so more air is coming in, but there is not time for the air to be exhaled. Large volumes of air can get trapped in the lungs, which causes increased feelings of shortness of breath and panic. The goal with these patients is to teach them to relax the neck and chest accessory muscles and use more diaphragmatic breathing (abdominal and lateral costal breathing) to reduce the work of breathing in combination with relaxed pursed-lip breathing and prolonged exhalation. Their treatment programs focus on energy conservation, relaxation, and pacing activity with breath control. In pulmonary rehabilitation programs, exercise is a key component. Patients learn to coordinate their breathing with their activities and find that they have less dyspnea with exertion (Gigliotti et al, 2003).

However, in patients with secondary pulmonary dysfunction such as SCI, there is a more restrictive component to inspiration. In these cases, accessory muscles may be intact, but they are not being used to facilitate deep breathing or coughing. Patients may have strong diaphragmatic breaths but the upper chest collapses on inspiration (paradoxical breathing; see Chapter 39). The goal is to teach the patients to use the accessory muscles to balance the upper and lower chest. This facilitates an increase in vital capacity that prevents atelectasis and pneumonia by increasing the volume of ventilation and improving the cough mechanism.

The choice of appropriate ventilatory strategies is determined by the individual patient's problem. The following questions should be considered when evaluating a patient:

- Does the patient have more difficulty in inspiration or exhalation?

- Is there a normal sequence to inspiration (i.e., abdominal wall rise, then lateral costal expansion, then upper chest expansion, with a full inspiration)? Or does the chest sink and the abdomen rise on inspiration?
- Does the patient appear to be working hard to breathe? Is the patient using the accessory muscles to an extreme?
- Does the patient have trouble coughing or frequently clear throat or have difficulty in speaking a normal volume and for the normal length of sentences?
- Is ventilation the limiting factor in accomplishing an activity (e.g., transfer, gait, or bed mobility)?

Patients with primary pulmonary disease generally benefit from ventilatory strategies that relax the accessory muscles and facilitate relaxed diaphragmatic breathing. On the other hand, patients with secondary pulmonary dysfunction usually benefit from the balanced use of the diaphragm and accessory muscles to increase vital capacity and breath support for activities.

PURSED-LIPS BREATHING

PLB is a strategy that is often spontaneously used by people with COPD during episodes of dyspnea. Many patients feel this breathing pattern helps to decrease their breathlessness. The effect of PLB is an increase in the time of exhalation, which results in a decrease in the end expiratory volume and an increase in the total time of the respiratory cycle. This results in a decreased respiratory rate and increased TV. There was also found to be a decrease in the Borg scale of perceived exertion when PLB was used (Bianchi et al, 2004).

When instructing a patient in PLB, emphasis should be placed on a relaxed, slow, prolonged, controlled exhalation. Often when patients initiate PLB spontaneously, they use a forceful exhalation, which tightens the neck musculature and oral area. This builds a significant pressure that can counteract the effectiveness of the technique and the subsequent relief of dysnpnea. A relaxed neck and mouth are essential.

If a patient has difficulty relaxing the mouth, he or she may be encouraged to try to making an sssss, or hissing, sound, which will still prolong exhalation and provide back pressure.

RELATIONSHIP OF THE DIAPHRAGM AND POSTURE

The respiratory action of the diaphragm and other respiratory muscles is normally coordinated with the need to provide postural control of the trunk during movement of the extremities (Temprado et al, 2002). The diaphragm acts both as a muscle of respiration and as a muscle in the group of muscles providing core stability to the trunk. However, when respiratory demand increases, the diaphragm may not be able to continue to provide both functions (Hodges, 1997, 2000a, 2000b, 2001, 2002; Saunders, 2004). Because the diaphragm is the primary muscle of respiration, postural control may be impaired. A complete discussion of this concept is provided in Chapter 39.

BOX 23-6

Diaphragmatic Facilitation Techniques

1. Relaxation technique
2. Repatterning techniques
   - Relaxed pursed-lips breathing
   - Exhalation, hold, and inhalation
3. Sniffing
4. Diaphragmatic scoop technique
5. Lateral costal facilitation technique
6. Upper chest inhibiting technique
7. Normal timing technique

FACILITATING DIAPHRAGMATIC BREATHING

In the initial phases of breathing retraining, the easiest intervention that facilitates diaphragmatic breathing is utilized; if it is not successful, there will be a progression of specific inhibition and facilitation techniques. A summary of methods of facilitating diaphragmatic ventilation patterns is given in Box 23-6.

DIAPHRAGMATIC CONTROLLED BREATHING

Diaphragmatic breathing is the normal mode of ventilation. The diaphragm and intercostals are the normal muscles of quiet inspiration. When evaluating a patient's breathing pattern, the use of accessory muscles during quiet breathing should be noted; the patient with primary pulmonary disease need to be instructed in relaxation of the accessory muscles to decrease the work of breathing. However, in a patient with a spinal cord injury or other neuromuscular disorder, these accessory muscles may assist in balancing ventilation and may be useful in increasing vital capacity, improving the ability to cough, improving breath support for speaking, and increasing the potential for functional activities.

In general, controlled diaphragmatic breathing should be emphasized in each posture and in all therapeutic activities because carry-over of the breathing pattern from one posture to another or one activity to another is not necessarily present. If the patient is shown the pattern only when in the supine position, it may not carry over to sitting or to a sliding-board transfer, when the activity becomes more complex. A helpful sequence might be to teach the breathing pattern in side-lying, supine, sitting, and standing positions and in walking, stair climbing, and other functional activities, especially in patients with COPD. Patients with neurological impairment may require modification of the breathing pattern so it conforms with their activity levels and capabilities.

POSITIONING CONCERNS

Position of Pelvis

The first step in facilitating any breathing pattern is to position the patient for ventilatory success. The details are discussed in this chapter and in Chapter 42. Often a patient's posture and pelvic position have dramatic effects on breathing. In general, a slight, relative posterior tilt of the pelvis facilitates diaphragmatic breathing, and a relative anterior tilt facilitates the opening of the anterior chest and upper chest breathing. It is helpful to see what difference a slight, relative change in pelvic position will do to a patient's ability to ventilate. This is especially true in secondary pulmonary problems related to neurological and neuromuscular dysfunction. A lumbar roll or a roll under the ischial tuberosities can facilitate an anterior pelvic tilt (see Chapter 42).

RELAXATION OF UPPER CHEST AND SHOULDERS

Jacobsen's progressive relaxation exercises are familiar to physical therapists. Jacobsen proposed that a maximal muscle contraction would yield a maximal muscle relaxation. This technique can be applied to the upper chest and shoulders. The therapist places his or her hands on the patient's shoulder girdle. The patient is asked to shrug his or her shoulders up into the therapist's hands and hold it. "Don't let me push your shoulders down," is the therapist's command. Then, "Let your shoulders relax, let them go." The emphasis is on the relaxation phase. Verbal commands can be very important with this procedure. A strong command to "Raise your shoulders into my hands" is followed by a quiet, calmer, "Now relax and let them go," repeating quietly, "That's it, let them go, feel them relax." The addition of counter-rotation of the shoulder girdle can make this intervention more effective. Patients can learn the techniques independently so they can relax their shoulders when they begin to feel tense. In addition, making shoulder circles in both directions, forward and backwards, can loosen the shoulder girdle. Sometimes the relaxation activity is all that it takes to resume a more natural pattern of breathing, and you can move on to other therapeutic activities. If the patient starts to use accessory muscles again, the technique is repeated. The patient learns to feel the difference between tension and relaxation of the shoulders and can self-monitor and perform the relaxation independently.

REPATTERNING TECHNIQUE

If a patient needs more support to gain control of breathing and is experiencing shortness of breath, a simple repatterning technique may be beneficial. An example might be a patient with asthma who has a high respiratory rate and is feeling panicky. When the patient is asked why he or she is breathing so fast the reply will usually be, "I am not getting enough air, I can't catch my breath." The patient is asked to start with exhalation. "Try to blow out easily with your lips pursed. Don't force it just let it come out." Suggesting that the patient visualize a candle with a flame which their exhalation makes flicker but not go out will help to produce a prolonged, easy exhalation. Doing this allows the respiratory rate to decrease automatically. When the patient feels some control of this step, then ask him or her to "hold your breath at the top of

inspiration just for a second or two." Make sure the patient does not hold his or her breath and bear down as in a Valsalva maneuver. Last, ask the patient to take a slow breath in, hold it, and let it go out through pursed lips. Patients learn that when they are short of breath, this technique often helps them to gain control, making them feel less panicky.

Sniffing

If working toward a generalized controlled-breathing pattern does not improve the patient's ventilatory pattern adequately, a technique that more specifically addresses the need to initiate breathing from the diaphragm can be attempted. Sniffing is a simple and effective means of teaching diaphragmatic breathing (Katagiri, 2003). Sniffing is accomplished primarily by the diaphragm. This technique can be utilized first when attempting more specific diaphragmatic training with patients who are capable of attempting sniffing because of its simplicity.

As with all procedures, the most important step is the first step: position the patient appropriately to increase the likelihood of increased diaphragmatic breathing resulting from musculoskeletal alignment. This includes the following: (1) choosing a gravity-eliminated position such as side-lying or a gravity-assisted position such as a supported semi-Fowler sitting position (supported spine); (2) choosing a relatively posteriorly tilted pelvis with flexed knees; (3) choosing the arms to be down below 90 degrees of flexion (in relative shoulder extension, adduction, and internal rotation); and (4) choosing to use a pillow or pillows under the head. (For details on positioning, see Chapter 40.) For each patient, choices will be different (e.g., the amount of knee flexion or the number of pillows). Find the right combination of positioning characteristics that best facilitates diaphragmatic movement for that particular patient. In this manner the therapist sets up the patient for ventilatory success before beginning the manual or verbal technique.

Initially, ask the patient to place his or her hands on the abdomen for increased proprioceptive feedback and the relative extension, adduction, and internal rotation position of the shoulders. In a quiet voice, ask the patient to "sniff in three times." Note whether the patient demonstrates more abdominal rise or lower chest expansion or both. If so, draw attention to this fact. During exhalation, tell the patient to "let it out slowly," which helps to prolong the exhalation and slow the respiratory rate (RR) and often encourages some relaxation. Progress the training by asking the patient to "now sniff in twice, a little deeper." Do you still see greater diaphragmatic excursion and less upper chest excursion? If so, continue by asking for "one long slow sniff." If successful, the therapist should follow with "now do it more quietly," then "now do it more slowly," "even more quietly," "less effort," and so forth. By this time, the patient should be demonstrating an easy-onset, slower RR and a diaphragmatic pattern with relaxed shoulders.

Clinical experience has shown this technique to be highly successful with about 80% of patients who have primary pulmonary pathologies or neurological impairments. The key to success seems to stem from the relaxed tones and words that the therapist uses, which decrease anxiety and imply relaxation and not "effort." Once the pattern has been established, the patient can easily be instructed to go through the training independently, as needed. The sequence (in whole or in part) may be appropriate for patients before getting out of bed if they become anxious and demonstrate excessive upper chest breathing during this activity. For other patients, it may be appropriate before or during eating or before climbing stairs. Obviously, the application of this technique will be individualized for each patient, depending on individual impairments.

PROCEDURE FOR TEACHING CONTROLLED DIAPHRAGMATIC BREATHING (SCOOP TECHNIQUE)

Minimal patient instruction is necessary to facilitate diaphragmatic breathing using the scoop technique. It allows the patient to feel the breathing pattern; then it is brought to the patient's cognitive awareness. The patient then learns to self-cue to incorporate the breathing pattern.

The following is a suggested sequence:

1. Position the patient for success, generally in a side-lying position in a semi-Fowler position or supine in a semi-Fowler position, with a bend in the knees to achieve a relative posterior pelvic tilt and relaxation of the abdominal muscles.
2. Place your hand on the patient's abdomen at the level of the umbilicus. Tell the patient you want to feel his or her breathing. Follow the patient's breathing pattern for a few cycles until you are in synchrony with his or her respiratory rhythm. Do not invade the patient's breathing pattern; rather, at first, follow its movement.
3. After the normal end of the patient's exhalation, give a slow stretch and "scoop" your hand up and under the anterior thorax as shown in Figure 23-4. The command, "Now, breathe into my hand," is given as the slow scoop stretch is done.

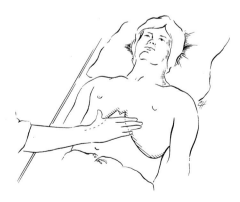

FIGURE 23-4 Therapist's hand placement for diaphragmatic breathing.

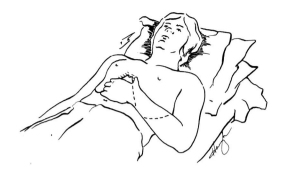

FIGURE 23-5 The patient is encouraged to continue practicing diaphragmatic breathing to become aware of his breathing pattern. This is usually the first position of the diaphragmatic breathing teaching sequence.

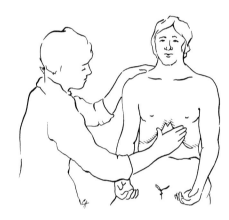

FIGURE 23-6 The patient advances to the sitting position for breathing retraining. Note the relaxed position of the patient's shoulders and hands.

4. As the scoop stretch is performed, instruct the patient to, "breathe into my hand" during the inspiration. Give a scoop at the end of exhalation with each breath. The verbal command can be effectively replaced after a few respiratory cycles with audible breathing to facilitate the ventilatory pattern.
5. After achieving some success, call the patient's attention to the awareness of the breathing pattern. For example, the therapist can ask, "Can you feel how your abdomen rises as you breathe in and your ribs go up to the side?" The patient's hand can be placed on the abdomen with the therapist's hand on top. Reinforce the breathing pattern, then remove your hand and allow the patient to feel independently the ventilatory pattern (Figure 23-5).

A few things should be taken into consideration. Don't ask patients to take too many deep breaths; they may begin to feel light-headed because they may hyperventilate and blow off too much CO_2. The fact that they are breathing more with their diaphragms is the important consideration. Note also the position of the pelvis and trunk.

When the patient has mastered the breathing pattern in the side-lying position, try supine. Then progress to sitting (Figure 23-6), standing (Figure 23-7), walking (Figure 23-8)

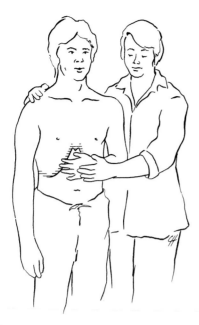

FIGURE 23-7 The third position in the sequence is standing. Full-length mirrors are helpful at this point.

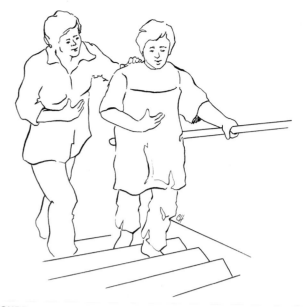

FIGURE 23-9 Stairs are important, especially if the patient has them at home. He is instructed to pause slightly as he breathes in and to exhale as he climbs one to two steps.

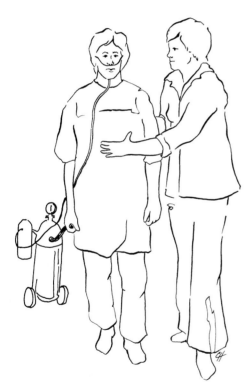

FIGURE 23-8 Walking is the fourth stage of retraining. The patient is encouraged to relax, control his breathing, take long steps, and slow down.

and, finally, stairs (Figure 23-9). Each position increases the difficulty in performing diaphragmatic breathing. In the side-lying or supine position, the patient is fully supported. The side-lying position is especially good for teaching diaphragmatic breathing initially because the diaphragm is in a gravity-

eliminated position. In the supine position, the patient must breathe against gravity. As he or she progresses to sitting, the patient must also provide trunk support and maintain stability against gravity as well as relax the shoulders. In standing, the entire body must be supported, and when walking and stairs are added, the element of breathing coordination as well as weight shifting and balance increase the complexity of the activity.

Coordination of breathing for walking involves being careful not to allow the patient to hold the breath. It is important to keep inspiration and exhalation regular at a ratio of at least 1 to 1, preferably exhaling a little longer—1 to 2 or 1 to 4. In some yoga breathing techniques the exhalation is significantly longer—1 to 6, 1 to 8, or at times even longer.

In general, the preferred pattern for a patient with primary pulmonary dysfunction is as follows: (1) Have the patient pause at the base of the stairs to gain control. (2) Have the patient take a breath in and move up one step as he or she exhales. (3) The patient then pauses to inspire and exhales as he or she walks up another step. (4) The patient should be encouraged to use the handrail and pace his or her movement slowly and with breath control.

In general, a patient with neuromusculoskeletal issues who has lower-extremity weakness may benefit from inspiration while ascending stairs and exhalation during descent. Going downstairs uses an eccentric muscle pattern and exhalation is a relatively eccentric contraction of the diaphragm. Refer to the section on ventilation and movement strategies in this chapter for additional information.

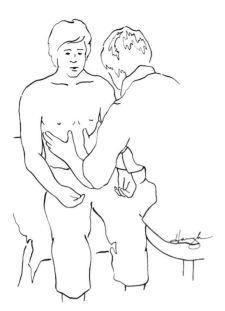

FIGURE 23-10 Bilateral lower lobe expansion (this also facilitates diaphragmatic movement).

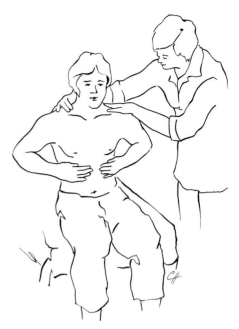

FIGURE 23-12 Self-assisted bilateral chest expansion exercise. Keep the patient's shoulders relaxed.

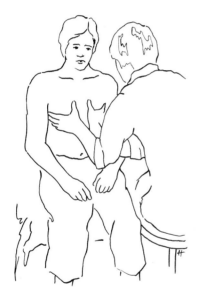

FIGURE 23-11 Bilateral midchest expansion exercise.

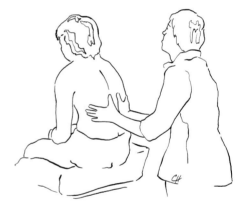

FIGURE 23-13 Bilateral posterior chest expansion exercise.

LATERAL COSTAL BREATHING

Lateral costal breathing also facilitates diaphragmatic excusion. It may be done bilaterally, as shown in Figures 23-10, 23-11, 23-12, 23-13, and 23-14, or unilaterally as shown in Figures 23-15, 23-16, and 23-17. Lower chest lateral costal expansion facilitates diaphragmatic and intercostal breathing in which the mid chest recruits primarily intercostal activity (DeTroyer et al, 2003).

Upper Chest Inhibition

If all other manual facilitation interventions do not produce the desired increase in diaphragmatic breathing, inhibiting the upper chest during inhalation may be effective.

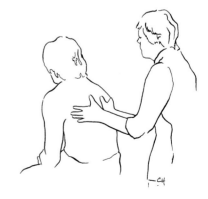

FIGURE 23-14 Bilateral posterior chest expansion exercise.

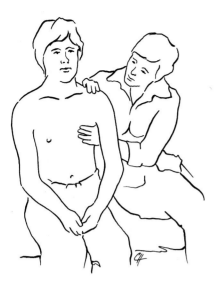

FIGURE 23-15 Unilateral (segmental) breathing, left mid-lung field.

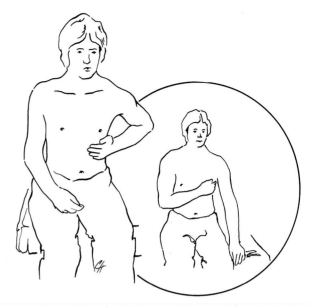

FIGURE 23-17 The patient can perform unilateral (segmental) breathing by placing either hand on the side of the chest to be emphasized. The patient can also perform mid-chest expansion by moving his hand up.

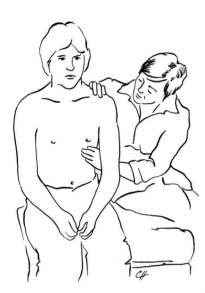

FIGURE 23-16 Unilateral (segmental) breathing emphasizing the left lower lobe. Note that the patient's shoulder must remain down, with hands placed on ulnar border or palms up in his lap.

First, position the patient appropriately in a side-lying, three quarter supine, or supine position. Begin by facilitating the diaphragm, usually with the diaphragm scoop. Slowly bring your other arm across the upper chest at about the level of the sternal angle. Leave it there for a couple of respiratory cycles without applying any pressure so as to feel the upper chest's movement.

After assessing this movement, gently allow your arm to follow the upper chest back to its resting position when the patient exhales. On the patient's next inspiratory effort, do not move your arm position. Thus your arm position will apply pressure or resistance to the expansion of the upper chest. This gentle pressure will cause postural inhibition to the

anterior and superior movement of the upper chest. After each expiratory cycle, add more pressure until the patient subconsciously increases the lower chest breathing out of necessity.

When you note more diaphragmatic or lower intercostal muscle excursion, mention it to the patient. Ask the patient to try to reproduce this pattern. With your other arm, continue to facilitate the desired response, such as with the diaphragm scoop. Slowly, during each of the next series of inhalations, release your inhibition as the patient tries to maintain the improved lower chest breathing pattern. If the patient is only partially successful, the inhibition can be partially reapplied to assist the patient. If the patient becomes anxious because the therapist's inhibition is preventing upper chest breathing, then decrease the inhibition to a comfortable level. This technique should never cause an increase in anxiety or it will only encourage more upper chest breathing rather than less. When the pressure is released on the upper chest, continue to facilitate diaphragmatic breathing and strive to have the patient do it independently.

Normal Timing

During normal quiet inspiration (controlled breathing), the diaphragm contracts, which is seen outwardly as a gentle rise of the abdomen. The second movement is seen as lateral costal expansion of the lower chest and, usually to a lesser extent, lower anterior chest expansion. Last, the upper chest rises slightly primarily in a superior-anterior plane, with less lateral expansion noted. A normal timing technique adapted from the physical therapy approach of proprioceptive neuromuscular facilitation (PNF) can help the patient work on this sequence. After the patient has learned to initiate inspiration with his or her diaphragm and lower chest wall muscles more consistently, this technique can help to put the whole sequence together. The diaphragm continues to be the primary mover, but the accessory muscles are encouraged to do what they should do, which is to assist the diaphragm for better overall ventilation.

Generally, the patient is positioned symmetrically in either a supine or a supported sitting position, with a neutral pelvic position. The therapist waits until the end of an expiratory cycle and then, using the hand placement of the diaphragm scoop, asks the patient to breathe in "here." With the other hand, the therapist moves up the chest wall to the lower sternum and touches the patient, giving instructions again to "now breathe here." Finally, the therapist uses the first hand to move up to the upper sternum (usually around the level of the sternal angle) and asks the patient to "now breathe here." It is important that the therapist smoothly transition from one hand to the next to assist the patient in developing a smooth motor transition from one area of the chest to the other. The manual cues provide tactile cuing rather than true motor facilitation. Because of this, the normal timing sequence is obviously a more advanced technique intended for use after success has been achieved in initial diaphragmatic training. It can address the functional need of the patient to take a quick deep breath to cough or a deeper breath in order to talk in longer sentences.

MOBILIZING THE THORAX

For some patients, controlled breathing alone may not alleviate inefficient ventilatory patterns, even with utilization of good positioning and appropriate ventilatory strategies. The thorax itself may be incapable of moving freely enough to allow for the adequate chest wall excursion necessary for that breathing pattern. For example, a patient with a spinal cord injury who is demonstrating an excessive diaphragmatic pattern that is unbalanced by the normal neuromuscular support of the intercostal and abdominal muscles can breathe using minimal chest wall expansion. This is often referred to as "belly breathing." It may be necessary to mobilize individual rib segments to gain the potential for chest wall expansion in all three planes of ventilation before facilitating a specific breathing pattern. If the potential for movement is not there, the breathing pattern cannot change. Likewise, a patient having primary pulmonary dysfunction and COPD, undergoing chest surgery, having chest tubes, or suffering from acute chest trauma may also find the rib cage stiff or sore and thus limited in its potential expansion. All these patients may benefit from the inclusion of rib cage mobilization in their therapy programs. The rib cage musculoskeletal limitation may be secondary to muscular atrophy or spasticity or to pain. Thus patients with either primary pulmonary dysfunction or secondary pulmonary dysfunction can benefit from the practice of chest mobilization.

It is beyond the scope of this textbook to detail all the numerous techniques involved in musculoskeletal mobilization

---

BOX 23-7

Techniques to Mobilize the Thorax

1. Use of towel rolls or pillows to mechanically open up the anterior or lateral chest wall
2. Use of upper-extremity patterns to facilitate the opening of individual rib segments
3. Counter-rotation of the trunk
4. Use of ventilatory-movement strategies to facilitate opening of the entire thorax
5. Specific rib mobilization to free up an individual segment
6. Myofascial release techniques to free up restrictive connective tissue on and around the thorax
7. Soft-tissue release techniques to lengthen individual tight muscles

---

of the thorax, but some simple techniques and suggestions for further study are presented. A summary of mobilization techniques is found in Box 23-7.

Once again the therapist should note that the initial step toward achieving success is positioning. Starting with the patient in the supine position, anterior chest wall mobility can be improved by placing a vertical towel roll down the length of the thoracic spine and allowing gravity to pull the shoulders back to the bed. In this position, the anterior chest is opened up, stretching the intercostal and pectoralis muscles for easier facilitation of upper chest expansion.

In the side-lying position, the lateral aspect of the chest can be passively mobilized with gravity's assistance by placing one or more towel rolls or pillows under the lower chest (ribs 8 to 10) on the weight-bearing side. To determine an appropriate amount of side-bending, make sure that the patient's shoulder and pelvis are still in direct contact with the surface, even with the towel rolls in place. This maximizes the stretch of the chest without placing the patient in a position that is too advanced for his or her current chest wall mobility. Patients vary from tolerating only a single thin towel roll to tolerating three pillows under the lower ribs.

In both postures, active or passive stretching can be added after positioning for success. In the supine position, the patient is asked to move arms directly up over his or her head (shoulder flexion) as far as possible while watching his or her hands. Using the appropriate ventilatory strategy, the patient is also instructed to inhale during this movement. Because both full shoulder flexion and inspiration require the opening of the individual rib segments, pairing them in this gravity-assisted position promotes a greater passive chest wall stretch then either technique alone. If straight flexion is not a viable option, use a butterfly position, raising the arms up in shoulder flexion, abduction, and external rotation with elbows bent (like butterfly wings), again pairing this with voluntary maximal inspiration and upward eye gaze. Pairing inspiration and shoulder flexion maximizes the stretch on the chest and encourages better ventilatory strategies.

Ask the patient, while in a side-lying position, to bring his or her arm up in straight flexion to maximize anterior chest expansion or to move the arm into abduction so as to maximize the lateral costal expansion. Pair either movement with inspiration and upward eye gaze. If upper extremity movement is not possible, the therapist can passively use counter-rotation of the trunk to mobilize the chest while the patient is in the side-lying position over a towel or pillow. Continue to ask the patient to follow the movement with his or her eyes.

The same concepts can be used in upright postures, such as sitting or standing. Use a vertical towel roll along the thoracic spine, either along the back of a chair or wheelchair or along a wall. Move the patient's arms passively or actively up into the most extreme flexion or butterfly position possible. The patient will experience a more significant stretch in the anterior chest wall using the towel roll than without it. Precautions must be taken in patients with musculoskeletal problems along the spine and in patients with impaired skin-tolerance.

If these general mobilization techniques do not produce enough chest wall mobility to allow freer breathing patterns to occur, more specific techniques must be considered, including the following: (1) specific rib mobilization; (2) myofascial release of tight connective tissues (e.g., scar tissue secondary to areas of surgery or trauma); and (3) soft tissue release in tight muscle groups. (Neurologically impaired patients often present with tightness in the pectoralis, intercostal, and quadratus lumborum muscle groups, whereas orthopedically impaired patients tend to have more tightness in the neck and back muscles.) Use the positioning and ventilatory strategies previously suggested (e.g., side-lying over a towel roll) during these specific interventions to maximize the potential gains in chest wall mobility. It is beyond the scope of this textbook to detail all the numerous techniques involved in musculoskeletal mobilization and release of the thorax. These three interventions are intended as suggestions for further study in other texts dealing primarily with musculoskeletal issues.

FACILITATING ACCESSORY MUSCLES IN VENTILATION

If the patient is still not demonstrating an optimal breathing pattern after experiencing appropriate positioning, appropriate ventilatory strategies, chest wall mobilization, and diaphragmatic retraining, specific facilitatory or inhibitory techniques should be initiated to stimulate the accessory muscles of ventilation. Specific techniques are discussed here in detail. A summary of interventions is listed in Box 23-8.

Because the diaphragm normally supplies the bulk of the inspired air during quiet breathing, diaphragmatic breathing is the preferred pattern of breathing. However, after certain neurological insults, strictly diaphragmatic breathing may not be possible or even preferred (Lissoni et al, 1998). Unlike pulmonary rehabilitation programs for people with COPD or asthma, in which diaphragmatic breathing is almost always encouraged and use of accessory muscles discouraged, the restoration of independent, efficient breathing patterns for

---

BOX 23-8

Accessory Muscle Facilitation Techniques

1. Pectoralis facilitation
2. Sternocleidomastoid and scalenes facilitation
3. Trapezius facilitation
4. Diaphragm-inhibiting technique
   - Manual inhibition
   - Postural inhibition
5. Lateral costal facilitation
6. Serratus push-up

---

people with neurological impairment may require the regular use of accessory muscles.

Positioning continues to be the single most important aspect of all ventilatory facilitation techniques. If the patient is positioned for success, the probability of a successful response is much more likely. By assessing the patient's head, upper-extremity, trunk, pelvic, and lower-extremity positions before every activity or technique, the therapist is empowered to use mechanical positioning and gravity to the patient's advantage rather than disadvantage. For example, a slightly posteriorly tilted pelvis tends to facilitate diaphragmatic breathing, whereas a slightly anteriorly tilted pelvis tends to facilitate upper chest breathing. Thus when the therapist is facilitating breathing with accessory muscles, the patient would be put in an advantageous posture by slightly tilting the pelvis anteriorly. In the supine position, this could be as simple as decreasing the amount of knee flexion that is present or using a small towel roll under the lumbar spine.

Pectoralis Facilitation

The pectoralis muscle group provides powerful anterior and lateral expansion of the upper chest and can substitute quite effectively for paralyzed intercostal muscles in the upper chest when trained to do so. Training usually begins in either a modified side-lying or a supine position. To increase the use of this muscle group during inspiration, the therapist should place his or her hand in the same direction as the contracting muscle fibers. Specific proprioceptive input is very important when facilitating a muscle, so make sure the hand is placed diagonally on the upper thorax (Figure 23-18).

The heel of the therapist's hand should be near the sternum and the fingers aligned up and out toward the shoulder in a diagonal pattern. The patient is asked to breathe into the therapist's hands while the therapist applies a quick manual stretch (as in repeated contractions in PNF) to the muscle fibers (down and in toward the sternum). This elicits the quick stretch reflex of the muscle and simultaneously provides added sensory input, which facilitates a stronger and more specific muscle contraction. To emphasize an increase in lateral expansion, facilitation should gradually be transferred from the sternal area out toward the therapist's fingertips by

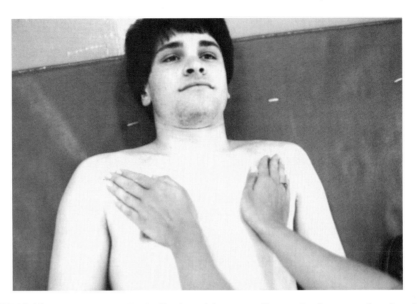

FIGURE 23-18 Hand placement for facilitation of the pectoralis muscles for upper chest breathing.

the patient's shoulder. The verbal cues are stronger and require more effort than the quieter verbal cues for diaphragmatic breathing.

Sternocleidomastoid and Scalene Facilitation

The same principle can be applied to the sternocleidomastoid and scalene muscles (Costa, 1994). When the patient is in the supine position, the therapist need change only the angle of hand alignment to more specifically facilitate the sternocleidomastoid and scalene muscles. Turning the hands parallel to the trunk so that the fingers are pointing up toward the neck rather than pointing out toward the shoulder, the therapist applies the same quick stretch and uses the same verbal cues. The altered hand position now specifically facilitates the sternocleidomastoid and scalene muscles and secondarily influences the pectoralis muscles. The sternocleidomastoid and scalene muscles expand the chest primarily in a superior and anterior plane, whereas the pectoralis muscles expand the chest primarily in a lateral and anterior plane, thus accounting for the slight difference in the facilitation positioning.

Trapezius Facilitation

The trapezius muscle assists in superior expansion of the chest. Facilitation can be initiated in the supine or side-lying position to decrease the resistance of gravity. It can be progressed to an upright posture in which the patient would have to work against gravity.

Placing the hands on top of the patient's shoulders, the therapist gives a quick stretch to the trapezius in a downward direction to facilitate a stronger elevation response. Repeated contractions can be added to facilitate the contraction throughout the full ROM. The shoulder-shrug motion should

be paired with inhalation and upward eye gaze to maximize the facilitation response.

Inhibition of the Diaphragm

Two techniques are described to inhibit the excessive use of the diaphragm during inspiration. Ideally, the therapist is venturing to balance the use of accessory muscles, especially the intercostal, sternocleidomastoid, scalene, and trapezius muscles, with the diaphragm's contraction. This is done to prevent paradoxical movements of the chest, or worse, to prevent adverse musculoskeletal changes in the chest wall, such as pectus excuvatum, which can result from muscle imbalance.

Inhibiting the diaphragm may be necessary during breathing retraining for some patients with spinal cord injuries, polio, spina bifida, developmental delays, head traumas, and cerebral palsy. The diaphragm may be too weak to produce an adequate TV or vital capacity without the assistance of accessory muscles. In these cases the diaphragm-inhibiting technique is used to encourage the use of the accessory muscles to assist in independent voluntary ventilation. Patients learn to use their weakened diaphragm muscles in concert with intact accessory muscles. Not only does this allow for increased TV and vital capacity, it also attempts to provide better aeration of all lung segments and better mobilization of the entire thorax.

In contrast to the first reason that this technique might be used, an unusually strong diaphragm, acting without support from surrounding musculature, specifically the intercostals and abdominal muscles, may also need to be inhibited. For example, patients with paraplegia or lower-level tetraplegia with intact diaphragm but absent abdominal and intercostal muscles may demonstrate a paradoxical breathing pattern (see compensatory breathing patterns, Chapter 37). In this case the accessory muscles must be encouraged to keep the diaphragm in check, attempting to avoid the development of a pectus excuvatum. The goal of this breathing retraining method is to stop the paradoxical movements of the upper chest during inspiration by balancing the use of the upper and lower chest. In some cases, spastic intercostal muscles, found in some spinal cord injuries, may intercede to prevent this paradoxical movement by maintaining the upper chest's position during inspiration in spite of the negative pressure within the chest and gravity's influence on the chest. Balancing the movement of the chest should produce an increase in TV and vital capacity potential and mobilize a greater portion of the chest.

To perform the diaphragm-inhibiting technique, the patient is positioned in a supine, semi-sitting, or side-lying position, with the top arm positioned overhead or pulled back at the waist to open up the upper chest. If patient can tolerate it, pillows are removed from under his or her head, the pelvis tilted anteriorly, and airway safety is assessed by checking to see if the patient can still swallow comfortably. The heel of the therapist's hand is placed lightly on the patient's abdomen at about the level of the umbilicus. No instructions are given to the patient at this point. As the patient begins to exhale a normal breath of air, the therapist gently allows the heel of his or her hand to move up and in toward the central tendon of the patient's diaphragm (see Figure 23-4). When the expiration of that breath is complete, the therapist strictly maintains the hand position in that shortened expiratory position. During the following inspiratory phase, the diaphragm will experience some gentle resistance to its inferior descent, causing inhibition to its full ROM. On the next expiration, the technique is repeated, with the therapist carefully pushing the heel of his or her hand further up and in, maintaining greater inhibition during each inspiratory phase. After two or three ventilatory cycles, a patient usually begins subconsciously to alter his or her breathing pattern to include more upper chest expansion so as to reconcile the diaphragm's transient inability to produce enough chest expansion to yield an adequate TV. The therapist should carefully observe which accessory muscles the patient spontaneously chooses. Are they used symmetrically? What is the general quality of the movement? Is the onset harsh or smooth? Does the patient appear fatigued or uncoordinated?

It is not until this point that the therapist should verbally acknowledge any alteration of the patient's breathing pattern. Without changing his or her hand position, the therapist tells the patient what it is that he or she likes about the new breathing pattern (e.g., balance between upper and lower chest expansion or less paradoxical motion of the sternum). Then the patient is asked if he or she notices any difference from before, bringing this breathing pattern to a conscious level. Only after some orientation to this pattern, usually no more than four to six breathing cycles in the full inhibiting pattern, should the therapist begin gradually to release the pressure being applied.

While slowly releasing pressure with each cycle of inspiration, the therapist asks the patient to attempt cognitively to reproduce the desired pattern. It should take the same number of cycles to release the pressure as it did to apply it. This technique easily allows for gradations of inhibition, from full inhibition, when the patient is forced to use upper accessory muscles or risk becoming short of breath, to a barely proprioceptive reminder to change his or her breathing pattern. It also allows for gradation of inhibition while the patient is learning to assume control over the new breathing pattern. If, during the releasing phase of this technique, the patient begins to lose control over the new pattern, the therapist can gently reapply some pressure during the next expiratory phase to help the patient regain that control. At that point, the therapist can release or reapply pressure as necessary until the desired pattern is obtained and full release of pressure is acceptable.

This technique is particularly effective in patients who are having difficulty cognitively altering their own breathing patterns, such as small children, brain-damaged patients, or slow motor learners, because it requires no cognitive effort until success has already been achieved. Extra care must be taken to avoid initiating any applied pressure quickly because of the likelihood of eliciting unwanted abdominal contractions or spasticity (Laffont et al, 2003) or eliciting a stronger diaphragmatic contraction resulting from the quick stretch reflex. The technique should never be painful. The therapist must keep his or her hand on the abdomen, not the rib cage, to properly influence the diaphragm. This technique can be progressed by changing postures, which requires greater trunk control. Can the patient still maintain the overall pattern? Can the patient breathe without paradoxical movements against gravity?

The second technique is for the more advanced patient and simply presents a physical block to diaphragmatic excursion. The patient is positioned in a prone-on-elbows position (Figure 23-19). In patients who are most severely impaired neurologically, the lower chest will be in direct contact with the surface, so lower anterior and inferior expansion is

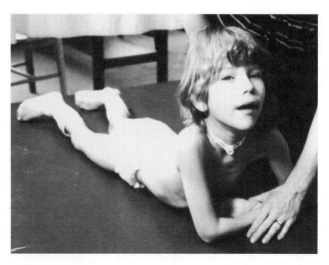

FIGURE 23-19 Diaphragm inhibiting in prone-on-elbows position.

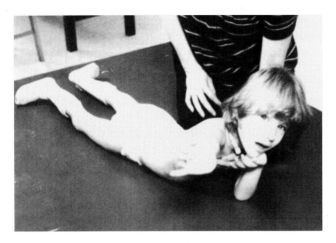

FIGURE 23-20 Static-dynamic upper extremity activities in prone-on-elbows position to encourage upper chest accessory muscle participation.

inhibited and lateral costal expansion is limited. The upper chest is positioned in extension and the upper extremities are fixed, optimizing the length-tension relationship of the anterior and superior accessory muscles for easy facilitation. In addition, anterior excursion of the upper chest is now in a gravity-assisted posture. Through the use of head and neck patterns, such as in PNF diagonals, or the use of static-dynamic activities, such as in weight shifting to one supporting limb while reaching out with the other extremity, the therapist can readily facilitate greater upper chest breathing (Figure 23-20). These are the same patterns the therapist can use to achieve other goals, such as increased head and neck control, increased shoulder stability, or increased upper body balance. Therefore, by helping patients to coordinate movement goals with ventilatory patterns, it becomes more likely that the patients will incorporate these patterns functionally into daily activities. This is the ultimate goal of any ventilatory retraining procedure.

The manual diaphragm-inhibiting technique is usually less threatening to the patient than the prone-on-elbows inhibition technique. Prone on elbows itself can inhibit the diaphragm so completely for neurological patients lacking spinal extensors that they become extremely short of breath. Consequently, do not position the patients in this more demanding posture until success appears likely.

Serratus Push-up

Facilitating greater posterior chest expansion can be achieved in a prone-on-elbows position. Gravity is now assisting anterior excursion of the chest and resisting posterior excursion. To emphasize the serratus anterior muscle's role in posterior expansion, the patient is instructed to perform an upper body push-up (with or without the therapist's assistance). The serratus anterior muscle causes lateral scapular movement, thereby facilitating maximal posterior excursion of the thorax.

The patient is instructed to take a deep breath in during the push-up and to exhale the air (passively or forcefully) when returning to the starting position. Forceful exhalation in this activity can be used as a forerunner to effective cough retraining. Gentle or controlled exhalation can be used to encourage greater breath support for vocalization or for eccentric trunk muscle training.

Emphasizing posterior chest expansion during inhalation is the only occasion in which inspiration would be paired with trunk flexion. In all other inspiratory situations, inspiration is paired with trunk extension, and exhalation is paired with trunk flexion.

PATIENTS WITH ASYMMETRICAL DYSFUNCTION

Patients with asymmetrical weakness need a different approach from the controlled or upper chest breathing patterns presented previously (Lanini, 2003). These patients need facilitation of the weaker side to promote symmetrical chest wall expansion in both the upper and lower chest. A summary of techniques is listed in Box 23-9.

Symmetrical Positioning

Symmetrical ventilatory patterns may be effortlessly achieved by altering the patient's position in each posture to maximize the chest wall's potential to move in a symmetrical pattern. This is especially true in an upright position in which asymmetry is generally more pronounced. For example, a patient with hemiplegia may lean toward the involved side when sitting because of weakness or spasticity. Likewise, after thoracic surgery, a patient with primary pulmonary impairment may lean toward the surgical side to splint the area so as to avoid the pain caused by chest movement around the incision and the chest tubes. Both situations cause asymmetrical breathing patterns and decrease ventilation on the involved side. Improving chest wall alignment may alleviate the ventilatory deficit on the involved side. This may be achieved by the use of towel rolls or pillows to support the affected side as well as by good pain management postoperatively.

Postural Inhibition

For some patients, more aggressive positioning must be used to achieve greater chest wall excursion and ventilation on the involved side. This can be accomplished by inhibiting the chest wall movements on the uninvolved, or stronger, side. Usually, the best position in which to achieve this inhibition is side-lying. When the patient lies on his or her uninvolved side, with his or her arms positioned below 90 degrees of shoulder flexion, lateral chest expansion into that side becomes inhibited because of the physical barrier. This forces the patient to find another way to meet his or her ventilatory needs, which indirectly facilitates chest expansion on the opposite side (the uppermost side). The therapist can then supply sensory and motor input through his or her hands to the patient's upper, middle, or lower chest on the involved or weaker side to facilitate increased ventilation on that side. Early in the rehabilitation process or soon after thoracic surgery, the patient may have difficulty performing lateral chest expansion against gravity when in a side-lying position (gravity-resisted movement). If so, place the patient in a three quarter supine position to lessen the workload imposed by gravity. Gradually, work the patient up to a full side-lying posture to achieve the greatest strengthening benefits.

Timing for Emphasis

Another technique to promote symmetrical chest wall movements is performed in numerous postures, such as supine, sitting, or standing. The therapist places his or her hand symmetrically on the lower lateral chest wall, on the mid chest, or on the upper anterior chest wall. At the end of exhalation, the therapist gives a quick stretch to the muscles being touched so as to facilitate a deep inspiratory effort in that area of the chest. Immediately after both sides begin to move into an inspiratory pattern, the therapist manually blocks (or inhibits) expansion of the chest on the stronger side while giving continued quick stretches to the weaker side. This facilitates greater expansion on the weak side by means of an overflow response. This technique, adapted from the PNFs timing-for-emphasis technique, uses the strength of the stronger side to facilitate movement on the weaker side. It can be applied to any area of the chest where symmetrical movements should be the norm.

REDUCING RESPIRATORY RATES

In addition to altering breathing patterns through facilitation and inhibition techniques, reducing RRs may also be necessary before arriving at an efficient breathing pattern for some patients. See Box 23-10 for a summary of techniques. Many patients with neurological impairment who have high neuromuscular tone increase their RRs to compensate for a decrease in their TVs or because of brainstem impairments tthat affect the respiratory centers. In addition, many patients who are anxious, such as people with asthma and those who

---

BOX 23-10

Techniques to Reduce High Respiratory Rates

1. Previous techniques that increased tidal volume
2. Counter-rotation technique
3. Butterfly technique in sitting
   - Straight planes
   - Counter-rotation
4. Relaxed pursed-lips breathing with inspiratory and expiratory pauses

---

have orthopedic or surgical conditions and are experiencing pain, may also demonstrate excessively high RRs. Attempting to restore ventilatory efficiency may require increasing TV while concurrently decreasing RR.

Previous Facilitation Techniques

The techniques previously described in this chapter promote an increase in TV by improving the overall ventilatory patterns and often cause a secondary reduction in RR. Interventions such as PLB and repatterning, mobilization of the thorax, and upper chest breathing facilitation for neurologically impaired patients are often helpful in accomplishing slower, deeper, more controlled breathing.

Counter-rotation

The technique described next has been developed specifically to promote a lower RR and improvement of chest wall mobility. The counter-rotation technique reduces high neuromuscular tone and increases thoracic mobility, thus often resulting in an increase in TV and a simultaneous reduction in RR. This intervention is extremely effective for the following: (1) patients with decreased cognitive functioning after a neurological insult or after surgery; (2) very young children because verbal cues cannot be used; and (3) patients with high neuromuscular tone. As described in Chapter 22, counter-rotation also can be easily adapted as a very effective assisted-cough technique. One medical contraindication for this technique, because of its rotary nature, is bony instability of the spine.

In bed or on a mat, place the patient in a side-lying position with knees bent and arms resting comfortably out in front of the head and shoulders. In this technique, the higher the upper extremities can be placed within a comfort zone, the better the result. Relaxed positioning of the patient is essential to the success of this technique, so the patient should be positioned in an open yet comfortable position. Normalizing neuromuscular tone is the first step in attempting to decrease a high RR. Patient discomfort is likely to elicit increased tone and an increased RR.

The therapist's own position is also important because it directs the force that is applied to the patient's chest. Initially, the therapist should stand behind the patient, perpendicular to his or her trunk. If the patient is lying on the left side, the therapist places his or her left hand on the patient's shoulder and his or her right hand on the patient's hip. The therapist then leaves his or her hands in place and simply follows the patient's respiratory cycle. This allows the therapist to assess the patient's subjective rate and rhythm and the patient's overall neuromuscular tone. Only after this assessment should the clinician begin the active phase of the technique. Using a PNF technique called rhythmic initiation, the patient is gently log-rolled in a small ROM in the side-lying position. The rolling is gradually increased achieving more ROM from side-lying toward prone. This progression of movement generally reduces high tone, which usually makes the second phase of the technique more effective.

During this phase, the therapist should audibly duplicate the patient's RR. As the patient moves into greater rolling ROM and begins to slow his or her RR, the therapist needs to use the patient's audible cuing as a facilitator for establishing a slower RR. Thus the therapist begins by having the patient establish the audible RR and then the therapist slowly takes over. Audible cues can be very strong facilitators of ventilatory rhythms.

Phase two requires the therapist to slowly change position. Transitioning to a diagonal posture, the therapist then stands or half kneels behind the patient near his or her hips, turning to a diagonal position until facing the patient's head at roughly at 45-degree angle. Here the hand placement begins to get more specific. Assume again that the patient is side-lying on the left. At the beginning of the expiratory cycle, the therapist's left hand slowly glides over the patient's shoulder on the right pectoral region, with care being taken not to unintentionally use the thumb or finger tips, and the right hand slowly glides back to the patient's right gluteal fossa (the hollow of the buttocks) (Figure 22-6, A). The therapist can then manually compress the rib cage on all three planes of ventilation at the end of exhalation by gently pulling the shoulder back and down, while simultaneously pushing the hip up and forward. This movement promotes more complete exhalation.

When the patient begins the next inspiration, the therapist switches hand placement to capitalize on the improved potential for TV. The therapist's left hand slides back to the patient's right scapula, and the therapist's right hand slides forward just anterior to the patient's right iliac crest (see Figure 22-6, B). As the patient inhales, the therapist slowly stretches the chest to maximize inspiration TVs. The therapist's left hand pushes the scapula (or the thorax if the scapula is unstable) up and away from the spine and the right hand pulls the pelvis back and down to maximize all three planes of ventilation, resulting in greater inspiration. The therapist should use the flat or heel of the hand whenever possible to avoid unintentional patient discomfort and to maximize the facilitated area.

Initially, the therapist begins and ends the respiratory cycle according to the patient's RR. However, as the patient's tone is relaxed and increased TVs are promoted by the effects of counter-rotation, the therapist gradually slows down the rate of rotation, giving the patient audible breathing cues to further facilitate a slower RR. The patient generally accommodates to a slower RR as the therapist gains more control over the patient's breathing pattern. With many patients, the results can be marked. If the patient can cognitively follow commands, he or she can be alerted to this change and encouraged to assist in voluntarily breathing at the slower rate.

The therapist can progress the technique by decreasing the manual input. The last facilitation to be removed should be the audible cues. As with the diaphragm-inhibiting technique, the therapist can reestablish control quickly if need be by simply reapplying stronger manual input. If the patient has an extremely fast RR (i.e., 50 to 60 breaths/min), the facilitation can be applied every two to three breaths so as to avoid fatiguing the patient or therapist.

It should be apparent that this technique need not be used exclusively for respiratory goals but rather can be incorporated into a patient's total rehabilitation program. It is a natural precursor to active rolling or it can be used as a vestibular stimulator.

Butterfly Technique

If a patient has good motor control, an upright version of this technique may be appropriate. In unsupported sitting, stand behind or in front of the patient, depending on his or her balance needs, and ask the patient to bring his or her arms up into a butterfly posture, or assist his or her arms into this posture. Starting from a comfortable ROM position for that patient, begin to breathe audibly in time with the patient's RR. When the patient inhales, raise the arms up into slightly more shoulder flexion. When the patient exhales, lower the arms slightly. Slowly begin to move in greater and greater increments of range, all the while breathing out loud with your patient. Through your audible breathing cues, begin to "ask" your patient to slow down the RR and take deeper slower breaths. The use of the following concurrent ventilatory strategies promotes deeper inhalations and exhalations: (1) shoulder flexion and trunk extension paired with inspiration; and (2) shoulder extension and trunk flexion paired with exhalation. Thus it becomes possible for the patient to increase TV and decrease RR.

As in the previous technique, the therapist begins by breathing loudly at the patient's respiratory rate and transitions to breathing audibly at a slower, more desirable pace. The patient picks up on this subtle cue and subconsciously reduces his or her own RR, even if unable to follow verbal commands.

This technique can be modified to encourage more intercostal and oblique abdominal muscle contractions by using a diagonal rather than a straight plane of movement. Have the patient look up and over one shoulder as he or she breathes in and brings arms up and behind his or her head. Then have the patient look down and away toward the opposite knee as he or

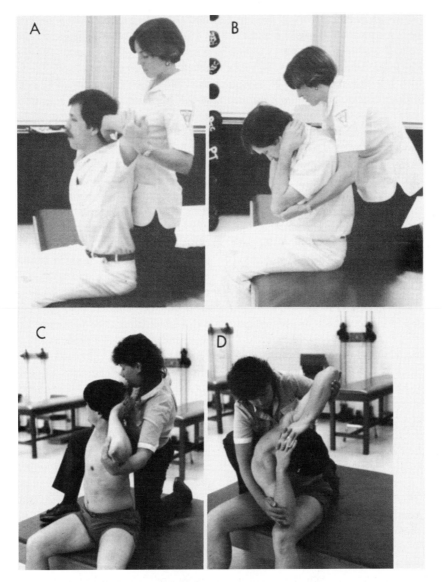

FIGURE 23-21 A, Butterfly technique facilitating inspiration. **B,** Butterfly technique facilitating exhalation. **C,** Butterfly with trunk rotation facilitating inspiration. All three planes of respiration are stretched on the patient's right side. **D,** Butterfly with trunk rotation facilitating exhalation. All planes are compressed on the right side.

she breathes out and brings arms down to the opposite knee (Figure 23-21).

Relaxed Pursed-Lip Breathing

Using a relaxed PLB pattern (as previously described) is also a technique that reduces RR. By prolonging the expiratory phase through pursed lips, the patient secondarily decreases his or her RR.

GLOSSOPHARYNGEAL BREATHING

A small population of patients with neurological impairments requires more than just promoting the use of accessory muscles or changing RR to meet basic ventilatory needs

(Warren, 2002). In the past decade, more people experiencing high-level SCIs (above C4) have survived the initial trauma because of advances in medical technology. However, the therapist in the rehabilitation setting is then faced with the difficult task of restoring quality of life. For these patients, as well as many elder polio patients, mastery of the glossopharyngeal breathing (GPB) technique allows for greater voluntary ventilation, which many patients state does improve the quality of their lives. This augmented breathing pattern allows patients to regain some control over their lives and to regain control over their ventilation, which was lost as a result of severe neurological insult.

GPB is a technique developed in the 1950s by polio patients looking for a way to reduce their dependence on the iron lung for ventilation. It was found that by using the lips, soft palate, mouth, tongue, pharynx, and larynx, a patient could actually inhale enough air to sustain life without mechanical ventilation. Only intact cranial nerves are required. This method is sometimes referred to as frog breathing because it uses the principles of inspiration common to the frog. The patient learns to create a pocket of negative pressure within the buccal cavity (mouth) by maximizing that internal space, thereby causing the outside air to rush in. At that point, the patient closes off the entrance (the lips) and proceeds to force the air back and down the throat with a stroking maneuver of the tongue, pharynx, and larynx.

Research has shown consistently that use of this technique in patients who have severe neurological impairment can increase pulmonary functions significantly, especially TV and vital capacity (VC). If GPB is the only means of ventilation possible when a patient has been disconnected from a ventilator or phrenic nerve stimulator, mastery of this technique is critical to the patient's survival in case of mechanical failure. All attempts should be made to teach GPB to this patient population.

A clinical example may help to illustrate its usefulness. A 14-year-old male sustained a C1 complete SCI while racing in front of a train. After he was medically stable, two phrenic nerve stimulators were implanted in his chest. The patient had no unassisted means of ventilation. Neuromuscularly, the patient had limited use of one trapezius, the sternocleidomastoid, and intrinsic neck muscles. The patient and family feared that long-term nursing home placement would be inevitable because of their fear that his phrenic nerve stimulator would malfunction or a battery would wear out, causing immediate respiratory distress. The family believed it could not bear the psychological burden placed on them if the patient went home to live. GPB instruction was suggested and was begun slowly because the patient stated that he learned motor skills slowly. After a painstaking 2-month period, the patient learned to breathe without the use of his phrenic nerve stimulator for 3 to 5 minutes before becoming fatigued and hypoventilating. Within the next 1 to 2 months, this same patient learned to breathe for up to 2 hours off of his stimulator, using GPB only. To the staff's surprise, he even learned to talk and operate his sip-and-puff wheelchair while using GPB. The patient was then successfully discharged to his home. This was not the only factor considered in his discharge planning, but it was perhaps the most significant.

Instruction in GPB takes time and concentration. It is best to start off in small time blocks of 10 to 15 minutes because it can be very fatiguing. However, it is important to successful learning of the technique that the patient get consistent, preferably daily, training. Once the patient has mastered the technique, practice sessions can be lengthened considerably, and the patient can be taught self-monitoring techniques. The specific goals of GPB training must be explained to the patient before the beginning of treatment so as to gain his or her support and cooperation. In addition to providing the ventilator- or stimulator-dependent patient with a TV

necessary for gaining independence from mechanical assists, GPB has many other benefits. For the tetraplegic patient who has a partially intact diaphragm (C3 to C4) or the loss of essential accessory muscles (C5 to C8), GPB can accomplish the following: (1) increase VC to produce a more effective cough; (2) assist in a longer and stronger phonation effort; and (3) act as an internal mobilizer of the chest wall.

The muscles used in this technique do not have the same internal proprioceptive, sensory, or visual feedback mechanisms as the trunk and limb muscles, so necessary adjustments in the technique are sometimes difficult to perceive. The patient cannot see his or her tongue pushing the air back or truly feel the pharynx swallowing the air into the lungs, so the therapist's external feedback system is very influential. Use of a mirror can greatly enhance the visual component of feedback. Small changes, like adjustments in posture or the suggestion of another sound to imitate, may be all that is needed for the patient to learn the stroking maneuver correctly. Success in GPB can be assessed objectively with a spirometer and a pulse oximeter. For patients incapable of breathing independently, any TV reading will indicate successful intake of air. For patients who are not ventilator dependent, a VC reading that is greater than 5% over the baseline indicates successful use of GPB. Low level tetraplegics (C5 to C8) have demonstrated increases in VC by as much as 70% to 100%.

Therapists can monitor their own successes with this technique by taking VC readings with and without GPB or by subjective analyses. Maximal inhalation, followed by three or four successful GPB strokes, will cause a feeling that the chest will burst if an attempt is made to inhale more air. Likewise, the sensation of "needing to cough" is another subjective indication of successful GPB. However, a feeling of indigestion is usually indicative that air has been swallowed into the stomach instead of the lungs.

During the initial treatment session, the therapist demonstrates several times what a stroking maneuver looks like give the patient an idea of the motion required. The therapist continues to mimic the pattern as the patient attempts to duplicate it. This gives the patient an active model to mimic and decreases feelings of uneasiness surrounding the necessary but somewhat silly facial grimaces. If the patient is able to breathe independently, his or her ability to breath hold and to close off the nasal passageway should be checked because air leakage is a common cause of failure. The patient is then instructed to take in a maximal inspiration before attempting the stroking maneuvers so as to eliminate the possibility of using other accessory muscles during the technique.

If possible, the patient is positioned in an upright or at least a symmetrical position. Specifically, the patient is instructed to bring the jaws down and then forward as if reaching the bottom lip up for a carrot dangling just in front and above the upper lip (Figure 23-22, *A*). Slight cervical hyperextension is necessary to allow for maximal temporal mandibular joint (TMJ) excursion. (A contraindication for this technique is a TMJ disorder.) The lips should be shaped as if they were to make the sound *oop*. The patient is then told to close the

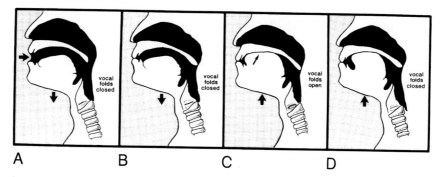

FIGURE 23-22 Glossopharyngeal breathing. **A,** Mouth opened to draw in air. **B,** Jaw closed to entrap the air. **C,** Air pushed back with tongue into trachea. **D,** Vocal folds closed to prevent passive air leaks. Entire maneuver is then repeated.

mouth, reaching the bottom lip up to the top lip (see Figure 23-22, *B*). The tongue and jaw are drawn back toward the throat, with the mouth and tongue formed as though saying *up* or *ell* (see Figure 23-22, *B*). The lower jaw is moving in a roughly rectangular pattern. Most patients learn the stroking maneuvers by making the sounds; as they become more proficient, the sounds and excessive head and neck motions diminish. Often, the students (patients) outperform the teachers (therapists) because through consistent use, they learn all of its finer subtleties.

Although this technique can be broken down into several stages as it has been here for the purpose of description, most of the literature cautions the therapist against doing so. (Zumwalt et al, 1956). Simple, minimal instructions seem to accomplish more, perhaps because the continuity of movement is so essential to the success of the inhalation. Specific instructions can be given later if necessary.

Common problems encountered with GPB instruction are as follows: (1) an open nasal passage or glottis that allows the air to escape; (2) a feeling of indigestion, indicating that the air is being swallowed into the esophagus rather than the trachea; (3) incorrect shape of the mouth as the air is being drawn in (usually not puckered enough); (4) uncoordinated backward movement of the tongue; (5) inadequate jaw mobility, TMJ dysfunction, or decreased cervical ROM; or (6) incorrect sounds while performing the technique, such as the word *gulp* or *em*. Avoiding any instruction for the tongue seems to produce better results. Concentrate on assisting the patient in learning the external physical movements.

Tolerance of GPB can be increased when mastery of a single stroke becomes consistent. For patients using it as an assist to their own voluntary ventilation, three to four strokes on top of a maximal inspiration is usually sufficient. Ventilator- or stimulator-dependent patients may need to use as many as 10 to 14 strokes per breath. These figures should be used only as rough guidelines. Each patient will use a slightly different technique and a different number of strokes; the only important factor is a method that works for the individual. Fatigue after long trials of GPB can be monitored effectively by an oximeter. The oxygen saturation level should stay above 90% to maintain adequate PaO$_2$ levels. For example, if the patient begins the GPB session with an oxygen saturation level in the upper 90s, fatigue can be monitored and anticipated by watching to see if the oxygen level decreases. If the level begins to fall to the mid 90s and then the low 90s, you can anticipate when they will reach 90%. At that point, end the GPB training and put the patient back on the previous ventilatory support system. Oximetry not only allows for accurate monitoring but also provides an objective means of monitoring progress over time. In addition, a spirometer objectively measures improvements in using GPB. It gives the patient concrete indications of success or failure in mastering the technique.

ENHANCING VOCALIZATION SKILLS

In contrast to procedures that assist a patient in inhalation, procedures intended to improve a patient's phonation skill must focus on elongating the expiration phase. Coughing is a gross-motor skill that relies more on force than on fine control of the ventilatory muscles for its effectiveness. Conversely, phonation requires precise, fine-motor control of these muscles and demands that the vocal folds provide a consistent air flow through the larynx. Both are expiration activities and they depend on the preceding inspiration for optimal performance; however, coughing uses concentric contractions of the expiratory muscles to force the air out, and quiet talking uses primarily eccentric contractions of the inspiratory muscles to slowly release the air during expiration. Because of these differences, procedures to improve coughing and phonation are different in focus. Looking at the relationship between speaking and breathing and the concepts of shared respiratory control, it is notable that speaking can lead to shortness of breath, and shortness of breath can alter speaking ability (Bailey & Hoit, 2002). Previous discussions of posture and use of abdominal binders in patients with spinal cord injury should also be considered when speaking is impaired (Hoit & Lohmeir, 2002). A summary of techniques is listed in Box 23-11. Coughing is covered in detail in Chapter 22.

BOX 23-11

Enhancing Vocalization Skills through Increased Breath Support

1. Position to achieve a neutral chin tuck and optimal vocal fold alignment
2. Manual techniques
   - Vibration or shaking
   - Percussion or tapping
3. Eccentric resistance
   - Agonistic reversal technique
   - Functional resistance
4. Verbal techniques to refine breath support
   - Singing and whistling
   - Games
   - Wind or brass instruments
   - Stopping and starting vocalizations

Because the patient's TV and total inspiratory capacity are the power source for phonation, they become important concerns in a phonation program. Generally, a normal TV is adequate for conversational speech. However, larger volumes of air, thus greater inspiratory capacities, are required for singing, loud talking, or professional speaking. Therefore, the breathing pattern facilitation techniques described earlier in this chapter are ideal for use before instructing the patient in better expiration control. For example, facilitating diaphragmatic and accessory-muscle breathing techniques, along with the use of quick stretches or repeated contractions, can facilitate the desired deeper inhalation.

Positioning Concerns

Consistent with all previous techniques, the first aspect of improving breath support for vocalization is to optimize the patient's position. The vocal folds have an ideal muscle length-tension relationship when the head is in a neutral chin tuck. In addition, an open anterior chest wall allows for the greatest potential for chest wall excursion and thus the largest VC. Use the previously described suggestions for positioning to determine whether a particular patient needs positioning to encourage a more diaphragmatic, upper chest, or unilateral breathing pattern.

Manual Techniques

Several simple techniques can be used to improve eccentric control of the diaphragm and intercostal muscles in preparation for speech. Vibration or shaking of the lower chest during expiration helps to produce a slower, more controlled recoil of the diaphragm. Why this occurs is not fully understood. It may be that the sensory and proprioceptive stimulation that the vibration or shaking provides augments the patient's concentration on those muscles, resulting in longer phonation. The patient is instructed to phonate an *ah* or

oh sound for as long as possible. The therapist simultaneously vibrates the patient's chest with an even and gentle force throughout and slightly beyond the full expiration phase, placing his or her hands on the lateral costal borders of the thorax, the mid chest, or the pectoral area, depending on which area of the chest needs the most help in controlling exhalation. This is very different from the rapid, forceful pressure that is applied to the patient's chest when promoting a deep cough. Be certain that the patient understands this important difference. The therapist must stress that the patient should not let air escape before vocalizing and should try to keep voice intensity consistent throughout the procedure. This will promote slow, eccentric release of the inspiratory muscles during the entire course of the vocalization. Progress can be readily monitored by timing the patient's vocalization before, during, and after this technique. About 10 to 12 seconds of vocalization at 8 to 10 syllables per breath is generally considered adequate for functional use in speech.

For a child, this technique can be modified. The child is asked to say *ah* or *oh* for as long as possible while the therapist percusses or taps lightly with his or her hands on the child's upper or lower chest so as to produce a series of staccato sounds. Usually, a child enjoys the new sound that this makes and tries repeatedly to phonate longer and louder to accentuate the different intensities.

Therapeutically, this requires the child to take a deeper inhalation before vocalizing, followed by an elongated expiratory phase, both of which are necessary for functional speech. As the child becomes more adept at it, the therapist can apply more pronounced clapping over the chest, accomplishing a wider range of voice intensities and doubling as a means of percussion for postural drainage.

Eccentric Resistance Techniques

More specific facilitation can be used to increase breath support. Ideally, the patient is positioned symmetrically in a supine or supported-sitting position, allowing for maximal chest wall expansion. The patient is instructed to visualize his or her chest being pulled up toward the ceiling and held there. They are then told to vocalize slowly trying not to let the chest "fall." Meanwhile, the therapist is applying consistent pressure to the patient's chest to try to force a quicker exhalation. The patient is told to resist this motion by trying to control and prolong expiration. Like the antagonistic reversal technique described in PNF, the therapist is resisting the patient's attempt to eccentrically contract and control the trunk muscles. This strengthens the eccentric phase of exhalation and promotes greater breath control for vocalization.

The same concept can be applied to functional tasks. Moving into gravity (i.e., coming down to sitting from a standing posture, lying down from a sitting posture, and bringing an arm down from reaching into a high cabinet) requires eccentric control of the muscles involved in that activity to slow the body's descent into gravity's influence. Because quiet speech uses a similar muscular contraction, teaching the patient to count out loud or to otherwise vocalize when performing an overall eccentric activity usually improves both activities. For example, the patient can be instructed to reach up to a high shelf while inhaling. Then, using gravity to provide the eccentric resistance, the patient is asked to bring his or her arm back down to his or her lap or side while slowly counting out loud and controlling the rate of the arm's descent. The activity can be progressed several ways. The activity can include lifting something heavy off the shelf and controlling it along with the arm and trunk while lowering the object to a table or to the patient's lap. Or the postural demands of the activity can be increased. The patient can still lift the heavy object but can now be required to do while standing, which increases the demands on the musculoskeletal system.

Verbal Techniques

Speech activities that do not require a therapist's physical assistance can be done in a group or individual setting. Singing, for instance, promotes strong and prolonged vocalization with maximal inspiration, which is a significant goal in a phonation program. Similarly, whistling or playing a kazoo or harmonica promotes long, even exhalations but is nonverbal. Both are easily incorporated into a group activity on the nursing floor, in therapy, or in the community.

Along recreational lines, games that promote controlled blowing further the refinement of motor control of the respiratory muscles. This can be accomplished by blowing bubbles, especially large ones, blowing out candles, especially trick candles, blowing a ping-pong ball through a maze, or blowing air hockey disks across the table rather than pushing them. Patients with musical inclinations should be encouraged to learn to play wind or brass instruments, in which refined breath control is mandatory for success. Obviously, the possibilities in recreational are endless and simply require imagination on the part of the therapist.

Further refinement of breath control for speech can be promoted by interrupting the outgoing air flow. This procedure is geared toward improving functional communication skills. Functional speech is a series of vocal stops and starts. The therapist tells the patient to take a deep breath and count out loud to 100. After a few numbers, the patient is told to "hold it" and is then told to start up where he or she left off; the therapist periodically interrupts. Because this activity requires the patient to stop and start the inhalation and exhalation phases at will in all aspects of the ventilatory cycle, it is more advanced and should be used only after some control of exhalation has been mastered.

SUMMARY

The use of appropriate choices in positioning, together with use of an appropriate ventilatory and movement strategy for any given task will make success in mastering that task all the more likely. If these simple, time-efficient methods of facilitation do not produce adequate ventilatory changes by themselves, it is then appropriate to add the next layer of facilitation—manual facilitation techniques. Specifically, the techniques that are described in this chapter assist in facilitating the following: (1) greater diaphragmatic breathing patterns (or controlled breathing); (2) increased chest wall mobility; (3) greater accessory-muscle breathing patterns (or primarily upper chest breathing); (4) more symmetrical breathing patterns (in unilateral disorders); (5) reduction in high respiratory rates; (6) auxillary techniques (GBP); and (7) improved phonation support. Obviously, not all techniques would be appropriate for any single patient. It is up to the therapist to determine which techniques would best address their patients' deficits.

Positioning is vital to increasing ventilation potential and functional skills. From the beginning of the patient's respiratory program, optimizing ventilation and breath control through passive and active positioning techniques should be used by all medical disciplines, not just physical therapy. As the patients progress, the clinician can and should, assist them in developing better and more efficient movement strategies for higher level activities by coordinating appropriate breathing patterns, such as trunk extension-inhalation or trunk flexion-exhalation strategies, into all activities. After these quick and easy suggestions are used, a therapist who has been exposed to numerous methods of manual facilitation and techniques to promote more effective and efficient breathing patterns can choose the most appropriate interventions. In some cases, increasing diaphragmatic breathing may be the desired outcome. In other patients, increased upper chest breathing or increased movement on one side of the chest may be more desirable. Some may benefit even more from techniques to reduce the high RR or to mobilize the thorax. For a select patient population, instruction in GPB may be necessary to support breathing without mechanical ventilatory support. Last, the therapist can now choose to use techniques to improve the patient in developing adequate breath support for vocalization and communication.

As therapists understand how profound the influence of effective ventilation can be on a patient's recovery from disease or trauma they will incorporate breathing and ventilation strategies into all patient treatment. Understanding that facilitating effective ventilation goes far beyond the old diaphragmatic exercises, therapists can be empowered to incorporate other techniques and strategies to help their patients become healthier more quickly and to assist them in reaching their highest potential and prevent future respiratory complications.

The take-home message is that the cardiovascular and pulmonary system will be either an asset or a detriment to patient function. Choosing to incorporate examination and evaluation of breathing patterns and breathing control will result in improved patient outcomes.

Review Questions

1. Why would a therapist want to try to change a patient's breathing pattern?
2. How can ventilatory strategies be incorporated into a treatment session?
3. When would a therapist not teach diaphragmatic breathing?
4. What is the role of relaxation in breathing control?
5. When would a therapist consider teaching the patient to use his upper chest more in breathing?
6. When would a unilateral breathing pattern be taught?

REFERENCES

Andreasson, B., Jonson, B., & Kornfralt, R. (1987). Long-term effects of physical exercise on working capacity and pulmonary function in cystic fibrosis. Acta Paediatrica Scandanavia 76:70-75.

Atrice, M., Backus, D.A., Gonter, M., & Morrison, S. (1993). Acute physical therapy management of individuals with spinal cord injury. Orthopedics & Physical Therapy Clinics of North America 2:53-70.

Bach, J.R. (1991). New approaches in the rehabilitation of the traumatic high level quadriplegic. American Journal of Physical Medicine and Rehabilitation 70:13-9.

Bailey, E.F., & Hoit, J.D. (2002). Speaking and breathing in high respiratory drive. Journal of Speech, Language & Hearing Research 45:89-99.

Beuret-Blanquart, F., & Boucand, M.H. (2003). Aging with spinal cord injury. Annals of Readaptive Medical Physiology 46:578-591

Bianchi, R., Gigliotti, F. Romagnoli, I., Lanini, B., Castellani, C., Grazzini, M., & Scano, G. (2004). Chest wall kinematics and breathlessness during pursed lip breathing in patients with COPD. Chest 125:459-465.

Boaventura, C.D., Gastaldi, A.C. (2003). Effect of an abdominal binder on the efficacy of respiratory muscles in seated and supine tetraplegic patients. Physiotherapy 89:290-295.

Boughton, A., & Ciesla, N. (1986). Physical therapy management of the head-injured patient in the intensive care unit. Topics in Acute Care Trauma Rehabilitation 1:1-18.

Boehme, R. (1992). Assessment and treatment of the respiratory system for breathing, sound production and trunk control. Teamtalk 2:2-8.

Braun, N.T. (1982). Force-length relationship of the normal human diaphragm. Journal of Applied Physiology 53:405-412.

Brown, J.C., Swank, S.M., Matta, J., & Farras, D.M. (1984). Late spinal deformity in quadriplegic children and adolescents. Journal of Pediatric Orthopedics 4:456-461.

Cash, J. (1977). Neurology for physiotherapists, ed 2. London: JB Lippincott.

Cheshire, D.J., & Flack, W.J. (1979). The use of operant conditioning techniques in the respiratory rehabilitation of the tetraplegic. Paraplegia 16:162-174.

Clough, P. (1983). Glossopharyngeal breathing: its application with a traumatic quadriplegic patient. Archives of Physical Medicine Rehabilitation 64:384-385.

Costa, D. (1994). Participation of the sternocleidomastoid muscle on deep inspiration in man, an electromyographic study. Electromyography & Clinical Neurophysiology 34:315-320.

Delgado, H.R., Braun, S.R., Skatrud, J.B., Reddan, W.G., & Pegelow, D.F. (1982). Chest wall and abdominal motion during exercise in patients with chronic obstructive pulmonary disease. American Review of Respiratory Disorders 126:200-205.

DeTroyer, A. (1983). Mechanical action of the abdominal muscles. Bulletin of European Physiopathology and Respiration 19:575.

DeTroyer, A., Kelly, S., Macklem, P.T., & Zin, W.A. (1985). Mechanics of intercostal space and actions of external and internal intercostal muscles. Journal of Clinical Investigation 5:850-857.

DeTroyer, A., Gorman, R.B., & Gandevia, S.C. (2003). Distribution of inspiratory drive to the external intercostal muscles in humans. Journal of Physiology 546:943-954.

Druz, W.S., & Sharp, J.T. (1982). Electrical and mechanical activity of the diaphragm accompanying body position in severe chronic obstructive pulmonary disease. American Review of Respiratory Disorders 125:275.

Estenne, M., & DeTroyer, A. (1990). Cough in tetraplegic subjects: an active process. Annals of Internal Medicine 112:22-28.

Fishburn, M.J., Marino, R.J., & Ditunno, J.F. (1990). Atelectasis and pneumonia in acute spinal cord injury. Archives of Physical Medicine Rehabilitation 71:197-200.

Gandevia, S.C. (2002). Balancing acts: respiratory sensations, motor control and human posture. Clinics in Experimental Pharmacology and Physiology 29:118-121.

Gigliotti, F., Coli, C., Bianchi, R., Romagnoli, I., Lanini, B., Binazzi, B., & Scano, G. (2003). Exercise training improves exertional dyspnea in patients with COPD: evidence of the role of mechanical factors. Chest 123:1794-1802.

Gigliotti, F., Romagnoli, I., & Scano, G. (2003). Breathing retraining and exercise conditioning in patients with chronic obstructive pulmonary disease (COPD): a physiological approach. Respiratory Medicine 97:197-204.

Goldman, J.M., Rose, L.S., William, S.J., Silver, J.R., & Denison, D.M. (1986). Effect of abdominal binders on breathing in tetraplegic patients. Thorax 41:940-945.

Gross, D., Ladd, H.W., Riley, E.J., Macklem, P.T., & Grassino, A. (1980). The effect of training on strength and endurance of the diaphragm in quadriplegia. American Journal of Medicine 68:27-35.

Hapy, M.J. (1992). Wheelchair seating and positioning: options and solutions. Physical Therapy Forum 4-8.

Hixon, T.J. (1991). Respiratory function in speech and song. San Diego: Singular Publishing Group.

Hodges, P.W., Gandevia, S.C., & Richardson, C.A. (1997). Contractions of specific abdominal muscles in postural tasks are affected by respiratory maneuvers. Journal of Applied Physiology 83:753-760.

Hodges, P.W., & Gandevia, S.C. (2000). Changes in intra-abdominal pressure during postural and respiratory activation of the human diaphragm. Journal of Applied Physiology 89:967-976.

Hodges, P.W., & Gandevia, S.C. (2000). Activation of the human diaphragm during a repetitive task. Journal of Physiology 522:165-175.

Hodges, P.W., Heijnen, I., & Gandevia, S.C. (2001). Postural activity of the diaphragm is reduced in humans when respiratory demand increases. Journal of Physiology 537:999-1008.

Hodges, P.W., Gurfinkel, V.S., Brumagne, S. Smith, T.C., & Cordo, P.C. (2002). Coexistence of stability and mobility in postural control: evidence from postural compensation for respiration. Experiments in Brain Research 144:293-302.

Hoit, J.D., & Lohmeir, H. (2002). Binding the abdomen can improve speech in men with phrenic nerve pacers. American Journal of Speech-Language Pathology 117:1-6.

Hornstein, S., & Ledsome, J. (1986). Ventilatory muscle training in acute quadriplegia. Physiotherapy Canada 38:145-149.

Huss, D. (1987). Seating for spinal cord clients. In Proceedings of the Third International Seating Symposium, Memphis, Tenn: 209-222.

Imle, P., & Boughton, A.C. (1987). The physical therapist's role in the early management of acute spinal cord injury. Topics in Acute Care Trauma Rehabilitation 1:32-47.

Jasper, M., Kruger, M., Ectors, P., & Sergysels, R. (1986). Unilateral chest wall paradoxical motion mimicking a flail chest in a patient with hemilateral C7 spinal injury. Intensive Care Medicine 12:396-398.

Johnson, E.W., Reynolds, H.T., & Staugh, D. (1985). Duchenne muscular dystrophy: a case of prolonged survival. Archives of Physical Medicine and Rehabilitation 66:260-261.

Katagiri, M. (2003). Neck and abdominal muscle activity during a sniff. Respiratory Medicine 97:1027-1035.

Kendall, F.P., McCreary, E.K., & Provance, P.G. (1993). Muscles testing and function. Baltimore: Williams and Wilkins.

Lafffont, I., Durand, M.C., Rech, C., De La Sotta, A.P., Hart, N., Dizien, O., & Lofaso, F. (2003). Breathlessness associated with abdominal spastic contraction in a patient with C4 tetraplegia: a case report. Archives of Phys Med Rehabilitation 84:906-908.

Lanini, B. (2003). Chest wall kinematics in patients with hemiplegia. American Journal of Respiratory & Critical Care Medicine 168:109-113.

Linn, W., Spungen, A.M., Gong, H. Jr., Bauman, W.A., Adkins, R.H., & Waters, R.L. (2003). Smoking and obstructive lung dysfunction in persons with chronic spinal cord injury. Journal of Spinal Cord Medicine 26:28-35.

Lissoni, A., Aliverti, A., Tzeng, A.C., & Bach, J.R. (1998). Kinematic analysis of patients with spinal muscular atrophy during spontaneous breathing and mechanical ventilation. American Journal of Physical Medicine & Rehabilitation 77:188-192.

MacLean, D., Drummond, G., Macpherson, C., McLaren, G., & Prescott, R. (1989). Maximum expiratory airflow during chest physiotherapy on ventilated patients before and after the application of an abdominal binder. Intensive Care Medicine 15:396-399.

Mahler, D.A. (1990). Therapeutic strategies. In Mahler, D.A. (Ed). Dyspnea. New York: Futura Publishing.

Maloney, F.P. (1979). Pulmonary function in quadriplegia: effects of a corset. Archives of Physical Medicine Rehabilitation 60:261-265.

Martinez, F.J., Couser, J.I., Celli, B.R. (1991). Respiratory response to arm elevation in patients with chronic airflow obstruction. American Review of Respiratory Diseases 143:476.

Massery, M.P. (1994). What's positioning got to do with it? Neurology Report 18:11-14.

Mazza, F.G., DiMarco, A.F., Altose, M.D., & Strohl, K.P. (1984). The flow-volume loop during glossopharyngeal breathing. Chest 85:638-640.

Mellin, G., & Harjula, R. (1987). Lung function in relation to thoracic spinal mobility and kyphosis, Scandanavian Journal of Rehabilitation Medicine 19:89-92.

Micheli, J. (1985). The use of the modified Boston orthosis sytem for back pain: clinical indications. Journal of Ortho Pros 39:41-46.

Mitchell, G.S., & Johnson, S.M. (2003). Neuroplasticity in respiratory motor control. Journal of Applied Physiology 94;358-374.

Montero, J.C., Feldman, D.J., & Montero, D. (1967). Effects of glossopharyngeal breathing on respiratory function after cervical cord transection. Archives of Physical Medicine and Rehabilitation 48:650-653.

Morris, K.F., Baekey, D.M., Nuding, S.C., Dick, T.E., Shannon, R., & Lindsey, B.G. (2003). Invited review: neural network plasticity in respiratory control. Journal of Applied Physiology 94: 1242-1252.

Mueller, R.E., Petty, T.L., & Filley, G.F. (1970). Ventilation and arterial blood gas changes induced by pursed lips breathing. Journal of Applied Physiology 28:784.

Roa, J., Epstein, S., Preslin, E., Shannon, T. & Celli, K.B. (1991). Work of breathing and ventilatory muscle recruitment during pursed lips breathing in patients with chronic airway obstruction. American Review of Respiratory Disorders 143:77.

Rood, M.S. (1962). The use of sensory receptors to activate, facilitate and inhibit motor response. In Sattely, G. Approaches to the treatment of patients with neuromuscular dysfunction. 3rd International Congress, World Confederation of Occupational Therapists.

Saumarez, R.C. (1986). An analysis of possible movements of human upper rib cage. Journal of Applied Physiology 2:678-689.

Saunders, S., Rath, D., & Hodges, P.W. (2004). Postural and respiratory activation of the trunk muscles changes with mode and speed of locomotion. Gait Posture 20:280-290.

Scheitzer, J.A. (1994). Specific breathing exercises for the patients with quadriplegia. Physical Therapy Practice 3:109-122.

Shaffer, T.H., Wolfson, M.R., & Bhutani, V.K. (1981). Respiratory muscle function, assessment and training. Physical Therapy 61:1711-1723.

Sharp, J.T., Drutz, W.S., Moisan, T., Foster, J., & Machnach, W. (1980). Postural relief of dyspnea in severe chronic obstructive pulmonary disease. American Review of Respiratory Disoders 122:201.

Sivak, E.D., Gipson, W.T., & Hanson, M.R. (1982). Long-term management of respiratory failure in amyotrophic lateral sclerosis. Annals of Neurology 12:18-23.

Sullivan, P.E., Markos, P.D., & Minor, A.D. (1982). An integrated approach to therapeutic exercise: theory and clinical application. Reston, Va: Reston Publishing

Temprado, J.J., Milliex, L., Grelot, L., Coyle, T., Calvin, S., & Laurent, M. (2002). A dynamic pattern analysis of coordination between breathing and rhythmic arm movements in humans. Neuroscience Letters 329:314-318.

Warren, V.C. (2002) Glossopharyngeal and neck accessory muscle breathing in a young adult with C2 complete tetraplegia resulting in ventilator dependency. Physical Therapy 82:590-600.

Zumwalt, M., Adkins, H.V., Dail, C.W., & Affeldt, J.E. (1956). Glossopharyngeal breathing. Physical Therapy Review 36: 455-459.

CHAPTER 24

Exercise Testing and Training: Primary Cardiopulmonary Dysfunction

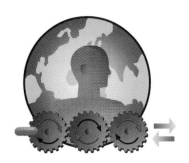

Elizabeth Dean and Donna Frownfelter

KEY TERMS
Cardiac rehabilitation
Central adaptation
Exercise testing and training principles
Lifelong health behavior change

Patient education
Peripheral adaptation
Pulmonary rehabilitation
Team work

The principles of physical therapy practice in the management of individuals with primary cardiovascular and pulmonary conditions can be applied in formally structured programs or in one-on-one sessions. Exercise testing and training are primary components of comprehensive physical therapy management, which is detailed in Chapter 31. This chapter describes these principles. Structured cardiac and pulmonary rehabilitation programs are therapeutic multidisciplinary programs that encompass the essentials of the best physical therapy practice (see definition in Box 24-1). The distinctions among structured programs lie in the primary patient populations they serve rather than in the principles of physical therapy management, which are comparable when applied on a one-to-one basis. The general principles of comprehensive care include teamwork, patient education, exercise testing and training, long-term sustainable lifestyle change, and follow-up, and these are common across patient groups. This chapter extends the basic principles of exercise testing and training outlined in Chapter 18. The chapter highlights state-of-the-art literature and the physical therapist's central role as clinical exercise physiologist in addressing the needs of individuals with primary cardiovascular and pulmonary conditions.

The role of the physical therapist as health coach and advocate to promote lifelong health and wellbeing is further emphasized in the management of these patient groups. These principles are also applied when primary cardiovascular and pulmonary dysfunction is a secondary diagnosis—that is, for example, in a patient whose primary diagnosis is a frozen shoulder but who has history of heart disease or its risk factors. This underlying condition has major implications for the modification of an exercise program for the frozen shoulder in addition to implementing management to specifically address it.

Over the past decade, there have been a plethora of published position statements, clinical practice guidelines, and consensus statements to guide contemporary practice in cardiac and pulmonary rehabilitation programs. The major benefit of these programs is to improve quality of life and tolerance of daily activities. An overriding objective is to institute lifelong healthy practices, including secondary prevention (Dafoe & Huston, 1997). The application of these principles is central to the management of cardiovascular and pulmonary conditions, whether they are primary or secondary conditions. In general practice today, patients (including children) presenting to the physical therapist with musculoskeletal or neuromuscular complaints have a high probability of having underlying cardiac or pulmonary pathology, or one or more associated risk factors (see Chapter 1). Established guidelines for cardiac and rehabilitation programs do not replace the expert clinical judgment of rehabilitation

---

Definition of Cardiopulmonary Rehabilitation

The goal of cardiopulmonary rehabilitation is to maintain or return an individual with cardiopulmonary dysfunction to full participation in life with a high level of life satisfaction.

Cardiopulmonary rehabilitation consists of a comprehensive interdisciplinary management program, including physical activity and exercise, education, and behavioral change designed to improve the physical and emotional status of individuals with cardiopulmonary dysfunction or their risk factors.

---

professionals and goal-directed, patient-centered service delivery (Stone et al, 2001). Consistent with the World Health Organization's definition of health (see Chapter 1), both programs focus on the enhancement and maintenance of cardiopulmonary health through individualized programs designed to optimize physical, psychological, social, vocational, and emotional status overall. In addition, they promote secondary prevention through risk-factor identification and modification in an effort to prevent disease progression and the recurrence of cardiopulmonary events (Stone et al, 2001).

This chapter extends the information in Chapter 31 concerning the management of chronic, primary cardiopulmonary dysfunction. In the review of the state-of-the-art literature, $\dot{V}O_2$max was often reported in studies and was used to mean $\dot{V}O_2$peak (see Chapter 18 for elaboration of this physiologic distinction). Despite this, the term used by the original investigators in each study is used in the summary of these studies.

A criticism of conventional cardiac and rehabilitation programs is that they are structured with little individualization (NHS Bulletin, 1998). The physical therapist, who is uniquely qualified as an applied clinical exercise physiologist and health coach, needs to ensure that the components, and in particular exercise, are prescribed to meet the specific needs and comorbidities of each individual.

CARDIAC AND PULMONARY REHABILITATION: EVIDENCE BASE, EFFICACY, AND PRACTICALITIES

Although a multidisciplinary team approach is fundamental to both types of programs, individuals who regularly participate in moderate exercise experience greater control of symptoms and increased functional capacity than do those treated with drugs alone (Rosenberg & Resnick, 2003). Self-management strategies learned in a pulmonary education program also contribute to perceived control of symptoms and to self-confidence (Klein et al, 2001). This sense of control is perhaps the single best argument supporting the exploitation of noninvasive interventions for the management of chronic conditions. This component may be singularly important in determining long-term outcomes, such as reduced demands for health care and lower health care costs (Michalsen et al, 1998).

The effectiveness of cardiac and pulmonary rehabilitation has been established at the highest level of evidence (ACC/AHA 2002 Guideline Update for Exercise Testing; AHA Scientific Statement, 2003; European Society of Cardiology, 2001; Fabbri & Hurd, 2003; Global Initiative for Chronic Obstructive Pulmonary Disease (GOLD), 2002, 2003; Grundy et al, 2002; O'Donnell et al, 2003; Smith et al, 2001; Stone, 2001; Suskind et al, 2003) and this is true irrespective of stage of disease (Gerald et al, 2001; Jungbauer & Fuller, 1999). These interdisciplinary programs have internationally recognized standards that are well described and are recommended for all patients with cardiovascular and pulmonary conditions. They specialize in patient education, including smoking cessation, nutrition and weight control, and promotion of self-management and training, that has sustained, lifelong, positive effects on cardiopulmonary status and sense of well being (Mayou et al, 2002; Ockene & Miller, 1997). The term *end stage* needs to be revisited, given the efficacy of rehabilitation in severely compromised individuals (Roche & Huchon, 1997). Given these benefits and the enormous economic implications of keeping people healthy and out of hospitals and doctors' offices, rehabilitation can be supported as a primary intervention rather than a secondary priority after suboptimal effects of pharmacotherapy or surgery (Celli, 1997).

Noninvasive cardiac and pulmonary rehabilitation is more cost-effective than medical and surgical treatments, and it offers long-term health benefits and reduced risk. However, there is a significant discrepancy between the actual provision and practice of cardiac rehabilitation and that advocated in published guidelines. These evidence-based, noninvasive, cost-effective interventions are being grossly underused, and participation rates are low (Campbell et al, 1996). Referral to cardiac rehabilitation has been reported to reflect selected groups, namely, younger age groups, those who have participated previously, those admitted to hospital with outpatient cardiac rehabilitation services, and those having a discharge diagnosis of myocardial infarction or coronary artery bypass surgery (Gassner et al, 2003; Johnson et al, 2004). Significant barriers also have been reported to exist with respect to availability, referral, and utilization of these programs; there are also payment issues (Womack, 2003). Only a small proportion of individuals are referred, and of those, only a small proportion can access the programs (Decramer et al, 2003; Fahy, 2004; Simonds, 2003). Inpatient cardiac rehabilitation Phase I has been reported to be a declining trend (Spencer et al, 2001). Physicians and surgeons may not have knowledge and awareness of the efficacy of noninvasive approaches to health problems that have been managed primarily with drugs and surgery, so suitable candidates are not always referred (De Busk, 1992). In addition, there are psychosocial reasons for underutilization of these resources. Women are referred less commonly than men, and their drop-out rates are higher (Blackburn et al, 2000; Halm et al, 1999). Thus, there is a selection bias in the individuals sampled for studies of cardiac rehabilitation (Lloyd-Williams et al, 2002). The participation of women is associated with insurance, level of education, bypass surgery, and transportation availability (Missik, 2001). Cost containment and increasing accessibility are two primary barriers to participation in cardiac rehabilitation (Gordon et al, 2002). Low participation rates, particularly by women, minority group members, and older people, and means of increasing access have become a primary focus of interest (Thomas et al, 1996).

Of the multiple facets of a cardiac rehabilitation program, different components may have different effects on individual heart health. In addition, physiologic differences between men and women lead to differences in the incidence and manifestation of cardiovascular conditions, and such differences may explain differences in the responses of the two genders to cardiac rehabilitation. Women tend to have lower systolic blood pressure and pulse pressure than men and to have more favorable lipid and homocysteine levels (Winer et al, 2001). The compliance of women's small blood vessels tends to be lower however, which may reflect female sex hormones and the higher mortality rates of premenopausal women hospitalized for myocardial infarction. Women also tend to have more silent heart disease than men, which is more often associated with sleep disturbance in women. The results of one descriptive study showed that women were less likely to adhere to diet and exercise modification guidelines compared with regimens for smoking cessation, medication, and stress management (Gallagher et al, 2003).

Special attention needs to be paid to motivating individuals to participate (identify facilitating factors and barriers to participation); to helping them to generalize their new skills to home activities and the community; and to continuing their new lifestyle behaviors beyond formal enrollment in the program (Rosenberg & Resnick, 2003). Given that education and exercise are core components of cardiac and pulmonary rehabilitation, physical therapy is uniquely positioned to implement care for individuals with cardiac or pulmonary conditions as primary or secondary diagnoses and to mobilize an interdisciplinary health care team for a given individual if no formal program exists. Education materials should be individualized to the learner's needs and capacities; otherwise, resources will be wasted. There is a marked disparity between the average American's reading ability (8th grade level) and the readability levels of cardiac rehabilitation materials (Johnson & Stern, 2004). The large number of polysyllabic words is a primary factor.

Cardiac and pulmonary rehabilitation programs are typically conducted in formal centers in large communities. The vast majority of patients however, do not have access to cardiac and pulmonary rehabilitation. Second, long-term participation and adherence to the principles of the program have been disappointing, particularly for women (Farley et al, 2003). The principles of these programs reflect fundamental physical therapy practice, which can be implemented on a one-to-one basis in a private practice (in a large or small community) or in a hospital that does not have a formal program in cardiac or pulmonary rehabilitation; in such settings, the outcomes are comparable to those in formal programs (Ilarraza et al, 2004;

Tyler 1997; Yohannes & Hardy, 2003). A close-to-home philosophy of care is emerging in the field of health care, including cardiac rehabilitation, so as to improve access to underserved people and groups (Suskin et al, 2003). Patients who are stable after bypass surgery do as well (in terms of improved exercise capacity and risk reduction) with an individualized detailed home program as those participating in a supervised center-based rehabilitation program (Kodis et al, 2001).

As patients become more active, their pharmacokinetics change. Medications must be reviewed on an ongoing basis and prescriptions modified accordingly (Persky et al, 2003). These changes reflect the long-term metabolic effects of exercise, in addition to improved health and potential weight loss. Close teamwork is needed to monitor a patient's medications and ensure that drug prescriptions are changed so that they promote weaning from medication commensurate with the benefits of noninvasive intervention, including education and exercise. Eliminating or reducing the needs for medication and pharmacological support is an important physical therapy outcome consistent with the philosophy of exploiting non-invasive care as much as possible.

Formal exercise testing and training—primary physical therapy skills—are warranted in patient diagnosis, evaluation, and exercise prescription. Early intervention with exercise for heart and lung conditions has become an established practice to counter the deleterious effects of deconditioning and the loss of cardiac and pulmonary function and to maximize remaining oxygen-transport reserve (Carter et al, 1993).

Addressing the psychosocial components of care in cardiac and pulmonary rehabilitation is an element of the internationally accepted definition of rehabilitation. Psychosocial factors, however, constitute few if any aspects of the workup and assessment of an individual with heart or lung disease. A structured assessment tool to assess and monitor psychosocial factors and changes in patients with heart disease has been proposed (Lau-Walker, 2004). Guidelines concerning the psychosocial component of cardiac rehabilitation are the sole focus of a position paper being developed in Europe; it is designed to promote active psychological as well as physical well-being (Sommaruga et al, 2003). Given the aging of the populations of high-income countries, cardiac rehabilitation programs must pay particular attention to the needs of older adults with respect to nutrition, physical activity and exercise, program adherence, smoking cessation, psychological issues, and methods of teaching the older learner (Williams et al, 2002). Doing so will help to reduce the high exclusion rate of this cohort of the population from cardiac rehabilitation programs.

Finally, with the advent of databases and outcome measures, projects such as the WISCVPR Web-based Outcomes Project, which focused on outcomes for cardiac rehabilitation, will help to develop benchmarks and further refine best practice guidelines (Vitcenda, 2003). Outcomes of pulmonary rehabilitation include quality of life which, for those with chronic lung disease, is reflected in the St George's Respiratory

Questionnaire and the 36-item Short-Form Health Survey. A simple linear analog quality-of-life scale has also been shown to be valid in terms of evaluating disease-specific, health-related quality-of-life issues in older individuals with chronic lung disease (Katsura et al, 2003). With databases and outcomes evaluation, physical therapists will be able to individualize programs to promote more immediate, more effective, and more long-lasting effects (Sanderson et al, 2004). In addition, programs are being evaluated that will enhance the quality of prevention strategies initiated by health care providers through hospital-based programs for patients at risk. Such a quality-improvement initiative, which involved interactive training of hospital teams and Web-based teaching tools, enhanced adherence to prevention guidelines in hospitalized patients with cardiac disease (LaBresh et al, 2004). From baseline to one year, marked improvements occurred in smoking cessation, lipid control, blood pressure control, and cardiac rehabilitation referral. Quality-improvement initiatives for activities related to cardiac rehabilitation produce marked benefits. In addition to structured exercise, cardiac rehabilitation focuses on counseling and teaching about risk reduction so as to promote lifelong health; however, long-term studies are needed to address the issue of deterioration with respect to risk factors and lifestyle behaviors over time (Lear et al, 2002). A multistate outcome program for cardiopulmonary rehabilitation was shown to be feasible; it was possible to benchmark data across programs (Jungbauer & Fuler, 1999). Outcomes included the SF-36 Health Survey, a patient knowledge test, and a 6-minute-walk test distance. All outcomes improved in both cardiac and pulmonary rehabilitation programs. Such outcomes are useful for judging the effects of cardiac and pulmonary rehabilitation programs.

Although cardiac rehabilitation reduces cardiac deaths, whether exercise alone or the comprehensive range of interventions associated with cardiac rehabilitation is responsible remains unclear (Jolliffe et al, 2001). The answer to this question is singularly important in refining the principles and practices of cardiac rehabilitation programs.

Studies of the efficacy of cardiac rehabilitation are methodologically marred by selection bias: subjects tend to be low-risk, middle-aged men, and those who might benefit most are often excluded, namely, those who are older, at high risk, and have multiple comorbidities (Jolliffe et al, 2001). Also, ethnicity is rarely reported. Given the needs of the aging population, the number of people with multiple conditions, and the increasingly ethnically diverse society in the United States and Canada, the reports on the effects of cardiac rehabilitation, to date, have relatively limited generalizability.

PATIENTS WITH CHRONIC CARDIAC DYSFUNCTION: EXERCISE RESPONSES

Cardiac dysfunction includes a range of types of pathology, causes (acquired or congenital), and severity, that may be managed medically, surgically, or in both ways (see Chapter 31 for the principles of comprehensive physical therapy manage-

ment). The most common cause is ischemic heart disease and myocardial infarction. The muscle that is infarcted never recovers, so remodeling of the heart occurs, and that alters the electrical (as shown on an electrocardiogram [ECG]) and the mechanical functions of the heart (evidenced by ECG and echocardiogram). Remodeling takes place over time and with exercise. Ejection fraction (right ventricle) at rest is a poor indicator of cardiac function and exercise capacity (Hacker et al, 2003). In fact, heart failure can occur in the presence of a normal ejection fraction (Klapholz et al, 2004), a form of disorder that typically occurs in women who have histories of hypertension and increased left ventricular mass.

Patients can range from being asymptomatic and having risk factors to being in severe distress and having minimal functional capacity, requiring high levels of supplemental oxygen and pharmacologic support and awaiting heart transplantation. Patients with extremely severe disease may require mechanical ventilation. To be able to classify patients' functional capacity in a semiquantitative manner, the New York Heart Association classification of function is commonly used (see Box 31-2). Exercise is now considered an essential component in the management of individuals with stable heart failure and in those who have undergone transplantation (Braith, 1998). Surgical options include keyhole surgery, open-heart surgery (e.g., coronary artery bypass surgery, valve repair, and aneurysm repair), and heart transplantation.

There is an interaction between circadian rhythms and the pathogenesis of heart rate and blood pressure variability. These rhythms are under the influence of adrenal, autonomic, hypothalamic, and pituitary activity. Thus, physical exertion, sleep deprivation, emotional stress, and high-fat meals are major triggers of myocardial ischemia, angina, infarction, sudden cardiac death, and stroke, which have a higher incidence in the second quarter of the day, between 0600 and 1200 (Singh et al, 2001). Heart rate and blood pressure variation have been implicated in the pathogenesis and progression of atherosclerosis, heart failure, and thrombosis, and are independent risk factors. During this period, vitamins C and E are lower than during the rest of the day; it has been postulated that regulating the intake of these vitamins and exercising may minimize the variability of heart rate and blood pressure. Whether such regulation can then modulate cardiovascular events warrants further study.

Although dyspnea is a common limiter to exercise in cardiac failure, the other factors that contribute to exercise limitation are multiple. In addition to central hemodynamic impairments, exercise capacity is affected by impaired ventilatory control, lung function, peripheral circulation, and skeletal muscle function (Harrington & Coats, 1997). Exertional dyspnea has been attributed to the regulation of arterial pH during exercise (Koike et al, 1993). Pulmonary hypertension and systemic hypotension can also limit exercise performance (Mabee et al, 1994). Explanations for these limiters include baroreceptor dysfunction, beta-receptor downregulation, abnormal vascular adaptation, and poor cardiac output in relation to elevated right ventricular afterload. The delayed $\dot{V}O_2$ responses (delayed oxygen kinetics or time constant for this variable) are associated with lactate production and early anaerobiosis (Zhang et al, 1993). Maladaptive gait changes have been ruled out as a factor influencing ventilation in patients with chronic heart failure (Clark et al, 1997b).

The physiologic capacity of patients with cardiac dysfunction to adapt to exercise depends on the type and severity of impairment in the heart and in other steps in the oxygen transport pathway. Reduced alveolar-capillary membrane diffusing capacity (Puri et al, 1995) and a ventilation to perfusion mismatch have been proposed (Banning et al, 1995) and may reflect chronically elevated pulmonary capillary pressure. A primary ventilation-perfusion mismatch defect in patients with heart failure may explain their increased ventilatory response to exercise, but this theory has been questioned (Clark et al, 1995). Patients with severe left ventricular dysfunction enhance their aerobic capacity primarily by improving oxygen extraction at the tissue level rather than by means of central adaptation. Similarly, with aerobic exercise, these patients improve the collateralization of peripheral capillaries so as to improve blood flow to working muscles and increase nitric oxide production in the blood vessels, which mediates endothelium-dependent relaxation (Belardinelli & Perna, 2002). This effect is correlated with functional capacity. Thus, evaluation of vasomotor reactivity has been proposed as a means of explaining the effects of interventions, including exercise and medications. Aortic wall elasticity modulates left ventricular function and coronary blood flow. Pulse wave velocity is a marker of arterial stiffness and is an independent predictor of $\dot{V}O_2$peak (Bonapace et al, 2003). The exercise intolerance observed in individuals with dilated cardiomyopathy may be explained by an increase in arterial stiffness.

Individuals with Chronic Cardiac Dysfunction and Failure

The cardiac dysfunction managed by physical therapists can range from mild to severe. With increasing severity of disease, an individual's response and adaptation to exercise are altered markedly, which has major implications for exercise testing and training.

Chronic heart failure is usually hallmarked by left ventricular dysfunction. In health, normal left stroke volume coupled with increased heart rate leads to greater cardiac output and greater metabolic demand, as during exercise. As the left ventricle becomes increasingly compromised, the individual with heart failure becomes more dependent on heart rate to increase cardiac output and peripheral oxygen extraction. Left ventricular ejection fraction during exercise is not consistently associated with resting ejection fraction (Verberne et al, 2003), even in those with objective signs of myocardial ischemia and increased heart rates during exercise. Thus, the left ventricular ejection fraction at rest must be interpreted cautiously in the context of exercise and predicted exercise responses.

Determining which patients will benefit from a rehabilitation program has been the subject of debate. Goebbels and colleagues (1998) reported that patients with depressed left ventricular function benefit, whereas patients whose left ventricular function has been preserved, such as may occur after myocardial infarction and coronary artery bypass surgery, tend to improve spontaneously within 3 months (Dubach et al, 1995). Proponents of selecting patients for cardiac rehabilitation however, have failed to address the past history of patients, their comorbidities, access to rehabilitation, return to work, and secondary prevention strategies to maximize their care and long-term outcomes. Noninvasive practices need to be exploited before, during, as well as after a myocardial event or surgery to maximize long-term gains, including reduced recurrence of the problem and need for doctor- and hospital-based care, reduced risk factors and morbidity, and prolonged productive and quality of life. Physical therapy has a commitment to long-term outcomes, including reduced doctor- and hospital-based care, reduction or elimination of medications, and reduced probability of repeat surgeries.

Conservative management of patients with heart failure who exploit physical therapy has emerged as a major focus in the literature, in part because of the cost of surgery and an inadequate supply of organ donors. The benefits include reduction of deconditioning, including restoration of normal autonomic balance and, potentially, some primary effects on the underlying pathology (Coats et al, 1992). Patients with chronic heart failure respond to aerobic exercise favorably, showing improvement in functional class as defined by the New York Heart Association (Killavuori et al, 1996). Both $\dot{V}O_2$max and anaerobic threshold improve. In addition, the exaggerated ventilatory response at maximal and submaximal work rates that is observed in these patients is reduced. As a result, symptoms are reduced. Exercise benefits persist after patients shift from a supervised-center-based to a home-based program. This finding has important practical and economic implications.

Over recent years attention has turned to exercise training of patients with cardiac failure and the role of ventilatory changes in exercise-induced dyspnea. The periodic breathing of patients with cardiovascular disease is well known clinically; however, the mechanism underlying the cycling hyperpnea and hypopnea is not clear. Fluctuations in pulmonary blood flow have been proposed as a mechanism for this periodic breathing (Yajima et al, 1994). With respect to other ventilatory correlates of heart failure, ventilatory efficency, the ratios of $\dot{V}_E$ and $\dot{V}CO_2$, have yielded important prognostic information (Tabet et al, 2003). When used in combination with $\dot{V}O_2$ (≥ 15ml/kg/min), $\dot{V}_E/\dot{V}CO_2$ (≥ 50 L/L) can be useful in defining a high-risk group that should be prioritized for heart transplantation (MacGowan et al, 1997b).

At rest, individuals with more severe heart failure have more restrictive lung pathology and impaired gas exchange (Tomkiewicz-Pajak et al, 2002). During exercise, these patients have increased dead space, impaired gas exchange, and greater submaximal ventilatory responses than individuals whose disease is less severe. Exercise limitation in patients with chronic heart failure correlates with reduced FEV_1 and FVC, implicating airway resistance in the increased work of breathing in exercise intolerance (Witte et al, 2002). In addition, an exercise-induced diffusion defect has been identified (Agostoni et al, 2002). Alveolar-capillary membrane conductance has been identified as the best lung function predictor of $\dot{V}O_2$peak in patients with chronic heart failure (Guazzi, 2000). The impairment in ventilatory efficiency is associated with reduced exercise tolerance and pulmonary artery pressures (Reindl et al, 1998). Pulmonary vasoconstriction has been implicated in leading to pulmonary hypertension and alveolar hypoperfusion. Overall, exertional dyspnea observed in patients with heart failure is not the result of abnormal ventilatory function (Russell et al, 1998).

Ventilatory exercise parameters, including $\dot{V}O_2$peak, $\dot{V}_E/\dot{V}O_2$, and $\dot{V}_E/\dot{V}CO_2$, are strong predictors of mortality (Huelsmann et al, 2002; Mejhert et al, 2002). $\dot{V}O_2$peak, however, may be underestimated, given the slowed O_2 kinetics in this population (Cohen-Solal et al, 1997). Gas exchange, therefore, should continue to be monitored throughout recovery. Submaximal respiratory gas indexes have been proposed as being more sensitive than peak $\dot{V}O_2$ for assessing functional impairment (MacGowan et al, 2001a) and for predicting survival in ambulatory patients with chronic heart disease (Koike et al, 2002). Nonetheless, ventilatory capacity is not likely to limit exercise performance in patients with stable chronic heart failure (Clark et al, 2000). Ventilatory and heart rate responses are, however, strong and powerful predictors of mortality in these patients, and they are superior to the use of $\dot{V}O_2$peak (Robbins et al, 1999). Inspiratory capacity varies inversely with pulmonary capillary wedge pressure in individuals with chronic heart failure, and it is a strong independent predictor of functional capacity (Nanas et al, 2003).

Patients with severe chronic heart failure often have high ventilatory demands during exercise, and they have respiratory alkalosis, which is consistent with significant wasted ventilation on exertion (Al-Rawas et al, 1995), and increased respiratory drive (Bellone et al, 1999); only a relatively small effect is attributed to ventilation-perfusion mismatch. However, increased ventilatory drive, as evidenced by the ventilatory equivalent of carbon dioxide ($\dot{V}_E/\dot{V}CO_2$), has been reported to occur infrequently (MacGowan et al, 1997a). Knowledge and understanding of which patients exhibit this response and which do not would be clinically useful.

Patients with severe chronic heart failure have a reduced ratio of increase in $\dot{V}O_2$ to increase in work rate during incremental exercise (Tanabe et al, 2002). The reduced Do_2 due to severely compromised cardiac output is not fully compensated by an increase in oxygen extraction. These patients do tend to show improved exercise response through improved peripheral oxygen extraction. Changes in cardiac performance may reflect the Frank-Starling effect rather than changes in contractility (Tyberg et al, 2000). Low cardiac output, particularly in less intense exercise, does not necessarily

result in lower exercise capacity (Tanehata et al, 1998). This phenomenon has been attributed to a unique mechanism that regulates arteriovenous oxygen content difference to optimize Do_2 to the tissues in patients with severe heart failure. At peak exercise, fractional oxygen extraction in the muscle is greater in patients with chronic heart failure than in healthy people in proportion to the level of the patient's impairment (Katz et al, 2000). This observation supports the importance of peripheral adaptation to aerobic training in patients with heart failure.

Heart failure can be categorized as either diastolic or systolic; the former may be the dominant form in elderly people (Kitzman, 2002). In stable outpatients, mortality due to diastolic failure is about half that due to systolic failure. However, when patients are hospitalized, the rates are comparable. Because of its strong prevalence among the elderly, diastolic failure exceeds systolic failure in being the cause of mortality. In diastolic failure, the Frank-Starling mechanism is impaired, causing reduced maximal cardiac output, heart rate, stroke volume, and left ventricular filling pressure. Vascular stiffness is also increased. Acute exacerbations result in pulmonary edema and are associated with hypertension, sodium intake, and lack of adherence to medication schedule. A primary goal is to reduce blood pressure, which improves symptoms and reduces exacerbations.

Exercise testing is an important means of establishing the prognosis of an individual with chronic heart failure with respect to treatment response, morbidity, and mortality. Peak $\dot{V}O_2$ pulse, ($\dot{V}O_2$/heart rate), and lean body mass adjusted for O_2 pulse are useful prognosticators (Lavie et al, 2004). Post-exercise blood pressure response has shown to be a reliable and valid predictor of adverse cardiac events in individuals with dilated cardiomyopathy (Kitaoka et al, 2003). The post-exercise blood pressure response is defined as the ratio of systolic blood pressure at 3 minutes post exercise to that at peak exercise, with a criterion of 0.79 or greater to predict complications. The 6-minute walk test has been reported not to replace $\dot{V}O_2$peak as a prognosticator in individuals with advanced heart failure (Lucas et al, 1999).

Prediction of the prognosis of individuals with chronic heart failure can be improved with a two-step exercise-test protocol (Rickli et al, 2003). This test combines maximal and low-intensity exercise to improve accuracy and reproducibility. In addition, a distance of less than 300 meters walked in the 6 minute walk test (see Chapter 18) has been reported to be a useful prognostic marker of subsequent cardiac death in individuals with mild to moderate heart failure (Rostagno et al, 2003). Exercise testing has also been reported to provide good prognostic value in determining postoperative outcomes (mitral and aortic regurgitation) (Kim et al, 2003). An important role for exercise testing in prognosis is emerging.

Although tests of $\dot{V}O_2$max can be used to stratify patients with cardiac failure according to risk factors, these tests can be invalid due to premature termination by the tester or lack of motivation by the patient. Tests of anaerobic threshold may be less influenced by these factors in such a potentially compromised group (Gitt et al, 2002). Rather, the combination of a $\dot{V}O_2$ at an anaerobic threshold (gas exchange threshold) of less than 11 ml/kg/min and a $\dot{V}_E$ versus $\dot{V}CO_2$ slope of more than 34 is a better predictor of mortality at 6 months than is $\dot{V}O_2$max, and it may provide a guide when prioritizing patients for heart transplantation. Submaximal and endurance tests and determining the anaerobic threshold have been advocated over maximal tests for clinical evaluation of patients with heart failure because they are relatively easy to perform, are associated with less risk, and are more valid indexes of a patient's capacity for daily activity (Koike et al, 1996; Larsen et al, 2001).

Individuals with heart failure have a higher incidence of glucose intolerance compared with healthy individuals (20% lower) (Kemppainen et al, 2003). After an aerobic exercise program, glucose uptake can increase by 25%. The mechanism of the reduction in glucose tolerance in individuals with heart failure and the remediating effects of aerobic exercise has yet to be elucidated. Whether secondary improvement in insulin sensitivity from aerobic exercise occurs in these individuals comparable to healthy people warrants clarification.

Body position may be an important factor to consider when exercising patients with chronic heart failure who often complain of orthopnea. However, when exercise responses in the erect and supine positions were compared in one study, no change was reported in breathlessness, and no change occurred in $\dot{V}_E/\dot{V}CO_2$. However, $\dot{V}_E$peak was greater in the upright position (Armour et al, 1998).

Patients with chronic heart failure can benefit from aerobic training. Exercise training of patients with impaired left ventricular function is associated with improved ventilatory function (Myers et al, 1999). In addition to improved cardiac output, long-term high-intensity exercise resulted in reduced ventilatory dead space and improved ventilatory efficiency. Even high-intensity exercise (2 hours of walking daily in combination with high-intensity, monitored cycle ergometry at 70% to 80% of peak capacity for 40 minutes, four times a week for 8 weeks) can result in marked increases in $\dot{V}O_2$max secondary to increased cardiac output and widening of the A-aO_2 difference (Dubach et al, 1997). No improvement in myocardial contractility is observed in these patients after such an exercise program. High-intensity exercise does not impair hemodynamic status or lead to further myocardial damage. Low-intensity exercise in individuals with chronic heart failure has been shown to improve autonomic tone and reactivity to vagal and sympathetic stimulation (Malfatto et al, 2002).

The effects of exercise training on pulmonary function in individuals with heart failure are becoming better understood. After training, individuals with coronary artery disease have been reported to show no change in pulmonary function, with the exception of the respiratory exchange ratio at peak exercise (Stratmann, 1991). Also, alveolar-capillary diffusing capacity may contribute to improvement in exercise tolerance after training (Guazzi et al, 2004). Pretraining pulmonary function is not correlated with improvement in exercise performance.

With aerobic exercise training, respiratory muscle endurance improves, and that contributes to improved overall exercise capacity (McConnell et al, 2003). Breathlessness is also reduced. The reverse occurs too—that is, respiratory muscle training can improve $\dot{V}O_2$peak as well as respiratory muscle endurance in patients with chronic heart failure. The combination of muscle and endurance training is superior to endurance training alone in this patient cohort with respect to improved left ventricular function, $\dot{V}O_2$peak, and strength (Delagardelle et al, 2002; Radzewitz et al, 2002).

An understanding of skeletal muscle function in individuals with chronic heart failure is important because improvements in aerobic capacity may be largely dependent on maximizing peripheral oxygen extraction. Strength training in combination with aerobic training improves walking distance in the 6-minute walk test, which is an independent prognosticator in individuals with chronic heart failure (Hendrican et al, 2000). Regular endurance exercise increases oxidative enzymes in the working muscles and is associated with a shift from type II to type I fibers (Hambrecht et al, 1997). These skeletal muscle adaptations are independent of peripheral circulatory adaptations.

Adaptation to resistance muscle training reflects changes in the myosin heavy chain of peripheral skeletal muscle and a shift from slow aerobic to fast glycolytic and fast oxidative characteristics (Vescovo et al, 1998). These findings are associated with $\dot{V}O_2$peak, O_2pulse, and tidal volume. Reduced strength of the knee flexors and extensors in patients with chronic heart failure is associated with impaired ventilatory response to exercise; thus, muscle dysfunction has been proposed as a contributing factor to symptoms (Clark et al, 1997a). Improved functional outcomes, increase walking distance, and reduced muscle area with increased interstitial space after exercise training support the theory that these effects are mediated by improved capillary density and flow reserve to exercising muscle (Larsen et al, 2002).

Peripheral myopathy in individuals with chronic heart failure may contribute to exercise intolerance and training capacity (Gosker et al, 2003). Features include reduced proportion of type I fibers, shift to type II fibers, biochemical shift consistent with increased muscle fatiguability, reduced mitochondrial density, and reduced capillary density (Warburton & Mathur, 2004). However, some of these changes, such as altered capillary density, appear to be gender-specific, which may have implications for training (Duscha et al, 2001). Skeletal muscle appears to adapt to central impairment of oxygen transport in heart failure. There is histochemical and gas exchange evidence showing that physiologic recovery is delayed in patients with heart failure (Belardinelli et al, 1997). Markers of skeletal muscle oxygenation including myoglobin, and its derivatives are reduced during incremental aerobic exercise to maximum, and during the recovery. Inflammatory cytokines have been implicated in the myopathy associated with heart failure (Larsen et al, 2002). However, the possibility that this outcome reflected deconditioning could not be ruled out because the patients did not achieve exercise intensities comparable to those of the control group (Matsui et al, 1995). Inflammatory cytokines have been implicated in the myopathy associated with heart failure (Larsen et al, 2002).

The recovery process in these patients has important implications for optimizing exercise training parameters and, thereby, training effects. However, further study of differences in exercise recovery characteristics between patients with heart failure and healthy people is warranted (Riley et al, 1994; Yamani et al, 1995). Evidence supports the idea that exercise intolerance in these patients is characterized by slower adaptation to acute exercise and recovery and to reduced maximal exercise capacity compared with healthy people (Sietsema et al, 1994).

After angiography, positioning and mobilization have important roles after several hours of bed rest (Pollard et al, 2003). Limiting restricted mobility after cardiac catheterization to 2 hours from 6 hours has been reported to be safe, and it may limit complications (Vlasic & Almond, 1999).

Different types of exercise stress (aerobic or resistance) have differential effects on the heart and circulation (Longhurst & Stebbins, 1997). In health, for example, static exercise exerts a pressure load on the heart that can be distinguished from the normal hemodynamic response to dynamic exercise, which involves a volume load on the heart. Static exercise leads to concentric cardiac hypertrophy (left ventricular), and dynamic training is associated with eccentric hypertrophy. Static exercise can produce effects that have been associated with aerobic training. Isotonic exercise using hand weights has been reported to be associated with increases in systolic and diastolic blood pressure, rate pressure product, serum norepinephrine, and perceived exertion (King et al, 2000). Pulmonary capillary wedge pressure, incidence of dysrhythmias, and ST-segment changes do not differ from rates recorded at rest. Generally, isotonic exercise is tolerated well by individuals with heart failure, and no angina or dyspnea occurs.

Low to moderately intense strength training may cause fewer cardiovascular complications than aerobic exercise training in individuals who have undergone myocardial infarction (Daub et al, 1996). Resting blood pressure can be reduced, albeit to a lesser extent, suggesting reduced sympathetic and baroreceptor activity. In addition, lipid profiles may improve. These benefits can be observed in patients with cardiac and circulatory pathology without adverse effects. Even older, frail patients may tolerate weight training at 40% to 60% of maximal voluntary contraction. Qualitatively similar hemodynamic responses occur in response to resistance exercise, as in aerobic exercise in individuals with heart failure (Cheetham et al, 2002). In general, resistance training with multiple repetitions of moderate weight produces the most beneficial effects. To ensure that a patient is able to perform optimally the activities of daily living, which require a certain degree of muscle strength, strength training is considered an integral component of a cardiac rehabilitation program.

The effect of cardiac dysfunction on regional circulation has been of interest, particularly with respect to cerebral perfusion. A recent study has shown that patients with left ventricular dysfunction can have impaired cerebral perfusion. During exercise, the adequacy of cerebral perfusion is dependent upon the adequacy of cardiopulmonary function; it is compromised in patients whose cardiac output fails to increase appropriately in response to exercise (Koike et al, 2004).

Some individuals with chronic heart failure have been reported to have sick euthyroid syndrome in which serum-free triiodothyronine is reduced in the presence of normal free L-thyroxin and thyrotropin (Psirropoulos et al, 2002). Sick euthyroid syndrome is a poor prognostic sign in individuals in failure. Exercise, however, can normalize the free triiodothyronine levels and reverse the syndrome, in turn improving exercise capacity.

Individuals with persistent life-threatening cardiac rhythms may require artificial pacemakers. Advances in this area have included biventricular pacing for individuals with systolic left ventricular failure with prolonged duration of the QRS complex. Preliminary reports suggest that these pacemakers are safe and efficacious (Mortensen et al, 2004). Further, biventricular pacing can improve symptoms and quality of life by improving walking times and ejection fraction (Molhoek et al, 2002). These effects persisted at the 6-month follow-up, and the two-year survival rate was excellent. There are few specific guidelines for these individuals with respect to exercise testing and prescription. Similarly, there are few guidelines for individuals with automatic implantable cardioverter defibrillators (Friedman et al, 1996). Preliminary reports suggest that exercise and lifestyle recommendations are needed for individuals with pacemakers and implanted cardioverter defibrillators and that with due modification, exercise testing and training are feasible.

Ventricular dysrhythmias contribute to a significant number of deaths. Despite improved survival, this cohort of high-risk individuals may be considered inappropriate for cardiac rehabilitation. With careful patient screening and monitoring, however, some patients with ventricular dysrhythmias may safely participate in cardiac rehabilitation (Kelly, 1996).

Individuals After Heart Transplantation

Heart transplantation has become an accepted therapy for end-stage heart failure over the past 20 years, with its ultimate goal being the return of function and a good quality of life (see Chapter 1). Postoperatively, the resting heart rate for heart transplant recipients is higher than normal. In the early postoperative period, the peak $\dot{V}O_2$ and work rate of people who have had heart transplants are 50% of those for healthy people (Chen et al, 1999). At ventilatory threshold, the $\dot{V}O_2$ and work rate were also 50% of normal. Peak heart rate, which increases for up to 3 minutes after peak exercise, is also significantly lower. This evidence supports the need for mandatory rehabilitation so as to maximize the benefits of this high-risk surgery including optimizing functional work capacity, return to work, and life satisfaction.

Without training, exercise tolerance remains severely limited over the first 16 months postoperatively. This has been explained by the reduced capacity to respond to the Frank-Starling mechanism and the residual low cardiac index (Kao et al, 1994). Rehabilitation begins preoperatively and continues for one year after discharge (Braith & Edwards, 2000). The principles of cardiac rehabilitation are applied; however, response of the denervated heart to exercise requires an extended warm-up and cool-down, and limits the maximal heart rate and $\dot{V}O_2$ that can be achieved. Reinnervation of the sympathetic nerves to the heart is associated with improved heart rate response to exercise and contractile function (Bengel et al, 2001). Hemodynamic responses to exercise are initially dependent upon exogenous catecholamines rather than on the fast-responding sympathetic release from nerve endings. Systolic blood pressure is more appropriate than heart rate for assessing exercise response and recovery (Ehrman et al, 1992). Anaerobiosis is achieved early. The degree to which neuroplasticity can be influenced by exercise training to promote autonomic reinnervation to the heart after transplant has yet to be established.

When compared with patients after bypass surgery in postoperative cardiac rehabilitation programs (phase II; up to 3 months postoperatively), patients with heart transplants have comparable functional outcomes (Daida et al, 1996). However, after graduation from this program and being on a home-based program for 9 months, patients with transplants had lower $\dot{V}O_2$peak, and were significantly more limited at the 1-year follow-up. Thus, phase I only, combined with recommendations for a home program, may be inadequate for patients after heart transplantation; they may benefit from long-term supervised training programs.

Persistently low $\dot{V}O_2$max after transplant reflects in part intrinsic skeletal muscle abnormalities (Gullestad et al, 1996; Mettauer et al, 1996). In addition to intensive aerobic exercise, resistance muscle training, too, has an important role in countering the effects of corticosteroid-related osteoporosis and peripheral myopathy. With respect to predicting the prognosis of patients with heart failure who undergo heart transplantation, $\dot{V}O_2$peak is considered a superior indicator of submaximal indexes of exercise capacity (Pardaens et al, 2000).

Isometric exercise and activities requiring postural stabilization are largely avoided in people who have had heart transplants because of potential hemodynamic stress. Light isometric exercise (handgrip) attenuates increases in heart rate, blood pressure, and systemic vascular resistance. Whole-body isometric exercise also attenuates these hemodynamic variables (Auerbach et al, 2000). At rest, heart rate, blood pressure, and rate pressure product are higher in individuals after transplants than in healthy people.

Some patients who receive heart transplants have low pulmonary diffusion capacity, and this is associated with lower exercise tolerance than is found in patients who do not have this impairment (Ville et al, 1998). Poor diffusion capacity, however, is not associated with exercise-induced hypoxemia, thus is not considered a primary contributor to impaired exercise tolerance.

Individuals with Left Ventricular Assist Devices

Left ventricular assist devices have become more common as an interim intervention for an individual awaiting heart transplant. The donor pool is small, so many individuals may not survive the wait for surgery. The Jarvik heart is a left ventricular device designed as a long-term solution for heart failure. In an initial case study describing a patient with a Jarvik heart, exercise tolerance, myocardial function, and end-organ function all improved 6 weeks after surgery (Westaby et al, 2000). The Jarvik heart shows some promise for the management of end-stage heart failure; however, its success will depend on its mechanical dependability.

Individuals with Congenital Heart Disease

Guidelines for individuals with congenital heart disease warrant development. Barriers to exercise in this cohort have been reported to be their perceived physical limitations, lack of interest, and fear (Swan & Hillis, 2000). Currently, guidelines are suboptimal.

Individuals with Intermittent Claudication

Intermittent claudication (IC) is the symptom of exercise-induced muscle ischemia of peripheral arterial disease. IC is a systemic complication of atherosclerosis with or without overt ischemic heart disease. The disabling pain during walking results from muscle ischemia. The risk of cardiovascular morbidity and mortality far exceeds that of severe limb ischemia or limb loss (Schmieder & Comerota, 2001). A patient with IC must be managed as a patient with heart disease as well as peripheral arterial disease. Conservative management is a priority and should include physical activity and exercise programs, smoking cessation, weight loss, and optimal nutrition, and stress management.

Claudication symptoms may mask cardiac symptoms. In addition, a comorbidity such as arthritis can complicate the clinical picture such that the disease may be manifested neither peripherally nor centrally. Alternatively, during exercise testing and training, conditions such as arthritis may limit the patient's tolerance (Tan et al, 2000). Without such limitation, exercise can improve exercise tolerance in the absence of improved peripheral blood flow (Tan et al, 2000). Exercise effects include reduced submaximal heart rates and oxygen cost and reduced post-exercise lactate levels. In addition, lipid profiles can be improved.

The exercise responses of patients with IC also exhibit a slowed $\dot{V}O_2$ response related to impaired muscle perfusion (Haouzi et al, 1997). The associated delayed ventilatory response has been associated with the hyperemic response in the exercising muscle rather than with ischemia.

Individuals with Anemia

The exercise responses of patients with anemia have not been well described. The capacity of the blood to transport oxygen is determined by the hemoglobin concentration and the binding characteristics of the hemoglobin. Patients who develop acute anemia are more likely to complain of dyspnea than patients who develop anemia gradually. Rather than a primary cardiac, pulmonary, or muscle compensatory mechanism, this adaptation is mediated by increased diphosphoglycerate, which decreases the affinity of hemoglobin for oxygen in the tissue. Patients with sickle cell anemia have a low $\dot{V}O_2$peak and a low anaerobic threshold in the presence of a high heart rate reserve but no gas exchange abnormalities (Callahan et al, 2002). The disease is characterized by restrictive lung pathology, increased alveolar dead space, and hypoxemia (Pianosi et al, 1991). Increased dead space may reflect impaired pulmonary capillary perfusion due to the sickle cells. Exercise hyperventilation is thought to be associated with increased anaerobiosis.

Individuals with Hypertension

Hypertension remains the silent killer for which efficacious nonpharmacologic interventions are underused. Hypertension is associated with sedentary lifestyle, diet, obesity, smoking, and stress. Modifying one or more of these factors can reduce high blood pressure and its lethal sequelae and eliminate or at least reduce the need for medication. Regular physical activity and a formal exercise program reduce the risk of hypertension or modify it. This effect is likely mediated through a decrease in total peripheral vascular resistance. African American men are particularly at risk for hypertension, and this risk can be detected by an exaggerated blood pressure response to exercise (Bond et al, 2002). Endurance training reduces this exaggerated response and thereby may reduce the risk in African American men for developing hypertension.

Individuals with Type 2 Diabetes

Type 2 diabetes mellitus is a strong risk factor for coronary artery disease and sudden cardiac death. This condition is associated with reduced baroreceptor sensitivity and heart rate variability, which are also risk factors for morbidity and mortality. Exercise training improves baroreceptor sensitivity in people with type 2 diabetes as well as glucose sensitivity, exercise tolerance, and muscle strength (Loimaala et al, 2003). Prognosis may well be improved with exercise.

Type 2 diabetes mellitus results in multiple deficits to exercise capacity, both central and peripheral. Muscle blood flow may be impaired at the level of microcirculation in the absence of overt peripheral vascular disease (Young et al, 1991). In patients with chronic diabetes, exercise capacity is compromised by reduced oxygen delivery. A reduction in the arteriovenous oxygen difference may contribute to a reduction in $\dot{V}O_2$ peak (Baldi et al, 2003). When smoking is controlled, individuals with diabetes mellitus who are insulin dependent and have complications have been reported not to exhibit impaired pulmonary gas exchange during exercise despite thickening of the alveolar basal lamina (Minette et al, 1999).

Individuals with non-insulin-dependent diabetes mellitus have reduced glucose transport in skeletal muscles, and this may contribute to exercise intolerance.

Diabetes mellitus is an independent risk factor for reduced left ventricular ejection fraction during exercise as is severity of coronary artery disease (Yamagishi et al, 2003).

ROLE OF MEDICATIONS: AUGMENTERS AND ATTENUATORS OF OUTCOME

Among the factors that can confound exercise responses of patients are medications. Medications can enhance, limit, or have no effect on exercise performance. Patients with cardiovascular dysfunction, particularly those under a physical therapist's care, are likely to be taking one or more potent medications. The timing of their ingestion of these medications in relation to their performing an exercise test should be recorded in order to standardize testing procedures from one time to the next; at least it is important to be aware of the confounding effects of a medication that could explain improved or worsened responses. Beta blockers are commonly taken by patients with cardiac dysfunction to improve the rhythm and contractile force of the heart. Long-term use of beta blockers causes no significant improvement in delayed heart rate recovery, which is a predictor of mortality in patients with heart failure (Racine et al, 2003). These drugs can contribute to fatigue and exercise intolerance. Many patients are taking angiotensin-converting enzyme (ACE) inhibitors to enhance cardiac function. This classification of drug improves diffusion capacity and exercise capacity, an effect mediated through prostaglandin activity. However, this activity can be mitigated by aspirin, another drug commonly taken by patients with heart failure (Guazzi et al, 1999). Thus, a change in aspirin administration in combination with ACE inhibitors can worsen exercise tolerance. Captopril, a commonly prescribed ACE inhibitor, has a demonstrable beneficial effect on exercise responses in patients after myocardial infarction (McConnell et al, 1998). Ventilatory efficiency is improved, as is evidenced by a reduction in $\dot{V}_E/\dot{V}CO_2$ at submaximal workloads. Reduced perception of exertion and improved capacity to perform the activities of daily living may result from a reduction in ventilatory demand. Concurrent with physical therapy management, an inventory of the patient's medications and medication changes should be maintained and considered when conducting an exercise test or interpreting exercise test data.

INDIVIDUALS WITH CHRONIC PULMONARY DYSFUNCTION: EXERCISE RESPONSES

Of individuals who participate in pulmonary rehabilitation programs, the largest proportion is made up of those with emphysema. Smoking is the primary cause of emphysematous changes in the lungs and the associated systemic complications (see Chapter 5). Patients with moderate or severe pulmonary distress may be referred to pulmonary rehabilitation. Other groups that may be referred are individuals with cystic fibrosis, asthma, interstitial lung disease, and alpha$_1$-antitrypsin deficiency. Patients with lung cancer are typically under-represented in rehabilitation programs and warrant being targeted as a group that could benefit.

Like patients with chronic cardiac dysfunction, patients with chronic pulmonary dysfunction may have a history of being managed pharmacologically or surgically. Surgical options include lung volume reduction surgery, segmentectomies, lobectomies, pneumonectomies, and lung transplantation.

Individuals with Chronic Obstructive Lung Disease

Deconditioning in patients with chronic lung disease is an anticipated consequence of the downward spiral of pathophysiologic compensation for the structural and functional damage to the lungs. In individuals with severe disease, exercise intolerance may reflect limited peripheral perfusion and oxygen extraction due to the disproportionate demand on the respiratory muscles. (Simon et al, 2001). These individuals are unable to exercise at an intensity that induces a high level of aerobic conditioning, and they experience early onset of dyspnea. On experiencing dyspnea with exercise, a person with chronic obstructive pulmonary disease (COPD) reduces his or her activity level, which leads to deconditioning. With impaired aerobic capacity, anaerobic glycolysis has an increasingly important role in supporting physical activity. This leads to increased blood lactate which needs to be buffered with bicarbonate, thereby producing additional carbon dioxide. This further increases ventilatory load and dyspnea and leads to further inactivity and deconditioniong. These individuals frequently have secondary cardiac and hematological changes. The goal of physical therapy is to relieve dyspnea and increase exercise tolerance, hence, quality of life. After smoking cessation, exercise is the single best intervention for controlling dyspnea in individuals with COPD.

Exercise testing has become an established component of the workup of an individual with impaired functional capacity including patients with chronic lung disease. Although estimating the ventilatory capacity of patients with COPD on the basis of whether they can climb one or two flights of stairs is no a longer tenable test, symptom-limited stair climbing can be used to evaluate cardiopulmonary reserve (Pollack et al, 1993). Stairs climbed in a symptom-limited stair-climbing test correlate with $\dot{V}O_2$peak, $\dot{V}_E$, heart rate, and respiratory rate in response to a maximal cycle ergometer test.

During acute exercise, patients with COPD have elevated heart rates and blood pressures and show increased hypoxemia and desaturation with incremental or prolonged constant work-rate exercise. Impaired exercise capacity reflects physical damage to the lungs, including impaired pulmonary vasculature (Fujii et al, 1996) as well as cardiac and skeletal muscle abnormalities. Exercise capacity is marked by a disproportionate ventilatory response and differences in FEV$_1$ but these responses explain only a fraction of the variability in $\dot{V}O_2$max (Bauerle & Younes, 1995). Variability in the ventilatory

response to exercise is a primary determinant of variability in the exercise capacity of patients with COPD. In the absence of right heart failure, right ventricular end diastolic volume is highly correlated with $\dot{V}O_2$max and cardiac index in patients with COPD, suggesting that right ventricular end diastolic volume compensates optimally (Keller et al, 1995).

As in other conditions, in the management of patients with COPD, individualized training programs based on heart rate as the gas exchange threshold (anaerobic threshold), as opposed to standard protocols based on 50% of heart rate reserve, produce superior therapeutic outcomes; that is, they reduce ventilatory requirements and are safer (Vallet et al, 1997). Supervised training of individuals with COPD has been reported to have advantages over self-monitored exercise programs (Puente-Maestu et al, 2000). When two to eight programs were compared, the supervised treadmill program was superior to a community-based walking program with respect to training intensity in terms of improved $\dot{V}O_2$, $\dot{V}CO_2$, $\dot{V}_E$, and heart rate in response to moderate-intensity workloads. Research is needed to design home-based programs for selected patients so as to maximize the programs' effectiveness.

The 6-minute walk test is useful in the assessment and management of patients with COPD, for whom the test was originally developed. The discriminating capacity of the test can be increased by considering factors in addition to walking distance. Four factors based on an evaluation of 15 variables accounted for 78% of the variances in distance walked (van Stel et al, 2001). Factor 1 was heart rate; factor 2 was endurance; factor 3 was impaired oxygen transport; and factor 4 was perceived exertion. Based on a walking-distance test, the effect of an exercise program can be predicted on the basis of low pretraining walking distance and higher FEV$_1$ (Zu Wallack et al, 1991).

Symptom-limited tests are used to estimate the effects of training on patients with COPD. In patients with low functional work capacity, objective submaximal indexes of training effects are useful. With respect to oxygen kinetics during constant work rate, the time constant of $\dot{V}O_2$ after training is reduced, and it reverts after detraining (Otsuko et al, 1997). The O_2 pulse similarly increases and decreases with training and detraining, respectively, and serum lactate decreases with training and increases with detraining.

Rigorous training (80% of peak work rate, for 45 minutes, 3 times a week, for 6 weeks) results in significant training responses in individuals with severe COPD (Casburi et al, 1997). Peak work rate and exercise endurance increase. In response to constant work rate, the kinetics of O_2 uptake, CO_2 production, $\dot{V}_E$, and heart rate are reduced. Improved exercise tolerance may reflect changes in breathing pattern, specifically, increased tidal volume and reduced respiratory rate.

During the past decade, research that sought to elucidate the training responses of individuals with COPD and their adaptation to exercise has focused on peripheral muscle pathophysiology and adaptation. With refinement in exercise testing and training procedures and in measurement, changes in peripheral muscles have been found to be associated with the underlying disease. In addition, aerobic training responses reflect both central and peripheral adaptations.

Compared with healthy people matched for activity level, individuals with COPD have less muscle strength (70% to 80% of age-matched healthy people), which may be explained by deconditioning, a disease-related myopathy, or both (Storer, 2001). In addition, mechanical efficiency may be impaired. Patients have large numbers of less efficient type II muscle fibers, but cross-sectional fiber area, capillarization, and mitochondrial density are comparable or reduced (Gosker et al, 2003a; Richardson et al, 2004). Although metabolic capacity is unchanged, differences in fiber type in COPD may explain the reduced mechanical efficiency.

Systemic factors contributing to exercise intolerance have been identified in individuals with chronic lung disease, and they appear to resemble those observed in individuals with chronic heart disease (Gosker et al, 2003b). Some individuals with COPD have impaired peripheral perfusion and oxygen extraction, which may be explained by the redistribution of cardiac output from the peripheral to the respiratory muscles during increasing work rates (Simon et al, 2001). This may be a primary exercise limiter in these patients. In a study designed to distinguish central from peripheral limitations in the exercise responses of patients with COPD, central factors rather than peripheral muscle limitations were reported to be responsible (although not wholly) for their exercise intolerance (Richardson et al, 1999). Endurance training is associated with increased skeletal muscle activity and recruitment of slow-twitch fibers (Gosselin et al, 2003).

Individuals with cystic fibrosis have increasingly longer life expectancies. Exercise programs have an essential role in the management of every individual with cystic fibrosis for maintaining endurance and optimizing oxygen transport in the face of impaired mucociliary transport; exercise augments airway clearance and promotes coughing. A comprehensive program of aerobic exercise and resistance muscle training on a background of regular daily activity is prescribed and is modified in the event of an acute exacerbation.

Individuals with Primary Pulmonary Hypertension

Patients with primary pulmonary hypertension have impaired exercise responses that may resemble those of patients with COPD and secondary pulmonary hypertension. During incremental exercise, the lungs become less efficient as gas exchangers because of impaired lung perfusion (Riley et al, 2000).

Individuals After Lung Volume Reduction Surgery

Lung volume reduction surgery has been of increasing interest as an invasive means of correcting the hyperinflation in the lungs of patients with COPD. A good quality of life is correlated with reduced lung hyperinflation after surgery (Leyenson et al, 2000), and these improvements have been maintained for at least 18 months on follow-up (Cordova et al, 1997). A commensurate reduced work of breathing appears to facilitate performance of activities of daily living. Improvement in functional capacity after surgery has been attributed to improved breathing mechanics during exercise as well as at rest (Tschernko et al, 1998) and to improved respiratory muscle strength (Criner et al, 1998). Specifically, higher maximum levels of tidal volume and $\dot{V}_E$ are achieved; in turn, these lead to improvements in $\dot{V}O_2$ and $\dot{V}CO_2$.

Individuals with Interstitial Lung Disease

Performing exercise testing in individuals with interstitial lung disease can elucidate the extent of the pathology and its functional consequences—diffusing capacity and alveolar arterial oxygen tension difference (Hsia, 1999). These patients have less ability than healthy people to recruit the pulmonary capillary bed during increased exercise stress, so they can desaturate readily (Chung & Dean, 1989; Riley et al, 1997). $\dot{V}O_2$peak is correlated with impairment of gas exchange and circulation, rather than with ventilatory impairment. Thus, the pathophysiology of the pulmonary vasculature is considered more important than impaired ventilatory mechanics in patients with interstitial lung disease ((Hansen & Wasserman, 1996). Abnormal exercise responses in individuals with pulmonary sarcoidosis may reflect subclinical right heart dysfunction (Sietsema et al, 1992).

One study that examined the contribution of diffusion limitation to exercise performance in this patient group showed evidence of a ventilatory impairment that was manifested by a decrease in alveolar oxygen tension (Heller et al, 1998). Cardiac impairment such as impaired diastolic filling may occur secondary to pulmonary fibrosis during exercise or restriction of the pleurae and thoracic cavity. Changes in gas exchange during exercise may be the most sensitive indicator of physiologic limitation in patients with subclinical evidence of interstitial lung disease (Medinger et al, 2001; Schwaiblmair et al, 1997). However, in terms of prognostic capability, the results of an exercise test for evaluating gas exchange do not appear to augment standard pulmonary function testing (Erbes et al, 1997).

Individuals After Lung Transplantation

Lung transplantation improves pulmonary function and quality of life in individuals such as those with cystic fibrosis. When exercise responses before and after bilateral lung transplantation are compared, exercise capacity remains low, although improved (Mathur et al, 2004). This observation has been explained on the basis of poor oxygen extraction (Oelberg et al, 1998). Exercise conditioning is required in these patients postoperatively to maximize their functional capacity. However, maximum oxygen consumption may remain below that of healthy peers matched for age and gender, and anaerobiois during exercise is achieved earlier. These responses reflect inadequate adaptation of cardiac output in these patients as well as deconditioning.

Individuals with Asthma

There are several specific aspects to consider when testing and training individuals with exercise-induced asthma (NHLB Institute and National Asthma Education Program, 1991). For those who are managed with medication, a low-intensity warm-up prior to exercise can optimize its therapeutic effect. A longer cool-down may also be beneficial. Individuals with asthma are taught to monitor their unique responses to their medication and its coordination with physical activity and exercise. They also monitor the ambient air (humidity and temperature) to anticipate the potential for bronchoconstriction and respiratory distress. With good knowledge of conditions and medication, individuals with asthma can participate in high-intensity exercise safely.

Individuals with Cystic Fibrosis

General health and wellness have become primary goals for individuals with cystic fibrosis (CF). Twenty years ago, management of people with this condition, primarily children, was based largely on passive removal of excessive secretions by means of postural drainage and vigorous percussion. Now people with cystic fibrosis are living longer, and comprehensive physical therapy management, including a regular program of exercise, is recognized as a central component of promoting general health and airway clearance (Jaffe & Bush, 2001; Wagener & Headley, 2003).

Although life expectancy continues to improve in people with CF, end of life usually results from respiratory infection, so exacerbations have to be prevented. With a basis of good health resulting from proper nutrition and exercise, exacerbations may occur less often and last for a shorter time. The exercise program is adjusted during these times and then ramped up afterwards. Medications, including bronchodilators, are coordinated with exercise to produce the best effects both during sessions and over the long term (Weinberger, 2002).

CARDIAC AND PULMONARY REHABILITATION: COMMON COMPONENTS

Definition, Purpose, Goals, and Outcomes

Most individuals with heart or lung disease can benefit from the principles of healthful living that underlie the philosophies of conventional cardiac and pulmonary rehabilitation programs. In comparing patients participating in these programs with nonparticipants, cardiovascular deaths are reduced by 20% and sudden death by 37% in the year after infarction (Pashkow, 1993). Those who meet the criteria for admission and are within access of a center that offers these programs are evaluated by a multidisciplinary team that establishes the patient's short- and long-term goals and sets up an overall program that includes exercise prescription, a nutritional plan, a smoking cessation program if required, and life-skills and stress-management instruction. These programs are patient-focused, and the health care team, including the physical therapist, serves largely as health coaches and advisers. Fundamental to that program's success is establishing an individual's readiness to change lifestyle behaviors and participate in a lifelong program of health (see Chapter 1). The health education component of the program is then targeted to shift the individual to a higher level of readiness or to engage the individual immediately in an active rehabilitation program.

The preadmission workup for cardiac rehabilitation includes a complete history and a questionnaire related to current status and health behaviors and the individual's goals (Box 24-2). Because of the interdependence of heart and lung function, these questions are relevant to individuals being considered for admission to a pulmonary rehabilitation program as well as to a cardiac rehabilitation program.

A key component of the assessment on admission to a cardiac or rehabilitation program is an objective assessment of the patient's risk factors, which enables risk-factor-reduction interventions to be specifically targeted and a lifelong health plan designed and implemented.

The relative benefit of structured programs as opposed to community and home-based programs is being debated. Maximizing the potential benefits of the program is key, so the program has to be optimal in terms of the individual's needs, including the setting that will produce the best short- and long-term outcomes. Exercise gains have been demonstrated in healthy middle-aged people when programs are home-based (Marshall et al, 2001). This evidence supports the idea that individuals with cardiopulmonary dysfunction who are being managed one-on-one by a physical therapist may also demonstrate benefits when the exercise program is home-based. However, further study is needed to determine the safety and effectiveness of home-based programs for candidates for cardiopulmonary rehabilitation.

The core components of cardiac and pulmonary rehabilitation programs are shown in Box 24-3; they reflect the skills and expertise of the multidisciplinary team in addressing each individual's needs in a comprehensive manner. These components include awareness of the patient's condition and health education overall, nutrition and weight control, smoking cessation, general physical activity and exercise, and stress management. Psychological support is important with respect to the patient's adjustment to his or her condition, the management of anxiety, anger, hostility, and depression, and the maximization of adherence to recommendations and guidelines related to nutrition, physical activity and exercise, smoking cessation and so forth, and to a lifelong health plan. Such support is elicited from the individual's family and friends, as well as health care providers.

The exercise program focuses on improving flexibility and strength as well as aerobic capacity, with the goals of improving the patient's health and capacity to perform the activities of daily living and thus improving quality of life. Psychosocial and end-of-life issues are also an important part of rehabilitation programs and should be addressed, particularly in individuals who are severely ill and their families.

BOX 24-2

Preadmission Work-up for Cardiac Rehabilitation

Name: **Birth Date and Age:** **Gender:**

Weight: Height: Body Mass Index: Waist circumference:

Summary of History

List the dates and types of the medical and surgical procedures you have had over the years.

Medication

List the medications you are currently taking and the doses and frequencies.

Family History

Did your father or brothers have heart disease before 55 years of age?

Did your mother or sisters have heart disease before 65 years of age?

Current Status

Do you experience pain (tightness or heaviness) or angina in your chest on exercise?
If so, what specifically triggers it?
What relieves it?
How long does it take to go away?
Do you take medication for chest pain/angina?
If so, for how long?
How much?
Effect:
Do you every feel short of breath?
If so, what triggers it?
What relieves it?
How long does it take to go away?
Do you ever feel short of breath when you lie down?
Do you experience pain in your legs when you walk?
Have you had this investigated?
If so, what was the diagnosis?
Do your ankles swell?
Do you have high blood pressure?
If so, for how long, and how has it been managed?
Do you have normal blood pressure now?
Do you take medication for high blood pressure?
What?
How much?
Is your blood pressure controlled now?
Do you have glucose intolerance?

Type 2 diabetes?
If so, for how long and how is your blood sugar controlled?
Is your blood sugar within normal limits now?
Do you take insulin? Oral agents?
What?
How much?
Is your blood sugar controlled now?
Do you have thyroid disease?
If so, what, and for how long?
Do you take medication for your thyroid problem?
What?
How much?
Is your thyroid controlled now?
Do you have anemia?
Do you have gastrointestinal complaints?
If so, describe them.
Are you being medically treated for them?
Do you have any musculoskeletal or neurologic problems?
If so, describe them.
Are you being medically treated for them?
Do you have any balance problems?
If so, is there an explanation?
Are you being medically treated for them?
Is your vision normal with or without corrective lenses?
Is your hearing normal with or without hearing aids?

Health Behaviors

Describe your *weekly* food consumption in terms of whole grains, fruit and vegetables, beans and lentils, meat and fish, saturated and trans fats, refined sugar, and low fiber foods.
Do you have high cholesterol?
For how long?
Have you ever smoked?
When, how much, and for how long?
Do you smoke now?
If so, how much?
How much alcohol do you consume? Type, amount, and frequency:
What is your regular activity level (describe activity or exercise, intensity of exercise, duration, and frequency each week)?
How stressful is your life?
Identify life-event stressors.
Identify daily-hassle stressors.
What are your stress-management strategies?
How many hours a night do you sleep on average?
How many times do you wake up or get up during the night?

Health education is a major component of cardiac rehabilitation and constitutes a skill in its own right. The patient requires knowledge about health and the incentive to translate this information into his or her own life. Each learner's knowledge deficits are different and learning style is unique; these should be evaluated so that health education can be properly targeted so that it is the right type, the right level, the right format, and delivered at the right time (see Chapter 27). The knowledge deficit needs to be established so that education can be targeted specifically to meet this deficit.

Individuals with coronary artery disease typically have little awareness of some of the major risk factors. Generally, their knowledge about cholesterol, use of lipid-lowering medications, and achievement of cholesterol levels consistent with consensus-based guidelines is minimal (Bairey et al, 1996). Participation in structured cardiac rehabilitation programs improves knowledge related to heart disease, signs and symptoms, and self-management strategies. However, the learning and homework have to be evaluated on each visit to determine how well the knowledge has been internalized and

---

BOX 24-3

Core Components of Cardiac and Pulmonary Rehabilitation

Assessment
Entrance complaint
Height, weight, body mass index
Education
Occupation/Employment
Socioeconomic status
Family situation
Smoking history
Alcohol consumption

History

Present illness (medical and surgical details of management to date)
Multisystem review (e.g., cardiovascular, peripheral vascular, pulmonary, musculoskeletal, neuromuscular, gastrointestinal, endocrine, renal, liver, immune)
Medication status
Lab tests and investigations: blood work, ECG, x-rays and scans, exercise test
Learning assessment (education level, preferred learning styles, self-efficacy, and behavioral readiness to change.

Goals

Prevention
Short-term
Long-term

Interventions
Promotion of empowerment and self-efficacy through teaching
Smoking cessation
Nutritional counseling (optimal nutrition, lipid management, sodium control, salt control, weight control)
Hypertension management
Diabetes management
Psychosocial management
Physical activity counseling
Exercise training
Work simplification and energy conservation
Sleep and rest
Vocational rehabilitation
Recreational rehabilitation

Outcomes (monitored over the short and long term and consistent with the individual's goals)
Participation
Capacity to fulfill unique life roles, e.g., parent, spouse/partner, occupation/profession, worship and spiritual life, recreation and leisure, community activities
Abilities
ADLs and task-specific activities related to life roles, including work and home management

Structure and Function

Changes in physiologic dependent measures consistent with goal achievements

Modified from Balady, G.J., Ades, P.A., Comoss, P., Limacher, M., Pina, I.L., Southard, D., Williams, M.A., & Bazzarre, T. (2000). Core components of cardiac rehabilitation/secondary prevention programs. A statement for healthcare professionals from the American Heart Association and the American Association of Cardiovascular and Pulmonary Rehabilitation. Circulation 102:1069-1073.

---

put into practice in daily life. Lifestyle recommendations should be suitable for application to daily living. For example, healthy food choices should be described specifically. Energy utilization should be translated into terms that are meaningful for the individual, such as 1000 kilocalories (kcal) of energy per week (although 1500 kcal/wk has been identified as the threshold for reducing all-cause mortality risk [Schairer et al, 2003]). People least likely to achieve the latter threshold include women, those with a body mass index of 30 or more, and those who are 70 years of age or older. Weekly kilocalorie energy expenditure should be a component of the exercise prescription so as to ensure that maximum health benefits are achieved. The physical therapist's capacity to communicate and educate effectively will determine the long-term outcome of the program.

Many outcomes related to a sense of well being, a health-related quality of life, sickness impact, and life satisfaction are dealt with in conjunction with physiologic and clinical outcomes. The former variables are consistent with the International Classification of Function and the impact of disability on the individual, but noncardiac and nonpulmonary outcomes should also be considered.

Chronic disability is often associated with clinical depression, so management of depression alone may improve

functional capacity. With respect to pulmonary disease, 45% to 63% of deaths are attributable to advanced lung disease itself (Geraldi & Zu Wallack, 2001). Other factors that explain mortality include nutritional deficits, impaired exercise tolerance, functional performance, and social factors, including marital status. Thus, nutrition and exercise are essential elements of cardiopulmonary rehabilitation. Similar findings have been reported for cardiac disease. A negative emotional state is associated with high long-term mortality. Addressing the individual's psychological status may improve functional status (Denollet & Brutsaert, 2001).

The specific rehabilitation goals include the following.
- To serve as a health-promotion resource for the individual, community, and health care providers
- To increase aerobic capacity and muscle strength and endurance consistent with overall health and well-being
- To improve capacity to perform the activities of daily living and maintain gainful employment
- To promote self-efficacy in healthy lifestyle behaviors for long-term health and wellbeing as well as secondary prevention
- To shift an individual to a lower risk classification
- To reduce risk of revascularization procedures, medical intervention, and doctor and hospital visits

- To promote health and well-being in the patient's family and community
- To reduce direct and indirect health care costs over the short and long term

Setting and Team Members

In addition to the physical therapist, the team consists of physicians, nurses, a psychologist, a social worker, a pharmacist and, in some centers, an exercise physiologist. Typically, the physical therapist is involved with exercise testing and training, program modification and progression, and eventual discharge. An additional role is education and risk-factor modification. A physical therapist applies the principles and practices of cardiopulmonary rehabilitation to any patient in any setting and to patients who have cardiopulmonary dysfunction or its risk factors as a primary or secondary diagnosis or concern. The guidelines and standards for assessment and exercise testing and training must be adhered to if the best service and the best and safest outcomes are to be achieved (Pina et al, 1995).

Components of Physical Therapy

Assessment

Central to comprehensive physical therapy management is focusing on the individual rather than on the condition. Although this chapter emphasizes exercise testing and training in individuals with primary cardiopulmonary conditions, in reality, people present with comorbidities. Thus, individuals with secondary cardiopulmonary dysfunction (see Chapters 25 and 32) are likely to have a high incidence of primary cardiopulmonary dysfunction or risk for it (at least compared to the general population). Thus, underlying risk factors and disease must be examined in all patients, irrespective of their primary presenting diagnoses.

The history, lab tests, and investigations, including scans and ECGs, and the basic assessment of an individual with cardiopulmonary dysfunction are described in Part Two, but the aspects of the assessment that warrant particular attention in exercise testing and in training individuals with cardiovascular and pulmonary dysfunction are highlighted in this section. Although the cardiovascular and pulmonary systems may be the focus, a complete review of all systems is necessary to determine limitations imposed by musculoskeletal, neurologic, endocrine, hematologic, or other conditions. These need to be considered in both testing and training.

The assessment comprises the examination of risk factors, including profiles of the patient's nutrition intake, weight, smoking history, and stress management (including rest and sleep profiles) as well as physical activity and aerobic capacity. Prior to the onset of any intervention, a detailed history, examination, and lab data are accumulated to provide an objective baseline. Within 6 to 8 weeks, elements of the assessment are repeated and outcome measures recorded to determine the degree to which the patient has progressed with respect to achieving short-term goals.

Predictors of long-term survival of myocardial infarction include several factors that need to be identified so that patients can be stratified according to risk. These factors include age, left ventricular ejection fraction, diabetes, hypertension, and elevated resting heart rate (Lewis et al, 2003). Attention to these factors may help to detect changes in status early and avoid adverse exercise by judicious modification of an exercise program. Individuals who develop late-onset heart failure have a tenfold increased risk of mortality. Glucose abnormalities (hyperglycemia and hyperinsulinemia) in those who are not diabetic are common in individuals with heart failure (43%) (Suskin et al, 2000). Further, these findings are associated with greater functional deterioration than is found in individuals with heart failure without glucose abnormalities. Thus, knowledge of an individual's glucose tolerance is essential at baseline and over time within the rehabilitation program.

Well-being extends beyond physical health. Rehabilitation programs record and monitor outcomes related to the subjective sense of well-being, the health-related quality of life, the general quality of life, and life satisfaction. Many scales and questionnaires are available to provide outcomes and fluctuations in these variables over time.

Depression is an independent risk factor for cardiovascular disease and related increased morbidity and mortality (Thornton, 2001). Up to 45% of individuals exhibit symptoms of major depression after acute myocardial infarction. Thus, individuals referred to cardiac rehabilitation need to be screened for depression, and psychotherapy, counseling, or pharmacotherapy may be indicated. Remediation of depression associated with chronic disease may augment functional capacity independent of physical rehabilitation. Depression as well as peak aerobic capacity have been reported to be the best independent predictors of patient-reported physical function scores in older individuals with heart disease (Ades et al, 2002). These findings suggest a role for depression management that is independent of exercise training but augments functional capacity.

The general assessment must also include an assessment of the individual's learning style (see Chapter 27). Prochaska's Transtheoretical Model of readiness to change has important implications for rehabilitation programs that are formalized (e.g., cardiac and pulmonary rehabilitation) as well as for individual rehabilitation programs (see Chapter 1). Comparable to the goal of shifting an individual into a lower risk category, another objective is to shift an individual into a higher readiness-to-change category. An individual's readiness to change his or her health behavior is assessed, along with his or her intention to engage in the recommended risk-reduction behaviors, including dietary changes, physical activity and exercise, smoking cessation, and relaxation. Readiness to change may differ for each behavior. Barriers include time management, psychological adaptation, and laziness (Godin et al, 1991). Another component of the education is the assessment of the individual's knowledge deficits regarding his or her condition.

Interventions

In addition to the exercise program, the patient may also be in a smoking-cessation program and a weight-loss program. During the course of management, medications may change. Detailed records of the progress of the patient in these various programs warrant monitoring so that the perceived outcome of exercise can be explained in a valid manner. Other factors such as weight loss or smoking reduction (cessation) or change in medication could explain in whole or in part, the apparent effect of exercise.

Education

Education is the central component of cardiopulmonary rehabilitation. The patient is taught the basics of anatomy and the physiology of heart and lung health, basic nutrition, physical activity and exercise, analysis of lab tests, effects of smoking, effects of medications, and so on. In this way, the patient is empowered and, it is hoped, well motivated to be an agent of change in his or her own life. Lifestyle recommendations need to be reinforced irrespective of phase of the program. One report estimated that after a coronary event, 50% of smokers resume smoking on discharge from the hospital (van Berkel et al, 1999).

Like exercise, education can be tailor-made to suit the learning needs of each person (see Chapter 27). Individualization of the education considers age, literacy, preferred learning style, ethnic and cultural issues, and readiness to change. Smoking cessation is the most important intervention for patients with heart disease and pulmonary disease (Mokdad et al, 2004; Pierson, 2004).

Promoting self-efficacy and perceived control are central to education strategies developed by physical therapists. Follow-up is needed, however, to ensure self-treatment is sustained over time (Klein et al, 1997). Inadequate self-treatment behavior at follow-up suggests that new teaching and learning strategies should be developed to ensure that the quality of self-treatment is maintained.

Exercise Program

A reduction in respiratory rate in patients with chronic heart failure improves pulmonary gas exchange, reduces dyspnea, and increases exercise performance (Bernardi et al, 1998). Respiratory training involved 1 month of training to breathe at a rate of 6 breaths per minute. Slowing breathing rate may have some application for patients with chronic heart failure who have impaired gas exchange and breathlessness during exercise as well as at rest.

Goals: Short-term

A distinction is made between short- and long-term goals. Short-term goals are aimed at reducing cardiopulmonary risk factors, particularly those that are most life threatening, and at

---

BOX 24-4

Comprehensive Physical Therapy Management and Lifelong Health Plan

Patient's entry point to physical therapy

A primary diagnosis of cardiovascular or pulmonary dysfunction

A secondary diagnosis of cardiovascular or pulmonary dysfunction

A diagnosis of cardiovascular or pulmonary dysfunction secondary to dysfunction of systems other than primary oxygen transport dysfunction (i.e., the heart, circulation, or lungs) (Chapters 6, 25, and 32)

Assessment

Readiness to change (precontemplative, contemplative, preparation, action, maintenance)
Demographics, including literacy, culture, and education
Learning needs and style
Preventive goals and outcomes
Long-term goals and outcomes
Short-term goals and outcomes

Follow-up

Physical evaluation
Sustained adherence to behavioral-change programs
Visits to physician, clinic, hospital (details of when and why, and, if admitted to hospital, for how long)
Medication changes (what, when, why, and dose or discontinued) or new medications (what, when, why, dose)

---

developing and learning strategies for healthier living. Long-term strategies are an extension of short-term goals and address the sustainability of health and fitness consistent with the patient's needs, wants, and capabilities for the rest of their lives. These goals include sustained healthy diet and weight control, sustained high daily physical activity level, and aerobic exercise three times a week. In addition, if an individual is receiving medication that relates to cardiovascular dysfunction, a physical therapy outcome is to minimize, reduce, or eliminate the need for medication in the short and long terms.

Goals: Long-term

Long-term goals and outcomes are as important as the short-term physical therapy goals and outcomes. Intervention (drugs and surgery) has short-term benefits, as is evidenced by the apparently high number of repeated revascularization procedures performed, compared with the lifestyle behavioral changes inherent in physical therapy management, including education, smoking cessation, optimal nutrition, and exercise. At the point of entry into physical therapy (acute, subacute, or chronic, with cardiovascular dysfunction as a primary or secondary diagnosis), a long-term plan with goals, outcomes, and follow-ups is integral to the management plan overall (Box 24-4).

BOX 24-5

Rehabilitation Phases of Cardiac and Pulmonary Rehabilitation

Phase	Cardiac Rehabilitation	Pulmonary Rehabilitation
I*		
II		
Under supervision in hospital, center, or community-based program or one-on-one	6 weeks post acute episode or discharge, to 6 months Exercise retest Review of risk factors; lifestyle behaviors and changes Revision of lifestyle recommendations	≤6 weeks post acute episode or discharge, to 6 months Exercise retest Review of risk factors and lifestyle behaviors and changes Revision of lifestyle recommendations
III		
Under supervision in hospital, center, or community-based program or one-on-one	6 to 12 months Exercise retest Review of risk factors and lifestyle behaviors and changes Revision of lifestyle recommendations Exit retest for recommendations for self management phase IV	6 to 12 months Exercise retest Review of risk factors and lifestyle behaviors and changes Revision of lifestyle recommendations Exit retest for recommendations for self-management phase IV
IV	>12 months	>12 months
Self-management	Provision for follow-up	Provision for follow-up

*Phase I is described in Chapter 29, the management of Individuals with Acute Medical Conditions.

CARDIAC REHABILITATION: SPECIFIC COMPONENTS

Phases

Patients are referred to cardiac rehabilitation for management and secondary prevention of myocardial insufficiency and after revascularization procedures, including cardiac surgery (Pasquali et al, 2003). People can also benefit if they have significant risk for disease but are asymptomatic.

The phases of cardiac rehabilitation appear in Box 24-5 (with the exception of phase I, inpatient management, which is described in Chapter 29). Phase I refers to inpatient care (medical and surgical) and the predischarge exercise test.

Phase II refers to a supervised exercise program lasting 3 to 6 months. Phase II usually takes place in a community center where the patients can be monitored during exercise and education by the rehabilitation professions can be ongoing. However, a trial of home-based phase II programs for high-risk patients after cardiac surgery produced the same results as were found in the control group, which received general guidelines to increase activity levels (Brosseau et al, 1995). Further study is needed on the short- and long-term efficacy of home-based phase II programs as opposed to center-based programs with respect to symptom recurrence, indications for revascularization procedures, and risk-factor reduction.

Phase III refers to the maintenance phase during which the patient is responsible for exercising mostly at home. This phase lasts from 6 to 12 months.

Phase IV refers to an unsupervised community program. The patient is usually ready for this phase within 9 to 12 months. Patients may be referred to cardiac rehabilitation when they are stable and not in conjunction with an acute event.

Smoking Cessation

The risk of myocardial infarction is three times higher in patients who continue to smoke after a cardiac event (Serrano et al, 2003). On quitting, the risk of reinfarction is reduced to that of nonsmokers prior to the first infarction.

Nutrition and Weight Control

Optimal nutrition and weight control are priorities. Individuals with cardiovascular dysfunction are at risk for fluid and electrolyte imbalances and related ECG irregularities, so these aspects of nutrition need to be included. In addition, patients with chronic heart failure have some special considerations. These patients rely more on fat substrate during exercise than on carbohydrates, which may contribute to increased catecholamines and free fatty-acid levels (Riley et al, 1990). These changes may compensate to protect muscle glycogen stores. However, given that fat metabolism is not energy-efficient, this shift may contribute to exercise intolerance.

Psychosocial Issues

Stress management and life-skills training are fundamental to rehabilitation programs in minimizing undue sympathetic arousal and impact on the cardiovascular and pulmonary systems. Depression control and anger and hostility management are provided by the appropriate professional as indicated. Remediation of depression alone can enhance functional status.

Cardiac Risk Analysis

Estimate Your Risk for Developing Heart Disease

in the Next 10 Years

Step 1: Find your points based on your Age, Blood Pressure, LDL and HDL Cholesterol, and whether you Smoke or have Diabetes

AGE

Age	M	F
30-34	-1	-9
35-39	0	-4
40-44	1	0
45-49	2	3
50-54	3	6
55-59	4	7
60-64	5	8
65-69	6	8
70-74	7	9

CHOLESTEROL

LDL Cholesterol

	M	F
<100	-3	-2
100-129	0	0
130-159	0	0
160-189	1	2
>189	2	2

HDL Cholesterol

	M	F
<35	2	5
35-44	1	2
45-49	0	1
50-59	0	0
>59	-1	-3

DO YOU SMOKE?

	M	F
YES	2	2
No	0	0

Blood Pressure

	M	F
<120/<80	0	-3
120-129/80-84	0	0
130-139/85-89	1	0
140-159/90-99	2	2
>159/>99	3	3

DO YOU HAVE DIABETES?

	M	F
YES	2	4
No	0	0

FIGURE 24-1 Cardiac Risk Analysis: Estimate Your Risk for Developing Heart Disease in the Next 10 Years. *(Adapted from The Framingham Heart Study, www.nhlbi.nih.gov/about/Framingham/index.html; Wilson, P.W., D'Agostino, R.B., Levy, D., Belanger, A.M., Silbershatz, H., & Kannel, W.B. [1998]. Prediction of coronary heart disease using risk factor categories. Circulation 97:1837-1847.)*

Risk Reduction

Prevention and rehabilitation programs aim to reduce an individual's cardiac risk factor category. Figure 24-1 shows an example of a scale for assessing cardiac risk and categorizing an individual. Using such a scale provides objective markers for risk factor modification, and reduction of risk can be identified. Box 24-6 shows the distinctions among low, intermediate, and high risk for cardiac disease (American College of Sports Medicine, 2000). The overall purpose of management is to reduce an individual's risk factor categorization.

After angioplasty, bypass surgery, and medical therapy for fixed obstructions, individuals remain at risk, as judged by the proportion of patients who require further pharmacologic and surgical management. Risk-reduction interventions are priorities is this cohort of individuals; they can extend survival, improve quality of life, reduce the need for further invasive procedures such as angioplasty and bypass surgery, and reduce the incidence of myocardial infarction (Smith, 1997). Secondary risk reduction should be a routine component of both medical and surgical management, and it is as important as primary risk reduction.

Physical Activity and Exercise: Special Considerations

The principles and practice of exercise prescription are described in detail in Chapter 18. However, special

Step 2: Add up your points for Age, LDL-Cholesterol, HDL-Cholesterol, Blood Pressure, Smoking & Diabetes

Age	
LDL-Cholesterol	
HDL-Cholesterol	
Blood Pressure	
Diabetes	
Smoking	
TOTAL POINTS	

Step 3: Find Your Risk Level Based on Your **Point Total**

Total Points	<-2	-2	-1	0	1	2	3	4	5	6	7	8	9	10	11	12	13	14	15	16	>17
% Risk Male	1	2	2	3	4	4	5	7	8	10	13	17	21	26	32	38	46	54	54	54	54
% Risk Female	1	1	2	2	2	3	3	4	5	6	7	8	9	11	12	14	16	20	22	25	30

Your **Framingham Risk** for developing Heart Disease including a <u>Heart Attack</u> over the next <u>10 years</u> is denoted by the **%RISK Male or Female** corresponding to your **Total Points Score**

Step 4: Compare Your Risk to Others. For comparison purposes, **Low Risk** is the risk of developing heart disease within the next 10 years for a Man or Woman of the same age with normal blood pressure and cholesterol who does not smoke or have diabetes

COMPARATIVE RISK

MALES				FEMALES		
AGE	AVERAGE RISK	LOW RISK		AGE	AVERAGE RISK	LOW RISK
30-34	3%	2%		30-34	<1%	<1%
35-39	5%	3%		35-39	1%	<1%
40-44	7%	4%		40-44	2%	2%
45-49	11%	4%		45-49	5%	3%
50-54	14%	6%		50-54	8%	5%
55-59	16%	7%		55-59	12%	7%
60-64	21%	9%		60-64	12%	8%
65-69	25%	11%		65-69	13%	8%
70-74	30%	14%		70-74	14%	8%

Note that there is no risk estimate for patients < 30 or older than 74 because this analysis is based on real data collected from Framingham

FIGURE 24-1 Cont'd Cardiac Risk Analysis: Estimate Your Risk for Developing Heart Disease in the Next 10 Years. *(Adapted from The Framingham Heart Study, www.nhlbi.nih.gov/about/Framingham/index.html; Wilson, P.W., D'Agostino, R.B., Levy, D., Belanger, A.M., Silbershatz, H., & Kannel, W.B. [1998]. Prediction of coronary heart disease using risk factor categories. Circulation 97:1837-1847.)*

BOX 24-6

Risk Stratification

Low Risk

After uncomplicated myocardial infarction or bypass surgery
Functional capacity below 8 METs on 3-week exercise test
Asymptomatic at rest, with exercise adequate for most vocational and recreational activities
No ECG evidence of ischemia, left ventricular dysfunction, or complex dysrhythmias

Intermediate Risk

Functional capacity below 8 METs on 3-week exercise test.
Shock or congestive heart failure during recent myocardial infarction (<6 months)
Inability to self-monitor heart rate
Failure to adhere to exercise prescription

High Risk

Severely depressed left ventricular function (ejection fraction <30%)
Resting complex ventricular dysrhythmias (low-grade IV or V)
Premature ventricular contractions appearing or increasing with exercise
Exertional hypotension (≥15 mm Hg)
Recent myocardial infarction (<6 months) complicated by serious ventricular dysrhythmias
Exercise-induced ischemia of more than 2 mm ST depression
Survivors of cardiac arrest

MET, Metablic equivalents (1 MET = 3.5 ml O_2/kg of bodyweight/minute, which is the metabolic rate at rest).
Adapted from American College of Sports Medicine (2000). ACSM's Guidelines for Exercise Testing and Prescription (ed 6). Philadelphia: Lippincott Williams & Wilkins.

considerations for individuals with chronic heart conditions with respect to monitoring, exercise testing and training are detailed below.

Monitoring

Assessment and monitoring considerations for the individual with heart disease are described in Part Two and Chapter 31. At the onset of the program, a baseline assessment is made of the subjective sense of well-being, including health-related quality of life, impact of sickness and disability, quality of life, and life satisfaction. Related assessments are made throughout the program to observe the program's effects on these outcomes and to assess the impact of the program on its completion.

An individual with primary cardiovascular dysfunction or its risk factors requires particular attention to his or her hemodynamic status. Risk factors, however, do not necessarily predict complications during supervised exercise (Paul-Labrador et al, 1999). Serial lipid profiles, blood pressure, resting heart rate,

and body weight are monitored regularly, and interventions are modified accordingly (Allison et al, 1999). Blood pressure, however, can be abnormal in individuals with exercise-induced left ventricular systolic dysfunction, which leads to unstable hemodynamic status (Ciampi et al, 2002). Blood pressure may not be a valid measure of exercise stress in such individuals. Further study is needed before exercise risk stratification guidelines can be used with any assurance to monitor supervised rehabilitation programs.

The absolute and relative changes in heart rate, blood pressure, rate pressure product, arterial saturation, and perceived exertion are particularly important. ECGs may be performed intermittently throughout exercise or continuously, as indicated. Recent evidence has questioned the conventional guideline of an ST-segment depression of >1 mm in favor of a more conservative guideline, >.5 mm during or after exercise (Bodegard et al, 2004). This value is associated with risk for myocardial infarction, requiring bypass surgery, and risk for cardiac mortality.

Exercise-induced silent myocardial ischemia is an important indicator of increased risk for cardiovascular disease (3.5-fold) and stroke (2.2-fold) in men when they are compared to those without silent ischemia, along with other risk factors such as smoking, hypercholesteremia, hypertension, and being overweight (Kurl et al, 2003).

Recovery data are important components of the exercise testing assessment and interpretation. Delayed heart rate recovery is a predictor of mortality (Racine et al, 2003), irrespective of angiographic evidence of disease severity (Vivekananthan et al, 2003). Heart rate recovery is calculated as the difference in heart rate from peak exercise to that recorded at 1, 2, and 3 minutes after exercise. Women have been reported to be more susceptible to postexercise hypotension than men, which may be offset with an active cool-down period (Carter et al, 2001).

Signs and symptoms of overexertion must be monitored; they are summarized in Box 24-7.

Each individual is taught to monitor his or her baseline, exercise, and recovery responses in a logbook at each visit, after the parameters have been prescribed and it is considered safe for the patient to self-monitor in the supervised setting. Commonly, the individual is taught to record heart rate and a rating of perceived exertion. In addition, data sheets are logged with respect to stretching and warm-up, the parameters used for each day's exercise, including the aerobic exercise prescription, and for the cool-down and recovery periods. Also, completion of the resistance muscle training prescription is logged.

Exercise Testing

Exercise testing is used for diagnosis, assessment of functional work capacity, assessment of the outcome of one or more interventions, including a training program, and prognosis. A poor response to exercise after percutaneous transluminal coronary angioplasty can identify restenosis (Lan et al, 2003). The graded exercise test, or maximal stress test, is usually a short (8 to 12 minutes, ideally), progressively ramped, symptom-limited exercise test conducted on a treadmill or cycle ergometer. There are several established cardiac stress test protocols, such as the Bruce and the Balke. In some situations, a submaximal test is preferred because a maximal test may be risky or difficult to conduct in a valid manner because of a secondary problem. Recently, the prognostic superiority of a two-step exercise test that combines a low-intensity, steady-work-rate phase and a maximal exercise phase has been reported (Rickli et al, 2003). An exercise test may answer questions about an individual's status and thus obviate or reduce the need for more invasive and costly testing (Mahler & Franco, 1996).

The exercise testing protocol is designed to stress the patient's oxygen transport system—ventilation, heart, circulation, and muscles—progressively and in an integrated manner. Exercise is the single best way to assess the integrated function of these systems and their capacity for oxygen transport. Assessment of $\dot{V}O_2$peak is preferable for detailed evaluation and prognosis of a patient with advanced heart failure to the use of submaximal exercise tests such as the 6-minute walk test (Lucas et al, 1999). Walking on a treadmill has been reported to have greater diagnostic sensitivity than cycling in asymptomatic men with coronary artery disease (Hambrecht et al, 1992).

Valid testing of functional capacity in individuals with cardiac failure is necessary because of the discordance of the results of various tests in the same individual (Rostagno et al, 2000). The 6-minute walk test distance has been reported to be highly reproducible in patients with heart failure

(Demers et al, 2001). Distance walked is somewhat correlated to the New York Heart Association functional classification and quality of life, and this correlation is stronger for individuals with mild and moderate disease severity (New York Heart Association classifications II and III; Rostagno et al, 2000). Compared with more sophisticated and more invasive testing, the 6-minute walk test can serve to stratify individuals in terms of functional status, which is of therapeutic and prognostic importance.

Chapter 18 describes indications for and relative and absolute contraindications to conducting an exercise test. It also notes the importance of maximizing test validity and reliability by adhering to strict standards for pretest conditions in the patient, including medications, testing standards, and monitoring recovery data. In addition, the chapter describes basic and advanced measures that can be taken, depending on the needs of the patient and the specific purpose of the test. In most individuals with cardiac dysfunction, an ECG is monitored continuously, as is heart rate; blood pressure and ratings of perceived exertion and dyspnea (PE) are monitored intermittently. Additional measures are taken as indicated. For example, a patient may be limited by arthritic pain, so it is important to monitor discomfort and pain using a standardized scale (see Chapters 15 and 18). The medications are reviewed and the time at which they were last taken is noted so as to determine their impact on responses during the exercise test and to establish which measures will be most valid in terms of assessment of exercise response.

Potential complications that could occur during exercise in patients with heart failure need to be anticipated and appropriate monitoring instituted so as to maximize the safety of exercise testing and training. Adverse responses include dysrhythmias and hypotension (Hanson, 1994).

Individuals with unexplained dyspnea are at risk for ischemia and cardiac events. Exercise echocardiography provides independently derived information that identifies patients at risk (Bergeron et al, 2004). In individuals with suspected or known heart disease, dyspnea requires investigation.

Exercise testing has a role in predicting surgical outcomes. $\dot{V}O_2$peak and exercise duration are good parameters for evaluating functional class and postoperative status in people who have undergone valve repairs or valvuloplasty (Kim et al, 2003). Patients who have a $\dot{V}O_2$peak of at least 19 ml/kg/min preoperatively achieve a higher functional class 1 year after surgery.

Of particular importance is identifying and recording why the test was stopped: a pre-determined sign or symptom in the patient was reached, or the patient wished to discontinue. Although the patient may be being tested for oxygen transport capacity, a comorbidity may have terminated the test, such as musculoskeletal strain, muscle weakness, or pain or discomfort of musculoskeletal origin.

Exercise Training

The parameters of exercise training are based on the assessment and on the short- and long-term objectives of the exercise program, and these differ for each individual. The training session begins with a warm-up defined by a work rate intermediate between the target training zone and rest. Warm-up exercise has a protective effect against left ventricular dysfunction in individuals with angina (Kelion et al, 2001). In a repeat test 30 minutes after the first, the threshold for angina, ST-segment depression, has been reported to increase along with the rate pressure product. No threshold intensity has been identified for aerobic training in individuals with cardiac disease (Swain & Franklin, 2002). Even though a lower limit of 45% of $\dot{V}O_2$ reserve is commonly reported in the literature, intensities below this level cannot be ruled out, particularly in extremely deconditioned people. The absence of such a limit supports the need to consider individual differences and to prescribe exercise on an individual basis (see the components in Box 24-8).

Many types of exercise can be considered in the exercise prescription. Improving walking tolerance and distance is a primary goal in that it is a hallmark of independence and mobility, particularly with advancing age, and it is coupled with the upright position and its associated gravitational stress. Walking has multiple physiologic benefits in individuals with coronary artery disease (Gaenzer et al, 2000) as well as in healthy people. Decisions are made based on the specificity principle: activities that are closest to the functional needs of the patient, if that is the goal, or exercise that involves more limbs, if improving aerobic fitness and maximum functional capacity is the goal.

Hydrotherapy and aquacize have been prominent in Europe. Another application that has been reported to have beneficial effects on the exercise responses of individuals with chronic heart failure is thermal hydrotherapy, which involves the passive application of heat and cold (Michalsen et al, 2004). A 6-week program of home-based hydrotherapy was reported to improve resting and submaximal heart rates and in addition to reduce symptoms and improve quality of life. These effects were attributed to physiologic adaptations to alternating hot and cold body stimulation. Further study of this application and its mechanisms is necessary; its indications may prove to be positive in individuals challenged by even minimal amounts of exercise.

Conventionally, the exercise intensity for patients with heart disease is set at a proportion of oxygen uptake reserve or heart rate reserve, which suggests a critical threshold for training effects. No intensity threshold for aerobic training has been identified, however, so intensities below the accepted standard probably provide training stimulus, particularly for patients with low functional capacity (Swain & Franklin, 2002).

It has been suggested that interval training leads to more marked improvement in hemodynamics in individuals with heart failure than does steady-rate work (Nechwatal et al, 2002). Another suggestion is that steady-rate aerobic exercise contributes to greater well-being and quality of life. Further study is needed to examine the effects of various parameters in training protocols in this cohort.

BOX 24-8

Guidelines for Exercise Prescription for Individuals with Heart Conditions

Aerobic Exercise

Type

Large muscle groups

Intensity

Percentage of functional capacity ($\dot{V}O_2$) based on HR, RPE, or METs
50% to 85% of HR reserve
RPE 3 to 6 (0-10 scale) or 12 to 16 (18-20 scale)
METs (40%-85% peak METs)

Duration

20 to 40 minutes continuous
Three 10-minute sessions per day

Frequency

Less than 2 to 3 METs short sessions several times daily
3 to 5 METs once daily
5 to 8 METs 3 to 5 times weekly

Resistance Muscle Training

Type

Peripheral muscle groups

Intensity

Progressively increasing loads 10% to 50% of maximum

Duration

Three sets of 12 to 15 repetitions

Frequency

Three times weekly

HR, Heart rate; *MET*, metabolic equivalent; *RPE*, rating of perceived exertion

---

Peak functional capacity depends on muscle strength and endurance in individuals with chronic heart failure (Suzuki et al, 2004). Improvement in subjective symptoms reported in daily activities, especially dyspnea on exertion, however, depends largely on muscle endurance.

Resistance muscle training has an important role in cardiac rehabilitation programs; it allows a patient to regain lost strength, and it facilitates avocational activities and return to work soon after a cardiac event (Verrill & Ribisl, 1996). Resistance muscle training in the form of circuit weight training can be integrated into the cardiac rehabilitation program. Muscle training can be safe and therapeutic even at relatively high workloads in properly selected individuals, including the elderly (Braith & Vincent, 1999). The hemodynamic response depends on the isometric and postural stabilization component, in addition to the load or resistance used, the muscle mass activated, the number of repetitions in the set, and the duration of each contraction, as well as the involvement of the Valsalva maneuver. Upper-body work has been viewed conservatively as an exercise option for individuals with cardiac problems, and it warrants greater emphasis (Kay, 1991). Despite caveats regarding isometric exercise for individuals with coronary artery disease, one study compared the hemodynamic responses of brief and sustained isometric exercise and dynamic exercise in individuals with heart disease and healthy people (Li et al, 2000). The incidence of myocardial ischemia was reported to be lower during isometric exercise than during dynamic exercise in patients at the same level of perceived exertion. The investigators postulated that isometric exercise generates high perfusion pressure in the coronary arteries and prolongs perfusion, thereby potentially protecting the myocardia from ischemia. Further study is needed to examine this hypothesis.

Lengthening (eccentric) muscle contractions as opposed to shortening (concentric) muscle contractions have distinct energetic and metabolic properties that may make them well suited for certain patient populations (Chung et al, 1999; Dean, 1988; Dean et al, 1989). Eccentric muscle contractions are associated with higher muscle tension and less metabolic demand. For low-risk individuals who have cardiac disease without angina, inducible ischemia, or left ventricular dysfunction, eccentric exercise can be recommended; they can perform high-load resistance exercise with minimal cardiovascular stress (Meyer et al, 2003).

Electrical stimulation of the quadriceps has been examined as a form of exercise for individuals with chronic heart failure (Harris et al, 2003). Although the improvement in muscle performance and exercise capacity was comparable to that of individuals in an ergometer exercise program, the use of electrical stimulation should be considered in the overall context of the individual's needs. Active exercise has many multisystem benefits that electrical stimulation does not provide. In addition, electrical stimulation is a more passive modality than active exercise, and that may be counter to the goal of self-efficacy that cardiac rehabilitation promotes.

Hydrotherapy in a home-based program has shown some interesting applications to individuals with chronic heart failure (Michalsen et al, 2003). In a study of individuals with mild heart failure, an intensive 6-week program of home-based repeated brief cold stimuli appeared to improve peripheral circulation and, in turn, improve heart-failure symptoms, heart rate response to exercise, and quality of life.

Long-term Plan

Long-term planning, in which regular physical activity and a structured program of exercise are components, is detailed in Chapter 31 for individuals with chronic, *primary* cardiovascular and pulmonary conditions.

PULMONARY REHABILITATION: SPECIFIC COMPONENTS
Phases

Although less well defined than cardiac rehabilitation with respect to a formal inpatient phase after an acute episode,

followed by progressively less closely supervised phases, the phases of pulmonary rehabilitation can generally be considered comparable (see Box 24-5). A patients with chronic lung disease is more likely to be referred when stable than in conjunction with an acute event. The first graded exercise test may be in the supervised program rather than in the hospital before discharge after an admission for acute symptoms.

Smoking Cessation

Smoking cessation is essential for the health and well-being of all people, in particular those with pulmonary disease. The physical therapist has a responsibility to address this modifiable risk as a priority of management (see Chapters 1 and 31).

Nutrition and Weight Control

The connection between nutrition and lung health has become a focus of research interest, and that research supports the role of good nutrition (in particular, the consumption of fruits, vegetables, and fish) in optimal lung health (Jones et al, 2005; Romieu & Trenga, 2001). Diet may be an important cofactor in the development of COPD. Whether good nutrition improves damaged lungs has not been substantiated, but good nutrition improves general health, thus should be a primary recommendation when managing these patients.

Psychosocial Issues

Individuals with chronic conditions have higher incidences of depression and poorer psychosocial adjustment than do the general population. Although chronically poor blood gases can affect psychological and cognitive function, the remediation of any depression can independently improve function. Thus, depression and other psychological issues must be assessed and managed independently.

Risk Reduction

Lifestyle modification and risk factor modification are fundamental components of the pulmonary rehabilitation program; they include risk factor modification with respect to smoking cessation, nutrition and weight control, and stress management, in conjunction with physical activity and exercise. Optimal nutrition is encouraged as a lifelong change in patients with COPD, whose nutritional status is often suboptimal (Olopade et al, 1992). Carbohydrate-rich foods, known to increase carbon dioxide production, have been targeted as a food group that should be limited in patients with COPD. Small changes in the carbohydrate constituents of diet have been reported to have a major effect on $\dot{V}CO_2$, exercise tolerance, and breathlessness (Efthimious et al, 1992). Smoking cessation is essential to limit further lung damage and has the potential for some reversal of impaired pulmonary function, improved oxygen transport capacity, and helping to reduce or reverse smoking-related risk factors as the period of non-smoking lengthens. Reduction of pulmonary and cardiac risk factors in an individual with primary lung dysfunction is essential.

Physical Activity and Exercise: Special Considerations

The principles and practice of exercise prescription are described in detail in Chapter 18. However, special considerations for this patient group, with respect to monitoring, testing, and training are detailed below.

Monitoring

The objective and subjective measures used to monitor patients with pulmonary dysfunction during exercise are comparable to those used in patients with cardiac dysfunction, because the heart and lung are interdependent. However, ventilatory parameters, such as breathing pattern, arterial saturation as gauged by pulse oximetry, and subjective sense of breathlessness, are particularly important, as are heart rate, blood pressure, and ECG readings.

Exercise Testing

The indications for and contraindications to testing are established (see Chapter 18). The goals of an exercise test are determined beforehand for each given individual. The exercise test may be selected to evaluate aerobic capacity or the strength and endurance of peripheral or respiratory muscles. The demands of upper-body work may compete with breathing demands in some patients, so upper-body work is integrated into the overall program judiciously and monitored accordingly.

The exercise test may be maximal or submaximal and may involve a modality such as a treadmill or ergometer, depending on the device's suitability for the patient and on the best means of maximizing the test's validity and reliability. Depending on the purpose of the test, a decision is made beforehand about the patient's medications and when they are taken in relation to the timing of the test. Some patients may be tested with oxygen or purposely without oxygen, or with or without bronchodilators, depending on whether the effect of such interventions is being evaluated. It is essential to monitor dyspnea in these patients and to correlate the dyspnea rating with objective measures. Some patients may have invasive blood work done before, during, and after the test to monitor serial arterial blood gases. Pulse oximetry is routinely monitored along with heart rate and blood pressure. Some patients may require ECG monitoring. Invasive procedures such as arterial blood gas measurement are done as indicated. Respiratory muscle testing and training are based on similar principles. (Detailed descriptions appear in Chapter 26.)

Oxygen consumption studies provide a metabolic and ventilatory profile of the patient's response to progressive exercise and recovery. Submaximal and peak levels of $\dot{V}O_2$ can be examined along with their physiologic and clinical correlates. The ventilatory efficiency can be determined on the basis of the ventilatory equivalent of CO_2 (minute ventilation [$\dot{V}_E$] divided by CO_2 production [$\dot{V}CO_2$]). The limitation of oxygen consumption studies is the difficulty of ensuring a valid and reliable test. The test requires that a face mask or mouthpiece be worn and these can distort the patient's breathing. The patient may feel anxious when wearing these devices or may alter his or her breathing pattern because of the increased dead space in the expiratory hose.

Exercise testing can be used to diagnose exercise-limiting factors. For example, exercise testing in a patient with pulmonary fibrosis can distinguish cardiovascular and pulmonary limitations. Exercise-induced hypoxemia in this cohort has been closely related to survival (Miki et al, 2003).

Choice of exercise testing and training modalities is determined by the indications for the test and for training. Patients with COPD show different responses to walking and to cycling (Palange et al, 2000). Aerobic capacity in walking is less than in cycling and is associated with excessive ventilatory demand during peak exercise supported by increased ventilatory dead space, reduced ventilatory efficiency, and arterial hypoxemia. Arm ergometry is associated with greater dyssynchronous breathing than is leg work, so it may be an inappropriate modality for patients with severe disease (Celli et al, 1986).

Low-flow oxygen is a common intervention for hypoxemia in patients with severe COPD. Although long-term oxygen therapy improves survival (Chapman, 1996; Wilkinson & Rees, 1996), there remain many unanswered questions regarding the use of the modality and its efficacy during exercise training (MacIntyre, 2000). Further study is needed to establish its efficacy in improving exercise capacity in patients with hypoxemia as well as without hypoxemia and to establish the characteristics of responders versus nonresponders, which will allow for the refinement of exercise prescription in this patient cohort. A study of patients with cystic fibrosis showed that supplemental oxygen speeded recovery after a short bout of maximal exercise and preserved subsequent exercise performance (Shah et al, 1997).

In individuals with COPD and mild exercise hypoxemia, relief of breathlessness with supplemental oxygen has been explained by a commensurate reduction in ventilatory demand and reduced blood lactate levels (O'Donnell et al, 1997). Short-term use of oxygen before or after exercise has not been supported (Nandi et al, 2003).

As in exercise testing any patient, it is essential to record why an exercise test was terminated—whether it was a sign or symptom predetermined by the tester or a symptom of the patient. If it was a symptom reported by the patient, was it shortness of breath or another or unrelated cause, such as dizziness, muscle strain, plantar fasciitis, arthritic discomfort or pain, or imbalance?

Exercise Training

Training involves flexibility and strengthening, as well as aerobic exercise. Patients learn to self-monitor and pace their exercise based on their responses. Walking is particularly useful for patients with pulmonary dysfunction. Pulse oximetry may have to be used to guide the training session.

Lengthening (eccentric) muscle contractions are associated with reduced energy cost, so such exercise has important therapeutic implications for individuals with poor aerobic capacity (Dean, 1999). However, eccentric-muscle work in the form of downhill walking or cycling on a negative-work ergometer alters breathing patterns toward a tendency to breathe rapidly and shallowly (Chung et al, 1999; Dean & Ross, 1989). Thus, patients require stringent monitoring when performing this type of energy-efficient exercise.

Although resistance muscle training has been receiving some attention for individuals with chronic lung disease, the prescriptive parameters for optimal benefit have yet to be defined. They should become clear when the role of deconditioning as opposed to a disease-specific myopathy is better understood with respect to the reduced strength observed in these individuals.

CARDIAC AND PULMONARY REHABILITATION: FUTURE DIRECTIONS

The effects of cardiac and pulmonary rehabilitation have been well established on the basis of the highest levels of evidence. However, without the access to people that would allow for primary prevention of heart and lung disease and for management and secondary prevention, the impact of this knowledge has not been maximized for at risk or affected individuals or for the health of the community. Health policies must be structured to enable individuals to take advantage of the resources of such programs. Physical therapists need to be well trained in the principles and practice of cardiac and pulmonary rehabilitation so that these can be applied on a one-on-one basis across areas of specialty practice. This is essential because most individuals under the care of a physical therapist have one or more risk factors. These risk factors need to be addressed, irrespective of whether the individual is presenting with cardiac or pulmonary risk factors or with a diagnosis that is primary or secondary. Further, this knowledge is essential to ensure that physical therapy interventions are modified accordingly in patients with these conditions or their risk factors.

Based on epidemiologic indicators, behavioral strategies have the greatest potential for long-term improvement in the abilities and participation of individuals with lung conditions (see Chapter 1). When effectively administered and adhered to, these interventions are not associated with the risks of invasive management, which must be minimized as much as possible commensurate with the individual's functional improvements; rather, they help to ensure reduced long-term morbidity (and thus, reduced health care needs) and increased health overall, therefore potentially increased longevity.

Finally, research is needed to establish how best to structure the principles of cardiac and pulmonary rehabilitation on an individual basis so as to maximize sustainable benefit for life. Some have argued for inclusion and exclusion criteria to maximize the success of the program (Balady et al, 2000). Identifying and reducing barriers to access and participation and maximizing adherence through motivational interviewing and cognitive therapeutic interventions may maximize the impact of these services on society.

SUMMARY

Based on state-of-the-art literature, this chapter extends the general exercise testing and training principles described in Chapter 18 to specific considerations vis-à-vis principles of best physical therapy practice in cardiac and pulmonary rehabilitation programs, regardless of whether delivered in a structured group format or one-on-one. Structured formal programs are often available only in large urban areas and thus have low access rates. The principles, however, are fundamental to physical therapy practice overall and can be readily applied in a one-on-one setting in private practice or in a health care facility. These principles should be applied not only to patients with primary heart and lung conditions but also in the physical therapy management of patients being treated for musculoskeletal and neuromuscular conditions who have secondary diagnoses of chronic heart and lung conditions or who have associated risk factors. In these cases, the physical therapy program must be adapted to the requirements of these underlying conditions or possibly managed independently if they have not been previously identified as a priority. In this way, the patient's more serious underlying cardiopulmonary problem is being addressed and the interventions, including exercise prescribed for the musculoskeletal or neuromuscular problems, are modified according to the more serious life-threatening condition. Exercise testing and training is but one component of the comprehensive management of individuals with chronic, primary cardiopulmonary dysfunction; the comprehensive approach is described in Chapter 31.

The common components of cardiac and pulmonary rehabilitation are described and then differentiated based on their distinct underlying pathophysiologies and impacts on individuals. Lifelong health behavior change and reduced need for invasive care in the short and long terms are primary outcomes.

The goal of the physical therapist, who is uniquely qualified as an applied clinical exercise physiologist and health coach, is to ensure that the proper components, in particular exercise, are prescribed to meet the specific needs and comorbidities of each individual. One criticism of structured cardiac and pulmonary rehabilitation programs has been that they are regimented and insufficiently individualized in accordance with contemporary principles of exercise prescription to produce optimal results. Physical therapists have a unique perspective that considers each individual based on a detailed multisystem assessment and prescribes a program and evaluates it accordingly.

The principles of exercise testing and training in individuals with cardiopulmonary dysfunction secondary to conditions other than primary cardiopulmonary dysfunction are described in the following chapter.

Review Questions

1. Describe how the principles and practices of cardiac and pulmonary rehabilitation are included within the fundamental principles and practices of physical therapy.

2. Describe how the principles and practices of physical therapy, which include cardiac and pulmonary rehabilitation programs, can be applied in a one-on-one setting as well as in a formally structured program.

3. Describe how the goals of physical therapy management in these programs are consistent with the philosophy and framework of the International Classification of Function.

4. Describe the rationale for assessing an individual's readiness to change with respect to participating in a rehabilitation program; discuss its clinical implications. Consider the limitations of this construct.

5. Describe how individuals with chronic cardiovascular conditions can adapt physiologically and psychologically to exercise.

6. Describe how individuals with chronic pulmonary conditions can adapt physiologically and psychologically to exercise.

7. Contrast and compare measurements and outcomes used in individuals with chronic cardiac conditions as opposed to chronic pulmonary conditions.

8. Describe the rationale for goal setting with patients at three levels: prevention, short term, and long term.

REFERENCES

Ades, P.A., Savage, P.D., Tischler, M.D., Poehlman, E.T., Dee, J., & Niggel, J. (2002). Determinants of disability in older coronary patients. American Heart Journal 143:151-156.

Agostoni, P.G., Bussotti, M., Palermo, P., & Guazzi, M. (2002). Does lung diffusion impairment affect exercise capacity in patients with heart failure? Heart 88:453-459.

Allison, T.G., Squires, R.W., Johnson, B.D., & Gau, G.T. (1999). Achieving National Cholesterol Education Program goals for low-density lipoprotein cholesterol in cardiac patients: importance of diet, exercise, weight control, and drug therapy. Mayo Clinic Proceedings 74:466-73.

Al-Rawas, O.A., Carter, R., Richens, D., Stevenson, R.D., Naik, S.K., Tweddel, A., & Wheatley, D.J. (1995). Ventilatory and gas exchange abnormalities in exercise in chronic heart failure. European Respiratory Journal 8:2022-2028.

American College of Cardiology/American Heart Association Task Force on Practice Guidelines. (2002). ACC/AHA 2002 guideline update for exercise testing: summary article. Journal of the American College of Cardiology 40:1531-1540.

American College of Sports Medicine. (2000). ACSM's guidelines for exercise testing and prescription, ed 6. Philadelphia: Lippincott Williams & Wilkins.

American College of Sports Medicine. (1993). Resource manual for guidelines for exercise testing and prescription, ed 2. Philadelphia: Lea & Febiger.

American Heart Association. (2003). Exercise and physical activity in the prevention and treatment of atherosclerotic cardiovascular disease. Circulation 107:3109-3116.

Armour, W., Clark, A.L., McCann, G.P., & Hillis, W.S. (1998). Effects of exercise position on the ventilatory responses to exercise in chronic heart failure. International Journal of Cardiology 66:59-63.

Auerbach, I., Tenebaum, A., Motro, M., Stroh, C.I., Har-Zahav, Y., & Fisman, E.Z. (2000). Blunted responses of Doppler-derived aortic flow parameters during whole-body heavy isometric exercise in heart transplant recipients. Journal of Heart and Lung Transplantation 19:1063-1070.

Bairey Merz, C.N., Felando, M.N., & Klein, J. (1996). Cholesterol awareness and treatment in patients with coronary artery disease participating in cardiac rehabilitation. Journal of Cardiopulmonary Rehabiliatation 16:117-122.

Balady, G.J., Ades, P.A., Comoss, P., Limacher, M., Pina, I.L., Southard, D., Williams, M.A., & Bazzarre, T. (2000). Core components of cardiac rehabilitation/secondary prevention programs. A statement for healthcare professionals from the American Heart Association and the American Association of Cardiovascular and Pulmonary Rehabilitation. Circulation 102:1069-1073.

Baldi, J.C., Aoina, J.L., Oxenham, H.C., Bagg, W., & Doughty, R.N. (2003). Reduced arteriovenous O_2 difference in type 2 diabetes. Journal of Applied Physiology 94:1033-1038.

Banning, A.P., Lewis, N.P., Northridge, D.B., Elborn, J.S., & Hendersen, A.H. (1995). Perfusion/ventilation mismatch during exercise in chronic heart failure: an investigation of circulatory determinants. British Heart Journal 74:27-33.

Bauerle, O., & Younes, M. (1995). Role of ventilatory response to exercise in determining exercise capacity in COPD. Journal of Applied Physiology 79:1870-1877.

Bellardinelli, R., Barstow, T.J., Nguyen, P., & Wasserman, K. (1997). Skeletal muscle oxygenation and oxygen uptake kinetics following constant work rate exercise in chronic congestive heart failure. American Journal of Cardiology 80:1319-1324.

Bellardinelli, R., & Perna, G.P. (2002). Vasomotor reactivity evaluation in cardiac rehabilitation. Monaldi Archives of Chest Diseases 58:79-86.

Bellone, A., Rusconi, F., Frisinghelli, A., Aliprandi, P., Castelli, C., Confalonieri, M., & Palange, P. (1999). Gas exchange response to exercise in patients with chronic heart failure. Monaldi Archives of Chest Diseases 54:3-6.

Bengel, F.M., Ueberfuhr, P., Schiepel, N., Nekolla, S.G., Reichart, B., & Schwaiger, M. (2001). Effect of sympathetic reinnervation on cardiac performance after heart transplantation. New England Journal of Medicine 345:731-738.

Bergeron, S., Ommen, S.R., Bailey, K.R., Oh, J.K., McCully, R.B., & Pellikka, P.A. (2004). Exercise echocardiograpic findings and outcome of patients referred for evaluation of dyspnea. Journal of the American College of Cardiology 16:2242-2246.

Bernardi, L., Spadacini, G., Bellwon, J., Hajric, R., Roskamm, H., & Frey, A.W. (1998). Effect of breathing rate on oxygen saturation and exercise performance in chronic heart failure. Lancet 351:1308-1311.

Blackburn, G.G., Foody, J.M., Spreecher, D.L., Park, E., Apperson-Hansen, C., & Pashkow, F.J. (2000). Cardiac rehabilitation participation patterns in a large, tertiary care center: evidence for selection bias. Journal of Cardiopulmonary Rehabilitation 20:189-195.

Bodegard, J., Erikssen, G., Bjornholt, J.V., Gjesdal, K., Thell, D., & Erikssen, J. (2004). Symptom-limited exercise testing, ST depressions and long-term coronary heart disease mortality in apparently healthy middle-aged men. European Journal of Cardiovascular Prevention and Rehabilitation 11:320-327.

Bonapace, S., Rossi, A., Cicoira, M., Franceschini, L. Golia, G., Zanolla, L., Marino, P, & Zardini, P. (2003). Aortic distensibility independently affects exercise tolerance in patients with dilated cardiomyopathy. Circulation 107:1603-1608.

Bond, V., Stephens, Q., Adams, R.G., Vaccaro, P., Demeersman, R., Williams, D., Obisesan, T.O., Franks, B.D., Oke, L.M., Coleman, B., Blakely, R., & Millis, R.M. (2002). Aerobic exercise attenuates an exaggerated exercise blood pressure response in normotensive young adult African-American men. Blood Pressure 11: 229-234.

Braith, R.W. (1998). Exercise training in patients with CHF and heart transplant recipients. Medicine and Science and Sports and Exercise 30 (Suppl 10):S367-S378.

Braith, R.W., & Edwards, D.G. (2000). Exercise following heart transplantation. Sports Medicine 30:171-192.

Braith, R.W., & Vincent, K.R. (1999). Resistance exercise in the elderly person with cardiovascular disease. American Journal of Geriatric Cardiology 8:63-70.

Brosseau, R., Juneau, M., Sirard, A., Savard, A., Marchand, C., Boudreau, M.H., Bradley, S., & Bleau, L. (1995). Safety and feasibility of a self-monitored, home-based phase II exercise program for high risk patients after cardiac surgery. Canadian Journal of Cardiology 11:675-685.

Callahan, L.A., Woods, K.F., Mensah, G.A., Ramsey, L.T., Barbeau, P., & Gutin, B. (2002). Cardiopulmonary responses to exercise in women with sickle cell anemia. American Journal of Respiratory and Critical Care Medicine 165:1309-1316.

Campbell, N.C., Grimshaw, J.M., Ritchie, L.D., & Rawles, J.M. (1996). Outpatient cardiac rehabilitation: are the potential benefits being realized? Journal of the Royal College of Physicians London 30:514-519.

Carter, R., Nicotra, B., Blevins, W., & Holiday, D. (1993). Altered exercise gas exchange and cardiac function in patients with mild chronic obstructive pulmonary disease. Chest 103:745-750.

Carter, R., 3rd, Watenpaugh, D.E., & Smith, M.L. (2001). Gender differences in cardiovascular regulation during recovery from exercise. Journal of Applied Physiology 91:1902-1907.

Casaburi, R., Porszasz, J., Burns, M.R., Carithers, E.R., Chang, R.S., & Cooper, C.B. (1997). Physiologic benefits of exercise training in rehabilitation of patients with severe chronic obstructive pulmonary disease. American Journal of Respiratory and Critical Care Medicine 155:1541-1551.

Celli, B.R. (1997). ATS standards for the optimal management of chronic obstructive pulmonary disease. Respiratory 2 (Suppl 1): S1-S4.

Celli, B.R., Rassulo, J., & Make, B.J. (1986). Dyssynchronous breathing during arm but not leg exercise in patients with chronic airflow obstruction. The New England Journal of Medicine 314:1485-1490.

Chapman, K.R. (1996). Therapeutic approaches to chronic obstructive pulmonary disease: an emerging consensus. American Journal of Medicine 100:5S-10S.

Cheetham, C., Green, D., Collis, J., Dembo, L., & O'Driscoll, G. (2002). Effect of aerobic and resistance exercise on central hemodynamic responses in severe chronic heart failure. Journal of Applied Physiology 93:175-180.

Chen, S.Y., Lan, C., Ko, W.J., Chou, N.K., Hsu, R.B., Chen, Y.S., Chu, S.H., & Lai, J.S. (1999). Cardiorespiratory responses of heart transplantation recipients to exercise in the early postoperative period. Journal of the Formosan Medical Association 98:165-170.

Chung, F., Dean, E., & Ross, J. (1999). Cardiopulmonary responses of middle-aged men without cardiopulmonary disease to steady-rate positive and negative work performed on a cycle ergometer. Physical Therapy 79:476-487.

Ciampi, Q., Betocchi, S., Lombardi, R., Manganelli, F., Storto, G., Losi, M.A., Pezzalla, E., Finizio, F., Cuocolo, A., & Chiariello, M. (2002). Hemodynamic determinants of exercise-induced abnormal blood pressure response in hypertrophic cardiomyopathy. Journal of the American College of Cardiology 40:278-284.

Clark, A.L., Davies, L.C., Francis, D.P., & Coats, A.J. (2000). Ventilatory capacity and exercise tolerance in patients with chronic stable heart failure. European Journal of Heart Failure 2:47-51.

Clark, A.L., Rafferty, D., & Arbuthnott, K. (1997a). Relationship between isokinetic muscle strength and exercise capacity in chronic heart failure. International Journal of Cardiology 59:145-148.

Clark, A.L., Rafferty, D., & Arbuthnott, K. (1997b). Exercise dynamics at submaximal workloads in patients with chronic heart failure. Journal of Cardiac Failure 3:15-19.

Clarke, A.L., Volterrani, M., Swan, J.W., & Coats, A.J. (1995). Ventilation-perfusion matching in chronic heart failure. International Journal of Cardiology 48:259-270.

Coats, A.J., Adamopoulos, S., Radaelli, A., McCance, A., Meyer, T.E., Bernardi, L., Solda, P.L., Davey, P., Ormerod, O., Forfar, C., Conway, J., & Sleight, P. (1992). Controlled trial of physical training in chronic heart failure. Exercise performance, hemodynamics, ventilation, and autonomic function. Circulation 85:2119-2131.

Cohen-Solal, A., Czitrom, D., Geneves, M., & Gourgon, R. (1997). Delayed attainment of peak oxygen consumption after the end of exercise in patients with chronic heart failure. International Journal of Cardiology 27:23-29.

Cordova, F., O'Brien, G., Furukawa, S., Kuzma, A.M., Traveline, J., & Criner, G.J. (1997). Stability of improvements in exercise performance and quality of life following bilateral lung volume reduction surgery in severe COPD. Chest 112:907-915.

Corriveau, M.L., Rosen B.J., & Dolan, G.F. (1989). Oxygen transport and oxygen consumption during supplemental oxygen administration in patients with chronic obstructive pulmonary disease. American Journal of Medicine 87:633-637.

Criner, G.J., & Celli, B.R. (1988). Effect of unsupported arm exercise of ventilatory muscle recruitment in patients with severe chronic airflow obstruction. American Review of Respiratory Disease 138:856-861.

Criner, G., Cordova, F.C., Leyenson, V., Roy, B., Traveline, J., Sudarshan, S., O'Brien, G., Kuzma, A.M., & Furokawa, S. (1998). Effect of lung volume reduction surgery on diaphragm strength. American Journal of Respiratory and Critical Care Medicine 157:1578-1585.

Dafoe, W., & Huston, P. (1997). Current trends in cardiac rehabilitation. Canadian Medical Association Journal 156:527-532.

Daida, H., Squires, R.W., Allison, T.G., Johnson, B.D., & Gau, G.T. (1996). Sequential assessment of exercise tolerance in heart transplantation compared with coronary artery bypass surgery after phase II cardiac rehabilitation. American Journal of Cardiology 77:696-700.

Daub, W.D., Knapik, G.P., & Black, W.R. (1996). Strength training early after myocardial infarction. Journal of Cardiopulmonary Rehabilitation 16:100-108.

Dean, E. (1988). The physiology of negative work and therapeutic implications. Physical Therapy, 68:233-237.

Dean, E., & Ross, J. (1989). Downhill walking induces rapid shallow breathing. Pflugers Archives 415:351-354.

De Busk, R.F. (1992). Why is cardiac rehabilitation not widely used? Western Journal of Medicine 156:206-208.

Decramer, M., Bartsch, P., Pauwels, R., & Yernault, J.C. (2003). Management of COPD according to guidelines. A national survey among Belgian physicians. Monaldi Archives of Chest Diseases 59:62-80.

Delagardelle, C., Feiereisen, P., Autier, P., Shita, R., Krecke, R., & Beissel, J. (2002). Strength/endurance training versus endurance training in congestive heart failure. Medicine and Science in Sports and Exercise 34:1868-1872.

Demers, C., McKelvie, R.S., Negassa, A., & Yusuf, S. Reliability, validity, and responsiveness of the six-minute walk test in patients with heart failure. American Heart Journal 142:698-703.

Denollet, J., & Brutsaert, D.L. (2001). Reducing emotional distress improves prognosis in coronary heart disease: 9-year mortality in a clinical trial of rehabilitation. Circulation 104:2018-2023.

Dubach, P., Myers, J., Dziekan, G., Goebbels, U., Reinhart, W., Muller, P., Buser, P., Stulz, P., Vogt, P., & Ratti, R. (1997). Effect of high-intensity exercise training on central hemodynamic responses to exercise in men with reduced left ventricular function. Journal of the American College of Cardiology 29:1591-1598.

Dubach, P., Myers, J., Dziekan, G., Goerre, S., Buser, P., & Laske, A. (1995). Effect of residential cardiac rehabilitation following bypass surgery. Observations in Switzerland. Chest 108:1434-1439.

Duscha, B.D., Annex, B.H., Keteyian, S.J., Green, H.J., Sullivan, M.J., Samsa, G.P., Brawner, C.A., Schachat, F.H., & Kraus, W.E. (2001). Differences in skeletal muscle between men and women with chronic heart failure. Journal of Applied Physiology 90:280-286.

Efthimious, J., Mounsey, P.J., Benson, D.N., Madgwick. R., Coles, S.J., & Bension, M.K. (1992). Effect of carbohydrate rich versus fat rich loads on gas exchange and walking performance in patients with chronic obstructive lung disease. Thorax 47:451-456.

Ehrman, J., Keyeyian, S., Fedel, F., Rhoads, K., Levine, T.B., & Shepard, R. (1992). Cardiovascular responses of heart transplant recipients to graded exercise testing. Journal of Applied Physiology 73:260-264.

Erbes, R., Schalberg, T., & Loddenkemper, R. (1997). Lung function tests in patients with idiopathic pulmonary fibrosis. Are they helpful for predicting outcome? Chest 111:51-57.

European Society of Cardiology. (2001). Recommendations for exercise training in chronic heart failure patients. (2001). European Heart Journal 22:125-135.

Fabbri, L.M., & Hurd, S.S. (2003). Global strategy for the diagnosis, management, and prevention of COPD 2003 update (editorial). European Respiratory Journal 22:1-2.

Fahy, B.F. (2004). Pulmonary rehabilitation for chronic obstructive pulmonary disease: a scientific and political agenda. Respiratory Care 49:28-36.

Farley, R.L., Wade, T.D., & Birchmore, L. (2003). Factors influencing attendance at cardiac rehabilitation among coronary heart disease patients. European Journal of Cardiovascular Nursing 2:205-212.

Friedman, A.W., Lipman, R.C., Silver, S.J., Minella, R.A., & Hoover, J.L. (1996). Cardiac rehabilitation/exercise in patients with implantable cardioverter defibrillators. Journal of the National Medical Association 88:374-378.

Fujii, T., Kurihara, N., Fujimoto, S., Hirata, K., & Yoshimkawa, J. (1996). Role of pulmonary vascular disorder in determining exercise capacity in patients with severe chronic obstructive pulmonary disease. Clinical Physiology 16:521-533.

Gaenzer, H., Sturm, W., & Neumayr, G. (2000). Effects of walking on coronary artery disease in elderly men. Circulation 102:E16.

Gallagher, R., McKinley, S., & Dracup, K. (2003). Predictors of women's attendance at cardiac rehabilitation programs. Progress in Cardiovascular Nursing 18:121-126.

Gassner, L.A., Dunn, S., & Piller, N. (2003). Aerobic exercise and the post myocardial infarction patient: a review of the literature. Heart & Lung 32:258-265.

Gerald, L.B., Sanderson, B., Redden, D., & Bailey, W.C. (2001). Chronic obstructive pulmonary disease stage and 6-minute walk outcome. Journal of Cardiopulmonary Rehabilitation 21:296-299.

Geraldi, D., & Zu Wallack, R. (2001). Non-pulmonary factors affecting survival in patients completing pulmonary rehabilitation. Monaldi Archives of Chest Diseases 56:331-335.

Gitt, A.K., Wasserman, K., Kilkowski, C., Kleemann, T., Kilkowski, A., Bangert, M., Schneider, S., Schwarz, A., & Senges, J. (2002). Exercise anaerobic threshold and ventilatory efficiency identify heart failure patients for high risk of early death. Circulation 106:3079-3084.

Global Initiative for Chronic Obstructive Pulmonary Disease. GOLD Patient Guide. May 2002. http:/www.goldcopd.com. Retrieved January 2005.

Global Initiative for Chronic Obstructive Pulmonary Disease. Pocket Guide to COPD Diagnosis, Management, and Prevention: A Guide for Physicians and Nurses. July 2003. http:/www.goldcopd.com; retrieved January 2005.

Godin, G., Valois, P., Jobin, J., & Ross, A. (1991). Prediction of intention to exercise of individuals who have suffered from coronary artery disease. Journal of Clinical Psychology 47:762-772.

Goebbels, U., Myers, J., Dziekan, G., Muller, P., Kuhn, M., Ratte, R., & Dubach, P. (1998). A randomized comparison of exercise training in patients with normal vs. reduced ventricular function. Chest 113:1387-1393.

Gordon, N.F., English, C.D., Contractor, A.S., Salmon, R.D., Leighton, R.F., Franklin, B.A., & Haskell, W.L. (2002). Effectiveness of three models for comprehensive cardiovascular disease risk reduction. American Journal of Cardiology 89:1263-1268.

Gosselin, N., Lambert, K., Poulain, M., Martin, A., Prefaut, C., & Varray, A. (2003). Endurance training improves skeletal muscle electrical activity in active COPD patients. Muscle Nerve 28:744-753.

Grundy, S.M., Garber, A., Goldberg, R., Havas, S., Holman, R., Lamendola, C., Howard, W.J., Savage, P., Sowers, J., & Vega, G.L. (2002). Lifestyle and medical management of risk factors. Circulation 105:153-158.

Guazzi, M. (2000). Alveolar-capillary membrane dysfunction in chronic heart failure: pathophysiology and therapeutic implications. Clinical Science (London) 98:633-641.

Guazzi, M., Pontone, G., & Agostini, P. (1999). Aspirin worsens exercise performance and pulmonary gas exchange in patients with heart failure who are taking angiotensin-converting enzyme inhibitors. American Heart Journal 138:254-260.

Guazzi, M., Reina, G., Tumminello, G., & Guazzi, M.D. (2004). Improvement of alveolar-capillary membrane diffusing capacity with exercise training in chronic heart failure. Journal of Applied Physiology 97:1866-1873.

Gullestad, L., Haywood, G., Ross, H., Bjornerheim, R., Geiran, O., Kjekshus, J., Simonsen, S., & Fowler, M. (1996). Exercise capacity of heart transplant recipients: the importance of chronotropic incompetence. Journal of Heart and Lung Transplantation 15:1075-1083.

Hacker, M., Stork, S., Stratakis, D., Angermann, C.E., Huber, R., Hahn, K., & Tausig, A. (2003). Relationship between right ventricular ejection fraction and maximum exercise oxygen consumption: a methodological study in chronic heart failure patients. Journal of Nuclear Cardiology 10:644-649.

Halm, M., Penque, S., Doll, N., & Beahrs, M. (1999). Women and cardiac rehabilitation: referral and compliance patterns. Journal of Cardiovascular Nursing 13:83-92.

Hambrecht, R., Fiehn, E., Yu, J., Niebauer, J., Weigl, C., Hilbrich, L., Adams, V., Riede, U., & Schuler, G. (1997). Effects of endurance training on mitochondrial ultrastructure and fiber type distribution in skeletal muscle of patients with stable chronic heart failure. Journal of the American College of Cardiology 29:1067-1073.

Hambrecht, R., Schuler, G.C., Muth, T., Grunze, M.F., Marburger, C.T., Niebauer, J., Methfessel, S.M., & Kubler, W. (1992). Greater diagnostic sensitivity of treadmill versus cycle exercise testing of asymptomatic men with coronary artery disease. American College of Cardiology 70:141-146.

Hansen, J.E., & Wasserman, K. (1996). Pathophysiology of activity limitation in patients with interstitial lung disease. Chest 109:1566-1576.

Hanson, P. (1994). Exercise testing and training in patients with chronic heart failure. Medicine and Science in Sports and Exercise 26:527-537.

Harrington, D., & Coats, A.J. (1997). Mechanisms of exercise intolerance in congestive heart failure. Current Opinions in Cardiology 12:224-232.

Haouzi, P., Hirsch, J.J., Marchal, F., & Huszczuk, A. (1997). Ventilatory and gas exchange response during walking in severe peripheral vascular disease. Respiratory Physiology 107:181-190.

Harris, S., LeMaitre, J.P., Mackenzie, G., Fox, K.A., & Denvir, M.A. (2003). A randomized study of home-based electrical stimulation of the legs and conventional bicycle exercise training for patients with chronic heart failure. European Heart Journal 24:871-878.

Heller, H., Konen-Bergmann, M., Overlack, A., & Schuster, K.D. (1998). Decreasing diffusion limitation on exercise in lower-graded interstitial lung disease. Pflugers Archives 435:762-766.

Hendrican, M.C., McKelvie, R.S., Smith, T., McCartney, N., Pogue, J., Teo, K.K., & Yusuf, S. (2000). Functional capacity in patients with congestive heart failure. Journal of Cardiac Failure 6:214-219.

Hsia, C.C. (1999). Cardiopulmonary limitations to exercise in restrictive lung disease. Medicine and Science in Sports and Exercise 31suppl:S28-S32.

Hueslmann, M., Stefenelli, T., Berger, R., Frey, B., & Pacher, R. (2002). Prognostic impact of workload in patients with congestive heart failure. American Heart Journal 143:308-312.

Ilarraza, H., Myers, J., Kottman, W., Rickli, H., & Dubach, P. (2004). An evaluation of training responses using self-regulation in a residential rehabilitation program. Journal of Cardiopulmonary Rehabilitation 24:27-33.

Jaffe, A., & Bush, A. (2001). Cystic fibrosis: review of the decade. Monaldi Archives of Chest Diseases 56:240-247.

Johnson, N., Fisher, J., Nagle, A., Inder, K., & Wiggers, J. (2004). Factors associated with referral to outpatient cardiac rehabilitation services. Journal of Cardiopulmonary Rehabilitation 24:165-170.

Jolliffe, J.A., Rees, K., Taylor, R.S., Thompson, D., Oldridge, N., & Ebrahim, S., (2001). Exercise-based rehabilitation for coronary artery disease. Cochrane Database Systematic Reviews 1:CD001-800.

Jones, A.Y.M., Dean, E., Lam, P.K.W., & Lo, S.K. (2005). Discordance between lung function of Chinese university students and 20-year-old established norms. Chest: in press.

Jungbauer, J.S., & Fuller, B. (1999). Feasibility of a multi-state outcomes program for cardiopulmonary rehabilitation. Journal of Cardiopulmonary Rehabilitation 19:352-359.

Katsura, H., Yamada, K., & Kida, K. (2003). Usefulness of a linear analog scale questionnaire to measure health-related quality of life in elderly patients with chronic obstructive pulmonary disease. Journal of the American Geriatric Society 51:1131-1135.

Katz, S.D., Maskin, C., Jondeau, G., Cocke, T., Berkowitz, R., & LeJemtel, T. (2000). Near-maximal fractional oxygen extraction by active skeletal muscle in patients with chronic heart failure. Journal of Applied Physiology 88:2138-2142.

Kaw, A.C., Van Trigt, P., 3rd, Shaeffer-McCall, G.S., Shaw, J.P., Kuzil, B.B., Page, R.D., & Higginbotham, M.B. (1994). Central and peripheral limitations to upright exercise in untrained cardiac transplant patients. Circulation 89:2605-2615.

Kay, G.L. (1991). Athletic participation after myocardial revascularization. Possibilities and benefits. Clinics in Sports Medicine 10:371-389.

Kelion, A.D., Webb, T.P., Gardner, M.A., Ormerod, O.J., & Banning, A.P. (2001). The warm-up effect protects against ischemic left ventricular dysfunction in patients with angina. Journal of American College of Cardiology 37:705-710.

Keller, C.A., Ohar, J., Ruppel, G., Wittry, M.D., & Goodgold, H.M. (1995). Right ventricular function in patients with severe COPD evaluated for lung transplantation. Chest 107:1510-1516.

Kelly, T.M. (1996). Exercise testing and training of patients with malignant ventricular arrhythmias. Medicine and Science in Sports and Exercise 28:53-61.

Kemppainen, J., Tsuchida, H., Stolen, K., Karlsson, H., Bjornholm, M., Heinonen, O.J., Nuutila, P., Krook, J., & Zierath, J.R. (2003). Insulin signaling and resistance in patients with chronic heart failure. Journal of Physiology 550:305-315.

Killavuori, K., Sovijarvi, A., Naveri, H., Ikonen, T., & Leinonen, H. (1996). Effect of physical training on exercise capacity and gas exchange in patients with chronic heart failure. Chest 110:985-991.

Kim, H.J., Park, S.W., Cho, B.R., Hong, S.H., Park, P.W., & Hong, K.P. (2003). The role of cardiopulmonary exercise test in mitral and aortic regurgitation: it can predict post-operative results. The Korean Journal of Internal Medicine 18:35-39.

King, M.L., Dracup, K.A., Fonarow, G.C., & Woo, M.A. (2000). The hemodynamic effects of isotonic exercise using hand-held weights in patients with heart failure. Journal of Heart and Lung Transplantation 19:1209-1218.

Kitaoka, H., Hitoma, N., Okawa, M., Furuno, T., & Doi, Y. (2003). Prognostic significance of post-exercise blood pressure response in patients with dilated cardiomyopathy. Journal of Cardiology, 42:165-171.

Kitzman, D.W. (2002). Diastolic failure in the elderly. Heart Failure Review 7:17-27.

Klapholz, M., Maurer, M., Lowe, A.M., Messineo, F., Meisner, J.S., Mitchell, J., Kalman, J., Phillips, R.A., Steingart, R., Brown, E.J., Jr., Berkowitz, R., Moskowitz, R., Soni, A., Mancini, D., Bijou, R., Sehhat, K., Varshneya, N., Kukin, M., Katz, S.D., Sleeper, L.A., Le Jemtel, T.H.; New York Heart Failure Consortium. (2004). Hospitalization for heart failure in the presence of a normal left ventricular ejection fraction: results of the New York Heart Failure Registry. Journal of the American College of Cardiology 43:1432-1438.

Klein, J.J., van der Palen, J., Uil, S.M., Zielhuis, G.A., Seydel, E.R., & van Herwaarden, C.L. (2001). Benefit from the inclusion of self-treatment guidelines to a self-management programme for adults with asthma. European Respiratory Journal 17:386-394.

Klein, J.J., van der Palen, J., van den Hof, S., & Rovers, M.M. (1997). Self-treatment by adults during slow-onset exacerbations of asthma. Patient Education and Counseling 32 (Suppl 1): S61-S66.

Kodis, J., Smith, K.M., Arthur, H.M., Daniels, C., Suskin, N., & McKelvie, R.S. (2001). Changes in exercise capacity and lipids after clinic versus home-based aerobic training in coronary artery bypass graft surgery patients. Journal of Cardiopulmonary Rehabilitation 21:31-36.

Koike, A., Hiroe, M., Taniguchi, K., & Marumo, F. (1993). Respiratory control during exercise in patients with cardiovascular disease. American Review of Respiratory Disease 147:425-429.

Koike, A., Itoh, H., Kato, M., Sawada, H., Aizawa, T., Fu, L.T., & Watanabe, H. (2002). Prognostic power of ventilatory responses during submaximal exercise in patients with chronic heart disease. Chest 121:1581-1588.

Koike, A., Itoh, H., Oohara, R., Hoshimoto, M., Tajima, A., Aizawa, T, & Fu, L.T. (2004). Cerebral oxygenation during exercise in cardiac patients. Chest 125:182-190.

Koike, A., Yajima, T., Kano, H., Koyama, Y., Marumo, F., & Hiroe, M. (1996). Relation between oxygen uptake and carbon dioxide output during constant work rate exercise in patients with mild congestive heart failure. American Journal of Cardiology 77:602-605.

Kurl, S., Laukkanen, J.A., Tuomainen, T.P., Rauramaa, R., Lakka, T.A., Salonen, R., Eranen, J., Sivenius, J., & Salonen, J.T. (2003). Association of exercise-induced, silent ST-segment depression with the risk of stroke and cardiovascular diseases in men. Stroke 34:1760-1765.

LaBresh, K.A., Ellrodt, A.G., Gliklich, R., Liljestrand, J., & Peto, R. (2004). Get with the guidelines for cardiovascular secondary prevention: pilot results. Archives of Internal Medicine 164: 203-209.

Lan, C., Chen, S.Y., Chui, S.F., Hsu, C.J., Lai, J.S., & Kuan, P.L. (2003). Poor functional recovery may indicate restenosis in patients after coronary angioplasty. Archives of Physical Medicine and Rehabilitation 84:1023-1027.

Larsen, A.I., Aarsland, T., Kristiansen, M., Haugland, A., & Dickstein, K. (2001). Assessing the effect of exercise training in men with heart failure: comparison of maximal, submaximal and endurance exercise protocols. European Heart Journal 22:684-692.

Larsen, A.I., Lindal, S., Aukrust, P., Toft, I., Aarsland, T., & Dickstein, K. (2002). Effect of exercise training on skeletal muscle fibre characteristics in men with chronic heart failure. Correlation between muscle alterations, cytokines, and exercise capacity. International Journal of Cardiology 83:25-32.

Lau-Walker, M. (2004). Cardiac rehabilitation: the importance of patient expectations—a practitioner survey. Journal of Clinical Nursing 13:177-184.

Lavie, C.J., Milani, R.V., & Mehra, M.R. (2004). Peak exercise oxygen pulse and prognosis in chronic heart failure. American Journal of Cardiology 93:588-593.

Lear, S.A., Ignaszewski, A., Linden, W., Brozie, A., Kiess, M., Spinelli, J.J., Pritchard, P.H., & Frohlich, J.J. (2002). A randomized controlled trial of an extensive lifestyle management intervention (ELMI) following cardiac rehabilitation: study design and baseline data. Current Controlled Trials in Cardiovascular Medicine 12:9.

Lewis, E.F., Moye, L.A., Rouleau, J.L., Sacks, F.M., Arnold, J.M., Warnica, J.W., Flaker, G.C., Braunwald, E., & Pfeffer, M.A. Predictors of late development of heart failure in stable survivors of myocardial infarction; the CARE study. Journal of the American College of Cardiology 42:1446-1453.

Leyenson, V., Furukawa, S., Kuzma, A.M., Cordova, F., Traveline, J., & Criner, G.J. (2000). Correlation of changes in quality of life after lung volume reduction surgery with changes in lung function, exercise, and gas exchange. Chest 18:728-735.

Li, J., Zhao, W., Zhou, S., Lu, X., & Zhang, Q. (2000). Relationship between isometric exercise and myocardial ischemia in patients with coronary artery disease: an Echo-Doppler study. Chinese Medical Journal (English abstract) 113:493-497.

Lloyd-Williams, F., Mair, F.S., & Leitner, M. (2002). Exercise training and heart failure: a systematic review of current evidence. British Journal of General Practice 52:47-55.

Loimaala, A., Huikuri, H.V., Koobi, T., Rinne, M., Nenonen, A., & Vuori, I. (2003). Exercise training improves baroreflex sensitivity in type 2 diabetes. Diabetes 52:1837-1842.

Longhurst, J.C., & Stebbins, C.L. (1997). The power athlete. Cardiology Clinics 15:413-429.

Lucas, C., Stevenson, L.W., Johnson, W., Hartley, H., Hamilton, M.A., Walden, J., Lem, V., & Eagen-Bengsten, E. (1999). The 6-minute walk and peak oxygen consumption in advanced heart failure: aerobic capacity and survival. American Heart Journal 138: 618-624.

Mabee, S.W., Metra, M., Reed, D.E., Dei Cas, L., & Cody, R.J. (1994). Pulmonary hypertension and systemic hypotension as limitations to exercise in chronic heart failure. Journal of Cardiac Failure 1:27-33.

MacGowan, G.A., Cecchetti, A., & Murali, S. (1997). Ventilatory drive during exercise in congestive heart failure. Journal of Cardiac Failure 3:257-262.

MacGowan, G.A., Janosko, K., Cecchetti, A., & Murali, S. (1997). Exercise-related ventilatory abnormalities and survival in congestive heart failure. American Journal of Cardiology 79:1264-1266.

MacGowan, G.A., Panzak, G., & Murali, S. (2001). Exercise-related ventilatory abnormalities are more specific for functional impairment in chronic heart failure than reduction in peak exercise oxygen consumption. Journal of Heart and Lung Transplantation 20:1167-1173.

MacIntyre, N.R. (2000). Oxygen therapy and exercise response in lung disease. Respiratory Care 45:194-200.

Mahler, D.A., & Franco, M.J. (1996). Clinical application of cardiopulmonary exercise testing. Journal of Cardiopulmonary Rehabilitation 16:357-365.

Malfatto, G., Branzi, G., Riva, B., Sala, L., Leonetti, G., & Facchini, M. (2002). Recovery of autonomic responsiveness with low-intensity physical training in patients with chronic heart failure. European Journal of Heart Failure 4:159-166.

Marshall, P., Al-Timman, J., Riley, R., Wright, J., Williams, S., Hainsworth, R., & Tan, L.B. (2001). Randomized controlled trial of home-based exercise training to evaluate cardiac functional gains. Clinical Science (London) 101:477-483.

Matsui, S., Tamura, N., Hirakawa, T., Kobayashi, S., Takekoshi, N., & Murakami, E. (1005). Assessment of working skeletal muscle oxygenation in patients with chronic heart failure. American Heart Journal 129:690-695.

Mayou, R.A., Thompson, D.R., Clements., A., Davies, C.H., Goodwin, S.J., Normington, K., Hicks, N., & Price, J. (2002). Guideline-based early rehabilitation after myocardial infarction. A pragmatic randomized controlled trial. Journal of Psychosomatic Research 52:89-95.

McConnell, T.R., Mandak, J.S., Sykes, J.S., Fesniak, H., & Dasgupta, H. (2003). Exercise training for heart failure patients improves respiratory muscle endurance, exercise tolerance, breathlessness, and quality of life. Journal of Cardiopulmonary Rehabilitation 23:10-16.

McConnell, T.R., Menapace, F.J., Jr., Hartley, L.H., & Pfeffer, M.A. (1998). Captopril reduces the V_E/V_{CO_2} ratio in myocardial infarction patients with low ejection fraction. Chest, 114:1289-1294.

McGavin, C.R., Gupta, S.P., & McHardy, G.J.R. (1976). Twelve-minute walking test for assessing disability in chronic bronchitis. British Medical Journal 1:822-823.

Medinger, A.E., Khouri, S., & Rohatgi, P.K. (2002). Sarcoidosis: the value of exercise testing. Chest 120:93-101.

Mejhert, M., Linder-Klingsell, E., Edner, M., Kahan, T., & Persson, H. (2002). Ventilatory variables are strong prognostic markers in elderly patients with heart failure. Heart 88:239-243.

Mettauer, B., Lampert, E., Petitjean, P., Bogui, P., Epailly, E., Schnedecker, B., Geny, B., Eisenmann, B., Haberey, P., & Lonsdorfer, J. (1996). Persistent exercise intolerance following cardiac transplantation despite normal oxygen transport. International Journal of Sports Medicine 17:277-286.

Meyer, K., Steiner, R., Lastayo, P., Lippuner, K., Allemann, Y., Eberli, F., Schmid, J., Saner, H., & Hoppeler, H. (2003). Eccentric exercise in coronary patients: central hemodynamic and metabolic responses. Medicine and Science in Sport and Exercise 35:1076-1082.

Michalsen, A., Ludtke, R., Buhring, M., Spahn, G., Langhorst, J., & Dobos, G.J (2003). Thermal hydrotherapy improves quality of life and hemodynamic function in patients with chronic heart failure. American Heart Journal 146:1-6.

Miki, K., Maekura, R., Hiraga, T., Okuda, Y., Okamoto, T., Hirotani, A., & Ogura, T. (2003). Impairments and prognostic factors for survival in patients with idiopathic pulmonary fibrosis. Respiratory Medicine 97:482-490.

Minette, P., Buysschaert, M., Rahier, J., Veriter, C., & Frans, A. (1999). Pulmonary gas exchange in life-long nonsmoking patients with diabetes mellitus. Respiration 66:20-24.

Missik, E. (2001). Women and cardiac rehabilitation: accessibility issues and policy recommendations. Rehabilitation Nursing 26:141-147.

Molhoek, S.G., Bax, J.J., Erven, L., Bootsman, M., Boersma, E., Steendijk, P., van der Wall, E.E., & Schalij, M.J. (2002). American Journal of Cardiology 90:379-383.

Mortensen, P.T., Sogaard, P., Mansour, H., Ponsonaille, J., Gras, D., Lazarus, A., Reiser, W., Alonso, C., Linde, C.M., Lunati, M., Kramm, B., & Harrison, E.M. (2004). Sequential biventricular pacing: evaluation of safety and efficacy. Pacing and Clinical Electrophysiology 27:339-345.

Myers, J., Dziekan, G., Goebbels, U., & Dubach, P. (1999). Influence of high-intensity exercise training on the ventilatory response to exercise in patients with reduced ventricular function. Medicine and Science in Sports and Exercise 31:929-937.

Nanas, S., Nanas, J., Papazachou, O., Kassiotis, C., Papamichalopoulos, A., Milic-Emili, J., & Roussos, C. (2003). Resting lung function and hemodynamic parameters as predictors of exercise capacity in patients with chronic heart failure. Chest 123:1386-1393.

Nandi, K., Smith, A.A., Crawford, A., MacRae, K.D., Garrod, R., Seed, W.A., & Roberts, C.M. (2003). Oxygen supplementation before or after submaximal exercise in patients with chronic obstructive lung disease. Thorax 58:670-673.

NHLB Institute and National Asthma Education Program. Expert Panel Report. (1991). Journal of Allergy and Clinical Immunology 88 3:425-534.

Nechwatal, R.M., Duck, C., & Gruber, G. (2002). Physical training as interval or continuous training in chronic heart failure for improving function capacity, hemodynamics and quality of life: a controlled study (English abstract). Zeitschrift fur Kardiologie 91:328-337.

National Health Service. (1998). Cardiac rehabilitation: effective health care 4:1-12.

Ockene, I.S., & Miller, N.H. (1997). Cigarette smoking, cardiovascular disease, and stroke: a statement for healthcare professionals from the American Heart Association. Circulation 96:3243-3247.

O'Donnell, D.E., Aaron, S., Bourbeau, J., Hernandez, P., Marciniuk, D., Balter, M., Ford, G., Gervais, A., Goldstein, R., Hodder, R., Maltais, F., & Road, J. Canadian Thoracic Society recommendations for management of chronic obstructive pulmonary disease: 2003. Canadian Respiratory Journal 10 (Suppl A): 11A-65A.

O'Donnell, D.E., Bain, D.J., & Webb, K.A. (1997). Factors contributing to relief of exertional breathlessness during hyperoxia in chronic airflow limitation. American Journal of Respiratory and Critical Care Medicine 155:530-535.

Oelberg, D.A., Systrom, D.M., Markowitz, D.H., Zorb, S.L., Wright, C., & Wain, J. (1998). Exercise performance in cystic fibrosis before and after bilateral lung transplantation. Journal of Heart and Lung Transplantation 17:1104-1112.

Olopade, C.O., Beck, K.C., Viggiano, R.W., & Staats, B.A. (1992). Exercise limitation and pulmonary rehabilitation in chronic obstructive lung disease. Mayo Clinic Proceedings 67:144-157.

Otsuka, T., Kurihara, N., Fujii, T., Fujimoto, S., & Yoshikawa, J. (1997). Effect of exercise training and detraining on gas exchange kinetics in patients with chronic obstructive lung disease. Clinical Physiology 17:287-297.

Palange, P., Forte, S., Onorati, P., Manfredi, F., Serra, P., & Carlone, S. (2000). Ventilatory and metabolic adaptations to walking and cycling in patients with COPD. Journal of Applied Physiology 88:1715-1720.

Pardaens, K., Van Cleemput, J., Vanhaecke, J., & Fagard, R.H. (2000). Peak oxygen uptake better predicts outcome than submaximal respiratory data in heart transplant candidates. Circulation 101:1152-1157.

Pashkow, F.J. (1993). Issues in contemporary cardiac rehabilitation: a historical perspective. Journal of the American College of Cardiology 21:822-834.

Pasquali, S.K., Alexander, K.P., Coombs, L.P., Lytle, B.L., & Peterson, E.D. (2003). Effect of cardiac rehabilitation on functional outcomes after coronary revascularlization. American Heart Journal 145:445-451.

Paul-Labrador, M., Vongvanich, P., & Merz, C.N. (1999). Risk stratification for exercise training in cardiac patients: do the proposed guidelines work? Journal of Cardiopulmonary Rehabilitation 19:118-125.

Persky, A.M., Eddington, N.D., & Derendorf, H. (2003). A review of the effects of chronic exercise and physical fitness level on resting pharmacokinetics. International Journal of Clinical Pharmacological Therapy 41:504-516.

Pianosi, P., D'Souza, S.J., Esseltine, D.W., Charge, T.D., & Coates, A.L. (1991). Ventilation and gas exchange during exercise in sickle cell anemia. American Review of Respiratory Disease 143:226-230.

Pierson, D.J., (2004). Translating new understanding into better care for the patient with chronic obstructive lung disease. Respiratory Care 49:99-109.

Pina, I.L., Balady, G.J., Hanson, P., Labovitz, A.J., Madonna, D.W., & Myers, J. (1995). Guidelines for clinical exercise testing laboratories. A statement for healthcare professionals from the Committee on Exercise and Cardiac Rehabilitation, American Heart Association. Circulation 91:912-921.

Pollard, S.D., Munks, K., Wales, C., Crossman, D.C., Cumberland, D.C., Oakley, G.D., & Gunn, J. Position and mobilization post-angiography study (PAMPAS): a comparison of 4.5 hours and 2.5 hours bed rest. Heart 89:447-448.

Pollack, M., Roa, J., Benditt, J., & Celli, B. (1993). Estimation of ventilatory reserve by stair climbing. A study in patients with chronic airflow limitation. Chest 104;1378-1383.

Psirropoulos, D., Lefkos, N., Boudonas, G., Efthimiadis, A., Vogas, V., Keskilidis, C., & Tsapas, G. (2002). Heart failure accompanied by sick euthyroid syndrome and exercise training. Current Opinions in Cardiology 17:266-270.

Puente-Maestu, L., Sanz, M.L., Sanz, P., Ruiz de Ona, J.M., Rodriguez-Hermosa, J.L., & Whipp, B.J. (2000). Effects of two types of training on pulmonary and cardiac responses to moderate exercise in patients with COPD. European Respiratory Journal 15:1026-1032.

Puri, S., Baker, B.L., Dutka, D.P., Oakley, C.M., Hughes, J.M., & Cleland, J.G. (1995). Reduced alveolar-capillary membrane diffusing capacity in chronic heart failure. Its pathophysiological relevance and relationship to exercise performance. Circulation 91:2769-2774.

Racine, N., Blanchet, M., Ducharme, A., Marquis, J., Boucher, J.M., Juneau, M., & White, M. (2003). Decreased heart rate recovery after exercise in patients with congestive heart failure: effect of beta-blocker therapy. Journal of Cardiac Failure 9:296-302.

Radzewitz, A., Miche, E., Herrmann, G., Nowak, M., Montanus, U., Adam, U., Stockmann, Y., & Barth, M. (2002). Exercise and muscle strength training and their effect on quality of life in patients with chronic heart failure. European Journal of Heart Failure 4:627-634.

Reindl, I., Wernecke, K.D., Opitz, C., Wensel, R., Konig, D., Dengler, T., Schimke, I., & Kleber, F.X. (1998). Impaired ventilatory efficiency in chronic heart failure: possible role of pulmonary vasoconstriction. American Heart Journal 136:778-785.

Reis, A.L., Ellis, B., & Hawkins, R.W. (1988). Upper extremity exercise training in chronic obstructive pulmonary disease. Chest 93:688-692.

Richardson, R.S., Leek, B.T., Gavin, T.P., Haseler, L.J., Mudaliar, S.R., Henry, R., Mathieu-Costello, O., & Wagner, P.D., (2004). Reduced mechanical efficiency in chronic obstructive pulmonary disease but normal peak V_{O_2} with small muscle mass contraction. American Journal of Critical Care Medicine 169: 89-96.

Richardson, R.S., Sheldon, J., Poole, D.C. Hopkins, S.R., Ries, A.L., & Wagner, P.D. (1999). Evidence of skeletal muscle metabolic reserve during whole body exercise in patients with chronic obstructive pulmonary disease. American Journal of Respiratory and Critical Care Medicine 159:881-885.

Rickli, H., Kiowski, W., Brehm, M., Weilenmann, D., Schalcher, C., Bernheim, A., Oecslin, E., & Brunner-La Rocca, H.P. (2003). Combining low-intensity and maximal exercise test results improves prognostic prediction in chronic heart failure. Journal of the American College of Cardiology 42:116-122.

Riley, M.S., Elborn, J.S., Bell, N., Stanford, C.F., & Nicholls, D.P. (1990). Substrate utilization during exercise in chronic cardiac failure. Clinical Science (London) 79:89-95.

Riley, M.S., Porszasz, J., Engelen, M.P., Brundage, B.H., & Wasserman, K. (2000). European Journal of Applied Physiology 83:63-70.

Riley, M.S., Porszasz, J., Miranda, J., Engelen, M.P., Brundage, B., & Wasserman, K. (1997). Exhaled nitric oxide during exercise in primary pulmonary hypertension and pulmonary fibrosis. Chest 111:44-50.

Riley, M., Stanford, C.F., & Nicholls, D.P. (1994). Ventilatory and heart rate responses after exercise in chronic cardiac failure. Clinical Science (London) 87:231-238.

Robbins, M., Francis, G., Pashkow, F.J., Snader, C.E., Hoercher, K., Young, J.B., & Lauer, M.S. (1999). Ventilatory and heart rate responses to exercise: better predictors of heart failure mortality than peak oxygen consumption. Circulation 100:2411-2417.

Roche, N., & Huchon, G.J. (1997). Current issues in the management of chronic obstructive pulmonary diseases. Respirology 2:215-229.

Romieu, I., & Trenga, C. (2001). Diet and obstructive lung diseases. Epidemiological Reviews 23:268-287.

Rosenberg, H., & Resnick, B. (2003). Exercise intervention in patients with chronic obstructive pulmonary disease. Geriatric Nursing 24:90-95.

Rostagno, C., Galanti, G., Comeglio, M., Boddi, V. Olivo, G., & Gatone Neri Serneri, G. (2000). Comparison of different methods of functional evaluation in patients with chronic heart failure. European Journal of Heart Failure 2:273-280.

Rostagno, C., Olivo, G., Comeglio, M., Boddi, V., Banchelli, M., Galanti, G., & Gensini, G.F. (2003). Prognostic value of 6-minute walk corridor test in patients with mild to moderate heart failure: comparison with other methods of functional evaluation. European Journal of Heart Failure 5:247-252.

Russell, S.D., McNeer, F.R., & Higginbotham, M.B. (1998). Exertional dyspnea in heart failure: a symptom unrelated to pulmonary function at rest or during exercise. Duke University Clinical Cardiology Studies (DUCCS) Exercise Group. American Heart Journal 135:398-405.

Sanderson, B.K., Southard, D., & Oldridge, N. (2004). AACVPR consensus statement. Outcomes evaluation in cardiac rehabilitation/ secondary prevention programs; improving patient care and program effectiveness. Journal of Cardiopulmonary Rehabilitation 24:68-79.

Schairer, J.R., Keteyian, S.J., Ehrman, J.K., Brawner, C.A., & Berkebile, N.D. (2003). Leisure time physical activity of patients in maintenance cardiac rehabilitation. Journal of Cardiopulmonary Rehabilitation 23:260-265.

Schmieder, F.A., & Comerota, A.J. (2001). Intermittent claudication: magnitude of the problem, patient evaluation, and therapeutic strategies. American Journal of Cardiology 87:3D-13D.

Schwaiblmair, M., Beinert, T., Vogelmeier, C., & Fruhmann, G. (1997). Cardiopulmonary exercise testing following hay exposure challenge in farmer's lung. European Respiratory Journal 10:2360-2365.

Serrano, M., Madoz, E., Ezpeleta, I., San Julian, B., Amezqueta, C., Perez Marco, J.A., & de Irala, J. (2003). Smoking cessation and risk of myocardial reinfarction in coronary patients: a nested case-control study. Revue Espanole Cardiologie (English abstract). 56:445-451.

Sietsema, K.E., Kraft, M., Ginzton, L., & Sharma, O.P. (1992). Abnormal oxygen update responses to exercise in patients with mild pulmonary sarcoidosis. Chest 102:838-845.

Simon, M., LeBlanc, P., Jobin, J., Desmeules, M., Sullivan, M.J., & Maltais, F. (2001). Limitation of lower limb V_{O_2} during cycling exercise in COPD patients. Journal of Applied Physiology 90:1013-1019.

Shah, A.R., Keens, T.G., & Gozal, D. (1997). Effect of supplemental oxygen on supramaximal exercise performance and recovery in cystic fibrosis. Journal of Applied Physiology 83:1641-1647.

Sietsema, K.E., Ben-Dov, I., Zhang, Y.Y., Sullivan, C., & Wasserman, K. (1994). Dynamics of oxygen uptake for sub-maximal exercise and recovery in patients with chronic heart failure. Chest 105:1693-1670.

Simonds, A.K. (2003). Ethics and decision making in end-stage lung disease. Thorax 58:272-277.

Singh, R.B., Weydahl, A., Otsuka, K., Watanabe, Y., Yano, S., Mori, H., Ichimaru,Y., Misutake, G., Sato, Y., Fanghong, L., Zhao, Z.Y.,

Kartik, C., & Gvozdjakova, A. (2001). Can nutrition influence circadian rhythm and heart rate variability? Biomedical Pharmacotherapy 55 suppl 1:115S-124S.

Sommaruga, M., Tramarin, R., Angelino, E., Bettinardi, O., Cauteruccio, M.A., Miglioretti, M., Monti, M., Pierobon, A., & Sguazzin, C. Guidelines on psychological interventions in cardiac rehabilitation: methodological process. Monaldi Archives of Chest Diseases (English abstract) 60:40-44.

Smith, S.C., Jr., Blair, S.N., Bonow, R.O., Brass, L.M., Cerqueira, M.D., Dracup, K., Fuster, V., Gotto, A., Grundy, S.M., Miller, N.H., Jacobs, A., Jones, D., Krauss, R.M., Mosca, L., Ockene, I., Pasternak, R.C., Pearson, T., Pfeffer, M.A., Starke, R.D., & Taubert, K.A. (2001). AHA/ACC guidelines for preventing heart attack and death in patients with atherosclerotic heart disease: 2001 update: a statement for healthcare professionals from the American Heart Association and the American College of Cardiology. Journal of the American College of Cardiology 38:1581-1583.

Smith, S.C., Jr. (1997). The challenge of risk reduction therapy for cardiovascular disease. American Family Physician 55:491-500.

Spencer, F.A., Salami, B., Yarzebski, J., Lessard, D., Gore, J.M., & Goldberg, R.J. (2001). Temporal trends and associated factors of inpatient cardiac rehabilitation in patients with acute myocardial infarction: a community-wide perspective. Journal of Cardiopulmonary Rehabilitation 21:377-384.

Stone, J.A. (2001). Canadian guidelines for cardiac rehabilitation and cardiovascular disease prevention are available. Journal of Cardiopulmonary Rehabilitation 21:344-345.

Stone, J.A., Cyr, C., Friesen, M., Kennedy-Symonds, H., Stene, R., & Smilovitch, M. (2001). Canadian guidelines for cardiac rehabilitation and atherosclerotic heart disease prevention: a summary. Canadian Journal of Cardiology 17 (Suppl B):3B-30B.

Storer, T.W. (2001). Exercise in chronic pulmonary disease: resistance exercise prescription. Medicine and Science in Sport and Exercise 33 (Suppl 7):S680-692.

Stratmann, H. (1991). Effect of exercise training on multiple respiratory variables in patients with coronary artery disease: correlation with changes in exercise capacity. Angiology 42:948-956.

Suskind, N., McKelvie, R.S., Burns, R.J., Latini, R., Pericak, D., Probstfield, J., Rouleau, J.L., Sigouin, C., Solymoss, C.B., Tsuyuki, R., White, M., & Yusuf, S. (2000). Glucose and insulin abnormalities related to functional capacity in patients with congestive heart failure. European Heart Journal 21:1368-1375.

Suskind, N., MacDonald, S., Swabey, T., Arthur, H., Vimr, M.A., & Tihaliani, R. (2003). Cardiac rehabilitation and secondary prevention services in Ontario: recommendations from a consensus panel. Canadian Journal of Cardiology 19:833-838.

Suzuki, K., Omiya, K., Yamada, S., Kobayashi, T., Suzuki, N., Osada, N., & Miyake, F. (2004). Relations between strength and endurance of leg skeletal muscle and cardiopulmonary exercise testing parameters in patients with chronic heart failure. Journal of Cardiology 43:59-68.

Swain, D.P., & Franklin, B.A. (2002). Is there a training intensity for aerobic training in cardiac patients? Medicine and Science in Sport and Exercise 34:1071-1075.

Swan, L., & Hillis, W.S. (2000). Exercise prescription in adults with congenital heart disease: a long way to go. Heart 83:685-687.

Tabet, J.Y., Beauvais, F., Thabut, G., Tartiere, J.M., Logeart, D., & Cohen-Solal, A. (2003). European Journal of Cardiovascular and Preventive Rehabilitation 10:267-272.

Tan, K.H., Cotterrell, D., Sykes, K., Sissons, G.R., de Cossart, L., & Edwards, P.R. (2000). Exercise training for claudicants: changes in blood flow, cardiorespiratory status, metabolic functions, blood rheology and lipid profile. European Journal of Vascular and Endovascular Surgery 20:72-78.

Tanabi, Y., Nakagawa, I., Ito, E., and Suzuki, K. (2002). Hemodynamic basis of the reduced oxygen uptake relative to work rate during incremental exercise in patients with chronic heart failure. International Journal of Cardiology 83:57-62.

Tanehato, M., Adachi, H., Oshima, S., Taniguchi, K., Itoh, H., Hasegawa, A., & Nagai, R. (1998). Improved oxygen utilization during mild exercise in heart failure. Japanese Circulation Journal 62:741-747.

Tangri, S., & Woolf, C.R. (1973). The breathing pattern in chronic obstructive lung disease during the performance of some common daily activities. Chest 63:126-127.

Thoman, R.L., Stroker, G.L., & Ross, J.C. (1966). The efficacy of pursed-lips breathing in patients with chronic obstructive pulmonary disease. American Review of Respiratory Disease 93:100-106.

Thomas, R.J., Miller, N.H., Lamendola, C., Berra, K., Hedback, B., Durstine, J.L., & Haskell, W. (1996). National survey of gender differences in cardiac rehabilitation programs: patient characteristics and enrollment patterns. Journal of Cardiopulmonary Rehabilitation 16:402-412.

Tomkiewicz-Pajak, L., Podolec, P., Tracz, W., Olszowska, M., & Plazak, W. (2002). Evaluation of the respiratory system in patients with heart failure based on spiro-ergometric exercise test parameters. Przegl Lek 59:568-571.

Tschernko, E.M., Gruber, E.M., Jaksch, P., Jandrasits, O., Jantsch, U., Brack, T., Lahrmann, H., Klepetko, W., & Wanke, T. (1998). Ventilatory mechanics and gas exchange during exercise before and after lung volume reduction surgery. American Journal of Respiratory and Critical Care Medicine 158:1424-1431.

Thornton, L.A. (2001). Depression in post-acute myocardial infarction patients. Journal of the American Academy of Nursing Practice 13:364-367.

Tyberg, J.V., Grant, D.A., Kingma, I., Moore, T.D., Sun, Y., Smith E.R., & Belenkic, I. (2000). Effects of positive intrathoracic pressure on pulmonary and systemic hemodynamics. Respiratory Physiology 119:171-179.

Tyler, D.O. (1997). Activity progression in acute cardiac patients. Journal of Cardiovascular Nursing 12:16-32.

Vallet, G., Ahmaidi, S., Serres, I., Fabre, C., Bourgouin, D., Desplan, J., Varray, A., & Prefaut, C. (1997). Comparison of two training programmes in chronic airway limitation patients: standardized versus individualized protocols. European Respiratory Journal 10:114-122.

van Berkel, T.F., Boersma, H., De Basquer, D., Deckers, J.W., & Wood, D. (1999). Registration and management of smoking behaviour in patients with coronary heart disease. The EUROASPIRE survey. European Heart Journal 20:1630-1637.

van Stel, H.F., Bogaard, J.M., Rijssenbeek-Nouwens, L.H., & Colland, V.T. (2001). Multivariable assessment of the 6-minute walking test in patients with chronic obstructive pulmonary disease. American Journal of Critical Care Medicine 163:1567-1571.

Verrill, D.E., & Ribisl, P.M. (1996). Resistive muscle training in cardiac rehabilitation. An update. Sports Medicine 21:347-383.

Vescovo, G., Serafini, F., Dalla Libera, L., Leprotti, C., Facchin, L., Tenderini, P., & Ambrosio, G.B. (1998). Skeletal muscle myosin heavy chain in heart failure: correlation between magnitude of the isozyme shift, exercise capacity, and gas exchange measurements. American Heart Journal 135:130-137.

Ville, N., Mercier, J., Varray, A., Albat, B., Messner-Pellenc, P., & Prefaut, C. (1998). Exercise tolerance in heart transplant patients with altered pulmonary diffusion capacity. Medicine and Science in Sport and Exercise 30:339-344.

Vitcenda, M. (2003). The Wisconsin outcomes experience: baseline outcomes of the WISCVPR Web-based Outcomes Project. Journal of Cardiopulmonary Rehabilitation 23:290-298.

Vivekananthan, D.P., Blackstone, E.H., Pothier, C.E., & Lauer, M.S. (2003). Heart rate recovery after exercise is a predictor of mortality, independent of the angiographic severity of coronary disease. Journal of the American College of Cardiology 42:831-838.

Vlasic, W., & Almond, D. (1999). Research-based practice: reducing bed rest following cardiac catheterization. Canadian Journal of Cardiovascular Nursing 10:19-22.

Wagener, J.S., & Headley, A.A. (2003). Cystic fibrosis: current concepts in respiratory care. Respiratory Care 48:234-245.

Warburton, D.E.R., & Mathur, S. (2004). Skeletal muscle training in people with chronic heart failure or chronic obstructive pulmonary disease. Physiotherapy Canada 56:143-157.

Weber, K.T., & Szidon, J.P. (1986). Exertional dyspnea. In Weber, K.T., Janicki, J.S. (Eds.). Cardiopulmonary exercise testing. Philadelphia: WB Saunders.

Weinberger, M. (2002). Airways reactivity in patients with CF. Clinical Review of Allergy and Immunology 23:77-85.

Westaby, S., Banning, A.P., Jarvik, R., Frazier, O.H., Pigoyy, D.W., Jin, X.Y., Catarino, P.A., Saito, S., Robson, D., Freeland, A., Myers, T.J., & Poole-Wilson, P.A. (2000). First permanent implant of the Jarvik 2000 Heart. Lancet 356:900-903.

Wilkinson, J., & Rees, J. (1996). Domiciliary oxygen. British Journal of Clinical Practice 50:151-153.

Williams, M.A., Fleg, J.L., Ades, P.A., Chaitman, B.R., Miller, N.H., Mohiuddin, S.M., Ockene, I.S., Taylor, C.B., & Wenger, N.K. (2002). Secondary prevention of coronary heart disease in the elderly (with an emphasis on patients > or = 75 years of age): An American Heart Association scientific statement from the Council on Clinical Cardiology Subcommittee on Exercise, Cardiac Rehabilitation, and Prevention. Circulation 105:1735-1743.

Wilson, P.W., D'Agostino, R.B., Levy, D., Belanger, A.M., Silbershatz, H., & Kannel, W.B. (1998). Prediction of coronary heart disease using risk factor categories. Circulation 97:1837-1847.

Winer, N., Sowers, J.R., & Weber, M.A. (2001). Gender differences in vascular compliance in young, healthy subjects assessed by pulse contour analysis. Journal of Clinical Hypertension (Greenwich) 3:145-152.

Witt, K.K., Morice, A., Clark, A.L., & Cleland, J.G. (2002). Airway resistance in chronic heart failure measured by impulse oscillometry. Journal of Cardiac Failure 8:225-231.

Womack, L. (2003). Cardiac rehabilitation secondary prevention programs. Clinical Sports Medicine 22:135-160.

Yajima, T., Koike, A., Sugimoto, K., Miyahara, Y., Marumo, F., & Hiroe, M. (1994). Mechanism of periodic breathing in patients with cardiovascular disease. Chest 106:142-146.

Yamagishi, H., Yoshiyama, M., Shirai, N., Akioka, K., Takeuchi, K, & Yoshikawa, J. (2003). Impact of diabetes mellitus on worsening of the left ventricular ejection fraction in exercise-gated 201T1 myocardial single photon emission computed tomography in patients with coronary artery disease. Circulation Journal 67:839-845.

Yamani, M.H., Sahgal, P., Wells, L., & Massie, B.M. (1995). Exercise intolerance in chronic heart failure is not associated with impaired recovery of muscle function or submaximal exercise performance. Journal of the American College of Cardiology 25:1232-1238.

Yohannes, A.M., & Hardy, C.C. (2003). Treatment of chronic obstructive pulmonary disease in older patients: a practical guide. Drugs and Aging 20:209-228.

Young, J.L., Pendergast, D.R., & Steinbach, J. (1991). Oxygen transport and peripheral microcirculation in long-term diabetes. Proceedings of the Society of Experimental and Biological Medicine 196:61-68.

Zhang, Y.Y., Wasserman, K., Sietsema, K.E., Ben-Dov, I., Barstow, T.J., Mizumoto, G., & Sullivan, C.S. (1993). O₂ kinetics in response to exercise: a measure of tissue anaerobiosis in heart failure. Chest 103:735-741.

Zu Wallack, R.L., Patel, K., Reardon, J.Z., & Clark, B.A. 3rd, & Normandin, E.A. (1991). Predictors of improvement in the 12-minute walking distance following a six-week outpatient pulmonary rehabilitation program. Chest 99:805-808.

C H A P T E R   2 5

Exercise Testing and Training: Secondary Cardiopulmonary Dysfunction

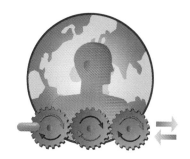

Elizabeth Dean and Donna Frownfelter

KEY TERMS

Anorexia nervosa
Connective tissue conditions
Diabetes
Endocrine conditions
Gastrointestinal conditions
Hematological conditions
Immunodeficiency conditions

Liver conditions
Musculoskeletal conditions
Neuromuscular conditions
Obesity
Renal conditions
Thyroid conditions

This chapter extends the general principles of exercise testing and training presented in Chapter 18 and describes special considerations concerning exercise testing and training individuals with *secondary* cardiopulmonary dysfunction. These special considerations are also important when managing an individual with primary cardiopulmonary dysfunction who, in addition, has cardiopulmonary dysfunction *secondary* to other conditions. In this case, management is modified based on this combination of comorbidities. Individuals with progressive degenerative conditions are often older and debilitated, thus the combination of problems is common. Exercise testing and training is one component of the comprehensive physical therapy management of individuals with chronic, secondary cardiovascular and pulmonary dysfunction, which is described in Chapter 32.

Secondary cardiopulmonary dysfunction refers to dysfunction of the cardiopulmonary system that is a consequence of pathology other than primary chronic heart and lung disease. Examples of such secondary conditions are described in Chapter 6. These conditions include dysfunction of the musculoskeletal, connective tissue, neurological, gastrointestinal, hepatic, renal, hematological, endocrine, and

immunological systems, or some combination thereof. Nutritional disorders, specifically obesity and starvation (anorexia nervosa), also have cardiopulmonary manifestations. Conditions leading to secondary cardiopulmonary dysfunction impact on one or more steps in the oxygen transport pathway such that the capacity for oxygen delivery is reduced, oxygen consumption is increased, or both (Dean, 1997). Often oxygen delivery is further compromised by restricted mobility. Oxygen transport limitations resulting from secondary cardiopulmonary dysfunction can present subtly, yet have significant clinical implications. Exercise has a primary role in the management of these conditions, along with the elements of comprehensive multidisciplinary prevention and long-term rehabilitation programs.

Contemporary approaches to the rehabilitation of individuals with stroke serve as a prime example of conventional practice aligning with contemporary exercise physiology principles. Over the past 20 years, stroke rehabilitation has shifted from a focus on Bobath and Brunstrum interventions to structured exercise training. Exercise training in the management of stroke has the potential for driving brain reorganization and exploiting the property of neuroplasticity to maximize functional capacity (Shepherd, 2001a). Exercise can exploit the potential for neural reorganization, optimize functional capacity, and address deconditioning. A focus on endurance and strengthening exercise, task-specific training, and treadmill walking in the rehabilitation of individuals with stroke, in addition to the conventional focus on cognitive engagement, sensorimotor integration, skill acquisition, and social readjustment has been an exciting advance in the rehabilitation of people with strokes.

Another prime example of exercise testing and training being prescribed for noncardiopulmonary conditions is their inclusion as a component of prehabilitation in preparation for surgery for a range of conditions. Before orthopedic surgical procedures, for example, improvements in functional capacity have been advocated to reduce perioperative complications and speed recovery (Ditmyer et al, 2002). Such programs include warm-up, aerobic training, resistance training, flexibility, and daily functional activities.

ASSESSMENT AND GOALS

Assessment

Knowledge of the cardiovascular and pulmonary consequences of conditions other than those of the cardiovascular and pulmonary systems enables the physical therapist to assess oxygen transport status, limitations, and risk factors in these individuals, in addition to ensuring their safety when undergoing physical activity and exercise. Such knowledge enables the physical therapist to prescribe exercise to optimize oxygen transport, maximize functional capacity and life participation, and maintain optimal long-term health.

Goals: Prevention

Many individuals with systemic conditions (see Chapter 6), the focus of this chapter, have manifestations of oxygen transport limitations or one or more risk factors. The risk factors must be identified and considered in a preventive management plan that includes exercise prescription to exploit the preventive effects of activity described in Chapter 18. Preventive goals for individuals with chronic, secondary cardiopulmonary conditions include optimizing central and peripheral adaptations to exercise, reducing biomechanical stress and strain and hence minimizing oxygen cost of exercise at submaximal work rates, optimizing fluid dynamics and hemodynamics, and optimizing lung health (e.g., alveolar ventilation, flow rates, mucociliary transport, and lymphatic drainage).

Another consideration with respect to prevention is that many chronic conditions lead to deterioration over time, and this may be exacerbated further with aging and unhealthy lifestyles. Exercise training is modified over time to accommodate each individual's needs and to help offset further deterioration and associated disability. Further, optimal training effects will benefit the individual's health overall and help

prevent contracting illnesses whose effects may be more devastating than in the healthy population.

Mobility aids and devices may be indicated for people with progressive functional deterioration. These adjuncts are titrated to the individual's needs to avoid their overuse. Overuse can lead to loss of remaining musculoskeletal function, which must be preserved as much as possible. Thus an individual can use these adjuncts to optimize functional performance throughout the day (e.g., use a wheelchair for activities in which symptoms are anticipated, or use an ankle foot orthosis in the afternoon when the tibial anterior muscle tends to be fatigued and needs support).

Goals: Short-term

When oxygen transport limitations occur, a regime of physical activity and exercise can be prescribed to elicit the acute effects of exercise (see Chapter 18). Prescription of the acute effects of exercise has a primary role in the management of individuals during acute episodes and set backs.

Goals: Long-term

When an individual has recovered from an acute episode, or an individual requires subacute and long-term management, a regime of physical activity and exercise can be prescribed to elicit the long-term effects of exercise described in Chapter 18. The capacity of each individual to respond to an exercise stimulus and the individual's oxygen transport reserve capacity are both assessed in detail. Knowledge of the reserve capacity is essential for optimal exercise prescription.

INDIVIDUALS WITH MUSCULOSKELETAL CONDITIONS

Exercise is prescribed for a broad range of conditions affecting the musculoskeletal system with favorable outcomes and no documented deleterious effects. With increased understanding of exercise pathophysiology, physical therapists can prescribe therapeutic exercise that has the greatest benefit in terms of improved activities of daily living and life satisfaction with the least risk. Individuals with mitochondrial myopathies and nonmetabolic myopathies experience typical aerobic responses to low intensity training (i.e., improved aerobic capacity and reduced submaximal heart rate and blood lactate) (Taivassalo et al, 1999). The extent of these training effects, however, is less in individuals with non-metabolic myopathies compared to those with mitochondrial myopathies. Improved aerobic capacity is associated with improved self-reported functional status and quality of life in both groups.

Exercise is central to the prevention and management of osteopenia and osteoporosis. In addition to weight bearing exercise, relatively intense exercise promotes bone density as well as a high volume of activity (Shepherd, 2001b). Muscle stress across joints appears to be a critical component for osteogenesis, thus torsion around joints such as in racket sports is favorable provided risk of falling is minimized. Tai Chi Chuan may reduce bone loss in postmenopausal women and may have some role in the management of osteoporosis (Qin et al, 2002).

Individuals with idiopathic scoliosis and associated restrictive ventilatory disorder can improve pulmonary function with exercise (Weiss, 1991). Selected exercise can improve both vital capacity and chest wall expansion by almost 20%. The role of exercise for remediation of restrictive lung dysfunction associated with other spinal and chest wall deformities warrants further investigation.

INDIVIDUALS WITH NEUROMUSCULAR CONDITIONS

Individuals with Stroke

Because the pathoetiology of stroke involves atherosclerosis and hypertension, individuals with stroke need to be managed comparably to individuals with systemic atherosclerosis and circulatory dysfunction. Appropriate precautions must be taken when exercising these individuals or conducting other physical therapy interventions. Within weeks after a stroke, cardiorespiratory deconditioning complicates the clinical picture along with muscle weakness, spasticity, incoordination, and abnormal gait (Kelly et al, 2003). In the subacute stage of stroke, individuals who undergo aerobic training can improve aerobic and functional abilities (Katz-Leurer et al, 2003b); however, these benefits may not be reflected in the long-term by indexes such as the Frenchay Activities Index (Katz-Leurer et al, 2003a; Meek et al, 2003). Although research is necessary to refine exercise testing and training procedures for individuals with stroke (Saunders et al, 2004), there is no reason to believe they would not respond to aerobic conditioning to counter the deconditioning that occurs post stroke or that this intervention would not augment gait reeducation and sensorimotor integration. Evidence supports that the application of a modified treadmill training protocol, based on exercise physiology principles, can be superior to conventional approaches to the rehabilitation of people with strokes (Pohl et al, 2002).

Although individuals with physical impairment secondary to stroke present methodological challenges during exercise testing and training, submaximal oxygen consumption ($\dot{V}O_2$) has good agreement with maximum $\dot{V}O_2$ ($\dot{V}O_2$max) when the test is tightly standardized (Eng et al, 2004). The high degree of reliability of these tests supports their use as outcome measures in this population. Metabolic assessment during short, submaximal tests, such as a five-minute walk, can provide supplemental information for evaluating gait in individuals with stroke (Teixeira da Cunha-Filho et al, 2003). Individuals with mild-to-moderate impairment from chronic stroke who require hand rail support on the treadmill also have been reported to have good reliability with respect to heart rate and oxygen pulse in peak effort treadmill testing (Dubrovolny et al, 2003). Hand rail support, however, is an important variable that can increase or decrease work

intensity and thus must be described and recorded to facilitate comparison of exercise results across tests. Hand rail support can be described on the data sheet with respect to side or front support, one or two hands, finger support or grasp support, and heavy or light support.

Treadmill training has proven to be a useful means of improving fitness and offsetting deconditioning in individuals with stroke. Individuals with impaired gait can improve their oxygen transport reserve capacity with a regular program of treadmill walking (Macko et al, 2001). Peak $\dot{V}O_2$ and walking workload increase and the energy cost associated with abnormal gait is reduced. These changes may enhance functional capacity in individuals with stroke comparable to other individuals with neurological deficits.

Treadmill training and weight support with a body harness for walking after stroke is showing promise in terms of a conditioning strategy and gait reeducation (Moseley et al, 2003). Patients with severe impairments after stroke who retrain their gait with a portion of their body weight (up to 40%) supported during exercise have better outcomes after training than those who carry their full weight (Barbeau & Visintin, 2003). Individuals with the most impairment as well as older individuals benefit the most. They walk more symmetrically on a treadmill compared with ground walking, with less spasticity and improved movement economy (Hesse et al, 2003). Furthermore, improvement in treadmill walking speed in these individuals generalizes to balance, trunk control, functional activities, and ground locomotion (Mudge et al, 2003; Barbeau & Visintin, 2003). Training at speeds comparable to an individual's normal velocity over ground is more effective than training at speeds above or below that velocity (Sullivan et al, 2002). Also, when different treadmill walking protocols are compared, structured speed-dependent treadmill training, as performed in sports training, improves walking ability more than either modified progressive treadmill training or conventional gait training (Pohl et al, 2002).

Despite the compelling results of studies on partial body weight support in the rehabilitation of individuals with stroke, these and related studies often fail to address the principles of physical therapy for management of individuals with systemic atherosclerosis, which include hemodynamic monitoring and possibly electrocardiogram (ECG) screening. One exception was a study by Eng et al (2002) that recommended that actual exertion (defined as a physiology measure; specifically, rate pressure product or heart rate) be measured in conjunction with walking distance in functional walk tests when testing people with stroke. When performance on several functional walk tests was compared, performance was associated with level of impairment rather than perceived exertion or intensity as measured by rate pressure product or heart rate. Thus debility may limit aerobic training capacity.

Aerobic exercise may have a preventive effect for stroke mediated by endothelium-dependent vasodilatation in the cerebral arterioles (McCarty, 2000). Several risk factors are associated with impairment of this mechanism. Exercise stimulates the expression of endothelial nitric oxide synthase, which promotes vascular dilatation and thereby exercise's potential protective and preventive effect.

Community ambulation is a meaningful outcome for people with stroke (Lord et al, 2004). A discrepancy exists, however, between mobility outcomes on standardized measures of community-based individuals and the extent to which they actually get out in the community. Gait velocity is an important variable in determining community ambulation capacity.

Resistance muscle training has been of interest as a component of physical therapy management of individuals with stroke. Strength training augments the benefits of aerobic exercise with respect to functional strength (Carr & Jones, 2003) without reinforcing abnormal movement patterns (Riolo & Fisher, 2003). One study, however, reported no difference between leg exercise training programs with and without resistance (Moreland et al, 2003). Inadequate exercise prescription to explain the absence of an effect of resistance training cannot be ruled out.

When prescribing exercise for individuals with stroke it must be remembered that stroke results from a hemodynamic insult—usually high blood pressure. Aerobic exercise and resistance muscle training elicit unique hemodynamic responses, thus the hemodynamic status of individuals with stroke must be assessed in the initial baseline review, considered carefully in the exercise prescription, and assessed in the outcomes of these programs. If blood pressure is being pharmacologically managed, then an objective of exercise will be to augment oxygen transport efficiency and normalize blood pressure. Medications must be followed so that these can be reduced or withdrawn in response to an overall effect of a comprehensive exercise and management program.

Individuals with Spinal Cord Injury

Spinal cord injury (SCI) can afflict anyone at any age. Most often, however, SCI results from trauma incurred in young adulthood, and it is more prevalent in men. Depending on the level of the injury, individuals with SCI have altered hemodynamic response to exercise and positional stress. Life expectancy has increased in recent decades for these individuals, which correspondingly has increased their incidence of cardiac risk factors and disease (Vidal et al, 2003). An active lifestyle and regular exercise are imperative to ensure that these risk factors and related cardiac morbidity are reduced. Heart rate is highly correlated with respiratory minute volume, $\dot{V}O_2$, and workload, which enables exercise to be prescribed in a predictable manner for this group. Exercise capacity is a function of the capacity of the patient to increase heart rate (Barstow et al, 1996). Significant aerobic gains in peak $\dot{V}O_2$ and work rate peak result from aerobic exercise in combination with functional electrical stimulation of the lower extremity muscles performed, on average, twice a week. Recovery times also improve with training.

Individuals with SCI have a higher heart rate and lower stroke volume during exercise compared with individuals without SCI (Jacobs et al, 2002). Cardiac output is lower at rest. Peak exercise responses are greater for those without SCI with the exception of heart rate. Despite higher heart rates for a given work load, stroke volume and cardiac output are lower. An intact autonomic nervous system is necessary for a large increase in cardiac output and blood flow to working muscles. Thus, depending on the level of the lesion, the heart and peripheral circulation and their capacity to respond to increased work demand are affected (Dela et al, 2003).

Arm ergometry can be used to test the aerobic capacity of individuals with SCI. Because of the small muscle mass of the arms compared with the legs, the pressure of contracting upper extremity muscles over blood vessels, and the need for postural stabilization, hemodynamic responses are disproportionately elevated compared with the same work intensity performed by the legs. With training, $\dot{V}O_2$ *on-off* kinetics, but not heart rate, is accelerated in individuals with SCI (Fukuoka et al, 2002). Cardiac output during exercise also tends to be lower for these individuals. Thus $\dot{V}O_2$ kinetics may be a prime limiter of exercise capacity in people with SCI, which could contribute to their lower anaerobic threshold with deconditioning.

Wheelchair athletes with SCI show cardiovascular adaptation to exercise. Echocardiographic evidence shows an increase in left ventricular volume compared with individuals without SCI, but this adaptation is less than in healthy runners (Price et al, 2000). Both long-term arm and leg exercise produce morphometric changes in cardiac mass and volume; however, these changes are less pronounced in wheelchair athletes compared with runners. Also, submaximal heart rates are greater for the wheelchair athletes than runners.

Movement economy varies depending on how a specific activity is performed mechanically. Wheelchair propulsion is more mechanically and energetically efficient using a pumping motion rather than the traditional semi-circular motion (de Groot et al, 2004). This has implications for energy conservation and minimization of upper extremity overload in individuals with SCI and for optimizing energy-efficient wheelchair design.

Movement economy (i.e., energy cost in relation to workload) is a concern in managing individuals with physical deformity related to musculoskeletal impairments because of the increased energy cost associated with physical activity associated with tasks and exercise in general. The degree to which spasticity contributes to increased energy cost is unclear. In individuals with acquired brain injury, for example, $\dot{V}O_2$ increases with exercise in a predictable, linear manner, although energy cost does not increase disproportionately with spasticity (Dawes et al, 2003).

Lastly, unlike able-bodied individuals, those with SCI do not show comparable cardiac adaptation. The typical left ventricular enlargement is not observed (Gates et al, 2002), suggesting that peripheral factors are responsible for conditioning with training in this cohort.

Individuals with the Chronic Effects of Poliomyelitis

The last poliomyelitis epidemic this century in the western world was in the 1950s. Individuals who had poliomyelitis as children at that time are now older adults. The delayed effects of having lived for years with poliomyelitis and its associating limitations may begin to manifest with or without post polio syndrome (PPS). The chronic effects of poliomyelitis impact functional capacity, exercise tolerance, and cardiovascular and cardiopulmonary risk. Some 50% of individuals who had poliomyelitis develop PPS. The exercise principles are distinct for those survivors of poliomyelitis with or without PPS (Dean & Dallimore, 2004; Dean & Dallimore, 2005).

PPS is hallmarked by new fatigue, muscle weakness, and pain (see overview Dean, 1991). In addition, survivors of poliomyelitis with PPS may experience exercise intolerance, choking and swallowing dysfunction, temperature sensitivity, and psychological problems. Patients who did not have ventilatory involvement at onset, as well as those who had bulbar involvement at disease onset, may have impaired pulmonary function with PPS. During exercise, ventilatory involvement may be evidenced by impaired blood gases that are not apparent at rest (Weinberg et al, 1999). This has been proposed as a mechanism for delaying diaphragmatic fatigue. In addition to the chronic effects of poliomyelitis, survivors of poliomyelitis are also afflicted with the same health challenges faced by their peers who have no history of poliomyelitis. This clinical picture may be further super-imposed with weight gain and reduced activity, hence, deconditioning, which is associated with aging in western cultures.

Overuse abuse has been proposed as a mechanism of the delayed onset effects of poliomyelitis (Perry et al, 1988). Injudicious prescription of strengthening or aerobic exercise can be deleterious to the patient because it contributes to the overuse abuse of affected as well as unaffected muscle (Dean & Dallimore, 2005). A reduced motor unit pool has less capacity to recover with prolonged demands, and this pool is further reduced with advancing years. With a prescribed program of rest and activity that augments muscle and endurance capacity without contributing to the patient's symptoms, an individual can show improved tolerance to activities of daily living (Dean & Dallimore, 2004).

Because of the overuse abuse phenomenon associated with PPS, an injudicious exercise program (aerobic or muscle strengthening) can lead to further overuse and progressive deterioration (Dean et al, 1989). Thus reserve capacity for exercise is assessed based on a detailed assessment so that overuse is not worsened.

An exercise test can be used to assess conditioning and movement economy, which are distinct entities (Dean & Ross, 1991). Modified aerobic training can be prescribed within the limits of subjective complaints of fatigue and discomfort/pain rather than conventional indexes of exercise intensity (i.e., heart rate and blood pressure). Although conventional sub-maximal indexes of conditioning may not be apparent after several weeks of training, walking tolerance at subthreshold levels, measured by walking duration, may improve, as may movement economy (Dean & Ross, 1991). Thus some patients with a history of poliomyelitis can respond favorably to a modified walking program.

Individuals with postural malalignment experience biomechanical stress over joints during ambulation, which in turn can contribute to increased energy cost (Dean & Ross, 1993). An individual's overall energy cost must be considered when prescribing exercise. Activities normally associated with low energy cost for an individual with normal posture and muscle strength can have significantly higher metabolic demand in an individual with postural deformity, limb length discrepancy, and strength asymmetry. Because fatigue and pain are symptoms associated with PPS, these subjective parameters must be monitored before, during, and between exercise sessions to monitor immediate and delayed effects and capacity to recover after exercise. In this way deleterious exercise workloads may be minimized. Overall, objective measures of walking performance are reported to be associated with subjective reports of functional capacity (Noonan et al, 2000).

New muscle weakness is a marker of PPS. Modified strengthening programs may have some benefit in individuals whose muscles are not showing signs of progressive muscular atrophy and fatigue versus weakness (Dean & Dallimore, 2005). Stronger muscles may help improve peripheral extraction of oxygen at the peripheral level and thus contribute to an aerobic training effect and improved endurance.

Individuals with Down Syndrome

Down syndrome is an example of a condition marked by mental as well as physical challenges. People with the syndrome vary widely with respect to the severity of the condition and their functional capacity, which ranges from living totally independently and being gainfully employed to being somewhat dependent in these domains. Many individuals with the syndrome benefit from physical therapy that includes a lifelong exercise program, usually commencing in child-hood during growth and development. Longevity has improved as a result of improved detection and management of heart defects and prevention of respiratory complications. With greater life expectancy, individuals with the syndrome encounter many of the same acute and chronic conditions that individuals without the syndrome encounter over their lifecycle, such as the diseases of civilization. Cardiac defects and sleep apnea are more common in persons with Down syndrome than the general population (Bosch, 2003). These may impact exercise capacity, thus exercise and monitoring must be individualized to each person's unique needs. Obesity and deconditioning can further complicate the clinical presentation. Communication style must be adapted with respect to the exercise prescription and health maintenance program. Optimal health is necessary to maximize function and long-term self-care. A care giver may need to be involved to promote a sustained program of regular physical activity and exercise.

INDIVIDUALS WITH CONNECTIVE TISSUE CONDITIONS

The exercise limitations of individuals with connective tissue conditions result in part from the restrictive component of lung dysfunction associated with these conditions. They may have normal chest x-ray and conventional pulmonary function yet have histochemical abnormalities of their lungs (e.g., shrinking lung associated with scleroderma).

Resting data are limited in predicting responses to activities of daily living and exercise. Thus exercise testing is a primary tool to assess pulmonary function dynamically and thereby unmask abnormalities that can compromise daily function (Schwaiblmair et al, 1996). Women with systemic lupus erythematosus (SLE) have a several-fold increase in incidence of heart disease than other women, corresponding to an increased number of cardiac risk factors (Bruce et al, 2003). In addition, hypertension and diabetes are also more prevalent in this group.

INDIVIDUALS WITH RHEUMATOID CONDITIONS

Individuals with rheumatoid arthritis (RA) have a higher incidence of cardiovascular disease and related mortality. Despite normal left ventricular systolic function, left ventricular diastolic function is impaired without clinical evidence of cardiovascular disease, which may place this group at risk (Mustonen et al, 1993). At maximal exercise, heart rate, systolic blood pressure, and peak $\dot{V}O_2$ are comparable for individuals with RA and healthy people.

Contemporary approaches to the management of people with RA include exercise prescription for strength, endurance, and emotional well-being (Forrest & Rynes, 1994). Joint inflammation may be reduced with judiciously prescribed exercise.

INDIVIDUALS WITH GASTROINTESTINAL CONDITIONS

Conditions such as irritable bowel syndrome and Crohn's disease are characterized by disturbed homeostasis related to gut motility and function. Because these conditions are chronic and medical care is noncurative, physical deconditioning and debility are common. Few studies have examined the acute or chronic effects of exercise in this population, so specific guidelines for testing and training are lacking. One study examined the effects of moderately intense exercise (60% of $\dot{V}O_2$max for one hour) on gastrointestinal function in individuals with Crohn's disease who were in remission (D'Inca et al, 1999). The conventional measures of gastrointestinal function were unchanged. It may be necessary to observe caution because of oxygen metabolite production and potential zinc deficiency. Individuals with gastrointestinal conditions have nutritional deficits that must be considered when placing increased metabolic demands on energy substrate stores. The capacity of these individuals to respond to exercise appropriately will fluctuate with exacerbations and remissions of their conditions. It is hoped that with improved health and functional capacity, the duration between exacerbations will be increased, the severity of exacerbations will be reduced, and speed of recovery will be increased.

INDIVIDUALS WITH LIVER CONDITIONS

The exercise responses of individuals with hepatopulmonary syndrome (HPS) are not well understood, which has hampered defining mobilization and exercise testing and training guidelines. One study, however, has shown that individuals with HPS have markedly reduced aerobic capacity and exercise-induced hypoxemia that exceeds the limitations of patients with liver disease but without the syndrome (Epstein et al, 1998). Hypoxemia and increased ventilatory dead space at peak exercise support impairment in the pulmonary circulation.

Exercise capacity and maximum oxygen consumption are impaired by cirrhosis. This can be explained by an associated cirrhotic cardiomyopathy. Myocardial thickening and ventricular stiffness lead to decreased diastolic function and inotropic and chronotropic incompetence when the oxygen transport system is stressed during exercise (Wong et al, 2001).

INDIVIDUALS WITH RENAL CONDITIONS

Limitation of mitochondrial oxidative capacity has been ruled out as a limiter of exercise capacity in patients with chronic renal failure (Sala et al, 2001). Muscle oxygen conductance, however, is low.

Exercise has a role in the management of individuals undergoing hemodialysis. One study examined the role that normalizing hemoglobin has on exercise response of these individuals (McMahon et al, 1999). Although both young and old subjects showed evidence of improved oxygen transport and exercise tolerance, exercise responses were not normalized completely. Further, impaired potassium regulation appeared related to hemoglobin concentration and was thought to contribute to exercise limitation.

Patients with end-stage renal disease can also benefit from exercise. Minimally, deconditioning may be prevented, but alternatively, functional status will be improved. An ideal exercise program should have both aerobic exercise and resistance muscle training components, and the prescription for both should be designed to minimize cardiovascular and musculoskeletal risks. Exercise is initiated at a low level to ensure the exercise responses are normal and the patient responds favorably before progression of the prescription. With respect to exercising patients who are severely ill, the consequences of not exercising must be considered (Copley & Lindberg, 1999). Regular physical activity, particularly when the patient is relatively stable and well, must be encouraged. This ensures that the patient is as well as possible when a change in his or her condition occurs, which in turn speeds recovery and minimizes associated challenges to aerobic and strength status.

Erythropoietin therapy in the management of patients with chronic renal failure fails to augment peak $\dot{V}O_2$ as much as might be predicted from a corresponding increase in hemoglobin (Marrades et al, 1996). Lactate differences may explain abnormal muscle oxygen transport and reduced exercise tolerance in these patients. Erythropoietin-mediated increases in hemoglobin, however, reduce the respiratory exchange ratio at submaximal exercise (comparable to activities of daily living), reflecting a decrease in anaerobic metabolism and reduced exercise stress (Lundin et al, 1991).

Chronic renal insufficiency is strongly associated with exercise-induced ischemia in individuals with atherosclerosis. The greater the severity of atherosclerosis in these individuals with chronic renal insufficiency reflects their increased cardiovascular risk (Ix et al, 2003).

Frequent exercise for patients with renal disease has been proposed as a means of maximizing effective use of their anemia-imposed reduced oxygen delivery capacity (Williams, 1995).

INDIVIDUALS WITH HEMATOLOGICAL CONDITIONS

Sickle cell anemia is a common hematological condition in the United States with a high prevalence in the African American population. Patients with sickle cell disease have reduced hemoglobin and oxygen transport capacity. On maximal exercise testing and endurance testing they have lower exercise tolerance; however, their responses relative to deconditioned individuals without sickle cell anemia are generally comparable (Oyono-Enguelle et al, 2000). Thus exercise performance of these individuals must be interpreted in this context.

INDIVIDUALS WITH ENDOCRINE CONDITIONS

Individuals with diabetes warrant special consideration with respect to exercise testing and training. Exercise imposes demands on energy substrates and their utilization. Blood sugar abnormalities associated with diabetes necessitate monitoring blood sugar fluctuations before, during, and after exercise. The physical therapist must ensure that the individual eats appropriate foods and at appropriate times in relation to physical activity and exercise. Obesity management is fundamental to the goals of an exercise program as well as normalizing blood sugar metabolism.

Autonomic neuropathies, myopathies, and angiopathies contribute to abnormal exercise responses. Acute exercise responses (e.g., heart rate and blood pressure) may be blunted, as may subjective response to exercise. People with diabetes have a higher incidence of silent ischemia. Heart rate and blood pressure may be less valid indexes of work load. Peripheral vascular disease may result from the direct effect of diabetes, as well as vascular occlusive disease, which is accelerated in individuals with diabetes compared with those

without this condition. Altered glucose transfer may also interfere with normal exercise responses. Weight control and nutrition are important to optimize training responses. The capacity to exhibit an optimal training response depends on disease severity, management of the disease, and complications (HbA1c provides an index of potential complications). Limb perfusion and skin perfusion are monitored before and after exercise. Well fitting, smooth, clean socks must be worn at all times.

Special considerations include monitoring blood sugar before, during, and after exercise (immediate and delayed), at least initially when prescribing exercise for a person with diabetes. Exercise is postponed if blood sugar is extremely high and in the presence of ketone bodies. Daily regular exercise is recommended to maintain health and optimal blood sugar regulation. Intensity should be mild to moderate for a given individual (American College of Sports Medicine, 2000). Exercise is judiciously timed with the intake of both foods of optimal glycemic index for the person's needs and insulin or oral agents, as indicated. With improved glucose tolerance and insulin sensitivity and a long-term aerobic exercise program, the need for insulin or oral agents will be affected. The need for these will be eliminated ideally, or at least reduced.

Individuals with thyroid disease warrant close monitoring. Those who are hypothyroid will be more easily fatigued. Their medical management warrants close monitoring to ensure that their condition is normalized as much as possible. If it is, these individuals should have generally normal exercise responses. Those with hyperthyroidism will have high resting heart rates and blood pressure and exaggerated exercise responses.

INDIVIDUALS WITH IMMUNODEFICIENCY CONDITIONS

The pharmaceutical drugs that have been developed to improve the survival of individuals with human immunodeficiency virus (HIV) and acquired immune deficiency syndrome (AIDS) (e.g., highly active antiretroviral therapy [HAART]) can impair oxygen transport and, hence, functional capacity. At peak exercise heart rate has been reported to be lower and stroke volume higher in individuals with HIV taking HAART when compared with individuals with HIV not taking the drug (Cade et al, 2003). The $a-vO_2$ difference was lower at peak exercise for those on the drug. HAART is a primary contributor to decreased muscle oxygen extraction-utilization in individuals infected with HIV. The physical therapist must be highly knowledgeable about the combined response of exercise and the potent medications used to control the disease in these individuals. This is important in order to build on an individual's exercise reserve capacity when health is best, and maintain health and social participation. It is hoped that with improved health and conditioning, morbidity and its severity is reduced.

Immunodeficiency has been implicated in chronic fatigue syndrome (CFS). This syndrome, currently of unknown etiology, appears to run its course over time. Guidelines for exercise testing, particularly maximal testing and training, have been uncertain. In one study individuals with CFS were maximally exercise tested. Exercise responses were comparable to individuals with reduced conditioning without CFS, supporting the theory that the physiological responses of individuals with CFS were not abnormal and that exercise testing resulted in no harmful or deleterious effects (Mullis et al, 1999).

INDIVIDUALS WITH NUTRITION-RELATED CONDITIONS

Individuals Who Are Obese

In preparation for exercise prescription, the individual who is obese requires a comprehensive multisystem assessment to establish all factors that may limit exercise tolerance. These individuals require high volumes of physical activity and exercise (see physical activity and exercise pyramid in Chapter 1) in conjunction with a nutritious dietary program. Introducing more exercise, however, must be done gradually so that it is not only enjoyable and nonaversive but reduces musculoskeletal strain and injury. Biomechanics change with weight loss, and exercise becomes biomechanically less stressful and better tolerated.

Prescriptive parameters for optimal weight loss remain a matter of debate with respect to prolonged, low-intensity aerobic exercise versus short, high-intensity exercise. Moderate relative intensities of effort, however, have been reported to be more effective at mobilizing fat, whereas heavy relative exercise promotes energy expenditure post exercise (Shepherd, 2001b). The critical factor is the number of calories expended, and burning calories is best achieved with a regularly active lifestyle supplemented with additional formal exercise sessions. Lower intensity exercise may be favored to avoid musculoskeletal strain, or for psychological and motivational reasons. Aerobic training increases lipid oxidation during exercise in fasting conditions (Thalamus et al, 2003). Such a regimen maintains glucose homeostasis as well as facilitates fat oxidation. Additional benefits of endurance training for individuals who are obese include reduced cholesterol and insulin concentrations in the blood.

Some individuals may benefit from a structured program (see Chapter 32) and the social support of others in the program.

Individuals with Anorexia Nervosa

The malnutrition and weight loss due to catabolism associated with anorexia nervosa predisposes individuals with the condition to deconditioning and impaired oxygen transport reserve capacity. Such capacity is vital to optimally respond and adapt to exercise and the physical demands of daily life in the short- and long-term (Rowland et al, 2003). Fluid and electrolyte imbalance can complicate the clinical picture and

is the primary cause of death in extreme cases. Although quantitatively abnormal, responses to exercise may be appropriate in the absence of abnormal myocardial performance. Exercise is prescribed in conjunction with an optimal nutritional plan so that further catabolism is not precipitated.

SUMMARY

This chapter extends the general exercise testing and training principles described in Chapter 18 and describes special considerations for exercise testing and training individuals with cardiopulmonary dysfunction *secondary* to conditions *other* than primary chronic heart and lung disease. Exercise testing and training is one component of a comprehensive physical therapy management program that is described in Chapter 32.

Conditions that can lead to secondary cardiopulmonary dysfunction include dysfunction of the musculoskeletal, connective tissue, neurological, gastrointestinal, hepatic, renal, hematological, endocrine, and immunological systems, or some combination thereof. Nutritional disorders, specifically obesity and starvation (anorexia nervosa), also have cardiopulmonary manifestations. Exercise has a primary role in the management of these conditions along with the elements of a comprehensive multidisciplinary prevention and rehabilitation program. Knowledge of the potential cardiopulmonary consequences of conditions other than primary cardiovascular and pulmonary disease is essential to prescribe mobilization and exercise safely and therapeutically for individuals with these conditions to maintain their health and well-being (capacity for activity and participation in life with least physiological risk). Individuals with these conditions are often managed by physical therapists. Thus the cardiovascular and pulmonary manifestations must be considered with respect to physical activity recommendations, and the prescription of optimal and safe exercise programs.

Individuals with the potential for cardiopulmonary dysfunction secondary to noncardiopulmonary conditions are at significant health risk. Even minor illnesses can have a major impact on their functional capacity. Further, many of these conditions have a progressive degenerative component. This, coupled with aging, can result in apparently sudden functional decline. Thus oxygen transport of these individuals can benefit from the general health benefits of a lifelong program that includes an exercise program that is modified based on changes in their condition. Finally, individuals with chronic, secondary cardiopulmonary conditions likely have underlying risk factors for primary cardiopulmonary conditions comparable to the general population, if not to a greater extent. Thus both types of pathoetiology must be considered when evaluating limitations in life participation and related activities and their remediation, as well as when evaluating preventive measures for lifelong health and well-being.

Review Questions

1. Describe how chronic, *secondary* cardiovascular and pulmonary dysfunction associated with the following conditions can limit participation in life and associated activities in the absence of chronic, *primary* cardiopulmonary conditions.
   - Musculoskeletal (osteoporosis, ankylosing spondylitis, muscular dystrophy, osteroarthritis)
   - Connective tissue (systemic lupus erythematosus, scleroderma) and autoimmune conditions (rheumatoid arthritis)
   - Neurological (stroke, spinal cord injury, chronic effects of poliomyelitis)
   - Gastrointestinal
   - Hepatic
   - Renal
   - Hematological
   - Endocrine
   - Immunological
   - Obesity
   - Anorexia nervosa
2. Describe special considerations for exercise testing and training individuals with the conditions above.

REFERENCES

American College of Sports Medicine. (2000). Guidelines for exercise testing and prescription, ed 6. Philadelphia: Lippincott Williams & Wilkins.

Barbeau, H., & Visintin, M. (2003). Optimal outcomes obtained with body-weight support combined with treadmill training in stroke subjects. Archives of Physical Medicine and Rehabilitation 84:1458-1465.

Barstow, T.J., Scremin, A.M., Mutton, D.L., Kunkel, C.F., Cagle, T.G., & Whipp, B.J. (1996). Changes in gas exchange kinetics with training in patients with spinal cord injury. Medicine and Science in Sports and Exercise 28:1221-1228.

Bosch, J.J. (2003). Health maintenance throughout the life span for individuals with Down syndrome. Journal of the American Academy of Nurse Practitioners 15:5-17.

Bruce, I.N., Urowitz, M.B., Gladman, D.D., Ibanez, D., & Steiner, G. (2003). Risk factors for coronary heart disease in women with systemic lupus erythematosus: the Toronto Risk Factor Study. Arthritis and Rhematism 48:3159-3167.

Cade, W.T., Fantry, L.E., Nabar, S.R., Shaw, D.K, & Keyser, RE. (2003). A comparison of Qt and a-v O_2 in individuals with HIV taking and not taking HAART. Medicine and Science in Sports and Exercise 35:1108-1117.

Carr, M., & Jones, J. (2003). Physiologic effects of exercise on stroke survivors. Topics in Stroke Rehabilitation 9:57-64.

Copley, J.B., & Lindberg, J.S. (1999). The risks of exercise. Advances in Renal Replacement Therapy 6:165-171.

Dawes, H., Bateman, A., Culpan, J., Scott, O., Wade, D.T., Roach, N., & Greenwood, R. (2003). The effect of increasing effort on movement economy during incremental cycling exercise in individuals early after acquired brain injury. Clinical Rehabilitation 17:528-534.

Dean, E. (1991). Clinical decision making in the management of the late sequelae of poliomyelitis. Physical Therapy 71:757-761.

Dean, E. (1997). Oxygen transport deficits in systemic disease and implications for physical therapy. Physical Therapy 77:187-202.

Dean, E., & Dallimore, D. (2004). Physical therapy in the management of chronic poliomyelitis and postpolio syndrome. In Silver, J.K., & Gawne, A.C. (Eds). Postpolio syndrome. Philadelphia: Elsevier.

Dean, E., & Dallimore, D. (2005). Muscle function and training of individuals with the chronic effects of poliomyelitis with and without post polio syndrome. Physiotherapy Canada 57:1-14.

Dean, E., & Ross, J. (1991). Effect of modified aerobic training on movement energetics in polio survivor. Orthopedics 14: 1243-1246.

Dean, E., & Ross, J. (1993). Movement energetics of individuals with a history of poliomyelitis. Archives of Physical Medicine and Rehabilitation 74:478-483.

Dean, E., Ross, J., & MacIntyre, D. (1989). A rejoinder to "Exercise programs for patients with post-polio syndrome: a case report": a short communication. Physical Therapy 69:695-699.

Dean, E., Ross, J., Road, J., Courtney, L., & Madill, K. (1991). Lung function in individuals with a history of poliomyelitis. Chest 100:118-123.

de Groot, S., Veeger, H.E., Hollander, A.P., & van der Woude, L.H. (2004). Effect of wheelchair stroke pattern on mechanical efficiency. American Journal of Physical Medicine and Rehabilitation 83:640-649.

Dela, F., Mohr, T., Jensen, C.M., Haahr, H.L., Secher, N.H., Biering-Sorensen, F., & Kjaer, M. (2003). Cardiovascular control during exercise: insights from spinal cord-injured humans. Circulation 107:2127-2133.

D'Inca, R., Varnier, M., Mestriner, C., Martines, D., D'Odorico, A., & Sturniolo, G.C. (1999). Effect of moderate exercise on Crohn's disease patients in remission. Italian Journal of Gastroenterology and Hepatology 31:205-210.

Ditmyer, M.M., Topp, R., & Pifer, M. (2002). Prehabilitation in preparation for orthopedic surgery. Orthopedic Nursing 21:43-51.

Dubrovolny, C.L., Ivey, F.M., Rogers, M.A., Sorkin, J.D., & Macko, R.F. (2003). Reliability of treadmill exercise testing in older patients with chronic hemiparetic stroke. Archives of Physical Medicine and Rehabilitation 84:1308-1312.

Eng, J.J., Chu, K.S., Dawson, A.S., Kim, C.M., & Hepburn, K.E. (2002). Functional walk tests in individuals with stroke: relation to perceived exertion and myocardial exertion. Stroke 33:756-761.

Eng, J.J., Dawson, A.S., & Chu, K.S. (2004). Submaximal exercise in persons with stroke: test-retest reliability and concurrent validity with maximal oxygen consumption. Archives of Physical Medicine and Rehabilitation 85:113-118.

Epstein, S.K., Zilberberg, M.D., Jacoby, C., Ciubotaru, R.L., & Kaplan, L.M. (1998). Response to symptom-limited exercise in patients with hepatopulmonary syndrome. Chest 114:736-741.

Forrest, G., & Rynes, R.I. (1994). Exercise for rheumatoid arthritis. Contemporary Internal Medicine 6:23-28.

Fukuoka, Y., Endo, M., Kagawa, H., Itoh, M., & Nakanishi, R. (2002). Kinetics and steady-state of V O_2 responses to arm exercise in trained spinal cord injured humans. Spinal Cord 40:631-638.

Gates, P.E., Campbell, I.G., & George, K.P. (2002). Absence of training-specific cardiac adaptation in paraplegic athletes. Medicine and Science in Sports and Exercise 34:1699-1704.

Gorman, D. The body moveable. Guelph, Ontario, Canada: Ampersand Printing Co.

Hesse, S., Werner, C., von Frankenberg, S., & Bardeleben, A. (2003). Treadmill training with partial body weight support after stroke.

Physical Medicine Rehabilitation Clinics of North America 14(Suppl 1):S111-S123.

Ix, J.H., Shlipak, M.G., Liu, H.H., Schiller, N.B., & Whooley, M.A. (2003). Association between renal insufficiency and inducible ischemia in patients with coronary artery disease: the heart and soul study. Journal of the American Society for Nephrology 14:3233-3238.

Jacobs, P.L., Mahoney, E.T., Robbins, A., & Nash, M. (2002). Hypokinetic circulation in persons with paraplegia. Medicine and Science in Sports and Exercise 34:1401-1407.

Katz-Leurer, M., Carmeli, E., & Shochina, M. (2003a). The effect of early aerobic training on independence six months post stroke. Clinical Rehabilitation 17:735-741.

Katz-Leurer, M., Shochina, M., Carmeli, E., & Friedlander, Y. (2003b). The influence of early aerobic training on the functional capacity in patients with cerebrovascular accident at the subacute stage. Archives of Physical Medicine and Rehabilitation 84:1609-1614.

Kelly, J.O., Kilbreath, S.L., Davis, G.M., Zeman, B., & Raymond, J. (2003). Cardiorespiratory fitness and walking ability in subacute stroke patients. Archives of Physical Medicine and Rehabilitation 84:1780-1785.

Lord, S.E., McPherson, K., McNaughton, H.K., Rochester, L., & Weatherall, M. (2004). Community ambulation after stroke: how important and obtainable is it and what measures appear predictive? Archives of Physical Medicine and Rehabilitation 85:234-239.

Lundin, A.P., Akerman, M.J., Chesler, R.M., Delano, B.G., Goldberg, N., Stein, R.A., & Friedman, E.A. (1991). Exercise in hemodialysis patients after treatment with recombinant human erythropoietin. Nephron 58:315-319.

Macko, R.F., Smith, G.V., Dobrovolny, C.L., Sorkin, J.D., Goldberg, A.P., & Silver, K.H. (2001). Treadmill training improves fitness reserve in chronic stroke patients. Archives of Physical Medicine and Rehabilitation 82:879-884.

Marrades, R.M., Roca, J., Campistol, J.M., Diaz, O., Barbera, J.A., Torregrosa, J.V., Masclans, J.R., Cobos, A., Rodriguez-Roisin, R., & Wagner, P.D. (1996). Effects of erythropoietin on muscle O_2 transport during exercise in patients with chronic renal failure. Journal of Clinical Investigation 97:2092-2100.

McCarty, M.F. (2000). Up-regulation of endothelial nitric oxide activity as a central strategy for prevention of ischemic stroke - just say NO to stroke. Medical Hypotheses 55:386-403.

McMahon, L.P., McKenna, M.J., Sangkabutra, T., Mason, K., Sostaric, S., Skinner, S.L., Burge, C., Murphy, B., & Crankshaw, D. (1999). Physical performance and associated electrolyte changes after haemoglobin normalization: a comparative study in haemodialysis patients. Nephrology, Dialysis, and Transplant 14:1182-1187.

Meek, C., Pollack, A., Potter, J., & Langhorne, P. (2003). A systematic review of exercise trials post stroke. Clinical Rehabilitation 17:6-13.

Moreland, J.D., Goldsmith, C.H., Huijbregts, M.P., Anderson, R.E., Prentice, D.M, Brunton, K.B., O'Brien, M.A., & Torresin, W.D. (2003). Progressive resistance strengthening exercises after stroke: a single-blind randomized controlled trial. Archives of Physical Medicine and Rehabilitation 84:1433-1440.

Moseley, A.M., Stark, A., Cameron, I.D., & Pollack, A. (2003). Treadmill training and body weight support for walking after stroke. Stroke 34:3006.

Mudge, S., Rochester, L., & Recordon, A. (2003). The effect of treadmill training on gait, balance and trunk control in a hemiplegic subject: a single system design. Disability and Rehabilitation 25:1000-1007.

Mullis, R., Campbell, I.T., Wearden, A.J., Morriss, R.K., & Pearson, D.J. (1999). Prediction of peak oxygen uptake in chronic fatigue syndrome. British Journal of Sports Medicine 33:352-356.

Mustonen, J., Laakso, M., Hirvonen, T., Mutru, O., Pirnes, M., Vainio, P., Kuikka, J.T., Rautio, P., & Lansimies, E. (1993). Abnormalities in left ventricular diastolic function in male patients with rheumatoid arthritis without clinically evident cardiovascular disease. European Journal of Clinical Investigation 23:246-253.

Noonan, V., Dean, E., & Dallimore, M. (2000). Are objective measures of disability related to self-reports in individuals with the late effects of poliomyelitis? A validation study. Archives of Physical Medicine and Rehabilitation 81:1422-1427.

Oyono-Enguelle, S., LeGallais, D., Lonsdorfer, A., Dah, C., Freund, H., Bogui, P., & Lonsdorfer, J. (2000). Cardiorespiratory and metabolic responses to exercise in HbSC sickle cell patients. Medicine and Science in Sports and Exercise 32:725-731.

Perry, J., Barnes, G., & Gronley, J.K. (1988). The postpolio syndrome: an overuse phenomenon. Clinical Orthopedics 233:145-162.

Pohl, M., Mehrholz, J., Ritschel, C., & Ruckriem, S. (2002). Speed-dependent treadmill training in ambulatory hemiparetic stroke patients: a randomized controlled trial. Stroke 33:553-558.

Price, D.T., Davidoff, R., & Balady, G.J. (2000). Comparison of cardiovascular adaptations to long-term arm and leg exercise in wheelchair athletes versus long-distance runners. American Journal of Cardiology 85:996-1001.

Qin, L., Au, S., Choy, W., Leung, P., Neff, M., Lee, K., Lau, M., Woo, J., & Chan, K. (2002). Regular Tai Chi Chuan exercise may retard bone loss in postmenopausal women: a case-controlled study. Archives of Physical Medicine and Rehabilitation 83:1355-1359.

Riolo, L., & Fisher, K. (2003). Is there evidence that strength training could help improve muscle function and other outcomes without reinforcing abnormal movement patterns or increasing reflex activity in a man who has had a stroke? Physical Therapy 83:844-851.

Rowland, T., Koenigs, L., & Miller, N. (2003). Myocardial performance during maximal exercise in adolescents with anorexia nervosa. Journal of Sports Medicine and Physical Fitness 43:202-208

Sala, E., Noyszewski, E.A., Campistol, J.M., Marrades, R.M., Dreha, S., Torregrossa, J.V., Beers, J.S., Wagner, P.D., & Roea, J. (2001). Impaired muscle oxygen transfer in patients with chronic renal failure. American Journal of Physiology. Regulatory, Integrative and Comparative Physiology 280:R1240-R1248.

Saunders, D.H., Greig, C.A., Young, A., & Mead, G.E. (2004). Physical fitness training for stroke patients. Cochrane Database Systematic Reviews 1, CD003316.

Schwaiblmair, M., Behr, J., & Fruhmann, G. (1996). Cardiorespiratory responses to incremental exercise in patients with systemic sclerosis. Chest 110:1520-1525.

Shepherd, R.B. (2001a). Exercise and training to optimize functional motor performance in stroke: driving neural reorganization? Neural Plasticity 8:121-129.

Shepherd, R.J. (2001b). Absolute versus relative intensity of physical activity in a dose response context. Medicine and Science in Sports and Exercise 33(Suppl 6):S400-S418.

Sullivan, K.J., Knowlton, B.J., & Dobkin, B.H. (2002). Step training with body weight support: effect of treadmill speed and practice paradigms on poststroke locomotor recovery. Archives of Physical Medicine and Rehabilitation 83:683-691.

Taivassalo, T., De Stefano, N., Chen, J., Karpati, G., Arnold, D.L., & Argove, Z. (1999). Short-term aerobic training response in chronic myopathies. Muscle Nerve 22:1239-1243.

Teixeira da Cunha-Filho, I., Henson, H., Qureshy, H., Williams, A.L., Holmes, S.A., & Protas, E.J. (2003). Differential responses to measures of gait performance among healthy and neurologically impaired individuals. Archives of Physical Medicine and Rehabilitation 84:1774-1779.

Thalamus, C., Stich, V., Riviere, D., Lafontan, M., & Berlan, M. (2003). Effects of a longitudinal training program on responses to exercise in overweight men. Obesity Research 11:247-256.

Vidal, J., Javierre, C., Segura, R., Lizarraga, A., Barbany, J.R., & Perez, A. (2003). Physiologic adaptations to exercise in people with spinal cord injury. Journal of Physiology and Biochemistry 59:11-18.

Weinberg, J., Borg, J., Bevegard, S., & Sinderby, C. (1999). Respiratory response to exercise in postpolio patients with severe inspiratory muscle dysfunction. Archives of Physical Medicine and Rehabilitation 80:1095-1100.

Weiss, H. (1991). The effect of an exercise program on vital capacity and rib mobility in patients with idiopathic scoliosis. Spine 16:88-93.

Williams, C. (1995). Haemoglobin - is more better? Nephrology, Dialysis, Transplantation 10(Suppl 2):48-55.

Wong, F., Girgrah, N., Graba, J., Allidina, Y., Liu, P., & Blendis, L. (2001). The cardiac response to exercise in cirrhosis. Gut 49:268-275.

C H A P T E R 2 6

Respiratory Muscle Training

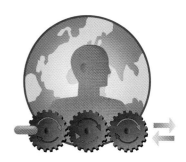

Rik Gosselink and Simone Dal Corso

The capacity of the respiratory muscle pump is vital for the movement of air to the level of gas exchange in the respiratory system. Impairment of the respiratory pump compromises ventilation, gas exchange, and tissue respiration. The respiratory muscles drive ventilation. In conditions where the load on the respiratory muscles is increased or the capacity of the respiratory muscles is decreased, muscle weakness can occur. Adaptations in breathing pattern (i.e., rapid shallow breathing), however, help counter muscle fatigue (Bellemare & Grassino, 1982). Although this adaptation decreases the efficacy of gas exchange, prevention of muscle fatigue will facilitate an alteration in breathing pattern to a lower tidal volume and higher breathing rate.

Although the adaptation in breathing pattern affects the efficacy of gas exchange, prevention of muscle fatigue and respiratory arrest modify breathing pattern (i.e., there is a decrease in tidal volume and an increase in breathing rate). Figure 26-1 illustrates this adaptation in patients at risk for respiratory failure. Respiratory muscle weakness increases the relative load for breathing (inspiratory pressure/maximum inspiratory pressure [PI/PI$_{max}$] ratio, see Figure 26-1) and this can lead to clinical consequences such as dyspnea, impaired exercise performance, ineffective coughing, respiratory insufficiency, weaning failure, and death. Dysfunction of the respiratory muscles is observed in several conditions, such as

chronic obstructive pulmonary disease, asthma, cystic fibrosis, neuromuscular disease including spinal cord injury, congestive heart failure, and in critical illness. This chapter describes the clinical relevance of respiratory muscle weakness, the assessment and testing of respiratory muscle function, and the application and effectiveness of respiratory muscle training for the conditions above, and its role in weaning some patients from mechanical ventilation.

RESPIRATORY MUSCLE ASSESSMENT

Respiratory Muscle Strength Testing

Clinically, respiratory muscle strength is measured as PI$_{max}$ and maximum expiratory pressure (PE$_{max}$). These pressures are measured using a small cylinder that fits to the patient's mouth with a circular mouthpiece (Figure 26-2). A small leak in the cylinder (two mm diameter and 15 mm length) prevents high pressures due to the contraction of the cheek muscles (Black & Hyatt, 1969). Standardizing the lung volume at which the pressures are measured is crucial (Coast & Weise, 1990). To prevent chest wall and lung recoil pressures from contributing to the pressure generated by the inspiratory muscles, measurements are recorded at functional residual capacity (FRC). This lung volume, however, is difficult to

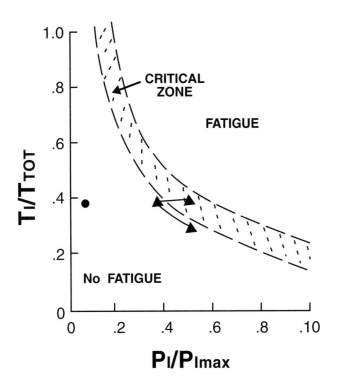

FIGURE 26-1 The relationship between relative contraction force (PI/PI_{max}) and relative contraction duration (T_I/T_{TOT}) in a healthy subject (●) and a patient with COPD (▲). The hatched area represents the critical zone in which fatigue develops. With progressive mechanical loading (e.g., exercise and acute exacerbation), the patients with COPD needs to increase PI and, therefore, might fall into the fatiguing zone (*dashed arrow*). This is generally avoided by a concomitant reduction in the duration of inspiration, T_I/T_{TOT} (*solid arrow*). This results in a decrease in tidal volume and a consequent increase in respiratory rate to maintain constant minute ventilation. Interventions aimed at reducing the load on the inspiratory muscles (PI) or increasing the maximum capacity of the inspiratory muscles (PI_{max}) reduce the relative contraction force of the inspiratory muscles. This prevents muscle fatigue and, thus, respiratory insufficiency. (*Adapted from Bellemare, F., & Grassino, A. [1982]. Effect of pressure and timing of contraction on human diaphragm fatigue. Journal of Applied Physiology 53:1190-1195).*

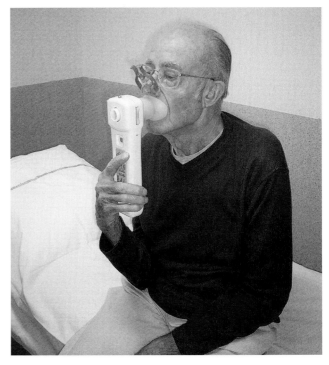

FIGURE 26-2 Assessment of respiratory muscle strength with measurement of mouth pressure.

standardize. In clinical practice, PI_{max} is measured from residual volume whereas PE_{max} is measured at total lung capacity (TLC). At least five repetitions should be performed. Respiratory muscle testing is described in detail in a recent American Thoracic Society/European Respiratory Society position statement (2002).

Several groups of investigators have published norms for PI_{max} and PE_{max} (Black & Hyatt, 1969; Rochester & Arora, 1983; Wilson et al, 1984) (Table 26-1). Regardless of the norms used, the standard deviation is typically large. Therefore, weakness is not easy to define (Polkey et al, 1995). Inspiratory weakness is defined as a PI_{max} lower than 50% of predicted (DeVito & Grassino, 1995) in the presence of clinical signs (e.g., dyspnea, impaired cough, and orthopnea) consistent with reduced respiratory muscle strength.

Other methods, such as the sniff maneuver, have been developed as tools to quantify global respiratory muscle function (Koulouris et al, 1989). The results of the sniff maneuver have been reported to be highly reliable in children with neuromuscular disease. More invasive methods such as electric or magnetic diaphragm stimulation can provide more accurate and detailed information on diaphragmatic function (Yan et al, 1992) and are useful in the diagnosis of diaphragmatic paresis. For most clinical applications, however, the assessment of inspiratory and expiratory mouth pressures is sufficient.

Respiratory Muscle Endurance Testing

Tests

Several tests for assessing respiratory muscle endurance capacity have been described. Most commonly the patient breathes against a submaximal inspiratory load (60% to 75% PI_{max}) for as long as possible (Rochester, 1988; Wanke et al, 1994). This test can detect changes in inspiratory muscle endurance after training. Incremental threshold loading, breathing against an incremental load (approximately five cm H_2O) every two minutes is also reproducible (Johnson et al, 1997). The highest load that can be sustained for two minutes is termed the sustainable pressure and is expressed as a percentage of the maximal load (Johnson et al, 1997; Martyn et al, 1987). Healthy people can usually sustain 70% of the PI_{max} for two minutes (Martyn et al, 1987). Johnson et al (1997) reported large intra individual variations in this percentage,

TABLE 26-1

Reference Values for Maximal Inspiratory and Expiratory Mouth Pressures in Healthy Adults

REFERENCE		PI_{max}	PE_{max}
Black & Hyatt (1969)	M	124 ± 22	233 ± 42
	F	87 ± 16	152 ± 27
Rinqvist (1966)	M	130 ± 32	237 ± 46
	F	98 ± 25	165 ± 30
Leech et al (1983)	M	114 ± 36	154 ± 82
	F	71 ± 27	94 ± 33
Rochester & Arora (1983)	M	127 ± 28	216 ± 41
	F	91 ± 25	138 ± 39
Wilson et al (1984)	M	106 ± 31	148 ± 17
	F	73 ± 22	93 ± 17
Vincken et al (1987)	M	105 ± 25	140 ± 38
	F	71 ± 23	89 ± 24
Bruschi et al (1992)	M	120 ± 37	140 ± 30
	F	84 ± 30	95 ± 20

M, Male; *F*, female.

which tends to decrease with age. The sustainable pressure has been shown to be more reduced than maximal inspiratory and expiratory pressures in individuals with chronic obstructive pulmonary disease (COPD) (Van't Hul et al, 1997). A third method (McKenzie & Gandevia, 1986, 1987; Gandevia et al, 1983) is a repetitive maximal inspiratory or expiratory maneuver performed against an occluded airway with a well-defined contraction duration (10 seconds) and relaxation time (five seconds). The relative decline in maximal pressure after 18 contractions is a measure of the endurance capacity of the respiratory muscles.

Modalities

Comparable to muscle training of the peripheral skeletal muscles, training of the respiratory muscles aims to improve specific characteristics of inspiratory or expiratory muscle contraction force, endurance, or velocity (Leith & Bradley, 1976; Tzelepis et al, 1994; Tzelepis et al, 1994).

Inspiratory Muscle Training

Because the inspiratory muscles are mainly involved in repetitive contractions with low intensity, training strategies emphasize enhancing inspiratory muscle endurance. Three types of training (i.e., inspiratory resistive training [Figure 26-3], threshold loading [Figure 26-4], and normocapnic hyperpnea [NCH] [Figure 26-5]) are currently practiced. During NCH, the patient is asked to breathe at a high proportion (>60%) of the maximal voluntary ventilation for 15 to 20 minutes (Leith & Bradley, 1976; Scherer et al, 2000). In the past the equipment used for this type of training was complicated, but recently a simpler, partial rebreathing system has been developed (Boutellier & Piwko, 1992).

During inspiratory resistive breathing the patient inhales through a mouthpiece with an adapter fitted with an adjustable diameter. This resistance is flow-dependent. Adequate training intensity is only achieved by feedback of the target pressure if flow and pressure are tightly coupled (Belman & Shadmehr, 1988). Recently a flow-independent resistance has been developed, the so-called 'threshold loading' valve, a valve that opens at a critical pressure (Nickerson & Keens, 1982; Gosselink et al, 1996). Training intensity varies across studies, from as high as maximal sustained inspiratory (Müller) maneuvers (Wanke et al, 1994) to 50% to 80% PI_{max} (Wanke et al, 1994; Dekhuijzen et al, 1991; Heijdra et al, 1996; Preusser et al, 1994) to a low intensity of 30% PI_{max} (Preusser et al, 1994; Larson et al, 1988; Lisboa et al, 1994; Lisboa et al, 1997). All these studies carefully controlled the target pressure or the threshold loading during training (Gosselink et al, 1996).

To date there are no data to support resistive or threshold loading as the training method of choice. The disadvantage of resistive breathing through a small hole is that the inspiratory pressure is flow dependent (Belman & Shadmehr, (1988). Threshold loading has the advantage of being independent of inspiratory flow rate (Gosselink et al, 1996) but requires a build-up of negative pressure before flow is initiated, hence, it is inertive in nature. Belman et al (1994) showed that similar work loads were obtained during resistive loading and threshold loading. The fact that threshold loading enhances velocity of inspiratory muscle shortening (Villafranca et al, 1998) could provide additional benefit because this shortens inspiratory time and increases time for exhalation and relaxation. Whether resistive loading or this inertive loading produces differential training effects remains to be studied (Gosselink & Decramer, 1994). Increased relaxation time may prevent the development of muscle fatigue in patients who are at risk.

Expiratory Muscle Training

Explosive expiratory maneuvers and low intensity contractions of abdominal muscles are similar to those involved

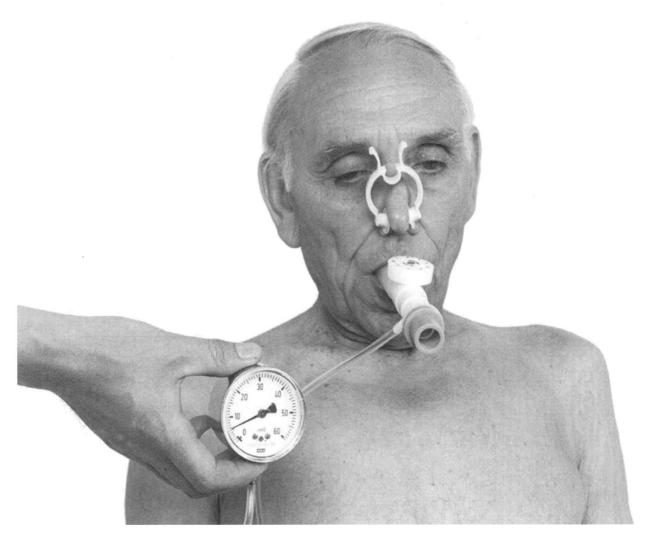

FIGURE 26-3 Resistive breathing device.

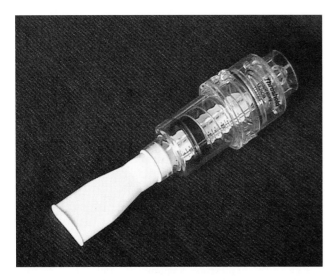

FIGURE 26-4 Threshold loading device.

in coughing, the Vasalva maneuver, and exercise. Consequently, training parameters for expiratory muscle training can be either high intensity strength training or moderate to low intensity endurance training. An example of the parameters for endurance expiratory muscle training is 30 minutes of continuous training at 15% to 45% of PE_{max} (Weiner et al, 2003). An example of strength training parameters is 15 Vasalva maneuvers at 60% of PE_{max} (Gosselink et al, 1998). Both training programs can be implemented using expiratory resistance at the mouth, such as threshold loading (Weiner et al, 2003; Gosselink et al, 1998).

RESPIRATORY MUSCLE TRAINING IN HEALTH

Because diaphragm fatigue can occur during sustained high intensity exercise (Johnson et al, 1993; Babcock et al, 1995), it is rational to improve the strength and endurance of the respiratory muscles in order to improve exercise performance.

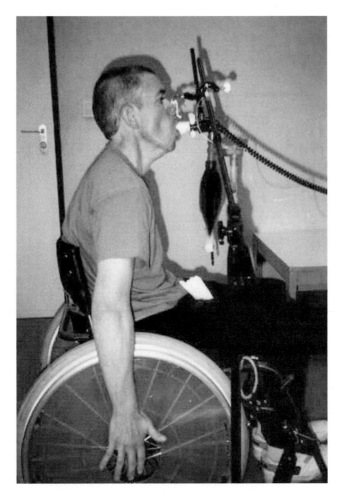

FIGURE 26-5 Normocapnic hyperpnea equipment.

TABLE 26-2

Effect Size of Inspiratory Muscle Training Based on Meta-analyses

	EFFECT SIZE	P VALUE
PI$_{max}$ (cm H$_2$O)	11	.001
Endurance (s)	154	.01
Endurance (cm H$_2$O)	10	.001
6M WD (m)	48	.11
Dyspnea (Borg)	-1.5	.01
Dyspnea (TDI)	+2.7	.01

PI$_{max}$, Maximal inspiratory pressure; *6MWD,* 6-minute walk distance; *Borg,* Borg scale of breathlessness; *TDI,* total dyspnea index.
From Lotters, F., van Tol, B., Kwakkel, G., & Gosselink, R. (2002). Effects of controlled inspiratory muscle training in patients with COPD: a meta-analysis. European Respiratory Journal 20:570-576.

Several uncontrolled studies (Boutellier & Piwko, 1992; Boutellier et al, 1992) have reported improved exercise performance after respiratory muscle endurance training. These were not randomized, controlled studies in which group responses were compared (Sonetti et al, 2001; Morgan et al, 1987). Markov et al (2001), however, observed an increase in endurance time but not in maximal exercise performance in an experimental group that was compared to a control group. In addition, Romer et al (2002) reported a decrease in the cycle time needed to cover 20 and 40 km and a decrease in perceived respiratory and peripheral exertion after respiratory muscle training compared to a placebo group. Based on our current understanding, the capacity to meet high ventilatory demands improves with inspiratory muscle training in healthy subjects. This does not, however, appear to be associated with improved maximal oxygen uptake or other physiological variables.

RESPIRATORY MUSCLE TRAINING IN DISEASE

COPD

Respiratory muscle weakness is often observed in patients with COPD (Decramer et al, 1980; Rochester & Braum, 1985;

Perez et al, 1996; Polkey et al, 1980; Polkey et al, 1996). Adaptation of the diaphragm results in greater fatigue resistance and improved muscle function (Levine et al, 1997; Orozco-Levi et al, 1999). The diaphragm is remodeled in part by the transformation of fast fiber types to slow fiber types (Levine et al, 2003; Levine et al, 2002). Despite these adaptations, both functional inspiratory muscle strength (Rochester & Braun, 1985) and endurance (Perez et al, 1996) remain compromised in patients with COPD and contribute to hypercapnia (Begin & Grassino, 1991), dyspnea (Killian & Jones, 1988; Hamilton et al, 1995), nocturnal oxygen desaturation (Heijdra et al, 1996), and reduced walking distance (Gosselink et al, 1996). During exercise, patients with COPD use a larger proportion of their maximal inspiratory pressure than healthy people (O'Donnell et al, 1997). This pattern of breathing is closely related to dyspnea during exercise (O'Donnell et al, 1997) and may induce respiratory muscle fatigue. The diaphragm, however, does not appear to fatigue after exhaustive exercise (Polkey et al, 1995). There is compelling evidence to suggest that breathing against an inspiratory load increases both maximal inspiratory pressure (Wanke et al, 1994; Belman & Shadmehr, 1988; Dekhuijzen et al, 1991; Heijdra et al, 1996; Preusser et al, 1994; Larson et al, 1988; Lisboa et al, 1994; Lisboa et al, 1997; Patessio et al, 1989) and endurance of the inspiratory muscles (Belman & Shadmehr, 1988; Heijdra et al, 1996; Preusser et al, 1994; Patessio et al, 1989). Respiratory muscle training has been reported to produce hypertrophy of predominantly type I and IIA fibers in the diaphragms of hamsters (Bisschop et al, 1997; Rollier et al, 1998). The proportion of type I fibers and size of type II fibers in the external intercostals after inspiratory muscle training (IMT) has been recently reported to increase in a study of patients with COPD (Ramirez-Sarmiento et al, 2002). Dyspnea (Lisboa et al, 1994; Lisboa et al, 1997; Harver et al, 1989) and nocturnal desaturation time (Heijdra et al, 1996) also decreased, while exercise performance tended to improve (Lotters et al, 2002) (Table 26-2).

Inspiratory muscle training in addition to exercise training can improve exercise capacity more than exercise training alone (Wanke et al, 1994; Dekhuijzen et al, 1991; Larson et al, 1988; Lisboa et al, 1997). In a recent meta-analysis, the additional effect of IMT on exercise performance appeared related to inspiratory muscle weakness (Lotters et al, 2002). Long-term effects were shown for exercise performance and dyspnea in patients with COPD who continued performing their training program three times per week at high training intensity (60% PI_{max}) (Weiner et al, 2002).

NCH was applied in one randomized controlled trial and resulted in enhanced respiratory muscle endurance and exercise capacity as well as quality of life in patients with COPD (Scherer et al, 2000).

Well-controlled inspiratory muscle training for people with inspiratory muscle weakness secondary to COPD can improve inspiratory muscle function and lead to further improvement in exercise capacity and decreased dyspnea and nocturnal desaturation time. Training intensity should be at least 30% of the maximal inspiratory pressure for 30 minutes per day. Threshold loading, resistive breathing, and normocapnic hyperpnea have not been shown to be superior to one another.

Asthma

Respiratory muscle weakness is not frequently observed in patients with asthma (Weiner et al, 2002; De Bruin et al, 1997; Lavietes et al, 1988). Although some studies report a moderate reduction in inspiratory muscle strength (De Bruin et al, 1997), other studies have not found inspiratory muscle strength to be affected (Perez et al, 1996; McKenzie & Gandevina, 1986). Inspiratory muscle endurance has been shown to be increased in people with asthma (McKenzie & Gandevina, 1986) but reduced in those who are steroid dependent (Perez et al, 1996). In patients with asthma, dyspnea has been observed to be greater in woman than man, resulting in their greater need for beta-2 agonists. This may reflect sex differences in inspiratory muscle strength (Weiner et al, 2002). IMT has been studied in people with asthma, and evidence from randomized trials support that, in addition to improvements in inspiratory muscle strength, dyspnea and beta-2 agonist consumption was reduced in those with high dyspnea and high utilization of beta-2 agonists (Weiner et al, 2000), especially among women (Weiner et al, 2002). A recent Cochrane review, however, concluded that the evidence supporting a role for inspiratory muscle training for people with asthma was inconclusive (Ram et al, 2003).

Cystic Fibrosis

Reports on the inspiratory muscle strength of people with cystic fibrosis (CF) have also been contradictory. Some have shown that inspiratory muscle strength is decreased (Pradal et al, 1994; Szeinberg et al, 1985; Mier et al, 1990; Lands et al, 1990), some have shown that it is normal (Lands et al, 1993; Hanning et al, 1993), and others have shown it is supranormal (Asher et al, 1982; O'Neill et al, 1983; Marks et al, 1986). The discrepancy across studies can be attributed to methodo-

logical inconsistencies such as age, degree of pulmonary dysfunction, nutritional status, and the assessment of PI_{max}. Normal or supranormal PI_{max} in this population can be explained physiologically. For example, abnormalities in pulmonary function (e.g., airflow obstruction, hyperinflation, and airway resistance) could produce a training effect (Lands et al, 1993; De Jong et al, 2001; Enright et al, 2004).

There are few reports on IMT in patients with CF (Asher et al, 1982; De Jong et al, 2001; Enright et al, 2004; Keen et al, 1977; Sawyer & Clanton, 1993). The protocols to train inspiratory muscle in these patients are similar to those used in the management of other conditions, such as COPD and asthma. As yet there is no consensus by experts regarding the optimal training intensity for patients with CF. Even though training at low intensity improves inspiratory endurance (De Jong et al, 2001), high intensity training can further augment inspiratory muscle function, pulmonary function, and exercise capacity (Enright et al, 2004).

IMT may have a role in the management of some patients with CF because of its benefits on respiratory strength, endurance, and exercise performance in individuals with other types of chronic lung dysfunction.

Quadriplegia

Several studies have reported that inspiratory or expiratory muscle training is a means of enhancing inspiratory or expiratory muscle function in individuals with quadriplegia, reducing dyspnea, and improving exercise performance (Uijl et al, 1999; Liauw et al, 2000; Estenne et al, 1989). There is some controversy in the literature. Although limited, some evidence supports that pulmonary function and expiratory muscle strength are improved. Based on evidence from randomized controlled trials, however, inspiratory muscle strength, endurance, exercise capacity, and clinical symptoms do not appear to improve.

Neurological and Neuromuscular Disease

Independent of the site of the pathology (e.g., the central nervous system, peripheral nerves, neuromuscular junction and/or muscles themselves), respiratory muscle weakness associated with other factors (e.g., pulmonary dysfunction and immobility) plays a role in increasing the risk of ventilatory failure and respiratory complications, and hence of morbidity and mortality.

In patients with amyotrophic lateral sclerosis (ALS), involvement of inspiratory muscle weakness is prominent and underlies ventilatory insufficiency and symptoms, while expiratory muscle weakness is mainly present in symptomatic patients and affects cough (Polkey et al, 1998). Patients with Parkinson syndrome can exhibit respiratory muscle weakness even if the severity is mild, but the syndrome is less associated with dyspnea (Weiner et al, 2002). The weakness is associated with impaired exercise performance while quality of life appears unaffected (Haas et al, 2004). Respiratory muscle function is affected in patients with acute ischemic stroke but it is not related to dyspnea (Lanini et al, 2002). Diaphragm contractility is affected on the contralateral side, which may be related to an increased incidence of pneumonia (Urban et al, 2002). To our knowledge there are no published reports evaluating the outcomes of respiratory muscle training in patients with stroke, ALS, or Parkinson syndrome. Although inspiratory muscle function is commonly affected in neurological disease, expiratory muscle function can, in contrast, be preferentially impaired such as in multiple sclerosis; thus expiratory muscle training has been shown to be beneficial (Gosselink et al, 1999).

In patients with neuromuscular disease (NMD), the mechanisms underlying respiratory muscle dysfunction are complex and dependent on the particular disease and its stage. The indications for IMT in NMD are based on the benefits of strengthening the respiratory muscles, which may delay pulmonary complications and the onset of respiratory failure (McCool & Tzelepis, 1995). Studies have reported improved respiratory muscle function after IMT in different types of NMD (DiMarco & Kelling, 1985; Winkler et al, 2000; Gozal & Thiriet, 1999). A correlation exists between training intensity and improvement of respiratory muscle capacity (Winkler et al, 2000). Patients with NMD who have more than 25% of predicted pulmonary function can respond to training (Wanke et al, 1994; Gozal & Thiriet, 1999). Patients with severe impairment of ventilatory function, however, may show less improvement in respiratory strength because they are not able to achieve the critical training intensity, respiratory muscle weakness may predispose their muscle to damage rather than the benefits of training, and their muscle mass may be insufficient. In the long term the progression of most neuromuscular diseases affecting muscle probably impedes an optimal training effect.

Inspiratory and expiratory training enhances the respiratory muscle performance in patients with NMD. The transfer of these gains to increased cough effectiveness, reduced respiratory infection, and delayed ventilatory failure remains unclear.

Chronic Heart Failure

Although impairment of cardiac function is the principal factor associated with reduced functional capacity in people with chronic heart failure (CHF), abnormal respiratory muscle function plays an important role in premature exercise termination and contributes to sensory consequences, especially breathlessness on exertion. Exertional dyspnea can result from respiratory muscle weakness, increased respiratory muscles activity, or both (Killian & Jones, 1988).

An impressive body of literature supports the notion that reduced respiratory muscle strength in patients with CHF results from both volitional (Ambrosino et al, 1994; Hammond et al, 1990; McParland et al, 1992) and non-volitional (twitch transdiaphragmatic pressure) (Hughes et al, 1999) measurements. Changes in pulmonary function secondary to ventricular dysfunction, increased left ventricular size, chronic pulmonary congestion, reduced lung compliance, and increased airway resistance (Evans et al, 1995) result in an altered breathing pattern in which patients breathe at rest near residual volume and are expiratory-flow limited with little or minimal exercise (Johnson et al, 1999). Therefore the ventilatory muscles are subjected to increased work of breathing (WOB) (Evans et al, 1995; Clark & Coasts, 1992), which may lead to respiratory muscle fatigue. As a positive consequence of the high WOB in people with heart failure, however, the diaphragm exhibits a predominance of slow myosin heavy chain isoforms with an increase in oxidative enzymes and a decrease in glycolitic capacity (Tikunov et al, 1997). These adaptations are similar to those observed after endurance training of the limb muscles in healthy people. These observations are consistent with the well preserved endurance of the inspiratory muscles when expressed as a function of endurance time, and the inspiratory muscle load-to-capacity ratio in patients with CHF (Hart et al, 2004).

The effects of inspiratory muscle training in patients with CHF have been well documented (Mancini et al, 1995; Cahalin et al, 1997; Johnson et al, 1998; Weiner et al, 1999; Darnley et al, 1999; Martinez et al, 2001; Laoutaris et al, 2004). There is no consensus in the literature related to types of training, intensity, and duration of IMT, which can explain the wide variation in the responses of patients with CHF to IMT. Based on the literature, the recommended intensity is at least 30% of PI_{max} (Mancini et al, 1995; Johnson et al, 1998; Martinez et al, 2001), but an intensity of 60% of PI_{max} (Laoutaris et al, 2004) has also been also recommended. In the majority of studies, patients performed IMT three times per week (Mancini et al, 1995; Cahalin et al, 1997; Darnley et al, 1999; Laoutaris et al, 2004). The duration of each session was between 15 and 30 minutes.

IMT in CHF increases inspiratory strength (Mancini et al, 1995; Cahalin et al, 1997; Johnson et al, 1998; Weiner et al, 1999; Martinez et al, 2001; Laoutaris et al, 2004) and endurance (Weiner et al, 1999; Darnley et al, 1999; Laoutaris et al, 2004; Mancini et al, 1995; Martinez et al, 2001), increases maximal exercise capacity as reflected by improvement of exercise duration (Darnley et al, 1999) or oxygen consumption (Mancini et al, 1995; Martinez et al, 2001; Laoutaris et al, 2004), increases submaximal exercise capacity evaluated by the 12-minute walking test (Weiner et al, 1999) and six-minute walking distance (Mancini et al, 1995; Martinez et al, 2001; Laoutaris et al, 2004), and improves dyspnea (Cahalin et al, 1997; Weiner et al, 1999; Darnley et al, 1999; Martinez et al, 2001; Laoutaris et al, 2004) and quality of life (Laoutaris et al, 2004).

Based on its capacity to improve respiratory muscle performance and exercise capacity, IMT can be considered an additional tool that is safe and effective in the comprehensive management of respiratory muscle dysfunction in patients with CHF.

Weaning Failure

The majority (75% to 80%) of patients who are mechanically ventilated can be weaned to breathe spontaneously without difficulty (Nava & Rubini, 2001). Patients who experience difficulty weaning have poorer prognoses that include increased mortality, longer intensive care unit (ICU) stay, and prolonged rehabilitation. Several factors contribute to weaning failure, such as the underlying disease, age, muscle weakness, malnutrition, hypoxemia and hypercapnia, and medications (e.g., corticosteroids and muscle relaxants). The method of weaning affects the outcome (Nava & Rubini, 2001). Current expert opinion supports that familiarity and skill are the most important determinants of the choice of weaning. The specific method seems less important. Weaning based on bedside assessment and the use of standardized protocols is effective. Daily screening of respiratory function and trials of spontaneous breathing result in shortening of the period of mechanical ventilation and thus the costs and complications associated with an ICU stay (Cohen et al, 1991; Horst et al, 1998; Ely et al, 1996; Kollef et al, 1997; Nava et al, 1997). These therapist-driven protocols are action plans based on consensus and expert opinion. Physical therapists contribute to the assessment and treatment of patients who have difficulty being weaned from mechanical ventilation. Respiratory muscle weakness is a frequent cause of weaning failure. Uncontrolled trials suggest that inspiratory muscle training during the weaning period could facilitate the weaning process (Aldrich et al, 1989; Aldrich & Uhrlass, 1987; Martin et al, 2002; Sprague & Hopkins, 2003). Biofeedback of the pattern of breathing to the patient can also enhance the weaning process of patients receiving long-term mechanical ventilation (Holiday & Hyers, 1990).

SUMMARY

Respiratory muscle weakness and fatigue have been identified in a variety of conditions and associated with clinically important symptoms such as dyspnea, impaired cough, exercise impairment, respiratory insufficiency, weaning failure, and survival. Respiratory muscle training is a treatment option for weak respiratory muscles seen in a wide range of conditions. However, its indications, contraindications, and the specific criteria that determine the type of testing and training, intensity of training, and potential side-effects warrant elucidation. Regardless, tools have emerged that are enabling physical therapists to identify and assess the severity of respiratory muscle weakness and thereby intervene in a timely and effective manner.

Review Questions

1. Define respiratory muscle weakness and how it is measured. How does it clinically manifest?
2. Distinguish respiratory muscle weakness from respiratory muscle fatigue.
3. How are respiratory muscle strength and endurance related to exercise capacity, and how is exercise capacity related to respiratory muscle strength and endurance?
4. Describe current concepts and principles related to respiratory muscle strength testing.

5. Describe how respiratory muscle endurance testing differs from respiratory muscle strength training. What are the training implications?
6. Distinguish between inspiratory and expiratory muscle training, how they are assessed, and how their different training programs are prescribed.
7. Explain what the differences in inspiratory and expiratory muscle strength and endurance indicate about individuals with each of the following conditions: asthma, cystic fibrosis, quadriplegia, and chronic heart failure.
8. How might respiratory muscle training augment weaning? How would the indications be established?
9. What remains to be elucidated in the area of respiratory muscle testing and training?

REFERENCES

Aldrich, T. K., Karpel, J.P., Uhrlass, R.M., Sparapani, M.A., Eramo, D., & Ferranti, R. (1989). Weaning from mechanical ventilation: adjunctive use of inspiratory muscle resistive training. Critical Care Medicine 17:143-147.

Aldrich, T. K., & Uhrlass, R.M. (1987). Weaning from mechanical ventilation: successful use of modified inspiratory resistive training in muscular dystrophy. Critical Care Medicine 15:247-249.

Ambrosino, N., Opasich, C., Crotti, P., Cobelli, F., Tavazzi, L., & Rampulla, C. (1994). Breathing pattern, ventilatory drive and respiratory muscle strength in patients with chronic heart failure. European Respiratory Journal 7:17-22.

Asher, M.I., Pardy, R.L., Coates, A.L., Thomas, E., & Macklem, P.T. (1982). The effects of inspiratory muscle training in patients with cystic fibrosis. American Review of Respiratory Disease 126:855-859.

American Thoracic Society/European Respiratory Society. (2002). ATS/ERS Statement on respiratory muscle testing. American Journal of Respiratory Critical Care Medicine 166:518-624.

Babcock, M.A., Pegelow, D.F., McClaran, S.R., Suman, O.E., & Dempsey, J.A. (1995). Contribution of diaphragmatic power output to exercise-induced diaphragm fatigue. Journal of Applied Physiology 78:1710-1719.

Begin, P., & Grassino, A. (1991). Inspiratory muscle dysfunction and chronic hypercapnia in chronic obstructive pulmonary disease. American Review of Respiratory Disease 143:905-912.

Bellemare, F., & Grassino, A. (1982). Effect of pressure and timing of contraction on human diaphragm fatigue. Journal of Applied Physiology 53:1190-1195.

Belman, M.J., & Shadmehr, R. (1988). Targeted resistive ventilatory muscle training in chronic pulmonary disease. Journal of Applied Physiology 65:2726-2735.

Belman, M.J., Warren, C.B., Nathan, S.D., & Chon, K.H. (1994). Ventilatory load characteristics during ventilatory muscle training. American Journal of Respiratory Critical Care Medicine 149:925-929.

Bisschop, A., Gayan-Ramirez, G., Rollier, H., Gosselink, R., de Bock, V., & Decramer, M. (1997). Intermittent inspiratory muscle training induces fiber hypertrophy in rat diaphragm. American Journal of Respiratory Critical Care Medicine 155:1583-1589.

Black, L.F., & Hyatt, R.E. (1969). Maximal respiratory pressures: normal values and relationship to age and sex. American Review of Respiratory Disease 99:696-702.

Boutellier, U., & Piwko, P. (1992). The respiratory system as an exercise limiting factor in normal sedentary subjects. European Journal of Applied Physiology 64:145-152.

Boutellier, U., Buchel, R., Kundert, A., & Spengler, C. (1992). The respiratory system as an exercise limiting factor in normal trained subjects. European Journal of Applied Physiology 65:347-353.

Bruschi, C., Cerveri, I., & Zoia, M.C. (1992). Reference values of maximal respiratory mouth pressures: a population-based study. American Review of Respiratory Disease 146:790-793.

Cahalin, L.P., Semigran, M.J., & Dec, G.W. (1997). Inspiratory muscle training in patients with chronic heart failure awaiting cardiac transplantation: results of a pilot clinical trial. Physical Therapy 77:830-838.

Clark, A., & Coats, A. (1992). The mechanisms underlying the increased ventilatory response to exercise in chronic stable heart failure. European Heart Journal 13:1698-1708.

Coast, J. R., & Weise, S.D. (1990). Lung volume changes and maximal inspirator pressure. Journal of Cardiopulmonary Rehabilitation 10:461-464.

Cohen, I.L., Bari, N., Strosberg, M.A., Weinberg, P.F., Wacksman, R.M., Millstein, B.H., & Fein, I.A. (1991). Reduction of duration and cost of mechanical ventilation in an intensive care unit by use of a ventilatory management team. Critical Care Medicine 19:1278-1284.

Darnley, G.M., Gray, A.C., McClure, S.J., Neary, P., Petrie, M., McMurray, J.J., & MacFarlane, N.G. (1999). Effects of resistive breathing on exercise capacity and diaphragm function in patients with ischaemic heart disease. European Journal of Heart Failure 1:297-300.

DeBruin, P.F., Ueki, J., Watson, A., & Pride, N.B. (1997). Size and strength of the respiratory and quadriceps muscles in patients with chronic asthma. European Respiratory Journal 10:59-64.

Decramer, M., Demedts, M., Rochette, F., & Billiet, L. (1980). Maximal transrespiratory pressures in obstructive lung disease. Bulletin European Physiopathological Respiration 16:479-490.

DeJong, W., van Aalderen, W.M., Kraan, J., Koeter, G.H., & van der Schans, C.P. (2001). Inspiratory muscle training in patients with cystic fibrosis. Respiratory Medicine 95:31-36.

Dekhuijzen, P.N., Folgering, H.T., & van Herwaarden, C.L. (1991). Target-flow inspiratory muscle training during pulmonary rehabilitation in patients with COPD. Chest 99:128-133.

DeVito, E., & Grassino, A. (1995). Respiratory muscle fatigue. Rationale for diagnostic tests. In Roussos, C. (Ed). The thorax, ed 2. New York: Marcel Dekker Inc.

DiMarco, A.F., & Kelling, J.S. (1985). The effects of inspiratory resistive training on respiratory muscle function in patients with muscular dystrophy. Muscle Nerve 8:284-290.

Ely, E.W., Baker, A.M., Dunagan, D.P., Burke, H.L., Smith, A.C., Kelly, P.T., Johnson, M.M., Browder, R.W., Bowton, D.L., & Haponik, E.F. (1996). Effect on the duration of mechanical ventilation of identifying patients capable of breathing spontaneously. New England Journal of Medicine 335: 1864-1869.

Enright, S., Chatham, K., Ionescu, A.A., Unnithan, V.B., & Shale, D.J. (2004). Inspiratory muscle training improves lung function and exercise capacity in adults with cystic fibrosis. Chest 126: 405-411.

Estenne, M., Knoop, C., Vanvaerenbergh, J., Heilporn, A., & De Troyer, A. (1989). The effect of pectoralis muscle training in tetraplegic subjects. American Review of Respiratory Disease 139:1218-1222.

Evans, S.A., Watson, L., Cowley, A.J., Johnston, I.D., & Kinnear, W.J. (1995). Static lung compliance in chronic heart failure: relation with dyspnoea and exercise capacity. Thorax 50:245-248.

Gandevia, S.C., McKenzie, D.K., & Neering, I.R. (1983). Endurance capacity of respiratory and limb muscles. Respiratory Physiology 53:47-61.

Gosselink, R., Wagenaar, R.C., & Decramer, M. (1996). The reliability of a commercially available threshold loading device. Thorax 51:601-605.

Gosselink, R., Kovacs, L., & Decramer, M. (1999). Respiratory muscle involvement in multiple sclerosis. European Respiratory Journal 13:449-454.

Gosselink, R., Kovacs, L., Ketelaer, P., Carton, H., & Decramer, M. (2000). Respiratory muscle weakness and respiratory muscle training in severely disabled multiple sclerosis patients. Archives of Physical Medical Rehabilitation 81:747-751.

Gosselink, R., & Decramer, M. (1994). Inspiratory muscle training: where are we? European Respiratory Journal 7:2103-2105.

Gosselink, R., Troosters, T., & Decramer, M. (1996). Peripheral muscle weakness contributes to exercise limitation in COPD. American Journal of Respiratory Critical Care Medicine 153:976-980.

Gozal, D., Thiriet, P. (1999). Respiratory muscle training in neuro-muscular disease: long-term effects on strength and load perception. Medical Science of Sports Exercise 31:1522-1527.

Haas, B.M., Trew, M., & Castle, P.C. (2004). Effects of respiratory muscle weakness on daily living function, quality of life, activity levels, and exercise capacity in mild to moderate Parkinson's disease. American Journal of Physical Medical Rehabilitation 83:601-607.

Hamilton, N., Killian, K.J., Summers, E., & Jones, N.L. (1995). Muscle strength, symptom intensity, and exercise capacity in patients with cardiorespiratory disorders. American Journal of Respiratory Critical Care Medicine 152:2021-2031.

Hammond, M.D., Bauer, K.A., Sharp, J.T., & Rocha, R.D. (1990). Respiratory muscle strength in congestive heart failure. Chest 98:1091-1094.

Hanning, R.M., Blimkie, C.J., Bar-Or, O., Lands, L.C., Moss, L.A., & Wilson, W.M. (1993). Relationships among nutritional status and skeletal and respiratory muscle function in cystic fibrosis: does early dietary supplementation make a difference? American Journal of Clinical Nutrition 57:580-587.

Hart, N., Kearney, M.T., Pride, N.B., Green, M., Lofaso, F., Shah, A.M., Moxham, J., & Polkey, M.I. (2004). Inspiratory muscle load and capacity in chronic heart failure. Thorax 59:477-482.

Harver, A., Mahler, D.A., & Daubenspeck, J.A. (1989). Targeted inspiratory muscle training improves respiratory muscle function and reduces dyspnea in patients with chronic obstructive pulmonary disease. Annals of Internal Medicine 111:117-124.

Heijdra, Y.F., Dekhuijzen, P.N., van Herwaarden, C.L., & Folgering, T.H. (1996). Nocturnal saturation improves by target-flow inspiratory muscle training in patients with COPD. American Journal of Respiratory Critical Care Medicine 153:260-265.

Holliday, J.E., & Hyers, T.M. (1990). The reduction of weaning time from mechanical ventilation using tidal volume and relaxation biofeedback. American Review of Respiratory Disease 141: 1214-1220.

Horst, H.M., Mouro, D., Hall-Jenssens, R.A., & Pamukov, N. (1998). Decrease in ventilation time with a standardized weaning process. Archives of Surgery 133:483-488.

Hughes, P.D., Polkey, M.I., Harrus, M.L., Coats, A.J, Moxham, J., & Green, M. (1999). Diaphragm strength in chronic heart failure. American Journal of Respiratory Critical Care Medicine 160:529-534.

Johnson, B.D., Weisman, I.M., Zeballos, R.J., & Beck, K.C. (1999). Emerging concepts in the evaluation of ventilatory limitation during exercise: the exercise tidal flow-volume loop. Chest 116:488-503.

Johnson, B.D., Babcock, M.A., Suman, O.E., & Dempsey, J.A. (1993). Exercise-induced diaphragmatic fatigue in healthy humans. Journal of Physiology 460:385-405.

Johnson, P.H., Cowley, A.J., & Kinnear, W.J. (1997). Incremental threshold loading: a standard protocol and establishment of a reference range in naive normal subjects. European Respiratory Journal 10:2868-2871.

Johnson, P.H., Cowley, A.J., & Kinnear, W.J. (1998). A randomized controlled trial of inspiratory muscle training in stable chronic heart failure. European Heart Journal 19:1249-1253.

Keens, T.G., Krastins, I.R.B., Wannamaker, E.M., Levison, H., Crozier, D.N., & Bryan, A.C. (1977). Ventilatory muscle endurance training in normal subjects and patients with cystic fibrosis. American Review of Respiratory Disease 116:853-860.

Killian, K.J., & Jones, N.L. (1988). Respiratory muscles and dyspnea. Clinical Chest Medicine 9:237-248.

Kollef, M.H., Shapiro, S.D., Silver, P., St. John, R.E., Prentice, D., Sauer, S., Ahrens, T.S., Shannon, W., & Baker-Clinkscale, D. (1997). A randomized, controlled trial of protocol-directed versus physician-directed weaning from mechanical ventilation. Critical Care Medicine 25:567-574.

Koulouris, N., Mulvey, D.A., Laroche, C.M., Sawicka, E.H., Green, M., & Moxham, J. (1989). The measurement of inspiratory muscle strength by sniff esophageal, nasopharyngeal, and mouth pressures. American Review of Respiratory Disease 139:641-646.

Lands, L., Desmond, K.J., Demizio, D., Pavilanis, A., & Coates, A.L. (1990). The effects of nutritional status and hyperinflation on respiratory muscle strength in children and young adults. American Review of Respiratory Disease 141:1506-1509.

Lands, L.C., Heigenhauser, G.J.F., & Jones, N.L. (1993). Respiratory and peripheral muscle function in cystic fibrosis. American Review of Respiratory Disease 147:865-869.

Lanini, B., Gigliotti, F., Coli, C., Bianchi, R., Pizzi, A., Romagnoli, I., Grazzini, M., Stendardi, L., & Scano, G. (2002). Dissociation between respiratory effort and dyspnoea in a subset of patients with stroke. Clinical Science (London) 103:467-473.

Laoutaris, I., Dritsas, A., Brown, M.D., Manginas, A., Alivizatos, P.A., & Cokkinos, D.V. (2004). Inspiratory muscle training using an incremental endurance test alleviates dyspnea and improves functional status in patients with chronic heart failure. European Journal of Cardiovascular Prevention and Rehabilitation 11: 489-496.

Larson, J.L., Kim, M.J., Sharp, J.T., & Larson, D.A. (1988). Inspiratory muscle training with a pressure threshold breathing device in patients with chronic obstructive pulmonary disease. American Review of Respiratory Disease 138:689-696.

Lavietes, M.H., Grocela, J.A., Maniatis, T., Potulski, F., Ritter, A.B., & Sunderam, G. (1988). Inspiratory muscle strength in asthma. Chest 93:1043-1048.

Leech, J.A., Ghezzo, H., Stevens, D., & Blecklake, M.R. (1983). Respiratory pressures and function in young adults. American Review of Respiratory Disease 128:17-23.

Leith, D.E., & Bradley, M.E. (1976). Ventilatory muscle strength and endurance training. Journal of Applied Physiology 41:508-516.

Levine, S., Gregory, C., Nguyen, T., Shrager, J., Kaiser, L., Rubinstein, N., & Dudley, G. (2002). Bioenergetic adaptation of individual human diaphragmatic myofibers to severe COPD. Journal of Applied Physiology 92:1205-1213.

Levine, S., Kaiser, L., Leferovich, J., & Tikunov, B. (1997). Cellular adaptations in the diaphragm in chronic obstructive pulmonary disease. New England Journal of Medicine 337:1799-1806.

Levine, S., Nguyen, T., Kaiser, L.R., Rubinstein, N.A., Maislin, G., Gregory, C., Rome, L.C., Dudley, G.A., Sieck, G.C., & Shrager, J.B. (2003). Human diaphragm remodeling associated with chronic obstructive pulmonary disease: clinical implications. American Journal of Respiratory Critical Care Medicine 168:706-713.

Liauw, M.Y., Lin, M.C., Cheng, P.T., Wong, M.K., & Tang, F.T. (2000). Resistive inspiratory muscle training: its effectiveness in patients with acute complete cervical cord injury. Archives of Physical Medical Rehabilitation 81:752-756.

Lisboa, C., Villafranca, C., Leiva, A., Cruz, E., Pertuze, J., & Borzone, G. (1997). Inspiratory muscle training in chronic airflow limitation: effect on exercise performance. European Respiratory Journal 10:537-542.

Lisboa, C., Munoz, V., Beroiza, T., Leiva, A., & Cruz, E. (1994). Inspiratory muscle training in chronic airflow limitation: comparison of two different training loads with a threshold device. European Respiratory Journal 7:1266-1274.

Lotters, F., van Tol, B., Kwakkel, G., & Gosselink, R. (2002). Effects of controlled inspiratory muscle training in patients with COPD: a meta-analysis. European Respiratory Journal 20:570-576.

Mancini, D.M., Henson, D., La Manca, J., Donchez, L., & Levine, S. (1995). Benefit of selective respiratory muscle training on exercise capacity in patients with chronic congestive heart failure. Circulation 91:320-329.

Markov, G., Spengler, C.M., Knopfli-Lenzin, C., Stuessi, C., & Boutellier, U. (2001). Respiratory muscle training increases cycling endurance without affecting cardiovascular responses to exercise. European Journal of Applied Physiology 85:233-239.

Marks, J., Pasterkamp, H., Tal, A., & Leahy, F. (1986). Relationship between respiratory muscle strength, nutritional status, and lung volume in cystic fibrosis and asthma. American Review of Respiratory Disease 133:414-417.

Martin, A.D., Davenport, P.D., Franceschi, A.C., & Harman, E. (2002). Use of inspiratory muscle strength training to facilitate ventilator weaning: a series of 10 consecutive patients. Chest 122:192-196.

Martinez, A., Lisboa, C., Jalil, J., Munoz, V., Diaz, O., Casanegra, P., Corbalan, R., Vasquez, A.M., & Leiva, A. (2001). Selective training of respiratory muscles in patients with chronic heart failure. Revista medica de Chile 129:133-139.

Martyn, J.B., Moreno, R.H., Pare, P.D., & Pardy, R.L. (1987). Measurement of inspiratory muscle performance with incremental threshold loading. American Review of Respiratory Disease 135:919-923.

McCool, F.D., & Tzelepis, G.E. (1995). Inspiratory muscle training in patients with neuromuscular disease. Physical Therapy 75:1006-1014.

McKenzie, D.K., & Gandevia, S.C. (1986). Strength and endurance of inspiratory, expiratory and limb muscles in asthma. American Review of Respiratory Disease 134:999-1004.

McKenzie, D.K., & Gandevia, S.C. (1987). Influence of muscle length on human inspiratory and limb muscle endurance. Respiratory Physiology 67:171-182.

McParland, C., Krishnan, B., Wang, Y., & Gallagher, C.G. (1992). Inspiratory muscle weakness and dyspnea in chronic heart failure. American Review of Respiratory Disease 146:467-472.

Mier, A., Redington, A., Brophy, C., Hodson, M., & Green, M. (1990). Respiratory muscle function in cystic fibrosis. Thorax 45:750-752.

Morgan, D.W., Kohrt, W.M., Bates, B.J., & Skinner, J.S. (1987). Effects of respiratory muscle endurance training on ventilatory and endurance performance of moderately trained cyclists. International Journal of Sports Medicine 8:88-93.

Nava, S., & Rubini, F. (2001). Noninvasive mechanical ventilation to facilitate weaning from mechanical ventilation. In Hill, N.S., & Levy, M. (Eds). Ventilator management strategies for critical care. New York: Marcel Dekker.

Nava, S., Evangelisti, I., Rampulla, C., Compagnoni, M.L., Fracchia, C., & Rubini, F. (1997). Human and financial costs of noninvasive mechanical ventilation in patients affected by COPD and acute respiratory failure. Chest 111:1631-1638.

Nickerson, B.C., & Keens, T.G. (1982). Measuring ventilatory muscle endurance in humans as sustainable inspiratory pressure. Journal of Applies Physiology 52:768-772.

O'Donnell, D.E., Bertley, J.C., Chau, L.K., & Webb, K.A. (1997). Qualitative aspects of exertional breathlessness in chronic airflow limitation: pathophysiologic mechanisms. American Journal of Respiratory Critical Care Medicine 155:109-115.

O'Neill, S., Leahy, F., Pasterkamp, H., & Tal, A. (1983). The effects of chronic hyperinflation, nutritional status, and posture on respiratory muscle strength in cystic fibrosis. American Review of Respiratory Disease 128:1051-1054.

Orozco-Levi, M., Gea, J., Lloreta, J.L., Félez, M., Minguella, J., Serrano, S., & Broquetas, J.M. (1999). Subcellular adaptation of the human diaphragm in chronic obstructive pulmonary disease. European Respiratory Journal 13:371-378.

Patessio, A., Rampulla, C., Fracchia, C., Ioli, F., Majani, U., DeMarchi, A., & Donner, C.F. (1989). Relationship between the perception of breathlessness and inspiratory resistive loading: a report on a clinical trial. European Respiratory Journal 7:587S-591S.

Perez, T., Becquart, L.A., Stach, B., Wallaert, B., & Tonnel, A.B. (1996). Inspiratory muscle strength and endurance in steroid-dependent asthma. American Journal of Respiratory Critical Care Medicine 153:610-615.

Polkey, M.I., Kyroussis, D., Hamnegard, C.H., Mills, G.H., Green, M., & Moxham, J. (1996). Diaphragm strength in chronic obstructive pulmonary disease. American Journal of Respiratory Critical Care Medicine 154:1310-1317.

Polkey, M.I., Kyroussis, D., Keilty, S.E., Hamnegard, C.H., Mills, G.H., Green, M., & Moxham, J. (1995). Exhaustive treadmill exercise does not reduce twitch transdiaphragmatic pressure in patients with COPD. American Journal of Respiratory Critical Care Medicine 152:959-964.

Polkey, M.I., Green, M., & Moxham, J. (1995). Measurement of respiratory muscle strength. Thorax 50:1131-1135.

Polkey, M.I., Lyall, R.A., Green, M., Nigel, L.P., & Moxham, J. (1998). Expiratory muscle function in amyotrophic lateral sclerosis. American Journal of Respiratory Critical Care Medicine 158:734-741.

Pradal, U., Polese, G., Braggion, C., Poggi, R., Zanolla, L., Mastella, G., & Rossi, A. (1994). Determinants of maximal transdiaphragmatic pressure in adults with cystic fibrosis. American Journal of Respiratory Critical Care Medicine 150:167-173.

Preusser, B.A., Winningham, M.L., & Clanton, T.L. (1994). High vs. low intensity inspiratory muscle interval training in patients with COPD. Chest 106:110-117.

Ram, F.S., Wellington, E.R., & Barnes, N.C. (2003). Inspiratory muscle training for asthma. Cochrane Database Syst Rev CD003792.

Ramirez-Sarmiento, A., Orozco-Levi, M., Guell, R., Barreiro, E., Hernandez, N., Mota, S., Sangenis, M., Broquetas, J.M., Casan, P., & Gea, J. (2002). Inspiratory muscle training in patients with chronic obstructive pulmonary disease: structural adaptation and physiologic outcomes. American Journal of Respiratory Critical Care Medicine 166:1491-1497.

Rinqvist, T. (1966). The ventilatory capacity in healthy adults: an analysis of causal factors with special reference to the respiratory forces. Scand Journal of Clinical Laboratory Investigation 18(Suppl):1-111.

Rochester, D.F., & Braun, N.M.T. (1985). Determinants of maximal inspiratory pressure in chronic obstructive pulmonary disease. American Review of Respiratory Disease 132:42-47.

Rochester, D.F. (1988). Tests of respiratory muscle function. Clinical Chest Medicine 9:249-261.

Rochester, D., & Arora, N.S. (1983). Respiratory muscle failure. The Medical Clinics of North America 67:573-598.

Rollier, H., Bisschop, A., Gayan-Ramirez, G., Gosselink, R., & Decramer, M. (1998). Low load inspiratory muscle training increases diaphragmatic fiber dimensions in rats. American Journal of Respiratory Critical Care Medicine 157:833-839.

Romer, L.M., McConnell, A.K., & Jones, D.A. (2002). Effects of inspiratory muscle training on time-trial performance in trained cyclists. Journal of Sports Science 20:547-562.

Sawyer, E.H., & Clanton, T.L. (1993). Improved pulmonary function and exercise tolerance with inspiratory muscle conditioning in children with cystic fibrosis. Chest 104:1490-1497.

Scherer, T.A., Spengler, C., Owassapian, D., Imhof, E., & Boutellier, U. (2000). Respiratory muscle endurance training in chronic obstructive pulmonary disease. Impact on exercise capacity, dyspnea, and quality of life. American Journal of Respiratory Critical Care Medicine 162:1709-1714.

Similowski, T., Fleury, B., Launois, S., Cathala, H.P., Bouche, P., & Derenne, J.P. (1989). Cervical magnetic stimulation: a new painless method for bilateral phrenic nerve stimulation in conscious humans. Journal Applied Physiology 67:1311-1318.

Sonetti, D.A., Wetter, T.J., Pegelow, D.F., & Dempsey, J.A. (2001). Effects of respiratory muscle training versus placebo on endurance exercise performance. Respiratory Physiology 127:185-199.

Sprague, S.S., & Hopkins, P.D. (2003). Use of inspiratory strength training to wean six patients who were ventilator-dependent. Physical Therapy 83:171-181.

Szeinberg, A., England, S., Mindorff, C., Fraser, I.M., & Levison, H. (1985). Maximal inspiratory and expiratory pressures are reduced in hyperinflated, malnourished, young adult male patients with cystic fibrosis. American Review of Respiratory Disease 132:766-769.

Tikunov, B., Levine, S., & Mancini, D. (1997). Chronic congestive heart failure elicits adaptations of endurance exercise in diaphragmatic muscle. Circulation 95:910-916.

Tzelepis, G.E., Vega, D.L., Cohen, M.E, Fulambarker, A.M., Patel, K.K., & McCool, F.D. (1994). Pressure-flow specificity of inspiratory muscle training. Journal of Applied Physiology 77:795-801.

Tzelepis, G.E., Vega, D.L., Cohen, M.E., & McCool, F.D. (1994). Lung volume specificity of inspiratory muscle training. Journal of Applied Physiology 77:789-794.

Uijl, S.G., Houtman, S., Folgering, H.T., & Hopman, M.T. (1999). Training of the respiratory muscles in individuals with tetraplegia. Paraplegia 37:575-579.

Urban, P.P., Morgenstern, M., Brause, K., Wicht, S., Vukurevic, G., Kessler, S., & Stoeter, P. (2002). Distribution and course of cortico-respiratory projections for voluntary activation in man. A transcranial magnetic stimulation study in healthy subjects and patients with cerebral ischemia. Journal of Neurology 249:735-744.

Van't Hul, A.J., Chadwick-Straver, R.V.M., Wagenaar, R.C., Sol, G., & de Vries, P.M. (1997). Inspiratory muscle endurance is reduced more than maximal respiratory pressures in COPD patients. European Respiratory Journal 10:168S.

Villafranca, C., Borzone, G., Leiva, A., & Lisboa, C. (1998). Effect of inspiratory muscle training with intermediate load on inspiratory power output in COPD. European Respiratory Journal 11:28-33.

Vincken, W., Ghezzo, H., & Cosio, M.G. (1987). Maximal static respiratory pressures in adults: normal values and their relationship to determinants of respiratory function. Bulletin of European Physiopathology of Respiration 23:435-439.

Wanke, T., Formanek, D., Lahrmann, H., Brath, H., Wild, M., Wagner, C., & Zwick, H. (1994). The effects of combined inspiratory muscle and cycle ergometer training on exercise performance in patients with COPD. European Respiratory Journal 7:2205-2211.

Wanke, T., Toifl, K., Merkle, M., Formanek, D., Lahrmann, H., & Zwick, H. (1994). Inspiratory muscle training in patients with Duchenne muscular dystrophy. Chest 105:475-482.

Weiner, P., Waizman, J., Magadle, R., Berar-Yanay, N., & Pelled, B. (1999). The effect of specific inspiratory muscle training on the sensation of dyspnea and exercise tolerance in patients with congestive heart failure. Clinical Cardiology 22:727-732.

Weiner, P., Berar-Yanay, N., Davidovich, A., Magadle, R., & Weiner, M. (2000). Specific inspiratory muscle training in patients with mild asthma with high consumption of inhaled beta(2)-agonists. Chest 117:722-727.

Weiner, P., Inzelberg, R., Davidovich, A., Nisipeanu, P., Magadle, R., Berar-Yanay, N., & Carasso, R.L. (2002). Respiratory muscle performance and the perception of dyspnea in Parkinson's disease. Canadian Journal of Neurological Science 29:68-72.

Weiner, P., Magadle, R., Massarwa, F., Beckerman, M., & Berar-Yanay, N. (2002). Influence of gender and inspiratory muscle training on the perception of dyspnea in patients with asthma. Chest 122:197-201.

Weiner, P., Magadle, R., Beckerman, M., Weiner, M., & Berar-Yanay, N. (2003). Comparison of specific expiratory, inspiratory, and combined muscle training programs in COPD. Chest 124:1357-1364.

Weiner, P., Magadle, R., Beckerman, M., Weiner, M., & Berar-Yanay, N. (2004). Maintenance of inspiratory muscle training in COPD patients: one year follow-up. European Respiratory Journal 23:61-65.

Weiner, P., Magadle, R., Beckerman, M., Weiner, M., & Berar-Yanay, N. (2003). Specific expiratory muscle training in COPD. Chest 124:468-473.

Wilson, D.O., Cooke, N.T., Edwards, R.H.T., & Spiro, S.G. (1984). Predicted normal values for maximal respiratory pressures in caucasian adults and children. Thorax 39:535-538.

Winkler, G., Zifko, U., Nader, A., Frank, W., Zwick, H., Toifl, K., & Wanke, T. (2000). Dose-dependent effects of inspiratory muscle training in neuromuscular disorders. Muscle Nerve 23:1257-1260.

Yan, S., Gauthier, A.P., Similowski, T., Macklem, P.T., & Bellemare, F. (1992). Evaluation of human contractility using mouth pressure twitches. American Review of Respiratory Disease 145:1064-1069.

Complementary Therapies as Cardiopulmonary Physical Therapy Interventions

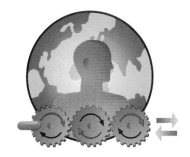

Meryl I. Cohen and Carol M. Davis

What does the literature say about a possible role for complementary and alternative therapies in helping to achieve common therapeutic goals for patients with cardiac, pulmonary, and/or vascular pathology? Believe it or not, there is a wealth of literature available, with some articles reflecting greater scientific rigor than others. Cardiopulmonary pathology is highly correlated with increased stress, and many complementary therapies are designed specifically to help people modify stress related behaviors.

WHAT ARE COMPLEMENTARY THERAPIES?

Complementary therapies are often viewed as holistic, mind/body, or energy-based therapies, and are categorized in a variety of different ways. Sometimes they are referred to as alternative therapies or alternative medicine, and sometimes as integrated therapies. Complementary therapies are used by physical therapists to complement (usually not replace) traditional therapies from the allopathic model of health care and are viewed as energy-based therapies that stress the importance of vibration or energy flow, both in the application of the technique and in the response by the client or patient.

The goal of most of these therapies is to "unblock" blocked body energy (or chi) so that the body can heal itself (Davis, 2004). It is hypothesized that homeostasis, balance, and self-regulation (the highly advanced ability of the body/mind to supply optimum conditions for metabolism, such as proper pH, body temperature, etc.) result from the unrestricted flow of body energy. A system in balance thus becomes resistant to inflammation. Some suggest that inflammation is the foundation of all diseases and disorders (Oschman, 2003). Two large studies, one in men and one in women, demonstrated that higher levels of C-reactive protein correlate with a higher

risk of heart attack and stroke and treatments that reduce C-reactive protein level reduce heart disease risk (Ridker, 1997; Ridker, 2000). Therefore complementary therapies are used to facilitate the flow of body energy, or chi, and thus help the body restore balance and return to a healthier state.

Examples of Complementary and Alternative Therapies

The following are examples of complementary and alternative therapies that have been found to be useful in health care. A list and brief description of these therapies can be found in Appendix A at the end of this chapter.

Manual Therapies

Manual therapies, also known as body work, include myofascial release, craniosacral therapy, Rosen method, Rolfing, Hellerwork, soma, neuromuscular therapy, massage, and osteopathic and chiropractic medicine. The manual therapies involve the use of hands on the body/mind surface to stimulate bioelectromagnetic force. How this occurs remains a mystery. Interestingly, research by Hunt and others is currently being conducted to measure energy flow from the body (Hunt, 1989; Rubik, 1995). Perhaps both mechanical and energetic forces stimulate response from the tissue in several ways. It has been hypothesized that mechanical force may be transformed into a chemical response within the collagen of the myofascia, causing a flow of the polyglycoid layer of the collagen by way of a piezoelectric effect (Oschman, 2000). For patients with cardiopulmonary pathology, the manual therapies can assist in opening up the ribcage and vertebral spine to allow increased ventilation and better posture and thereby support cardiorespiratory health.

Mind/Body Interventions

Mind/body intervention include psychotherapies, support groups, meditation, imagery, hypnosis, dance and music therapy, art therapy, prayer, neurolinguistic psychology, biofeedback, yoga, Pilates, and t'ai chi. These mind/body interventions are examples of how movement and verbal and nonverbal communication with the mind/body open up new pathways for thought and thereby unblock what might be blocked energy flow or chi. These interventions are quite prevalent in the treatment of cardiorespiratory and pulmonary disorders. Stress is positively affected by being aware of thoughts and habits that affect the mind/body in a negative way. These interventions put the patient back in control of negative behaviors, and often focusing on the breath is an integral part of furthering relaxation.

Movement Awareness Techniques

Movement awareness techniques include Feldenkrais method, the Alexander technique, and the Trager approach. It is postulated that movement awareness techniques help people bring to consciousness the way in which they tend to move habitually so that they can practice new ways of moving and holding themselves posturally, thus freeing up blocked energy that gets trapped in fascia and soft tissue as a result of maintaining habitual postures. Those people who walk around with protracted scapulae and forward heads are revealing fascial restrictions around the thoracic inlet, lungs, and mediastinum. It is hypothesized that tight fascia, revealed in extremes of posture, restricts blood flow and nerve conduction critical to the maintenance of healthy heart tissue.

Energy Work

Traditional Chinese Medicine

Traditional Chinese medicine includes acupuncture, acupressure, reflexology, and qi gong. These approaches within the system of traditional Chinese medicine focus on enhancing the flow of chi along body pathways or meridians, but the concept of meridians and energy flow is just one part of this complex, centuries-old system of health care. The acupuncture or acupressure or reflexology point is a specific point where access to the flow of chi on a meridian is most available. One analogy is that an acupuncture point is to a flow of chi as the entrance to a subway access is to the train tracks below the surface

Bioelectromagnetics

Bioelectromagnetics include thermal applications of nonionizing radiation such as radio frequency hyperthermia laser and pulsed electromagnetic field therapy, as well as magnets. Credible research exists on the effects of electromagnetic energy for wound healing and bone repair. Biomicroelectro-magnetics is the term applied to the energy that seems to emanate from the hands of people who have

proven to be healers (Rubik, 1995). Ultrasound and diathermy have been used in physical therapy for decades as deep heat mechanisms, and although there is not a clear understanding of the mechanism of action, it undoubtedly involves a stimulation of energy flow; therefore, this therapeutic approach falls in the bioelectromagnetic category. The use of magnets in physical therapy is very controversial, but there are some very compelling results from case studies that make it important to include in this category.

Personal Transmission of Healing Energy

Methods of personal transmission of healing energy include Reiki, noncontact therapeutic touch, and distant healing prayer. The practitioner goes through a period of training in order to learn how to focus attention and intention on transmitting the universal life force for healing and well-being, either though touch (Reiki), manipulation of bioenergy fields (noncontact therapeutic touch), or thorough focusing the mind for distant healing effects (intercessory prayer and Reiki).

Herbal Approaches

Naturopathy and homeopathy represent the use of plants and animal substances to fight off disease and the use of wise nutrition to combat illness. Naturopathy, like osteopathic medicine, represents an entire system of health care that uses homeopathy, osteopathy, proper nutrition and other means to bring about healing. Naturopathic physicians complete four years of medical school. Homeopathy involves the use of minute chemicals in diluted solution to resolve chemical imbalances in the body. Proper nutrition has long been associated with cardiac and pulmonary health, especially in Dean Ornish's plan for healing from cardiac pathology (Ornish, 1990).

MIND/BODY LINK

Mind/body health care has brought about a way of linking the traditional linear research methods with the more contemporary, complementary, and alternative health-care practices. The influence of the mind on the body was first introduced in the Western hemisphere by Herbert Benson, a well known Harvard cardiologist, through his research on Tibetan monks who were able to control their autonomic nervous system to the extent that they could lower their body temperatures and respiration rates and enter a wakeful, hypometabolic physiological state by will (Wallace, 1971). This information shocked the western world, and Benson presented his data most dramatically by videotaping the actual sessions of the monks taking control of their bodies with their minds.

The proof that the mind and body are inextricably linked has since been well documented in various studies. There is even a basic science now devoted to the study of the effect of the mind on the body: psychoneuroimmunology. Ader and Cohen are credited with coining the term psychoneuroimmunology, and such studies have shown that the mind affects the immune system by way of the autonomic nervous system and by way of the "fluid" nervous system, or the nonadrenergic and noncholinergic nervous system (Ader, 1991). Candice Pert has clearly articulated the physiological functioning of the fluid nervous system, which manifests by way of the effects of thought on the neurotransmitters, the neuropeptides and the steroids of the body (Pert, 1997). The neurotransmitters and the neuropeptides communicate with most all of the cells of the body. This science has been termed psychoneuroendocrinology. It is no longer correct to assume that the mind resides in the cranium or brain. In truth, the mind has been shown to reside in every cell in the body. According to Pert and others, the science clearly reveals that all cells have memory (Pert, 1997).

The biochemistry of psychoneuroendocrinology reflects a flow of a different sort than microelectro-potentials or the exchange of energy from the hands of the therapist, but illustrates, none the less, that the mind and the body are inseparable and the mind communicates with every cell of the body.

Complementary and alternative therapies are energy-based therapies that require belief that there is such a phenomenon as vital flow of energy in the body, and that the natural state of the body is to be healthy. (Kaptchuk, 1996) Illness is an aberration set up by an imbalance caused by restriction in flow. The body has many energies, and the ways that we can observe energy at work in the body are varied. For example, electrocardiograms, electroencephalograms, and electromyograms all measure the energy output from various body organs. The piezoelectric effect, another energy phenomenon, enables osteoblastic activity, which keeps our bones strong. Mechanical energy in gravity is transformed to chemical energy to allow the osteoblasts to deposit calcium appropriately in our skeleton.

Biomicroelectro-potentials, or the subtle energies in electromagnetic fields that emanate from the hands of "healers," are currently being researched (Rubik, 1995; Waechter, 2004). It is believed that complementary and alternative therapies have an effect on patients by way of the energy that emanates from the healer's hands. This energy is of a frequency of 0.3 to 30 Hz, which is usually centered around eight to 10 Hz (Zimmerman, 1990; Seto, 1992).

As we move into this new century, many researchers and practitioners in health care are seriously exploring and publishing studies that reveal new ways of viewing reality. What we know about quantum physics and systems theory and what we have observed and experienced, both the inadequacies of traditional allopathic medicine in overcoming chronic illness and autoimmune disease and the growing tendency of patients and clients to seek out complementary and alternative therapies, positions us well into a paradigm shift, a revolution in the linear and materialistic view of reality. A common perspective is that current medicine falls short because it is designed on the infectious disease model, or mechanistic model, in which it is hoped that a single drug or intervention will be able to cure and save lives.

Most current diseases, especially the chronic diseases that affect people, do not lend themselves to single-purpose cures. Chronic illness is most adequately addressed if the patient is involved in the healing process as an active partner, if the patient is willing to make certain lifestyle changes to eliminate choices that interfere with wellness, and when illness is perceived by both patients and practitioners not as a simple biophysiological event but as a system or contextual event. We are all consciously and unconsciously influenced by a variety of systems that we are embedded within that mandate our reactions to inflammation and illness. No two people react to illness in the exact same way, and no two people heal from illness in the exact same way. Any physical therapist or health care professional will admit that how a person thinks or perceives has everything to do with how he or she responds to health and illness. A variety of systems impacting on each of us include a broad range such as our birth order, our identity, how we feel about ourselves and our family members, how well we enjoy our work and our recreation, how meaningful our relationships are, the weather, who won the Super Bowl, and what we had for breakfast, for example (Mehl-Madrona, 2005).

TRADITIONAL THERAPIES APPLIED FROM A HOLISTIC APPROACH—INTENTION

Patients with cardiovascular and pulmonary complications often present with comorbidities of acute and chronic diseases that challenge our interventions. The application of energy medicine or holistic approaches in treating these patients and clients is becoming more commonplace. There are traditional therapies that can be applied from a holistic approach. In working with patients with cardiopulmonary pathology, for example, treatments such as massage, exercise, and relaxation can be approached by a therapist in a traditional manner in which the intention is a mechanical, linear effect, or it can be approached in a holistic or mind/body manner in which the intention is to attempt to influence the flow of vital energy. When massage and exercise are offered as treatments from a holistic perspective, the idea is to enhance the flow of body energy and bring about homeostasis.

Researchers confirm the importance of hope and faith in one's physician and practitioners, including physical therapists (Jonas, 2003). The fact that the patient believes that the practitioner has hope that they will improve seems to help, but exactly how this facilitates healing remains unclear. It seems to be related to the concept of intention and the effects of consciousness and nonlocal mind (Jonas, 2003).

One more important point: to ignore the positive effect of therapeutic presence is to neglect a powerful intervention. How practitioners are with their patients, not just what they do, is the important thing (Davis, 2004). The exchange of energy in the form of the positive response to being truly listened to as a patient is, time and again, mentioned by patients to be critical to their healing response. Now the research is finally documenting the effects of this positive intention (Jonas, 2003).

THE PROBLEM OF SCIENTIFIC PROOF

Should physical therapists use complementary therapies that have shown good clinical results but have not been proven scientifically to be efficacious?

Yes. But it's not a simple yes. At the foundation of this question are two ethical questions. What right do we have, as professionals, to subject patients to treatments that have not been proven to be efficacious by way of scientific evidence? Conversely, what right do we have to deny patients holistic treatments that have been shown for centuries to benefit patients and have a negligible chance of causing harm? Physical therapy has a long history of using therapeutic agents for the good of patients without any science to explain efficacy or mechanism of action. And now that we are finally doing this important research on ultrasound, heat, exercise, and electrical modalities, along come t'ai chi, yoga, transcendental meditation, and craniosacral therapy.

SCIENTIFIC EVIDENCE

Reductionistic science tries to show evidence of cause and effect by reducing the experimental variables (ideally to just one) and by reducing all possible outcomes so as to eliminate the effects of chance (or other causes) on the evidence that is collected. Unlike single cells or molecules, human beings and their illnesses do not lend themselves to being reduced in such a manner. People are whole systems of interacting needs and functions (physical, intellectual, emotional, spiritual, and social) that cannot be fully understood by separation from one another or by reduction. Systems theory, from the life sciences, is foundational to holistic or complementary therapies and states that the whole can never be fully understood by reducing it to its parts because the whole is always more than the sum of the parts. How the parts interact with one another is critical to understanding the whole. Reductionism tries to control for this confounding variable.

Complementary therapies such as t'ai chi, acupuncture, biofeedback, meditation, cognitive behavioral therapy, music therapy, hypnosis, electrical stimulation, prayer and distant healing efforts, yoga, and qi gong have been shown, as a matter of fact, to be effective in the relief of pain and anxiety and in the improvement of balance by way of the randomized controlled trial (RCT) (Luskin, 2000). Literature reviews of mind/body therapies in the treatment of musculoskeletal disorders with implications for the elderly have been conducted (Spencer, 1999; Wolf, 1997). But the fact remains that many complementary therapies, especially those manual therapies designed to assist in the release of fascial restrictions in order to restore the flow of the body's self-regulating energy, or chi, do not lend themselves to study by the RCT because energy itself cannot be measured or seen. Only the results of energy can be measured (heat, work, movement,

etc), and we cannot yet validate what results occur from what intervention, except by way of anecdote and measuring the effects of treatment on impairments and function. Scientists such as Valerie Hunt, James Oschman, Gary Schwartz and Linda Russek, Candace Pert and others, however, are busy working out the biochemical, quantum physics, and systems theories that postulate physiological and biochemical mechanisms of action that allow us to hypothesize basic cellular energy theory (Hunt, 1996; Oschman, 2000; Schwartz, 1997; Pert, 1985). This basic theory or cellular energetic theory can then be tested to describe the evidence that we yearn for. If we can hypothesize a basic mechanism of action of myofascial release, for example, then we can examine whether that action does indeed take place in the way that the theory postulates. But we will never be able to see energy any more than we can see velocity.

Demonstration of efficacy and safety is paramount to professional care. But is this goal actually achievable to the satisfaction of the scientific community? Not as long as reductionism remains the gold standard in the search for reality. In 1997, the Council on Scientific Affairs of the American Medical Association suggested that "physicians should evaluate the scientific perspectives of unconventional theories for treatment and practice, looking particularly at potential utility, safety and efficacy of these [holistic] modalities" (Luskin, 2000).

Holistic approaches should not be exempt from careful study. Complementary therapies must be researched by way of case studies, single case designs, and other methods of systematic examination of intervention and results. And as we build the body of evidence justifying the positive benefits of the restored flow of healing energy that help the body/mind self-regulate and heal itself, we may just come to realize that complementary therapies have done more to restore healing to health care than had been anticipated. What follows is a review of the evidence of how complementary therapies influence normal cardiopulmonary responses and the effect that they have on patients with cardiopulmonary conditions.

USE OF SPECIFIC COMPLEMENTARY THERAPY TECHNIQUES IN CARDIOPULMONARY CONDITIONS

As described throughout Part III of this book, the goal of physical therapy intervention is to improve the efficiency of the oxygen transport and gas exchange systems. The decision to use a specific complementary therapy and integrate it into more traditional cardiopulmonary treatments is often dependent on the practitioner's familiarity with the technique. Rehabilitation practitioners without specialized training in a complementary therapeutic technique frequently do not realize that they are already incorporating components of complementary therapies in established, traditional therapeutic interventions. Patient education, including behavioral and biofeedback techniques used to alter breathing patterns and reduce sympathetic nervous system stimulation, are forms of mind/body therapies. These techniques have been studied extensively, reported in the literature, and are widely used and accepted in clinical practice (Lescowitz, 2003; Astin, 2003; Spencer & Jacobs, 2003).

Physical therapy practitioners with expertise in a specific complementary technique may decide to focus their treatment on cardiopulmonary impairments. T'ai chi and yoga are mind/body therapies that emphasize coordinated breathing with movement. These techniques may be used as the primary approach to treat the impairment, or they may complement traditional physical therapy. The body of evidence addressing the usefulness of these techniques in improving oxygen transport has expanded in both quantity and quality in recent years (Luskin, 1998; Levy, 1993).

Other interventions that have not been subjected to rigorous, scientific study may still be worthy of clinical application. For example, the Alexander technique, which emphasizes posture and movement, intuitively suggests an improvement in oxygen transport. An improvement in posture optimizes muscle function, thoracic cage efficiency, and hence oxygen transport; however, there is limited research published on this technique in relation to the cardiopulmonary systems (Ives, 2000).

The increasing consumer demand for complementary and alternative medical (CAM) therapies has occurred despite the lack of rigorous or acceptable scientific investigation into many of them. In an attempt to protect the general public from unethical and unsafe practices, the National Heart, Lung and Blood Institute and the National Center for Complementary and Alternative Medicine have proposed large-scale clinical trials to determine standards of practice and safety standards (Lin, 2001). It is important for all health-care practitioners to become familiar with some of the more popular CAM therapies, recognize that our patients are using them, and be especially aware of the effects of these therapies on the cardiovascular and pulmonary systems.

The following section reviews the normal cardiovascular and pulmonary responses to various CAM techniques in healthy individuals. A presentation of the evidence for using specific complementary and alternative medicine therapies to treat major cardiovascular and cardiopulmonary pathologies follows. A discussion of naturopathic and homeopathic therapies is outside the scope of this chapter. Breathing exercises will be discussed in relation to a specific CAM therapy. Traditional breathing exercises (e.g. diaphragmatic, purse-lip, etc.) are addressed elsewhere in this book.

Normal Cardiovascular and Pulmonary Responses to CAM Therapies

T'ai Chi

T'ai chi is one of the most well-studied mind/body therapies. Cardiovascular responses have been documented during T'ai chi sessions in novice as well as in master practitioners, and in the many forms of practice (see Appendix A). In several of these studies responses have been compared to cardiovascular and pulmonary responses observed in other forms of exercise (e.g. bicycle ergometry and treadmill ambulation). Most investigations are small and have methodological shortcomings. A brief sampling of the results of several studies addressing the cardiovascular and pulmonary responses found during t'ai chi practice can be found in Table 27-1. In general, in these studies of healthy individuals, sex and experience level do not seem to influence the responses. It is reasonable to conclude that t'ai chi is a low to moderate intensity exercise that stresses the oxygen transport system. Investigators generally conclude that t'ai chi is a safe activity for healthy individuals. Prescreening for mind/body techniques is recommended, however, just as would be expected for any other exercise intervention (Ives, 2000).

Several authors have investigated the cardiovascular and pulmonary benefits of a prolonged program of t'ai chi. In contrast to the studies reported in Table 27-1, several studies demonstrate that experienced t'ai chi chuan practitioners achieve significantly higher maximum oxygen consumption (VO_2max) levels than sedentary subjects (Jin, 1989; Lai, 1993; Lai, 1995; Lan, 1996; Lan, 1998). These authors conclude that t'ai chi is a form of aerobic exercise, it has benefits for health-related fitness, and it may slow the decline in cardiorespiratory fitness in older, healthy individuals.

In a small study (n = 32), Wang et al (2002) studied endothelium-dependent dilation in skin vasculature in healthy, older (69.9 ± 1.5 years), male t'ai chi practitioners and a control group. Their results demonstrate that when compared to older sedentary men (67.0 ± 1.0 years), long-time, experienced practitioners of t'ai chi have more favorable arterial and venous hemodynamics. In some cases these vascular findings were comparable with a group of younger, healthy, sedentary men (23.5 ± 0.68 years).

Young et al (1999) compared the effects of aerobic exercise and t'ai chi on blood pressure responses in older individuals (79% women). In this RCT of 62 sedentary older adults (66.7 ± 5.2 years), subjects participated in 12 weeks of either aerobic exercise or t'ai chi. Baseline systolic blood pressure (BP) was 130 to 159 mm Hg. Subjects were not on antihypertensive medication and results indicated similar statistically significant reductions in systolic BP occurred in both intervention groups. Of note, the aerobic exercise group demonstrated a significant increase in predicted VO_2 max while the t'ai chi group did not. The authors concluded that both light and moderate intensity exercise programs can have an important effect on systolic blood pressure.

Yoga

Another popular mind/body technique is yoga. The cardiovascular responses to several types of yoga in healthy individuals have been investigated. General conclusions are difficult to make given the weaknesses of the studies and the different characteristics of the types of yoga studied. Table 27-2 lists cardiovascular and pulmonary responses before and after a single yoga session or a period of yoga practice. Overall it appears that those forms of yoga that primarily involve meditation show minimal changes in cardiovascular

TABLE 27-1

Cardiovascular and Pulmonary Responses Found During Continuous T'ai Chi Exercise

STUDY AUTHORS	T'AI CHI FORM	SAMPLE CHARACTERISTICS AND METHODS	CARDIOVASCULAR AND PULMONARY RESPONSES
Schneider, 1991	Wing Chun (WG) T'ai Chi Chuan (TCC)	Experienced practitioners VO_2 max measured on treadmill	TCC: 36.4% VO_2 max, 59.8% HRmax, VE/ VO_2 21.7 WG: 52.4% VO_2 max, 70.5% HR max, VE/VO_2 24.2
Lan, 2001	Yang T'ai Chi Chuan	15 Men Age 26-56 years Experienced practitioners (>1 year) VO_2 measured on cycle ergometer	TCC: 58% HR max (max on cycle was 186 ± 8), 55% VO_2 max (max on cycle was 39.1 ± 7.7)
Brown, 1989	T'ai Chi Chuan (long form Yang style, Cloud H)	6 Men Experienced practitioners VO_2 measured on cycle ergometer	TCC: Vf 11.3, VE/VO_2 23.47, VD/VT 20% Cycle: Vf 15.7, VE/VO_2 27.41, VD/VT 27% Cardiac output, stroke volume, and HR were not significantly different between TCC and ergometry at the same VO_2
Fontana, 2000	T'ai Chi C'hi in slow and fast movements in sitting and standing	26 Healthy adults Age 21-50 years Convenience sample Novice and experienced practitioners	METS: Sitting 1.5 ± 0 .2, Slow standing 2.3 ± 0.3, Fast standing 2.6 ± 0.5, Breathing exercises 3-3.6, 43%-49% predicted HR max
Chao, 2002	T'ai-Chi-Qui- Gong (54 motions divided into 3 sets)	47 Adults Age 32-76 years Experienced practitioners (mean 3.6 ± 2.6 years)	50% VO_2 max in elderly (≥65 years) 60% VO_2 max in women Each motion ≈3 METS

VO_2 max, Maximum oxygen uptake (in L/min or ml/kg/min); VE/VO_2, ventilatory equivalent for oxygen; Vf, ventilatory frequency in breaths per minute; VD/VT, ratio of dead space ventilation to tidal volume; METS, metabolic equivalents (1 MET = 3.5 ml of oxygen/kilogram/weight).

and pulmonary parameters when compared to those forms that include stimulation phases.

Other Mind/Body Therapies

Although social support is not typically considered a mind/body therapy, part of the success of many of the CAM techniques has been attributed to group interactions or those interactions between subject and practitioner. In a review of 81 studies, Uchino et al (1996) investigated the benefits of social support on the cardiovascular, endocrine, and immune systems. Social support includes individual, family, or group interactions. There is strong evidence correlating a decrease in cardiovascular reactivity in healthy individuals when social support is increased.

Manual Therapies/Body Work Therapies

There is a paucity of literature addressing cardiovascular and pulmonary responses to body work techniques in healthy individuals. One study of therapeutic massage demonstrated statistically significant reductions in cardiovascular parameters after a three-day intervention of slow stroke back massage on individuals in a rehabilitation setting (Holland, 2001). Twenty-four adults (age range 52 to 88 years) underwent daily intervention. Statistically significant decreases in systolic and diastolic BP were noted each day; this was true

for heart rate (HR) and respiratory rate only on days one and three. Subjects also reported improved perception and less anxiety.

Cottingham et al (1988b) investigated the effects of the Rolf method of soft tissue mobilization on parasympathetic nervous system (PNS) tone in 32 young, healthy men. This RCT compared a group that performed 45 minutes of Rolfing with pelvic mobilization (pelvic lift) to a control group that received a 45-minute durational touch without Rolfing (pelvic lift intervention). At baseline all subjects had an anterior pelvic tilt. PNS tone was measured before, immediately after, and 24 hours after intervention. Results demonstrated a significant increase in PNS tone and decreased standing pelvic tilt angle in the intervention group. Earlier, Cottingham et al (1988a) demonstrated an increase in PNS tone with the pelvic lift technique unrelated to the "durational touch" used simultaneously in the technique. The authors concluded that this technique of soft tissue pelvic manipulation (i.e., durational touch plus pelvic lift) can help individuals with muscle dysfunction and conditions associated with reduced PNS activity and increased sympathetic nervous system activity. The latter condition can be representative of deconditioning.

In a small study of 12 children and adults, investigators attempted to examine the reliability of craniosacral technique

TABLE 27-2

Cardiovascular and Pulmonary Responses to Yoga Practices in Healthy Individuals

STUDY AUTHORS	TYPE OF YOGA	SAMPLE CHARACTERISTICS AND METHODS	CARDIOVASCULAR AND PULMONARY RESPONSES
Telles, 1993	Brahmakumaris Raja yoga meditation	18 Males Age 20-52 years (34.1 ± 8.1) Experienced practitioners Subjects served as own control in sessions of random thinking	Yoga: HR increased compared to baseline and control Yoga and control: no difference in measures of autonomic function
Schell, 1994	Hatha yoga	Experienced practitioners Control group volunteers	Yoga: HR decreased during practice compared to controls Yoga and control: no difference in BP or endocrine measures
Ray, 2001	Hatha yoga	40 Men Age 19-23 years Vo_2 max measured on cycle ergometer Both yoga and conventional physical exercise groups performed 1 hour of activity every morning for 6 months	Yoga: Vo_2max increased from baseline; perception of exertion decreased from baseline Conventional physical exercise: Vo_2 increased from baseline; no change in perception of exertion (no information was given regarding differences between group outcomes)
Telles, 2000	Cyclic meditation (calming and stimulating) Shavasana (calming)	40 Male volunteers Age 27 ± 5.7 years Experienced practitioners Measurements taken before and after yoga session	CM: Vo_2 decreased 32.1%, RR rate decreased 18%, TV decreased 28.8 % SH: Vo_2 decreased 10.1%, RR decreased 15.2%, TV decreased 15.9% Results were significantly different from baseline and decreases were significantly greater in CM than SH
Knowles, 2003	Asanas (yoga poses) Pranayama (breathing exercises)	Single case study Age 42 years Healthy male Performed 6 days per week for 10 weeks 5 Poses and 2 breathing exercises	Vital capacity: increased 9% Chest circumference measures: increased in all regions Chest flexibility measures: increased in forward bending

Vo_2, Oxygen consumption (ml/min); *RR*, respiratory rate (breath rate); *TV*, tidal volume (breath volume), *CM*, cyclic meditation; *SH*, shavasana.

interpretation among three expert practitioners of craniosacral therapy (Wirth-Pattullo, 1994). They also investigated the relationship of the craniosacral rate to HR and BP of subject and practitioner. Results demonstrated no inter-rater reliability between the three practitioners. Results also demonstrated no relationship between HR and BP and the craniosacral rates. Although this study did not attempt to report on the effects of craniosacral therapy on cardiovascular parameters, the results do shed light on potential considerations for future study design.

More recently, Green et al (2004) conducted a rigorous review of the evidence for using craniosacral therapy. Nine of the 34 studies reviewed looked at whether movement of cranial bones was possible, and 10 of the 34 studies looked at whether cerebrospinal fluid moves rhythmically. The authors concluded that evidence supports the belief that there is a cranial "pulse" or rhythm that is separate from the cardiac or respiratory rhythms.

Energy Work Techniques

A few studies addressing the cardiovascular and pulmonary responses to energy work in healthy subjects have been conducted. Some of these are summarized in Table 27-3. In most cases, methodological weaknesses limit generalizations about the results. Studies of Reiki demonstrate trends toward increased relaxation and improved immune system markers (Wetzel, 1989; Wardell, 2001; Olson, 2003). In the study of qi-training, the authors provide a detailed description of the intervention facilitating replication of the study with a larger sample (Lee, 2000). The two studies investigating responses to magnets demonstrate no significant differences from control (Hinman, 2002; Martel, 2002). Of interest, in a study investigating the safety of prosthetic mini-magnets in individuals with cardiac pacemakers, the authors found no electrocardiographic changes in nine of 12 subjects. When the magnets were moved at least one cm away from the pacemaker implant, these changes no longer existed (Hiller, 1995).

In a well-written and well-designed paper, investigators reported on the effects of acupuncture on autonomic nervous system (ANS) function (Haker, 2000). Twelve healthy volunteers, six men and six women, aged 23 to 48 years, underwent randomized needle insertion into three distinct acupuncture sites. Measures of ANS function were monitored during the 25-minute intervention period and for the 60

TABLE 27-3

Cardiovascular and Pulmonary Responses to Energy Work in Healthy Individuals

STUDY AUTHORS	ENERGY WORK	SAMPLE CHARACTERISTICS AND METHODS	CARDIOVASCULAR AND PULMONARY RESPONSES
Hinman, 2002	Magnets Negative polarity Positive polarity	Double blind RCT 75 Adults, 25 in each group Age 21-57 years Measurements at rest, 1, 5, 10, 15 minutes on magnet mattress and 5 min after exposure	BP and HR responses were not significantly different between positive polarity, negative polarity, and control groups
Martel, 2002	Magnets	Prospective RCT 20 Healthy men Age 25 ± 2 years Magnets worn for 30 min on 2 separate occasions Measurements at 10, 20, 30 min	Forearm blood flow responses were not significantly different from placebo
Wardell, 2001	Reiki	Convenience sample 23 Healthy subjects Age 29-55 years Treatment consisted of 30 min of Reiki by expert practitioner Measurements before, during, and after session	Pretreatment to post-treatment: significant decrease in anxiety, BP; trend to decrease in EMG (muscle tension) and salivary cortisol; significant increase in salivary IgA; trend to increase galvanic skin temperature, indicating relaxation
Wetzel, 1989	Reiki	48 Healthy individuals (plus 10 controls) Monitored over 24 hours	Pretreatment to post-treatment: significant improvement in hemoglobin and hematocrit
Olson, 2003	Reiki	24 Subjects with cancer pain Treated 1.5 hours with Reiki or 1.5 hours of rest for 4 consecutive days	Significant decrease in HR, DBP, on day 1 Significant decrease in pain on days 1 and 3 Trend to decrease in DBP on day 3 Significant increase in psychological quality of life from day 1 to day 7 No change in SBP or RR day 1-4
Lee, 2000	Qi-training (3 stages): Sound 10 min Motion 10 min Meditation 10 min	12 Healthy volunteers Age 19-37 years 1 Hour per day, 6 times per week 1.3 ± 0.2 years of training	After 10 min: significant decrease in SBP and RPP, trend in decrease HR, RR After 60 min: significant decrease in HR, SBP, RR, and RPP from baseline

RCT, Randomized control trial; *DBP,* diastolic BP; *SBP,* systolic BP; *RPP,* rate-pressure product.

minutes after intervention at each insertion site. An interesting combination of results was found depending on the needle insertion site. Stimulation of the ear site resulted in increased PNS activity during both the needle insertion and the post-stimulation periods. Stimulation of the skin over the left thenar muscle resulted in increased sympathetic nervous system (SNS) and PNS activity during both measurement periods. Stimulation of the right thenar muscle resulted in an increase in SNS and PNS activity during the poststimulation period but no changes were seen during the needle insertion period. These results begin to shed light on which acupuncture techniques may be cardiosuppressive and possibly account for the calmness and relaxation often reported after treatment. Delayed responses may have a therapeutic effect as well.

In a controversial study by Rosa et al (1998), the investigators failed to demonstrate that those practitioners of noncontact therapeutic touch were able to perceive a "human energy field." Significant limitations to the study have been noted, including experimenter bias, inconsistent conclusions,

and incomplete statistical analysis (Lescowitz, 1998). Although this study does not address cardiovascular and pulmonary responses to therapeutic touch, it does provoke discussion about the difficulties of conducting research on this technique.

A study by Haas et al (1986) is worthy of mention in this discussion of energy techniques. These authors were able to demonstrate the ability of musical rhythm to "pace" respirations. In a sample of 20 healthy volunteers (half musically trained), breathing rhythms were correlated with metronome and tapping rhythms. This ability of musical rhythms to entrain respiration may have potential benefits in managing stress-induced respiratory patterns.

Cardiovascular Conditions

Much of the pathophysiological basis for applying CAM therapies to cardiovascular conditions rests in the relationship between the cardiovascular system and the ANS (Haskell, 2003). Stimulation of the ANS, specifically the SNS, can cause both an increase in circulating levels of catecholamines and damage to endothelial cells lining arterial walls. Often triggered by psychological factors, the resulting increase in metabolic and myocardial oxygen demand has a negative impact on the oxygen transport system (Rozanski, 1999). Interventions that can reduce or reverse these responses to SNS stimulation have a potential positive effect on cardiovascular conditions.

Risk Factors for Coronary Artery Disease

Numerous complementary therapies have been studied and shown efficacious in the management of known risk factors for coronary artery disease (CAD). Specifically, interventions addressing psychological stress and hypertension have been extensively examined.

Stress Reduction

First studied in the late 1970s and early 1980s, Benson et al (1977) recognized the benefits of meditation and the "relaxation response." They postulated that when properly applied, these techniques facilitated downregulation of the SNS and upregulation of the PNS.

During 15 to 30 minutes of practicing the relaxation response, changes in cardiopulmonary parameters have been noted. These include a decrease in respiratory rate (RR) and oxygen consumption (VO_2) and an increase in cardiac output (CO) without a concurrent increase in BP, reflecting a reduction in peripheral vascular resistance. In addition, skilled practitioners of the relaxation response demonstrate a decrease in VO_2 at a constant workload during treadmill activity (Schiller, 2003).

In an important paper addressing the impact of psychological factors on the development of cardiovascular disease, researchers related CAD to depression, anxiety, personality factors and character traits, social isolation, and chronic life stress (Rozanski, 1999). Several authors have addressed behavioral interventions effective in the management of these psychosocial stresses.

In a comprehensive meta-analysis of 70 articles, the treatment of trait anxiety with transcendental meditation (TM), progressive relaxation, relaxation response, and electromyographic (EMG) biofeedback were reviewed. Sources for the reviewed articles included journals, dissertations, and books. All interventions had a positive effect on self-reports or physiological measures of anxiety. Transcendental meditation had the strongest effect of the four interventions studied. In general, subjects who received more frequent interventions initially and who were followed the longest received the most benefit. It was recommended that future studies measure performance outcomes, and that subjects be closely followed-up in an attempt to reduce loss due to attrition (Eppley, 1989).

Miller et al (1995) reported on 22 subjects with anxiety disorders who participated in a noncontrolled clinical trial. Subjects were trained in mindfulness meditation, participated in a once-a-week group program for eight weeks, and were followed-up for three years. Significant reductions in medications and counseling requirements were noted. The authors concluded that "mindfulness training… may be able to provide medical patients suffering from anxiety with a set of tools for achieving effective long-term non-pharmacological self-regulation… and be used as a complement to more conventional medical interventions." Conversely, Astin (2003) reported an increase in anxiety levels in 17% to 31% of subjects practicing relaxation techniques, and an increase in anxiety levels in up to 53.8% of subjects practicing TM. No negative medical consequences were reported as a result of the increased anxiety levels. Several causes for this negative response were postulated, including subject's fear of loosing control, general restlessness, intrusive thoughts, and feelings of vulnerability.

Several small, noncontrolled clinical studies examining the effects of TM on blood levels related to cardiovascular disease have been reported. Infante et al (2001) measured plasma catecholamine levels (epinephrine, norepinephrine, and dopamine) in 19 skilled practitioners of TM. Resting values were compared with catecholamine levels in nonmatched controls. Results demonstrated lower values in the skilled practitioners when compared to the controls. The authors concluded TM may have been responsible for the lower catecholamine levels and consequent downregulation of the SNS. Similarly, Schneider et al (1998) concluded that TM may have been responsible for lower serum lipid peroxide levels found in 18 practitioners of TM compared with higher levels found in 23 nonmatched, nonpracticing control subjects. Lipid peroxide has been implicated in the pathophysiology of atherosclerosis.

Cognitive approaches to the reduction of stress have been subjected to clinical study. McCrone et al (2001) compared the effectiveness of psychoeducational interventions on 33 male subjects with risk factors for CAD. In addition to nutrition counseling and exercise training, educational sessions addressing cardiovascular disease, risk factors, and stress reduction were offered to 25 participants. These subjects were also trained to use specific skills to improve their responses to stress and were given audiotapes to practice progressive muscle relaxation. Eight subjects in the non-randomized control group received weight management counseling and health education only. They did not participate in any discussions related to stress management. Subjects, ranging in age from 57 to 79 years, participated in the interventions for six months. Although both groups showed improvements in risk factor profiles, there was greater improvement in the group trained in stress management techniques. Significant improvements were noted in BP, lipid profile, obesity indices, and fitness level.

In spite of a positive theoretical basis for the use of CAM therapies in stress management, many techniques have not been subjected to systematic investigation. Table 27-4 summarizes the effects of t'ai chi, Feldenkrais method, yoga, and therapeutic massage in stress management. Although these

TABLE 27-4

Effect of Selected CAM Therapies in Stress Management in Healthy Individuals

STUDY AUTHORS	CAM THERAPY	SAMPLE CHARACTERISTICS AND METHODS	OUTCOMES
Jin, 1992	T'ai chi	48 Male and 48 female Experienced practitioners Subjected to mental stress before intervention Randomized to 4 groups (t'ai chi, brisk walking, meditation, neutral reading) Measurements before and after intervention	Pretreatment to post-treatment: significant decrease in salivary cortisol levels; improved mood states; reduction in HR, BP, for t'ai chi were similar to walking at 6 km/h
Kolt, 2000	Feldenkrais	54 Volunteers College age Followed-up for 2 weeks Randomized to 3 groups (Feldenkrais, relaxation, or control) Measurements taken 4 times (baseline, before 4th session, after 4th session, 1 day after 4th session)	Feldenkrais and relaxation groups: significantly reduced anxiety scores in females after 4th session when compared to anxiety scores before 4th session and to controls Reduction maintained 1 day later
Hanley, 2003	Therapeutic massage	69 Subjects Randomized to 3 groups (6 sessions of therapeutic massage, 6 sessions of relaxation tape used in surgery, relaxation tape to use at home)	Pretreatment to post-treatment: significant improvements in sleep scale and index of well-being scores in all 3 groups; strong patient preference for therapeutic massage
Kalayil, 1989	Yoga meditation and progressive relaxation	80 Middle-grade students Randomly assigned to 4 groups (YM, PR, reading control, and catnap)	At baseline all 4 groups were similar in HR and state anxiety Results included: YM and PR decreased state anxiety, headaches, and general tension; YM decreased HR; catnap decreased headache when compared to reading control

YM, Yoga meditation; *PR*, progressive relaxation.

four studies have significant methodological weaknesses, the number of subjects participating in each study is formidable. These initial attempts at providing efficacy of the respective technique help suggest a launching ground for future study.

Hypertension

There is a large body of literature addressing the benefits of CAM interventions in the management of hypertension (HTN). The majority of the larger studies address mind/body interventions, with most demonstrating positive effects on BP. In 1999 The Canadian Hypertension Society and the Heart and Stroke Foundation of Canada published guidelines recommending "individualized cognitive behavior modification to reduce the negative effects of stress" (Spence, 1999).

Eisenberg et al (1993) performed a meta-analysis addressing the effectiveness of cognitive behavioral therapies on HTN. Techniques accepted in this review were biofeedback, meditation, the relaxation response, progressive relaxation techniques, and stress management interventions such as

imagery. They collected more than 800 published papers; however, due to methodological problems of the majority of papers, their limited inclusion criteria of adult subjects with diastolic BP of 90 to 114 mm Hg, randomized control design, detailed description of the study, and detailed reporting of BP values, only 26 studies were entered for detail review. Results of this comprehensive analysis of 1264 patients indicated superior outcomes in the group receiving cognitive intervention techniques when compared to controls. No one intervention demonstrated more favorable outcomes than another. In addition, when control groups were subjected to a placebo intervention (i.e. sham biofeedback), no significant differences in outcomes were noted. This is consistent with the belief that an intervention effect is inherent in the concept of placebo (Spencer & Jacobs, 2003).

In two RCTs of African American subjects, investigators examined the effects of stress reduction approaches on HTN. In one study, 111 males and females with mean BP of 147/92 mm Hg and mean age of 67 years were randomized to

TABLE 27-5

Effect of Selected CAM Therapies in the Management of HTN

STUDY AUTHORS	CAM THERAPY	SAMPLE CHARACTERISTICS AND METHODS	OUTCOMES
Paran, 1996	Biofeedback	38 Patients (15 white-coat HTN; 23 essential HTN) Random assignment Biofeedback given 1 time per week for 4 weeks	Pretreatment to post-treatment: both groups had statistically significant reductions in BP in the clinic; white-coat HTN had significantly lower SBP and DBP at home than essential HTN
Patel, 1975	Yoga (and biofeedback) "psychophysical relaxation exercise"	40 Patients with HTN Followed-up for 9-12 months 20 Received intervention; 20 remained as controls	Statistically significant reductions in BP and anti-HTN medication requirements in intervention group
Brownstein, 1989	Yoga relaxation	Case report Age 46 years Male History of mild essential HTN 6-Week program	Discontinuation of anti-HTN medications; normalization of DBP; return to full flight status (aviator in US Air Force)
Zucker, 1997	Qi gong (breathing, meditation, movement)	22 Patients with HTN (15 in intervention group, 7 control) Intervention classes 2 times per week for 8 weeks	Pretreatment to post-treatment: significant decreases in SBP, DBP, MAP, RR in intervention group; significant increases in QOL in intervention group

MAP, Mean arterial blood pressure; *QOL,* quality of life.

a three-month trial of TM and progressive muscle relaxation (PMR) or a lifestyle modification education control program (Schneider, 1995). Results demonstrated that TM had a greater effect at lowering both systolic and diastolic BP than PMR and that both intervention groups had a significantly greater impact on BP reduction than the control group. In a small but well-designed study, Barnes et al (2001) recruited 34 African American adolescents (aged 15 to 18 years) with high normal BP (>85th and <95th percentile for age and sex, respectively). After randomization, 17 subjects participated in two months of daily, 15-minutes sessions of TM. The control group attended seven weekly, one-hour lessons on health education. Measures of cardiovascular function were collected at rest and during performance of a stressful activity, at baseline and again at the end of the intervention period. Although no significant changes were noted in resting values, results indicated that individuals in the TM group responded more favorably to stressor activities. Blood pressure increased appropriately during the activity in both groups; however, the degree of elevation was reduced in the TM group when compared to controls.

Reduction in antihypertensive medication requirements has been reported when mind/body therapies are added to the management regimen of HTN. In an RCT, Shapiro et al (1997) studied 39 individuals with medically treated HTN. Subjects trained in cognitive behavior therapies (i.e. PMR, biofeedback, deep diaphragmatic breathing, and imagery) showed a 73% reduction of BP medication requirements during the study follow-up period compared to a 35%

reduction in the control group. In addition, 55% of subjects in the intervention group were completely free of medication compared to only 30% of subjects in the control group. The reduction in BP levels was consistent across clinical, ambulatory, and home settings.

Yucha et al (2004) reviewed 20 RCTs investigating the effects of biofeedback on HTN. Several forms of biofeedback. including thermal, EMG, and electrodermal, resulted in reductions in blood pressure when the intervention was combined with related cognitive therapy and relaxation training. When biofeedback was the sole intervention, significant reductions in BP were not demonstrated.

In addition to the mind/body therapies discussed above, several additional studies investigating the effects of select CAM therapies in individuals with HTN are summarized in Table 27-5. Although the evidence presented in these studies is weak, these investigations provide valuable insights to consider when structuring future research protocols. Several review articles addressing effects of other interventions are summarized in Table 27-6. In general, the results of these investigations assist in providing evidence for the benefit of the intervention in the management of HTN. In one review, Levin and Vanderpool (1989) consider the beneficial effects of religious commitment and affiliation in the management of HTN. Possible explanations offered for lower blood pressure in individuals with HTN include the psychosocial effects of membership in an organized religious community, the inherent health promotion behaviors and preferences often supported by religious traditions, and the psychodynamics of

TABLE 27-6

Select CAM Therapies and their Effects on HTN: Summary of Review Papers

STUDY AUTHORS	CAM THERAPY	NUMBER OF ARTICLES REVIEWED	OUTCOME VARIABLES	OUTCOME
Levin, 1989	Religion*: RC, RA	20	SBP, DPB, HTN, heart disease mortality, HTN-related mortality, history of HTN	RC: 19 studies demonstrate intervention is associated with lower BP or lower rates of HTN; 5 studies demonstrate protective effects of intervention RA: significantly lower rates of HTN-related morbidity and mortality in highly devout, behaviorally strict groups (e.g., Mormons, Buddhists, Seventh-Day Adventists, clergy)
Sancier, 1999; Mayer, 1999	Qi gong	30	BP, measures of blood flow, CHF, acute MI, stroke, total mortality rate	Decreased stroke and mortality; decreased anti-HTN medication requirements

RC, Religious commitment; *RA*, religious affiliation.
*Measures of religion include religious attendance, church membership, religious affiliation, ethnic traditions within Judaism, monastic orders, clergy status, religious education, and subjective religiosity.

religious rites, faith, and belief systems. In the review articles of the effects of qi gong in HTN, authors acknowledge significant methodological weaknesses in many of the studies reviewed (Sancier, 1999; Mayer, 1999). Some of the reported weaknesses include selection biases, lack of randomization, noncompliance with the intervention, concerns regarding BP measurement reliability, and the differences amongst the many styles of qi gong, which were not typically considered.

CAD

Beneficial effects of CAM techniques in the use of CAD management are documented throughout the published literature (Luskin, 1998; Astin, 2003; Lescowitz, 2003). Although significant methodological problems are apparent in many papers, numerous large, well-designed studies can be found. Much of the evidence supporting the use of these techniques in individuals with CAD demonstrates improvement in exercise tolerance, reduction of ischemia, and reduction of anxiety and depression. Mind/body techniques including cognitive behavioral interventions, yoga, t'ai chi, guided imagery, and music therapy have been successfully used in patients with CAD. The benefits of energy work including distant healing prayer and qi gong in patients with CAD have been reported.

In 1959, Friedman and Rosenman first documented the relationship between certain emotional behaviors and the prevalence of CAD (Friedman, 1986). They defined the Type A behavior pattern as "an emotional syndrome characterized by a continuously harrying sense of time urgency and easily aroused free-floating hostility." In subsequent decades, the study of interventions aimed at modifying the behavior of

individuals with Type A behavior pattern and CAD was undertaken.

In a large study of post-myocardial infarction (MI) patients with Type A behavior, 1013 subjects were randomized into three groups (Friedman, 1986). Two hundred and seventy subjects received group cardiac counseling, 592 subjects received both cardiac counseling and Type A behavioral counseling, and the remaining 151 individuals did not receive any counseling. Subjects were followed-up for four-and-a-half years to determine the impact of Type A behavior counseling on recurrent coronary events (both nonfatal infarctions and cardiac deaths). Cardiac counseling sessions consisted of 90-minute group meetings where topics concerning diet, exercise, medications, cardiovascular pathophysiology, and possible surgical procedures were discussed. Type A behavioral counseling sessions included progressive muscle relaxation as well as specific psychotherapeutic interventions. Results indicated statistically significant reductions in recurrence rates of cardiac events in both intervention groups, with a greater reduction in the rate of recurrent events in those subjects who received both forms of counseling.

In a landmark study of 48 patients with known CAD, Ornish et al (1990) analyzed the number of coronary artery lesions detected at angiography before and after a year long lifestyle intervention. In addition to a low-fat vegetarian diet, smoking cessation, and a moderate exercise program, subjects participated in a stress management training program of guided imagery. At the end of the year, the 28 subjects in the intervention group demonstrated statistically significant fewer coronary lesions than the 20 subjects in the usual-care control group. The regression in coronary atherosclerosis was attributed to the comprehensive lifestyle changes, brought about without the assistance of lipid-lowering medications. Clinical reports of angina were reduced as well.

Upon recognition of the impact of emotions on the recurrence rate of cardiac events in individuals with CAD, behavioral interventions became routine therapies in cardiac care (Levy, 1993). Dusseldorp et al (1999) published a meta-analysis of the results of 37 studies investigating the effects of psychoeducational programs on patients with known CAD. All studies were conducted between 1974 and 1997 and were categorized according to stress management (SM) and health education (HE) interventions. Techniques used included various combinations of education, cognitive-behavioral therapies, relaxation, imaging, and emotional support. A number of studies included SM and HE interventions in combination with standard exercise training programs typically found in traditional cardiac rehabilitation programs. Results from studies administering either SM or HE intervention suggested a 34% reduction in fatal cardiac events and a 29% reduction in recurrent MI. The authors concluded that although psychoeducational therapies should be encouraged in cardiac rehabilitation programs, future research focusing on specific SM or HE interventions is warranted. In another meta-analysis addressing the effects of psychosocial interventions with subjects with CAD, Linden et al (1996) reviewed 23 studies of 2024 patients and 1156 control subjects. In addition to the typical education component of cardiac rehabilitation programs, almost half of the studies included in this analysis had an intervention of some form of CAM treatment. These included relaxation, breathing relaxation, and music therapy. Just as in the aforementioned meta-analysis, the benefits of adding a psychosocial component to these cardiac rehabilitation programs significantly reduced morbidity and mortality and psychological distress.

In 2000, in a scientific statement presented by the American Heart Association and the American Association of Cardiovascular and Pulmonary Rehabilitation, psychosocial management was identified as a "core component of cardiac rehabilitation/secondary prevention programs." Suggested interventions included "individual and/or small group education and counseling regarding adjustment to Coronary Heart Disease, stress management, and health-related lifestyle change… supportive rehabilitation environment and community resources to enhance patient's and family's level of social support" (Balady, 2000).

The relationship between mental stress and myocardial ischemia in men with CAD has been well studied. Investigators have documented greater mental–stress-induced ischemia in individuals experiencing daily life ischemia than in those without mental–stress-induced ischemia (Stone, 1999). Individuals with chronic anxiety and depression also exhibit more episodes of myocardial ischemia than those without documented anxiety and depression (Sullivan, 2000). In a five-year, nonrandomized controlled study of 94 men with documented mental–stress-induced ischemia, researchers reported on the usefulness of a stress management program

(Blumenthal, 1997; Blumenthal, 2002). In addition to educational classes, the intervention group received instruction aimed at reducing the physiological effects of stress. This included instruction in progressive muscle relaxation and individual sessions of EMG biofeedback. Outcomes of recurrent cardiac events were significantly reduced in the stress management group when compared to the control group at one-, two-, and five-year follow-up. Overall reductions in hostility and clinical depression were also reported as statistically and clinically significant. The five-year financial burden, including hospitalization and physician costs, was also significantly less in the stress management group. Similar results were reported by Zamarra et al (1996) in a small, nonrandomized controlled study of the effects of an eight-month trial of TM. At follow-up bicycle exercise testing, participants demonstrated increases in exercise duration and maximal workload achieved and a delay in the onset of ST depression. In an early paper, Benson et al (1975) reported on the beneficial effects of the relaxation response in reducing the number of premature ventricular contractions (PVC) in individuals with stable CAD. Subjects in this report practiced the relaxation response for 20 minutes, twice a day. Frequency of PVCs was documented by Holter monitor at baseline and again after four weeks.

Several studies have demonstrated no or limited improvements in cardiovascular outcomes with the intervention of specific behavioral therapies. In a large (n = 2328), RCT of early post-MI intervention, investigators reported limited benefit of psychological counseling (Jones, 1996). In this two-year follow-up study, patients with acute MI returned within 28 days of the acute event to participate in seven weeks of outpatient counseling, including PMR and skills to reduce stress. Subjects in the intervention group experienced significantly fewer episodes of angina; however, mortality, clinical complications, and clinical sequelae of CAD did not differ between groups. The authors concluded the intervention was conducted too soon after the cardiac event, possibly accounting for the reduced treatment effect. In a study of patients participating in a Phase II cardiac rehabilitation program, progressive muscle relaxation and guided imagery interventions failed to result in beneficial outcomes (Collins, 1997). Although there were methodological limitations in this paper, the authors similarly concluded the timing of the interventions may have contributed to the absence of benefit.

Results of the effects of selected mind/body therapies in CAD are summarized in Table 27-7. Manchanda et al (2000) investigated the effects of yoga on numerous cardiovascular measures. Although improved outcomes were documented in the intervention group when compared to controls, the demonstrated benefits may be due to the moderate exercise component of the intervention and not necessarily the yoga component.

T'ai chi practice has been recommended as a therapeutic intervention in balance disorders and fall prevention in the elderly (Wolf, 1997; Lee, 2004; Wayne, 2004). Its potential benefits as an adjunct therapy in cardiac rehabilitation

TABLE 27-7

Effect of Selected Mind/Body Therapies in CAD

STUDY AUTHORS	MBT THERAPY	SAMPLE CHARACTERISTICS AND METHODS	OUTCOMES
Manchanda, 2000	Yoga	Prospective RCCT 42 Men with CAD 2 Groups Intervention: yoga, RF control, diet control, moderate exercise Control: RF control, AHA step 1 diet control	Yoga group: (compared to controls) significant decrease in number of anginal episodes per week; improved exercise capacity; decreased body weight, total cholesterol, LDL cholesterol, triglycerides; fewer revascularization procedures; more lesion regression and less lesion progression (angiographic findings); improved functional class, symptomatic status, and RF profile
Friedlander, 1986	Religion (Orthodox Jewish)	Had first MI: 454 Men (51% secular) 85 Women (50% secular) Healthy, no CAD 295 Men (21% secular) 391 Women (16% secular)	Higher risk of first MI if: older, smoker, less education; European born; secular; men and women; results persisted 2-3 months after acute event
Strawbridge, 1997	Religion	5286 Survey respondents Followed-up for 28 years Analyzed for association between attendance at religious services and mortality	Frequent attenders compared to infrequent attenders: lower mortality rates; results were stronger for females; improved health practices (stop smoking, increase exercising, increase social contacts, stay married)

MBT, Mind/body therapy; *RCCT*, randomized control clinical trial; *RF*, risk factors; *AHA*, American Heart Association.

programs have been suggested as well (Taylor-Piliae, 2003). In an interesting commentary in 1992, Ng stated that t'ai chi "has many similarities with...walking exercise—the most recommended aerobic exercise for coronary artery disease" (Ng, 1992). Further clinical study is warranted to provide evidence of the benefit of t'ai chi in the population with CAD.

There is minimal evidence available investigating the effects of energy work on patients with CAD. Several studies compared acupuncture to sham acupuncture in individuals with angina (Heidenrich, 1999). Although no significant differences were noted in the number of anginal episodes or nitroglycerin use, the use of sham acupuncture has been questioned. As noted earlier, not all practitioners agree on proper needle location, hence what one practitioner thinks is an active acupuncture site may be considered a sham site to another practitioner.

Another role for CAM therapies that address stress reduction in patients with CAD is based on the relationship between chronic stress and reduced immune system function. Individuals with depressed immune systems are more vulnerable to inflammatory processes, the latter recently implicated in CAD (Ross, 1999; Ridker, 2002; Ehrenstein, 2005).

Other Cardiovascular Conditions and Considerations

Cardiac Surgery. The Complementary Care Center (CCC) at Columbia-Presbyterian Medical Center is a "multi-faceted program dedicated to evaluating and researching the effects of new modalities in health care" (Whitworth, 1998). Since 1995, practitioners at this center have been evaluating

and researching the effects of various types of CAM therapies. One area of intervention involves patients having cardiac surgery. Upon initial evaluation, these patients are offered several options to help with recovery and healing. Some of these modalities include meditation, music therapy, yoga, massage, and therapeutic touch. Audiotapes can be used at different times in the perioperative period. This includes five to 10 days preoperatively, intraoperatively, immediately postoperatively, and during the recuperation phase. Therapeutic touch has been offered on the day of surgery and on postoperative days two and three. Group yoga classes are offered to those patients who are medically stable as early as the third postoperative day. In addition, patients are encouraged to contact a religious leader of their choice. Continuation of these therapies is offered to the patient after hospital discharge. Patients can choose to attend sessions at the center or at a more convenient site.

The innovative approach used at the CCC resonates with the philosophy of increasing the patient's participation in his or her health and healing. Liu et al (2000) have reported on the use of CAM therapies in 376 consecutive patients undergoing cardiac surgery. Patients were surveyed before surgery, and 75% reported using CAM therapies. When prayer and vitamins were excluded, 44% reported using CAM therapies. Seventy-two percent of subjects were male, 76% were white, and 59% were well educated. No differences in overall CAM use were found among sex, age, race, or education level. The authors did offer an important recommendation. They noted that only 17% of patients had discussed their use of CAM therapies with their physicians, and 48% of patients did not

TABLE 27-8
Effects of Selected CAM Therapies on Outcomes of Cardiovascular Surgery

STUDY AUTHORS	CAM THERAPY	SAMPLE CHARACTERISTICS AND METHOD	OUTCOME
Lan, 1999	T'ai chi	Prospective, 1-year program, 20 Patients >3 months since CABG Age 53-64 years All males T'ai chi group: (20 min w/up, 24 min t'ai chi, 10 min c/d); daily program Control group: (walking program 10 min w/up,30 min walking, 10 min c/d); 3 times per week VO_2max measured on cycle ergometer	T'ai chi: increased VO_2max; increased compliance with attendance
Barnason, 1995	Music therapy	Prospective, random, repeated measures 96 Subjects underwent elective CABG Age 37-84 years 65% Male Three groups (music therapy, music-video therapy, rest group) 30-Minute intervention on postoperative days 2 and 3 (inpatient)	Music therapy: improved mood; decreased heart rate; decreased SBP or DBP
Oxman, 1995	Social support Religion	232 Patients 21 Deaths within 6 months of elective open heart surgery	Predictors of mortality: history of previous cardiac surgery; greater impairment in presurgery ADL; older age; lack of participation in social or community groups; absence of strength and comfort from religion

CABG, Coronary artery bypass graft surgery; *w/up*, warm-up; *c/d*, cool down; *ADL*, activities of daily living.

want to discuss the topic at all. Since the frequency of CAM use found in this sample was consistent with the frequency of CAM use reported in the general population, the authors reinforced the importance of questioning patients about their use of CAM therapies (Eisenberg, 2001).

Evidence supporting the use of selected CAM therapies perioperatively is found in Table 27-8. Although methods were not always comprehensive in these studies, all demonstrated improvement in cardiovascular outcomes. In the study by Barnason et al (1995) the authors concluded that effects of the music therapy on outcomes were consistent with a relaxation response.

In another small but clinically important study, Miller and Perry (1990) examined the benefit of a deep-breathing relaxation technique on pain tolerance in patients undergoing cardiac surgery. On the evening before surgery, 15 subjects were taught a slow, rhythmic, deep-breathing relaxation technique in addition to traditional preoperative instruction. The remaining 14 subjects only received the traditional preoperative instruction. All subjects were visited by the investigators on the day of surgery and on postoperative day one for conversation; however, only subjects in the intervention group were encouraged to perform the relaxation technique. Patients in the relaxation group had significant decreases in systolic and diastolic BP, HR, respiratory rate, and self-report of pain (on visual descriptor scale) when compared to controls. The authors concluded that "relaxation techniques may interrupt the pain-anxiety cycle" and that, although there were methodological problems with their study, this "may be an effective non-narcotic, noninvasive pain-relieving modality after" cardiac surgery. Additional study of the relaxation response has demonstrated a reduction in postoperative arrhythmias, as well as reduced tension and anger in patients undergoing cardiac surgery (Luskin 1998).

Congestive Heart Failure. There are a limited number of published investigations on the effects of CAM therapies in patients with congestive heart failure (CHF). Results of three papers are summarized in Table 27-9. It is of interest that most of these papers utilized several techniques to achieve improved outcomes. This may be of value given the multiplicity of systems affected in CHF. Unfortunately, the degree of ventricular impairment was not documented in these studies. In addition, care must be taken when interpreting results of single case studies of patients with cardiac disease. The placebo effect evoked by the investigator's enthusiasm and expectation of success has been well studied in this

TABLE 27-9

Effects of Selected CAM Therapies in CHF

STUDY AUTHORS	CAM THERAPY	SAMPLE METHOD AND CHARACTERISTICS	OUTCOME
Moser, 1997	Skin-temperature biofeedback relaxation Guided imagery	40 Patients with advanced CHF Randomized to intervention (BFR) or control (C) BFR included 1 session of skin-temperature biofeedback, guided imagery of hand warmth, and progressive muscle relaxation. C group underwent measurement session but no intervention	Baseline: comparable measurements between groups When comparing BFR to C, BFR showed: increased skin temperature in finger and foot; increased cardiac output; decreased systemic vascular resistance; decreased RR No changes in oxygen consumption or catecholamines were found in either group
Bernardi, 1998	Complete yoga breathing	15 Patients with CHF; 11 healthy volunteer controls (C) CHF patients were randomized to intervention (YB) or rest (R) YB included reduction of RR through controlled breathing (CB) and altered breathing pattern within each breath to include diaphragm, lower chest, then upper chest in inspiration and expiration, 1 hour per day for 1 month Measurements at baseline, end of 1 month and 1 month after completion Maximum symptom-limited cycle ergometer exercise test	Baseline: SaO_2 was lower during spontaneous breathing (SB) in CHF compared to C; SaO_2 instability was higher during SB in CHF compared to C At 1 month: SaO_2 decreased during SB in YB compared to R, and approximated C during CB R results compared to YB: decreased sensation of dyspnea; decrease SB rate 13.4 ± 1.5 to 7.6 ± 1.9 bpm; SaO_2 (%) increased 92.5 ± 0.3 to 93.2 ± 0.4; VO_2 max increased 13.9 to 15.9 ± 0.8; maximum cycle workload increased 92 ± 6 to 100 ± 4 watts
Shinnick, 2002	Meditation Acupuncture Qi gong	Case report 97-Year-old terminally ill male Utilized techniques PRN	Qi gong used to increase body temperature Acupuncture to help sleep and improve appetite Meditation increased peacefulness, lucidity, and ability to control breathing

SaO2, Oxygen saturation; *bpm*, breaths per minute; *PRN*, whenever needed.

population (Benson, 1979; Bienenfeld, 1996). Symptomatic and objective improvements have been documented in angina outcomes related to pharmacological interventions, and after sham cardiac surgical procedures.

Patients in Coronary Care Unit. In two interesting, detailed, and well-designed studies, investigators examined the effects of intercessory prayer (praying for others) on outcomes of patients admitted to a coronary care unit (Byrd, 1988; Harris et al, 1999). With only slight differences in design, Harris et al attempted to replicate the results that Byrd demonstrated a decade earlier. Both studies were large, randomized controlled, blinded trials (Byrd with 393 subjects, Harris with 990 subjects). Patients were admitted to the coronary care unit (CCU) with a wide variety of diagnoses in both studies. In addition to common cardiac diagnoses, patients had conditions such as pneumonia, chronic obstructive lung disease, diabetes mellitus, renal failure, sepsis, liver disease, and gastrointestinal bleeding. Patients were monitored for new problems, new diagnoses, and new therapeutic interventions that occurred after hospital admission through discharge. This information contributed to the scoring

systems used by investigators to determine distinctions between recovery rates and severity of complications during hospitalization. Intercessors in the Byrd study were "born again" Christian individuals, while intercessors in the Harris study represented a variety of Christian traditions, including 35% nondenominational, 27% Episcopalian, and Protestant and Roman Catholic observers. In the original study, Byrd assigned three to seven intercessors to each patient in the intervention group. Intercessors were asked to pray daily (until hospital discharge) for the individual's rapid recovery and prevention of complications, as well as contribute other prayers they believed would be beneficial to the patient. They were provided the patient's first name, diagnosis, general condition, and pertinent updated information. Harris et al randomly assigned a five-member team to pray for each patient. Intercessors were not given any information about the patient. They were asked to pray daily for 28 days for a "speedy recovery with no complications" and anything else the intercessor believed appropriate. Results from both studies demonstrated statistically significant better outcomes in patients who were prayed for when compared to those not prayed for. Although in both studies the length of hospital stay was not significantly different between control and intervention groups, the CCU course severity scores were significantly different between control and intervention groups. Control subjects in the Byrd study required more frequent ventilatory assistance, antibiotics, and diuretics than subjects in the intervention group. Control subjects in the Harris et al study received higher scores on a scale quantifying severity of clinical outcomes from excellent to catastrophic than did subjects in the intervention group.

The basis of this therapeutic effect of distance healing remained unexplained by the authors. The outcomes provided by these two randomized controlled clinical trials, however, warrants continued exploration into the possible benefits of intercessory prayer in medical outcomes. McCullough et al (2000) reported data from 42 publications in a meta-analysis examining the association of religious involvement to all-cause mortality. Their results resonate with those of the Byrd and Harris studies, and concluded, from sampling more than 126,000 participants, that religious involvement was significantly associated with lower mortality rates. Similarly, they recommend that "elucidating the nature of this robust but poorly understood association could be a fruitful topic for future research at the interface of psychology and health."

Pulmonary Conditions

The basis for using CAM therapies in the management of individuals with cardiopulmonary disease is two-fold. In addition to focusing treatment goals on the reduction of SNS stimulation and metabolic demands, CAM therapies also alter the mechanics of the musculoskeletal pump of the thorax. As addressed earlier in Part III of this book, improvements in thoracic mobility and movement efficiency contribute to reduced metabolic demands and improved oxygen transport.

Asthma

Numerous factors have been implicated as causative agents of asthma. In addition to respiratory infection and allergens, emotional stress has been identified as a trigger. Generalized panic symptoms have been found to be both a cause of asthma as well as a response to an exacerbation of asthma. Panic and anxiety states correlate with hyperventilation, a symptom closely related to a hyperactive respiratory drive. A heightened respiratory drive is not always favorable in individuals with known asthma because it can further challenge airways that are already bronchoconstricted (Lehrer, 1998). Hyperventilation itself may exacerbate asthma because the rapid movement of cooler and dryer air into the airways can trigger further bronchoconstriction.

Repressive-coping styles have also been associated with asthma morbidity (Lehrer, 1998). Individuals with this behavior pattern typically ignore their symptoms, including dyspnea, and fail to seek timely health care. These individuals tend to have relatively high levels of endogenous opioids, neurochemicals that can depress unpleasant sensations.

Consequently these substances may limit an individual's ability to recognize early signs of bronchoconstriction. Additional evidence suggests that reduced immune system responsiveness in the setting of chronic emotional stress heightens inflammatory and infective processes, both of which are implicated in asthma exacerbation.

Numerous CAM therapies have been studied in attempts to reverse a number of these factors associated with asthma morbidity. Many of these studies have methodological shortcomings; however, several are well designed and provide insights into possible mechanisms of intervention efficacy. Relaxation therapy has been widely investigated; however, the results are inconsistent. In a meta-analysis of six studies on the effects of relaxation training in children with emotionally triggered asthma, McQuaid and Nassau (1999) concluded that "relaxation training is probably efficacious intervention" in this population. They noted concern regarding methods used in the articles reviewed and noted that only three of the studies reviewed in this analysis used appropriate controls, and only one examined maintenance of post-treatment effect. Although statistical significance was achieved in these investigations, the reduction of symptoms was less than 10% of baseline values, leading the authors to believe that the changes would not be clinically significant. Lehrer (1998) also concluded that relaxation therapy may only be effective with specific asthma patients. His results indicate significant improvement in asthma exacerbation in individuals with emotionally-triggered events when relaxation techniques are used. He noted worsening of symptoms when they were acute, however, and concluded that "relaxation training may provide protection from emotionally induced asthma" when symptoms are chronic. Some theories regarding the failure of relaxation therapy to benefit individuals with asthma relate to its effect on the ANS. Evidence demonstrates relaxation therapy downregulates the beta receptors of the SNS and thus reduces bronchodilation, an unfavorable outcome for individuals with asthma.

In a meta-analysis of 31 studies published between 1972 and 1993, Devine reported on the effects of psychoeducational care on adults with asthma. Psychoeducational interventions were defined as "education, behavioral skill development, cognitive therapy, and/or nonbehavioral support/counseling" (Devine, 1996). The author concluded that, despite methodological flaws primarily due to small numbers of subjects, education and relaxation-based behavioral interventions demonstrated improvement in clinical measures of pulmonary function. These measures included peak expiratory flow rate (PEFR), functional status, regimen compliance, use of medications, psychological well-being, and ability to use an inhaler properly. Similarly, a review of 12 well-designed studies investigating the effects of limited asthma education (information only) demonstrated a significant improvement in perceived asthma symptoms and reduced visits to the emergency department in adults with asthma (Gibson, 2004). In a controlled study of 35 children aged five to six years, researchers investigated the effects of a six-month psychoeducational program that included guided imagery on several clinical and immunological outcomes associated with asthma control (Castes, 1999). In addition to education classes and workshops for parents, daily instruction was given to the children to imagine visual images of unobstructed airways, mast cells and immunoglobulin E (IgE) suppression. The results demonstrated significant reductions in the number of asthmatic episodes requiring medical attention, and reduced bronchodilator requirements in the intervention group when compared to the control group. Spirometric values, specifically forced expiratory volume in one second (FEV_1), improved in the intervention group despite reduction in bronchodilator utilization. In addition, markers associated with immune system function (specific IgE levels, leukocyte surface markers, B cells) demonstrated improved efficiency. Conversely, a review of eight clinical trials investigating the effects of a limited asthma education program on over 1400 children with asthma failed to demonstrate any reduction in emergency department visits or hospital admissions (Haby, 2001). It appears that the addition of a guided imagery program to an asthma education program improves outcomes in children.

In a well-designed, RCT of the effects of guided imagery on a group of adult patients with asthma, outcome measures failed to reveal statistically significant differences between intervention and control groups (Epstein, 2004). Measures of FEV_1, anxiety, depression, quality of life scales, and the number of visits to the emergency department were not different between groups. Those subjects who practiced mental imagery, however, demonstrated statistically significant decreases in medication usage and reported more power and control in their ability to change the course of their disease. Authors stressed the pilot nature of this study and concluded that if a larger sample was studied, more significant outcomes may have been achieved because there were trends favoring the mental imagery group in all outcome measures.

Preliminary study of the effects of the Alexander technique on measures of pulmonary function warrants further investigation (Austin & Ausubel, 1992; Dennis & Cates, 2004). No controlled studies investigating the effects of this technique on individuals with asthma have been published. Although performing artists (musicians, singers, actors) reportedly benefit from this intervention, systematic study is lacking. In addition, individuals with asthma are reportedly helped with this technique. Austin and Ausubel documented improved pulmonary function measures in 10 healthy adults after 20 private sessions of therapy with the Alexander technique. No such improvement was found in 10 adults in a matched control group. Significant increases were demonstrated in PEFR, maximum voluntary ventilation (MVV), maximal inspiratory pressure (MIP), and maximal expiratory mouth pressure (MEP).

Both EMG and thermal biofeedback interventions have been studied in the management of asthma. Several of these interventions have been aimed at increasing HR. It has been postulated that by increasing HR, the accompanying increase in beta SNS activity produces increased bronchodilation. The

few studies investigating this intervention have not been able to validate this theory due to design flaws (Lehrer, 1998). Other trials of biofeedback have focused on general muscle relaxation and facial muscle relaxation. In a comprehensive review, McQuaid and Nassau (1999) concluded that studies investigating biofeedback with general muscle relaxation demonstrate similar results as those trials using relaxation without biofeedback. These results are inconclusive and conflicting in individuals with asthma. There is, however, strong evidence supporting the use of EMG biofeedback on the frontalis muscle of children with asthma (McQuaid & Nassau, 1999; Kotses et al, 1991). Tension in this muscle has been correlated with increased airway resistance, presumably a consequence of a trigeminal-vagal reflex. Well-designed, carefully detailed studies examining reduced tension in facial muscles have demonstrated improvements in clinical measures of pulmonary function, including PEFR and asthma severity. (Kotses et al, 1991)

The effects of yoga on asthma have been investigated by several authors. A summary of selected studies is found in Table 27-10. Results of these studies are still insufficient to draw sound conclusions. These initial trials, however, provide reasonable evidence supporting the use of yoga as complementary in the management of asthma. Although a discussion of breathing techniques is outside the scope of this chapter, there is evidence suggesting the value of certain techniques in asthma management (Ernst, 2000). Yoga breathing overlaps with some of these breathing exercises (e.g. slow, deep breathing mimics pranayama yoga exercise).

Writing about emotionally traumatic events has been shown to have physical and psychological benefits. Smyth et al (1999) studied 58 adults with asthma (mean age 41 years). Subjects were randomized to an intervention group that was instructed to write about the most stressful event in their lives, while the control group wrote about an emotionally neutral event. Subjects were instructed to write for 20 minutes, on three consecutive days. At two weeks follow-up, mean FEV_1 in the intervention group increased significantly from 63.9% of predicted values to 76.3% of predicted values. These statistically significant improvements were maintained at two- and four-month follow-up testing. No changes in FEV_1 were noted in the control group. Although the results of this study are complicated by the inclusion of subjects with rheumatoid arthritis, the authors offer strong preliminary evidence for the value of this writing intervention.

Most of the CAM therapies discussed thus far in the management of asthma have been mind/body techniques. Although there is a paucity of publications addressing the effects of body work on asthma, a review of five RCTs investigating the effects of manual therapy on asthma was recently published (Hondras et al, 2004). In general, the methodological differences between all studies and the shortcomings of each individual study preclude any strong recommendation supporting the use of manual therapy in the treatment of asthma. Two of the studies reported on chiropractic manipulation as compared to sham maneuvers,

TABLE 27-10			
Effect of Yoga on Asthma			
STUDY AUTHORS	TYPE OF YOGA	SAMPLE CHARACTERISTICS AND METHOD	OUTCOMES
Tandon, 1978	Yogic breathing exercises and posture	22 Patients with severe chronic airway obstruction Matching groups of 11 subjects Yoga group (YG) and control group (CG) followed-up monthly for 9 months; CG received physiotherapy breathing	Compared to CG, the YG showed: significant increase in maximum work by 60.55 kpm; symptomatic improvement
Jain, 1991	Yoga	46 Young individuals with asthma Age 11-18 years All had history of childhood asthma Subjects acted as their own controls	Compared to baseline, significant increase in pulmonary function and exercise capacity At 2 year follow-up, reduced symptoms and drug requirements
Vedanthan, 1998	Slow breathing (pranayama) Postures (asanas) Meditation	Adults with asthma Age 19-52 years 17 Volunteers randomly divided into yoga (YG) and nonyoga groups (NYG) YG practiced 3 times per week for 16 weeks Both groups maintained daily symptom and medication diaries; AM and PM PEFR; weekly spirometry and questionnaires	Compared to NYG, the YG showed: significant degree of relaxation and positive attitude; better yoga exercise tolerance; trend towards decrease use of beta adrenergic inhalers; no difference in pulmonary function measures

and a third compared massage therapy with a relaxation control group. Significant improvement in measures of lung function was found in the massage therapy study. The final two studies found no differences between intervention and control groups when chest physiotherapy was compared to placebo and when footzone (reflexology) therapy was compared to a no-treatment control.

Acupuncture, a form of energy work, has been discussed extensively in the management of asthma. Several review studies and meta-analyses have been published addressing the effects of acupuncture on various outcomes related to asthma (Jadad et al, 2000; Martin et al, 2002; McCarney et al, 2004). Inclusion criteria for an article to be reviewed in one of these publications consisted of randomized control design and measurement of objective pulmonary function outcomes, most often FEV_1. Significant disagreement exists among investigators regarding details of acupuncture techniques, including proper location of needles, depth of needle penetration, and frequency and duration of treatment (Biernacki & Peake, 1998; Birch, 2002; Medici et al, 2002; Shapira et al, 2002). There is general agreement, however, that strong evidence exists to support the *process* of inserting acupuncture needles into individuals with asthma. Medici et al (2002) have demonstrated that whether or not the actual point of needle insertion is considered proper is unessential. They successfully demonstrated that regardless of the site of needle insertion, certain physiological responses occur that improve pulmonary function in patients with asthma. They attribute

this to a direct physiological release of substances in response to the invasiveness of inserting the needles into the body, or to a physiological response triggered by the interaction between practitioner and subject (including the intention of the practitioner to heal the subject), or to some other unknown, as yet undefined factor. Hence, most investigators conclude that more research is necessary to understand the complexities of acupuncture as a technique and how it can best be prescribed in the treatment of asthma.

There is preliminary evidence that qi gong may be an effective adjunct to medical management of asthma (Sancier, 1999). When pharmacological intervention is combined with qi gong, reported benefits include symptom reduction, improved immune system function, decreased sick leave and hospitalization days, decreased emergency department visits, and decreased antibiotic requirements for bronchial infections. These would result in a reduction in asthma-related morbidity and a substantial cost savings.

Chronic Obstructive Pulmonary Disease

Pulmonary rehabilitation programs have been traditionally used as adjuncts to pharmacological management of chronic obstructive pulmonary disease (COPD). These programs generally consist of exercise training and a variety of educational and supportive interventions. Strong evidence has been shown to support pulmonary rehabilitation interventions in improving outcomes in patients with COPD (Ries, 1990). These outcomes include reduction of perception of dyspnea,

TABLE 27-11

Effect of various Psychoeducational Interventions on Outcomes in Individuals with COPD

OUTCOME VARIABLE AND MEASUREMENT	NUMBER OF STUDIES	STATISTICALLY SIGNIfiCANT BENEfiCIAL INTERVENTIONS	NONSTATISTICALLY BENEfiCIAL INTERVENTIONS
Psychological well-being (e.g., anxiety, mood questionnaires)	26	Relaxation-type therapy Pulmonary rehabilitation	Education only
Endurance (e.g., time/ distance able to exercise)	16	Pulmonary rehabilitation	Education only
Oxygen uptake (VO$_2$ max)	8	Vigorous exercise (e.g., 60 minutes of supervised exercise 3 times per week for 9 weeks)	Mild exercise (e.g., 10 minutes of exercise 3 times per day)*
Functional status (e.g., sickness impact profile)	–	Pulmonary rehabilitation Breathing exercise and large muscle exercises	Education only
Dyspnea (visual analogue scales)	–	Pulmonary rehabilitation Progressive muscle relaxation	Guided imagery
Pulmonary function (static volumes and FEV$_1$)	–	Static volumes improved Pulmonary rehabilitation	FEV$_1$ no change Education only relaxation/imagery Pulmonary rehabilitation
Knowledge of psychomotor skills (e.g., accurate inhaler use)	–	Education only	
Adherence (self-reports, provider assessed compliance)	–	Pulmonary rehabilitation	Education only
Utilization of health care (e.g., ED visits, hospitalizations and LOS)	–	Pulmonary rehabilitation	Education only

ED, Emergency department; *LOS*, length of stay.
*Significant negative effect
Based on data from Devine, E.C., & Pearcy, J. (1996). Meta-analysis of the effects of psychoeducational care in adults with chronic obstructive pulmonary disease. Patient Education and Counseling 29:167-178.

increased work tolerance, and increased physical conditioning. Results, however, are inconsistent with regards to improvements in pulmonary function measures.

Devine and Pearcy (1996) performed a meta-analysis of 65 studies investigating the effects of psychoeducational therapies in adults with COPD. For purposes of their analysis, they included education, exercise, and/or psychosocial support as psychoeducational therapies. The majority of articles were found in journals (66%) and dissertations (29%) and were published between 1954 and 1994. Thirty-four percent of the studies were RCTs, 54% included a control group, and 15% had a placebo-type control. Data were included on 3642 individuals with 72% reported as having COPD, 25% reported as having COPD or asthma, and 3% as having COPD, asthma, or other chronic pulmonary disease. Subjects ranged in age between 43 and 70 years, 81% of the studies had more men than women, and 19% had men only. Almost half of the studies were conducted in an outpatient setting, and about one quarter were conducted in the inpatient

hospital setting. The remaining studies involved various settings including home.

Although the results of Devine and Pearcy's analysis revealed significant benefits of various interventions, the authors noted methodological weaknesses in many of the studies, including no mention of the duration of intervention in almost half of them. Statistically significant benefits of the various interventions are listed in Table 27-11. In general, education-only interventions were of benefit in improving the subject's knowledge of psychomotor skills. Relaxation-type interventions were effective in improving dyspnea and psychological well-being. An overwhelming benefit of pulmonary rehabilitation interventions was demonstrated in many studies. One hundred percent of the pulmonary rehabilitation programs included in this analysis had education and large-muscle exercise components. Seventy-five percent had breathing retraining, 57% had relaxation training, 54% had physical therapy, 43% had psychosocial support, 40% had occupational therapy, 29% had nutritional education, and 18% had vocational counseling. Although the results of this analysis begin to shed light on the benefits of individual interventions, more research is warranted. Recognition of the contribution of each of the specific CAM therapies offered within the umbrella of pulmonary rehabilitation may be difficult. This is consistent with Devine and Pearcy's conclusion that further research efforts to break down interventions within pulmonary rehabilitation may not be clinically wise given the complex needs of these patients.

Intuitively, yoga would seem a beneficial adjunct to the medical management of COPD. Components of yoga include slow breathing, or pranayama, and body positions, or asanas. At times meditation is included as well. Unfortunately, investigation of the effects of yoga on COPD is in its infancy and is still mostly anecdotal (Crawford, 2004). The reports include improved perceptions of dyspnea and decreased anxiety.

SUMMARY

The purpose of this chapter is to introduce the reader to complementary therapies in general, to define several of the common complementary therapies found in rehabilitation and then examine the literature on the effects of various complementary therapies on the normal cardiopulmonary system and, finally, to discuss the efficacy of their use with patients with cardiopulmonary pathologies. The quality of evidence found in the literature is inconsistent, with designs representative of the entire research spectrum, from case studies to large and well-designed RCTs. The most sophisticated studies found were in the testing of the efficacy of t'ai chi, yoga, acupuncture, intercessory prayer, and psychoeducational group work on various cardiopulmonary conditions including CAD, CHF, cardiac surgery, COPD, asthma, and HTN.

Given the widespread presence of cardiopulmonary illness in our society and the reality that people are using complementary therapies, it is essential that therapists are adequately prepared to understand, administer, and correctly interpret responses to these techniques and conduct and publish the required research to establish efficacy.

Review Questions

1. Describe the cardiovascular and pulmonary responses to mind/body therapies in healthy individuals and discuss how these responses may be helpful or harmful to patients with cardiac or pulmonary diseases.
2. Identify three CAM therapies that include components of traditional physical therapy (e.g., yoga, t'ai chi, biofeedback, massage, Alexander method) and compare and contrast goals of the CAM therapies with goals of traditional physical therapy relative to the cardiovascular and pulmonary systems.

3. Choose three forms of energy work therapies and discuss their (possible) effects on the cardiovascular and pulmonary systems.
4. Design a study investigating the effects of one energy work technique and one manual therapy/body work technique on cardiovascular and pulmonary responses in individuals with cardiac or pulmonary disease.
5. Choose a cardiopulmonary diagnosis and describe how you would plan a program using CAM therapies to help treat a patient with the diagnosis.

REFERENCES

Ader, R., & Cohen, N. (1991). The influence of conditioning on immune responses. In Ader R., Felten, D.L., & Cohen, N. (Eds). Psychoneuroimmunology, ed 2. San Diego: Academic Press.

Astin, J.A., Shapiro, S.L., Eisenberg, D.M., & Forys, K.L. (2003). Mind-body medicine: state of the science, implications for practice. Journal of the American Board of Family Practice 16:131-147.

Austin, J.H., & Ausubel, P. (1992). Enhanced respiratory muscular function in normal adults after lessons in proprioceptive musculoskeletal education without success. Chest 102:486-490.

Balady, G.J., Ades, P.A., Comoss, P., Limacher, M., Pina, I.L., Southard, D., Williams, M.A., & Bazzarre, T. (2000). Core components of cardiac rehabilitation/secondary prevention programs: a statement for healthcare professionals from the American Heart Association and the American Association of Cardiovascular and Pulmonary Rehabilitation. Circulation 102:1069-1073.

Barnason, S., Zimmerman, L., & Nieveen, J. (1995). The effects of music interventions on anxiety in the patient after coronary artery bypass grafting. Heart and Lung Journal of Acute and Critical Care 24:124-132.

Barnes, V.A., Treiber, F.A., & Davis, H. (2001). Impact of transcendental meditation on cardiovascular function at rest and during acute stress in adolescents with high normal blood pressure. Journal of Psychosomatic Research 51:597-605.

Benson, H., Alexander, S., & Feldman, C.L. (1975). Decreased premature ventricular contractions through use of the relaxation response in patients with stable ischemic heart-disease. Lancet 306:380-382.

Benson, H., Kotch, J.B., & Crassweller, K.D. (1977). The relaxation response: a bridge between psychiatry and medicine. Medical Clinics of North America 61:929-938.

Benson, H., & McCallie, D.P. (1979). Angina pectoris and the placebo effect. The New England Journal of Medicine 300:1424-1429.

Bernardi, L., Spadacini, G., Bellwon, J., Hajric, R., Roskamm, H., & Frey, A.W. (1998). Effect of breathing rate on oxygen saturation and exercise performance in chronic heart failure. Lancet 351:1308-1311.

Bienenfeld, L., Frishman, W., & Glasser, S.P. (1996). The placebo effect in cardiovascular disease. American Heart Journal 132:1207-1221.

Biernacki, W., & Peake, M.D. (1998). Acupuncture in treatment of stable asthma. Respiratory Medicine 92:1143-1145.

Birch, S. (2002). Acupuncture and bronchial asthma: a long-term randomized study. The Journal of Alternative and Complementary Medicine 8:751-754.

Blumenthal, J.A., Jiang, W., Babyak, M.A., Krantz, D.S., Frid, D.J., Coleman, R.E., Waugh, R., Hanson, M., Appelbaum, M., O'Connor, C., & Morris, J.J. (1997). Stress management and exercise training in cardiac patients with myocardial ischemia. Archives of Internal Medicine 157:2113-2223.

Blumenthal, J.A., Babyak, M., Wei, J., O'Connor,C., Waugh, R., Eisenstein, E., Mark, D., Sherwood, A., Woodley, P.S., Irwin, R.J. & Reed, G. (2002). Usefulness of psychosocial treatment of mental stress-induced myocardial ischemia in men. American Journal of Cardiology 89:164-168.

Brown, D.D., Mucci, W.G., Hetzler, R.K., & Knowlton, R.G. (1989). Cardiovascular and ventilatory responses during formalized tai chi chuan exercise. Research Quarterly for Exercise and Sport 60:246-250.

Brownstein, A.H., & Dembert, M.L. (1989). Treatment of essential hypertension with yoga relaxation therapy in a USAF aviator: a case report. Aviation, Space, and Environment Medicine 60:684-687.

Burton Goldberg Group. (Eds) (1995). Alternative medicine - the definitive guide. Fife, WA: Future Medicine Publishing, Inc.

Byrd, R.C. (1988). Positive therapeutic effects of intercessory prayer in a coronary care unit population. Southern Medical Journal 81:826-829.

Castes, M., Hagel, I., Palenque, M., Canelones, P., Corao, A., & Lynch, N.R. (1999). Immunological changes associated with clinical improvement of asthmatic children subjected to psychosocial intervention. Brain, Behavior, and Immunity 13:1-13.

Chao, Y.F., Chen, S.Y., Lan, C., & Lai, J.S. (2002). The cardio-respiratory response and energy expenditure of tai-chi-qui-gong. American Journal of Chinese Medicine 30:451-462.

Collins, J.A., & Rice, V.H. (1997). Effects of relaxation in phase II cardiac rehabilitation: replication and extension. Journal of Acute and Critical Care 26:31-44.

Cottingham, J.T., Porges, S.W., & Lyon, T. (1988a). Effects of soft tissue mobilization (rolfing pelvic lift) on parasympathetic tone in two age groups. Physical Therapy 68:352-356.

Cottingham, J.T., Porges, S.W., & Richmond, K. (1988b). Shifts in pelvic inclination angle and parasympathetic tone produced by rolfing soft tissue manipulation. Physical Therapy 68:1364-1370.

Crawford, J. (2004). Yoga holds potential as COPD therapy. ADVANCE for Physical Therapists & PT Assistants. August 2. p 55.

Davis, C.M. (Ed) (1997). Complementary therapies in rehabilitation/ holistic approaches for prevention and wellness. Thorofare, NJ: SLACK, Inc.

Davis, C.M. (Ed) (1997). Complementary therapies in rehabilitation. Evidence for efficacy in therapy, prevention and wellness, ed 2. Thorofare, NJ: SLACK, Inc.

Dennis, J., & Cates, C. (2004). Alexander technique for chronic asthma. The Cochrane Library 2:CD00)995.

Devine, E.C., & Pearcy, J. (1996). Meta-analysis of the effects of psychoeducational care in adults with chronic obstructive pulmonary disease. Patient Education and Counseling 29: 167-178.

Dusseldorp, E., van Elderen, T., Maes, S., Meulman, J., & Kraaij, V. (1999). A meta-analysis of psychoeducational programs for coronary heart disease patients. Health Psychology 18:506-519.

Ehrenstein, M.R., Jury, E.C., & Mauri, C. (2005). Statins for atherosclerosis - as good as it gets? New England Journal of Medicine 352:73-75.

Eisenberg, D.M., Delbanco, T.L., Berkey, C.S., Kaptchuk, T.J., Kupelnick, B., Kuhl, J., & Chalmers, T.C. (1993). Cognitive behavioral techniques for hypertension. Annals of Internal Medicine 118:964-972.

Eisenberg, D.M., Kessler, R.C., Van Rompay, M.I., Kaptchuk, T.J., Wilkey, S.A., Appel, S., & Davis, R.B. (2001). Perceptions about complementary therapies relative to conventional therapies among adults who use both: results from a national survey. Annals of Internal Medicine 135:344-351.

Eppley, K.R., Abrams, A.I., & Shear, J. (1989). Differential effects of relaxation techniques on trait anxiety: a meta-analysis. Journal of Clinical Psychology 45:957-974.

Epstein, G.N., Halper, J.P., Barrett, E.A.M., Birdsall, C., McGee, M., Baron, K.P., & Lowenstein, S. (2004). A pilot study of mind-body changes in adults with asthma who practice mental imagery. Alternative Therapies 10:66-71.

Ernst, E. (2000). Breathing techniques - adjunctive treatment modalities for asthma? A systematic review. European Respiratory Journal 15:969-972.

Fontana, J.A. (2000). The energy costs of a modified form of tai chi exercise. Nursing Research 49:91-96.

Friedlander, Y., Kark, J.D., & Stein, Y. (1986). Religious orthodoxy and myocardial infarction in Jerusalem - a case control study. International Journal of Cardiology 10:33-41.

Friedman, M., & Rosenman, R.H. (1959). Association of specific overt behavior pattern with blood and cardiovascular findings. Journal of the American Medical Association 169:1286.

Friedman, M., Thoresen, C.E., Gill, J.J., Ulmer, D., Powell, L.H., Price, V.A., Brown, B., Thompson, L., Rabin, D.D., Breall, W.S., Bourg, E., Levy, R., & Dixon, T. (1986). Alteration of type A behavior and its effect on cardiac recurrence in post myocardial infarction patients: summary results of the recurrent coronary prevention project. American Heart Journal 112:653-665.

Gibson, P.G., Powell, H., Coughlan, J., Wilson, A.J., Hensley, M.H., Abramson, M., Bauman, A., & Walters, E.H. (2002). Limited (information only) patient education programs for adults with asthma. Cochrane Database Systematic Reviews 2:CD001005.

Green, C., Martin, C.W., Bassett, K., & Kazanjian, A. (2004). A systematic review and critical appraisal on the scientific evidence in craniosacral therapy. Database of Abstracts of Reviews of Effectiveness 2.

Haas, F., Distenfeld, S., & Axen, K. (1986). Effects of perceived musical rhythm on respiratory pattern. Journal of Applied Physiology 61:1185-1191.

Haby, M.M., Waters, E., Robertson, C.F., Gibson, P.G., & Ducharme, F.M. (2001). Interventions for educating children who have attended the emergency room for asthma. Cochrane Database of Systematic Reviews 1:CD001290.

Haker, E., Egekvist, H., & Bjerring, P. (2000). Effect of sensory stimulation (acupuncture) on sympathetic and parasympathetic activities in healthy subjects. Journal of the Autonomic Nervous System 79:52-59.

Hanley, J., Stirling, P., & Brown, C. (2003). Randomized controlled trial of therapeutic massage in the management of stress. British Journal of General Practice 53:20-25.

Harris, W.S., Gowda, M., Kolb, J.W., Strychacz, C.P., Vacek, J.L., Jones, P.G., Forker, A., O'Keefe, J.H., & McCallister, B.D. (1999). A randomized, controlled trial of the effects of remote, intercessory prayer on outcomes in patients admitted to the coronary care unit. Archives of Internal Medicine 159: 2273-2278.

Haskell, W.L., Luskin, F.M., & Marvasti, F.F. (2003). Atheroscleortic vascular disease. In Spencer, J., Jacobs, J., (Eds). Complementary and alternative medicine: an evidence-based approach, ed 2. St. Louis: Mosby.

Heidenreich, P.A., McDonald, K.M., Hastie, T., Fadel, B., Hagan, V., Lee, B.K., & Hlatky, M.A. (1999). An evaluation of beta-blockers, calcium antagonists, nitrates, and alternative therapies for stable angina. Agency for Healthcare Research and Quality, Publication # 00-E003, November 1999.

Hiller, H., Weissberg, N., Horowitz, G., & Ilan, M. (1995). The safety of dental mini-magnets in patients with permanent cardiac pacemakers. Journal of Prosthetic Dentistry 74:420-421.

Hinman, M.R. (2002). Comparative effect of positive and negative static magnetic fields on heart rate and blood pressure in healthy adults. Clinical Rehabilitation 16:669-674.

Holland, B., & Pokorny, M.E. (2001). Slow stroke back massage: its effect on patients in a rehabilitation setting. Rehabilitation Nursing 26:182-186.

Hondras, M.A., Linde, K., & Jones, A.P. (2004). Manual therapy for asthma (Cochrane Review). The Cochrane Library 2. Chichester, UK: John Wiley & Sons, Ltd.

Hunt, V. (1989). Infinite mind - the science of the human vibrations of consciousness. Malibu, CA: Malibu Publishing Co.

Infante, J.R., Torres-Avisbal, M., Pinel, P., Vallejo, J.A., Peran, F., Gonzalez, F., Contreras, P., Pacheco, C., Roldan, A., & Latre, J.M. (2001). Catecholamine levels in practitioners of the transcendental meditation technique. Physiology and Behavior 72:141-146.

Ives, J.C., & Sosnoff, J. (2000). Beyond the mind-body exercise hype. The Physician and Sportsmedicine 28:67-83.

Jadad, A.R., Moher, M., Browman, G.P., Booker, L., Sigouin, C., Fuentes, M., & Stevens, R. (2000). Systematic reviews and meta-analyses on treatment of asthma: critical evaluation. British Medical Journal 320:537-540.

Jain, S.C., Rai, L., Valecha, A., Jha, U.K., Bhatnagar, S.O., & Ram, K (1991). Effect of yoga training on exercise tolerance in adolescents with childhood asthma. Journal of Asthma 28: 437-442.

Jin, P. (1989). Changes in heart rate noradrenaline, cortisol and mood during tai chi. Journal of Psychosomatic Research 33:197-206.

Jin, P. (1992). Efficacy of tai chi, brisk walking, meditation, and reading in reducing mental and emotional stress. Journal of Psychosomatic Research 36:361-370.

Jonas, W.B., & Crawford, C.C. (2003). Science and spiritual healing: a critical review of spiritual healing, 'energy medicine' and intentionality. Alternative Therapy 9:56-61.

Jones, D.A., & West, R.R. (1996). Psychological rehabilitation after myocardial infarction: multicentre randomized controlled trail. British Medical Journal 313:1517-1521.

Kalayil, J.A. (1989). A controlled comparison of progressive relaxation and yoga meditation as methods to relieve stress in middle grade school children. Dissertation Abstracts International 49:3626.

Kaptchuk, T.J. (1996). Historical context of the concept of vitalism in complementary and alternative medicine. In Micozzi, M.S. (Ed). Fundamentals of complementary and alternative medicine. New York: Churchill Livingstone.

Knowles, C., & Hamilton, K. (2003). Effects of yoga poses and breathing exercises on vital capacity in a healthy middle-aged man. Cardiopulmonary Physical Therapy 14:25.

Kolt, G.S., & McConville, J.C. (2000). The effects of a Feldenkrais™ awareness through movement program on state anxiety. Journal of Bodywork and Movement Therapies 4:216-220.

Kotses, H., Harver, A., Segreto, J., Glaus, K.D., Creer, T.L., & Young, G. (1991). Long-term effects of biofeedback-induced facial relaxation on measures of asthma severity in children. Biofeedback and Self-Regulation 16:1-21.

Lai, J.S., Wong, M.K., Lan, C., Chong, C.K., & Lien, I.N. (1993). Cardiorespiratory responses of tai chi chuan practitioners and sedentary subjects during cycle ergometry. Journal of the Formosan Medical Association Taiwan Ti Zhi 92:894-899.

Lai, J.S., Lan, C., Wong, M.K., & Teng, S.H. (1995). Two-year trends in cardiorespiratory function among older tai chi chuan practitioners and sedentary subjects. Journal of American Geriatrics Society 43:1222-1227.

Lan, C., Lai, J.S., Wong, M.K., & Yu, M.L. (1996). Cardio-respiratory function, flexibility, and body composition among geriatric tai chi chuan practitioners. Archives of Physical Medical Rehabilitation 77:612-616.

Lan, C., Lai, J.S., Chen, S.Y., & Wong, M.K. (1998). 12-month tai chi training in the elderly: its effect on health fitness. Medicine and Science in Sports and Exercise 30:345-351.

Lan, C., Ssu-Yuan, C., Lai, J.S., & Wong, M.K. (1999). The effect of tai chi on cardiorespiratory function in patients with coronary artery bypass surgery. Medicine and Science in Sports and Exercise 31:634-638.

Lan, C., Chen, S.Y., Lai, J.S., & Wong, M.K. (2001). Heart rate responses and oxygen consumption during tai chi chuan practice. American Journal of Chinese Medicine 29:403-410.

Lee, K.M. (2004). The use of tai chi for improving the health status of older adults. GeriNotes: Section on Geriatrics. American Physical Therapy Association 11:9-14.

Lee, M.S., Kim, B.G., Huh, H.J., Rya, H., Lee, H.S., & Chung, H.T. (2000). Effect of qi-training on blood pressure, heart rate and respiration rate. Clinical Physiology 20:173-176.

Lehrer, P.M. (1998). Emotionally triggered asthma: a review of research literature and some hypotheses for self-regulation therapies. Applied Psychology and Biofeedback 23:13-41.

Lescowitz, E. (1998). Un-debunking therapeutic touch. Alternative Therapies 4:101-102.

Leskowitz, E., & Marcozi, M. (2003). Complimentary and alternative medicine in rehabilitation. New York: Churchill Livingstone.

Levin, J.S., & Vanderpool, H.Y. (1989). Is religion therapeutically significant for hypertension? Social Science Medicine 29:69-78.

Levy, J.K. (1993). Standard and alternative adjunctive treatments in cardiac rehabilitation. Texas Heart Institute Journal 20:198-212.

Lin, M.C., Nahin, R., Gershwin, E., Longhurst, J.C., & Wu, K.K. (2001). State of complementary and alternative medicine in cardio-vascular, lung, and blood research. Circulation 103:2038-2041.

Linden, W., Stossel, C., & Maurice, J. (1996). Psychosocial interventions for patients with coronary artery disease. Archives of Internal Medicine 156:745-752.

Liu, E.H., Tuner, L.M., Lin, S.X., Choi, L.Y., Whitworth, J., Ting, W., & Oz, M.C. (2000). Use of alternative medicine by patients undergoing cardiac surgery. Journal of Thoracic Cardiovascular Surgery 120:335-341.

Luskin, F.M., Newell, K.A., Griffith, M., Holmes, M., Telles, S., Marvasti, F.F., Pelletier, K.R., & Haskell, W.L. (1998). A review of mind-body therapies in the treatment of cardiovascular disease. Part I: Implications for the elderly. Alternative Therapy Health Medicine 4:46-61.

Luskin, F.M., Newell, K.A., Griffith, M., Holmes, M., Telles, S., DiNucci, E., Marvasti, F.F., Hill, M., Pelletier, K.R., & Haskell, W.L. (2000). A review of mind/body therapies in the treatment of musculoskeletal disorders with implications for the elderly. Alternative Therapies 6:46-56.

Manchanda, S.C., Narang, R., Reddy, K.S., Sachdeva, U., Prabhakaran, D., Dharmanand, S., & Rajani, M. (2000). Retardation of coronary atherosclerosis with yoga lifestyle intervention. Journal of the Association of Physicians of India 48:687-694.

Martel, G.F., Andrews, S.C., & Roseboom, C.G. (2002). Comparison of static and placebo magnets on resting forearm blood flow in young, healthy men. Journal of Orthopaedic and Sports Physical Therapy 32:518-524.

Martin, J., Donaldson, A.N.A., Villarroel, R., Parmar, M.K.B., Ernst, E., & Higginson, I.J. (2002). Efficacy of acupuncture in asthma: systematic review and meta-analysis of published data from 11 randomized controlled trials. European Respiratory Journal 20:846-852.

Mayer, M. (1999). Qigong and hypertension: a critique of research. The Journal of Alternative and Complementary Medicine 5:371-382.

McCarney, R.W., Linde, K., & Lasserson, T.J. (2004). Homeopathy for chronic asthma (Cochrane Review). The Cochrane Library 2:CD000353.

McCrone, S.H., Brendle, D., & Barton, K. (2001). A multibehavioral intervention to decrease cardiovascular disease risk factors in older men. American Association of Critical-Care Nurses 12:5-16.

McCullough, M.E., Hoyt, W.T., Larson, D.B., Koenig, H.G., & Thoresen, C. (2000). Religious involvement and mortality: a meta-analytic review. Health Psychology 19:211-222.

McQuaid, E.L., & Nassau, J.H. (1999). Empirically supported treatments of disease-related symptoms in pediatric psychology: asthma, diabetes, and cancer. Journal of Pediatric Psychology 24:305-328.

Medici, T.C., Grebski, E., Wu, J., Hinz, F., & Wuthrich, B. (2002). Acupuncture and bronchial asthma: a long-term randomized study of the effects of real versus sham acupuncture compared to controls in patients with bronchial asthma. The Journal of Alternative and Complementary Medicine 8:737-750.

Mehl-Madrona, L. (2005). Connectivity and healing: some hypotheses about the phenomenon and how to study it. Advances in Mind Body Medicine 21:12-28.

Miller, J.J., Fletcher, K., & Kabat-Zinn, J. (1995). Three-year follow-up and clinical implications of a mindfulness meditation-based stress reduction intervention in the treatment of anxiety disorders. General Hospital Psychiatry 17:192-200.

Miller, K.M., & Perry, P.A. (1990). Relaxation technique and postoperative pain in patients undergoing cardiac surgery. Pain Management 19:136-146.

Moser, D.K., Dracup, K., Woo, M.A., & Stevenson, L.W. (1997). Voluntary control of vascular tone by using skin-temperature biofeedback-relaxation in patients with advanced heart failure. Alternative Therapy Health Medicine 3:51-59.

Ng, R.K. (1992). Cardiopulonary exercise: a recently discovered secret of tai chi. Hawaii Medical Journal 51:216-217.

Olson, K., Hanson, J., & Michaud, M. (2003). A phase II trial of reiki for the management of pain in advanced cancer patients. Journal of Pain and Symptom Management 26:990-997.

Ornish, D., Brown, S.E., Billings, J.H., Scherwitz, L.W., Armstrong, W.T., Ports, T.A., McLanahan, S.M., Kirkeeide, R.L., Gould, K.L., & Brand, R.J. (1990). Can lifestyle changes reverse coronary heart disease? Lancet 336:129-133.

Oschman, J.L. (2000). Energy medicine - the scientific basis. New York: Churchill Livingstone.

Oschman, J.L. (2003). Breakthrough in subtle energies and energy medicine. Bridges 16:5-9.

Oxman, T.E., Freeman, D.H., & Manheimer, E.D. (1995). Lack of social participation or religious strength and comfort as risk factors for death after cardiac surgery in the elderly. Psychosomatic Medicine 57:5-15.

Paran, E., Amir, M., & Yaniv, N. (1996). Evaluating the response of mild hypertensives to biofeedback-assisted relaxation using a mental stress test. Journal of Behavior Therapy and Experimental Psychiatry 27:157-167.

Patel, C. (1975). 12-month follow-up of yoga and bio-feedback in the management of hypertension. Lancet 1:62-64.

Pert, C.B., Ruff, M.R., Weber, R.J., & Herkenham, M. (1985). Neuropeptides and their receptors: a psychosomatic network. Journal of Immunology 35(Suppl 2):820s-826s.

Pert, C. (1997). Molecules of emotion. New York: Scribner.

Ray, U.S., Sinha, B., Tomer, O.S., Pathak, A., Dasgupta, T., & Selvamurthy, W. (2001). Aerobic capacity and perceived exertion after practice of hatha yoga exercises. Indian Journal of Medical Research 114:215-221.

Ridker, P.M., Cushman, M., Stampfer, M.J., Tracy, R.P., & Hennekens, C.H. (1997). Inflammation, aspirin, and the risk of cardiovascular disease in apparently healthy men. New England Journal of Medicine 336:973-979.

Ridker, P.M., Hennekens, C.H., Buring, J.E., & Rifai, N. (2000). C-Reactive protein and other markers of inflammation in the prediction of cardiovascular disease in women. New England Journal of Medicine 342:836-843.

Ridker, P.M., Rifai, N., Rose, L., Buring, J., & Cook, N. (2002). Comparison of C-reactive protein and low-density lipoprotein cholesterol levels in the prediction of first cardiovascular events. New England Journal of Medicine 347:1557-1565.

Ries, A.L. (1990). Position paper of the American Association of Cardiovascular and Pulmonary Rehabilitation: scientific basis for pulmonary rehabilitation. Journal of Cardiopulmonary Rehabilitation 10:418-444.

Rosa, L., Rosa, E., Sarner, L., & Barrett, S. (1998). A close look at therapeutic touch. Journal of the American Medical Association 279:1005-1010.

Ross, R. (1999). Atherosclerosis - an inflammatory disease. New England Journal of Medicine 340:115-126.

Rozanski, A., Blumenthal, J.A., & Kaplan, J. (1999). Impact of psychological factors on the pathogenesis of cardiovascular disease and implications for therapy. Circulation 99:2192-2217.

Rubik, B. (1995). Energy medicine and the unifying concept of information. Alternative Therapies in Health and Medicine 1:34-39.

Sancier, K.M. (1999). Therapeutic benefits of qigong exercises in combination with drugs. The Journal of Alternative and Complementary Medicine 5:383-389.

Schell, F.J., Allilio, B., & Schonecke, O.W. (1994). Physiological and psychological effects of hatha-yoga exercise in healthy women. International Journal of Psychosomatics 41:46-52.

Schiller, A.D. (2003). Meditation. In Lescowitz, E., Marcozi, M., (Ed). Complementary and alternative medicine in rehabilitation. New York: Churchill Livingstone.

Schneider, D., & Leung, R. (1991). Metabolic and cardiorespiratory responses to the performance of wing chun and tai chi chuan exercises. International Journal of Sports Medicine 12:319-323.

Schneider, R.H., Staggers, F., Alexander, C.N., Sheppard, W., Rainforth, M., Kondwani, K., Smith, S., & King, C.G. (1995). A randomized controlled trail of stress reduction for hypertension in older African Americans. Hypertension 26:820.

Schneider, R.H., Nidich, S.I., Salerno, J.W., Sharma, H.M., Robinson, C.E., Nidich, R.J., & Alexander, C.N. (1998). Lower lipid peroxide levels in practitioners of the transcendental meditation program. Psychosomatic Medicine 60:38-41.

Schwartz, G., & Russek, L. (1997). Dynamical energy systems and modern physics: fostering the science and spirit of complementary and alternative medicine. Alternative Therapies 3:46-56.

Seto, A., Kusaka, C., Nakazato, S., Huang, W.R., Sato, T., Hisamitsu, T., & Takeshige, C. (1992). Detection of extraordinary large bio-magnetic field strength from human hands. Acupuncture and Electro-therapeutics Research International Journal 17:75-94.

Shapiro, D., Hui, K.K., Oakley, M.E., Pasic, J., & Jamner, L.D. (1997). Reduction in drug requirements for hypertension by means of a cognitive-behavioral intervention. American Journal of Hypertension 10:9-17.

Shapira, M.Y., Berkman, N., Ben-David, G., Avital, A., Bardach, E., & Breuer, R. (2002). Short-term acupuncture therapy is of no benefit in patients with moderate persistent asthma. Chest 121:1396-1400.

Shinnick, P., & Freed, S. (2002). A case study of the synchronization of human energy in an acute condition of chronic heart disease through complementary treatment. Subtle Energies and Energy Medicine 13:209-232.

Smyth, J.M., Stone, A.A., Hurewitz, A., & Kaell, A. (1999). Effects of writing about stressful experiences on symptom reduction in patients with asthma or rheumatoid arthritis. Journal of the American Medical Association 282:1304-1309.

Spence, J.D., Barnett, P.A., Linden, W., Ramsden, V., & Taenzer, P. (1999). Recommendations on stress management. Canadian Medical Association Journal 160:S46-S50.

Spencer, J.W. (2003). Essential issues in complementary and alternative medicine. In Spencer, J.W., Jacobs, J.J. (Eds). Complementary and alternative medicine: an evidence-based approach, ed 2. St. Louis: Mosby.

Spencer, J.W., & Jacobs, J.J. (Eds) (1999). Complementary and alternative medicine - an evidence based approach. St Louis: Mosby.

Spencer, J.W., Jacobs, J.J. (Eds) (2003). Complementary and alternative medicine: an evidence-based approach, ed 2. St. Louis: Mosby.

Stone, P.H., Krantz, D.S., McMahon, R.P., Goldberg, A.D., Becker, L.C., Chaitman, B.R., Taylor, H.A., Cohen, J.D., Freedland, K.E., Bertolet, B.D., Coughlan, C., Pepine, C.J., Kaufmann, P.G., & Sheps, D.S. (1999). Relationship among mental stress-induced ischemia and ischemia during daily life and during exercise: the psychophysiologic investigations of myocardial ischemia study. Journal of the American College of Cardiology 33:1476-1484.

Strawbridge, W.J., Cohen, R.D., Shema, S.J., & Kaplan, G.A. (1997). Frequent attendance at religious services and mortality over 28 years. American Journal of Public Health 87:957-961.

Sullivan, M.D., LaCroix, A.Z., Spertus, J.A., & Hecht, J. (2000). Five-year prospective study of the effects of anxiety and depression in patients with coronary artery disease. American Journal of Cardiology 86:1135-1138.

Tandon, M.K. (1978). Adjunct treatment with yoga in chronic severe airways obstruction. Thorax 33:514-517.

Taylor-Piliae, R.E. (2003). Tai chi as an adjunct to cardiac rehabilitation exercise training. Journal of Cardiopulmonary Rehabilitation 23:90-96.

Telles, S., & Desiraju, T. (1993). Autonomic changes in Brahmakumaris Raja yoga meditation. International Journal of Psychophysiology 15:147-152.

Telles, S., Reddy, S.K., & Nagendra, H.R. (2000). Oxygen consumption and respiration following two yoga relaxation techniques. Applied Psychophysiology and Biofeedback 25:221-227.

Uchino, B.N., Cacioppo, J.T., & Kiecolt-Glaser, J.K. (1996). The relationship between social support and physiological processes: a review with emphasis on underlying mechanisms and implications for health. Psychological Bulletin 119:488-531.

Vendanthan, P.K., Kesavalu, L.N., Murthy, K.C., Duvall, K., Hall, M.J., Baker, S., & Nagarathna, S. (1998). Clinical study of yoga techniques in university students with asthma: a controlled study. Allergy and Asthma Proceedings 19:3-9.

Waechter, R.L., & Sergio, L. (2004). Manipulation of the electromagnetic spectrum via fields projected from human hands: a Qi energy connection? Subtle Energies and Energy Medicine 13:233-250.

Wallace, R.K., Benson, H., Wilson, A.F. (1971). A wakeful hypometabolic physiologic state. American Journal of Physiology 221:795-799.

Wardell, D.W., & Engebretson, J. (2001). Biological correlates of Reiki Touch healing. Journal of Advanced Nursing 33:439-445.

Wang, J.S., Lan, C., Chen, S.Y., & Wong, M.K. (2002). Tai chi chuan training is associated with enhanced endothelium-dependent dilation in skin vasculature of healthy older men. Journal of American Geriatrics Society 50:1024-1030.

Wayne, P.M., Krebs, D.E., Wolf, S.L., Gill-Body, K.M., Scarborough, D.M., McGibbon, C.A., Kaptchuk, T.J., & Parker, S.W. (2004). Can tai chi improve vestibulopathic postural control? Archives of Physical Medical Rehabilitation 85:142-152.

Wetzel, W. (1989). Reiki healing: a physiologic perspective. Journal of Holistic Nursing 7:47-54.

Whitworth, J., Burkhardt, A., & Oz, M. (1998). Complementary therapy and cardiac surgery. Journal of Cardiovascular Nursing 12:87-94.

Wirth-Pattullo, V., Hayes, K.W., Echternach, J.L., & Ottenbacher, K. (1994). Interrater reliability of craniosacral rate measurements and their relationship with subjects' and examiners' heart and respiratory rate measurements. Physical Therapy 74:16-29.

Wolf, S.L., Barnhart, H.X., Ellison, G.L., & Coogler, C.E. (1997). The effect of tai chi quan and computerized balance training on postural stability in older subjects. Physical Therapy 77:371-383.

Young, D.R., Appel, L.J., Jee, S.H., & Miller, E.R. (1999). The effects of aerobic exercise and tai chi on blood pressure in older people: results of a randomized trails. Journal of American Geriatrics Society 47:277-284.

Yucha, C.B., Clark, L., Smith, M., Uris, P., LaFleur, B., & Duval, S. (2004). The effect of biofeedback in hypertension (structured abstract). Database of Abstracts of Reviews of Effectiveness 2.

Zamarra, J.W., Schneider, R.H., Besseghini, I., Robinson, D.K., & Salerno, J.W. (1996). Usefulness of the transcendental meditation program in the treatment of patients with coronary artery disease. American Journal of Cardiology 77:867-870.

Zimmerman, J. (1990). Laying on of hands healing and therapeutic touch: a testable theory. BEMI Currents, Journal of the Bio-Electro-Magnetics Institute 2:8-17.

Zucker, P.B. (1997). The effects of qi gong on resting systemic blood pressure and quality of life in hypertensive adults. Cardiopulmonary Physical Therapy 8:24.

APPENDIX A

BRIEF DESCRIPTION OF COMMON COMPLEMENTARY THERAPIES

Manual Therapies

Myofascial Release

Myofascial release is a manual therapy that utilizes energy from the therapist along with mechanical pressure of the hands to "release" fascia that is constricted. As taught by John F. Barnes, PT, this therapy includes release, unwinding and rebounding as a triad of approaches that releases "stuck" fascia to further enhance the flow of chi, which is thought to travel over the fascia much like electrons of energy travel over copper wire.

Craniosacral Therapy

Developed by John Upledger, DO, FAAO, craniosacral therapy is a manual therapy that uses light touch to balance energy flow, in part by balancing the flow of the cerebral spinal fluid as it circulates around the meninges of the cranium and down the spinal column. Those who have attempted to criticize this technique by asserting that the cranial plates are fused in adulthood and thus cannot move are conceding that electron microscope pictures of the cranial sutures reveal blood vessels and fascia that may indicate that the plates are not fused.

Rosen Method Body Work

Founded by Marion Rosen, PT, Rosen method body work is a form of hands-on therapy, the goal of which is to enhance relaxation and emotional awareness by helping the patient identify holding patterns, and assisting in the release of the physical and emotional tension, thereby allowing more of the true self to emerge, and facilitating healing.

Rolfing, Soma, Neuromuscular Therapy, Hellerwork

Rolfing was first developed by Ida Rolf, PhD, and is sometimes referred to as Structural Integration. This approach uses a deep connective tissue massage to loosen fascial restrictions and line up the structure of bones, muscles and organs so that the body mind has a more vertical relation to gravity. After 10 prescribed sessions, it is reasoned that the body is more in alignment and can heal itself. Soma, Hellerwork, and neuromuscular therapy are slight variations on this main theme.

Massage

Massage is the manipulation of tissue through the skin with the intention of bringing about a change in the present condition of the mind/body. Massage from a mechanistic perspective may be intended to move fluid from the extremities to the core, or simply to mechanically break up fibrocystic nodules in muscle. Massage from an energy-based intention is carried out with similar physical maneuvers, but the intention of the practitioner is to influence the body energy or chi to flow so that the mind/body can then heal itself, thus manual techniques are less vigorous, more gentle.

Osteopathic Medicine

In contrast to allopathic medicine, osteopathic medicine stresses the importance of holistic health, nutrition, and joint mobilization to maintain proper balance and homeostasis. At one time, curricula in osteopathic medical schools were quite different than that in allopathic schools and thus deemed inferior. Over time, osteopathic schools have become more rigorous and similar to allopathic medical schools and have increased in stature and reputation in Western medicine.

Chiropractic Medicine

Chiropractic medical education is oriented toward the belief that illness and disease result from vertebral misalignment, and regular manipulation can maintain flow of energy to organs and the body/mind, and thus maintain health.

Mind/Body Interventions

Psychotherapies, Hypnosis

The approach to healing taken by psychotherapies and hypnosis suggests that bringing to awareness incorrect or harmful ways of thinking about something and using this insight to change the way one thinks can remove blocks in energy flow and open up, for example, improved neurotransmitter flow. PET scans have shown that cognitive therapy and serotonin reuptake inhibitors work in similar ways to change synaptic transmission, resulting in the patient feeling better.

Meditation

With meditation the emphasis is on purposely shifting awareness away from logical, left brain thought (some call the ceaseless left brain chatter "monkey mind") to the rhythmical flow of the breath, or the peace of a pleasant sound, and thus closing off the stream of worry about the past and fear about the future. Meditation lowers stress by lowering cortisol levels, and thus balancing blood pressure and other physiological responses to stress.

Mindfulness meditation is sometimes called Vipassana meditation and has been developed very successfully as a stress reducer by Jon Kabat-Zinn. It comes from the Buddhist tradition.

Transcendental meditation is from the Hindu tradition and emphasizes focused concentration on a mantra that is given to a person after a period of initiation. Marharishi University in Fairfield, Iowa was founded by the person most known for bringing TM to the United States, and all of the campus personnel meditate regularly.

Imagery

Imagery purposefully replaces stressful thought with images that enhance relaxation, and thus affects the ANS. One can use imagery alone or participate in a group led by a person suggesting an imagery exercise.

Prayer for Self

Prayer for the self involves quieting the mind and purposefully intending communication with the transcendent, or God, for the well-being of self.

Support Groups

Support groups allow the individual to meet with others and share experiences to lessen the feeling of powerlessness. Religious groups can be included here.

Dance and Music Therapy, Art Therapy

Dance, music, and art therapy work by altering the existing flow of energy by movement and pulling up creative feelings and unleashing stuck energy by focusing concentration outward.

Neurolinguistic Psychology

Originally named neurolinguistic programming, neurolinguistic psychology is a psychotherapeutic approach that brings to awareness ways in which the use of certain words, body postures, and eye movement reveal "stuck" energy, thus allowing a person to choose a way in which to think and move that will enhance energy flow and bring a more relaxed state.

Biofeedback

Biofeedback involves the use of external monitoring devices that record autonomic and cortical nervous system and muscle action, such that a person can, through thought, change the reading on the monitor and thus alter the body/mind function. External monitors include EMG and oscilloscopes that quantify thermal energy.

Yoga

Yoga is an eight-fold path, comprising eight separate activities that emphasize physical, mental, and spiritual elements that enhance union of body and mind. Yoga means union. The most widely known yogic practice is hatha yoga, which features a variety of physical postures and exercises called asanas. Meditative asanas stress alignment of the spine with the head and focus on proper breathing. Therapeutic asanas, such as the cobra and shoulder stand, feature elongation of fascia and soft tissue. Both are done with discipline, awareness, and relaxed openness and thus help to stimulate prana—or life energy or chi.

Pilates

Named for its founder, Joseph Pilates, Pilates is an exercise system that aims to facilitate successful movement with less effort, less fatigue, and greater movement awareness retention. Often using equipment such as the Clinical Reformer and the Cadillac, the practitioner can manipulate gravity, the base of support, the length of levers, and the center of gravity with a series of springs and slings to assist or resist smooth movement.

T'ai Chi

T'ai chi is a mind/body exercise that features slow, controlled, nonimpact movement that gently moves the center of the mind/body mass over the base of support without loss of balance. It is an ancient physical art form that was developed by families in China as a way of defending the household from attack and passed on from generation to generation. The form of t'ai chi used would carry the family name, such as Chin, Yang, Wu, Chuan, etc. These are further condensed, at times, into short forms. T'ai chi develops both mind and body as the movement and breath facilitate the proper balance between the Yin and Yang energies, reducing Yang and increasing Yin and thus contributing to the healthy flow of chi.

Movement Awareness

Feldenkrais Method

The Feldenkrais method was developed by Moshe Feldenkrais, a physicist and Judo expert athlete. When told an injury he sustained would require fusing his knee, he developed a way of thinking that emphasized being able to purposely choose how he might move to protect his knee and avoid fusion. He adapted. He then identified habitual movements, and helped others to recognize endless options for adapting to a particular blockage or restriction in a movement, avoiding pain or perception of strain and thus avoiding reflex muscle splinting. Two strategies, awareness through movement (ATM) and functional integration (FI), are used in class "lessons." ATM is mainly verbal and visual and FI adds positioning, contact, and pressure.

Alexander Technique

The Alexander technique was developed by Frederick Matthias Alexander, who used himself in a single-case research design. Alexander discovered how habitual positions in the body affect movement and organ function. Through consciously inhibiting automatic ways of holding positions, we can choose to act in healthier ways. By integrating proper awareness and attention, movement can bring the mind and body into harmony and meet goals of efficient function. Alexander teachers assist students to learn by using touch to bring the student's awareness to areas of tension, inhibiting habitual use and facilitating a redistribution of postural tone, thus providing a different kinesthetic experience. In this way it is somewhat similar to the Feldenkrais method, without words.

Trager Approach

Developed by Milton Trager, MD, the Trager Approach uses a process of rhythmical "rocking, fluffing, jiggling, lengthening, and shimmering" motions to trigger tissue relaxation reflexively.

Energy Work

Traditional Chinese Medicine

Traditional Chinese medicine is an entire health-care system made up of various specific practices or approaches. Rather than treating disease, this approach looks for underlying systems of imbalance and patterns of disharmony in each individual and treats the whole patient by influencing the flow of chi along meridians. It features pulse and tongue diagnosis, acupuncture, qi gong, herbal medicine and tui na, a form of massage that combines acupressure, massage, and deep tissue manipulation.

Acupuncture, Acupressure

Acupuncture and acupressure are a part of traditional Chinese medicine in which various points along meridians or pathways are stimulated by way of very fine needles (acupuncture) or by way of touch or tapping (acupressure). This mechanical stimulation of the point is hypothesized to facilitate the flow of electrons along the fascia, thus opening up blocked energy and facilitating the flow of chi.

Reflexology

Organs and body parts are represented on zones on the feet, and reflexology works by way of stimulating the corresponding zone with a constant deep pressure for one or two minutes. Energy, circulation, and nerve impulses are stimulated, raising the vitality of the body and restoring homeostasis and flow of chi.

Qi Gong

An aspect of traditional Chinese medicine, qi gong (pronounced chee-kung) ranges from simple positions to rather complicated movements stressing, at the same time, rhythmic breathing and deep relaxation in order to facilitate the flow of chi. In external qi gong a master projects or emits his or her own chi to serve to heal another. Internal qi gong is breathing without movement to enhance self healing and self maintenance, and meditation is sometimes referred to as internal or quiescent qi gong. Dynamic qi gong includes movement, and, as such, t'ai chi is often classified as dynamic qi gong.

Therapeutic Touch

Developed by Delores Krieger and Dora Kunz, therapeutic touch is sometimes referred to as an energetic therapy and sometimes as a manual therapy. The therapists hands are used, but they do not come in contact with the skin. Instead the therapist "smoothes" the energy field surrounding the mind/body, thus gaining access to the flow of energy by way of the ethereal body or energetic field surrounding the mind/body.

Bioelectromagnetics/Energy Work

Laser

Cold laser or soft laser uses a beam of low intensity laser to initiate a series of enzymatic reactions and bioelectrical events that stimulate natural healing process at the cellular level. It is often used to stimulate acupuncture points.

TENS Units

Although transcutaneous electrical neuromuscular stimulation (TENS) is most commonly used to block noxious pain stimulus in physical therapy, TENS units have been shown to stimulate the production of the neurotransmitters and thus increase flow.

Pulsed Electromagnetic Field Therapy

Pulsed electromagnetic filed therapy uses small, battery-powered pulse generators to produce a magnetic field that induces currents to flow in nearby tissues, "jump starting" bone repair.

Magnets

The use of magnets involves magnetized substances against the skin or close to the skin (as in a cloth packet) to bring about a physiochemical or physiological effect. Monopolar magnets have only one pole (north or south) in contact with the skin whereas bipolar magnets have both north and south poles in contact. Strength of the magnets is measured in units called Gauss. The literature on magnets has been confusing, in part because of inconsistent meanings of the terms north and south poles, and inadequate true measures of magnet strength by manufacturers.

Reiki

Reiki is a healing system from Japan (pronounced ray-kee; Ray meaning universal, omnipresent, Ki meaning life force or energy). A Reiki practitioner channels the universal life force through the hands to promote energy balancing, healing, and a state of well-being. The universal life force energy can be transmitted through direct touch or by intending its transmission from a distance. The life force has intelligence and will flow to where it is needed.

Distant Healing Prayer

In distant healing prayer, focused attention is given to the person being prayed for with the intention of causing a positive outcome to result. In intercessory prayer, healing is requested for the self or for others. Directed prayer specifies a particular outcome that is desired. Nondirected prayer intends only that God's will be done in the life of the subject. At the heart of this method is the concept of nonlocal mind, or the belief that a person's consciousness is not limited to distance or time and that we can influence the world at a distance through our focused thought.

Herbal Approaches

Homeopathic Medicine

Homeopathic medicine is an approach to health and healing developed by Samuel Hahnemann, MD, that suggests that reactions to diluted tinctures of natural substances (herbs that cause symptoms like the disease) can be used to treat disease.

Naturopathy

Naturopathy is a holistic system of healing that features a four-year medical degree. Naturopathic doctors study herbal medicine, homeopathy, osteopathy, nutrition, and some forms of physical therapy as part of their curriculum, which is geared to prepare holistic diagnosticians and therapists.

This appendix is summarized from the following texts.

Davis, C.M. (Ed) (1997). Complementary therapies in rehabilitation/holistic approaches for prevention and wellness. Thorofare, NJ: SLACK, Inc.

Davis C.M. (Ed) (2004). Complementary therapies in rehabilitation/ evidence for efficacy in therapy, prevention and wellness, ed 2. Thorofare, NJ: SLACK, Inc.

Burton Goldberg Group. (Eds) (1995). Alternative medicine - the definitive guide. Fife, WA: Future Medicine Publishing, Inc.

C H A P T E R   2 8

Patient Education

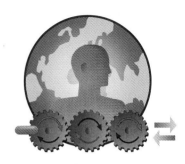

Alexandra J. Sciaky

KEY TERMS

Education
Effectiveness
Health behaviors
Health consequences
Learning theory

Methods
Needs assessment
Resources
Wellness

According to the *Guide to Physical Therapist Practice*, patient/client-related instruction is one of the three major components of physical therapist intervention (APTA, 2001). In cardiopulmonary physical therapy, choosing an effective procedural intervention is based on the physiological evaluation of the patient. Similarly, choosing effective patient instruction or education methods is based on the learning needs assessment of the patient (Rankin & Stallings, 1990). The overall goal of patient education is for the patient to practice health behaviors that promote health, well-being, and independence in self-care. Cardiopulmonary patient education can pose a significant challenge to the physical therapist. Patient education interventions can range from teaching a hospitalized patient about cardiac risk factor modification to designing a series of community-based exercise classes for children with asthma. Meeting this challenge is important because the benefits of patient education include reduced health-care costs, reduced disability, enhanced patient decision making, improved patient knowledge, and increased quality of life. In addition, physical therapists share the responsibility with other health-care providers of ensuring that patients have the opportunity to make informed choices in their care. Unless effective patient education is implemented, this opportunity will be lost.

The overall objective of this chapter is to provide the clinician with an understanding of the principles and practice of effective patient education. To meet this objective, patient education is defined and pertinent learning theories with examples of how they relate to cardiopulmonary patient education are presented. The learning needs assessment of the patient is explained, followed by a description of patient education methods and materials. Because the effectiveness of patient education efforts is important to evaluate, methods to determine it are addressed. Finally, interdisciplinary considerations and educational resources are discussed.

DEFINING PATIENT EDUCATION

Physical therapists believe that patient education is an important part of patient care (Chase et al, 1993). The teaching role of the physical therapist has been reported as highly valued by patients as well (Grannis, 1981). According to The Consumer and Patient Health Information Section of the Medical Library Association (1996), patient education is "a planned activity, initiated by a health professional, whose aim is to impart knowledge, attitudes and skills with the specific goal of changing behavior, increasing compliance with therapy and, thereby, improving health."

Several factors make patient education unique when compared with other types of teaching. The patient may have limited or no access to the teaching because of financial and/or geographical barriers to health care. The learner may lack a sense of well-being because of signs and symptoms of an acute illness, making learning more difficult. The relationship between the teacher and the learner in patient education may be perceived as hierarchical—a medical authority figure instructing a lay person. The learner's emotional status may be fearful or anxious, depending on the medical situation. There may be superimposed time constraints, such as length of hospital stay or clinic appointment, which have a direct impact on patient education. The physical therapist and the patient may be from different cultures. Any of these factors may pose barriers to learning. In addition, the patient's family dynamics may be altered as they try to cope with the patient's illness or disability. The physical therapist's responsibility extends to determining readiness to learn and including the family in the education process.

Objectives

The overall objective of patient education is to affect a durable cognitive improvement that results in a positive change in an individual's or group's health behavior. In most cases the physical therapist must embark on a process to meet this objective in the course of procedural interventions. The education process consists of assessing the learning needs of the patient, identifying measurable, realistic objectives, planning and implementing the patient education program, and finally evaluating its effectiveness. Specific examples of patient education learning objectives are listed in Box 28-1.

Achieving these objectives will lead to the achievement of a host of documented benefits of patient education. These include reduced length of hospital stay (Devine & Cook, 1983), reduced patient anxiety (O'Rourke et al, 1990), improved health-related knowledge (Rowland et al, 1994), increased quality of life (Manzetti et al, 1994), and improved response to and adherence with medical treatment (Mazzuca, 1982). Patient education has also been shown to empower patients to take more active roles in their health care (Smith, 1987). Patients who are educated partners in their care are able to be smart consumers in the health-care system and adapt more

readily to the changes in their lifestyles that result from illness. They learn the health consequences of their behaviors and choices.

Learning Theory: Concepts Pertinent to Cardiopulmonary Patient Education

Twentieth century behavioral scientists have developed a variety of learning theories and models that attempt to explain the complexities of human behavior. Subsequent models have emerged that specifically address health behavior. Although a comprehensive discussion of these models is beyond the scope of this chapter, a list of references for further reading may be found at the end of this chapter (see Bibliography). The discussion of the three theoretical concepts that follows is designed to provide the clinician with a rationale for patient education practice in terms of its basis in learning theory. The concepts are social-cognitive theory, the health-belief model, and the behavior-modification approach.

The social-cognitive theory as developed by Bandura (1986) posits that human behavior can be explained and predicted using the following key regulators: incentives, outcome expectations, and efficacy expectations. For example, a myocardial infarction patient perceives value in following the exercise program (incentive). This patient will attempt to exercise if he or she believes his or her current sedentary lifestyle poses a threat to health. The patient also believes exercise will reduce that threat (outcome expectation) and that he or she is personally capable of performing the exercise program (efficacy expectation). Outcome and efficacy expectations directly relate to patients' beliefs about their capabilities and the relationship of their behaviors to successful outcomes. In essence then, behavior is influenced by perceptions that create expectations for similar outcomes over time.

To function competently in a given environment requires a belief in one's ability to attain a certain level of performance. Bandura terms this self-efficacy (Bandura, 1977). He argues that perceived self-efficacy influences all aspects of behavior including learning new skills and inhibiting or stopping current behaviors. Self-efficacy has the following four primary determinants: (1) performance accomplishments, the strongest determinant, refers to acting out the desired behavior and mastering the task, resulting in increased self-efficacy; (2) vicarious experience involves learning through observing the actions of others, especially those with clear, rewarding outcomes; (3) verbal persuasion; and (4) one's physiological state as it relates to perceived ability to perform a given task. For example, a pulmonary rehabilitation program increases a patient's self-efficacy when he or she successfully completes multiple exercise sessions (performance accomplishments), learns how to deal with dyspnea by consulting fellow program graduates (vicarious experience), receives counseling on energy conservation techniques from the staff (verbal persuasion), and notes that oxygen saturation measured 95% before exercising (physiological state).

BOX 28-1

Patient Education Objectives

1. Enhanced patient-clinician rapport
2. Increased knowledge of health disorder/condition
3. Increased adherence to physical therapy treatment plan
4. Decreased health-care costs
5. Increased self-efficacy
6. Increased ability to make informed health-care choices

The health-belief model, developed in the early 1950s, theorizes that patients are likely to take a health action in the following situations: they believe they are at risk of illness; they believe that the disease poses a serious threat to their lives should they contract it; they desire to avoid illness and believe that certain actions will prevent or reduce the severity of the illness; and they believe that taking the health action is less threatening than the illness itself (Roenstock, 1974). This model was originally developed in an attempt to understand why large numbers of people failed to accept preventative care or screening tests for early disease detection. Subsequent studies have used the model to analyze compliance with regimes for hypertension, asthma, and diabetes (Becker, 1985).

The health-belief model conveys that in the context of health behavior some stimulus or "cue to action" is necessary to initiate the decision-making process. These cues can be internal (i.e., a productive cough) or external (i.e., instructional video tape on pulmonary hygiene techniques). Once the behavior commences, it is understood that many demographic, structural, personal, and social elements are capable of influencing the behavior. In addition, perceived barriers (i.e., unpleasant side effects) may limit or prevent undertaking the recommended behavior.

The behavior-modification approach has its roots in operant-learning theory and consists of techniques that manipulate environmental rewards and punishments in relationship to a specified behavior (Redman, 1993). The theme of this approach is that an individual's behavior can gradually be shaped to meet a set objective. According to Becker (1990), the behavior-modification approach frequently follows a general plan: "identify the problem; describe the problem in behavioral terms; select a target behavior that is measurable; identify the antecedents and consequences of the behavior; set behavioral objectives; devise and implement a behavior change program; and evaluate the program." This plan is similar to the Patient/Client Management model (APTA, 2001) that physical therapists use to achieve optimal patient care outcomes. The physical therapist examines the patient, describes the problem(s) in functional terms (evaluation and diagnosis), sets short-term and long-term functional goals, designs a plan of care to meet those goals (prognosis), implements the plan (intervention), and reevaluates the patient. These similarities may facilitate the use of the behavioral-modification approach by physical therapists.

Health-care contracts can be useful in implementing the behavior-modification approach. An example of such a contract may be seen in Box 28-2. The contract should be realistic, measurable, and renewable (Herje, 1980). Specific goals, time frames, behaviors, and contingencies are written in the contract. The clinician and patient discuss and then sign the contract. Positive and negative reinforcements are used to facilitate the desired behaviors in the patient. Ideally, once the contract expires, the patient feels competent and is able to continue the desired behaviors without the external reinforcements.

BOX 28-2

Health Care Contract

Date: _____

Contract goal: (specific outcome to be attained)

   I, (client's name), agree to (detailed description of required behaviors, time, and frequency limitations)

   in return for (positive reinforcements contingent upon completion of required behaviors; timing and mode of delivery of reinforcements).

   I, (provider's name), agree to (detailed description of required behaviors, time, and frequency limitations).

   (Optional) I, (significant other's name), agree to (detailed description of required behaviors, time, and frequency limitations).

   (Optional) Aversive consequences: (negative reinforcements for failure to meet minimum contract requirements).

   We will review the terms of this agreement, and will make my desired modifications, on (date). We hereby agree to abide by the terms of the contract describe above.

Signed: (Client) _____

Signed: (Significant other, if relevant).

_____

Signed: (Provider) _____

Contract effective from (date) _____ to (date)

From Janz, N.K., Becker, M.H., & Hartman, P.E. (1984). Contingency contracting to enhance patient compliance: a review. Patient Education Counseling 5:165-178.

NEEDS-BASED APPROACH TO PATIENT EDUCATION

The most important aspect of planning for patient education is assessing the learner. The process of patient education requires assessment of the total patient and family, including an understanding of the psychosocial, socioeconomic, educational, vocational, and cultural qualities of the patient and family unit (Nemshick, 1997). Assessing educational needs of the patient allows the physical therapist to determine what the patient needs to know to meet the desired cognitive and behavioral teaching objectives. This assessment also increases patient-teacher rapport and allows the physical therapist to individualize the learning experience.

LEARNING NEEDS ASSESSMENT

Tools

The American Physical Therapy Association's Commission on Accreditation of Physical Therapy Education (2004) requires that the graduate physical therapist be able to "effectively educate others using culturally appropriate teaching methods that are commensurate with the needs of the learner." Learning needs can be assessed in a variety of ways. These include

<table>
<tr><td>

BOX 28-3

Learning Needs Assessment Areas

Perceptual

Ability to receive input (vision, hearing, and touch)
Comprehension of symbols (figures, numbers, words, and
  pictures)

Cognitive

Knowledge and analytical skills
Memory

Motor

Fine- and gross-motor skills
Physical adaptations and responses to illness or stimuli

Affective

Attitudes
Value-belief system
Motivation (readiness to learn)
Perception of overall wellness

Environmental

Personal and societal resources
Amount of instructor contact and setting
Cultural influences (language, traditions, roles, religion, and
  lifestyle)

</td></tr>
</table>

patient and family interviews, questionnaires and surveys, written tests, and observation of patient performance (Haggard, 1989). Interviews allow the physical therapist to ask questions directed at determining the patient's view of the illness, including associated beliefs and attitudes. Questionnaires and surveys can be used in conjunction with the interview to document the patient's responses to specific questions about his or her condition. Open-ended questions such as "What are the major problems your illness has caused for you and your family?" elicit more information than a multiple-choice format. Written tests can be helpful in determining what patients already know when the tests are given, before any teaching. These tests can also identify problems with reading and comprehension skills. Observing patients as they perform a skill, such as diaphragmatic breathing, reveals whether the patient can demonstrate the correct technique. The physical therapist can also pose questions to the patient during the demonstration to determine whether the patient knows the rationale for the exercise.

Areas to Assess

The learning needs assessment encompasses the following five major areas: perceptual, cognitive, motor, affective, and environmental (Box 28-3). By addressing these five areas, the physical therapist will obtain an accurate picture of the patient's learning abilities, knowledge level, performance skills, attitudes, and cultural influences.

The perceptual area encompasses the learner's ability to receive information via the senses. If the learner's sight, hearing, or sense of touch is impaired, the instructor may need to make modifications so that the information can be received by the learner. The comprehension of symbols, such as numbers, words, or pictures, also needs to be assessed in the perceptual area. The instructor needs to know what meaning the learner attributes to the symbols that will be used in the education program to ensure clarity.

The cognitive area addresses the learner's knowledge and problem-solving skills. The instructor needs to know how much the learner already knows and what needs to be learned. The instructor also needs to know if the learner has any problems with memory. Short- or long-term memory deficits may require that the instructor integrate a prompting system into the education plan.

The patient's fine- and gross-motor skills and functional mobility are covered in the motor area. The instructor needs to be aware of the physiological changes in the patient that affect abilities to perform activities necessary for a given education program. For example, if patients who are wheelchair users are interested in attending a support group, the physical therapist would insure that it is being held in a room that is wheelchair accessible.

The affective area comprises the learner's attitudes, beliefs, and readiness to learn. Identifying the learner's value-belief system will assist the instructor in determining what is important to the learner and facilitate motivation. The patient's perception of wellness may vary from the absence of disease to an enhanced healthy state. What the instructor feels is important to learn may not be what the patient feels is important to learn. Identifying what the patient values early on will prevent instructor (and patient) frustration later.

Cultural influences and personal and societal resources are included in the environmental area. It is important for the instructor to be aware of the patient's lifestyle, religion, traditions, roles, and primary language in order to individualize the patient's learning experience. Presence or absence of the patient's resources may affect consistency in and access to patient education.

All five of these areas can be addressed with the use of a learning needs assessment survey. See Box 28-4 for an example. By using a survey in combination with the physical therapy patient evaluation, the therapist can gather all the necessary information to create an optimal patient education experience. The survey in Box 28-4 consists of three parts, which can be adapted to any patient-care setting. In the pediatric setting, some of the questions could be asked of the parent(s) or rephrased to address elementary-school-aged children. Part I primarily assesses the patient's perception of the illness or disability and its impact on the patient's life. Part II lists a wide variety of teaching methods and asks the patient to indicate which methods he or she personally feels are most useful. Part III identifies specific topics about which the patient would like to know more. This part is also helpful in alerting the therapist that referrals to other members of the

---

BOX 28-4

Learning Needs Assessment Survey

Your physical therapist would like to help you learn what you need to know to function as independently as possible and manage your illness/disability. Please answer the following questions.

Part I

Name:

Please describe your illness and/or disability here:
1. Do you have any problems seeing or hearing?
2. Do you have any body areas which are numb (can't feel)?
3. How long have you had this illness/disability?
4. What problems has it caused you?
5. Are you able to care for yourself at home?
6. Are you responsible for the care of any others at home?
7. Do you have someone at home to help you? If so, whom?
8. What questions or concerns do you have?
9. Do you practice a religion? If so, which?
10. What language(s) do you understand best?
11. How much education/schooling have you had?
12. What is your occupation?

Part II

There are many different ways to learn. Please read the list of ways to learn below and circle the ones which help you learn best.

Reading   Group discussion

Listening to lectures   Reflecting by myself

Watching demonstrations   Playing games

Using interactive videos/computer programs

Attending seminars

Practicing a skill or doing a simulation   Role playing

Taking written tests   Other

Part III

I would like to know more about: (check all that apply to you.)

_____ How to clear mucus from my lungs
_____ What causes heart disease

_____ How to avoid shortness of breath
_____ What I should eat

_____ Exercise _____ My medications

_____ Monitoring myself
_____ Planning my social life and/or work life

_____ What to do if I have chest pain
_____ Planning for sexual intimacy

_____ What causes lung disease
_____ Coping with my feelings

_____ How to stay well _____ How to quit smoking

_____ How to sleep better
_____ How to access community resources

Other things I would like to know:

The three most important things I need to know are:

---

interdisciplinary health-care team may be required. For example, if the patient checked off "what I should eat," the therapist would make a referral to the dietician.

Interpretation of Findings

The next important step after gathering information with the learning needs assessment survey is to interpret the findings. The physical therapist looks at the answer to each item on the survey and uses that information in the process of designing the content and method for teaching that patient. Primary and secondary prevention can be integrated into the content to promote overall wellness. Interpretation of the survey findings means applying the patient's current health concerns, learning abilities, and knowledge deficits to future learning activities. By identifying the patient's needs, the physical therapist is able to make informed choices in the planning and implementation of each patient's education experience.

Formulation and Prioritization of Goals

As physical therapists set intervention goals for their patients, they should include educational goals. Intervention goals usually describe functional outcomes (e.g., the patient will perform a stand and pivot transfer from bed to chair, independently), and they are written in behavioral terms. Educational goals should also be written in behavioral terms. For example, "Mr. J will safely perform percussion and postural drainage to Mrs. J's right lower lobe." The stated behavior must be observable and measurable. Motor skills can be observed, knowledge skills can be tested, and safety can be documented.

Prioritizing the patient's educational goals in conjunction with other intervention goals enhances the therapist's efficiency. Referring again to the learning needs assessment survey (see Box 28-4) to determine what knowledge is important to the patient will guide the therapist in creating the most appropriate prioritization of goals. Simplicity is usually best. Overwhelming patients with a huge list of items to be accomplished may discourage them before they even start. If the patient's learning needs are very great, start by breaking down the list of goals into smaller groups. Choose the most important goals and try to accomplish them first. If you run into a series of failures, tackle the next group. Build on each success the patient experiences.

TABLE 28-1		
Comparison Chart for Education Methods (Adults and Children Unless Otherwise Noted)		
TYPE	**ADVANTAGES**	**DISADVANTAGES**
Reading	Patient can refer back to material. Low effort for instructor.	Requires instructor follow-up for comprehension.
Lecture	Time-efficient for instructor. Cost-efficient.	Low interaction. May pacify rather than engage.
Demonstration	Adds sensory data to learning. Allows for problem solving and modification.	Instructor needs proficiency in skill to be demonstrated.
Video	Access to restricted areas. Portrays events that are infrequent, costly, and difficult to reproduce. Portable.	Noninteractive. May pacify rather than engage. Costly, requiring electronic equipment. Difficult to control quality.
Audiotape	Portable. Useful for sight-impaired learner.	Requires electronic equipment.
Group discussion	Effective use of instructor time. Enlarges pool of real-life experiences. Nonthreatening to some learners. Mutual support possible.	Not as much individual attention given. Group may be hard to control (e.g., too talkative, shy, hostile). Strong facilitator skills needed.
Clubs, camps, and retreats	Draws on community and individual resources. Needs less professional input and time.	Same as above. Some risk of perpetuating myths and false information.
Individual instruction	Instructor can tailor learning to student's needs and desires. More one-on-one time.	Inefficient use of instructor time. Limited pool of experience on which to draw.
Games and directed activities	Helpful for children. Reduces anxiety. Uses repetition. Fun. Unexpected experiences can lead to new understandings or insights.	Scheduling space. Finding participants.
Computer programs	Interactive, self-paced. Large information capacity. Time-efficient for instructor.	Expensive. Special equipment and space needed. May require expert help.
Seminars and workshops	Diversity of instructors and formats. Pool of experts and community resources. Can tailor content broadly or narrowly.	Expense, scheduling, and space.
Role-playing	Trial runs, problem-solving, simulated experiences.	Threatening to some. Can be time-consuming. Instructor needs to be skilled in techniques and dealing with effects on participants.
Oral and written tests	Can provide instructor with evidence of what learner needs to be taught and what has been learned.	Literacy and supplies required, if written. May be time-consuming.

EDUCATIONAL METHODS

Method Selection

Using the learning needs assessment survey (see Box 28-4) will allow the clinician to choose education methods that will facilitate optimal learning in a given patient or group. The patient(s) can self-select the available learning methods that have the greatest learning potential. A combination of methods may be necessary to achieve the educational goals that have been set. If a patient is not sure which methods to indicate, the therapist can base the choice on the other information provided in the survey (e.g., sensory deficits, literacy level, or type of information desired). Surveys generally require regular updates to ensure that all of the offered methods are listed and the discontinued methods are removed from the list. In addition, the physical therapist should assess potential learning materials for readability, age-appropriateness, accuracy of content, intended audience, and clarity (Nemshick, 1996).

Advantages and Disadvantages

Each education method has its own advantages and disadvantages. Table 28-1 shows 13 education methods listed

with their key advantages and disadvantages. The table is designed to assist the physical therapist in determining the settings and populations in which the methods will be most useful. This is not a comprehensive list. In fact, some health education challenges require truly innovative approaches.

In Boston, Massachusetts, for example, community health-care providers were faced with a dilemma. The incidence of acquired immune deficiency syndrome (AIDS) among women of color was increasing. Latino, African-American, and Haitian women were not receiving vital information about how to prevent the transmission of the human immunodeficiency virus (HIV). These communities were largely distrustful of the health-care establishment and were not mobilized to stop the spread of HIV. How could they be reached? The Boston Women's AIDS Information Project (BWAIP) trained lay women to educate other women in the places where they congregate, such as beauty salons. Informational brochures, condoms, and posters were distributed in a number of beauty salons in communities where women were at highest risk for contracting HIV. Lay and professional educators would give presentations, show videos, and answer questions from the staff and patrons of these establishments to empower them to disarm myths about AIDS, encourage other women to make appropriate behavior changes, and to make referrals to neighborhood health centers for testing and evaluation.

Teaching young children about their bodies and health may also require unique approaches. In 1993, members of the interdisciplinary team caring for children with cystic fibrosis (CF) at Texas Children's Hospital, Houston, held a CF Education Day for the children and their parents. The children ranged in age from seven to 11 years. To teach them about anatomy, a special anatomy apron was fabricated. The apron had life-sized removable organs made of stuffed fabric. The children took turns wearing the apron and learned to identify and locate the organs by removing and replacing the apron's heart, lungs, intestines, and pancreas.

By evaluating the advantages and disadvantages of available education methods, the physical therapist can choose the methods that are most effective and use them to his or her best advantage. Consideration must be given to cost, equipment, scheduling, labor, time, site, flexibility, and reusability. For example, videotaped presentations may be easy for the instructor to schedule, present, and reuse, but they can be costly to purchase and require expensive equipment to view.

Content

The specific content of patient education materials and programs should be determined by the needs of the individual or group being taught. There are, however, topics common to many cardiopulmonary education efforts. These topics are listed in Box 28-5. The physical therapist can use the topics

BOX 28-5

Cardiopulmonary Patient Education Content

Health promotion/wellness
Smoking cessation
Infection control
Risk-factor awareness and modification
Benefits and effects of exercise
Resumption of sexual activity
Normal cardiopulmonary anatomy and physiology, oxygen transport
Cardiopulmonary disease process
Airway clearance techniques and suctioning
Energy conservation and pacing techniques
Stress management
Resumption of school activities (children)
Instructions geared for parents of children with cardiopulmonary conditions
Cardiopulmonary resuscitation (CPR), basic life support
Heart rate, blood pressure, and dyspnea self-monitoring
Nutrition
Medications (schedules, actions, and side effects)
Use of oxygen and other respiratory equipment
Medical procedures (e.g., cardiac catheterization, bronchoscopy, cardiopulmonary transplantation)
Community resources
Emergency procedures

listed in the table as a checklist to explore the content covered (or to be covered) in a given cardiopulmonary education experience. Although the physical therapist may not be responsible for teaching on all these topics, he or she should be familiar with them because they are taught by others on the health-care team. Educational materials on all of these topics have already been developed by a variety of health-care providers, educators, and organizations and may be available for use by physical therapists (see Interdisciplinary Considerations and Resources).

DETERMINATION OF EFFECTIVENESS

Determining the effectiveness of patient education efforts involves evaluating what the patient learned as well as how the teacher taught. Sometimes patients learn in spite of educational efforts. Physical therapists need to examine their effectiveness at teaching and strive to improve their teaching skills just as they strive to improve their other clinical skills. Being able to communicate ideas and receive feedback from patients from diverse racial, ethnic, vocational, religious, and generational backgrounds is crucial for physical therapists. Formal or informal surveys of patients and families who have participated in education efforts can provide the physical therapist with information on teaching effectiveness from the patient and family perspective.

Physical therapists are responsible for evaluating and documenting the results of their patients' education activities. Observing a patient or family perform a skill (such as paced breathing) will give the physical therapist the opportunity to determine whether the patient/family has learned and properly performed the skill. Once the physical therapist has observed the skill being properly performed, he or she can document it as such in the medical record. The amount of supervision and equipment required, if any, should also be included in the documentation.

Teacher-Learner Relationship

According to Locke (1986), the primary step to understanding others is an awareness of one's self. Acknowledging one's own personal values, interests, and biases will significantly increase one's sensitivity toward others. The skilled teacher is aware of his or her own communication style and its limitations and can convey the desire to help despite those limitations.

The teacher-learner relationship that develops between physical therapist and patient is largely due to communication between the two in the context of culture. Communication is a two-way process consisting of verbal and nonverbal messages. The interpretation of these messages depends on the cultural cues operating in the educational setting. Fairchild (1970) defines culture as all social behavior, such as customs, techniques, beliefs, organizations, and regard for material objects, including behaviors transmitted by way of symbols. "The primary mode of transmission of culture is language, which enables people to learn, experience, and share their traditions and customs" (Locke, 1992). In addition, culture can be expressed or experienced via economic and political practices, art, and religion. Health care and medicine have their own cultures. To meet the needs of culturally diverse populations and engage in positive, productive relationships, physical therapists must operate from a framework of cross-cultural understanding. This understanding and knowledge can then be reflected in patient education efforts.

For example, in a large, urban, acute-care hospital, two physical therapy staff members were working together to treat an elderly Jewish woman who was critically ill. The clinicians worked carefully to reposition the woman without disturbing the many tubes and lines that were present. Later the woman expressed that she did not want to have two physical therapy clinicians working with her at the same time. She confided to the nurse that it was because she felt it was too much like the Jewish ritual washing of the body after death, which is traditionally performed by two people. This interpretation of the therapy surprised the physical therapy staff members who treated the woman because they were also Jewish and the thought never occurred to them. The next time the clinicians went to see the woman, they explained why it was necessary for both of them to be present during the treatment. They also encouraged the woman to have other supportive people present and to play her favorite recorded music during the therapy session.

Patient Adherence

The effectiveness of physical therapy treatment, or of any medical treatment, depends on the patient following the health-care provider's recommendations (adherence). Unfortunately there is often a gap between what the patient is asked to do and what the patient actually does. This gap, or nonadherence, has an incidence rate estimated to be between 18% and 35% (Banzer, 2004; Pasternak, 2004). Factors affecting patient adherence include knowledge of and course of the illness, complexity of the recommendations, convenience, availability of support system, financial resources, and the patient's beliefs.

Patient education can improve adherence when the information given includes what behaviors are expected, when they should be performed, and what to do should problems arise. Plans for patient education sessions should strive to remove or avoid barriers to patient adherence. These efforts include simplifying and individualizing treatment regimens, fostering collaborative teacher-learner relationships, enlisting family support, making use of interdisciplinary and community resources, and providing continuity of care (Meichenbaum & Turk, 1987). By using an approach that integrates these efforts, the physical therapist can optimize patient adherence to the prescribed physical therapy program.

INTERDISCIPLINARY CONSIDERATIONS AND RESOURCES

The interdisciplinary health-care team has evolved as the complexity and number of available medical treatments has grown. Physical therapists are trained to function as part of an interdisciplinary team and are responsible for learning the areas of responsibility and expertise covered by each member of their team. The team concerned with cardiopulmonary care consists of licensed and nonlicensed health-care providers and may include any or all of the following.

- Physician
- Nurse
- Physical therapist
- Occupational therapist
- Exercise physiologist
- Dietician
- Laboratory technologist
- Pharmacist
- Social worker
- Chaplain or pastoral care associate
- Clinical psychologist
- Speech therapist
- Vocational rehabilitation counselor
- Home-care personnel

All of the above providers may not be present on every team, but their services should be available for patients who need them. By understanding what services and patient education materials are provided by each discipline, the physical therapist can reinforce previously presented concepts and avoid giving conflicting information. This also allows the physical therapist to make referrals to the appropriate discipline when other knowledge deficits are identified.

Interdisciplinary team members can also provide the physical therapist with important patient feedback and information. Teaching methods found to be successful with a given patient by the nurse, for example, could be communicated to the physical therapist. The therapist can then use similar methods with that patient for physical therapy education objectives. Communication between team members is enhanced by regular team meetings or rounds and by having a central location to document completed patient education experiences (i.e., the medical record).

Health-related organizations can also be rich resources for patient education information. The American Heart Association and the American Lung Association, for example, have many cardiopulmonary materials available to health-care providers for little or no cost. State public health and local community service agencies may also be sources for printed or audiovisual materials. The Health and Human Services Department of the Federal government has numerous divisions and institutes that address health education and research. Catalogs listing cardiovascular and pulmonary publications can be obtained from the Federal Consumer Information Center, Pueblo, Colorado 81009 or via the Internet at www.nhbli.nih.gov.

Community organizations such as YMCA, YWCA, and the American Red Cross offer a wealth of health-education materials and classes. Many of these agencies also have catalogs of their educational offerings, which can be obtained by telephoning their local offices. Local public, medical, and hospital libraries are also useful for seeking out available health-education materials. Many Chambers of Commerce keep lists of local support groups or clubs, such as Breather's Club or Heartbeats. Regional state colleges or universities have departments dedicated to health education and may have cardiopulmonary materials to share.

SUMMARY

This chapter defined patient education and described selected learning theories as they relate to cardiopulmonary patient education. The evaluation of the patient's learning needs was emphasized and the advantages and disadvantages of a variety of educational methods were discussed. The role of the teacher-learner relationship and patient adherence were explained in reference to the determination of patient education and treatment effectiveness. Finally, interdisciplinary health-care team interactions and resources for patient education materials were considered.

Review Questions

1. Discuss the benefits of patient education, including impact on health-care costs and the patient's perception of wellness.
2. Contrast and compare a variety of teaching methods used in patient education.
3. Explain the rationale for patient education using concepts of adult learning theories or models.
4. Describe the aspects of planning for patient education.
5. Discuss the components of a learning needs assessment survey and ways to modify it for specific patient populations.
6. Critique a variety of patient education materials using criteria specific to patients with cardiopulmonary conditions.
7. Explain how to determine the effectiveness of patient education activities from both the patient's and the physical therapist's point of view.

REFERENCES

American Physical Therapy Association. (2001). Guide to physical therapist practice, ed 2. Physical Therapy 81:9-744.

Bandura, A. (1986). Foundations of thought and action: a social cognitive theory. Englewood Cliffs, NJ: Prentice-Hall.

Bandura, A. (1977). Self-efficacy: toward a unifying theory of behavioral change. Psychological Review 84:191-215.

Banzer, JA. (2004). Results of cardiac rehabilitation in patients with diabetes mellitus. American Journal of Cardiology 93:81-84.

Becker, M.H. & Janz, N.K. (1985). The health belief model applied to understanding diabetes regimen compliance. Diabetes Education 11:41-47.

Becker, M.H. (1990). Theoretical models of adherence and strategies of improving adherence. In Shumaker, S.A., Schron, E.R. &

Ockene, J.K. (Eds). The handbook of health behavior change. New York: Springer Publishing.

Chase, L., Elkins, J.A., Readinger, J., & Shepard, K.F. (1993). Perceptions of physical therapists toward patient education. Physical Therapy 73:787-795.

Commission of Accreditation of Physical Therapy Education. (2004). Evaluative criteria for accreditation of education programs for the preparation of physical therapists. Alexandria, VA: American Physical Therapy Association.

Devine, E., & Cook, T. (1983). A meta-analysis of effects of psycho-educational interventions on length of post surgical hospital stay. Nursing Research 32:333-339.

Fairchild, H.P. (Ed) (1970). Dictionary of sociology and related sciences. Totowa, NJ: Rowan & Allanheld.

Grannis, C.J. (1981). The ideal physical therapist as perceived by the elderly patient. Physical Therapy 61:479-486.

Haggard, A. (1989). Handbook of patient education. Rockville, MD: Aspen Publishers.

Herje, P.A. (1980). Hows and whys of patient contracting. Nursing Education 5:30-34.

Hoffman, S. (1987). Planning for patient teaching based on learning theory. In Smith, C.E. (Ed). Patient education nurses in partnership with other health professionals. Orlando: Grune & Stratton.

Liedekerken, P.C., Jonkers, R., DeHaes, W.F., Kok, G.J., & Saan, J. (Eds) (1990). Effectiveness of health education: review and analysis. Assen, Netherlands: Van Gorcum.

Locke, D.C. (1992). Increasing multicultural understanding: a comprehensive model. Newberry Park: Sage Publications.

Locke, D.C. (1986). Cross-cultural counseling issues. In Palmo, A.J., & Weikel, W.J., et al (Eds). Foundations of mental health counseling. Springfield, IL: Charles C. Thomas.

Manzetti, J.D., Hoffman, L.A., Sereika, S.M., Sciurba, F.C., & Griffith, B.P. (1994). Exercise, education, and quality of life in lung transplant candidates. Journal of Heart and Lung Transplantation 13:297-305.

Mazzuca, S. (1982). Does patient education in chronic disease have therapeutic value. Journal of Chronic Disease 35:521-529.

Meichenbaum, D., & Turk, D.C. (1987). Facilitating treatment adherence: a practitioner's guidebook. New York: Plenum Press.

Miller, P., Johnson, N.L., Garrett, M.J., Wickoff, R., & McMahon, M. (1982). Health beliefs of and adherence to the medical regimen by patients with ischemic heart disease. Heart Lung 11:332-339.

Nemshick, M.T. (1997). Designing educational interventions for patients and families. In

O'Rourke, A., Lewin, B., Whitcross, S., & Pacey, W. (1990). The effects of physical exercise training and cardiac education on levels of anxiety and depression in the rehabilitation of CABG patients. International Disability Studies 12:104-106.

Pasternak, R.C. (2004). Understanding physician and consumer attitudes concerning cholesterol management: results from the National Lipid Association surveys. American Journal of Cardiology 94:9F-15F.

Rankin, S.H., & Stallings, K.D. (1990). Patient education: issues, principles and practices, ed 2. Philadelphia: JB Lippincott.

Redman, B.K. (1993). The process of patient education. St. Louis: Mosby.

Roenstock, I.M. (1974). Historical origins of the health belief model. Health Education Monographs 2:328-335.

Rowland, L. Dickinson, E.T., Newman, P., & Ebrahim, S. (1994). Look After Your Heart Programme: impact on health status, exercise knowledge, attitudes and behavior of retired women in England. Journal of Epidemiology and Community Health 48:123-128.

Smith, C.E. (1987). Nurses' increasing responsibility for patient education. In Smith, C.E. (Ed). Patient education: nurses in partnership with other health professionals. Orlando: Grune & Stratton.

BIBLIOGRAPHY

Ajzen, I. (1985). From intentions to actions: a theory of planned behavior. In Kuhl, J., & Beekman, J. (Eds). Action control: from cognition to behavior. New York: Springer-Verlag.

Bandura, A. (1977). Social learning theory. Englewood Cliffs, NJ: Prentice-Hall.

Eraker, S.A., Becker, M.H., Strecher, V.J., & Kirscht, J.P. (1985). Smoking behavior, cessation techniques and the health decision model. American Journal of Medicine 78:817-825.

Fabrega, H. (1973). Toward a model of illness behavior. Medical Care 11:470-484.

Janz, N.K., & Becker, M.H. (1984). The health belief model: a decade later. Health Education Quarterly 11:1-47.

Leventhal, H., Meyer, D., & Gutman, M. (1980). The role of theory in the study of compliance to high blood pressure regimens. In Haynes, R.C., Mattson, M.E., & Engebretson, T.O. Jr. (Eds). Patient compliance to prescribed antihypertensive medication regimes: a report to the National Heart, Lung, and Blood Institute. (NIH Publication No. 81-2102). Washington, DC: US Department of Health and Human Services.

Lorig, K. (2000) Patient education. A practical approach, ed 2. Thousand Oaks, CA: Sage Publications.

Shepard, K.F. & Jensen, G.M. (Eds). Handbook of teaching for physical therapists. Newton, MA: Butterworth-Heinemann.

Marlatt, G.A., & Gordon, J.R. (Eds). (1985). Relapse prevention: maintenance strategies in addictive behavior change. New York: Guilford.

Stetchen, V.J., Devellis, B.M., Becker, M.H., & Rosenstock, I.M. (1986). The role of self-efficacy in achieving health behavior change. Health Education Quarterly 13:73-92.

PART IV

Guidelines for the Delivery of Cardiovascular and Pulmonary Physical Therapy

Acute Conditions

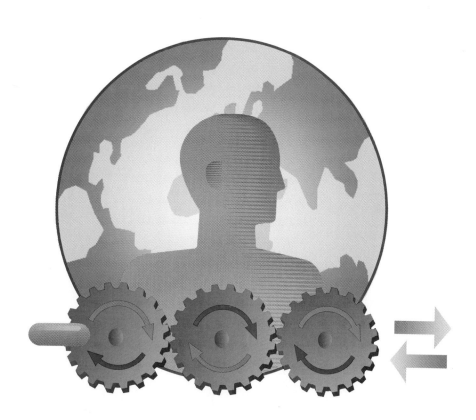

CHAPTER 29

Individuals with Acute Medical Conditions

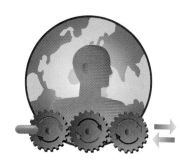

Elizabeth Dean

KEY TERMS

Acute exacerbations of chronic airflow
  limitation
Alveolar proteinosis
Alveolitis
Asthma
Atelectasis
Bronchiolitis
Bronchitis

Cystic fibrosis
Hypertension
Interstitial pulmonary fibrosis
Pneumonia
Stable angina
Stable myocardial infarction
Tuberculosis

The purpose of this chapter is to review the physical therapy management of individuals with *primary*, acute cardiopulmonary dysfunction. Such dysfunction may limit participation in life and its related activities in the short- or long-term. Furthermore, such dysfunction can constitute life threat in the absence of limitations to life participation and quality of life (e.g., hypertension and dysrhythmias). Management principles for people with several types of common acute medical conditions are described. Although medical conditions are usually classified as either *primary* lung disease or *primary* cardiovascular disease, the heart and lungs work synergistically to effect gas exchange and cardiac output and in series with the peripheral vascular circulation to effect tissue perfusion (Dantzker, 1983; Dantzker, 1988; Pryor et al, 2002; Wasserman & Whipp, 1975). Thus impairment of one organ invariably has implications for the function of the other. Threat to or impairment of oxygen transport has implications for all other organ systems, thus a multisystem approach is essential for overall management (see Chapters 1 and 5). The primary, *acute* pulmonary conditions that are presented include atelectasis, pneumonia, bronchitis, bronchiolitis,

alveolitis, alveolar proteinosis, acute exacerbations of chronic airflow limitation, asthma, cystic fibrosis, interstitial pulmonary fibrosis, and tuberculosis. For further epidemiological and pathophysiological detail on these conditions refer to Bates (1989), the *Epidemiological Standardization Project* of the American Thoracic Society (1989), Murray and Nadel (2000), and West (2003). The *primary*, acute cardiovascular conditions presented include hypertension, medically-stable angina, and uncomplicated myocardial infarction. For further details on these conditions refer to Cheitlin (2004), Kasper et al (2004), and Woods (2004).

The pathophysiology underlying the medical management of each condition extends the pathophysiology content of Chapter 5 and in turn provides a basis for each condition's physical therapy management. The management principles presented are not intended to serve as treatment prescriptions for a particular patient. The treatment priorities presented are not only based on the underlying pathology but on the complexity of its manifestation in a given patient. Without discussion of a specific patient and knowledge of other significant factors (i.e., the effects of restricted mobility,

---

BOX 29-1

Pathophysiological Mechanisms Contributing to Atelectasis

Central Mechanisms

Breathing at low lung volumes (e.g., when in pain or after certain medications)
Inability to generate adequate inspiratory pressure and volume
Central disruption of breathing centers controlling normal periodic and rhythmic breathing pattern

Extramural Mechanisms

Chest wall deformity
Asymmetry of intrathoracic structures
Respiratory muscle weakness (e.g., neuromuscular disease)
Phrenic nerve inhibition (e.g., secondary to upper abdominal or cardiovascular thoracic surgery)
Compression of lung parenchyma secondary to pleural fluid accumulation, blood, plasma, and pus
Compression of lung parenchyma during surgery
Reduced lung expansion secondary to reduced movement
Compression of lung parenchyma secondary to static body positioning
Compression of lung parenchyma secondary to prolonged static body positioning
Mechanical ventilation
Increased alveolar surface tension

Mural Mechanisms

Airway narrowing secondary to increased bronchial smooth muscle tone

Calcification or altered anatomical integrity of airways
Edema of the bronchial wall and epithelium

Intramural Mechanisms

Impaired mucociliary transport
Increased pulmonary secretions
Inspissated pulmonary secretions
Altered distribution of pulmonary secretions
Mucous plug

Space-Occupying Lesions

Exudative and transudative fluid in the lung parenchyma
Foreign-body aspiration
Inflammation

Other Factors

Increased compliance and dynamic airway compression secondary to age-related changes to the lung
Increased time constants because of increased airway resistance, reduced compliance, or both
Splinting or casting of chest wall restricting normal three-dimensional chest wall movement
Pain and altered breathing pattern
Medications including narcotics, sedatives, and relaxants
Supplemental oxygen

---

recumbency, and the effects of extrinsic and intrinsic factors) (see Chapter 17), however, the specific parameters of the treatment prescription cannot be completely established. Integration of patient-specific information is essential for treatment to be specific and maximally efficacious. Chapter 31 extends the principles involved with the management of many of the acute medical conditions described in this chapter, detailing their subacute and chronic stages.

Individuals with Atelectasis

Pathophysiology and Medical Management

Atelectasis refers to partial collapse of lung parenchyma. The pathophysiological mechanisms contributing to atelectasis are multiple (Box 29-1). These mechanisms include physical compression of the lung tissue (e.g., resulting from increased pleural fluid, pus, pneumothorax, or adjacent areas of lung collapse) or obstruction of an airway (e.g., due to secretions or tumor) with subsequent reabsorption of oxygen from the trapped air by the pulmonary capillaries resulting in a collapse of the lung tissue distal to the obstruction (i.e., reabsorption atelectasis).

There are two primary types of atelectasis: microatelectasis and segmental and lobar atelectasis. Microatelectasis is characterized by a diffuse area of lung units that are perfused but not ventilated, leading to a right-to-left shunt. Ill and

hospitalized patients who are deprived of being regularly upright and moving have reduced lung volumes and are prone to breathing at low lung volumes, which leads to microatelectasis. Thus such patients require prophylactic measures to avoid significant effects of atelectasis on oxygen transport and gas exchange. When the conditions for normal lung inflation are removed, alveolar collapse occurs instantly.

Microatelectasis is associated with reduced lung compliance because of reduced lung expansion. Patients who are mechanically ventilated are prone to microatelectasis because the normal mechanics of breathing are violated. This may be explained in part by restricted mobility, recumbency, and reduced arousal, in addition to reduced functional residual capacity (FRC). Positive end-expiratory pressure (PEEP) is routinely added to minimize these effects. High ventilator system pressure is required to counter reduced lung compliance, which indicates that atelectatic lung tissue it not readily re-expandable.

Microatelectasis is not detected readily with chest x-ray but is on the basis of clinical findings. Nonetheless, microatelectasis can be anticipated in every ill and hospitalized patient whose normal respiratory mechanics are disrupted, particularly in recumbent, relatively immobile patients. These effects are further exacerbated in patients who are older, overweight, have abdominal masses, spinal deformities, or chest wall asymmetry, smokers, and sedated patients.

Commensurate with its distribution, atelectasis presents with reduced chest wall movement and reduced breath sounds over the involved area. A chest x-ray shows increased density over the involved areas with a shift of the trachea and mediastinum toward the collapsed lung tissue. The patient may be tachypneic and cyanotic because of shunting. Segmental atelectasis results from significant progression of microatelectasis and obstruction of airways with reabsorption of gas in the distal lung units of a bronchopulmonary segment or lobe.

The patient who is dependent on a mechanical ventilator to breathe is predisposed to developing atelectasis because of an unnatural, monotonous breathing pattern, restricted movement, and abnormal and prolonged recumbent body positions. These factors contribute to reduced mucociliary transport, abnormal distribution of pulmonary mucus, and the accumulation of mucus in the dependent lung fields. Furthermore, production of mucus may be increased due to tracheostomy or the presence of an endotracheal tube. Mucociliary clearance is further compromised by reduced ciliary activity resulting from high concentrations of oxygen, medication, and loss of an effective cough due to an artificial airway.

The effect of atelectasis on oxygen transport reflects its type and distribution. Hypoxemia, right-to-left shunt, reduced lung compliance, and increased work of breathing are common clinical manifestations. An increased temperature reflects an inflammatory or infective process and not atelectasis per se.

Principles of Physical Therapy Management

Because it can develop instantaneously when respiratory mechanics are disrupted, microatelectasis should be anticipated and prevented. Those factors that contribute to atelectasis for a given patient are countered accordingly with aggressive prophylactic management. Many of the causes of atelectasis outlined in Box 29-1 can be readily reversed. The assessment includes a detailed analysis of the underlying cause(s) and mechanism(s) so that these may be addressed directly.

Atelectasis is always treated aggressively because it has the potential to worsen, develop into a severe clinical manifestation, and lead to pneumonia. Treatment is primarily directed at reversing the underlying contributing mechanisms whenever possible (Don et al, 1971; Glaister, 1967; Leblanc et al, 1970; Lewis, 1980; Ray et al, 1974; Remolina et al, 1981). For example, atelectasis resulting from restricted mobility is remediated with mobilization. Atelectasis resulting from prolonged static positioning and monotonous tidal ventilation is managed with mobilization, manipulating body position to increase alveolar volume of the atelectatic area, manipulating body position to optimize alveolar ventilation, or some combination of these interventions. Atelectasis arising from reduced arousal is managed by reducing the causative factors contributing to reduced arousal coupled with frequent sessions of mobilization and the upright position to increase arousal, promote greater tidal volumes and alveolar ventilation, increase zone two (area of optimal ventilation and perfusion matching), increase FRC, and minimize closing volume.

Breathing control and coughing maneuvers augment the cardiopulmonary physiological effects of mobilization and body positioning. Coordinating these interventions distributes ventilation more uniformly rather than directing gas to already open alveoli, which over-distends these units. The distribution of ventilation is primarily altered by body positioning and not by deep breathing (Roussos et al, 1977). Sustained maximal inspiratory efforts may augment alveolar ventilation; however, the parameters necessary for such efforts to be maximally therapeutic have not been studied in detail.

If impaired mucociliary transport or excessive secretions are obstructing airways and contributing to atelectasis, mobilization of pulmonary secretions is the goal that may be affected by mobilization and a stir-up regimen (Dripps & Waters, 1941; Ross & Dean, 1989). In addition, postural drainage coordinated with breathing control and coughing maneuvers can facilitate airway clearance. The addition of modified manual techniques may be indicated in some patients.

Individuals with Pneumonia

Pathophysiology and Medical Management

Pneumonia is a common complication and cause of morbidity and mortality in the hospitalized patient, particularly in the very young and very old (Bartelett & Gorbach, 1976). Comparable with other systemic infections, pneumonia results when the normal defense mechanisms of the respiratory system fail to adequately protect the lungs from infection.

Air inspired through the nasal passages is cleansed of particulate matter by filtration (cilia sweep it to the nasopharynx); impaction (irregular contour of the chamber causes particles to rain out); swelling of hygroscopic droplet nuclei, which are either filtered or become impacted; and defense factors located in the mucous blanket, such as immunoglobulins (IgA), lysozymes, polymorphonuclear leukocytes, and specific antibodies. Particles that escape one of these defense mechanisms in the nasopharynx may be prevented from entering the lower airways of the larynx. The mucosa of the larynx is sensitive to chemical irritation or mechanical deformation and responds by eliciting the cough reflex. The high velocities created by the cough are sufficient to clear several branches of the tracheobronchial tree of particulate matter. The cough reflex is frequently absent or depressed in patients who are unconscious from drug overdose, epilepsy, alcohol ingestion, or head injury. Patients with artificial airways are more susceptible to infection because the normal defense mechanisms are bypassed, causing organisms to be deposited directly in the lower airways. In the lower airways the cough mechanism is rendered ineffective by endotracheal tubes, which prevent approximation of the vocal cords, and by tracheostomy tubes, which cause air to bypass the cords altogether.

The trachea and the tracheobronchial tree to the level of the respiratory bronchioles are protected by the cough reflex, filtration (again by cilia, which transport particles to the pharynx), impaction, and chemical factors (IgA). Below the level of the respiratory bronchioles, the cough reflex is ineffective and filtration and transportation of particles by cilia cannot occur because cilia are absent. The alveolar macrophages play an important role in protecting these airways from particulate matter. Macrophages ingest organisms and transport them to the lymphatic system or higher in the tracheobronchial tree to where cilia can sweep them to the pharynx. This process of phagocytosis can be slowed or stopped by hypoxia, alcohol ingestion, air pollutants, corticosteroids, immunosuppressant agents, starvation, cigarette smoke, and supplemental oxygen.

Routes of Infection

A patient who has impaired or ineffective defense mechanisms of the respiratory tract becomes susceptible to a variety of organisms. The major routes of infection include airborne organisms, circulation, contiguous infection, and aspiration.

CLASSIFICATION OF PNEUMONIA

Viral Pneumonias

Most respiratory viral infections are contracted by droplets from the respiratory tracts of infected persons. These viruses are responsible for interstitial pneumonias, tracheobronchitis, bronchiolitis, and the common cold. The ciliated cells of the respiratory tract are the most frequent site of infection. They become paralyzed and degenerate with areas of necrosis and desquamation. The mucociliary blanket becomes interrupted because destruction of the cilia leaves a thin layer of non-ciliated basal replacement cells. Inflammatory responses cause exudation of fluid and erythrocytes in both the alveolar septae and airways. Congestion and edema become predominant with the formation of intraalveolar hyaline membranes. These changes in the normal mucosal structure and cilia increase the susceptibility of the involved lung to superimposed bacterial infections. This is the most common complication associated with viral infections and is usually responsible for the fatalities that occur.

The patient with viral pneumonia presents with fever, dyspnea, loss of appetite, and a persistent, nonproductive cough. On auscultation, normal breath sounds are heard throughout both lung fields with scattered inspiratory crackles. X-ray changes range from minor infiltrates to severe bilateral involvement. Consolidation and pleural effusions occur less frequently. Secondary bacterial infections occur frequently, causing patients to develop productive coughs.

Influenza may lead to viral pneumonia in 1% to 5% of cases. Influenza includes acute viral respiratory tract infection and is characterized by a sudden onset of headache, myalgia, and fever. The route of infection is by inhalation of airborne particles from an infected person. The incubation period is 24 to 72 hours.

Pulmonary lesions include edema of the respiratory epithelium with necrosis and hemorrhage. At the alveolar level, interstitial edema, proliferation of type I cells, hemorrhage, and an increased number of macrophages are seen. In patients with pneumonia, secondary bacterial infections are frequent and are the cause of most fatalities.

Medical management of viral infections is supportive and preventative. Patients should receive vaccines whenever possible to build up antibodies against specific viruses. Once the patient has contracted the organism, treatment becomes supportive, with rest, salicylates, and high fluid intake being the main treatment priorities. Patients who become more acutely ill with viral pneumonia should be on a vigorous preventative program to lessen the possibility of bacterial infection.

Recovery also depends on good nutrition, hydration, sleep, rest, and reduced stress.

Principles of Physical Therapy Management

Patients may respond to mobilization coordinated with breathing control exercises and positional rotation for enhancing alveolar ventilation, mucociliary transport, and gas exchange overall (Orlava, 1959). Extreme body positions may enhance alveolar volume and ventilation as well as ventilation and perfusion matching (Dean, 1985; Douglas et al, 1977; Grimby, 1974; Piehl & Brown, 1976). Vigorous treatment should be initiated at the first sign of a superimposed bacterial infection, which is often accompanied by a productive cough. The appropriate devices should be prescribed at this time (e.g., ultrasonic or medication nebulizers to loosen secretions). Postural drainage may be indicated in addition to mobilization for airway clearance. Treatments, particularly mobilization, must be paced to minimize undue tiring the patient or increasing oxygen demand beyond the patient's capacity to adequately deliver oxygen. Increasing oxygen demands excessively may compromise the patient's gas exchange. Patient education is also fundamental to the treatment that is to be instituted between treatments (i.e., mobilization and positional rotation coordinated with breathing control and coughing maneuvers).

The focus of cardiopulmonary physical therapy in the management of viral pneumonia is to augment alveolar ventilation, increase perfusion, increase diffusion, and improve ventilation and perfusion matching and thereby reduce the threat to oxygen transport and gas exchange. Treatments are prescribed to optimize oxygen transport and gas exchange and minimize fatigue and lethargy.

Bacterial Pneumonia

Bacterial pneumonia causes the largest number of deaths per year by an infective agent and is the fifth most common cause of all deaths in North America. The patient presents with an abrupt onset of a severe illness characterized by fever, tachypnea, dyspnea, hypoxemia, tachycardia, and a cough producing bloody or purulent sputum. The clinical findings depend on the organism involved and the extent of the pneumonia in the lungs. The infective process may cease with the use of chemotherapeutic agents, aerosols, and physical therapy, or it may spread to contiguous areas, causing pleural effusions and empyemas.

Bacterial pneumonia can occur as either primary or secondary infections. Primary pneumonias arise in otherwise healthy individuals and are usually pneumococcal in origin. Secondary pneumonias occur when the patient's defense system becomes ineffective.

Pneumococcal pneumonia is caused by pneumococcal bacteria, a gram-positive organism. It occurs most frequently in the winter months among adults between 15 and 40 years of age with a predilection for males. Patients present clinically with an abrupt onset of illness characterized by fever, cough, purulent or rust-colored sputum, and pleuritic chest pain over the affected lung field. Physical examination may reveal decreased expansion of the chest over the affected area and muscle splinting. On auscultation, there may be bronchial breath sounds (indicating consolidation), decreased or absent breath sounds, and wheezes or crackles over the affected lung. Chest x-rays may show atelectasis, infiltrates, and consolidation.

There are four stages associated with bacterial infection of lung tissue: engorgement, red hepatization, gray hepatization, and resolution. The engorgement stage occurs within the first few days of infection and is characterized by vascular engorgement, serous exudation, and evidence of bacteria colonization. Red hepatization occurs within two to four days as a result of diapedesis of the red blood cells. The alveoli are full of polymorphonuclear leukocytes, fibrin, and red blood cells. The organism continues to multiply within the fluid exudate. Areas of consolidation become evident. Gray hepatization occurs within four to eight days and is characterized by evidence of abundant fibrin, decreased poly-morphonuclear leukocytes, and dead bacteria. Consolidation continues to be a problem in this stage. Resolution occurs after eight days as areas of consolidation begin to resolve. Many macrophages are seen and evidence of enzymatic digestion of exudate is present. The affected tissue becomes softer with large amounts of grayish-red fluid present within the alveoli. This process continues for two to three weeks with the lung gradually assuming a more normal appearance.

Pleural involvement occurs frequently, with the pleural spaces filling with the same type of fluid seen within the alveoli. Resolution is much slower because there are few surfaces available for phagocytosis. Complications that may occur in patients with pneumococcal involvement include empyema, superinfections (occur when large numbers of new organisms invade the lung), abscesses, atelectasis, and delayed resolution (defined as taking more than four weeks to resolve).

Treatment of pneumococcal pneumonia involves the use of chemotherapeutic agents, with penicillin being the antibiotic of choice. Thoracentesis is performed when pleural fluid is present. The patient should also receive ultrasonic nebulization and physical therapy. Supplemental oxygen therapy may be indicated.

Staphlococcal pneumonia is caused by a gram-positive organism. It rarely occurs in the healthy adult but is a frequent cause of pneumonia in children, infants, and patients with chronic lung diseases, especially carcinoma, tuberculosis, and cystic fibrosis. Clinically the patient presents with the same picture as the patient with pneumococcal pneumonia. There are some differences in the chest x-ray (e.g., patchy areas of infiltrate). Consolidation occurs infrequently in this type of pneumonia. Pleural effusions, empyema, abscesses, broncho-pleural fistulas, and pneumatoceles (subpleural cyst-like structures) occur frequently. Treatment includes chemothera-peutic agents, rest, increased fluid intake, ultrasonic nebulization or medication nebulizers, and aggressive physical therapy.

Streptococcal pneumonia is caused by a gram-positive organism, *Streptococcus pyogenes*. It occurs most frequently in very young, very old, and debilitated patients. The clinical picture is very similar to that of staphlococcal pneumonia. Again consolidation is rare and chest x-rays usually show one or more areas of patchy infiltrates. Complications are rare but empyema does occasionally occur. Treatment for this organism is the same as that for pneumococcal pneumonia.

Hemophilus influenzae pneumonia is caused by a gram-negative organism and occurs primarily in children as bronchiolitis and in adults who have chronic bronchitis. The clinical picture is the same as for the other bacterial pneumonias, with numerous areas of infiltration evident on x-ray. On auscultation, breath sounds are generally good, with crackles heard at the end of inspiration. Treatment of this pneumonia includes chemotherapeutic agents (ampicillin), oxygen, ultrasonic nebulization, and physical therapy.

Other gram-negative organisms causing pneumonia include *Escherichia coli* and *Pseudomonas aeruginosa*. They are seen most frequently in patients with underlying disease, especially pulmonary disease, or in those who are debilitated. They are frequently the cause of superinfections in individuals who have received massive doses of broad-spectrum anti-biotics. Clinically these patients present with cough, fever, and dyspnea. On auscultation, crackles, bronchial breathing, and diminished or absent breath sounds can be noted. X-ray changes frequently show bibasilar infiltrates, with the amount of involvement being widely variable. As for other bacterial pneumonias, treatment includes chemotherapeutic agents, ultrasonic nebulization, and physical therapy.

Principles of Physical Therapy Management

The goals of management of bacterial pneumonia include reversing alveolar hypoventilation, increasing perfusion, reducing right-to-left shunt, increasing ventilation and perfusion matching, minimizing the effects of impaired mucociliary transport, minimizing the effects of increased mucous production, and optimizing lymphatic drainage. Bacterial pneumonia is frequently associated with increased mucous production. With respect to airway clearance, management focuses on augmenting mucociliary clearance overall, reducing excess mucous accumulation, and reducing mucous stasis. Patients are often mobile and should be encouraged to be so to promote mucociliary transport and enhance lymphatic drainage (Dean & Ross, 1992a; Orlava, 1959; Wolff et al, 1977). The oxygen demands of mobilization and exercise, however, must be within the patient's capacity to delivery oxygen. These interventions are prescribed such that they avoid jeopardizing this balance and unduly fatiguing the patient (Dean and Ross, 1992b). Deep breathing and effective coughing are singularly important maneuvers for clearing airways with special attention to the avoidance of airway closure (Bennett et al, 1990). Prescriptive body positioning can be used to optimize ventilation and perfusion matching (Clauss et al, 1968; Douglas et al, 1977; Hietpas et al, 1974; Hasani et al, 1991; Ross & Dean, 1992; Ross et al, 1992b; Zack et al, 1974) (see Chapter 19). A secondary goal is offsetting aerobic deconditioning.

Individuals with Acute Exacerbation of Chronic Bronchitis

Pathophysiology and Medical Management

Chronic bronchitis is a common condition in smokers and is characterized by a cough that produces sputum for at least three months overall, and recurs for two consecutive years. Pathological changes include an increase in the size of the tracheobronchial mucous glands and goblet cell hyperplasia. Mucous cell metaplasia of bronchial epithelium results in a decreased number of cilia. Ciliary dysfunction and disruption of the continuity of the mucous blanket are common. In the peripheral airways, bronchiolitis, bronchiolar narrowing, and increased amounts of mucus are observed.

Chronic bronchitis results from long-term irritation of the tracheobronchial tree. The most common cause of irritation is cigarette smoking. Inhaled smoke stimulates the goblet cells and mucous glands to secrete excessive mucus. Smoke also inhibits ciliary action. The hypersecretion of mucus and ciliary damage and dyskinesis lead to impaired mucous transport and a chronic productive cough. The fact that smokers secrete an abnormal amount of mucus increases the risk of respiratory infections and increases the length of the recovery time from these infections. Although smoking is the most common cause of chronic bronchitis, other factors that have been implicated are air pollution, certain occupational environments, and recurrent bronchial infections.

Patients with chronic bronchitis have been referred to as blue bloaters because of a tendency to have a dusky appearance and be stocky in build. Although many patients have a high partial pressure of carbon dioxide on arterial blood ($PaCO_2$), the pH is normalized by renal retention of bicarbonate. Over the long term the bone marrow produces more red blood cells, leading to polycythemia. The work of the heart is increased due to increased blood viscosity. Long-term hypoxemia leads to increased pulmonary artery pressure and right ventricular hypertrophy.

Patients with chronic bronchitis have tenacious, purulent sputum that is difficult to expectorate. In an exacerbation, usually because of inflammation, infection, or both, these patients produce even more sputum, which tends to be retained and stagnate. Retained secretions obstruct airways and thus air flow, and reduce alveolar volume. The resulting ventilation and perfusion inequality increases hypoxemia, carbon dioxide (CO_2) retention, accessory muscle use, metabolic demand, and breathing rate. Partial arterial oxygen tension (PaO_2) is further reduced and $PaCO_2$ tends to increase. Hypoxemia and acidemia increase pulmonary vasoconstriction, which increases pulmonary artery pressure and predisposes the patient to right heart failure (cor pulmonale) over time.

A patient with an acute exacerbation of chronic bronchitis tends to have the following characteristics: (1) The patient is often stocky in build and dusky in color. (2) The patient exhibits significant use of accessory muscles of respiration and has audible wheezing or wheezing that is audible on auscultation. (3) Intercostal or sternal retraction of the chest wall may be noted. (4) Edema in the extremities, particularly around the ankles, and neck vein distention reflect decompensated right heart failure. (5) The patient may report that breathing difficulty began with increased amounts of secretions (with a change in their normal color), which is often difficult to expectorate, and increased cough productivity. (6) PaO_2 is reduced, $PaCO_2$ increased, and pH reduced. Pulmonary function tests indicate reduced vital capacity, forced expiratory volume in one second (FEV_1), maximum voluntary ventilation, and diffusing capacity, and increased FRC and residual volume. Debility and deconditioning contribute to suboptimal health, accentuated symptoms, and compromised function.

Principles of Physical Therapy Management

During an exacerbation requiring hospitalization, patients with chronic bronchitis are usually treated with intravenous fluids, antibiotics, bronchodilators, and low-flow supplemental oxygen. Diuretics and digitalis are often given to treat associated right heart failure. Airway clearance interventions are selected (i.e., mobilization, body positioning, and postural drainage). These interventions are coordinated with breathing control and coughing maneuvers to facilitate secretion removal and optimize coughing and expectoration while minimizing dynamic airway compression and alveolar collapse. During recovery, exercise with supplemental oxygen may also benefit the patient. It is important for these patients to avoid bronchial irritants (e.g., cigarette smoking, second-hand smoke, and air pollutants) and be adequately hydrated to thin secretions to facilitate mucociliary transport and expectoration.

Patients with chronic bronchitis can benefit from a comprehensive rehabilitation program designed specifically for patients with chronic pulmonary disease (Murray, 1993; Oldenburg et al, 1979). Components of acute management are shown in Box 29-2 and are comparable to cardiac rehabilitation Phase I. Specific details of exercise prescription in the management of chronic lung disease and of a comprehensive pulmonary rehabilitation program are described in Chapters 24 and 31. Risk factor reduction is a principal goal to minimize further pulmonary pathological changes including irreversible emphysema. High priority strategies include targeted education, smoking cessation, and nutritional and exercise counseling.

BOX 29-2

Phase I of Cardiac and Pulmonary Rehabilitation

Phase I*	Cardiac Rehabilitation	Pulmonary Rehabilitation
Inpatient, <7-10 days admission	Post anginal attack, myocardial infarction, operative procedures including bypass surgery and valve surgery Optimize oxygen transport by directing treatment to the underlying limitations of structure and function (impairments) Risk factors assessment Assessment of knowledge deficits and learning style Readiness to change assessment Predischarge submaximal exercise test Discharge lifestyle recommendations: • Smoking cessation • Nutrition and weight control • Physical activity and exercise • Stress management Plan for follow up	After acute exacerbation or thoracic surgery (e.g., lung resection) Optimize oxygen transport by directing treatment to the underlying limitations of structure and function (impairments) Risk factor assessment Assessment of knowledge deficits and learning style Readiness to change assessment Predischarge submaximal exercise test Discharge lifestyle recommendations: • Smoking cessation • Nutrition and weight control • Physical activity and exercise • Stress management Plan for follow up

*Phases II, III, and IV are related to subacute and chronic care (see Chapter 31).

From Leon, A.S., Certo, C., Comoss, P., Franklin, B.A., Froelicher, V., Haskell, W.L., Hellerstein, H.K., Marlye, W.P., Pollock, M.L., Pies, A., Sivarajan, E.F., & Smith, L.K. (1990). Scientific evidence of the value of cardiac rehabilitation services with emphasis on patients following myocardial infarction - Section 1: Exercise conditioning component. Position paper of the American Association of Cardiovascular and Pulmonary Rehabilitation. Journal of Cardiopulmonary Rehabilitation 10:79-87.

Individuals who do not have access to such formal structured pulmonary programs (the majority do not) can be managed by the physical therapist, who applies the same principles of practice on an individual basis.

Individuals with Bronchiolitis

Pathophysiology and Medical Management

Bronchiolitis results from peripheral airway inflammation. In people with severe bronchiolitis, the exudate in the peripheral airways becomes organized into a connective tissue plug extending into the peripheral airway. The inflammatory process resembles that in other tissues (i.e., an inflammatory stage followed by a proliferative healing stage). Such inflammation is associated with vascular congestion, increased vascular permeability, formation of exudate, mucous hypersecretion, shedding of the epithelium, and narrowing of the bronchioles. Fluid is exudated out of the circulation onto the alveolar surfaces replacing the surfactant. This in turn increases the surface tension and promotes airway closure. The secretion production associated with airway irritants and inflammation results from the excess mucous production in combination with the inflammatory exudate consisting of fluid protein and cells of the exudate. The underlying pathophysiological cascade contributes to both a restrictive and an obstructive component of pulmonary limitation. Airway obstruction results if these exudative substances are not removed. The airway epithelium has the capacity to repair and reline the lumen. A rapid turnover of cells may contribute to cell sloughing and further airway obstruction and a thickened basement membrane. The obstruction associated with bronchiolitis leads to ventilation and perfusion abnormalities and diffusion defect. Clinically the patient presents with a productive cough. Obliterative bronchiolitis has been reported to be the most significant long-term complication of heart-lung transplantation (Burke et al, 1987). Medical management is directed at inflammation control with pharmacological agents, fluid management, and oxygen administration if necessary. Prevention of infection is a priority.

Principles of Physical Therapy Management

The principal pathophysiological deficits of bronchiolitis include ventilation and perfusion inequality and a diffusion defect. These deficits result from secretions produced by inflammation and increased mucous production and from atelectasis of adjacent alveoli. Physical therapy promotes mucociliary transport and the removal of secretions and mucus to central airways, promotes alveolar expansion and ventilation, optimizes ventilation and perfusion matching and gas exchange, and reduces the risk of infection.

Bronchiolitis is common in babies and young children. The effects of inflammation and obstruction in small children are always serious because the anatomical and physiological components of the cardiopulmonary system are smaller, respiratory muscle tone is less well developed, the anatomical configuration of the chest wall is cylindrical, breathing is less efficient until after two years of age, spontaneous movement and body positioning are more restricted (infants in particular spend more time in non-upright positions), and children are at greater risk of infection (see Chapter 37).

Individuals with Alveolitis

Pathophysiology and Medical Management

Aloveolitis or bronchioalveolitis is an inflammatory disorder of the peripheral airways that is often associated with an extrinsic allergic reaction. Comparable with bronchiolitis, alveolitis is prevalent in young children. In adults, chronic alveolitis may be a precursor to interstitial pulmonary fibrosis. Acute bouts of alveolitis are reversible; however, chronic inflammation can lead to fibrosis of the alveolar wall and complete obstruction of the airway by organization of the exudate. Chronic inflammation can lead to permanent irreversible parenchymal changes and chronic pulmonary restriction.

Principles of Physical Therapy Management

The principles of physical therapy management are comparable to that for the management of bronchiolitis. Principles of the management of cardiopulmonary dysfunction in children are presented in Chapter 37. Because children and infants in particular are physically immature, the principles of management are different from those for adults.

Individuals with Alveolar Proteinosis

Pathophysiology and Medical Management

Alveolar proteinosis is a condition of unknown etiology, characterized by alveoli filled with lipid-rich proteinaceous material and no abnormalities in the alveolar wall, interstitial spaces, conducting airways, or pleural surfaces. Most often it is observed in men between 30 and 50 years of age, although it has been reported in both men and women of all ages.

The most common symptoms are progressive dyspnea and weight loss, with cough, hemoptysis, and chest pain reported less frequently. Chest x-rays reveal diffuse bilateral (commonly perihilar) opacities (see Figure 5-10). Physical findings include fine inspiratory crackles and, in the later stages, cyanosis and clubbing. Pulmonary function studies usually show decreased vital capacity, FRC, and diffusing capacity. Arterial blood gases indicate a low partial pressure of oxygen (PO_2), especially during exercise, often with normal PCO_2 and pH.

Principles of Physical Therapy Management

Bronchopulmonary lavage is one treatment for patients with moderate-to-severe dyspnea on exertion due to alveolar proteinosis. The patient is taken to the operating room. After general anesthesia and placement of a tube that can isolate each lung, the patient is turned in the lateral decubitus position with the lung to be lavaged downward. The tube enables the patient to be ventilated by the uppermost lung while the lower lung is carefully filled with saline to FRC. Then an additional 300 to 500 ml of saline is alternately allowed to run into and out of the lung by gravitational flow. As the saline flows out, manual percussion over the affected lung being lavaged has been reported to increase the amount of proteinaceous material washed from the lung (see Figure 5-11) (Hammon, 1987).

Individuals with Acute Exacerbation of Chronic Airflow Limitation

Pathophysiology and Medical Management

Chronic airflow limitation (chronic obstructive lung disease) is a leading cause of preventable death from smoking. There are two principal types of emphysema: centrilobular and panlobular. Both types can coexist; however, centrilobular emphysema is 20 times more common than panlobular emphysema. Centrilobular is characterized by destruction of respiratory bronchioles (see Figure 5-1) as well as edema, inflammation, and thickened bronchiolar walls. These changes are more common and more marked in the upper portions of the lungs. This form of emphysema is found more often in men than in women, is rare in nonsmokers, and is common among individuals with chronic bronchitis. Panlobular emphysema is characterized by destructive enlargement of the alveoli distal to the terminal bronchioles (see Figure 5-1). This type of emphysema is also found in individuals with alpha$_1$ antitrypsin deficiency. Airway obstruction in these individuals is caused by loss of elastic recoil or radial traction on the bronchioles. When individuals with normal lungs inhale, the airways are stretched open by the enlarging elastic lung, and during exhalation the airways are narrowed due to the decreasing stretch of the lung. The lungs of individuals with panlobular emphysema, however, have decreased elasticity because of disruption and destruction of surrounding alveolar walls. This in turn leaves the bronchioles unsupported and vulnerable to collapse during exhalation. This form of emphysema can be local or diffuse. Lesions are more common in the bases than the apices and tend to be more prevalent in older people.

Bullae, emphysematous spaces larger than one cm in diameter, may be found in patients with emphysema (see Figure 5-2). It is thought that they develop from an obstruction of the conducting airways that permits the flow of air into the alveoli during inspiration but does not allow air to flow out again during expiration. This causes the alveoli to become hyperinflated and eventually leads to destruction of the alveolar walls with a resultant enlarged air space in the lung parenchyma. These bullae can be more than 10 cm in diameter and, by compression, can compromise the function of the remaining lung tissue (see Figure 5-3). If this happens, surgical intervention to remove the bulla is often necessary. Pneumothorax, a serious complication, can result from the rupture of bullae.

Both types of emphysema can lead to chronic chest wall changes. The loss of elastic recoil of the lung parenchyma disturbs the balance between the normal lung recoil pulling the chest wall in and the natural tendency of the chest wall to spring out. This balance is essential in maintaining normal FRC (i.e., the air in the lungs at the end of a normal tidal breath). Because the residual volume of the lungs is increased, FRC is correspondingly increased. This increase is not functional, however, because it reflects increased dead space. These patients are still prone to dynamic airway compression and airway closure because of the loss of the normal elastic recoil of the lung parenchyma (i.e., increased compliance). This contributes to uneven distribution of ventilation and decreased diffusing capacity. The pressure volume curve is shifted and ventilation is less efficient.

With loss of elastic recoil and the normal tethering of the alveoli maintaining them patent, the chest wall tends to expand outward, thereby contributing to the hyperinflated chest associated with the patient with chronic airflow limitation. The alveolar units are structurally less uniform and the distribution of ventilation becomes even less homogeneous. Inspiratory and expiratory times of the alveolar units also become significantly heterogeneous. The alveoli require long inspiratory filling times (i.e., long time constants). For this reason, the patient with chronic airflow limitation adopts a characteristic breathing pattern in which inspiration and expiration tend to be prolonged. On expiration the patient may spontaneously adopt a pursed-lip breathing pattern, which is believed to augment alveolar patency and promote collateral ventilation and gas exchange in the lungs by creating positive back pressures (Muller et al, 1970). In addition, the patient may actively expire to compensate for the loss of the passive elastic recoil that normally empties the lungs at end tidal volume. Overall the work of breathing is increased. As the lungs become more chronically hyperinflated the chest wall becomes increasingly barrel-shaped and rigid. Loss of both the normal shape of the chest wall and the bucket and pump handle motions further compromises efficient respiratory mechanics and breathing (Bake et al, 1976).

The most common complaint of the patient with emphysema is dyspnea. Physically these individuals appear thin and have an increased anteroposterior chest wall diameter. Depending on disease severity, they breathe using the accessory muscles of inspiration (Chapter 5). These patients may be observed leaning forward, resting their forearms on their knees, or sitting with their arms extended at their sides, pushing down against the bed or chair to elevate their shoulders and improve the effectiveness of the accessory muscles of inspiration.

Patients with emphysema have been referred to as pink puffers because of the increased respiratory work they must perform to maintain relatively normal blood gases. On auscultation, decreased breath sounds can be noted throughout most or all of the lung fields. Radiologically, the emphysema patient has over-inflated lungs, flattened hemidiaphragms, and a small, elongated heart (see Figure 5-4). Pulmonary function tests show a decreased vital capacity, FEV_1, maximum voluntary ventilation, and a greatly reduced diffusing capacity. The total lung capacity is increased and the residual volume and FRC are even more increased. Arterial blood gases reflect a mildly or moderately lowered PaO_2, a normal or slightly raised $PaCO_2$, and a normal pH. Emphysema patients, unlike patients with chronic bronchitis, tend to develop cardiac insufficiency with progression of the condition, leading to failure at the end stage of the disease (see Figure 5-5). At this stage, cardiac hypertrophy may be evident.

Hypoxemia leads to hypoxic pulmonary vasoconstriction, which shunts blood from under-ventilated to better-ventilated areas of the lung. The afterload against which the right heart has to pump is increased. This elevates pulmonary vascular resistance and pulmonary artery blood pressure (i.e., pulmonary hypertension). Over the long term, the right heart hypertrophies to work against this increased resistance and eventually may fail (right ventricular failure or cor pulmonale). Heart enlargement secondary to any cause alters the electrical conduction pattern effecting electromechanical coupling and cardiac output. The altered size and heart position within the chest wall can be detected by electrocardiogram (ECG) changes as well as on an echocardiogram.

Treatment of emphysema that requires hospitalization often includes intravenous fluids, antibiotics, and low-flow supplemental oxygen (Geddes, 1984; Make, 1983). Some patients require bronchodilators, diuretics, and digitalis. Patients with chronic airflow limitation can adapt to high $PaCO_2$ levels and thus become dependent on their hypoxic drives to breathe. Therefore, low-flow supplemental oxygen is administered to these patients to avoid abolishing their O_2-dependent drive to breathe.

The incidence of emphysema increases with age. It is most often found in patients with chronic bronchitis and is significantly more prevalent in smokers than nonsmokers. There appears to be a hereditary factor. Severe panlobular emphysema can develop in patients with an alpha$_1$ antitrypsin deficiency relatively early in life even though they never smoked. Repeated lower respiratory tract infections may also play a role in the pathology of emphysema.

Chronic bronchitis and emphysema are marked by a progressive loss of lung function and corresponding cardiac dysfunction. At the end of five years, patients with chronic airflow limitation have a death rate four to five times greater than the normal expected value. Death rates reported by various studies depend on the methods of selection of patients, types of diagnostic tests, and other criteria. In general the death rates five years after diagnosis are 20% to 55%. The five-year survival rates based on FEV_1 have been reported as follows: 80% in patients with a FEV_1 greater than 1.2 L, 60% in patients with a FEV_1 close to 1 L, and 40% for patients with a FEV_1 less than 0.75 L. If these flow rates, however, are found in patients with complications of resting tachycardia, chronic hypercapnia, and a severely impaired diffusing capacity, the survival rates are reduced by 25%. Other factors that have been associated with a poor prognosis are right ventricular failure, weight loss, radiological evidence of emphysema, a dyspneic onset, polycythemia, and Hoover's sign (inward movement of the ribs on inspiration). The most frequent causes of death in patients with airflow limitation are congestive heart failure (secondary to right ventricular failure), respiratory failure, pneumonia, bronchiolitis, and pulmonary embolism.

As emphysema becomes chronic, the hemidiaphragms become increasingly horizontally positioned, placing the muscle fibers at a less efficient position on their length tension curve (Druz & Sharp, 1982). Breathing when the muscle fibers of respiration are mechanically disadvantaged increases the work of breathing and therefore energy demands and oxygen cost. Respiratory muscle weakness and fatigue are serious complications of chronic lung disease that predispose the patient to respiratory muscle failure (Rochester & Arora, 1983) (Chapters 6 and 33).

The net effects of the pathological changes on gas exchange are hypoxemia, hypercapnia, and reduced pH consistent with respiratory acidosis. Long-term respiratory insufficiency leads to chronically impaired oxygen transport and gas exchange. To compensate for hypercapnia, production of bicarbonate is increased to buffer retained CO_2 (i.e., compensated respiratory acidosis). Red blood cell production (i.e., polycythemia) is increased to increase the oxygen-carrying capacity of the blood. The negative effect of polycythemia, however, is increased viscosity of the blood, leading to increased risk of circulatory stasis, thromboses, and increased work of the heart.

Principles of Physical Therapy Management

The patient with emphysema is prone to chronic pulmonary infections and respiratory insufficiency. The clinical picture is hallmarked by alveolar collapse and destruction, ventilation and perfusion mismatch, and diffusion defect. These defects result in impaired or threatened oxygen transport if the physiological compensations are unable to maintain adequate blood gases. Shortness of breath is exacerbated and breathing is labored. Increased work of breathing reflects airway obstruction and inefficiency of respiratory mechanics and the respiratory muscles. Because of long-term airway disease, mucociliary transport is disrupted. Therefore, in the presence of a pulmonary infection and increased production of pulmonary secretions, secretion removal can be a significant problem for the patient.

Box 29-2 shows the primary components of care in the acute phase of management, which can be compared with acute cardiac care (Phase I of cardiac rehabilitation). Specific treatments are prescribed for the patient based on the specific clinical findings (i.e., the type and severity of the cardio-pulmonary dysfunction and the presence of infection). Therefore treatments include mobilization coordinated with breathing control and coughing maneuvers, which are effective in enhancing alveolar ventilation, mobilizing secretions, and in ventilation and perfusion matching. Body positioning can be prescribed to alter the distribution of ventilation, to aid mucociliary transport, and to remove pulmonary secretions. Although "pure" emphysema is typically dry, postural drainage positions can facilitate the removal of pulmonary secretions from specific bronchopulmonary segments if indicated. In any given body position, alveolar volume is augmented in the uppermost lung fields and alveolar ventilation is augmented in the lowermost lung fields. The type and extent of pathology will determine the degree of benefit these physiological effects will have on oxygen transport. In addition, body positioning is essential to optimize respiratory mechanics and enhance pulmonary gas exchange, thereby reducing the work

of breathing and the work of the heart. The assessment will define the parameters of the treatment prescription that will be effective in relieving the work of breathing and the work of the heart. This information is essential not only for prescribing beneficial positions but also for avoiding deleterious positions. A sitting, leaned-forward position will assist ventilation secondary to the gravitational effects of the upright position on cardiopulmonary function. If the arms are supported, this position stabilizes the upper chest wall and rib cage, thereby facilitating inspiration. Some patients with horizontal diaphragms and significant respiratory distress benefit from recumbent positions in which the diaphragm is elevated within the chest wall by the viscera falling against the underside of the diaphragm in this position (i.e., viscerodiaphragmatic breathing) (Barach, 1974). The muscle fibers of the diaphragm are mechanically placed in a more favorable position with respect to their length-tension characteristics. This effect may further be augmented in the head-down position in some patients (Barach & Beck, 1954). Other patients, however, cannot tolerate recumbent positions; in fact, respiratory distress may be increased. If optimal treatment outcome has not been achieved with mobilization and body positioning coordinated with breathing control and coughing maneuvers, conventional physical therapy procedures may offer additional benefit in some patients (e.g., postural drainage and manual techniques).

Because of the tendency toward dynamic airway compression resulting from the highly compliant airways of individuals with emphysema, open-glottis coughing maneuvers are indicated. Specific outcome measures are recorded before, during, and after treatment to assess short- and long-term treatment effects. In addition, between-treatment treatments are central to maximizing overall treatment efficacy. Conveying information effectively and specifically to the patient, nursing staff, and possibly family members is therefore crucial to achieve an optimal treatment outcome.

Comparable to the individual with chronic bronchitis, a lifelong health program for people with chronic airflow limitation due to emphysema should be prescribed by the physical therapist and include smoking cessation along with nutritional and exercise counseling (see Chapters 24 and 29). Improved aerobic conditioning may reduce the frequency and severity of subsequent acute exacerbations.

Individuals with Acute Exacerbation of Asthma

Pathophysiology and Medical Management

Asthma is a condition characterized by an increased responsiveness of bronchial smooth muscle to various stimuli and is manifested by widespread narrowing of the airways that changes in severity either spontaneously or as a result of treatment (Hogg, 1984; Rees, 1984). During an asthma attack, the lumen of the airways is narrowed or occluded by a combination of bronchial smooth muscle spasm, inflammation of the mucosa and an overproduction of viscous, tenacious mucus.

Asthma is a widespread disorder affecting 1% of the population. It is common in children under 15 years of age; its prevalence is estimated to be 5% to 15%. It is estimated that 80% of asthmatic children do not have symptoms after the age of 10 years.

Asthma that begins in patients under the age of 35 years is usually allergic or extrinsic. These asthma attacks are precipitated when an individual comes into contact with a given substance to which he or she is sensitive, such as pollens or household dust (see Box 29-2). Patients with asthma can be allergic to a number of substances as opposed to only one or two.

If a patient's first asthma attack occurs after the age of 35, often there is evidence of chronic airway obstruction with intermittent episodes of acute bronchospasm. These individuals, whose attacks are not triggered by specific substances, are referred to as having nonallergic or intrinsic asthma (Box 29-3). Chronic bronchitis is commonly found in this group, and this is the type of asthma seen in the hospital setting.

The patient with asthma presents with the following picture during an attack. Lung volumes and expiratory flow rates are reduced, and the distribution of ventilation is less homogeneous (Ross et al, 1992b). The patient has a rapid rate of breathing

and uses the accessory respiratory muscles (see Figure 5-6). The expiratory phase of breathing is prolonged, with audible wheezing. The patient may cough frequently, although unproductively, and may complain of tightness in the chest. Radiologically the lungs may appear hyperinflated or show small atelectatic areas (reabsorption atelectasis). Early in the attack arterial blood gases reflect slight hypoxemia and a low PCO_2 (from hyperventilation). If the attack progresses, the PO_2 continues to fall as the PCO_2 increases above normal. As obstruction becomes severe, deterioration of the patient is evidenced by a high CO_2, a low PO_2, and a pH of less than 7.3.

Patients who are hospitalized are treated with intravenous fluids, bronchodilators, supplemental oxygen, and corticosteroids. Breathing control in the acute attack relaxes the patient, helps manage the attack more effectively, and also provides a means of helping to reduce subsequent attacks. Airway clearance procedures may have a role should the cough become productive. Patients should avoid bronchial irritants and substances that worsen or induce significant bronchospasm or an attack.

An asthmatic attack that persists for several hours and is unresponsive to medical management is referred to as status asthmaticus. This condition constitutes a medical emergency, necessitating admission to the intensive care unit (see Chapter 34).

Principles of Physical Therapy Management

The hallmark of an acute exacerbation of asthma is bronchospasm, an increased responsiveness of airway smooth muscle to various stimuli (i.e., reversible airway obstruction). Although bronchospasm can be a feature of chronic bronchitis and emphysema, the primary cause of airway obstruction in these conditions results from anatomical and physiological changes that are not usually reversible.

Box 29-2 shows the primary components of care in the acute phase of management, which are comparable to acute cardiac care (Phase I of cardiac rehabilitation). Physical therapy is directed at improving gas exchange without aggravating bronchospasm and other symptoms and reversing these when possible. Thus promoting more effective and efficient breathing with relaxed controlled breathing maneuvers and controlled unforced coughing maneuvers in optimal body positions is a priority. Overall oxygen demand, including that associated with an increased work of breathing, must be reduced during an exacerbation of asthma. This may require reduced activity, body positioning that improves breathing efficiency, judicious rest and sleep periods, altered diet or restricted diet, adequate hydration, maintenance of a thermoneutral environment, rest, reduced arousal, reduced social interaction and excitement, and reduced environmental stimulation. Although general relaxation does not directly relax bronchial smooth muscle, relaxation will assist breathing control, reduce arousal and metabolic demands, and promote more efficient breathing.

Airway narrowing and obstruction is a hallmark of this condition secondary to increased bronchial smooth muscle tone and airway edema. Even small amounts of pulmonary secretions can obstruct the lumen of narrowed airways, which leads to reabsorption atelectasis distal to the site of obstruction, impaired gas exchange, and reduced PaO_2. Thus mucociliary transport is a priority. Mucous clearance can be further impeded by the addition of serous fluid to pulmonary mucus, resulting from airway irritation and inflammation. Cilia are less effective at clearing mucoserous fluid compared with mucus alone. In addition, sheets of ciliated epithelium are shed into the bronchial lumen, further contributing to the stasis of secretions. Thus optimizing the mobilization of secretions and their removal is a priority even in the presence of scant secretions. Interventions that optimize mucociliary transport are selected to minimize exacerbating bronchospasm and further increases in airway resistance.

The primary goals in the management of asthma include reducing airway narrowing, improving alveolar ventilation, reducing the work and energy cost of breathing, reducing hypoxemia or minimizing its threat, and optimizing lung compliance.

Treatment outcome is assessed with indices of oxygen transport overall and of the function of the individual steps in the pathway (Epstein & Henning, 1993). Bedside spirometry, including peak expiratory flow rate, is a sensitive indicator of ensuing compromise in oxygen transport. Some patients use a peak expiratory flow rate meter at home to detect such changes and as an early indicator of the need for medical attention.

Individuals with asthma can often learn to control their condition effectively with optimal health education and an overall lifelong health program (see Chapters 24 and 31).

Individuals with Acute Exacerbation of Cystic Fibrosis

Pathophysiology and Medical Management

Cystic fibrosis (CF) is a complex multisystem disorder transmitted by an autosomal-recessive gene that affects the exocrine glands (Landau, 1973). CF involves all of the major organ systems in the body and is characterized by increased electrolyte content of the sweat, chronic airflow limitation, ventilation inhomogeneity, and pancreatic insufficiency. Definitive diagnosis of CF includes positive family history, clinical symptoms of poor digestion, growth or recurrent pulmonary infection, and, most importantly, a positive sweat chloride test. Survival has increased dramatically since 1940 when survival was reported to be approximately two years of age. In 1980, patient survival was estimated to be 20 years of age and increasing (Hunt & Geddes, 1985). Thus although CF is congenital and manifests in childhood, this condition has now become an adult disorder. Adult patients with CF often have an upper lobe infiltrate, with evidence of atelectasis and bronchiectasis, and chronic staphlococcal infections. The beat frequency of the cilia is often slowed to approximately three mm per minute, compared with 20 mm per minute in age-matched, healthy, control subjects (Wood et al, 1975). Patients can be categorized into three general groups: those

with no significant pulmonary signs, those with pulmonary signs and occasional cough and sputum, and those with pulmonary signs and constant cough and sputum. Those patients in the last group tend to have significantly impaired pulmonary function test results, reduced diffusing capacity, and increased hemoptysis, particularly in the presence of an abnormal chest x-ray and hyperinflation. Airway hyperreactivity appears to be variable.

Peripheral airways are often abnormal either anatomically or functionally because of mucous plugging. The lungs of patients with CF may be excessively stiff at maximal lung capacity, with a loss of elastic recoil at low lung volumes (Mansell et al, 1974). Regional ventilation is nonuniform and contributes to ventilation and perfusion mismatch and hypoxemia (Cotton et al, 1985; Ross et al, 1992a).

The chronic pulmonary limitation in CF is related to increased secretion of abnormally viscous mucus, impaired mucociliary transport resulting in airway obstruction, bronchiectasis, hyperinflation, infection, and impaired regional ventilatory function, leading to impaired ventilation and perfusion matching and gas exchange. Radiologically changes are most pronounced in the upper lobes, especially the right upper lobe.

Principles of Physical Therapy Management

Prophylactic cardiopulmonary physical therapy, including facilitation of mucociliary transport and maximizing alveolar ventilation, in conjunction with the judicious use of antibiotics provides effective measures for controlling or slowing the effects of bronchial and bronchiolar obstruction. Involvement of the patient and caregivers in chronic care in the long term is particularly important. Understanding the pathology and course of CF is essential to modify treatment prescription during exacerbations and remissions of the disease.

Box 29-2 shows the primary components of care in the acute phase of management, which can be compared generally with acute cardiac care (Phase I of cardiac rehabilitation). The clinical deficits related to oxygen transport include impaired mucociliary transport, increased mucous production, increased difficulty clearing mucus, impaired ventilation and perfusion matching, right-to-left shunt, a diffusion defect, respiratory muscle weakness or fatigue, and reduced cardiopulmonary conditioning (Chatham et al, 1994). The increased production of mucus and the difficulty removing mucus increases the risk of bacterial colonization and chronic respiratory infections. These manifestations of CF are worsened with recumbency. Significant postural hypoxemia has been reported in patients with CF when moving from sitting to a supine position (Stokes et al, 1985). Thus the object of treatment is to optimize oxygen transport and pulmonary gas exchange. Given the pathophysiological deficits in an acute exacerbation of CF, the specific goals are to enhance mucociliary transport, promote airway clearance, optimize alveolar ventilation and therefore gas exchange, maximize the efficiency of oxygen transport overall, and prevent and minimize infection.

Although the degree to which patients with chronic lung conditions, and in particular CF, can respond to aerobic training may be limited, it is essential that their capacity to transport oxygen overall is optimized to compensate for deficits in specific steps of the oxygen transport pathway (Anonymous, 1988; Dean & Ross, 1989). Deconditioning severely impairs oxygen transport. Improved aerobic capacity and cardiopulmonary conditioning is central in the management of patients with CF. Prescriptive aerobic exercise enhances the efficiency of oxygen transport overall by reducing airway resistance by mobilizing secretions, improving the homogeneity of ventilation in the lungs and therefore ventilation and perfusion matching, optimizing oxygen extraction at the tissue level, and increasing respiratory muscle endurance (Keens et al, 1977; Zach et al, 1992). If optimal conditioning is maintained, oxygen transport is not as compromised during acute exacerbations given the improved efficiency of oxygen transport overall. These effects will be lost, however, as the patient deconditions secondary to restricted mobility and recumbency during the acute episode. Thus it is important that mobility is minimally restricted during an exacerbation (based on the clinical assessment and morbidity) and that exercise conditioning is a mainstay of management between exacerbations. An important additional effect of long-term exercise, which has particular importance for patients with CF, is improved immunity (Pyne, 1994; Shepard et al, 1991). This may minimize the risk of infection and perhaps minimize the severity of an infection once acquired.

In severe exacerbations the patient is extremely stressed physiologically and has significantly increased oxygen consumption because of the increased work of breathing and for the heart. In addition, the patient is prone to arterial desaturation. Thus minimizing undue oxygen demand and fatigue guides the selection of treatment interventions and their parameters in conjunction with stringent monitoring. These patients become hypoxemic and distressed readily. Treatment interventions are selected based on the assessment and the patient's ability to tolerate the treatment and derive optimal benefit. Gradual, paced, low-intensity mobilization and frequent body positioning enhance mucociliary transport and airway clearance and maximize the efficiency of the steps in the oxygen transport pathway. Postural drainage can offer additional benefit in these patients if further clearance is required. The addition of manual techniques may be indicated; however, stringent monitoring must be carried out given their potential deleterious effects on gas exchange (Kirilloff et al, 1985; Murray, 1979; Sutton et al, 1982).

Forced coughing and expiratory techniques can contribute to airway closure, whereas huffing and other forms of modified coughing with an open glottis minimize airway closure and can be more effective in removing secretions that have accumulated centrally without compromising ventilation and gas exchange (Hietpas et al, 1974; Nunn et al, 1965). Forceful coughing, in which the glottis closes, contributes to airway closure and thus should be avoided, particularly in patients with elevated pulmonary artery pressure, because of the concomitant increase in intrathoracic pressure and strain on the heart and lungs. Patients with CF have severe paroxysms of coughing. This significantly increases intrathoracic pressure, which in turn impedes venous return and cardiac output. Although coughing is an essential mechanism for mucociliary clearance in these patients, the untoward cardiac effects must be minimized.

Over the past decade, other interventions aimed at secretion clearance in the treatment of patients with CF have included autogenic drainage, the use of the positive expiratory pressure (PEP) mask, and the Flutter® valve (Pryor, 1993; Pryor et al, 2002). Autogenic drainage is based on the theory that the equal pressure point is shifted along the airways by altering the lung volume at which the patient breathes. The patient initially breathes slowly and deliberately at low lung volumes, then at mid and high lung volumes. Breathing at low lung volumes is believed to loosen secretions from the walls of the airways. This is followed by breathing at mid lung volumes, which is believed to help localize and collect the secretions. Finally, breathing at high lung volumes is believed to centralize and facilitate the removal of the secretions with coughing. Thus autogenic drainage may enhance the effectiveness of the patient's cough by manipulating lung volumes and flow rates and controlling coughing to avoid unproductive coughing and wasteful expenditure of energy. The patient is coached by the physical therapist to breathe slowly and deliberately at the volumes set by the therapist, who gauges the patient's ventilatory effort and work by placing his or her hands around the patient's chest. The patient is not encouraged to breathe below end-expiratory volume and is encouraged to suppress coughing until the expelling phase (i.e., the phase during which the patient is breathing at high lung volumes).

Autogenic drainage may be a useful adjunct for facilitating airway clearance in patients with CF. It is a procedure that patients may use independently and can be applied relatively unobtrusively. It helps optimize the patient's coughing efforts and minimizes the potential for significant airway closure in these patients. This procedure is designed to minimize exhaustive, metabolically costly coughing and preserve energy to expectorate most effectively.

The PEP mask and Flutter valve device are believed to reduce airway closure and thus optimize alveolar ventilation and enhance mucociliary clearance in patients with CF.

Individuals with CF can often learn to control their condition effectively with optimal health education and overall lifelong health program (see Chapters 24 and 31).

Individuals with Acute Exacerbation of Interstitial Pulmonary Fibrosis

Pathophysiology and Medical Management

Interstitial lung disease has been associated with various occupations and the inhalation of inorganic and organic dusts. Conditions associated with the inhalation of inorganic dusts include silicosis, asbestosis, talc coal dusts, and beryllium.

These conditions are most often seen in miners, welders, and construction workers. Workers exposed to organic material, such as fungal spores and plant fibers, may develop a serious pulmonary reaction known as extrinsic allergic alveolitis. Generally, interstitial lung disease is characterized by inflammation of the lung parenchyma, which may resolve completely or progress to fibrosis. Interstitial pulmonary fibrosis results from the deposition of connective tissue after repeated bouts of infection.

The pathophysiological deficits are commensurate with morphological changes of interstitial infiltration and fibrosis, intraalveolar exudate and alveolar replacement (see Figure 5-12). Lung compliance and lung volumes are reduced, expiratory flow at mid lung volume is increased (stiff, inelastic lungs), diffusing capacity is reduced, and hypoxemia can be present in the absence of hypercapnia (Chung & Dean, 1989; Jernudd-Wilhelmsson et al, 1986). The chest x-ray of a patient with interstitial pulmonary fibrosis secondary to sarcoidosis is shown in Figure 5-12. Other changes include increased resting heart rate, pulmonary hypertension, impaired gas exchange, and shortness of breath during exercise, as well as at rest in some cases. Symptoms can be reversed by removing the worker from the exposure through change of employment, modification of the materials handling process, or use of protective clothing and masks. Repeated exposure to these organic dusts may result in irreversible interstitial fibrosis.

Reaction to fumes and gases can also lead to chronic restrictive patterns of lung disease. Individuals exposed to plastics being heated at high temperatures are also exposed to gases that are toxic to the respiratory system. Chronic pathological changes and impaired gas exchange can result.

Medical management is directed at reducing inflammation, reducing pulmonary hypertension, and increasing arterial oxygenation. Pharmacological management may include corticosteroids for inflammation, immunosuppressive agents, and oxygen therapy. Removing the patient from the work environment contributing to interstitial pulmonary fibrosis is essential in managing the disease and its long-term consequences.

Principles of Physical Therapy Management

The primary clinical manifestations of an acute exacerbation of interstitial pulmonary fibrosis reflect an acute or chronic problem usually resulting from an inflammatory episode, pulmonary infection, or both. The mechanisms responsible include reduced alveolar ventilation, an inflammatory process and its manifestations, potential airway obstruction, and increased work of breathing and of the heart in severe cases. These patients are susceptible to desaturation during exercise and thus need to be monitored closely.

Box 29-2 shows the primary components of care in the acute phase of management, which are similar to those of acute cardiac care (Phase I of cardiac rehabilitation). In mild cases mobilization increases the homogeneity of ventilation and ventilation and perfusion matching (Jernudd-Wilhelmsson et al, 1986). Between treatments and in the management of the severely affected patient, body positioning is used to reduce the work of breathing and arousal, maximize alveolar ventilation, maximize ventilation and perfusion matching, and optimize coughing.

Patients with moderate-to-severe interstitial lung disease may desaturate during sleep (Perez-Padilla et al, 1985) and readily desaturate on physical exertion (Arita et al, 1981). Thus they warrant close monitoring during and between treatments. Increased pulmonary vascular resistance secondary to hypoxic vasoconstriction contributes to increased work of the right heart and potential cardiac insufficiency.

General debility and deconditioning warrant a modified exercise program that can optimize the function of all of the steps in the oxygen transport pathway (Arita et al, 1981; Chung & Dean, 1989).

Individuals with interstitial pulmonary fibrosis require health education and an overall health program to help manage their symptoms (see Chapters 24 and 31).

Individuals with Tuberculosis

Pathophysiology and Medical Management

Although the incidence of tuberculosis, a lifelong disease, has declined significantly over the past several decades, this disease has been experiencing a resurgence in the industrialized world in recent decades. This may reflect declining sanitation and health standards in some segments of the population and immigration patterns.

Most infections result from inhalation of airborne tubercle bacilli, which triggers an inflammatory response (Luce, 1986). This response includes flooding of the affected area with fluid leukocytes and later macrophages. The area becomes consolidated and pathologically the condition is considered a tuberculous pneumonia. The infiltrating macrophages become localized and fused, resulting in the characteristic tubercle. Within two to four weeks the central part of the lesion necroses. Tuberculosis is associated primarily with pulmonary infection that is comparable with other infectious pneumonias. Tuberculosis, however, is distinct in that it may affect other parts of the body. Symptoms include fatigue, fever, reduced appetite, weight loss, night sweats, hemoptysis, and a cough with small amounts of nonpurulent sputum with pulmonary involvement. The course of the disease is variable. Some lesions heal promptly whereas other patients experience progression and ensuing death. Other systems that can be involved include brain and meninges, kidney, reproductive, and bone. In some individuals the disease appears to remit, whereas in others tuberculosis progresses to affect other organ systems, or previously dormant foci can be reactivated.

The effects of tuberculosis on pulmonary function are variable, depending on the extent and type of lesions. Lesions may involve the lung parenchyma, the bronchi, the pleurae, and chest wall. Parenchymal involvement can reduce lung volumes, leading to hypoventilation of perfused lung units. Significant disease leads to impaired arterial blood gases, whereas areas of unaffected lung may adequately compensate in milder cases. If fibrosis has occurred, lung compliance will be correspondingly reduced. Airflow resistance may be increased from narrowing or distortion of the bronchioles because of fibrosis. Pleural involvement may result in effusions, empyema, pleural fibrosis, and spontaneous pneumothorax. Unlike parenchymal damage, small amounts of pleural restriction can produce significant changes in pulmonary function. Clinically, patients with significant pleural involvement have significant restrictive disease and correspondingly low lung volumes. The work and energy cost of breathing are markedly increased. Shortness of breath is a common complaint. Comparable with an interstitial pulmonary fibrosis patient, the patient adopts a rapid, shallow breathing pattern to reduce the high cost of elastic work of breathing. Thus the dead space tends to be hyperventilated and alveolar hypoventilation results.

In addition to alveolar hypoventilation, lung tissue and pulmonary vascular damage impairs ventilation and perfusion matching and diffusing capacity. In severe cases, hypoxemia and hypercapnia are present. Chronic adaptation includes polycythemia and hypervolemia. Right heart failure may ensue.

The lungs become shrunken and geometrically distorted because of fibrotic changes in the lungs. These changes can lead to kinking and obstruction of the pulmonary blood vessels and maldistribution of pulmonary blood flow, which further compromises ventilation and perfusion matching.

Tuberculosis may be associated with an obstructive component. An increase in airflow resistance comparable with emphysema can be present. This obstruction results from chronic infection, mucosal edema, retained secretions, and bronchospasm.

Antibiotics can be effective in managing the disease such that hospitalization is avoided. If detected early, the prognosis is favorable, provided the patient adheres to the medication schedule and the bacilli do not become resistant to the medications. Surgery may be indicated to resect lung segments that are chronically involved. The extent and severity of the disease determines the course of recovery.

Maintenance of good general health is particularly important in the management, control, and prevention of tuberculosis (e.g., sanitation, balanced diet, sleep, regular exercise, and stress control).

Principles of Physical Therapy Management

Although the acute presentation of tuberculosis is comparable with acute pneumonia (refer to pneumonia section), there are some important differences with respect to physical therapy management. First, tuberculosis is particularly infectious, thus special precautions should be taken by the physical therapist to prevent its spread during its infectious stage. Second, patients may be prone to fatigue; treatments should be selected to promote improved oxygen transport without exceeding the patient's capacity to deliver oxygen and without contributing to excessive fatigue. Stimulation of the oxygen transport system with exercise is necessary to

avoid the deleterious effects of deconditioning and further compromise of oxygen transport. The patient warrants being monitored closely.

Hypertension

Pathophysiology and Medical Management

Essential hypertension, the "silent killer" (of unknown etiology), is the most common type of hypertension (90% of all reported cases). Salt sensitivity has been implicated in hypertension in African Americans, and increased rennin production in the Hispanic population (Kramer et al, 2004). Generally hypertension is classified as mild, moderate, or severe. Hypertension is managed pharmacologically with vasodilators (i.e., afterload reducers), diuretics (i.e., volume reducers), and beta-blocking agents (i.e., inotrophic agents). Despite a primarily pharmacological orientation to the management of hypertension, a high proportion of individuals with hypertension still have high blood pressure and are at increased risk of its deadly complications. Hypertension is a significant health-care concern in that the condition is frequently associated with heart disease and stroke. Thus its consequences can be dire. As described in Chapter 1, hypertension often occurs in the presence of obesity and diabetes, which complicates the clinical picture further.

Pharmacological management may have a role in the control of hypertension given its serious consequences and the necessity of maintaining blood pressure within acceptable limits. Like all medication, its effects must be monitored closely to ensure that the desired outcomes are being achieved. The following decisions must be made.

1. To what degree is pharmacological intervention warranted given the patient's severity of hypertension and overall clinical picture?
2. To what degree could the hypertension be managed with nonpharmacological interventions?
3. To what degree could pharmacological and nonpharmacological interventions be used concurrently? What type of schedule might be anticipated to wean the patient off medication with time?

Principles of Physical Therapy Management

Physical therapists treat patients with hypertension as a primary or secondary diagnosis. If it is a secondary diagnosis, it is important that the diagnosis is not overlooked. What the physical therapist can do for the hypertension may be clinically much more significant than management of the primary diagnosis for which the patient is referred.

Physical therapy can be an effective intervention for the management of hypertension with the primary goal of eliminating the need for medication. Secondarily, physical therapy will aim to reduce the need for medication or reduce the potency of medication required. The foundation of management in a patient with hypertension is a lifestyle review and recommendations in consultation with the patient. Recommendations include nutrition, weight control, exercise, smoking cessation guidelines (APTA, 2001), and stress management. Medical management may include beta blockers and diuretics to reduce plasma volume or other antihypertensive medication. A prescription of regular aerobic exercise may control hypertension (Froelicher & Myers, 2000; Goldberger, 1990). The prescription is based on a consideration of the patient's coexistent problems and general health status. If obesity is a concurrent problem, an exercise program is prescribed to address both concerns.

More frequently physical therapists treat patients whose hypertension is a secondary condition. Thus, whether the patient is being treated for osteoarthritis, stroke, or cardiopulmonary dysfunction, treatment is modified accordingly. An exercise prescription includes generalized aerobic exercise at an intensity that is optimally therapeutic and not associated with any excessive or untoward hemodynamic responses (Blair et al, 1988).

Patients with labile hypertension are the most difficult patients to prescribe an exercise program for because of the irregularity of their blood pressure responses. The intensity is modified at each session to accommodate these variations. Because beta-blockers and other medications blunt heart rate responses to exercise, the exercise prescription parameters are defined on the basis of some other objective hemodynamic response or on subjective responses (e.g., the Borg scale of perceived exertion).

The benefits of a modified aerobic exercise prescription include elimination of medication, reduction of medication, and improved pharmacological control on the same dose of medication. In addition, the patient derives all the other multisystem health benefits of exercise. A program of aerobic exercise should be carried out in conjunction with other lifestyle changes associated with blood pressure control (e.g., nutrition, weight control, stress reduction, and smoking cessation program). Medications should be monitored by the physician during the training program. In addition to exercise having a direct effect on controlling hypertension, the effect of exercise on overall metabolism may alter the absorption and degradation of the medications, which in turn can reduce the prescriptive requirements of that medication. Those types of exercise that are associated with a disproportionate hemodynamic challenge (e.g., static movements and stabilizing postures) are not usually indicated. Rather, aerobic exercise that is rhythmic, involves the large muscles of the legs and possibly the arms, and is performed frequently is indicated (Blair et al, 1988). Physical therapy outcomes include reduction or elimination of antihypertensive medication with self-monitoring and optimal lifestyle management.

A patient who is being managed acutely with high blood pressure may benefit from relaxation strategies, breathing control, and stress management. Further, complementary therapies, as described in Chapter 28, may have an important role. For noninvasive physical therapy management of hypertension, see Chapter 31.

Individuals with Angina

Pathophysiology and Medical Management

Angina refers to pain resulting from ischemia of the myocardium and often precedes myocardial infarction. Coronary artery disease is the primary cause of myocardial infarction and is among the leading causes of death in the Western world. Lifestyle factors, including high-fat diet, stress, and low activity levels, contribute to atherosclerosis and fat deposition within the coronary blood vessels. When these deposits narrow or totally occlude the vessel lumen, blood flow is restricted or totally obstructed. As the heart continues to demand oxygen and nutrients to work, blood supply must be increased. If one or more of the myocardial blood vessels is stenosed, insufficient blood reaches the working myocardial fibers, and ischemia and pain result. Although the classic description of anginal pain is retrosternal, vice-like, gripping pain radiating to the left side and down the arm and up into the neck, anginal pain may occur bilaterally anywhere above the umbilicus. Furthermore, patients vary considerably with respect to the degree to which the severity of the pain correlates with the degree of myocardial ischemia and infarction. Thus even apparently minimal chest pain may be associated with significant ischemia and should not be minimized with respect to its clinical significance. Approximately 10% to 15% of individuals who have a myocardial infarction do not report chest pain. Chest pain can also be blunted in individuals with diabetes due to the autonomic neuropathy.

Principles of Physical Therapy Management

The management of patients with heart disease who are hemodynamically unstable and require intensive monitoring to assess and to monitor physical therapy treatment is described in Chapter 34. This chapter addresses management of the patient with a cardiac medical condition who is stable and uncomplicated. Physical therapists must be knowledgeable and proficient in management of the patient with cardiac conditions because these patients are referred with cardiac disease as a primary or secondary problem. The principles for physical therapy in management of patients with acute heart disease are subsumed within the principles of Phase I cardiac rehabilitation (Box 29-2). Because physical therapy invariably involves physically stressing a patient either with therapeutic exercise or with the application of a therapeutic modality, the physical therapist must address the following questions when managing a patient with heart disease.

1. Does the patient's cardiac status preclude treatment? Why?
2. Is additional information about the patient necessary before physical therapy assessment and treatment? What information?
3. How should treatment be modified? Why?
4. Is the patient using antianginal medication appropriately? Is the prescription current? Does the patient have the antianginal medication present at all times?

5. Are there other medications that may influence the patient's cardiopulmonary status and response to treatment? What are they?
6. What physiological parameters should be monitored before, during, and after treatment?
7. What is the patient's knowledge about his or her condition? Can the patient clearly identify what triggers the angina and what makes it worse and better? What lifestyle changes have been made? What should be reinforced and what education is necessary?

A key consideration in the management of any person with cardiovascular dysfunction is minimizing myocardial strain (Cheitlin, 2004). Thus mobilization and exercise prescription must incorporate appropriate warm-up, steady-rate, cool-down, and recovery phases, and the type of exercise should be rhythmic and involve the legs (i.e., areas of large muscle mass) and possibly the arms as well. Initially, low-intensity activity that restricts the heart rate to no more than 20 beats above resting heart rate may be indicated to minimize the work of the heart without immobilizing the patient completely. Ejection fraction is not necessarily a good indicator of exercise tolerance because these variables are not well correlated (Dean, 1993). Upper-extremity work alone is more hemodynamically demanding than lower extremity work and thus is prescribed cautiously if at all, at least in the early stage. Exercise or physical activity involving sustained static postures and isometric muscle contraction are contraindicated. Breathing should be coordinated with activity such that breath holding and straining are avoided.

An individual with a history of angina, regardless of whether he or she is taking antianginal medications, must be hemodynamically monitored (i.e., heart rate, blood pressure, rate pressure product, and subjective responses; ECG monitoring may also be indicated).

Individuals prone to angina may exhibit symptoms in certain body positions (Lange et al, 1988; Langou et al, 1977; Prakash et al, 1973). Usually this reflects an increased workload and increased work of the heart. Recumbent positions increase the mechanical work of the heart by increasing central blood volume (Kaneko et al, 1966). These patients are not encouraged to lie flat. Instead the head of bed is elevated 10 to 15 degrees. Side-lying positions, particularly left side-lying, increase the work of the heart by compressing the heart and impeding ventricular filling and ejection. Patients with impaired oxygen transport and without prior cardiac disease may exhibit myocardial stress and ischemia in these body positions. Thus patients with impaired or threatened oxygenation must be monitored closely, particularly during turning and activities in which oxygen demand is increased, during which oxygen delivery must be increased correspondingly.

The principles of the physical therapy management of patients with stabilized angina include health education, risk factor reduction, and a long-term health program (see Chapters 24 and 31).

Individuals with Uncomplicated Myocardial Infarction

Pathophysiology and Medical Management

Myocardial infarction, commonly referred to as a heart attack, refers to insufficient myocardial perfusion resulting in a macroscopic area of damage and necrosis of the heart. Infarction results most frequently from narrowing and occlusion of the coronary blood vessels secondary to atherosclerosis. Other causes include occlusion secondary to a thrombus or embolus, reduced blood pressure, or coronary vasospasm. Angina, or ischemic chest pain, often precedes or accompanies a myocardial infarction. Infarctions vary in severity from being silent (i.e., having no characteristic signs and symptoms), and thus going undetected, to being fatal. Most infarctions, when detected, require some hospitalization and monitoring to ensure that the infarction is not evolving further and that the patient is medically stable and in no danger. Chapter 34 describes the management of patients with complicated myocardial dysfunction who are admitted to a coronary care unit. This section focuses on the patient with mild heart disease, the patient with cardiac dysfunction who is discharged from hospital, the patient who has a history of ischemic heart disease, and the patient who is hospitalized for a condition other than heart disease but develops and is being managed for myocardial ischemia. Judicious movement and body positioning are essential elements in the management of the patient with myocardial infarction (Harrison, 1944). Because these interventions can place significant demands on cardiopulmonary function and oxygen transport, they must be prescribed specifically by physical therapists with considerable knowledge and expertise in the area.

Principles of Physical Therapy Management

Box 29-2 shows the primary components of care in the acute phase of management (Phase I of cardiac rehabilitation). Physical therapy constitutes a prime hemodynamic stress secondary to exercise and gravitational stress secondary to mobilization/exercise and body position changes (Weissman & Kemper, 1991). Thus it is essential to establish the adequacy of the patient's cardiopulmonary system to effect oxygen transport during and between treatments. The optimal treatment prescription is based on the patient's overall signs and symptoms of coronary insufficiency and hemodynamic instability. The physical therapist must be knowledgeable in detecting inadequate myocardial tissue perfusion and in reducing and preventing myocardial tissue damage. In addition, acute or chronic impaired heart pump function leads to reduced cardiac output and systemic tissue perfusion. Clinical manifestations include reduced mentation, reduced renal function, fatigue, malaise, and moist, cool, and cyanotic skin.

Regardless of whether the patient is being treated in hospital, either on the ward or in the department, or in the private physical therapy clinic, the patient must be hemodynamically monitored. Minimally, heart rate and blood pressure must be taken before, during, and after treatment, along with a subjective rating of anginal chest pain. ECG monitoring is usually continuous in the early stages of the infarction. The object of treatment is to have the patient remain below his or her anginal threshold so that anginal pain is avoided. Breathlessness or rating of perceived exertion may also be used. The rate pressure product (RPP) (i.e., the product of heart rate and systolic blood pressure) is highly correlated with myocardial oxygen uptake and work. Previous stress tests will establish the RPP at which angina occurs, and the intensity of the exercise dose should be set at 65% to 80% of this threshold. Patients on beta-blockers have a blunted hemodynamic response to exercise, particularly heart rate responses. In such cases, use of ratings of perceived exertion to define the upper and lower limits of an acceptable mobilization stimulus may be indicated.

In some cases, patients have labile angina (i.e., the onset of angina does not occur reliably at a given RPP). This patient and the patient who reports angina at rest are at higher risk and appropriate precautions must be taken. First, the patient must be assessed to establish that treatment is not precluded (see pertinent questions to be answered before treating a patient with angina). Second, monitoring is essential and may include ECG monitoring. Third, treatments are prescribed below symptom threshold, which is usually consistent with a low exercise intensity in these patients. Comparable with any patient experiencing low functional work capacity, exercise prescribed on an interval schedule enables the patient to achieve a greater volume of work.

Similar to the patient with angina, body positions are selected for the patient with a myocardial infarction that will minimize the work of breathing and of the heart (Sonnenblick et al, 1968). Significant central fluid shifts are minimized by encouraging the upright position as much as possible to reduce the work of the heart (Levine & Lown, 1952) and by raising the head of the bed 10 to 15 degrees when the patient is recumbent. Patients with elevated intracardiac pressures are less susceptible to orthostatism (see Chapter 19).

Comparable with the management of the patient who has a history of angina, body positions, static postures, activities, and respiratory maneuvers associated with increased hemodynamic strain (e.g., breath holding) are avoided.

Relaxation is central in the management of the cardiac patient who is prone to being anxious and apprehensive. Relaxation interventions include autogenic relaxation, progressive relaxation, Benson's relaxation response procedures, biofeedback, and meditation. Also, the patient needs to identify and minimize stress triggers and effective, individual-specific, nonpharmacological relaxants. Relaxation training with or without pharmacological support can be integrated into treatment (Wood, 2004; Pryor et al, 2002). Patients with heart disease are often apprehensive and anxious about the intensity of physical activity they can undertake. Thus performing physical activity and exercise while monitored and under the supervision of a physical therapist is often reassuring and gives the patient confidence to perform activity when unsupervised.

The quality and quantity of the patient's sleep and a profile of sleep-wake periods should be reviewed to ensure he or she is deriving maximal benefit. Rapid-eye-movement sleep with bursts of sympathetic activity during the early hours of the morning may constitute a period of increased risk for the patient with cardiac dysfunction.

Appropriate safety precautions must be taken in all settings where physical therapists practice, given that most physical therapy interventions physically stress patients and that coronary symptoms can occur regardless of whether the patient has a known underlying heart disease. In addition, because the population is aging, physical therapists are treating a growing number of older persons who are known to have a higher prevalence of cardiovascular disease as well as younger people.

Optimal lifestyle habits and a lifelong health plan are central to maximizing recovery and improving an individual's long-term prognosis. Good nutrition and hydration, good sleep habits, stress management, smoking cessation, and regular physical exercise are all salient to comprehensive physical therapy management (Wood, 2004) (see Chapters 24 and 31).

SUMMARY

Primary, acute medical conditions that affect the cardiopulmonary system can impact on an individual's participation in life and its composite physical activities. However, serious limitations of structure and function (impairments) may be present that do not impact on life participation and yet are life threatening. Both categories must be managed by the physical therapist. Principles for management of individuals with common acute medical conditions including *primary* lung dysfunction (i.e., atelectasis, pneumonia, bronchitis, bronchiolitis, alveolitis, alveolar proteinosis, acute exacerbations of chronic airflow limitation, asthma, cystic fibrosis, interstitial pulmonary fibrosis, and tuberculosis) and *primary* cardiovascular dysfunction (i.e., hypertension, uncomplicated angina, and myocardial infarction) are presented. This chapter focuses on the pathophysiology underlying these disorders and the mechanisms by which they threaten or impair an individual's heart-lung interaction and oxygen transport. Thus the bases for the principles of physical therapy are described rather than specific treatment prescriptions, which necessitate consideration of particular cases. Treatment prescription is based on the effects of restricted mobility, recumbency, and extrinsic and intrinsic factors in addition to the underlying pathology, on an *individual's* oxygen transport status. Management is directed at the underlying pathophysiological mechanisms resulting from these four factors wherever possible, secondarily to symptom reduction. To prioritize treatments, the most physiological interventions are exploited foremost because these address multiple steps in the oxygen transport pathway. Less physiological interventions (i.e., conventional cardiopulmonary physical therapy) are instituted after the most physiological interventions have been exploited or are instituted in conjunction with these. The challenge of clinical problem solving is determining the optimal treatment prescription for a given individual that will effect the *best* outcomes with respect to oxygen transport and eventual sustained return to full participation in life with the least risk in the shortest period of time.

Review Questions

1. Describe how *acute* limitations of structure and function of the cardiovascular and pulmonary systems can affect an individual's participation in life and related activities (from no relationship to extensive relationship). Discuss the role of physical therapy in both circumstances.
2. Describe the *primary* cardiopulmonary pathophysiology and how a patient is likely to present clinically with the following *acute* conditions: atelectasis, pneumonia, bronchitis, bronchiolitis, alveolitis, alveolar proteinosis, acute exacerbations of chronic airflow limitation, asthma, cystic fibrosis, interstitial pulmonary fibrosis, tuberculosis, hypertension, stable angina, and stable myocardial infarction.
3. Relate physical therapy management and treatment interventions for patients with each of the above acute conditions to the underlying pathophysiology, and provide the rationale for your choices.

REFERENCES

American Thoracic Society. (1989). Epidemiology standardization project. American Review of Respiratory Disease 118:1-120.

Anonymous. (1988). Cystic fibrosis and physical activity. International Journal of Sports Medicine 9(Suppl 1):1-64.

Arita, K.I., Nishida, O., & Hiramoto, T. (1981). Physical exercise in "pulmonary fibrosis." Hiroshima Journal of Medical Science 30:149-159.

Bake, B., Dempsey, J., & Grimby, G. (1976). Effects of shape changes of the chest wall on distribution of inspired gas. American Review of Respiratory Disease 114:1113-1120.

Barach, A.L. (1974). Chronic obstructive lung disease: postural relief of dyspnea. Archives of Physical Medicine and Rehabilitation 55:494-504.

Barach, A.L., & Beck, G.J. (1954). Ventilatory effects of head-down position in pulmonary emphysema. American Journal of Medicine 16:55-60.

Bartelett, J.G., & Gorbach, S.L. (1976). The triple threat of pneumonia. Chest 68:4-10.

Bates, D.V. (1989). Respiratory function in diseases, ed 3. Philadelphia: WB Saunders.

Bennett, W.D., Foster, W.M., & Chapman, W.F. (1990). Cough-enhanced mucus clearance in the normal lung. Journal of Applied Physiology 69:1670-1675.

Blair, S.N., Painter, P., Pate, R.R., Smith, L.K., & Taylor, C.B. (1988). Resource manual for guidelines for exercise testing and prescription. Philadelphia: Lea & Febiger.

Burke, C.M., Glanville, A.R., Theodore, J., & Robin, E.D. (1987). Lung immunogenicity, rejection, and obliterative bronchiolitis. Chest 92:547-549.

Challum J., Berkson, B., & Smith, M.D. (2000). Syndrome X. New York: John Wiley & Sons, Inc.

Chatham, K., Berrow, S., Beeson, C., Griffiths, L., Brough, D., & Musa, I. (1994). Inspiratory pressures in adult cystic fibrosis. Physiotherapy 80:748-752.

Chung, F., & Dean, E. (1989). Pathophysiology and cardiorespiratory consequences of interstitial lung disease-review and clinical implications. Physical Therapy 69:956-966.

Clauss, R.H., Scalabrini, B.Y., Ray, R.F., & Reed, G.E. (1968). Effects of changing body position upon improved ventilation-perfusion relationships. Circulation 37(Suppl 4):214-217.

Cotton, D.J., Graham, B.L., Mink, J.T., & Habbick, B.F. (1985). Reduction of the single breath diffusing capacity in cystic fibrosis. European Journal of Respiratory Diseases 66:173-180.

Dantzker, D.R. (1983). The influence of cardiovascular function on gas exchange. Clinics in Chest Medicine 4:149-159.

Dantzker, D.R. (1988). Oxygen transport and utilization. Respiratory Care 33:874-880.

Dean, E. (1985). Effect of body position on pulmonary function. Physical Therapy 65:613-618.

Dean, E. (1993). Advances in rehabilitation for older persons with cardiopulmonary dysfunction. In Katz, P.R., Kane, R.L., & Mezey, M.D. (Eds). Advances in long-term care, ed 2. New York: Springer.

Dean, E., & Ross, J. (1989). Integrating current literature in the management of cystic fibrosis: a rejoinder. Physiotherapy Canada 41:46-47.

Dean, E., & Ross, J. (1992a). Oxygen transport. The basis for contemporary cardiopulmonary physical therapy and its optimization with body positioning and mobilization. Physical Therapy Practice 1:34-44.

Dean, E., & Ross, J. (1992b). Mobilization and exercise conditioning. In Zadai, C. (Ed). Pulmonary management in physical therapy. New York: Churchill Livingstone.

Don, H.F., Craig, D.B., Wahba, W.M., & Couture, J.G. (1971). The measurement of gas trapped in the lungs at functional residual capacity and the effects of posture. Anesthesiology 35:582-590.

Douglas, W.W., Rehder, K., Beynen, F.M., Sessler, A.D., & Marsh, H. M. (1977). Improved oxygenation in patients with acute respiratory failure: the prone position. American Review of Respiratory Disease 115:559-566.

Dripps, R.D., & Waters, R.M. (1941). Nursing care of the surgical patient. 1. The "stir-up." American Journal of Nursing 41:23-34.

Druz, W.S., & Sharp, J.T. (1982). Electrical and mechanical activity of the diaphragm accompanying body position in severe chronic obstructive pulmonary disease. American Review of Respiratory Disease 125:275-280.

Epstein, C.D., & Henning, R.J. (1993). Oxygen transport variables in the identification and treatment of tissue hypoxia. Heart and Lung 22:328-348.

Froelicher, V.F., & Myers, J.N. (2000). Exercise and the heart, ed 4. Philadelphia: Elsevier.

Geddes, D.M. (1984). Chronic airflow obstruction. Postgraduate Medicine 60:194-200.

Glaister, D.H. (1967). The effect of posture on the distribution of ventilation and blood flow in the normal lung. Clinical Science 33:391-398.

Goldberger, E. (1990). Essentials of clinical cardiology. Philadelphia: J.B. Lippincott.

Grimby, G. (1974). Aspects of lung expansion in relation to pulmonary physiotherapy. American Review of Respiratory Disease 110:145-153.

Hammon, W.E. (1987). Pathophysiology of chronic pulmonary disease. In Frownfelter, D.L. (Ed). Chest physical therapy and pulmonary rehabilitation, ed 2. St. Louis: Mosby.

Harrison, T.R. (1944). The abuse of rest as a therapeutic measure for patients with cardiovascular disease. Journal of the American Medical Association 125:1075-1077.

Hasani, A., Pavia, D., Agnew, J.E., & Clarke, S.W. (1991). The effect of unproductive coughing/FET on regional mucus movement in the human lungs. Respiratory Medicine 85:23-26.

Hietpas, B.G., Roth, R.D., & Jensen, W.M. (1974). Huff coughing and airway patency. Respiratory Care 24:710.

Hogg, J.C. (1984). The pathology of asthma. Clinics in Chest Medicine 5:567-571.

Hunt, B., & Geddes, D.M. (1985). Newly diagnosed cystic fibrosis in middle and later life. Thorax 40:23-26.

Jernudd-Wilhelmsson, Y., Hornblad, Y., & Hedenstierna, G. (1986). Ventilation perfusion relationships in interstitial lung disease. European Journal of Respiratory Disease 68:39-49.

Kaneko, K., Milic-Emili, J., Dolovich, M.B., Dawson, A., & Bates, D.V. (1966). Regional distribution of ventilation and perfusion as a function of body position. Journal of Applied Physiology 21:767-777.

Kasper, D.L., Braunwald, E., Fauci, A., Hauser, S., Longo, D., & Jameson, J.L. (2004). Harrison's principles of internal medicine, ed 16. Boston: McGraw Hill.

Keens, T.G., Krastins, I.R.B., Wannamaker, E.M., Levison, H., Crozier, D.N., & Bryan, A.C. (1977). Ventilatory muscle endurance training in normal subjects and patients with cystic fibrosis. American Review of Respiratory Disease 116:853-860.

Kirilloff, L.H., Owens, G.R., Rogers, R.M., & Mazzocco, M.C. (1985). Does chest physical therapy work? Chest 88:436-444.

Kramer, H., Han, C., Post, W., Goff, D., Diez-Roux, A., Cooper, R., Jinagouda, S., & Shea, S. (2004). Racial/ethnic differences in hypertension and hypertension treatment and control in the multi-ethnic study of atherosclerosis (MESA). American Journal of Hypertension 17:963-70.

Landau, L.I., & Phelan, P.D. (1973). The spectrum of cystic fibrosis. American Review of Respiratory Disease 108:593-602.

Lange, R.A., Katz, J., McBride, W., Moore, D.M., & Hillis, L.D. (1988). Effects of supine and lateral positions on cardiac output and intracardiac pressures. American Journal of Cardiology 62:330-333.

Langou, R.A., Wolfson, S., Olson, E.G., & Cohen, L.S. (1977). Effects of orthostatic postural changes on myocardial oxygen demands. American Journal of Cardiology 39:418-421.

Leblanc, P., Ruff, F., & Milic-Emili, J. (1970). Effects of age and body position on "airway closure" in man. Journal of Applied Physiology 28:448-451.

Leon, A.S., Certo, C., Comoss, P., Franklin, B.A., Froelicher, V., Haskell, W.L., Hellerstein, H.K., Marlye, W.P., Pollock, M.L., Pies, A., Sivarajan, E.F., & Smith, L.K. (1990). Scientific evidence of the value of cardiac rehabilitation services with emphasis on patients following myocardial infarction - Section 1: Exercise conditioning component. Position paper of the American Association of Cardiovascular and Pulmonary Rehabilitation. Journal of Cardiopulmonary Rehabilitation 10:79-87.

Levine, S.A., & Lown, B. (1952). 'Armchair' treatment of acute coronary thrombosis. Journal of the American Medical Association 148:1365-1369.

Lewis, F.R. (1980). Management of atelectasis and pneumonia. Surgical Clinics of North America 60:1391-1401.

Make, B. (1983). Medical management of emphysema. Clinics in Chest Medicine 4:465-482.

Mansell, A., Dubrawsky, C., Levison, H., Bryan, A.C., & Crozier, D.N. (1974). Lung elastic recoil in cystic fibrosis. American Review of Respiratory Disease 109:190-197.

Muller, R.E., Petty, T.L., & Filley, G.F. (1970). Ventilation and arterial blood gas changes induced by pursed-lip breathing. Journal of Applied Physiology 28:784-789.

Murray, E. (1993). Anyone for pulmonary rehabilitation? Physiotherapy 79:705-710.

Murray, J.E., & Nadel, J.A. (2000). Textbook of respiratory medicine, ed 3. Philadelphia: Elsevier.

Murray, J.E. (1979). The ketchup-bottle method. New England Journal of Medicine 300:1155-1157.

Nunn, J.F., Coleman, A.J., Sachithanandan, T., Bergman, N.A., & Laws, J.W. (1965). Hypoxaemia and atelectasis produced by forced expiration. British Journal of Anaesthesia 37:3-12.

Oldenburg, F.A., Dolovich, M.B., Montgomery, J.M., & Newhouse, M.T. (1979). Effects of postural drainage, exercise, and cough on mucus clearance in chronic bronchitis. American Review of Respiratory Disease 120:739-745.

Orlava, O.E. (1959). Therapeutic physical culture in the complex treatment of pneumonia. Physical Therapy Review 39:153-160.

Perez-Padilla, R., West, P., & Lertzman, M. (1985). Breathing during sleep in patients with interstitial lung disease. American Review of Respiratory Disease 132:224-229.

Piehl, M.A., & Brown, R.S. (1976). Use of extreme position changes in acute respiratory failure. Critical Care Medicine 4:13-14.

Prakash, R., Parmley, W.W., Dikshit, K., Forrester, J., & Swan, H.J. (1973). Hemodynamic effects of postural changes in patients with acute myocardial infarction. Chest 64:7-9.

Pryor, J.A. (1993). Respiratory care. Edinburgh: Churchill Livingstone.

Pryor, J.A., Prasad, S.A., & Webber, B.A. (2002). Physiotherapy for respiratory and cardiac problems: adults and paediatrics. St. Louis: Harcourt Health Sciences Group.

Pyne, D.B. (1994). Regulation of neutrophil function during exercise. Sports Medicine 17:245-258.

Ray, R.F., Yost, L., Moallem, S. (1974). Immobility, hypoxemia, and pulmonary arteriovenous shunting. Archives of Surgery 109:537-541.

Rees, J. (1984). ABC of asthma. Definition and diagnosis. British Medical Journal 5:1370-1372.

Remolina, C., Khan, A.U., Santiago, T.V., & Edelman, N.H. (1981). Positional hypoxemia in unilateral lung disease. New England Journal of Medicine 304:523-525.

Rochester, D.F., & Arora, N.S. (1983). Respiratory muscle failure. Medical Clinics of North America 67:573-597.

Ross, J., Bates, D.V., Dean, E., & Abboud, R.T. (1992a). Discordance of airflow limitation and ventilation inhomogeneity in asthma and cystic fibrosis. Clinical and Investigative Medicine 15:97-102.

Ross, J., & Dean, E. (1989). Integrating physiological principles into the comprehensive management of cardiopulmonary dysfunction. Physical Therapy 69:255-259.

Ross, J., & Dean, E. (1992). Body positioning. In Zadai, C.C. (Ed). Pulmonary management in physical therapy. New York: Churchill Livingstone.

Ross, J., Dean, E., & Abboud, R.T. (1992b). The effect of postural drainage positioning on ventilation homogeneity in healthy subjects. Physical Therapy 72:794-799.

Roussos, C.S., Fixley, M., Geriest, J., Cosio, M., Kelly, S., Martin, R.R., & Engel, L.A. (1977). Voluntary factors influencing the distribution of inspired gas. American Review of Respiratory Disease 116:457-467.

Shephard, R.J., Verde, T.J., Thomas, S.G., & Shek, P. (1991). Physical activity and the immune system. Canadian Journal of Sports Science 16:163-185.

Cheitlin, M.D. (2004). Clinical cardiology, ed 7. Stamford: Appleton & Lange.

Sonnenblick, E.H., Ross, J. Jr., & Braunwald, E. (1968). Oxygen consumption of the heart. Newer concepts of its multifactorial determination. American Journal of Cardiology 22:328-336.

Stokes, D.C., Wohl, M.E.B., Khaw, K.T., & Strieder, D.J. (1985). Postural hypoxemia in cystic fibrosis. Chest 87:785-789.

Sutton, P.P., Pavia, D., Bateman, J.R.M., & Clarke, S.W. (1982). Chest physiotherapy-a review. European Journal of Respiratory Disease 63:188-201.

Weissman, C., & Kemper, M. (1991). The oxygen uptake-oxygen delivery relationship during ICU interventions. Chest 99:430-435.

Wasserman, K.L., & Whipp, B.J. (1975). Exercise physiology in health and disease. American Review of Respiratory Disease 112:219-249.

West, J.B. (2003). Pulmonary pathophysiology: The essentials, ed 6. Philadelphia: Lippincott Williams & Wilkins.

Wolff, R.K., Dolovich, M.B., Obminski, G., & Newhouse, M.T. (1977). Effects of exercise and eucapnic hyperventilation on bronchial clearance in man. Journal of Applied Physiology 43:46-50.

Wood, R.E., Wanner, A., Hirsch, J., & Farrell, P.M. (1975). Tracheal mucociliary transport in patients with cystic fibrosis and its stimulation by terbutlaine. American Review of Respiratory Disease 111:733-738.

Woods, S.L. (2004). Cardiac nursing, ed 5. Philadelphia: Lippincott Williams & Wilkins.

Zach, M., Oberwaldner, B., & Hausler, F. (1982). Cystic fibrosis: physical exercise versus chest physiotherapy. Archives of Diseases in Children 57:587-589.

Zack, M.B., Pontoppidan, H., & Kazemi, H. (1974). The effect of lateral positions on gas exchange in pulmonary disease. American Review of Respiratory Disease 110:149-153.

C H A P T E R   3 0

Individuals with
Acute Surgical Conditions

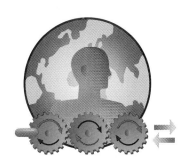

Elizabeth Dean

The overall success of surgery is not measured by its technical success alone. Rather, surgical success is based on the following.

- An individual's complete return to full participation in life and the capacity to perform its requisite activities
- Avoidance of recurrence of the problem for which the individual's surgery was indicated
- Reduced subsequent doctor- and hospital-based care
- Lifelong health

The physical therapist is involved at all stages of perioperative care as indicated and has a primary role in identifying individuals at risk of perioperative complications and preventing those complications as well as in ensuring true surgical success as defined above.

The decision as to whether and to what extent physical therapy is indicated is based on the individual's need rather than on his or her condition. The patient's condition is *one* factor that can determine perioperative risk, operative course, and long-term outcomes. Factors *other* than the primary indication for surgery, however, can have a more important effect on perioperative course and outcomes. Because of this, the preoperative assessment determines who requires management and who does not. Physical therapy prevents complications and addresses oxygen transport threats and

deficits. In the long-term, physical therapy helps ensure the individual returns to normal life and regains or surpasses premorbid presurgical functional status. In cases where recurrence of the underlying condition can occur, a prime physical therapy objective is to minimize this possibility. Surgical outcomes, based on the physical therapy perspective within the International Classification of Function (WHO, 2000), are shown in Box 30-1.

The specific purpose of this chapter is to review the identification of surgical risk in the individual, and the management of patients with cardiopulmonary risk factors and dysfunction *secondary* to acute surgical conditions. Surgery today has become more extreme in two ways. First, minimally invasive surgery has shortened the operative period, hastened discharge, and reduced risk (Toomasian et al, 1997). Second, with advances in instrumentation, monitoring, and anesthesia, more invasive, prolonged, and risky surgery is being performed with improved chances of survival.

The cardiopulmonary effects of anesthesia and surgery are described. The two types of surgery that have the greatest impact on cardiopulmonary function, namely thoracic and cardiovascular surgery, are highlighted. These surgeries are particularly invasive and lengthy, often require heavy and prolonged anesthesia and sedation, are typically performed on older people, and are generally associated with increased risk.

BOX 30-1

Surgical Outcomes and their Components Related to Physical Therapy

Long-Term Goals

Return of the individual to full participation in life and composite activities (WHO, 2000)

Sustained lifelong health

Patient empowerment vis a vis self-efficacy

Patient education and assessment of whether education goals are met/warrant modification

Avoid recurrence of the original problem

Reduce postoperative doctor- and hospital-based care

Reduced health care costs

Reduced burden of disease (suffering and cost) to the individual, family, community, and society

Perioperative Goals

Prevent perioperative complications (i.e., oxygen transport, musculoskeletal, neuromuscular, endocrine, gastrointestinal, renal, immunological, skin, and psychological)

Remediate oxygen transport limitations (limitations of structure and function)

Minimize the need for invasive intervention including mechanical ventilator support and supplemental oxygen, if these are required

Patient empowerment vis a vis self-efficacy

Patient education and assessment of whether education goals met/warrant modification

Educate team regarding physical therapy goals and how medical/surgical/nursing roles can augment noninvasive physical therapy outcomes

Minimize hospital stay

Seamless transition to the community

Follow-up in the community

BOX 30-2

Surgical Factors that Contribute to Perioperative Cardiopulmonary Risk and Dysfunction

Type of surgery

Surgical procedures

Anesthetics (general, with or without intubation, or regional) and sedation and reduced arousal

Muscle-relaxant agents and neuromuscular blockade

Supplemental oxygen and humidification

Static body position assumed

Duration of surgery and static body positioning

Incisions

Use of the cardiopulmonary bypass machine (CBM)

Use of the extracorporeal membrane exchanger (ECMO)

Dressings and binders

Splints and fixation devices

Lines and leads

Monitoring devices

Chest tube placement and number

Catheters

Perioperative anxiety, discomfort and pain

Perioperative pain control management

Perioperative fluid balance management

Perioperative blood and plasma transfusions

Thus they warrant intensive perioperative physical therapy. Patients are assessed with respect to their presurgical and surgical hemodynamic and oxygen transport status to establish oxygen transport capacity and the degree to which increased metabolic demands can be met. In particular, cardiac output and oxygen delivery (DO_2) will increase to compensate for these increased metabolic demands. Increased metabolic demands, however, are dependent on age, severity of illness, type or surgery, comorbidity, and complications (Shoemaker et al, 1993). Further, obesity can reduce arterial oxygen tensions and compliance of the respiratory system irrespective of the tidal volume or respiratory rate (Sprung et al, 2003). A detailed analysis of these factors can identify risks, expedite early intervention, and increase survival.

The four categories of factors that threaten or impair oxygen transport are described in Chapter 17. Specifically these factors include the underlying pathology, restricted mobility, and recumbency, extrinsic factors related to the patient's care, and intrinsic factors related to the patient. This chapter examines in detail the effects of surgery, such as anesthesia and other medications, on oxygen transport, as well as the impact that the underlying disease, restricted

mobility, recumbency, and factors associated with the patient have on an individual's status postoperatively.

Treatment principles are presented, though they are not intended to be a treatment prescription for a particular patient. The effects of surgery and anesthesia must be considered in addition to the underlying pathology, the effects of restricted mobility, body position, and intrinsic and extrinsic factors (see Chapter 17). All of these factors must be considered and integrated in the treatment prescription and in defining the precise parameters of the prescription. Such integration is essential for treatment to be specific and maximally efficacious.

PERIOPERATIVE COURSE

Surgery and its Cardiopulmonary Consequences

Those factors that put a patient at risk can contribute to perioperative cardiopulmonary dysfunction if preventive strategies fail (Box 30-2). Cardiovascular and pulmonary complications are the major cause of perioperative morbidity and mortality, particularly in patients undergoing thoracic or cardiovascular surgery (Kertai et al, 2003). The physical therapist must establish the risk factors based on premorbid health assessment including age, aerobic fitness, cardiac dysfunction, lung disease, smoking history, neuromuscular dysfunction, diabetes mellitus, and obesity (Hashimoto et al, 2003).

Anesthesia and Supplemental Oxygen

Anesthesia results in depression of breathing. Thoracic respiratory excursion is significantly reduced. The tone and pattern of contraction of the respiratory muscles, particularly the diaphragm and the intercostal muscles, change, which contributes to many of the secondary cardiopulmonary effects observed after surgery (Muller et al, 1979). The loss of end-expiratory diaphragmatic tone causes the diaphragm to ascend into the chest by two centimeters during anesthesia with or without paralysis (Froese & Bryan, 1974). Reductions in functional residual capacity (FRC) are correlated with this change and with altered chest wall configuration and increased thoracic blood volume (Hedenstierna et al, 1985; Hedenstierna et al, 1986). One of the most pervasive and predictable clinical effects observed in the postoperative period is alveolar collapse. Total lung capacity, FRC, and residual volume are significantly decreased. The FRC is significantly reduced in the supine position compared with the erect sitting position (Behrakis et al, 1983; Nunn, 1989) and is further reduced with the induction of anesthesia. Anesthesia, however, fails to reduce FRC in the sitting position (Nunn, 1989).

The consequences of reduced FRC with anesthesia and surgery have significant implications for postoperative complications and the course of recovery. Airway closure occurs with anesthesia and this likely contributes to intrapulmonary shunting. Compression atelectasis of the dependent lung fields occurs during surgery. In addition, compression atelectasis occurs when lung tissue and surrounding structures are being physically manipulated. Although reduced airway caliber in areas of low lung volume can be offset by the airway-dilating effect of many inhaled anesthetics, airway resistance is increased by obstruction of the breathing circuits, valves, and tracheal tubes. The airways may also be obstructed with foreign matter, such as blood and secretions, or from bronchospasm because of irritation of the airways. Because of the decrease in FRC, compliance is decreased and the work of breathing is increased. Hypoxemia secondary to transpulmonary shunting is usually maximal within 72 hours after surgery and often is not completely resolved for several days. Persistent reduction in FRC after surgery delays the restoration of the normal alveolar-arterial oxygen gradient (Alexander et al, 1973).

Anesthesia and tissue dissection contribute to major changes in lung volume, mechanics, and gas exchange. The extent and duration of these changes increase with the magnitude of the operative procedure and degree of anesthesia required. Tissue oxygenation can be threatened during the intraoperative period, and the relationship between oxygen consumption and delivery compromised (Lugo et al, 1993). Mismatch between DO_2 and oxygen consumption is associated with a complicated clinical course and prolonged intensive care unit stay in the absence of conventional indicators such as low ejection fraction and longer cardiopulmonary bypass time (Polonen et al, 1997). Oxygen extraction increases to compensate for reduced DO_2. Early optimization of the oxygen delivery/oxygen consumption ratio is indicated to reduce perioperative morbidity and mortality.

The fraction of inspired oxygen (FIO_2) depends on the mode of oxygen administration. Low-flow nasal oxygen reduces hypoxemia in the absence of hypercapnia and marked transpulmonary shunting in the postoperative patient. Low oxygen flows and low FIO_2 tend to be delivered via nasal cannulae, whereas higher flows can deliver higher FIO_2 via oxygen masks and masks with reservoir bags. FIO_2 and the body position of the patient at the time the blood sample was taken must always be considered when interpreting arterial blood gases. The FIO_2 is selected to provide adequate oxygenation with the lowest oxygen concentration possible.

After surgery the normal pattern of breathing is disrupted. Shallow, monotonous tidal ventilation without normal occasional, spontaneous deep breaths causes alveolar collapse within an hour (Nunn, 1989). Unless resolved, atelectasis becomes increasingly resistant to reinflation within a few hours. This complication is exacerbated in patients receiving narcotics.

Tachypnea and tachycardia are commonly observed with gross atelectasis secondary to hypoventilation. Breath sounds are decreased at the bases, and the coarse wheezes associated with mucus obstructing airflow are heard on auscultation. Large areas of atelectasis are present. Left lower lobe atelectasis is common after cardiac surgery.

Immediate Postoperative Period

After surgery the patient is detained in the recovery room until vital signs have stabilized, there is no apparent internal or external bleeding, and the patient is responding to his or her name. Patients recovering from minor surgery are usually transferred to a ward once discharged from the recovery room. A patient is transferred to the intensive care unit after surgery if complications arise during surgery, if the patient cannot be readily stabilized and requires close monitoring, or if the patient has had more serious surgery such as cranial, cardiovascular thoracic, or emergency surgery such as that resulting from multiple trauma (see Chapter 35).

Rest during the postoperative period is prescribed judiciously as treatment because rest is the time for healing, repair, and restoration. Sleep deprivation impairs recovery and healing. Sleep at night is biologically more restorative than daytime sleep. Thus daytime and nighttime cues are given to restore the patient's circadian rhythms. Although injudicious and excessive recumbency, bed rest, and prolonged periods in any given body position are deleterious, special attention is given to maximizing the amount of quality rest and sleep periods and minimizing disruption of nighttime sleep. Appropriate rest periods are interspersed within each treatment session, according to the patient's needs to avoid reaching suboptimal, suprathreshold physiological states. Suprathreshold states are associated with an inappropriate balance between oxygen delivery and demand such that the patient becomes compromised (e.g., hemodynamically unstable, cardiopulmonary distress is precipitated, or both).

Pharmacological Considerations

Common pharmacological agents prescribed for patients perioperatively are described in Chapter 45. Physical therapists need a thorough knowledge of these when managing the surgical patient so management can be optimized.

There are several factors that are particularly important in managing surgical patients that can affect their sensitivity to narcotic analgesics such as morphine (Gilman et al, 1990; Malamed, 2002). There is considerable intersubject response variability to these agents. Older patients can be expected to be more sensitive to narcotics. Diverse multisystem pathology has a significant effect on the degradation, absorption, biotransformation, and excretion of morphine. Exaggerated effects of morphine have been reported when administered in conjunction with other agents, such as other narcotic analgesics, phenothiazines, tranquilizers, or sedative-hypnotics; in addition, such exaggerated effects have been reported in patients with respiratory depression, hypotension, and sedation and in patients who are unconscious. These situations in which exaggerated drug effects have been reported are commonly encountered in the intensive care setting and can result in unpredictable responses. Finally, the physical dependence and abuse potential of these agents cannot be ignored.

The physical therapist must be familiar with the patient's medications and the indications, side effects, and contraindications of each. The physical therapist can determine to what extent oxygen transport may be compromised by medication effects, and whether some recommendation must be made to minimize untoward drug effects on arousal or some other factor that negatively affects oxygen transport and gas exchange. For example, although narcotics are excellent analgesics, they have widespread systemic effects including cardiopulmonary depression, gastrointestinal depression, and muscle relaxation, all of which compromise oxygen transport. Thus consideration must be given regarding whether other forms of analgesia can be used. For example, the following questions should be considered.

- Have nonpharmacological means of analgesia been exploited?
- If pharmacological analgesia is indicated, can analgesics other than narcotics be used?
- Can the dose of narcotic be reduced so that satisfactory pain control can be achieved in combination with nonpharmacological interventions?

The administration of narcotics has important implications for physical therapy. These powerful analgesics are the medications of choice for pain relief and comfort. Their secondary effects, however, which include reduced arousal and monotonous tidal ventilation, are primary physical therapy concerns. In addition, narcotics interfere with a patient's ability to cooperate with treatment. If narcotics impair the patient's ability to participate in treatment, analgesia with a less systemic effect is indicated. Patient controlled analgesia (PCA) is an effective means of having the patient regulate the amount of analgesia he or she is receiving. Interestingly, patients administer less medication to themselves than does a nurse. Intravenous administration prolongs the peak-effect time of analgesics and therefore helps the patient tolerate longer, more intense treatments.

Physical therapists have a range of noninvasive pain control interventions available to them, which should be considered in the acute surgical ward as well as in the outpatient clinic. These include relaxation, deep breathing, positioning, physical support, coordination of different treatments, and electrotherapeutics. Transcutaneous electrical nerve stimulation (TENS), for example, can be a useful adjunct in the management of postoperative pain in some patients. Pain control with TENS may enable the patient to participate more fully in mobilization, deep breathing, coughing, and bed mobility. Research is needed, however, to evaluate this technique in the management of acute pain and define the prescription parameters necessary to produce an optimal therapeutic effect. The role of nonpharmacological means of managing acute pain in place of or in conjunction with pharmacological means warrants greater exploitation clinically to produce the best analgesia with the least side effects and risks. Nonpharmacological analgesia enables patients to participate more fully in physical therapy treatments in the absence of the untoward side effects often associated with drug administration.

Although pharmacosedation is prescribed to make the patient more comfortable and reduce suffering, sedatives in particular reduce the patient's arousal and often the ability to cooperate actively with treatment. Thus these medications must be prescribed judiciously to ensure the patient is able to cooperate with physical therapy and other components of care. Over-sedation must be avoided if the patient is to derive maximal benefit from cardiopulmonary physical therapy treatments.

Prevention of Complications

Special attention in the postoperative period is given to the prevention or management of cardiopulmonary complications associated with reduced arousal, surgical pain, and restriction of lung capacity and secondary to dressings, binders, and diminished ability to cooperate, move spontaneously, and hyperventilate the lungs periodically. Patients are prone to aspiration in the immediate postoperative period, particularly while the sedation and anesthetic agents are wearing off. This risk is further increased if an airway is required or if an airway and mechanical ventilation is instituted. Postextubation atelectasis must be anticipated and avoided. To minimize this risk, patients are asked not to eat or drink fluids the day before surgery.

Endotracheal intubation and mechanical ventilation are indicated if blood gases fail to improve with conservative management. See Chapter 33 for treatment priorities for a patient during ventilation and the course of weaning from the mechanical ventilator.

A complication of thoracic and upper abdominal surgery, (e.g., cholecystectomy) is irritation or compression trauma of the phrenic nerve. This complication may be more common than expected. Inhibition of the phrenic nerve impairs the contraction of the affected hemidiaphragm, causing it to ascend into the thorax and contribute to atelectasis on that side. This inhibition may last for several days (Dureuil et al, 1986; Ford & Guenter, 1984).

The patient's position is changed frequently in the initial postoperative period. The patient is usually encouraged to change his or her body position frequently, transfer, sit in a chair, and ambulate as soon as possible after surgery. The importance of frequent postural changes and early ambulation in the initial postoperative period are stressed (Dull & Dull, 1983). Early ambulation is a priority in the management of all surgical patients unless contraindicated.

Factors Determining Surgical Response and Outcomes

A patient's response to and outcome after surgery, as well as potential complications depend on multiple factors (see Box 30-2). The type of surgery determines the degree of invasiveness, the type or types of anesthetics and sedatives, type and level of respiratory support, static body position assumed during surgery, approximate duration of the surgery and period of anesthesia, incisions that are required, dressings, lines, leads, catheters, and monitoring devices necessary, chest tubes, type and degree of pain, and the necessity for pain control after surgery.

Pathophysiology

The type and severity of underlying cardiopulmonary dysfunction increases a patient's risk of compromised oxygen transport and gas exchange perioperatively.

Restricted Mobility and Recumbency

Surgery imposes two nonphysiological states on the patient that impact significantly on oxygen transport.

1. Restricted mobility
2. Recumbency, specifically a prolonged period of static positioning with the patient breathing at monotonous tidal volumes

Extrinsic Factors

Surgery and related factors are the primary extrinsic factors contributing to cardiopulmonary dysfunction in the perioperative period.

Intrinsic Factors

Intrinsic factors that contribute to cardiopulmonary dysfunction in the surgical patient include a patient's premorbid status (e.g., preexisting cardiopulmonary, renal, endocrine, and hematological pathology). In addition, lifestyle factors are significant (i.e., preoperative conditioning level, nutrition, hydration, stress levels, weight, and smoking history).

PREOPERATIVE ASSESSMENT AND PREPARATION FOR SURGERY

To minimize risk, reduce perioperative morbidity and mortality, maximize healing, and shorten the postoperative recovery, patients need to be in the best physical and medical condition before anesthesia and surgery. In the case of elective surgery, patients often can be prescribed aerobic training (prescribed to meet the individual's needs and capacity), smoking cessation, and weight control programs beforehand. A preparatory preoperative role for physical therapy warrants greater attention and is currently underutilized in terms of improving the perioperative course and achieving optimal, sustainable surgical outcomes.

Preoperative physical therapy management includes the preoperative assessment and education; the primary components are shown in Box 30-2. During this time the physical therapist has an opportunity to develop rapport with the patient. The assessment establishes the risk of complications and prolonged hospital stay and the type and extent of perioperative physical therapy required. Postoperative neurological syndromes are common. Ongoing assessment helps ensure these are identified and addressed early (Weinstein et al, 1998). The assessment establishes what the postoperative priorities will be; however, these are modified based on the postoperative assessment. The surgical procedures are described and the effects of surgery and anesthesia and sedation on gas exchange are reviewed so that the patient understands the importance of being actively involved in physical therapy, both during and between treatments after surgery.

There are no strict guidelines about which patients should receive perioperative physical therapy. Rather, the need for physical therapy should be made on a case-by-case basis with the degree of the physical therapist's involvement determined on the basis of the patient's need. Although non-thoracic surgeries are generally associated with few cardiopulmonary complications (e.g., surgery of the extremities or lower abdomen), patients with preexisting cardiopulmonary, hematological or neuromuscular pathology, or musculoskeletal pathology of the chest wall are at greater risk even in these relatively low-risk types of surgeries. In addition, patients are at additional risk if they are older or younger, smoke, or are overweight or pregnant. Thus each surgical patient must be assessed individually to establish the degree of relative risk during surgery and the necessity of perioperative physical therapy. In this way perioperative complications can be anticipated and avoided or reduced, which is preferable to managing complications once they have developed. The cardiovascular and pulmonary assessment is particularly important in the older individual, and early mobilization is critical postoperatively (Daly, 1989).

Even though a patient may have had minimally invasive surgery and an uneventful perioperative course, the physical therapist still may have a critical role in helping to achieve long-term surgical outcomes. Recurrence is possible, particularly if surgery was related to lifestyle factors. The physical

---

BOX 30-3

Objectives of the Preoperative Physical Therapy Assessment and Teaching

Develop rapport with patient

Assess cognitive status, capacity to cooperate, language and communication skills, and cultural and ethnic beliefs and attitudes toward surgery and care

Assess the patient and estimate degree of surgical risk (e.g., age, smoking, previous cardiopulmonary dysfunction, neuromuscular dysfunction, musculoskeletal deformity, obesity, substance abuse, pregnancy, nutritional status, hydration status, and pain and discomfort)

Describe the general preoperative, intraoperative, and post-operative course

Review specific surgical procedures relevant to physical therapy (e.g., anesthesia, type of surgery, body position during surgery, airway, mechanical ventilation, duration, incisions, infusions, drainage systems, chest tubes, and recovery room)

Provide the rationale for, describe, demonstrate, and have the patient practice and provide feedback on the following breathing control maneuvers: maximal inspiratory hold, supported coughing maneuvers, relaxation, bed mobility and positioning, transfers, and mobilization

For patients at risk of postoperative cardiopulmonary dysfunction and complications, review the use of the incentive spirometer and conventional airway clearance interventions (e.g., postural drainage and manual techniques, if indicated)

Ask for any questions

---

therapist can take maximal advantage of contact with the patient and be actively involved in developing a program of sustained, lifelong health.

The importance of a thorough preoperative assessment and teaching by the physical therapist cannot be overstated. The components of preoperative assessment and teaching are summarized in Box 30-3. In cases of elective surgery, preoperative teaching includes a general description of the surgery to be performed, the effect of anesthesia and surgery on cardiopulmonary function, and the systemic effects of restricted mobility and recumbency. The lines, leads, and catheters usually associated with the surgery are explained. The patient is instructed in breathing control maneuvers, supported coughing, chest wall mobility exercises, mobility exercises for the limbs (e.g., hip and knee and foot and ankle exercises), turning in bed, sitting up, transferring, chair sitting, and walking erect postoperatively. In addition, the patient is taught methods of maximizing comfort with body positioning and supporting the surgical incision. If the bed has controls the patient can manipulate, he or she is taught how to make bed adjustments as required. The postoperative course is explained in general terms so the patient can anticipate this period. If the patient is well informed preoperatively, he or she will be better oriented and capable of cooperating when he or she wakes from the anesthetic.

Preoperative teaching is a central component of physical therapy management of the surgical patient. Such teaching

establishes rapport with the physical therapist who informs the patient about what to expect before and after surgery. In addition to reviewing the surgical procedures, the physical therapist reviews, and has the patient perform, deep breathing and supported coughing maneuvers, relaxation, bed mobility, positioning, transfers, and mobilization. Preoperative teaching reduces the patient's anxiety and encourages the patient to be as active as possible in his or her recovery. Preoperative teaching reduces postoperative complications and the length of the hospital stay. High-risk patients benefit from preoperative teaching, and their cooperation is more easily solicited after the surgery. Understanding the patient's perception of his or her condition, the surgery, expectations, and self-efficacy are also central to postoperative recovery.

The physical therapist may be consulted by the surgeon to help make a poor-risk patient into a better-risk patient. Patients with upper-respiratory tract infections before surgery may have their surgeries postponed, depending on the type and extent of surgery to be performed, level of anesthesia indicated, and other medical conditions including cardiopulmonary disease, age, and smoking history. Patients with preoperative lower-respiratory tract infections constitute a greater operative risk, hence these patients often have their surgeries postponed until the infection has resolved. Patients with chronic cardiopulmonary diseases require a prolonged period of preoperative physical therapy in preparation for surgery. Elective surgery is not usually considered during an exacerbation of chronic lung disease. Even minor surgery may be potentially hazardous for the patient with previous lung disease. The adverse effects of total anesthesia on these patients are magnified because of their reduced pulmonary reserve capacity. Smoking should be discontinued for as long as possible before surgery. The patient is placed on an exercise conditioning program, a regimen of bronchial hygiene, oxygen if necessary, and prophylactic antibiotics. Even patients with extremely low functional work capacity can enhance the efficiency of the steps in the oxygen transport pathway (see Chapter 18) with a modified aerobic exercise conditioning program. This preoperative preparation may take one to several weeks, depending on the patient and the indications for surgery. Patients who are overweight can reduce their risk of perioperative complications by losing weight. Body mass is a major determinant of lung function, respiratory mechanics, and oxygenation during anesthesia (Pelosi et al, 1998), and adverse effects of these can lead to major surgical complications and recovery.

POSTOPERATIVE MANAGEMENT

Goals

The goals of postoperative physical therapy management related to oxygen transport appear in Box 30-4. The patient is mobilized in a systematic sequence that progresses from supine to turning in bed to sitting over the bed to standing to sitting in a chair to walking (Box 30-5). Some patients progress

BOX 30-4

Goals of Postoperative Physical Therapy Related to Oxygen Transport

Maximize arousal
Control anxiety and pain
Maximize alveolar volume
Optimize alveolar ventilation
Optimize perfusion
Maximize lung volumes and capacities, especially functional residual capacity
Minimize closing volume
Minimize intrapulmonary shunting
Optimize lung compliance
Optimize mucociliary transport
Optimize mucous clearance
Optimize ventilation and perfusion matching and gas exchange
Maximize expiratory flow rates
Maximize chest tube drainage
Optimize fluid balance systemically (renal function)
Optimize lung water balance and distribution
Promote optimal lymphatic draining
Minimize third spacing and collection of fluid
Minimize the risk of aspiration
Minimize undue work of breathing
Minimize undue work of the heart
Maximize chest wall mobility and movement in three planes
Optimize body and posture alignment when sitting, standing, walking, and recumbent
Optimize circulatory status and tissue perfusion
Optimize peripheral blood flow and velocity
Optimize muscle pump action
Minimize effects of central fluid shifts with recumbency
Maintain fluid-volume regulating mechanisms
Minimize pain nonpharmacologically and coordinate with the patient's pain medications as indicated
Maximize cardiopulmonary endurance
Optimize relaxation and sleep
Provide instruction to patient regarding between-treatment treatment

1. Maximize the patient's ability to perform activities of daily living.
2. Maintain or increase general muscle strength and endurance.
3. Maximize muscle and soft tissue length and ligament integrity.
4. Maintain normal arousal and neurological function.
5. Maintain skin integrity.
6. Maintain normal cognitive function to avoid disorientation and hospital-related psychoses.
7. Prescribe secondary prevention.

These goals are achieved with the prescription of mobility exercises including hip and knee flexion and extension exercises, and foot and ankle exercises. These exercises are performed hourly regardless of whether the patient is sitting in the chair or resting in bed.

Finally, there are important preventive goals (e.g., minimizing the effects of restricted mobility and recumbency on all organ systems) (see Chapters 18 and 19). Of particular concern in the surgical patient is the risk of thromboemboli and pulmonary emboli and the risk of pressure points and skin breakdown. Thus mobilization and regular activation of the muscle pumps to minimize circulatory stasis and frequent body-position changes are essential to reduce risks, which can have serious consequences for the patient's recovery. Compression stockings are often put on the patient after surgery. These are not removed, except for cleaning and redistributing pressure, until the patient is consistently up and about. These stockings facilitate venous return and increase blood flow and velocity, thereby minimizing the risk of thrombus formation. Should thrombus formation be suspected, it may be necessary to attach an intermittent compression device to the legs to simulate muscle pump action.

With the exception of patients undergoing thoracic or cardiovascular surgery, patients are usually extubated before leaving the operating room or recovery area. Provided no complications develop, most other patients do not require an airway. Patients undergoing major thoracic surgery or cardiovascular surgery remain intubated and mechanically ventilated from several hours to 24 hours after surgery to minimize the work of breathing and hence the work of the heart required to meet the metabolic demands of respiration. These patients are informed that artificial airway and mechanical ventilation enables them to breathe more efficiently initially. A patient is also informed that he or she will not be able to speak while the airway is in place and may have a sore throat after its removal.

Patients are usually aroused and repositioned before leaving the operating room, although this is seldom remembered by patients. Not recalling the immediate postoperative course is common. Patients are likely to be receiving some form of pharmacological analgesia (e.g., morphine). If blood was required intraoperatively, whole blood, packed cells, or plasma may still be infused in the immediate postoperative period or for a longer period of time. Saline or other solutions

through these steps quickly, while others take longer. The rate at which patients are progressed depends on their responses. Pain medications are coordinated as needed with treatments to maximize treatment efficacy. This progressive sequence is comparable to that of phase I of cardiac rehabilitation, the inpatient phase for surgical as well as medical patients, and includes education, counseling, and treatment as indicated. These goals are addressed between as well as during treatments. The patient is instructed in mobilization and body positioning coordinated with deep breathing and supported coughing maneuvers between treatment sessions, and these interventions should be performed hourly during waking hours (Bennett et al, 1990; Blomqvist & Stone, 1983; Bourn & Jenkins, 1992; Hasani et al, 1991; Hietpas et al, 1974; Orlava, 1959).

In addition to the primary treatment goals related to oxygen transport, other postoperative goals include the following.

BOX 30-5

Template for Progressing Mobilization in Surgical Patients

Level	Date	Activity	Bathroom	Bathing
1		Confined to bed Assessment Body positioning	Portable toilet when possible	Personal care by nurse May wash hands and feet
2		Sit up in chair for 20 minutes, 3 times per day	Use portable toilet	May wash in bed (not legs, back, or feet)
3		Sit up in chair as much as possible		Bathe at bedside
4			Walk to bathroom	Bathe at sink (sitting)
5		Walk around room as able		Bathe at sink
6		Short walks in hall 2 to 3 times per day		
7		Walk in halls as able		Take shower (sitting) or tub bath
8		Walk one flight of stairs with assistance		
9		Discharge		

Adapted from Makrides, L. (1997). Cardiac rehabilitation manual. Halifax, Canada: Cardiac Prevention Research Centre, Dalhousie University.

are also infused for regulation of fluid balance until the patient is able to drink and eat normally. Once vital signs have stabilized, wounds are stable and not draining, and the patient reasonably alert, the patient is transferred to the ward. The patient is retained in the recovery area should further monitoring be required. If complications develop and oxygen transport and gas exchange are threatened, the patient may be transferred to the intensive care unit.

The physical therapist may be consulted to assess and treat the patient as soon as he or she leaves the operating room or while in the recovery room. Most frequently the physical therapist sees the patient once he or she has been transferred to the ward and has been settled. The first 24 hours are critical.

The risk of cardiopulmonary complications is greatest during the perioperative period and diminishes as the patient becomes increasingly upright and mobile. Atelectasis and aspiration after extubation are significant risks for the patient who has been intubated. The goal immediately after extubation is to promote optimal alveolar ventilation, maximize lung volumes and capacities (especially FRC), minimize closing volumes, and maximize expiratory flow rates and hence cough effectiveness. Areas most susceptible to atelectasis are those that may have been physically compressed during surgery (e.g., the left lower lobe of the cardiovascular surgical patient and areas adjacent to a lobectomy or segmentectomy).

Surgery constitutes a significant insult to the body. After the trauma of surgery, anesthesia, sedation, fluid loss, incisions, and the significant energy requirements for healing and repair, patients can be expected to be lethargic and difficult to arouse. The relaxed state induced by anesthesia, sedation, and narcotics

increases the risk of aspiration. This risk is exacerbated further in some patients by nausea and vomiting associated with anesthesia and narcotics. Moving and positioning the patient upright whenever possible and interacting with the patient stimulates the reticular activating system making the patient more responsive and aroused. The increased metabolic demands that this requires, along with increased catecholamine release, helps overcome the residual effects of anesthesia, sedation, and muscle relaxants and their threat to oxygen transport, provided the demands are not beyond the capacity of the oxygen transport system to deliver oxygen.

Alternatively, some patients are restless and agitated after the effects of anesthesia have worn off. Hypoxemia can lead to restlessness and agitation. Thus it is important that these patients are not inappropriately sedated. This compounds their need for treatment while making them less able to cooperate with treatment simultaneously (Dripps & Waters, 1941; Ross & Dean, 1989).

At the outset of any treatment the patient must be aroused as much as possible to cooperate fully and derive the maximum benefit from treatment. The physical therapist interacts continuously with the patient to arouse the patient fully, maintain arousal, stimulate normal cognitive function and orientation, and elicit feedback from the patient to assess his or her response to treatment. Narcotics depress respiratory status and arousal, and these effects are accentuated in patients whose metabolic states have been disrupted with illness and in older persons. Thus the physical therapist must be vigilant in detecting untoward residual effects of narcotics in the surgical patient.

EARLY POSTOPERATIVE PHYSICAL THERAPY

Rationale

The role of perioperative physical therapy has been debated. Some argue that the nursing staff can assume responsibility for the prevention of postoperative complications, particularly in patients with minimally invasive and short surgeries. The assessment and goals of the physical therapist, however, are unique and are not duplicated by the medical or nursing staff or respiratory therapist.

Physical therapists identify threats to oxygen transport as well as its limitations and prevent and remediate these by prescribing noninvasive interventions. Further, the physical therapist considers multiple factors that threaten the long-term health and function of the patient after discharge. The physical therapist has a primary commitment to returning the patient to full participation in the community and prolonged, sustained health. A decision to institute physical therapy for a given patient is not based on the type of surgery alone. Rather it is determined through a systemic assessment of age, weight, fitness, smoking status, comorbidities, anxiety and stress, and external factors related to the patient's response to anesthesia and surgery.

To sustain alveolar inflation and normal FRC postoperatively, mobilization and body positioning coordinated with breathing control and supported coughing must be carried out frequently (i.e., every one to two hours) to maintain optimal alveolar volume and distribution of ventilation. Maximal inspiratory maneuvers are coordinated with mobilization and body positioning at least every hour as tolerated. Maximal inspiratory maneuvers alone, however, are unlikely to be effective because the inspiratory pressure may be insufficient to inflate atelectatic alveoli. Rather patent alveoli will tend to be overexpanded. Mobilization and body positioning will directly alter the intrapleural pressure gradient and thereby optimize alveolar expansion (Roussos et al, 1977). In patients who are obese and anesthetized and paralyzed, the prone position increases FRC, lung compliance, and oxygenation (Pelosi et al, 1996; Pelosi et al, 1998). Prone may have some role in some patient who are obese postoperatively, but the hazards of recumbent positions must be weighed against the benefits of being upright.

Normal passive expiratory efforts to end tidal volume are encouraged and maximal or forced expiratory efforts are usually avoided to prevent airway closure and potential increase of atelectasis (Hasani et al, 1991; Hietpas et al, 1974; Nunn et al, 1965). Huffing (glottis open) rather than coughing (glottis closed) also minimizes airway closure. With huffing there is less risk of bronchospasm than with coughing, in which the glottis is closed, transpulmonary pressure is increased, and a compressive phase is involved. If indicated, coughing maneuvers are most effective in the sitting or slightly leaned-forward position in which lung volumes and forced expiratory flow are maximized and the respiratory muscles are at a mechanical advantage with respect to the length-tension characteristics of the muscle fibers. Airway closure is position-

dependent (Chapter 19); therefore the degree of expiration encouraged by the physical therapist should be based on the patient's body position. Airway closure is potentiated in patients who are older, smoke, or are obese and in patients who are in horizontal as opposed to upright body positions.

Mobilization and body positioning coordinated with breathing control and supported coughing maneuvers offer the greatest benefit to oxygen transport in the postoperative patient. Specific benefits are described in Chapters 18 and 19. They include maximizing FRC, reducing closing volume, maximizing expiratory flow rates, promoting mucociliary transport, promoting airway clearance, optimizing lymphatic drainage, minimizing the effects of increased thoracic blood volume, maintaining fluid-volume regulating mechanisms, and minimizing the work of breathing and of the heart. Sustained maximal inspiration is one intervention that promotes alveolar expansion. Each deep breath is performed to maximal inspiration (i.e., to total lung capacity) with a three- to five-second breath hold. This maneuver may reduce pulmonary complications by promoting alveolar inflation and gas exchange. The patient is encouraged to repeat this maneuver several times hourly, and frequently during mobilization, and before, during, and after body-position changes.

Incentive spirometry may be useful in patients who are resistant or unable to cooperate fully with maximal inspiratory efforts (Figure 30-1). Postoperative hypoxemia may be reduced with this technique, which uses the principle of sustained inspiration using a feedback device (either flow or volume feedback) to achieve maximal inflating pressure in the alveoli and maximal inhaled volume. The incentive spirometer can be used independently by the patient. This technique ensures that each inspiration is physiologically optimal and is reproduced precisely from one inspiration to the next. Patients who are surgical risks can benefit from being taught how to use the incentive spirometer preoperatively by the physical therapist in order to promote better inflation of the lungs with incentive spirometry postoperatively. The patient continues with a regimen of breathing control and coughing maneuvers until full mobility and activities of daily living are resumed.

The application of intermittent positive pressure breathing (IPPB) appears to be less effective for the postoperative patient than previously believed. The details of this modality are described in Chapter 42.

Exercise testing echocardiography performed early after coronary bypass surgery can identify individuals who are high risk and would benefit from intensive secondary prevention as a particular focus in a cardiac rehabilitation program (Sellier et al, 2003). Early exercise training improves autonomic nervous system function in addition to aerobic and functional capacity (Takeyama et al, 2000).

Getting the Surgical Patient "Upright and Moving"

Mobilization in the upright position coordinated with breathing control and supported coughing maneuvers is encouraged immediately after the patient is first aroused after

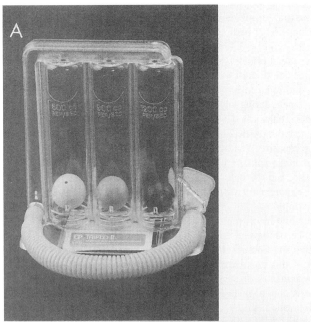

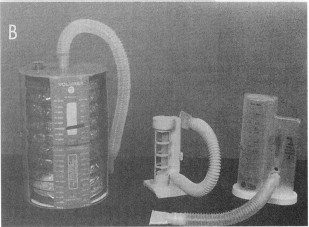

FIGURE 30-1 Incentive spirometers.

surgery, unless contraindicated, to help reverse and mitigate reduced arousal, atelectasis, FRC, and impaired mucociliary transport associated with surgery. Mobilization augments cardiopulmonary function (see Chapter 18), particularly when the patient is upright (Levine & Lown, 1952; Lewis, 1980). These beneficial effects are enhanced by improved three-dimensional chest wall motion, improved gut motility, and reduced intraabdominal pressure. Extremity movement during ambulation increases alveolar ventilation, enhances ventilation and perfusion matching by increasing zone two of the lungs, and optimizes diffusing capacity through stimulating dilatation and recruitment of alveolar capillaries. The upright position ensures that the spine is erect, upper body musculature is relaxed, and the chest wall is symmetrical. Slouching and leaning, particularly to the affected side, reduces alveolar ventilation and contributes to uneven distribution of ventilation and areas of atelectasis (Bake et al, 1976; Don et al, 1971;

Glaister, 1967). In addition, if this abnormal posture is maintained, mucociliary transport of the area is impaired and mucus collects and stagnates, increasing the risk of bacterial colonization and infection. Symmetrical posture is monitored at all times (i.e., during ambulation, sitting at bedside, bed mobility exercises, sitting up in bed, and lying in bed). Slouching and favoring the affected side will lead to cardiopulmonary complications and possibly musculoskeletal complications in the short and long term.

Mobilization and active exercise in upright postures whenever possible are prescribed based on the need to enhance multiple steps in the oxygen transport pathway (Dean & Ross, 1992; Ray et al, 1974). The priority is to perform as much activity as possible out of bed and upright (i.e., ambulation, transferring, sitting upright in a chair, and chair exercises with or without hand weights or exercise bands). When in bed, similar devices can be used, including a monkey bar to facilitate moving in bed for patients other than cardiovascular thoracic patients (e.g., the orthopedic patient with extremity fractures and traction). In addition, the use of the monkey bar is beneficial to perform repetitive bouts of exercises that maintain upper-extremity strength and some general endurance capacity, relieve pressure and stiffness, and facilitate frequent turning. Cycle pedals can be adapted to chairs for recumbent exercise in bed, if necessary. Patients whose positioning is restricted with fixation and traction devices require hand, wrist, or ankle weights, and possibly pulleys and other devices, to maintain muscle strength and power. Movements performed with moderately heavy weights for multiple sets (e.g., three sets of 10 repetitions) develop muscle strength. Movements performed with lighter weight for multiple sets (e.g., five to 10 sets of 10 repetitions) tend to develop endurance and aerobic capacity. Because of the restrictions imposed by these devices, maintaining joint range is essential (i.e., of the neck, spinal column, and chest wall, as well as the extremities). The rotation component of joint movement is readily compromised, thus this must be an integral component of joint range of motion exercises. Proprioceptive neuromuscular facilitation (PNF) movements of the extremities can be beneficial. PNF movements of the chest wall can be coordinated with breathing control and supported coughing maneuvers. Upper body and trunk mobility and strengthening are important goals, particularly in the patient with chest wall incisions. The prescription is progressed gradually in the patient with a chest wall incision, particularly in the patient with a median sternotomy who is usually restricted to unresisted, upper-extremity mobility exercises in the first several weeks.

Prescription of body positioning is essential in the management of the patient postsurgically for two reasons. First, without direction, the patient will tend to assume a deleterious body position (i.e., maintaining a restricted number of body positions that favor the affected side for prolonged periods of time with minimal movement and "stirring up"). Thus once the effects of mobilization have been exploited in a given treatment session, body positions are prescribed for "between-treatment" times that continue to enhance oxygen transport for a given patient and discourage excessive time in deleterious body positions. When not ambulating, patients are encouraged to assume a wide range of body positions (e.g., semi-prone) between treatments, as frequently as possible, (i.e., at least every one to two hours) (Dean, 1985; Douglas et al, 1977; Piehl & Brown, 1976; Remolina et al, 1981; Ross & Dean, 1992; Zack et al, 1974).

THORACIC AND CARDIOVASCULAR SURGERY

Thoracic Surgery

Thoracic surgery refers to surgery that necessitates opening the chest wall. By convention this term excludes specialized cardiovascular surgery (i.e., surgery of the heart and great vessels). Thoracic surgery is commonly performed for lung resections secondary to cancer (e.g., pneumonectomy, lobectomy, segmentectomy, and wedge resection). In addition, thoracic surgery is performed to remove an irreversibly damaged area of lung tissue secondary to bronchiectasis, benign tumors, fungal infections, and tuberculosis.

The most common incisions are posterolateral thoracotomy and median sternotomy. The posterolateral thoracotomy procedure requires the patient to assume the side-lying position with the involved side uppermost for the duration of the surgery. The uppermost arm is fully flexed anteriorly. The incision is made through an intercostal space, corresponding to the location of the lesion to be excised. The muscles incised include latissimus dorsi, serratus anterior, external and internal intercostals laterally, and trapezius and rhomboid posteriorly.

At the conclusion of the surgery, chest tubes are placed to evacuate air and fluid from the pleural space by means of an underwater chest tube drainage system. The chest tube and drainage system resolve the pneumothorax created by reestablishing negative pressure in the pleural space and help to reinflate the remaining atelectatic lung tissue. After thoracic surgery, two chest tubes are usually inserted, one at the apex of the lung to evacuate air and one at the base of the lung to drain serosanguinous fluid. The therapist should become familiar with the various drainage systems, how drainage can be facilitated with mobilization and body positioning coordinated with breathing control and supported coughing maneuvers, and certain precautions that must be observed to avoid impairing drainage or disconnecting the tubing.

Provided the chest tubes are not kinked, there is no contraindication to lying on the side of the chest tubes. Lying on this side, which is usually the side of the surgery and incision, is typically avoided by the patient. Consistent with the adage *down with the good lung*, a patient prefers to lie on the nonsurgical side. Prolonged periods in any position, however, particularly lying on the unaffected side, places these lung fields at risk. To minimize the risk of positional complications and hypoxemia, the patient is encouraged to turn to both sides (Leaver et al, 1994; Seaton et al, 1979;

Sutton et al, 1982). The specific positions and the duration of time spent within each, however, are based on a comprehensive assessment of the patient's condition and the indications and contraindications for each body position.

Patients may appear to splint themselves, thereby restricting chest wall motion, to avoid pain when moving and deep breathing. They also may resist maximal inspiratory efforts when coughing. Although pain likely contributes to breathing at low lung volumes and ineffective coughing, phrenic nerve inhibition in patients with thoracic and upper abdominal surgeries is likely a more important factor restricting lung expansion (Ford & Guenter, 1984).

Postoperative complaints of pain are both musculoskeletal and pleural in origin. The large number of muscles incised, particularly in the posterolateral thoracotomy incision, combined with the operative position, contributes to the patient's complaints of chest wall pain, shoulder soreness, and restricted movement. Deep breathing and coughing maneuvers may be associated with considerable discomfort after surgery. Pain is accentuated by apprehension and anxiety. Therefore treatments are coordinated with relaxation, noninvasive pain control modalities, and pain medication schedules to elicit the full cooperation of the patient.

Cardiovascular Surgery

Cardiovascular surgery is specialized thoracic surgery involving the heart and great vessels. Because the flow of blood through the cardiopulmonary system is interrupted, the patient is placed on a cardiopulmonary bypass machine or on a machine called an extracorporeal membrane oxygenator. Cardiovascular surgery is most commonly performed for coronary artery bypass grafting, valve replacements, and aneurysm repairs. Because patients acquire an oxygen debt during the bypass procedure, high oxygen demands are required postsurgically (Utoh et al, 1999).

After bypass surgery, patients in whom the saphenous vein is excised for graft material have the added complication of surgery and wound healing in one leg. Mobility exercises on that leg are often restricted until there is no risk of bleeding or interference with healing. Comparable with the thoracic surgical patient, a cardiovascular patient leaves the operating room with various monitoring lines and leads, intravenous fluid infusions, possible blood or plasma infusions, a Swan-Ganz catheter (see Chapter 16), a central venous pressure line, an arterial line, a Foley catheter, and oxygen cannulae.

The preoperative preparation and teaching and the postoperative physical therapy management is intensive. Because of the invasiveness of cardiovascular surgery, patients are usually treated postoperatively in a specialized intensive care unit (see Chapter 33). The preoperative and postoperative physical therapy management of patients in the intensive care unit is a specialized area and is described in Chapter 35. Providing the patient with information about what to expect during the perioperative course relieves fear and anxiety. In addition, relaxation procedures can be useful. Patients must be reassured that their incisions and suture lines will not be disrupted with movement and physical therapy and that supported coughing and supporting themselves when moving will maximize comfort. Until the patient has stabilized, the patient's mobility is restricted to low-intensity mobilization to promote its benefits on gas exchange and reduce metabolic demands and body positioning to optimize alveolar ventilation coordinated with deep breathing and supported coughing maneuvers. Conventional airway clearance interventions (e.g., postural drainage and manual techniques) may be prescribed in the presence of excessive secretions, difficulty in mobilizing secretions, and in the event of productive hydrostatic pneumonia.

Patients undergoing cardiovascular surgery are transferred from the cardiovascular intensive care unit to the ward as quickly as possible. From the ward, these patients should be referred to a physical therapist and a cardiac rehabilitation program in the community for continuity of care and to maximize the functional gains resulting from the surgery. Exercise is prescribed progressively to maximize oxygen transport at each step of the rehabilitation period (i.e., acute, before and immediately after discharge, and long-term). The conditioning effects of exercise enable the patient to resume various activities of daily living commensurate with an increasing oxygen transport system capacity. Activities involving straining and isometric contractions are avoided. Weight lifting may be introduced in a long-term rehabilitation program, but the weights are not sufficient to cause strain. Patients with median sternotomy incisions are usually prohibited from using their arms to support themselves when sitting or driving and during activities that may strain the incision site for several weeks or more.

SUMMARY

Optimal surgical outcome is a team effort that extends beyond the technical success of the surgery. It is based on the return of the individual to full participation in life and long-term health, including no recurrence of the patient's problem and reduced need for biomedical care and drugs in the short- and long-term; these also being primary physical therapy outcomes. This chapter reviews the principles of perioperative physical therapy management in individuals slated for surgery with a view to maximize both short- and long-term outcomes. The physical therapy has a key role in risk factor identification and early intervention. Although risk is increased with more invasive and prolonged surgeries, this should not be assumed. Even minor surgery with an apparently uneventful immediate post-operative period can have an untoward outcome because of underlying risk factors. Thus indication for physical therapy is based on risk factors rather than condition or type of surgery.

Teamwork is the essence of successful surgical outcomes. The physical therapist is highly involved from assessment of the patient preoperatively with respect to anticipated necessity of treatment afterwards based on a detailed assessment of perioperative risks, to treatment postoperatively, to, most importantly, postdischarge follow-up to ensure function is regained and the benefits of surgical and related management are sustained over the long-term. Physical therapy intervention for the surgical patient is based on indications for that individual rather than the type of surgery.

The four categories of factors contributing to or threatening oxygen transport were described in Chapter 16 and are evaluated in the preoperative and postoperative assessments. These factors include pathology, restricted mobility and recumbency, extrinsic factors related to the patient's care, and intrinsic factors related to the patient. This chapter examines in detail those factors related to surgery and anesthesia in particular, and the impact of underlying disease, restricted mobility, recumbency and intrinsic factors on the effects of surgery and anesthesia. The role of the physical therapist, an integral member of the surgical team, is to ensure optimal long-term outcomes well beyond the technical success of the surgery, particularly in individuals who have undergone cardiovascular and thoracic surgery. A prime physical therapy outcome of surgery in patients who have undergone thoracic or cardiovascular surgery is prevention of both recurrence of the patient's problem and repeated surgery.

Surgery and its physiological effects are described. Special reference is made to two specialized types of surgery that have the greatest impact on cardiopulmonary function, namely, thoracic and cardiovascular surgery.

Review Questions

1. Describe what in meant by "surgical outcome is a team effort."
2. Why is it that the decision for the physical therapist to treat a patient postoperatively cannot be made based on the type of surgery alone?
3. Describe the physiological effects of surgery including the specific surgical procedure; the type, depth, and duration of anesthesia; sedation; types of respiratory support; static body position assumed during surgery; length of surgery; number and type of invasive perioperative procedures; and incisions.
4. Describe surgical risk factors. Why are detection of these of primary importance in the physical therapy assessment and management of the surgical patient?
5. Relate cardiopulmonary physical therapy management and treatment interventions to the underlying pathophysiology associated with surgery and those factors listed in Question 3, and provide the rationale for your choice.
6. Differentiate the role of the physical therapist on the surgical team from the role of the medical/surgical staff and the nursing staff.
7. Describe the role of physical therapy follow-up in the management of the patient who has had surgery.

REFERENCES

Alexander, J.L., Spence, A.A., Parikh, R.K., & Stuart, B. (1973). The role of airway closure in postoperative hypoxaemia. British Journal of Anaesthesiology 59:1070-1079.

Bake, B., Dempsey, J., & Grimby, G. (1976). Effects of shape changes of the chest wall on distribution of inspired gas. American Review of Respiratory Disease 114:1113-1120.

Behrakis, P.K., Baydur, A., Jaeger, M.J., & Milic-Emili, J. (1983). Lung mechanics in sitting and horizontal body positions. Chest 83:643-646.

Bennett, W.D., Foster, W.M., & Chapman, W.F. (1990). Cough-enhanced mucus clearance in the normal lung. Journal of Applied Physiology 69:1670-1675.

Blomqvist, C.G., & Stone, H.L. (1983). Cardiovascular adjustments to gravitational stress. Handbook of physiology, ed 2. Washington, DC: American Physiological Society.

Bourn, J., & Jenkins, S. (1992). Post-operative respiratory physiotherapy: indications for treatment. Physiotherapy 78:80-85.

Daly, M.P. (1989). The medical evaluation of the elderly preoperative patient. Primary Care 16:361-376.

Dean, E. (1985). Effect of body position on pulmonary function. Physical Therapy 65:613-618.

Dean, E., & Ross, J. (1989). Integrating current literature in the management of cystic fibrosis: a rejoinder. Physiotherapy Canada 41:46-47.

Dean, E., & Ross, J. (1992). Mobilization and exercise conditioning. In Zadai, C.C. (Ed). Pulmonary management in physical therapy. New York: Churchill Livingstone.

Don, H.F., Craig, D.B., Wahba, W.M., & Couture, J.G. (1971). The measurement of gas trapped in the lungs at functional residual capacity and the effects of posture. Anesthesiology 35:582-590.

Douglas, W.W., Rehder, K., Beynen, F.M., Sessler, A.D., & Marsh, H.M. (1977). Improved oxygenation in patients with acute respiratory failure: the prone position. American Review of Respiratory Disease 115:559-566.

Dripps, R.D., & Waters, R.M. (1941). Nursing care of the surgical patient. 1. The "stir-up." American Journal of Nursing 41:530-534.

Dull, J.L., & Dull, W.L. (1983). Are maximal inspiratory breathing exercises or incentive spirometry better than early mobilization after cardiopulmonary bypass surgery? Physical Therapy 63: 655-659.

Dureuil, B., Viires, N., & Cantineau, J.P. (1986). Diaphragmatic contractility after upper abdominal surgery. Journal of Applied Physiology 61:1775-1780.

Ford, G.T., & Guenter, C.A. (1984). Toward prevention of postoperative complications. American Review of Respiratory Diseases 130:4-5.

Froese, A.B., & Bryan, A.C. (1974). Effects of anesthesia and paralysis on diaphragmatic mechanics in man. Anesthesiology 41:242-255.

Gilman, A.G., Goodman, L.S., & Gilman, A. (1990). Goodman and Gilman's the pharmacological basis of therapeutics, ed 8. New York: Macmillan Publishing.

Glaister, D.H. (1967). The effect of posture on the distribution of ventilation and blood flow in the normal lung. Clinical Science 33:391-398.

Hasani, A., Pavia, D., Agnew, J.E., & Clarke, S.W. (1991). The effect of unproductive coughing/FET on regional mucus movement in the human lungs. Respiratory Medicine 85:23-26.

Hashimoto, J., Suzuki, T., Nakahara, T., Kosuda, S., & Kubo, A. (2003). Preoperative risk stratification using stress myocardial perfusion scintigrapy with electrocardiographic gating. Journal of Nuclear Medicine 44:385-390.

Hedenstierna, G., Standberg, A., Brismar, B., Lundquist, H., Svenson, L., & Tokics, L. (1985). Functional residual capacity, thoracoabdominal dimensions and central blood volume during general anesthesia with muscle paralysis and mechanical ventilation. Anesthesiology 62:247-254.

Hedenstierna, G., Tokics, L., Strandberg, A., Lundquist, H., & Brismar, B. (1986). Correlation of gas exchange impairment to development of atelectasis during anesthesia and muscle paralysis. Acta Anaesthesiologica Scandinavica 30:183-191.

Hietpas, B.G., Roth, R.D., & Jensen, W.M. (1974). Huff coughing and airway patency. Respiratory Care 24:710.

Kertai, M.D., Poldermans, D., Bax, J.J, Klein, J., & Van Urk, H. (2003). Cardiac risk and perioperative management. Journal of Cardiovascular Surgery 44:431-435.

Leaver, H., Conway, J.H., & Holgate, S.T. (1994). The incidence of post-operative hypoxaemia following lobectomy and pneumonectomy: a pilot study. Physiotherapy 80:521-527.

Levine, R.D. (1984). Anesthesiology. A manual for medical students. Philadelphia: JB Lippincott.

Levine, S.A., & Lown, B. (1952). 'Armchair' treatment of acute coronary thrombosis. Journal of the American Medical Association 148:1365-1369.

Lewis, F.R. (1980). Management of atelectasis and pneumonia. Surgical Clinics of North America 60:1391-1401.

Lugo, G., Arizpe, D., Dominguez, G., Ramirez, M., & Tamariz, O. (1993). Relationship between oxygen consumption and oxygen delivery during anesthesia in high-risk surgical patients. Critical Care Medicine 21:64-69.

Makrides, L. (1997). Cardiac rehabilitation manual. Halifax, Canada: Cardiac Prevention Research Centre, Dalhousie University.

Malamed, S.F. (2002). Sedation. A guide to patient management, ed 4. Philadelphia: Elsevier.

Muller, N., Volgyesi, G., Becker, L., Bryan, M.H., & Bryan, A. C. (1979). Diaphragmatic muscle tone. Journal of Applied Physiology 47:279-284.

Nunn, J.F. (1989).The influence of anesthesia on the respiratory system. In Reinhart, K. & Eyrich, K. (Eds). Clinical aspect of O_2 transport and tissue oxygenation. New York: Springer-Verlag.

Nunn, J.F., Coleman, A.J., Sachithanandan, T., Bergman, N.A., & Laws, J.W. (1965). Hypoxaemia and atelectasis produced by forced expiration. British Journal of Anaesthesia 37:3-12.

Orlava, O.E. (1959). Therapeutic physical culture in the complex treatment of pneumonia. Physical Therapy Review 39:153-160.

Pelosi, P., Croci, M., Calappi, E., Mulazzi, D., Cerisara, M., Vercesi, P., Vicardi, P., & Gattinoni, L. (1996). Prone positioning improves pulmonary function in obese patients during general anesthesia. Anesthesia and Analgesia 83:578-583.

Pelosi, P., Croci, M., Ravagnan, I., Tredici, S., Pedoto, A., Lissoni, A., & Gattinoni, L. (1998). The effects of body mass on lung volumes, respiratory mechanics, and gas exchange, during general anesthesia. Anesthesia and Analgesia 87:654-660.

Piehl, M.A., & Brown, R.S. (1976). Use of extreme position changes in acute respiratory failure. Critical Care Medicine 4:13-14.

Polonen, P., Hippelainen, M., Takala, R., Ruokonen, E., & Takala, J. (1997). Relationship between intra- and postoperative oxygen transport and prolonged intensive care after cardiac surgery: a prospective study. Acta Anaesthesiologica Scandinavica 41:810-817.

Ray, R. F., Yost, L., Moallem, S., Sanoudos, G.M., Villamena, P., & Paredes, R.M. (1974). Immobility, hypoxemia, and pulmonary arteriovenous shunting. Archives of Surgery 109:537-541.

Remolina, C., Khan, A.U., Santiago, T.V., & Edelman, N.H. (1981). Positional hypoxemia in unilateral lung disease. New England Journal of Medicine 304:523-525.

Ross, J., & Dean, E. (1989). Integrating physiological principles into the comprehensive management of cardiopulmonary dysfunction. Physical Therapy 69:255-259.

Ross, J., & Dean, E. (1992). Body positioning. In Zadai, C.C. (Ed). Pulmonary management in physical therapy. New York: Churchill Livingstone.

Roussos, C.S., Fixley, M., Geriest, J., Cosio, M., Kelly, S., Martin, R.R., & Engel, L.A. (1977). Voluntary factors influencing the distribution of inspired gas. American Review of Respiratory Disease 116:457-467.

Seaton, D., Lapp, N.I., & Morgan, W.K.C. (1979). Effect of body position on gas exchange after thoracotomy. Thorax 34:518-522.

Sellier, P., Chatellier, G., D'Agrosa-Boiteux, M.C., Douard, H., Dubois, C., Goepfert, P.C., Monpere, C., & Saint Pierre, A. (2003). Use of non-invasive cardiac investigations to predict clinical endpoints after coronary artery bypass surgery in coronary artery disease patients: results from the prognosis and evaluation of risk in the coronary operated patient (PERISCOP) study. European Heart Journal 24:916-926.

Shoemaker, W.C., Appel, P.L., & Kram, H.B. (1993). Hemodynamic and oxygen transport responses in survivors and nonsurvivors of high-risk surgery. Critical Care Medicine 21:977-990.

Sprung, J., Whalley, D.G., Falcone, T., Wilks, W., Navratil, J.E., & Bourke, D.L. (2003). The effects of tidal volume and respiratory rate on oxygenation and respiratory mechanics during laparoscopy in morbidly obese patients. Anesthesia and Analgesia 97:268-274.

Sutton, P.P., Pavia, D., Bateman, J.R.M., & Clarke, S.W. (1982). Chest physiotherapy-a review. European Journal of Respiratory Disease 63:188-201.

Takeyama, J., Itoh, H., Kato, M., Koike, A., Aoki, K., Fu, L.T., Watanabe, H., Nagayama, M., & Katagiri, T. (2000). Effects of physical training on the recovery of the autonomic nervous activity during exercise after coronary artery bypass grafting: effects of physical training after CABG. Japan Circulation 64:809-813.

Toomasian, J.M., Peters, W.S., Siegel, L.C., & Stevens, J.H. (1997). Extracorporeal circulation for post-access cardiac surgery. Perfusion 12:83-91.

Utoh, J., Moriyama, S., Okamoto, K., Kunitomo, R., Hara, M., & Kitamura, N. (1999). The effects of cardiopulmonary bypass on postoperative oxygen metabolism. Surgery Today 29:28-33.

Weinstein, C.S., Woodard, W.J., & DeSilva, R.A. (1998). Late neurocognitive changes from neurological damage following coronary bypass surgery. Behavior Medicine 24:131-137.

World Health Organization. International Classification of Functioning, Disability and Health. (2002). www.sustainable-design.ie/arch/ICIDH-2PFDec-2000.pdf. Accessed December 2004.

Zack, M.B., Pontoppidan, H., & Kazemi, H. (1974). The effect of lateral positions on gas exchange in pulmonary disease. American Review of Respiratory Disease 110:149-153.

Guidelines for the Delivery of Cardiovascular and Pulmonary Physical Therapy

Chronic Conditions

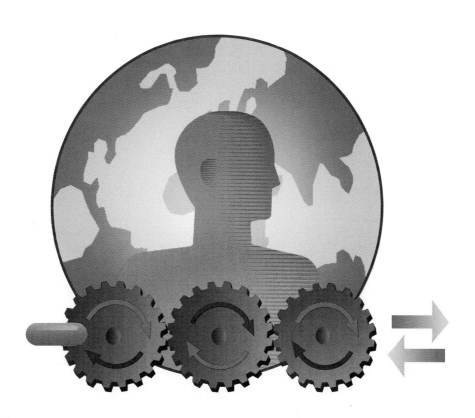

C H A P T E R 3 1

Individuals with Chronic Primary Cardiopulmonary Dysfunction

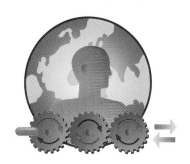

Elizabeth Dean and Donna Frownfelter

KEY TERMS

Angina
Asthma
Bronchiectasis
Chronic airflow limitation
Cystic fibrosis
Diabetes

Interstitial pulmonary fibrosis
Lung cancer
Myocardial infarction
Peripheral vascular disease
Valvular heart disease

The purpose of this chapter is to review the pathophysiology and medical management in relation to the comprehensive physical therapy management of individuals with chronic, *primary* cardiopulmonary pathology. Exercise testing and training is a major component of the comprehensive physical therapy management of individuals with chronic, primary cardiopulmonary conditions, and this topic is presented in detail separately in Chapter 24.

Because the heart and lungs are interdependent and function as a single unit, primary lung or heart disease must be considered with respect to the other organ and in the context of oxygen transport overall (Dantzker, 1983; Ross & Dean, 1989; Wasserman & Whipp, 1975). Despite a plethora of research and numerous official position statements and clinical practice guidelines, the definition and diagnoses of chronic heart disease and chronic lung disease and their management remain inconsistent in practice (Pierson, 2004). Although there is consensus regarding the efficacy of both cardiac and pulmonary rehabilitation (Ferguson, 2000), this inconsistent practice is associated with the under-use, overuse, and misuse of therapies regardless of their proven efficacy.

Although there is no clear line between obstructive and restrictive patterns of lung disease, the distinction is based on

the primary underlying pathophysiological problems. The primary conditions that are discussed include obstructive lung disease (i.e., chronic airflow limitation, asthma, bronchiectasis, and cystic fibrosis) and restrictive lung disease (i.e., interstitial pulmonary fibrosis). Lung cancer, which has the characteristics of both obstructive and restrictive patterns of pathology, is also presented.

The long-term cardiopulmonary management of people with heart disease is then presented with special attention to angina, myocardial infarction, and heart valve disease. Chronic vascular diseases including peripheral vascular disease, hypertension, and diabetes are also presented.

The principles of management of people with various chronic, primary cardiopulmonary conditions are presented rather than treatment prescriptions, which cannot be discussed without consideration of a specific patient. In this context, the general goals of the long-term management of people with each condition are presented, followed by the essential monitoring required, and the primary interventions for maximizing cardiopulmonary function and oxygen transport. The selection of interventions for any given patient is based on the physiological hierarchy. The most physiological interventions are exploited first followed by less physiological

---

BOX 31-1

Template of Principles of Comprehensive Physical Therapy Management for Chronic *Primary* Cardiopulmonary Dysfunction

Participation

Life participation (capacity to fulfill life's roles)
Empowerment and self-efficacy

Activities

Self care
Ambulation
Home management
Employment
Vocational activities

Structure and Function

Impairments of structure and function of oxygen transport and related factors (see Chapter 2)

Goals

Prevention

Preserve oxygen transport function and prevent threat to this system
Assess *readiness to change* health behavior

Short-term goals

Identify and treat limitations of structure and function of the oxygen transport system (associated with the greatest risk of future morbidity and mortality)
Identify other factors that impair participation and activity (see Chapters 1 and 17)

Long-term goals

Develop a lifelong health plan
Achieve *maintenance* stage of *readiness to change* (see Chapter 1)
Plan for follow-up

---

interventions and those whose efficacy is less well documented (see Chapter 17).

The principles outlined in this chapter also apply to the individual who has a secondary diagnosis of one or more chronic, primary cardiopulmonary conditions. These principles can be used to modify physical therapy management prescribed for some other condition or indicate the need for special monitoring.

A template of care is shown in Box 31-1. Although there are many commonalities of physical therapy management across patients, only a detailed knowledge of each specific patient, in terms of his or her underlying pathologies and other factors, will lead to the optimal management plan and treatment prescriptions.

INDIVIDUALS WITH PRIMARY PULMONARY DISEASE: OBSTRUCTIVE PATTERNS

Individuals with Chronic Airflow Limitation

Chronic airflow limitation is a descriptive term that refers to those disorders that previously have been termed chronic obstructive pulmonary disease (COPD) (e.g., chronic bronchitis, emphysema, bronchiectasis, and cystic fibrosis). Although there may be a reversible component, airflow obstruction associated with these disorders is largely irreversible. The pathophysiology of these conditions is reviewed in Chapter 5, and special considerations with respect to exercise testing and training are detailed in Chapter 24.

Bates (1989) described the syndrome of chronic airflow limitation as being caused by four external factors, mediated by four primary tissue responses, and modified by four physiological responses. The principal external causative factors include inhaled irritants, allergens, infections, and climate. The four principal tissue responses include large and small airway changes, airway hyperreactivity, bronchiolar damage, and alveolar destruction. The principal physiological responses include a reversible increased airway reactivity component, pulmonary vascular response to alveolar hypoventilation, control of breathing response to ventilation-perfusion imbalance and hypoxemia, and tissue defenses against elastase. Decline in pulmonary function and rate of development of the syndrome depend on the combination of causative factors and individual responses.

Management of chronic lung disease should be an integrated and comprehensive program that depends on team work, good communication, an approach focused on the individual, and his or her adherence to health recommendations (Pierson, 2004). Because of the primary contribution of lifestyle to most cases of heart and lung conditions, there is a long but variable latency before clinical signs and symptoms manifest (ACC/AHA 2002). Thus advocating healthy lifestyles and working with each individual to embrace such a lifestyle as health insurance will ultimately reduce the burden of the diseases of civilization.

Individuals with Chronic Bronchitis

Pathophysiology and Medical Management

Chronic bronchitis is usually associated with a history of smoking and is defined as mucous hypersecretion and cough producing sputum for three months or more over a two-year period (Murray & Nadel, 2000). Over the first few years of smoking, reversible airway changes occur. Over 10 to 15 years of smoking, mucous hypersecretion and chronic bronchitis become apparent. After 25 to 35 years of smoking, irreversible airway damage and chronic disability occur. Smoking is the major cause of emphysema and lung cancer.

The patient with chronic bronchitis is prone to infection and repeated periods of morbidity. Deterioration of aerobic capacity and functional capacity is related to the severity of the condition. Nutrition and hydration may be impaired particularly in severe cases because of neglect and the excessive energy cost of activities of daily living. Sleep may be irregular, thus the patient's symptoms are worsened (e.g., reduced endurance, fatigue, and lethargy) because of lack of normal physiological restoration from sleep.

The natural history of chronic bronchitis related to smoking includes mucous hypersecretion, reduction in forced expiratory volume in one second (FEV1), and increased heterogeneity of the distributions of ventilation, perfusion, ventilation perfusion matching, and diffusion (West, 2003). General debility and deconditioning ensue.

Smoking contributes to increased mucous production in the small airways, increased mucus in the large airways, respiratory bronchiolitis, reduced elastic recoil, increased airway reactivity, and vascular changes (Bates, 1989). These changes lead to nonuniformity of time constants in the lung, with consequent inhomogeneous distribution of inspired gas and premature small airway closure, and to nonuniformity of ventilation, perfusion, and diffusion distributions. Although variable among smokers, pulmonary function changes generally correspond to the amount smoked and duration of smoking history. Over time the pulmonary function profile becomes increasingly consistent with chronic airflow limitation (i.e., reduced FEV_1 and reduced FEV_1/forced vital capacity); however, these are late indicators of pulmonary changes. Signs of uneven distribution of ventilation and increased closing volumes, indicative of small airway involvement, are early pulmonary function changes in smokers. Exercise diffusing capacity is reduced, which explains in part the reduced maximal volume of oxygen utilization of smokers. Dynamic compliance with breathing frequency is also reduced. Residual volume is increased as a percent of total lung capacity (TLC). Tracheal mucous velocity is reduced and secretion clearance is impaired. Any patient with a smoking history, regardless of a diagnosis, has some degree of chronic airflow limitation, which must be considered when these patients receive medical or surgical care, as well as physical therapy.

The cardiac manifestations of chronic bronchitis stem from airway obstruction, secretion accumulation and reduced capacity to expectorate effectively, polycythemia, low arterial oxygen tension, and cardiopulmonary deconditioning. Increased airway resistance secondary to obstruction increases oxygen demand and hence the work of breathing. This increased demand is superimposed on an oxygen transport system that is already compromised. The cardiovascular system attempts to compensate for chronically reduced arterial oxygen tension by increasing cardiac output (i.e., stroke volume and heart rate). As blood gases deteriorate, the production of red blood cells increases (i.e., polycythemia) to enhance the oxygen-carrying capacity of the blood. Polycythemia increases the viscosity of the blood, however, and in turn, the work of the heart to pump blood to the pulmonary and systemic circulations. Furthermore, viscous blood is prone to circulatory stasis and clotting.

Low arterial oxygen tension leads to hypoxic pulmonary vasoconstriction and increased pulmonary vascular resistance (i.e., pulmonary hypertension). This also increases the work of the right heart in terms of ejecting blood to the lungs. Chronic overwork of the right ventricle leads to hypertrophy, insufficiency, and eventual failure of the right heart (cor pulmonale). Chronically reduced arterial oxygen can increase the demand on the left heart to maintain cardiac output. Similar to right-sided failure, the left heart may become hypertrophied, and over time, may fail.

The significantly increased intrathoracic pressures generated during chronic coughing reduce venous return, cardiac output, and coronary perfusion and increase blood pressure. These effects exert additional myocardial strain, lead to arterial desaturation, and increase the potential for cardiac dysrhythmias.

The complications of chronic bronchitis are exacerbated by cardiopulmonary deconditioning. Despite the pathology, the efficiency of oxygen transport along the steps in the pathway is suboptimal. This reduced efficiency increases the oxygen demands of the patient overall, who is unable to adequately supply oxygen.

Pharmacological support in the long-term management of chronic bronchitis includes bronchodilators (e.g., oral, metered-dose inhalant, inhaled powdered, or aerosol), corticosteroids (e.g., oral or inhaled), expectorants, antibiotics, inotropic agents (e.g., digitalis), beta-blockers, antidysrhythmic agents, and diuretics. Patients with chronic lung disease must be monitored closely during exercise because of the potential cardiac effects of disease and medications (e.g., beta-blocker agents attenuate the normal hemodynamic responses to exercise and bronchodilators, such as ventolin, elicit tachycardia).

Principles of Physical Therapy Management

Based on a comprehensive patient assessment, the goals of long-term management for the patient with chronic bronchitis may include the following.

- Maximize the patient's quality of life, general health, and well-being through maximizing his or her physiological reserve capacity
- Risk factor assessment
- Educate the patient about chronic bronchitis, self-management, effects of smoking, nutrition, weight control, smoking reduction or cessation, stress management, and other lifestyle factors, medications, infection control, and role of a long-term rehabilitation program
- Facilitate mucociliary transport
- Optimize secretion clearance
- Optimize alveolar ventilation
- Optimize lung volumes and capacities and flow rates
- Optimize ventilation and perfusion matching and gas exchange
- Reduce the work of breathing
- Reduce the work of the heart
- Maximize aerobic capacity and efficiency of oxygen transport
- Optimize physical endurance and exercise capacity
- Optimize general muscle strength and thereby peripheral oxygen extraction

• Design comprehensive lifelong health and rehabilitation programs with the patient

Patient monitoring includes dyspnea, respiratory distress, breathing pattern (depth and frequency), arterial saturation, cyanosis (delayed sign of desaturation), heart rate, blood pressure, and rate pressure product. Patients with cardiac dysfunction or low arterial oxygen tensions require electrocardiogram (ECG) monitoring, particularly during exercise. If supplemental oxygen is used, the fraction of inspired oxygen (FiO_2) administered is recorded. Subjectively, breathlessness is assessed using a modified version of the Borg scale of perceived exertion.

Medication that is needed to maximize treatment response is administered before treatment (e.g., bronchodilators). Knowledge of the type of medication, its administration route, and time to and duration of peak efficacy is essential if treatment is to be maximally efficacious.

The primary interventions for maximizing cardiopulmonary function and oxygen transport in patients with chronic bronchitis include some combination of education, aerobic exercises, strengthening exercises, chest wall mobility exercises, range of motion, body positioning, breathing control and coughing maneuvers, airway clearance interventions, relaxation, activity pacing, and energy conservation. An ergonomic assessment of the patient's work and home environments may be indicated to minimize oxygen demand and energy expenditure in these settings.

The use of supplemental oxygen depends on the severity of the disease. Some patients have no need for supplemental oxygen, some need it only during exercise, and some patients require continuous oxygen with proportionately more delivered during activity and exercise compared with rest. Supplemental oxygen is not usually required until lung damage becomes extreme (i.e., the morphological changes are consistent with the irreversible changes associated with emphysema).

Education is a principal focus of the long-term management of the patient with chronic bronchitis. Education includes the reinforcement of preventive health practices (e.g., smoking reduction and cessation, cold and flu prevention, flu shots, aerobic exercise, strengthening exercises, nutrition, weight control, hydration, pacing of activities, energy conservation, relaxation, and stress management). Chronic bronchitis and emphysema are often associated with sleep disturbances. Obstructive sleep apnea is increasingly prevalent with disease severity. Thus activity and sleep patterns must be assessed to ensure sleep is maximally restorative and not contributing to the patient's symptoms. Integral to an exercise prescription is the time of day it is to be performed. Exercise is prescribed when the patient is least fatigued, most energetic, and when performing such a program is most convenient.

Aerobic exercise is an essential component of the long-term management of the patient with chronic bronchitis to optimize the efficiency of oxygen transport overall including mobilizing and removing secretions (Oldenburg et al, 1979). The goal is to increase the exercise threshold intensity at which incapacitating dyspnea, perceived exertion, and desaturation occur.

Individuals with Emphysema

Pathophysiology and Medical Management

Emphysema is associated with a prolonged history of smoking and chronic bronchitis and indicates significant irreversible lung damage. A less common type of emphysema not associated with smoking is alpha$_1$ antitrypsin deficiency. Antitrypsin is essential in balancing elastin production and degradation and in preserving optimal lung compliance. A deficiency of antitrypsin reduces lung elasticity and contributes to the characteristic increase in lung compliance that is the hallmark of emphysema. The pathophysiology of emphysema is presented in detail in Chapter 5. The principal pathophysiological deficits include irreversible alveolar damage resulting from loss of elastic recoil and the normal tethering of the alveoli, which renders the lung parenchyma excessively compliant and floppy. Excessive distension and dilatation of the terminal bronchioles and destruction of alveoli reduce the surface area for gas exchange. Hence diffusing capacity is correspondingly reduced. The dead space in the lungs and TLC increase significantly. Breathing at normal tidal volume, the patient's airways close beyond that which normally occurs with aging, and this contributes to ventilation and perfusion mismatch and hypoxemia. Time constants are altered such that alveolar units are not evenly ventilated. In its nonacute, chronic stages the primary problems include inadequate and inefficient gas exchange resulting from the structural damage to the lungs and altered respiratory mechanics of the lungs, chest wall, and their interaction. The lungs are hyperinflated, the chest wall becomes rigidly fixed in a hyperinflated position, the normal bucket handle and pump handle motions of the chest wall are impaired, the hemidiaphragms are flattened, the mediastinal structures are shifted, and the heart is displaced and rotated, making it mechanically inefficient (Bake et al, 1974; Geddes, 1984; Murray & Nadel, 2003). The normal mucociliary transport system is ineffective because years of smoking destroy the cilia, reduce their number, and alter their configuration and orientation; thus their function is correspondingly obliterated or impaired. In addition, these patients are unable to generate high transpulmonary pressures and forced expiratory flow rates because of altered respiratory mechanics. Consequently, coughing is weak and ineffective. The administration of supplemental oxygen is limited because these patients rely on their hypoxic drive to breathe. This life-preserving drive can be attenuated with even moderate levels of oxygen. Thus oxygen administration is limited to low flows. The respiratory muscles are often weak, if not fatigued due to being in a flatened position, hence suboptimal on its length-tension curve (Rochester & Arora, 1983). The clinical consequences of hyperinflation include abnormal chest wall movement, impaired inspiratory muscle function, increased oxygen cost of breathing, impaired exercise capacity, hypoxemia and hypercapnia, and breathlessness. Overall, patients with emphysema, particularly severe emphysema, tend to be inactive and deconditioned, which further compromises the efficiency of the oxygen transport system and the capacity of other steps in the pathway to compensate.

There are several physiological compensations that occur in response to chronic hypoxemia. Stroke volume and cardiac output are increased. The red blood cell count increases (polycythemia); however, the blood becomes more viscous and requires more work to eject and distribute throughout the body. Thus the stroke work of the heart is further increased. This load on the heart occurs in addition to the increased afterload of the right ventricle because of an increase in pulmonary vascular resistance secondary to hypoxic vasoconstriction in the lungs. Over time, the heart becomes enlarged and pumps even less efficiently. In the long-term management of the patient with emphysema, impaired alveolar ventilation, impaired gas exchange, reduced oxygen transport efficiency, and the work of breathing and of the heart are the primary pathophysiological problems. Unlike chronic bronchitis, secretion accumulation may be less problematic in patients with emphysema during non-acute periods. Nonetheless, optimizing mucociliary transport is an ongoing goal of prevention in that the consequences of mucous retention and infection can be life threatening.

Noninvasive positive pressure mechanical ventilation (NPPV) has been an important advance in the management of individuals with chronic lung disease (Hill, 2000). Those with daytime hypercapnia with noctural hypoventilation may benefit most (Hill, 2004). The efficacy of NPPV, however, is jeopardized by poor adherence to its use. Predictors of successful use include ability to protect the airway, acuteness of illness, and a good initial response within the first couple of hours. Barriers include discomfort of the nose piece or face mask, patient-ventilator synchrony, sternocleidomastoid activity, vital signs, hours of ventilator use, problems with adaptation, symptoms, and gas exchange. In addition to immediate clinical benefits, NPPV may help avoid or postpone respiratory failure and invasive mechanical ventilation and weaning in this population. Other benefits that may be associated with NPPV include improved sleep and quality of life, and reduced hospitalization. The physical therapist needs to identify potential barriers and address these to maximize adaptation and adherence to NPPV. Patient subgroups of those who will benefit from NPPV must be identified. Technology research must improve comfort and adherence to NPPV.

Long-term outcome of lung volume reduction surgery for people with severe emphysema has been positive. Six months after surgery, right ventricular performance increases, particularly during exercise (Mineo et al, 2002).

Principles of Physical Therapy Management

The goals for long-term management of the patient with emphysema include the following.

- Maximize the patient's quality of life, general health, and well-being through maximizing his or her physiological reserve capacity

- Educate regarding emphysema, self-management, smoking reduction and cessation, medications, nutrition, weight control, stress management, infection control, and the role of a long-term rehabilitation program
- Optimize alveolar ventilation
- Optimize lung volumes and capacities and flow rates
- Optimize ventilation and perfusion matching
- Reduce the work of breathing
- Reduce the work of the heart
- Maximize aerobic capacity and efficiency of oxygen transport
- Optimize physical endurance and exercise capacity
- Optimize general muscle strength and thereby peripheral oxygen extraction
- Optimize respiratory muscle strength and endurance and overall respiratory muscle efficiency
- Ensure that sleep and rest are optimal
- Design comprehensive lifelong health and rehabilitation programs with the patient

Education focuses on teaching the patient about emphysema, self-management of the disease, the effect of smoking and smoking cessation, nutrition, weight control, hydration, relaxation, sleep and rest, stress management, activity pacing, energy conservation, and prevention (e.g., cold and flu prevention, flu shots, aerobic exercise, diet, sleep, and stress management).

Comparable to the patient with chronic bronchitis, sleep disturbances are common in the patient with emphysema. Activity and sleep patterns are assessed to ensure sleep is maximally restorative. If obstructive sleep apnea is disturbing the patient's sleep, recommendations can be made regarding optimal body positioning during sleep. Back elevation improves airway instability, and in some instances side-lying may reduce symptoms (Neill et al, 1997). If noninvasive mechanical ventilation (e.g., nasal continuous positive airway pressure) is necessary, these body positions may help reduce the amount of ventilatory support required.

Patient monitoring includes dyspnea, respiratory distress, breathing pattern (depth and frequency), arterial saturation, lightheadedness, discoordination, heart rate, blood pressure, and rate pressure product. Patients with cardiac dysfunction or low arterial oxygen tension require ECG monitoring, particularly during exercise. Subjectively, breathlessness is assessed using a modified version of the Borg scale of perceived exertion.

Medication that is necessary to maximize treatment response is administered before treatment (e.g., bronchodilator). Knowledge of the type of medication, its administration route, and time to and duration of peak efficacy is essential if treatment is to be maximally efficacious. When patients are on multiple medications, the interactions and implications on treatment response must be identified.

The primary interventions for maximizing cardiopulmonary function and oxygen transport in patients with emphysema include some combination of education, aerobic exercise, strengthening exercise, ventilatory muscle training (strength and endurance) or ventilatory muscle rest, low flow oxygen, mechanical ventilatory support for home use, chest wall mobility exercises, range of motion exercises, body positioning, breathing control and coughing maneuvers, airway-clearance techniques, relaxation, activity pacing, and energy conservation. An ergonomic assessment of work and home environments may be indicated to minimize oxygen demands in these settings.

The benefits of aerobic and strengthening exercise in the long-term management of airflow limitation to optimize oxygen transport in patients with compromised oxygen delivery is well established (Dean, 1993; Niederman et al, 1991; Ries et al, 1988; ZuWallack et al, 1991). Patients with severe limitations are often unable to exercise at a sufficient intensity to effect aerobic adaptations to the exercise stimulus. Benefits of exercise in these patients may be explained by desensitization of dyspnea, improved movement efficiency and hence movement economy, improved anaerobic capacity, improved ventilatory muscle strength and endurance, and increased motivation (Belman & Kengregan, 1981; Belman & Wasserman, 1981; Dean, 1993). Exercise intensity is prescribed based on rating of breathlessness (modified Borg scale) (Chapter 18), in conjunction with objective and other subjective responses from the exercise test. Objective and subjective responses to exercise in patient populations, however, reflect many factors in addition to pathophysiology (see Chapter 18 for guidelines to maximize test validity).

Patients with chronic airflow limitation alter their breathing patterns so that they breathe on the most metabolically efficient portion of the pressure relaxation curve (see Chapters 5 and 30). These patients tend to breathe with prolonged expiratory phases to maximize gas transfer and mixing in the lungs in order to minimize the effects of altered ventilatory time constants. To facilitate such a breathing pattern, the patient tends to breathe through pursed lips, which may create back pressure to maintain the patency of the airways (Muller et al, 1970). The metabolic efficiency of the patient's breathing pattern may be improved further by altering breathing mechanics rather than imposing a different breathing pattern that may be suboptimal (Jones et al, 2003). Altering breathing mechanics involves manipulating the patient's body position to promote alveolar ventilation, perfusion, and ventilation and perfusion matching, thereby reducing the work of the heart.

The increased intrathoracic pressures generated during chronic coughing limit venous return, cardiac output, and coronary perfusion. Blood pressure is also increased. These effects exert additional myocardial strain, lead to arterial desaturation, and increase the potential for cardiac dysrhythmias. Breathing control and coughing maneuvers coupled with body positioning and exercise are instructed such that the work of breathing is minimized (i.e., alveolar ventilation and gas transfer is as efficient as possible) and coughing is as efficient as possible (i.e., maximally productive with the least energy expenditure).

Physical therapy is one component of a comprehensive rehabilitation program in the long-term management of people with emphysema. Such a program also needs to include information on health promotion and maintenance, ongoing review and log of medications, respiratory support (e.g., oxygen aerosol therapy, and mechanical ventilatory support), occupational therapy, sexual rehabilitation, psychosocial rehabilitation, and vocational rehabilitation (Dean, 1993; Murray, 1993).

Breathing control maneuvers (breathing exercises) warrant special mention. Breathing control has been thought to reduce the work of breathing. Inadvertent use of breathing exercises, however, can increase the work of breathing. Diaphragmatic breathing can reduce ventilatory efficiency in people with COPD (Gosselink et al, 1995). Further, these exercises are associated with greater oxygen cost than spontaneous breathing in stable patients with COPD (Jones et al, 2003). The fact that patients do not breathe with the most energetically economic breathing pattern is of considerable clinical interest and suggests that biomechanical efficiency overrides economic efficiency. These findings support that an altered breathing pattern is the consequence of the underlying problem rather than the problem itself. Thus management should be focused on the factors that determine biomechanical efficiency and breathing pattern. Other than pursed-lip breathing, evidence for retraining breathing pattern in people with stable COPD is not well supported (Dechman & Wilson, 2004).

Body positioning is a primary determinant of pulmonary function. Thus patients should be encouraged to perform coughing and other forced expiratory maneuvers in upright positions (Badr et al, 2002). Leaning forward can increase intra-abdominal and intra-thoracic pressures, elevate the diaphragm, and increase expiratory flow rate.

Obstructive sleep apnea is often associated with COPD. This is complicated further with obesity in some patients. Upright positioning and weight loss can improve respiratory mechanics and oxygenation (Hakala et al, 2000). A more upright sleeping posture could improve nighttime oxygenation in this patient group.

Individuals with Asthma

Pathophysiology and Medical Management

Asthma is a common respiratory condition that is characterized by hypersensitivity of the airways to various triggers resulting in reversible airway obstruction (i.e., bronchospasm and bronchial edema) (Hogg, 1984; Murray & Nadel, 2000; Rees, 1984) (Chapter 5). In mild cases, no treatment other than prophylaxis may be needed. In severe cases, asthma can be life threatening. Once affected by the trigger, the airways narrow, increasing the resistance to airflow and reducing oxygen delivery. Breathing through narrowed airways contributes to wheezing, reduced alveolar ventilation, rapid shallow breathing, shortness of breath, increased work of breathing, desaturation, and cyanosis. Increased inhomogeneity of the distribution of ventilation is present in some patients with nonacute asthma (Ross et al, 1992). Expiratory flow-volume loops remain the cornerstone of monitoring asthma (Brand & Roorda, 2003). Although some triggers may produce mucous hypersecretion, even normal amounts of pulmonary secretions can obstruct narrowed airways and lead to atelectasis. Asthma that has well-defined triggers is easier to manage than cases in which the triggers are less specific.

Principles of Physical Therapy Management

The goals of long-term management of the patient with asthma include the following.

- Maximize the patient's quality of life, general health, and well-being through maximizing his or her physiological reserve capacity
- Educate regarding asthma, self-management, nutrition, weight control, air quality including smoking reduction and cessation, stress management, medications and their uses, prevention of asthmatic attacks, and infection control
- Reduce the work of breathing
- Maximize aerobic capacity and efficiency of oxygen transport
- Optimize physical endurance and exercise capacity
- Optimize general muscle strength and thereby peripheral oxygen extraction
- Design comprehensive lifelong health and rehabilitation programs with the patient

Patient monitoring includes dyspnea, respiratory distress, breathing pattern (depth and frequency), arterial saturation, cyanosis (delayed sign of desaturation), heart rate, blood pressure, and rate pressure product. Patients with cardiac dysfunction or low arterial oxygen tension require ECG monitoring, particularly during exercise. Subjectively, breathlessness is assessed using a modified version of the Borg scale of perceived exertion.

Medication that is needed to maximize treatment response is administered before treatment (e.g., bronchodilators and anti-inflammatories). Knowledge of the type of medication, its administration route, and time to and duration of peak efficacy is essential if treatment is to be maximally efficacious. When patients are on multiple medications, their interactions and the implications for management must be known.

The primary interventions for maximizing cardiopulmonary function and oxygen transport in patients with asthma include education, aerobic exercise, strengthening exercise, chest wall mobility exercises, range of motion, relaxation, activity pacing, and stress management.

Education is central to self-management of asthma (Wolf, 1991). The patient is taught the basic pathophysiology of the disease and its triggers. Other central topics, including preventive health practices, are also taught (e.g., cold and flu prevention; flu shots; medication types, administration, and effects; aerobic exercise; nutrition; weight control; hydration; air quality control including smoking reduction and cessation; relaxation and stress management; and the benefits of an integrative, lifelong, self-management rehabilitation program).

Special mention must be made regarding the use of medications and inhalers. These are frequently used unknowledgeably (i.e., the patient is unfamiliar with the basic

pharmacokinetics of the medications being used and thus is not deriving optimal effects). Inhalers are often used improperly; therefore the patient does not derive the full benefit of the medication. The instructions provided by the supplier of the inhalers should be strictly followed. There are numerous types of inhalers, all with different applications. By not adhering to the instructions, the patient's time and effort is wasted by using the inhaler ineffectively, the patient does not derive the full benefit of the medication, an excessive amount of inhaler may be used to compensate for ineffective application, there may be increased exposure of the patient to the side effects of the medication, and there is considerable economic waste.

Knowledge of the triggers of increased airway sensitivity enables the patient to exert control over bronchospastic attacks. The patient is taught to record the frequency of bronchospastic attacks and identify what triggers and relieves them. In this way, the patient learns to avoid or minimize their frequency, severity, and duration and minimizes the amount of medication required. In turn, doctor and hospital visits may be minimized. These are significant benefits.

The exercise prescription parameters are set below the bronchospasm threshold, which is established based on an exercise test (see Chapters 18 and 24). Specialized challenge tests are performed in a pulmonary function laboratory. Exercise training enables the patient to determine the balance between optimal aerobic capacity and medication and the optimal physical environment for exercise. Temperature and humidity can have significant effects on work output in patients with asthma.

Individuals with Bronchiectasis

Pathophysiology and Medical Management

Bronchiectasis is characterized by dilatation and anatomical distortion of the airways and obliteration of the peripheral bronchial tree (West, 2003). Bronchiectasis is often the sequelae of prolonged chronic lung infection. The associated inflammation leads to occlusion of the airways, which results in atelectasis of the parenchyma and consequent dilatation of central airways by increased traction on the peribronchial sheath (Bates, 1989). In addition, chronic inflammation weakens the walls of the airways, leading to further dilatation. Fibrotic, connective tissue changes in the wall contribute further to dilatation and airway distortion. These anatomical changes adversely affect normal respiratory mechanics and hence pressure volume characteristics of the lung. The chest wall becomes hyperinflated and assumes the barrel shape associated with chronic airflow limitation. The overall severity of bronchiectasis depends on the number of lung segments involved. There is often some reversible airflow limitation associated with bronchiectasis.

The patient with bronchiectasis has copious tenacious secretions, lung hyperinflation and impaired respiratory mechanics, inefficient breathing pattern, reduced ability to clear secretions, reduced aerobic capacity, and is generally debilitated.

The increased intrathoracic pressures generated during bouts of chronic coughing limit venous return, cardiac output, and coronary perfusion. Blood pressure is also increased. These effects exert additional myocardial strain, lead to arterial desaturation, and increase the potential for cardiac dysrhythmias and dysfunction.

Principles of Physical Therapy Management

The goals of long-term management of the patient with bronchiectasis include the following.

- Maximize the patient's quality of life, general health, and well-being through maximizing his or her physiological reserve capacity and function
- Educate regarding bronchiectasis, self-management, nutrition, weight control, smoking reduction and cessation, stress management, medications and their use, and infection control
- Facilitate mucociliary transport
- Optimize secretion clearance
- Optimize alveolar ventilation
- Optimize lung volumes and capacities and flow rates
- Optimize ventilation and perfusion matching
- Reduce the work of breathing
- Maximize aerobic capacity and efficiency of oxygen transport
- Optimize physical endurance and exercise capacity
- Optimize general muscle strength and thus peripheral oxygen extraction
- Design comprehensive lifelong health and rehabilitation programs with the patient

Patient monitoring includes dyspnea, respiratory distress, breathing pattern (depth and frequency), arterial saturation, cyanosis (a delayed sign of desaturation), heart rate, blood pressure, and rate pressure product. Patients with cardiac dysfunction or low arterial oxygen tension require ECG monitoring particularly during exercise. Subjectively, breathlessness is assessed using a modified version of the Borg scale of perceived exertion.

Medication that is needed to maximize treatment response is administered before treatment. Knowledge of the type of medication, its administration route, and time to and duration of peak efficacy is essential if treatment is to be maximally efficacious.

The primary interventions for maximizing cardiopulmonary function and oxygen transport in patients with bronchiectasis include some combination of education, aerobic exercises, strengthening exercises, chest wall mobility exercises, range of motion exercises, body positioning, breathing control and coughing maneuvers, airway clearance interventions, optimizing rest and sleep, relaxation, pacing, and energy conservation. Factors that trigger symptoms are identified and avoided. An ergonomic assessment of the patient's work and home environments may be indicated to maximize function in these settings.

Education is a central component of the patient's long-term, self-management rehabilitation program. Preventative health practices are taught (e.g., cold and flu prevention, flu shots, smoking cessation, sleep, aerobic exercise, nutrition, weight control, and hydration, relaxation, stress management, and the long-term benefits of an integrative, rehabilitation program).

Individuals with Cystic Fibrosis

Pathophysiology and Medical Management

Cystic fibrosis is a complex exocrine disease that has significant systemic effects (Landau & Phelan, 1973; Murray & Nadel, 2000). The disease is congenital and is hallmarked by nutritional deficits contributing to impaired growth and development. Pulmonary function shows progressive decline with commensurate reductions in homogeneity of ventilation and inspiratory pressures (Chatham et al, 1994; Cotton et al, 1985; Ross et al, 1992). Cardiopulmonary involvement can be classified into three groups: no physical signs in the chest; occasional cough and sputum; and constant cough, sputum, and other signs. Patients in each classification can benefit from physical therapy with respect to enhancing oxygen transport. Moderate and severe disease is characterized by significant airflow obstruction secondary to copious, tenacious secretions. In addition, pulmonary hypertension and right heart insufficiency may be manifested and eventual failure may ensue. Left ventricular diastolic failure may also be a feature of advanced disease (Koelling et al, 2003).

Between exacerbations, the medical priorities are to reduce the risk of infection and morbidity and promote optimal health, growth, and development.

Principles of Physical Therapy Management

The goals of long-term management of the patient with cystic fibrosis include the following.

- Maximize the patient's quality of life, general health, well-being, and growth and development through maximizing his or her physiological reserve capacity
- Educate the patient and family regarding cystic fibrosis, self-management, nutrition, avoidance of smokers, stress management and relaxation, prevention of acute exacerbations of the disease, infection control, and medication uses, modes of administration, pharmacokinetics, and times to peak efficacies
- Facilitate mucociliary transport
- Optimize secretion clearance
- Optimize alveolar ventilation
- Optimize lung volumes and capacities and flow rates
- Optimize ventilation and perfusion matching
- Reduce the work of breathing
- Reduce the work of and strain on the heart
- Maximize aerobic capacity and efficiency of oxygen transport
- Optimize physical endurance and exercise capacity
- Optimize general muscle strength and thereby peripheral oxygen extraction

- Design comprehensive lifelong health and rehabilitation programs with the individual (and the family if the patient is a child)

Patient monitoring includes dyspnea, respiratory distress, breathing pattern (depth and frequency), arterial saturation, cyanosis (a delayed sign of desaturation), heart rate, blood pressure, and rate pressure product. Patients with cardiac dysfunction or low arterial oxygen tension require ECG monitoring, particularly during exercise. Subjectively, breathlessness is assessed using a modified version of the Borg scale of perceived exertion.

Medication that is needed to maximize treatment response is administered before treatment. Knowledge of the type of medication, its administration route, and time to and duration of peak efficacy is essential if treatment is to be maximally efficacious.

The primary interventions for maximizing cardiopulmonary function and oxygen transport in patients with cystic fibrosis include some combination of education, aerobic exercises, strengthening exercises, ventilatory muscle training (strength and endurance), ventilatory muscle rest, supplemental oxygen, mechanical ventilation for home use, chest wall mobility exercises, range of motion exercises, body positioning, breathing control and coughing maneuvers, airway clearance interventions, relaxation, pacing, and energy conservation.

Education focuses on teaching preventative health practices and infection control (e.g., avoidance of cold and flu, flu shots, aerobic exercise, nutrition, hydration, relaxation, stress management, activity pacing, and energy conservation).

Physical activity and aerobic exercise must be integrated early into the lifestyle of the child with cystic fibrosis (Anonymous, 1988; Keens et al, 1977; Zach et al, 1992). As much as possible, the child is integrated into activities of his or her peer group. A prescribed aerobic exercise program is designed to optimize the efficiency of oxygen transport at all steps in the pathway and thereby enhance functional capacity overall. Physical activity and aerobic exercise enhances mucociliary transport and mucociliary clearance, maximizes alveolar ventilation and ventilation and perfusion matching, increases ventilatory muscle strength and endurance and airway diameter, and stimulates a productive effective cough. Furthermore, physical activity and exercise have been associated with improved immunity and reduced risks of infection (Pyne, 1994; Shephard et al, 1991). These are significant outcomes for patients with cystic fibrosis who have thick, copious secretions.

In addition, breathing control and coughing maneuvers are included as a component of a long-term, self-management rehabilitation program. Postural drainage and manual techniques have been the mainstay of airway clearance in the past. Exercise, however, has a primary role in secretion mobilization and as an airway clearance intervention (Dean & Ross, 1989). Breathing control and coughing strategies are coupled with exercise to facilitate secretion clearance. The principles of autogenic drainage can be integrated into breathing control.

This procedure focuses on eliciting coughing when it will be most productive, thereby minimizing less productive, exhaustive coughing. Patients with cystic fibrosis often cough so violently and uncontrollably that it leads to significant arterial desaturation, vomiting, and exhaustion and impedes venous return and cardiac output.

Ventilatory devices such as the positive expiratory pressure (PEP) mask and the flutter valve have shown benefit in some patients with cystic fibrosis with respect to reducing airway closure, clearing secretions, and enhancing gas exchange (Pryor, 1993; Pryor et al, 2002). Such aids may be useful adjuncts in some patients; however, they do not replace the multiple benefits (including mobilizing and removing secretions) of physical activity and exercise on optimizing oxygen transport.

INDIVIDUALS WITH PRIMARY PULMONARY DISEASE: RESTRICTIVE PATTERNS

Individuals with Interstitial Lung Disease

Pathophysiology and Medical Management

The pathophysiology of restrictive lung disorders and interstitial lung disease (ILD) in particular is described in Chapter 5. This classification of lung disease is associated with various occupations and the inhalation of inorganic and organic dust (Chung & Dean, 1989). As the disease progresses, TLC and vital capacity are reduced. Residual volume often remains the same. Maximal flow rates tend to be increased as compliance is reduced. The drive to breathe, breathing frequency, and the ratio of tidal volume to TLC are increased. Glandular hyperplasia may be present, leading to mucous hypersecretion in some patients. Diffusing capacity may be reduced but may only be apparent during exercise (i.e., arterial desaturation and dyspnea). Exercise-induced desaturation and reduction in partial pressure of arterial oxygen may also reflect shunt and ventilation and perfusion mismatch (Jernudd-Wilhelmsson et al, 1986).

Hemodynamic changes may be present (e.g., increased pulmonary artery pressure). Chronically increased pulmonary artery pressures and hence increased pulmonary vascular resistance, lead to increased right ventricular stroke work, hypertrophy, and right ventricular insufficiency. Partial pressure of oxygen in mixed venous blood may fall significantly during exercise, contributing to arterial hypoxemia.

Principles of Physical Therapy Management

The goals of long-term management of the patient with ILD include the following.

- Maximize the patient's quality of life, general health, and well-being through maximizing his or her physiological reserve capacity
- Educate regarding ILD, self-management, nutrition, weight control, smoking reduction and cessation, relaxation and stress management, medications and their uses, prevention, health promotion, and infection control

- Optimize alveolar ventilation
- Optimize lung volumes and capacities
- Optimize ventilation and perfusion matching
- Optimize mucociliary transport
- Reduce the work of breathing
- Reduce the work of the heart
- Maximize aerobic capacity and efficiency of oxygen transport
- Optimize physical endurance and exercise capacity
- Optimize general muscle strength and thereby peripheral oxygen extraction
- Design comprehensive lifelong health and rehabilitation programs with the patient

Patient monitoring includes dyspnea, respiratory distress, breathing pattern (depth and frequency), arterial saturation, heart rate, blood pressure, and rate pressure product. Patients with cardiac dysfunction or low arterial oxygen tension require ECG monitoring, particularly during exercise. Subjectively, breathlessness is assessed using a modified version of the Borg scale of perceived exertion.

Medication that is needed to maximize treatment response is administered before treatment. Knowledge of the type of medication, its administration route, and time to and duration of peak efficacy is essential if treatment is to be maximally efficacious.

The primary interventions for maximizing cardiopulmonary function and oxygen transport in patients with ILD include some combination of education, aerobic exercises, strengthening exercises, chest wall mobility exercises, range of motion exercises, body positioning, breathing control and coughing maneuvers, relaxation, pacing, and energy conservation. An ergonomic assessment of the patient's work and home environments may be indicated to maximize function in these settings.

Education is a central component of a comprehensive rehabilitation program for the management of ILD. Education includes information on preventative health practices (e.g., removal from the causative environment, cold and influenza prevention shots, triggers of disease exacerbations and their prevention, smoking reduction and cessation, nutrition, weight control, hydration, relaxation, activity pacing, and energy conservation).

During aerobic exercise, patients with ILD are prone to arterial desaturation (Arita et al, 1981). Patients who desaturate during sleep (Perez-Padilla et al, 1985) require supplemental oxygen during exercise. The intensity of the exercise prescribed is defined by arterial saturation, breathlessness, and work of the heart, in conjunction with other objective responses.

Individuals with Lung Cancer

Pathophysiology and Medical Management

Lung cancer is a leading cause of death for men and the incidence is increasing for women. Once diagnosed, 80% of patients survive one year. Lung cancer is highly correlated with a history of smoking and exposure to coal tars, asbestos, and radioactive dusts. The majority of primary malignant tumors are bronchogenic carcinomas. They are centrally located and thus contribute to bronchial obstruction, atelectasis, and pneumonia. Pathophysiologically, lung cancer has features of both obstructive and restrictive lung disease. The patient presents with airway obstruction, dyspnea, cough, and hemoptysis (Murray & Nadel, 2000). Treatment is limited to surgery, if metastasis has been ruled out, or conservative management with radiation and chemotherapy.

Bronchogenic carcinomas metastasize readily through the circulation and lymphatic channels to other organs including the brain, bone, liver, kidneys, and adrenal glands.

If detected early, thoracic surgery may be performed to excise the cancerous tumor (see Chapter 29). If inoperable, or in the case of metastases, a patient may be managed at home or in a hospice. Patients are debilitated, often undernourished, fatigued, short of breath, lethargic, depressed, and in pain (Saunders & McCorkle, 1985). Although these patients are often extremely ill, there is a growing trend to manage these patients in the community whenever possible. As the disease progresses, maintaining function and reducing the rate of deterioration become primary goals.

End-of-life issues and palliative care must be discussed. If the patient is managed at home, these principles of care can be practiced in this setting, and they are common to other conditions as well.

Principles of Physical Therapy Management

The goals of long-term management of the medical patient with lung cancer include the following.

- Maximize the patient's quality of life, general health, and well-being through maximizing his or her physiological reserve capacity
- Educate the patient and family about the benefits of a palliative program
- Promote self-determination and pay particular attention to being an active listener
- Provide supportive care
- Optimize pain control
- Facilitate mucociliary transport
- Optimize secretion clearance and protect the airways
- Optimize alveolar ventilation
- Optimize lung volumes and capacities and flow rates
- Optimize ventilation and perfusion matching
- Reduce the work of breathing
- Maximize aerobic capacity and efficiency of oxygen transport
- Optimize physical endurance and exercise capacity
- Optimize general muscle strength and thereby peripheral oxygen extraction
- Optimize the benefits of sleep and rest
- Minimize the effects of restricted mobility and recumbency

- Design a rehabilitation program with the patient that is suited to his or her fluctuating needs

Patient monitoring includes dyspnea, respiratory distress, breathing pattern (depth and frequency), arterial saturation, cyanosis (a delayed sign of desaturation), heart rate, blood pressure, and rate pressure product. Patients who can be mobilized but have cardiac dysfunction or low arterial oxygen tensions require ECG monitoring. Subjectively, breathlessness is assessed using a modified version of the Borg scale of perceived exertion.

Medication that is necessary to maximize treatment response is administered before treatment (e.g., analgesics or bronchodilators). Knowledge of the type of medication, its administration route, and time to and duration of peak efficacy is essential if treatment is to be maximally efficacious.

The primary interventions for maximizing cardiopulmonary function and oxygen transport in patients with lung cancer include some combination of education, mobilization, strengthening exercises, chest wall mobility exercises, body positioning, supplemental oxygen, mechanical respiratory support, breathing control and coughing maneuvers, airway clearance interventions, sleep and rest, relaxation, activity pacing, and energy conservation. Treatments are timed whenever possible to coincide with patients' peak energy level during the day.

Patients with lung cancer may benefit from the immunological effects, as well as oxygen transport effects, of mobilization and physical activity (Calabrese, 1990). The prescriptive parameters are adjusted each session given the rapid changes in these patients' conditions.

Patients with lung cancer often cough up and expectorate blood in their sputum. The airways must be as clear as possible to avoid obstruction, atelectasis, risk of infection, and pneumonia. Although airway clearance is an important goal, treatments should avoid contributing significantly to bleeding and blood loss, if possible. This blood loss may contribute to anemia and fatigue.

Manual airway clearance interventions may be indicated in some patients. Postural drainage may be coupled with percussion and manual vibration. The impact of manual interventions, however, may contribute to bleeding; thus the patient requires stringent monitoring. Despite lack of evidence, metastases to the thoracic cavity and the ribs in particular may preclude percussion in favor of manual vibration being performed over unaffected areas. Treatment duration may be limited by the patient's tolerance. Tolerance may be improved by modifying body position or by shortening treatments but increasing their frequency.

INDIVIDUALS WITH PRIMARY CARDIOVASCULAR DISEASE

Individuals with Angina

Pathophysiology and Medical Management

Angina pectoris refers to pain resulting from reduced blood flow to the myocardium. Even though it is usually

---

BOX 31-2

New York Heart Association Functional Classification

Classification	Characteristics
I	No symptoms and no limitation in ordinary physical activity.
II	Mild symptoms and slight limitation during ordinary physical activity.
III	Marked limitation in activity due to symptoms, even during less-than-ordinary activity. Comfortable only at rest.
IV	Severe limitations. Experiences symptoms even while at rest.

---

elicited during exercise, angina may be triggered by stress or, in severe cases, may occur at rest. Atherosclerosis of one or more of the coronary arteries is the principal cause. Coronary vasospasm is a less common cause of angina. The pathophysiology of angina is described in detail in Chapter 5. A history of angina necessitates further examination to establish the severity of the coronary artery occlusion. Individuals with manifestations of heart disease are categorized according to their limitation during physical activity based on the New York Heart Association (NYHA) Functional Classification (Box 31-2).

If angina is severe, the patient is scheduled for coronary bypass surgery (Chapter 29) to restore normal coronary blood flow. The acute and long-term management of the surgical cardiac patient is presented in Chapter 29. In less severe cases, angina is managed conservatively with medications (e.g., sublingual nitroglycerin, nitroglycerin patch, education, and physical therapy). After the patient has stabilized, a graded exercise tolerance test may be conducted under supervision in a cardiac stress testing facility where 12-lead ECG monitoring can be performed. The exercise intensity at which the patient exhibits angina (i.e., the anginal threshold) can be quantified and serve as the basis for the prescription of physical activity and exercise.

The body position in which exercise is performed is important in patients with heart disease. Positions of recumbency increase the volume of fluid shifted from the periphery to the central circulation. This increases venous return and the work of the heart. Thus upright body positions are selected for these patients to minimize cardiac work during exercise and when resting after exercise (Langou et al, 1977; Levine & Lown, 1952).

Principles of Physical Therapy Management

Patients may be referred to physical therapy with a history of angina as a primary or secondary problem. Regardless, angina is managed with the same care and vigilance because it can be a life-threatening condition either way. *A patient for whom antianginal medication is prescribed must have the medication present. The medication must not have expired and must be within visible access during treatment. The* physical therapist should examine the medication before treatment to ensure that the expiratory date has not passed and to take responsibility for positioning the medication near the patient for access to it should the patient develop angina during treatment.

The goals of long-term management of the patient with angina include the following.

- Maximize the patient's quality of life, general health, and well-being through maximizing physiological reserve capacity
- Educate regarding heart disease, self-management, nutrition, weight control, smoking reduction and cessation, anger and stress management, disease prevention, risk factors, medications and their use, physical activity, and exercise
- Maximize aerobic capacity and efficiency of oxygen transport of all steps in the pathway
- Optimize physical endurance and exercise capacity
- Optimize general muscle strength and thereby peripheral oxygen extraction
- Design comprehensive lifelong health and rehabilitation programs with the patient

Patient monitoring includes hemodynamic monitoring (i.e., heart rate, blood pressure, rate pressure product, and dyspnea). Subjective responses to treatment, particularly exercise, should also be recorded (e.g., Borg's rating of perceived exertion). Signs of chest pain, dyspnea, anxiety, light-headedness, dizziness, disorientation, discoordination, cyanosis, coughing, and chest sound changes (i.e., a gallop) must be monitored. *Angina is not an acceptable symptom under any circumstance.* Should it occur, treatment is immediately discontinued and emergency measures instituted as indicated. Treatments will be safer and more precisely prescribed with continuous ECG monitoring. Without ECG monitoring, treatments must be conservative. If there is any doubt at any time concerning the hemodynamic stability of a patient and his or her ability to tolerate treatment safely, the patient should be referred to a general practitioner or cardiologist for clearance before being treated.

Medication that is necessary to maximize treatment response is administered before treatment. Knowledge of the type of medication, its administration route, and time to as well as duration of peak efficacy is essential if treatment is to be maximally efficacious.

For the long-term management of patients with angina, interventions include some combination of education, aerobic exercises, strengthening exercises, chest wall mobility exercises, relaxation, activity pacing, and energy conservation. Education includes information about heart disease and risk factors (i.e., smoking, diet, stress, weight, alcohol, coffee, and being physically active in hot environments) and appropriate preventative strategies (i.e., smoking reduction and cessation, low-fat diet, reduced alcohol consumption, exercise, relaxation, activity pacing, and stress management).

Patients with angina are at risk of having an infarction; therefore, vigilance and stringent monitoring are necessary to detect angina or frank myocardial infarction. These patients are potentially hemodynamically unstable; thus their hemodynamic responses before, during, and after treatment, particularly aerobic and strengthening exercises, should be monitored and recorded. Minimally, heart rate, blood pressure, and rate pressure product should be recorded along with the patient's subjective responses to treatment. Heavy lifting, static exercise, straining, the Valsalva maneuver, and heavy, repetitive upper-extremity work are avoided during physical activity and exercise. These activities are associated with a disproportionate hemodynamic response. Physical activity and aerobic exercise are prescribed at a target heart rate or perceived exertion ranges that are below the anginal threshold based on a graded exercise tolerance test (see Chapter 18). Peak exercise tests in patients with cardiac dysfunction that may elicit angina or ST-segment changes are performed in a cardiac stress testing laboratory usually under the supervision of a cardiologist unless in a specialized facility where physical therapists perform such testing.

The body position in which aerobic exercise is performed is important in patients with heart disease. Positions of recumbency increase the volume of fluid shifted from the periphery to the central circulation. This increases venous return and the work of the heart. Thus upright body positions are selected for these patients to minimize cardiac work during exercise and during rest after exercise (Langou et al, 1977; Levine & Lown, 1952).

Sexual dysfunction is common in individuals with systemic atherosclerosis due in part to underlying pathology (dyslipidemia, vascular insufficiency, and diabetes), medication, and the psychological impact of heart disease (Jackson et al, 2002). In terms of energy demands, sexual activity is comparable to other daily activities (e.g., walking one mile on the level). Optimizing health in general with diet and exercise can contribute to regression of atherosclerosis and improved peripheral circulation. Breathing control, body positioning, and energy conservation strategies such as time of day may also help minimize symptoms comparable to other activities. Also, patients should be advised to avoid sexual activity within an hour of eating, and even then not to consume a heavy meal.

Individuals with Myocardial Infarction

Pathophysiology and Medical Management

Angina frequently precedes frank myocardial ischemia and infarction. Myocardial ischemia is reversible, whereas infarction denotes myocardial injury and cell death (i.e., necrosis). Injured myocardial cells either recover or die during the healing period. Thus minimizing further damage and maximizing the healing during this six-week period is critical. Myocardial infarctions can range from being silent and unnoticed by the patient to being life threatening. They can occur anywhere in the myocardium but occur primarily in the ventricles (in the left more frequently than in the right ventricle). The greater the severity, the greater the risk of ventricular insufficiency, acute pulmonary edema, and left ventricular failure. Because myocardial ischemia and infarction impair the pumping action of the heart and thus cardiac output, patients tend to be hypoxemic and in need of oxygen. Even after the oxygen has been discontinued and the myocardium has healed, the patient may continue to be vulnerable hemodynamically. The myocardium will have some scarring that will affect both the electrical excitability (producing dysrhythmias) and the mechanical function of the heart. In addition, the patient may continue to have low normal arterial blood gases. Hypoxemia is lethal in that it triggers dysrhythmias and predisposes tissues to hypoxia. Thus hypoxemia must be avoided. After myocardial infarction, patients are usually discharged home on several medications (e.g., nitroglycerin, calcium antagonists, beta-blockers, and diuretics). Depending on the severity of involvement, patients usually continue to require one or more of these medications over the long term. The need for oxygen is usually short term and restricted to the patient's hospital stay.

The patient's ECG will be important for determining the parameters of exercise, the level of monitoring required, and education. Dysrhythmias are described in Chapter 4, and basic ECG reading is presented in Chapter 12. Ventricular dysrhythmias can be lethal. Occasional premature ventricular contractions must be monitored to ensure their frequency remains low and that coupling does not occur. Atrial fibrillation is considered a relatively serious dysrhythmia. It is associated with a high incidence of coronary disease, stroke, and overall mortality (Aronow, 2002). Medication or a pacemaker may be necessary.

Central sleep-disordered breathing is highly prevalent in individuals with left ventricular dysfunction and is associated with abnormal cardiac autonomic control and increased dysrhythmias (Lanfranchi et al, 2003). Although sleep-disordered breathing may not be related to the severity of hemodynamic dysfunction, loss of recuperative sleep will impact on functional capacity as well as capacity and motivation to participate in an exercise program and be physically active.

Health related quality of life reported by individuals with chronic heart failure is associated with function and exercise capacity, not with ejection fraction (Mitani et al, 2003). Health related quality of life should be an outcome measure for all individuals managed for heart failure because it provides important supplemental information that is independent of physiological indices of cardiac function and the NYHA classification of function (see Box 31-2).

Nonpharmacological approaches to the management of individuals with heart failure are an essential component to the overall management of the condition (Gibbs et al, 2000). These measures are incorporated into an individualized program of health behavior change, and include the following.

- Promote adherence to the recommendations
- Maintain an adequate diet
- Maintain a normal weight
- Avoid added sodium (salt and preservatives)

- Maintain optimal blood cholesterol and triglyceride levels
- Maintain normal blood sugar
- Maintain normal blood pressure
- Restrict fluid in the presence of congestive heart failure
- Avoid smoking
- Exercise regularly
- Restrict alcohol use to a moderate amount, if any
- Receive flu and pneumococcal vaccinations

All patients with cardiovascular risk factors can benefit from cardiac rehabilitation. After a cardiac event, patients are typically discharged with drugs, the prospect of surgery, and rather infrequently with referral to an individual physical therapist or one who is a member of the cardiac rehabilitation team. There is a high incidence of recurrence and repeated surgery with further associated mortality and burden of disease. The physical therapist as a noninvasive practitioner has a primary responsibility to help avoid recurrence of symptoms and repeated surgeries. This is consistent with the physical therapist's overriding objective of reducing the need for invasive care (i.e, drugs and surgery) and developing a sustainable, lifelong health plan with the patient.

Risk factor modification is a major goal. A marker of inflammation such as C-reactive protein along with lipid testing may be a more discriminating risk factor than lipid profiling alone (Blake & Ridkner, 2002). Refining the risk factor definition on the basis of C-reactive protein level will help target management (for example, indicate necessity of intensified exercise programs, weight loss, and smoking cessation).

Principles of Physical Therapy Management

After discharge from hospital, many patients who have had a myocardial infarction see a physical therapist either privately or through a cardiac rehabilitation program. Patients may remain on a supervised rehabilitation program, including an exercise program, for six to 12 months in a specialized center (see Chapter 25).

Regardless of the setting, physical therapy includes education, psychosocial support, and a supervised setting for exercising safely and developing confidence during physical exertion. In addition, an exercise program is specifically prescribed for the patient to enhance oxygen transport (i.e., delivery, uptake, and utilization at the tissue level), thereby minimizing the metabolic demand on the heart.

Depression is a common symptom reported by individuals with coronary artery disease and is associated with an increased morbidity and mortality. Individuals with depressive symptoms are more likely to exhibit myocardial ischemia during mental stress testing and during activities of daily living (Jiang et al, 2003). Myocardial ischemia induced by mental stress may be a mechanism by which depression increases the risk of morbidity and mortality in individuals with coronary artery disease. Although aggressive Type A individuals are thought to have an increased incidence of heart disease compared with passive Type B personalities, anger and hostility have been identified as the toxic negative emotions most implicated in morbidity and mortality related to heart disease (Donker, 2000).

A graded exercise tolerance test is conducted before the patient leaves the hospital or when he or she is enrolled in an exercise program. The time between the exercise test and the exercise prescription and implementation of the exercise program should be minimal. Peak (formerly referred to as maximal) exercise tests are conducted in the presence of a cardiologist (unless in a specialized facility where physical therapists may do such testing) and provide the optimal basis for an exercise prescription. Submaximal exercise tests can be conducted by the physical therapist and can provide the basis for an exercise program; however, the prescription should be conservative compared with the prescription based on the peak exercise test. The principles and practice of exercise testing are described in Chapters 18, 24, and 25. Such testing is both an art and an exacting science and should be carried out in a rigidly standardized manner to ensure the test results are maximally valid, reliable, and useful.

Comparable to the patient with angina and no overt infarction, the following caution must be adhered to with the patient who has a history of myocardial infarction. *A patient for whom antianginal medication is prescribed must have the medication present. The medication must not have expired and must be within visible access during treatment.* The physical therapist should examine the medication before treatment to ensure that the expiratory date has not passed and take responsibility for positioning the medication near the patient for access to it should the patient develop angina during treatment.

The goals of long-term management of the patient with myocardial infarction include the following.

- Maximize the patient's quality of life, general health, capacity to return to work, and well-being through maximizing physiological reserve capacity
- Educate regarding myocardial infarction, self-management, nutrition, weight control, smoking reduction and cessation, relaxation and stress management, risk factors, disease prevention, medications, lifestyle, activities of daily living, and avoiding static exercise, straining, and the Valsalva maneuver
- Maximize aerobic capacity and efficiency of oxygen transport
- Reduce the work of the heart
- Optimize physical endurance and exercise capacity
- Optimize general muscle strength and thereby peripheral oxygen extraction
- Design comprehensive lifelong health and rehabilitation programs with the patient

Patient monitoring includes hemodynamic monitoring (i.e., heart rate, blood pressure, and rate pressure product). Subjective responses to treatment, particularly exercise, should also be recorded (e.g., Borg's rating of perceived exertion). *Angina is not an acceptable symptom under any*

circumstance. Should it occur, however, treatment is immediately discontinued and emergency measures instituted. Treatments will be safer and more precisely prescribed with continuous ECG monitoring. Without ECG monitoring, treatments must be conservative. If there is any doubt at any time about the hemodynamic stability of a patient and his or her ability to tolerate treatment safely, the patient should be referred to a general practitioner for clearance before being treated.

Medication that is needed to maximize treatment response is administered before treatment (e.g., antidysrhythmia agents). Knowledge of the type of medication, its administration route, and time to and duration of peak efficacy is essential if treatment is to be maximally efficacious.

The primary interventions for maximizing cardiopulmonary function and oxygen transport in patients with myocardial infarction include some combination of education, aerobic exercise, strengthening exercises, chest wall mobility exercises, body positioning, breathing control and coughing maneuvers, relaxation, activity pacing, and energy conservation. An ergonomic assessment of both work and home environments may be indicated to minimize myocardial strain.

Education focuses on teaching the basic pathophysiology of heart disease, its risk factors, and prevention. Health promotion practices are advocated (e.g., smoking reduction and cessation, good nutrition, weight control, hydration, quality rest, and sleep periods). In addition, types of physical activity that impose undue myocardial strain, increase intrathoracic pressure, and restrict venous return and cardiac output, such as heaving lifting, straining, or the Valsalva maneuver, are avoided. The patient is taught to monitor and practice vigilance in monitoring his or her own condition (e.g., new signs of infarction). These patients are potentially hemodynamically unstable and thus their hemodynamic responses before, during, and after treatments, particularly exercise, should be monitored and recorded (i.e., heart rate, blood pressure, and rate pressure product should be taken, along with their subjective responses to treatment).

Peak exercise tests in cardiac patients that may elicit angina or ST-segment changes are performed in a cardiac stress testing laboratory under the supervision of a cardiologist. The parameters of the exercise prescription are set based on a peak exercise test. Intensity is set within a heart rate, oxygen consumption, and exertion range (e.g., 70% to 85% of the anginal threshold) (see Chapter 18).

Aerobic exercise of large muscle groups rather than small muscle groups (e.g., arm ergometry) is selected to minimize the increased hemodynamic demand and strain and the increased work of the heart associated with working smaller, upper-body muscles. Hot and humid conditions also place additional stress on the heart, thus exercising under these conditions should be avoided.

The body position in which aerobic exercise is performed is important in patients with heart disease. Positions of recumbency increase the volume of fluid shifted from the periphery to the central circulation. This increases venous return and the work of the heart. Thus upright body positions are selected for these patients to minimize cardiac work during exercise and during rest after exercise (Langou et al, 1977; Levine & Lown, 1952; Prakash et al, 1973).

Individuals with Valve Disease

Pathophysiology and Medical Management

Valve dysfunction is either congenital or acquired and may require treatment as a primary condition or be present as a secondary condition. Any of the heart and pulmonary valves may be affected. Rheumatic fever was a common cause of rheumatic heart disease and in particular mitral valve insufficiency (Goldberger, 1990). Interconnecting lymphatic vessels between the tonsils and the heart are thought to be responsible. Calcification of valves that impairs opening and closing is another example of an acquired valve dysfunction.

Clinically, patients with valve disease may present with exertional dyspnea, excessive fatigue, palpitations, fluid retention, and orthopnea (Sokolow et al, 1990). These symptoms are often relieved when exertion is discontinued. Aerobic exercise, however, has been shown to reduce the symptoms of prolapsed valve (Scordo, 1991). Anxiety has been reported to decrease general well-being. If effectively managed, however, reduced anxiety can improve or reduce chest pain, fatigue, and dizziness.

Prophylactic antibiotics against endocarditis are administered to most patients with significant valvular involvement and in mild disease before procedures such as dental work.

Principles of Physical Therapy Management

The goals of long-term management of the patient with valvular heart disease include the following.

- Maximize the patient's quality of life, general health, and well-being through maximizing physiological reserve capacity
- Educate regarding cardiac valvular disease, self-management, nutrition, weight control, smoking reduction and cessation, relaxation and stress management, cardiac risk factors, disease prevention, medications, lifestyle, activities of daily living, and avoiding static exercise, straining, and the Valsalva maneuver
- Maximize aerobic capacity and efficiency of oxygen transport
- Optimize physical endurance and exercise capacity
- Reduce the work of the heart
- Optimize general muscle strength and thereby peripheral oxygen extraction
- Design comprehensive lifelong health and rehabilitation programs with the patient

Physical therapists are involved with the management of patients with valve defects in regards to both the medical aspects, either as a primary or secondary problem, and surgical aspects. After surgery, these patients progress well; the principles of their management are presented in Chapter 30.

With respect to the medical management of valve defects, the goal is to optimize oxygen transport in the patient for whom surgery is not indicated either because the defect is not sufficiently severe or because the patient cannot or refuses to undergo surgery. Although the mechanical defect cannot be improved, oxygen transport may be improved in some patients with judicious exercise prescription. The parameters of the exercise prescription are usually moderate in that inappropriate exercise doses can further disrupt the inappropriate balance between oxygen demand and supply and thus further exacerbate symptoms. In addition, there is the potential for further valvular dysfunction if the myocardium is mechanically strained.

The goal of the aerobic exercise prescription is to identify the exercise dose that will optimize the efficiency of other steps in the oxygen transport pathway such that the available oxygen delivered to the peripheral tissues is maximally used without constituting a significant mechanical strain on the heart. Maximizing work output over time is the goal. Thus the severely compromised patient will perform a significantly greater volume of functional work over time with short, frequent sessions of exercise rather than longer, less-frequent sessions.

If the valve defect is a secondary problem, the physical therapist must assess the severity of the defect and its functional consequences. The following questions must be addressed.

1. Does the defect preclude treatment?
2. Does the defect require that treatment be modified? If so, how?
3. What special precautions should be taken?
4. What signs and symptoms would indicate the patient is distressed?
5. What parameters should be monitored?
6. Is the patient taking medications as prescribed? How might these medications alter the patient's response to treatment?
7. Is there any evidence of heart failure? If so, what will the effects of exercise be?
8. If there is no evidence of heart failure at rest, what is the chance that insufficiency will develop with exercise?

Comparable with management of the patient with a history of angina with or without a history of myocardial infarction, body positions, activities, and respiratory maneuvers that are associated with increased hemodynamic strain are avoided.

Medication that is necessary to maximize treatment response is administered before treatment. Knowledge of the type of medication, its administration route, and time to and duration of peak efficacy is essential if treatment is to be maximally efficacious.

Patients with valve disease are potentially hemodynamically unstable; thus their hemodynamic responses before, during, and after treatments, particularly exercise, should be monitored and recorded. Monitoring includes hemodynamic monitoring (i.e., heart rate, blood pressure, and rate pressure product). Subjective responses to treatment (e.g., rating of perceived exertion) should also be recorded. Signs of dyspnea, chest pain, lightheadedness, dizziness, disorientation, discoordination, cyanosis, coughing, and chest sound changes (i.e., a gallop) must be monitored. Treatments will be safer and more precisely prescribed with continuous ECG monitoring. Without ECG monitoring, treatments must be conservative. If there is any doubt about the hemodynamic stability of a patient and his or her ability to tolerate treatment safely, the patient should be referred to his or her general practitioner for clearance before being treated.

The primary interventions for maximizing cardiopulmonary function and oxygen transport in patients with cardiac defects include some combination of education, aerobic exercise, strengthening exercises, chest wall mobility exercises, body positioning, breathing control, coughing maneuvers, relaxation, activity pacing, and energy conservation. An ergonomic assessment of both work and home environments may be indicated to minimize myocardial strain.

Exercise prescription for patients with valvular heart disease is modified to ensure that the energy demand is commensurate with oxygen supply. Otherwise excessive oxygen demand will worsen the patient's response to physical activity, lead to further distress, and possibly to reduced functional capacity. Aerobic exercise of large muscle groups rather than small muscle groups (e.g., arm ergometry) is selected to minimize the increased hemodynamic demand and strain and the increased work of the heart associated with working smaller, upper-body muscles. As for other types of cardiac conditions, exercising in hot and humid conditions should be avoided.

The body position in which aerobic exercise is performed is important in patients with heart disease. Positions of recumbency increase the volume of fluid shifted from the periphery to the central circulation. This increases venous return and the work of the heart. Thus upright body positions are selected for these patients to minimize cardiac work during exercise and during rest after exercise (Langou et al, 1977; Levine & Lown, 1952).

Individuals with Peripheral Vascular Disease

Pathophysiology and Medical Management

Peripheral vascular disease (PVD) refers to diseases of the arteries and the veins. Peripheral arterial disease results primarily from atherosclerosis and occlusion of the peripheral arteries (e.g., thoracic aorta, femoral artery, and political artery) (Spittell, 2003). The diagnosis may be overlooked until serious limb ischemia is evident (Dawson et al, 2002). Diabetes mellitus, which can result in microangiopathy and autonomic polyneuropathy, is another important cause of peripheral vascular disease in the lower extremities. Venous disease results in phlebitis, venous stasis, and thromboembolus and leads to valvular incompetence of the veins of the legs.

Arterial occlusion results in reduced blood flow to the extremities and hence reduced segmental blood pressure distal to the occlusion (i.e., lower ankle-brachial index). In mild cases of arterial stenosis the patient may be asymptomatic because considerable stenosis has to occur before there is significant reduction in peripheral blood flow. If atherosclerosis develops gradually, collateral circulation may develop sufficiently to offset progressive vessel narrowing. Clinically the patient presents with complaints of limb pain on exercise, coldness in the affected leg, and possibly numbness (Dean, 1987). The characteristic limb pain results from ischemia and is referred to as intermittent claudication. Mild to moderately severe cases are managed conservatively. Pain at rest is suggestive of severe stenosis and significant reduction of blood flow to the limb. Significantly reduced blood flow leads to ischemia color changes, skin breakdown, ulceration, and eventually gangrene. Bypass surgery is performed to revascularize a threatened limb. In severe cases in which gangrene has developed, amputation of the limb is indicated. The severity of peripheral vascular disease is a significant predictor of cardiovascular mortality. Individuals with PVD show a systemic endothelial dysfunction and an increase in the serum concentration of white blood cells, endothelin, and C-reactive protein that may trigger acute coronary syndromes.

Individuals with intermittent claudication can have a marked decrease in exercise tolerance and thus can benefit from aerobic exercise, which may stimulate the development of collateral blood vessels around the stenosed vessel. This condition can severely restrict mobility, which reduces function in addition to aerobic capacity and efficient oxygen transport overall.

Individuals with PVD from diffuse systemic atherosclerosis can be expected to have stenosis of the coronary arteries even though they may be asymptomatic. These individuals are monitored as stringently as if they had overt ischemic heart disease.

Venous insufficiency can lead to thromboemboli, skin lesions, and poorly healing ulcers of the lower extremities. Furthermore, the risk of infection and slow healing is increased.

Individuals with PVD secondary to diabetes mellitus have accelerated atherosclerosis compared with age-matched individuals without diabetes. Diabetes affects the macro and micro circulation; thus wounds must be prevented, particularly in the lower legs and feet, and managed aggressively should they occur. These individuals may be at risk for lower extremity lesions due to autonomic neuropathy and angiopathy. To restore insulin sensitivity and promote weight loss, activity levels must be significantly increased, and a formal exercise program instituted. Weight-bearing activities are safe for those individuals with poor sensation in the feet and do not increase the risk of re-ulceration (Lemaster et al, 2003).

Principles of Physical Therapy Management

It should be assumed that individuals with peripheral arterial disease have coronary and cerebral arterial disease necessitating aggressive risk factor management to reduce the risk of myocardial infarction, stroke, and death (Doyle & Creager, 2003). Primary interventions include smoking cessation, treatment of hypertension, glucose intolerance and diabetes, and management of low-density lipoprotein cholesterol.

The goals of long-term management of the patient with PVD secondary to atherosclerosis include the following.

- Maximize the patient's quality of life, general health, and well-being through maximizing physiological reserve capacity
- Educate regarding atherosclerosis, heart disease, and other sequelae, self-management, nutrition, weight control, smoking reduction and cessation, risk factors, disease prevention, medications, lifestyle, activities of daily living, and avoiding static exercise, straining, and the Valsalva maneuver
- If impaired peripheral perfusion of the limbs is present, educate regarding self-assessment of the skin; sock type, care and cleanliness; shoe fitting, and wound care if indicated
- Maximize aerobic capacity and efficiency of oxygen transport
- Optimize the work of the heart
- Optimize physical endurance and exercise capacity
- Optimize general muscle strength and thereby peripheral oxygen extraction
- Design comprehensive lifelong health and rehabilitation programs with the patient

The goals of long-term management of the patient with PVD secondary to diabetes mellitus must incorporate both the principles for the management of the patient with PVD secondary to atherosclerosis and secondary to diabetes mellitus.

Patient monitoring includes hemodynamic monitoring (i.e., heart rate, blood pressure, and rate pressure product). Subjective responses to treatment, particularly exercise, should also be recorded (e.g., pain scale and Borg's rating of perceived exertion). These patients have an increased risk of angina. *Angina is not an acceptable symptom under any circumstance.* Thus, before undertaking a therapeutic exercise program, patients should be cleared by their physicians or cardiologists. Individuals with diabetes are potentially hemodynamically unstable; thus their hemodynamic responses before, during, and after treatment, particularly exercise, should be monitored and recorded (i.e., heart rate, blood pressure, and rate pressure product should be taken) along with their subjective responses to exercise (e.g., pain and perceived exertion). If there is any doubt at any time about the hemodynamic stability of a patient and his or her ability to tolerate treatment safely, the patient should be referred to a general practitioner for clearance to begin or an okay to continue treatment.

Medication that is needed to maximize treatment response is administered before treatment. Knowledge of the type of medication, its administration route, and time to and duration of peak efficacy is essential if treatment is to be maximally efficacious.

The primary interventions for maximizing cardiopulmonary function and oxygen transport in patients with PVD secondary

to atherosclerosis include some combination of education, aerobic exercises, strengthening exercises, relaxation, activity pacing, and energy conservation. Exercise, in particular walking, is an important component of management to ameliorate symptoms and improve functional capacity and quality of life (Brevetti et al, 2002; Dawson et al, 2002). Pharmacotherapy may help relieve symptoms in the short term whereas exercise benefits are likely to be long term in terms of addressing systemic atherosclerosis. An ergonomic assessment of both work and home environments may be indicated to minimize myocardial strain.

Individuals with PVD may underestimate their increased risk of cardiovascular disease (McDermott et al, 2003); thus education focuses on teaching the basic pathophysiology of atherosclerosis, its risk factors, prevention, and reversal. Health promotion practices are advocated (e.g., smoking reduction and cessation, nutrition, weight control, and regular physical activity and exercise). In addition, types of physical activity that impose undue myocardial strain, increase intrathoracic pressure, and restrict venous return and cardiac output, such as heavy lifting, straining, or the Valsalva maneuver, are avoided. The patient is taught to practice vigilence in monitoring signs and symptoms of vascular insufficiency in the affected limb and intermittent claudication. Any sign of skin redness in the feet should be monitored closely. In the patient with diabetes, any threat of skin breakdown requires medical attention and discontinuation of exercise until medical clearance has been obtained. Patients with peripheral artery disease are taught to take special care of their feet before and after exercise. The feet and footwear should be kept clean. The inner surfaces of shoes and socks should be smooth.

During peak exercise tests, patients with PVD secondary to atherosclerosis have an increased risk of angina or ST-segment changes. Such tests therefore should be performed in a peripheral vascular laboratory or cardiac stress testing laboratory under the supervision of a peripheral vascular specialist or cardiologist. The parameters of the exercise prescription are based on a peak exercise test. Walking is the activity/exercise of choice because this activity is most severely limited by intermittent claudication, which has significant implications for function. Intensity of the training stimulus is based on pain rating in conjunction with hemodynamic and other subjective responses. The patient walks at a comfortable, even cadence within his or her pain tolerance (objectively defined on the pain scale) so that limping and gait deviation is avoided.

The body position in which aerobic exercise is performed is important in patients with PVD. Positions of recumbency eliminate the vertical gravitational gradient. This gradient significantly increases blood pressure in the lower extremities. Therefore the claudication threshold is lowered in recumbent positions. Recumbent positions also increase venous return and the work of the heart. Thus upright body positions are selected for these patients to maximize blood pressure in the lower extremities and to minimize cardiac work during exercise and during rest after exercise (Langou et al, 1977).

The management of venous stasis and disease requires patient involvement to promote healthy lifestyle (exercise and smoking cessation). Compression garments may help to facilitate venous return. Good foot and skin care and shoes that fit well are essential. The patient is taught to assess the skin of the lower extremities daily for signs of skin breakdown and abrasions. Because of impaired peripheral perfusion, skin lesions can occur quickly and then may be resistant to healing and at increased risk of infection.

Individuals with Hypertension

Pathophysiology and Medical Management

Systemic hypertension or high blood pressure is a serious condition. Most patients experience no symptoms; thus adherence to medication regimens is often poor. Approximately 90% of hypertension is termed essential hypertension (i.e., no known etiology). Hypertension predisposes a patient to stroke, myocardial infarction, hemorrhage, and infarction of other vital organs (Sokolow et al, 1990). Blood pressure tends to increase with age. With the aging of the population, the incidence of hypertension is increasing. Increased blood pressure results from increased peripheral vascular resistance; therefore medications are prescribed that reduce myocardial afterload and peripheral vascular resistance (Goldberger, 1990).

Patients with existing cardiovascular disease (i.e., hypertension) are at risk for multisystemic manifestations that must be assessed. In addition, this population tends to be older, and older populations are known to have a higher prevalence of cardiac dysrhythmias. Thus such patients' cardiac status, including ECG history, should be obtained.

Pulmonary hypertension may occur in the absence of primary cardiac disease. So-called primary pulmonary hypertension is often associated with altered resting lung function. Abnormal lung mechanics and diffusing capacity are directly associated with disease severity and may contribute to the dyspnea and fatigue reported by individuals with primary pulmonary hypertension (Sun et al, 2003).

Principles of Physical Therapy Management

Physical therapy contributes to increased metabolic demands and therefore imposes a hemodynamic load resulting in increased heart rate and blood pressure. The assessment should document the history of hypertension, its medical management, and the patient's response. Regardless of the condition being treated, the hypertensive patient's blood pressure must be monitored accurately and treatment modified accordingly (Zarnke et al, 2002). Blood pressure medications, however, are known to attenuate hemodynamic responses to exercise (Chapter 44); thus blood pressure as an index of hemodynamic status may be limited in some individuals.

Interventions for the physical therapy management of hypertension are cause-specific. Lifestyle factors are exploited to help reduce blood pressure and optimize long-term health. A program of aerobic exercise can effectively reduce high blood pressure in some patients (Blair et al, 1988; Sannerstedt, 1987). The parameters of the exercise prescription necessary to control hypertension include an aerobic type of exercise that is rhythmic and involves large muscle groups, an intensity of 60% to 75% of the patient's age-predicted maximal heart rate, 60 to 90 minutes in duration, and performed five to seven times weekly for three months to achieve an optimal effect. The exercise intensity should be equivalent to a perceived exertion rating of three to five on the Borg scale (the patient is able to speak while exercising without gasping), provided that blood pressure does not increase excessively. Only modest exercise intensities are prescribed if the patient has extremely high resting blood pressure to ensure that blood pressure does not rise excessively and is not maintained at a high pressure for a prolonged period. If the patient's hypertension responds to the exercise regimen, exercise must be included in the patient's lifestyle in order for the effects to be maintained. In addition to exercise, many patients lose weight, adopt healthier lifestyle habits, and learn stress management and coping skills concurrently. When exercise is combined with a weight loss program, both resting and stress-induced blood pressures are reduced. The resulting hemodynamic profile resembles that of successful control with pharmacotherapy (Georgiades et al, 2000).

Elderly individuals with hypertension may exhibit hypotension for almost 24 hours after exercise, along with lower cardiac output, stroke volume, and left ventricular end diastolic volume (Brandao Rondon et al, 2002). Thus such individuals should be examined for this effect, and exercise should be modified accordingly.

The goals of long-term management of the patient with hypertension include the following.

- Maximize the patient's quality of life, general health, and well-being through maximizing physiological reserve capacity
- Educate regarding hypertension, self-management, nutrition, weight control, smoking reduction and cessation, relaxation and stress management, risk factors, lifestyle factors, disease prevention, and medications and their applications and side effects
- Maximize aerobic capacity and efficiency of oxygen transport
- Optimize physical endurance and exercise capacity
- Optimize general muscle strength and thereby peripheral oxygen extraction
- With the effects of lifestyle changes (physical activity, weight loss, nutrition, smoking cessation, and potentially stress management), medication must be weaned correspondingly
- Design comprehensive, lifelong health and rehabilitation programs with the patient

Patient monitoring includes hemodynamic monitoring (i.e., heart rate, blood pressure, and rate pressure product).

Subjective responses to treatment, particularly exercise, should also be recorded. Signs of dyspnea, headache, lightheadedness, dizziness, disorientation, discoordination, cyanosis, coughing, and chest sound changes (i.e., a gallop) must be monitored. Blood pressure responses that fail to increase with increasing work load and power output may be indicative of congestive heart failure.

Treatments will be safer and more precisely prescribed with continuous ECG monitoring. Without ECG monitoring, treatments must be conservative. If there is any doubt about the hemodynamic stability of a patient and his or her ability to tolerate treatment safely, the patient should be referred to a general practitioner or cardiologist for clearance before being treated.

Medication that is necessary to maximize treatment response is administered before treatment (i.e., hypertension medications). Knowledge of the type of medication, its administration route, and time to and duration of peak efficacy is essential if treatment is to be maximally efficacious. A primary goal of noninvasive approaches to blood pressure control is to eliminate or minimize medication. The physical therapist monitors the blood pressure closely within and between visits. The patient is taught to log morning blood pressures at home, and to log medication. A close working relationship is needed with the patient's invasive practitioner during weaning of the medication.

The primary interventions in the long-term management of hypertension include education, aerobic exercise, general body strengthening, range of motion, body mechanics, relaxation, stress management, pacing, and energy conservation. The patient is instructed in self-monitoring blood pressure as well as recording his or her blood pressure, those factors associated with both high and low pressures, and blood pressure changes that occur after taking medication. Such monitoring enables the patient to self-manage his or her hypertension and thereby reduces, if not entirely eliminates, need for medication. Patients, however, should only alter their medications with their physicians' approval. Physical therapists work closely with both hypertensive patients and physicians.

Systemic blood pressure responses to dynamic exercise are greater for upper-extremity than lower-extremity work (Dean & Ross, 1992). Thus exercise prescription includes aerobic exercise of the large muscle groups. Avoiding small muscle group work avoids increases in peripheral vascular resistance and hence hemodynamic work, as well as the increased exertion, strain, and work of the heart experienced with upper-extremity work. Exercise is also performed in erect and upright rather than recumbent positions to minimize the increased work of the heart secondary to central fluid shifts that occur when the patient is lying in recumbent positions.

Self-monitoring is an important responsibility of the individual with hypertension given the need to establish valid measures on which interventions are based and modified (Zarnke et al, 2002). The most valid blood pressures are recorded by a well-trained individual with a reliable and accurate automatic blood pressure measurement system. The physical therapist can calibrate the home unit against a sphygmomanometer in the clinic or hospital. The individual is advised to measure his or her blood pressure first thing in the morning, and record it.

Individuals with Diabetes Mellitus and Metabolic Syndrome

Pathophysiology and Medical Management

Diabetes mellitus is a condition associated with impaired insulin metabolism that can result in serious long-term multisystem consequences (Guyton & Hall, 2000). The disease is classified as either insulin-dependent or non-insulin–dependent diabetes mellitus. Insulin is the carrier responsible for transporting glucose into the cells to undergo oxidation. Juvenile-onset diabetes is frequently the insulin-dependent type, whereas adult onset diabetes often is non-insulin–dependent. The underlying pathophysiology of juvenile and adult-onset diabetes, however, is distinct. Juvenile-onset (type 1) diabetes results from an inadequate number of islets of Langerhan in the pancreas, which are responsible for insulin production. Adult-onset (type 2) diabetes, on the other hand, results from reduced insulin sensitivity. In Western industrialized countries, adult-onset diabetes is associated with obesity, inactivity, diet, and stress. In addition, medications can contribute to blood sugar disturbances. The sequelae of diabetes mellitus that frequently result from poor regulation and management of the disease include angiopathy, peripheral neuropathy, autonomical neuropathy, gastrointestinal paresis, visual disturbance, and renal dysfunction (Bannister & Mathais, 2002; Ewing & Clarke, 1986).

Individuals with diabetes mellitus have an accelerated rate of atherosclerotic changes in the vasculature compared with age- and sex-matched individuals without diabetes. These individuals are also prone to peripheral vascular disease secondary to microangiopathy, macroangiopathy, and autonomic neuropathy. People with diabetes constitute a significant proportion of patients with peripheral vascular disease who require surgical amputation of affected limbs as a consequence of peripheral ischemia. Muscle infarction is a less common but clinically important complication of long-standing diabetes (Trujillo-Santos, 2003). Muscle infarction presents with pain and swelling over the affected area, and at times palpable mass and elevated creatine kinase levels. The symptoms resolve with conservative management including analgesics and relative immobility of the affected muscle.

Abnormalities of blood sugar metabolism can also be observed in individuals without diabetes. Diabetogenic factors, such as restricted mobility and stress, lead to glucose intolerance and insulin over-secretion (Lipman, 1972; Stannard & Johnson, 2003). In the individual without diabetes, these effects can be tolerated over the short term. These factors, however, may result in a critical situation for the individual with diabetes.

Metabolic syndrome is increasingly common and includes central obesity, low high-density lipoprotein cholesterol, hypertension, and often insulin resistance and hyper-triglyceridemia (Malloy & Kane, 2001).

Principles of Physical Therapy Management

Patients with diabetes may be referred to a physical therapist for several reasons. First, a newly diagnosed diabetic patient may be referred so that the physical therapist can expose the patient to a quantified exercise stimulus under supervised conditions and thereby help refine the prescription of insulin. Second, a patient may be referred for an exercise prescription to help minimize the insulin dose or avoid insulin administration entirely, depending on disease type and severity and the patient's response. Third but most frequently, patients are seen by a physical therapist for the treatment of some other condition and also report diabetes in their histories. A history of diabetes must be considered in the treatment of a patient who is referred for any reason to either improve or at least not contribute to abnormal blood glucose levels and late complications.

Patients with diabetes are treated cautiously. Exercise increases metabolic demand commensurate with intensity and hence cellular demand for glucose (American College of Sports Medicine, 2000; Blair et al, 1988). Usually insulin administration is increased in preparation for exercise. Many active individuals who have diabetes are closely attuned to their dietary and insulin needs, which permits them to be as physically active as people without diabetes. Individuals with diabetes seen by physical therapists, however are often labile and less well managed. Thus a readily available sugar source must be nearby for insulin regulation when a person with diabetes exercises or when the physical therapist exercises a diabetic patient on an ergometer after anterior cruciate ligament repair.

In addition, people with diabetes may have hemodynamic disturbances because of an autonomic neuropathy and may exhibit impaired fluid-volume regulation during exercise (Bannister & Mathais, 2002). Patients may experience postural hypotension and become dizzy and lightheaded. In addition, diabetic patients may require a longer cool-down period to adjust hemodynamically after exercise.

Hypoglycemia or low blood sugar is one of the most common complications of diabetes mellitus. This condition results from excess administration of insulin or oral hypoglycemic agent, insufficient food in relation to insulin dose, or an abnormal increase in physical activity or exercise. Hyperglycemia is common in patients who are obese and have adult-onset diabetes. High insulin levels are associated with a higher risk of coronary artery disease. Myocardial infarction and stroke are common causes of death. Another complication is cardiac hypertrophy secondary to hypertension and cardiomyopathy, which predisposes the patient to congestive heart failure. The incidence of peripheral vascular disease is also increased in diabetic patients.

The goals of the long-term management of diabetes mellitus and metabolic syndrome include the following.

- Maximize the patient's quality of life, general health and well-being through maximizing physiological reserve capacity
- Educate regarding diabetes mellitus or metabolic syndrome, self-management, nutrition (good nutrition with optimal lipid and triglyceride dietary control), weight control, blood sugar regulation and its management (i.e., the balance between nutrition, diet, exercise, stress and insulin requirements), medications, smoking reduction or cessation, relaxation, stress management, foot care, if necessary, in conjunction with hygiene and infection control
- Maximize aerobic capacity and efficiency of oxygen transport
- Optimize physical endurance and exercise capacity
- Optimize general muscle strength and thus peripheral oxygen extraction
- With the effects of lifestyle changes (physical activity, weight loss, nutrition, smoking cessation, and, potentially, stress management), medication must be weaned correspondingly
- Design comprehensive lifelong health and rehabilitation programs with the patient

Monitoring includes signs and symptoms of hypoglycemia (e.g., lightheadedness, weakness, fatigue, disorientation, and glucose tolerance test) or hyperglycemia (e.g., glucose tolerance test). Hemodynamic responses (i.e., heart rate, blood pressure, and rate pressure product) provide an index of the intensity of an exercise stimulus; however, these responses may be attenuated in the diabetic patient because of the autonomic neuropathy (both parasympathetic and sympathetic neuropathies).

Subjective responses to exercise, including the rating of perceived exertion, may be more valid indicators of exercise intensity than hemodynamic responses in the person with diabetes. The patient is taught to be vigilant in monitoring signs and symptoms of vascular insufficiency in the affected limb. Any sign of skin redness in the feet should be monitored closely. In individuals with diabetes, any threat of skin breakdown requires medical attention and discontinuation of exercise until medical clearance has been obtained. Healing is considerably delayed in the so-called diabetic foot. Without appropriate attention, infection and potential necrosis can ensue. Individuals with peripheral autonomic neuropathy are taught to monitor their footwear and socks diligently, to ensure the inner surfaces are clean and smooth before each exercise session, and to check for areas of redness or abrasion on their feet after exercise.

Medication that is necessary to maximize treatment response is administered before treatment (e.g., insulin or oral hypoglycemic agents). Knowledge of the type of medication, its administration route, and time to and duration of peak efficacy is essential if treatment is to be maximally efficacious. With lifestyle changes, including physical activity and weight loss, the physical therapist works closely with the invasive practitioner to monitor medication and the patient's changing requirements consistent with the medication weaning process.

The primary interventions in the long-term management of diabetes mellitus include education, maintenance of a log of diet and insulin regimens, activity and exercise, aerobic exercise, strengthening exercises, relaxation, stress management, activity pacing, and energy conservation (Leon, 2003). It may be necessary to consult a nutritionist to assist with promoting lifelong change.

Generally there are no contraindications to patients with diabetes mellitus being physically active and participating in an exercise program. Daily exercise is advocated for insulin-dependent and non-insulin–dependent diabetic patients to optimize glucose control. The exercise prescription parameters are set at 40% to 85% of peak functional work capacity (American College of Sports Medicine, 2000). If the patient is exercising daily, the exercise parameters are set at the lower end of this range. If the exercise sessions are less frequent (e.g., in the case of an individual with non-insulin–dependent diabetes whose blood glucose is well maintained and whose weight is acceptable), exercise intensity is set at the higher end of this range.

The risk of hypoglycemia can be reduced by observing the following precautions: frequently monitor blood glucose, decrease the insulin dose (in consultation with the physician) or increase carbohydrate intake before exercise, avoid injecting insulin into areas that are active during exercise, avoid exercise during peak insulin activity, consume carbohydrates before, during, and after prolonged aerobic activity, and be knowledgeable about the signs and symptoms of hypoglycemia (American College of Sports Medicine, 2000).

SUMMARY

This chapter reviews the pathophysiology, medical management, and comprehensive physical therapy management of individuals with chronic, primary cardiopulmonary pathology. Exercise testing and training is a major component of the comprehensive management of these conditions, and this topic is presented separately in Chapter 24. Given that the heart and lungs are interdependent and function as a single unit, *primary* lung or heart disease is considered with respect to the other organ and in the context of oxygen transport overall.

The principles of long-term management of people with chronic *primary* lung disease are presented first. Although there is no clear line between obstructive and restrictive patterns of lung disease as they often coexist, pathology can be generally defined based on the primary underlying pathophysiological problems. Thus the *primary* conditions presented included obstructive lung disease (i.e., chronic airflow limitation, asthma, bronchiectasis, and cystic fibrosis) and restrictive lung disease (i.e., interstitial pulmonary fibrosis). Lung cancer, which has the characteristics of both obstructive and restrictive patterns of pathology, is also presented.

The long-term cardiopulmonary management of people with chronic, *primary* heart disease is then presented with

special attention to angina, myocardial infarction, and heart valve disease. Chronic vascular diseases including peripheral vascular disease, hypertension, and diabetes are also presented.

The principles of management of people with various chronic, *primary* cardiopulmonary conditions are presented rather than treatment prescriptions, which cannot be discussed without consideration of a specific patient. These principles also are applied when one or more chronic, *primary* cardiopulmonary conditions are secondary diagnoses for a patient, as such dysfunction may necessitate either modifying the treatment prescription for some other condition or, minimally, indicate special monitoring.

Review Questions

1. Describe the chronic, *primary* cardiopulmonary pathophysiology associated with airflow limitation (i.e., COPD), asthma, bronchiectasis, cystic fibrosis, interstitial pulmonary fibrosis, lung cancer, angina, myocardial infarction, valvular heart disease, peripheral vascular disease, hypertension, and diabetes, and how such pathology may impact on an individual's participation in life or be a threat to it.

2. Relate cardiopulmonary physical therapy treatment interventions for individuals with each of the above chronic conditions and provide the rationale for your choice.

REFERENCES

ACC/AHA 2002 guideline update for exercise testing: summary article. A report of the American College of Cardiology/ American Heart Association Task Force on Practice Guidelines (Committee to Update the 1997 Exercise Testing Guidelines). Gibbons, R.J., Balady, G.J., Bricker, J.T., Chaitman, B.R., Fletcher, G.F., Froelicher, V.F., Mark, D.B., McCallister, B.D., Mooss, A.N., O'Reilly, M.G., Winters, W.L., Gibbons, R.J., Antman, E.M., Alpert, J.S., Faxon, D.P., Fuster, V., Gregoratos, G., Hiratzka, L.F., Jacobs, A.K., Russell, R.O., & Smith, S.C. (2002). American College of Cardiology/American Heart Association Task Force on Practice Guidelines. Available at:www.acc.org/ clinical/guidelines/exercise/exercise-clean.pdf. Retrieved September 28, 2005.

American College of Sports Medicine. (2000). ACSM's guidelines for exercise testing and prescription, ed 46. Philadelphia: Lippincott Williams & Wilkins.

Anonymous. (1988). Cystic fibrosis and physical activity. International Journal of Sports Medicine 9(Suppl 1):1-64.

Arita, K.I., Nishida, O., & Hiramoto, T. (1981). Physical exercise in "pulmonary fibrosis." Hiroshima Journal of Medical Science 30:149-159.

Aronow, W.S. (2002). Management of the older person with atrial fibrillation. Journal of Gerontology Series A. Biological Science and Medical Science 57:M352-M363.

Badr, C., Elkins, M.R., & Ellis, E.R. (2002). The effect of body position on maximal expiratory pressure and flow. Australia Journal of Physiotherapy 48:95-102.

Bake, B., Dempsey, J., & Grimby, G. (1976). Effects of shape changes of the chest wall on distribution of inspired gas. American Review of Respiratory Disease 114:1113-1120.

Bannister, R., & Mathais, C.J. (2002). Autonomic failure, ed 4. New York: Oxford University Press.

Bates, D.V. (1989). Respiratory function in diseases, ed 3. Philadelphia: WB Saunders.

Belman, M.J., & Kendregan, B.A. (1981). Exercise training fails to increase skeletal muscle enzymes in patients with chronic obstructive pulmonary disease. American Review of Respiratory Diseases 123:256-261.

Belman, M.J., & Wasserman, K. (1981). Exercise training and testing in patients with chronic obstructive pulmonary disease. Basics of Respiratory Diseases 10:1-6.

Blair, S.N., Painter, P., Pate, R.R., Smith, L.K., & Taylor, C.B. (1988). Resource manual for guidelines for exercise testing and prescription. Philadelphia: Lea & Febiger.

Blake, G.J., & Ridker, P.M. (2002). Inflammatory bio-markers and cardiovascular risk prediction. Journal of Internal Medicine 252:283-94.

Brand, P.L., & Roorda, R.J. (2003). Usefulness of monitoring lung function in asthma. Archives of Diseases in Children 88:1021-1025.

Brandao Rondon, M.U., Alves, M.J., Braga, A.M., Teixeira, O.T., Barretto, A.C., Krieger, E.M., & Negrao, C.E. (2002). Post-exercise blood pressure reduction in elderly hypertensive patients. Journal of the American College of Cardiology 39:676-682.

Brevetti, G., Annecchini, R., & Bucur, R. (2002). Intermittent claudication: pharmacoeconomic and quality of life aspects of treatment. Pharmacoeconomics 20:169-181.

Calabrese, L.H. (1991). Exercise, immunity, cancer, and infection. In Bouchard, C., Shepard, R.J., Stephens, T., Sutton, J.R., & McPherson, B.D. (Eds). Exercise, fitness, and health. A consensus of current knowledge. Champaign, IL: Human Kinetics Books.

Chatham, K., Berrow, S., Beeson, C., Griffiths, L., Brough, D., & Musa, I. (1994). Inspiratory pressures in adult cystic fibrosis. Physiotherapy 80:748-752.

Cheitlin, M.D. (2004). Clinical cardiology, ed 7. Stamford: Appleton & Lange.

Chung, F., & Dean, E. (1989). Pathophysiology and cardiorespiratory consequences of interstitial lung disease-review and clinical implications. Physical Therapy 69:956-966.

Cotton, D.J., Graham, B.L., Mink, J.T., & Habbick, B.F. (1985). Reduction of the single breath diffusing capacity in cystic fibrosis. European Journal of Respiratory Diseases 66:173-180.

Dantzker, D.R. (1983). The influence of cardiovascular function on gas exchange. Clinics in Chest Medicine 4:149-159.

Dawson, D.L., Hiatt, W.R., Creager, M.A., & Hirsch, A.T. (2002). Peripheral arterial disease: medical care and prevention of complications. Preventive Cardiology 5:119-130.

Dean, E. (1987). Assessment of the peripheral circulation: an update for practitioners. The Australian Journal of Physiotherapy 33:164-172.

Dean, E. (1993). Advances in rehabilitation for older persons with cardiopulmonary dysfunction. In Katz, P.R., Kane, R.L., & Mezey, M.D. (Eds). Advances in long-term care, ed 2. New York: Springer.

Dean, E., & Ross, J. (1989). Integrating current literature in the management of cystic fibrosis: a rejoinder. Physiotherapy Canada 41:46-47.

Dean, E., & Ross, J. (1992). Mobilization and exercise conditioning. In Zadai, C. (Ed). Pulmonary management in physical therapy. New York: Churchill Livingstone.

Dechman, G., & Wilson, C.R. (2004). Evidence underlying breathing retraining in people with stable chronic obstructive pulmonary disease. Physical Therapy 84:1189-1197.

Donker, F.J. (2000). Cardiac rehabilitation: a review of current developments. Clinical Psychology Review 20:923-943.

Doyle, J., & Creager, M.A. (2003). Pharmacotherapy and behavioral intervention for peripheral artery disease. Reviews in Cardiovascular Medicine 4:18-24.

Ewing, D.J., & Clarke, B.F. (1986). Autonomic neuropathy: its diagnosis and prognosis. In Watkins, P.J. (Ed). Clinics in endocrinology and metabolism. London: WB Saunders.

Ferguson, G.T. (2000). Recommendations for the management of COPD. Chest 117:23S-28S

Froelicher, V.F., & Myers, J.N. (2000). Exercise and the heart, ed 4. Philadelphia: Elsevier.

Geddes, D.M. (1984). Chronic airflow obstruction. Postgraduate Medicine 60:194-200.

Georgiades, A., Sherwood, A., Gullette, E.C., Babyak, M.A., Hinderliter, A., Waugh, R., Tweedy, D., Craighead, L., Bloomer, R., & Blumental, J.A. (2000). Effects of exercise and weight loss on mental stress-induced cardiovascular responses in individuals with high blood pressure. Hypertension 36:171-176.

Gibbs, C.R., Jackson, G., & Lip, G.Y.H. (2000). ABC of heart failure. Non-drug management. British Medical Journal 320:366-368.

Goldberger, E. (1990). Essentials of clinical cardiology. Philadelphia: JB Lippincott.

Guyton, A.C., & Hall, J.E. (2000). Textbook of medical physiology, ed 10. Philadelphia: Elsevier.

Hakala, K., Maasilta, P., & Sovijarvi, A.R. (2000). Upright body position and weight loss improve respiratory mechanics and daytime oxygenation in obese patients with obstructive sleep apnea. Clinical Physiology 20:50-55.

Hill, N.S. (2000). Noninvasive ventilation in chronic obstructive pulmonary disease. Clinics of Chest Medicine 21:783-797.

Hill, N.S. (2004). Noninvasive ventilation for chronic obstructive pulmonary disease. Respiratory Care 49:72-87.

Hogg, J.C. (1984). The pathology of asthma. Clinics in Chest Medicine 5:567-571.

Jackson, H.A. Jr. (1999). Sexual activity and the cardiovascular patient: guidelines. American Journal of Cardiology 84:6N-10N.

Jernudd-Wilhelmsson, Y., Hornblad, Y., & Hedenstierna, G. (1986). Ventilation perfusion relationships in interstitial lung disease. European Journal of Respiratory Disease 68:39-49.

Jiang, W., Babyak, M.A., Rozanski, A., Sherwood, A., O'Connor, C.M., Waugh, R.A., Coleman, R.E., Hanson, M.W., Morris, J.J, & Blumenthal, J.A. (2003). Depression and increased myocardial ischemic activity in patients with ischemic heart disease. American Heart Journal 146:55-61.

Jones, A.Y.M., Dean, E., & Chow, C.C.S. (2003). Comparison of the oxygen cost of breathing exercises and spontaneous breathing in patients with stable chronic obstructive pulmonary disease. Physical Therapy 83:424-431.

Keens, T.G., Krastins, I.R.B., Wannamaker, E.M., Levison, H., Crozier, D.N., & Bryan, A.C. (1977). Ventilatory muscle endurance training in normal subjects and patients with cystic fibrosis. American Review of Respiratory Disease 116:853-860.

Koelling, T.M., Dec, G.W., Ginns, L.C., & Semigran, M.J. (2003). Left ventricular diastolic function in patients with advanced cystic fibrosis. Chest 123:1488-1494.

Landau, L.I., & Phelan, P.D. (1973). The spectrum of cystic fibrosis. American Review of Respiratory Disease 108:593-602.

Lanfranchi, P.A., Somers, V.K., Braghiroli, A., Corra, U., Eleuteri, E., & Giannuzzi, P. (2003). Central sleep apnea in left ventricular dysfunction: prevalence and implications for arrhythmic risk. Circulation 107:727-732.

Langou, R.A., Wolfson, S., Olson, E.G., & Cohen, L.S. (1977). Effects of orthostatic postural changes on myocardial oxygen demands. American Journal of Cardiology 39:418-421.

Leon, A.S. (2003). Diabetes. In Skinner, J.S. (Ed). Exercise testing and exercise prescription for special cases. Theoretical basis and clinical application, ed 3. Philadelphia: Lippincott Williams & Wilkins.

Lemaster, J.W., Reiber, G.E., Smith, D.G., Heagerty, P.J., & Wallace, C. (2003). Daily weight-bearing activity does not increase the risk of diabetic foot ulcers. Medicine and Science in Sports and Exercise 35:1093-1099.

Levine, S.A., & Lown, B. (1952). 'Armchair' treatment of acute coronary thrombosis. Journal of the American Medical Association 148:1365-1369.

Lipman, R.L. (1972). Glucose tolerance during decreased physical activity in man. Diabetes 21:101-105.

Malloy, M.J., & Kane, J.P. (2001). A risk factor for atherosclerosis: triglyceride-rich lipoproteins. Advances in Internal Medicine 47:111-136.

McDermott, M.M., Mandapat, A.L., Moates, A., Albay, M., Chiou, E., Celic, L., & Greenland, P. (2003). Knowledge and attitudes regarding cardiovascular disease risk and prevention in patients with coronary or peripheral arterial disease. Archives of Internal Medicine 163:2157-2162.

Mineo, T.C., Pompeo, E., Rogliani, P., Dauri, M., Turani, F. Bollero, P., & Magliocchetti, N. (2002). Effect of lung volume reduction surgery for severe emphysema on right ventricular function. American Journal of Critical Care Medicine 165:489-494.

Mitani, H., Hashimoto, H., Isshiki, T., Kurokawa, S., Ogawa, K., Matsumoto, K., Miyake, F., Yoshino, H., & Fukuhara, S. (2003). Health-related quality of life of Japanese patients with chronic heart failure: assessment using the Medical Outcome Study Short From 36. Circulation Journal 67:215-220.

Muller, R.E., Petty, T.L., & Filley, G.F. (1970). Ventilation and arterial blood gas changes induced by pursed-lip breathing. Journal of Applied Physiology 28:784-789.

Murray, E. (1993). Anyone for pulmonary rehabilitation? Physiotherapy 79:705-710.

Murray, J.E., & Nadel, J.A. (2000). Textbook of respiratory medicine, ed 3. Philadelphia: Elsevier.

Neill, A.M., Angus, S.M., Sajkov, D., & McEvoy, R.D. (1997). Effects of sleep posture on upper airway stability in patients with obstructive sleep apnea. American Journal of Respiratory and Critical Care Medicine 155:199-204.

http:/encyclopedia.thefreedictionary.com (retrieved November 2004).

Niederman, M.S., Clemente, P.H., Fein, A.M., Feinsilver, S.H., Robinson, D.A., Howite, M.S., & Bernstein, M.G. (1991). Benefits of a multidisciplinary pulmonary rehabilitation program: improvements are independent of lung function. Chest 99:798-804.

Oldenburg, F.A., Dolovich, M.B., Montgomery, J.M., & Newhouse, M.T. (1979). Effects of postural drainage, exercise, and cough on mucus clearance in chronic bronchitis. American Review of Respiratory Disease 120:739-745.

Perez-Padilla, R., West, P., & Lertzman, M. (1985). Breathing during sleep in patients with interstitial lung disease. American Review of Respiratory Disease 132:224-229.

Pierson, D.J. (2004). Translating new understanding into better care for the patient with chronic obstructive pulmonary disease. Respiratory Care 49:99-109.

Prakash, R., Parmley, W.W., Dikshit, K., Forrester, J., & Swan, H.J. (1973). Hemodynamic effects of postural changes in patients with acute myocardial infarction. Chest 64:7-9.

Pryor, J.A. (1993). Respiratory care. Edinburgh: Churchill Livingstone.

Pryor, J.A., Prasad, S.A., & Webber, B.A. (2002). Physiotherapy for respiratory and cardiac problems: adults and paediatrics. St. Louis: Harcourt Health Sciences Group.

Pyne, D.B. (1994). Regulation of neutrophil function during exercise. Sports Medicine 17:245-258.

Rees, J. (1984). ABC of asthma. Definition and diagnosis. British Medical Journal 5:1370-1372.

Ries, A.L., Ellis, B., & Hawkins, R.W. (1988). Upper extremity exercise training in chronic obstructive pulmonary disease. Chest 93:688-692.

Rochester, D.F., & Arora, N.S. (1983). Respiratory muscle failure. Medical Clinics of North America 67:573-597.

Ross, J., Bates, D.V., Dean, E., & Abboud, J.T. (1992). Discordance of airflow limitation and ventilation inhomogeneity in asthma and cystic fibrosis. Clinical and Investigative Medicine 15:97-102.

Ross, J., & Dean, E. (1989). Integrating physiological principles into the comprehensive management of cardiopulmonary dysfunction. Physical Therapy 69:255-259.

Sannerstedt, R. (1987). Hypertension. In Skinner, J.S. (Ed). Exercise testing and exercise prescription for special cases. Theoretical basis and clinical application. Philadelphia: Lea & Febiger.

Saunders, J.M., & McCorkle, R. (1985). Model of care for persons with progressive cancer. Journal of Otolaryngology 14:365-378.

Scordo, K.A. (1991). Effects of aerobic exercise training on symptomatic women with mitral valve prolapse. American Journal of Cardiology 67:863-868.

Shephard, R.J., Verde, T.J., Thomas, S.G., & Shek, P. (1991). Physical activity and the immune system. Canadian Journal of Sports Science 16:163-185.

Spittell, J.A. (2003). Peripheral vascular disease for cardiologists. Armouk: Futura Publishing Co., Inc.

Stannard, S.R., & Johnson, N.A. (2004). Insulin resistance and elevated triglyceride in muscle: more important for survival than 'thrifty' genes? Journal of Physiology 554:595-607.

Sun, X.G., Hansen, J.E., Oudiz, R.J., & Wasserman, K. (2003). Pulmonary function in primary pulmonary hypertension. Journal of the American College of Cardiology 41:1028-1035.

Trujillo-Santos, A.J. (2003). Diabetic muscle infarction. An undiagnosed complication of long-standing diabetes. Diabetes Care 26:211-215.

Wasserman, K.L., & Whipp, B.J. (1975). Exercise physiology in health and disease. American Review of Respiratory Disease 112:219-249.

West, J.B. (2003). Pulmonary pathophysiology: The essentials, ed 6. Philadelphia: Lippincott Williams and Wilkins.

Wolf, S.I. (1991). Rehabilitation of asthmatic patients. Motivating your patient top improve their life-style. Postgraduate Medicine 90:93-96.

Zach, M., Oberwaldner, B., & Hausler, F. (1982). Cystic fibrosis: physical exercise versus chest physiotherapy. Archives of Diseases in Children 57:587-589.

Zarnke, K.B., McAlister, F.A., Campbell, N.R., Levine, M., Schiffrin, E.L. Grover, S., McKay, D.W., Myers, M.G., Wilson, T.W., Rabkin, S.W., Feldman, R.D., Burgess, E., Bolli, P., Honos, G., Lebel, M., Mann, K., Abbott, C., Tobe, S., Petrella, R., & Touyz, R. M. (2002). The 2001 Canadian recommendations for the management of hypertension: Part one—Assessment for diagnosis, cardiovascular risk, causes and lifestyle modification. Canadian Journal of Cardiology 18:604-624.

ZuWallack, R.L., Patel, K., Reardon, J.Z., Clark, B.A., & Normandin, E.A. (1991). Predictors of improvement in the 12-minute walking distance following a six-week outpatient pulmonary rehabilitation program. Chest 99:805-808.

C H A P T E R   3 2

Individuals with Chronic Secondary Cardiopulmonary Dysfunction

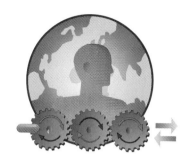

Elizabeth Dean and Donna Frownfelter

KEY TERMS

Ankylosing spondylitis
Cerebral palsy
Chronic renal insufficiency
Kyphoscoliosis
Multiple sclerosis
Muscular dystrophy
Osteoporosis

Parkinson syndrome
Post polio syndrome
Rheumatoid arthritis
Scleroderma
Spinal cord injury
Stroke
Systemic lupus erythematosus

The purpose of this chapter is to review the pathophysiology and medical management in relation to comprehensive physical therapy management of individuals with chronic, *secondary* cardiopulmonary pathology. Exercise testing and training is a major component of the comprehensive physical therapy management of individuals with chronic, secondary cardiopulmonary conditions, and this topic is presented separately in Chapter 25.

This chapter specifically addresses the comprehensive physical therapy management of chronic cardiopulmonary dysfunction secondary to neuromuscular, musculoskeletal, collagen vascular/connective tissue, and renal dysfunction. The neuromuscular conditions that are presented include stroke, Parkinson's syndrome, multiple sclerosis, cerebral palsy, spinal cord injury, chronic effects of poliomyelitis, and muscular dystrophy. The musculoskeletal conditions that are presented include thoracic deformity (kyphoscoliosis) and osteoporosis. The collagen vascular/connective tissue conditions that are presented include systemic lupus erythematosus, scleroderma, ankylosing spondylitis, and rheumatoid arthritis. Finally, management of the patient with chronic renal insufficiency and the person who is obese is presented. The principles of

management are presented rather than treatment prescriptions, which cannot be given without consideration of a specific patient. In this context the goals of long-term management of each condition are presented, followed by the essential monitoring required and the primary interventions for maximizing cardiopulmonary function and oxygen transport. The selection of interventions for any given patient is based on the physiological hierarchy. The most physiological interventions are exploited followed by less physiological interventions and those whose efficacy is less well documented (see Chapter 17). With respect to treatment prescription and monitoring, these principles must be considered when chronic, secondary cardiopulmonary dysfunction is the diagnosis.

INDIVIDUALS WITH NEUROMUSCULAR CONDITIONS

Individuals with Stroke

Pathophysiology and Medical Management

Stroke or hemiplegia affects cardiopulmonary function of the survivors either directly or indirectly (Fugl-Meyer & Grimby, 1984; Griggs & Donohoe, 1982). A cerebral infarct involving the vital centers of the brain can affect cardiopulmonary function. Such infarctions, however, are likely to be lethal. More commonly, after a stroke, chest wall movement and electrical activity on the ipsilateral side are reduced (DeTroyer et al, 1981; Fluck, 1966). Facial and pharyngeal weakness contribute to an inability to control oral secretions, swallow effectively, and protect the upper airway. Altered respiratory mechanics and efficiency reflect impaired chest wall movement, asymmetry, and the degree of muscle paresis and spasm.

Individuals with stroke have associated problems that contribute to cardiopulmonary dysfunction. These patients tend to be older, hypertensive, and have a high incidence of cardiac dysfunction. Muscle disuse and restricted mobility secondary to stroke lead to reduced cardiopulmonary conditioning and inefficient oxygen transport. Spasticity increases metabolic and oxygen demand. Hemiparesis results in gait deviations, which reduce movement efficiency and movement economy. Reduced movement economy results in an increased energy cost associated with ambulation, which may reduce exercise tolerance because of fatigue (Dean & Ross, 1993). In addition, ambulating with a walking aid is associated with a significantly increased energy cost compared with normal walking. This increased energy cost reduces the patient's exercise tolerance further and increases fatigue.

The notion of a motor recovery plateau in the management of individuals with stroke has been challenged (Bach-y-Rita et al, 2002; Page et al, 2004). It has been argued that individuals adapt to the training stimulus and plateau when that stimulus no longer changes. Thus individuals are deprived of therapy unless they are responding. Capacity to improve can be augmented with changes in type of activity and the introduction of new exercises, as well as changes in the intensity, duration, and frequency of the exercises. Computer-assisted motivating rehabilitation employs the use of games and unconscious limb activation and movement, rather than engaging the patient in specific limb exercises (Bach-y-Rita et al, 2002).

Individuals with stroke are at increased risk of having intercurrent heart disease, which compromises long-term survival and increases the risk of illness and inactivity (Roth, 1994). Further, concurrent congestive heart failure will adversely affect outcomes after stroke rehabilitation. Clinical assessment, even if patients are asymptomatic, must include a cardiac work-up to establish the degree to which cardiac insufficiency limits mobility, endurance, recovery, balance, and fatigue. An integrated multisystem approach will ensure improved rehabilitation outcomes and avoid complications.

Principles of Physical Therapy Management

The goals of long-term management for the patient with stroke include the following.

- Maximize the patient's quality of life, general health, and well-being through maximizing physiological reserve capacity

- Educate regarding cardiopulmonary manifestations of stroke, self-management, medications, smoking reduction and cessation, nutrition, weight control, and the role of a rehabilitation program
- Optimize aids and devices to reduce unnecessary energy demands by optimizing postural alignment
- Optimize chest wall excursion and ventilation
- Optimize alveolar ventilation
- Optimize lung volumes and capacities and flow rates
- Optimize ventilation and perfusion matching and gas exchange
- Reduce the work of breathing
- Reduce the work of the heart
- Protect the airways from aspiration
- Facilitate mucociliary transport
- Optimize secretion clearance
- Maximize aerobic capacity and efficiency of oxygen transport
- Optimize physical endurance and exercise capacity
- Optimize general muscle strength and thereby peripheral oxygen extraction
- Design lifelong health and rehabilitation programs with the patient

The management of people with stroke is shifting from a primary sensorimotor focus to an integrated management approach of which aerobic conditioning is an integral component. Structured, progressive rehabilitation programs for stroke produce greater therapeutic gains with respect to endurance, mobility, and balance than spontaneous recovery (Duncan et al, 2003). Body weight support has been examined to support an individual with stroke in the upright position to facilitate treadmill walking as a means of conditioning and gait reeducation (Moseley et al, 2003). Treadmill training with support appears to have a somewhat greater effect in ambulatory individuals with respect to improved walking speed than other interventions. In addition, traditional management approaches to stroke incorporate little exercise testing and monitoring. Given stroke results from dysfunction of the cerebral vessels secondary to the same common pathway as ischemic heart disease and intermittment claudication, comparable monitoring and precautions must be instituted during treatment.

Patient monitoring includes dyspnea, respiratory distress, breathing pattern (depth, symmetry, and frequency), arterial saturation, cyanosis (delayed sign of desaturation), heart rate, blood pressure, and rate pressure product. Patients with cardiac dysfunction require clearance from a cardiologist before participating in a rehabilitation program and may require electrocardiogram (ECG) monitoring, particularly during exercise. Subjectively, perceived exertion is rated using the Borg scale.

Medication that is needed to maximize treatment response is administered before treatment (e.g., antihypertensive and cardiac medications). Knowledge of the type of medication, its administration route, and time to and duration of peak efficacy is essential if treatment is to be maximally efficacious.

The primary interventions for maximizing cardiopulmonary function and oxygen transport in individuals with stroke include some combination of education, aerobic exercise, strengthening exercises, spasticity control, postural correction exercises, gait reeducation, chest wall mobility exercises, range of motion exercises, body positioning, breathing control and coughing maneuvers, airway clearance interventions, activity pacing, and energy conservation. An ergonomic assessment of the patient's work and home environments may be indicated to minimize oxygen demand and energy expenditure in these settings.

Education is a principal focus of the long-term management of the individual with stroke. Education includes the reinforcement of preventative health practices (e.g., infection control, smoking reduction and cessation, cold and flu prevention, flu shots, aerobic exercise, strengthening exercises, gait reeducation, nutrition, weight control, hydration, pacing of activities, and energy conservation). Stroke is often associated with sleep disturbances (e.g., obstructive sleep apnea). Thus activity and sleep patterns must be assessed to ensure sleep is maximally restorative and not contributing to the patient's symptoms.

Aerobic exercise is an essential component of long-term management of the individual with stroke to optimize the efficiency of oxygen transport overall. Maximizing ventilation with mobilization is limited if the patient has severe generalized muscular weakness and increased fatigue. Although aggressive mobilization can be supported in these patients (Malouin et al, 1992), appropriate selection of patients for such a regimen, judicious exercise prescription, and monitoring must be instituted to ensure the treatment is optimally therapeutic and poses no risk to a patient in this high-risk group. Chest wall exercises include movement in all planes combined with rotation. Body positioning to optimize lung volumes and airflow rates is a priority. Breathing control and coughing maneuvers are essential and should be coupled with body movement and positioning. Exercise is conducted in the upright positions to minimize the work of the heart and of breathing during physical exertion. Recumbent positions reduce lung volumes and expiratory flow rates, impair respiratory mechanics, increase closing volumes, increase thoracic blood volume, and increase compressive forces on both the lungs and the heart (Dean & Ross, 1992; Ross & Dean, 1992). Thus significant periods and intensities of aerobic exercise should be performed standing or sitting. Lower-extremity work is preferable to upper-extremity work in that the latter is associated with increased hemodynamic stress. Rhythmic exercise of large muscle groups is preferable to static exercise and exercise of small muscle groups, such as the arms, which produces smaller hemodynamic effects. Yoga-based exercise programs may be of some benefit for people with chronic stroke (Bastille & Gill-Body, 2004). Resistance muscle training for the limbs increases their muscle power in a dose-dependent relationship without increasing spasticity (Badics et al, 2002). Muscle training should be combined with aerobic training for optimal benefit and functional benefit (Anonymous, 2002).

Although social support is recognized clinically as an important component of the comprehensive management of people with chronic conditions, the literature in this area is scant. Family participation has been reported to improve the strength and mobility of an individual with stroke (Maeshima et al, 2003).

Ambulation or wheelchair locomotion should be as efficient as possible so that the metabolic demand of these functional activities is reduced. Performing these activities inefficiently on a frequent basis contributes to an excessive oxygen demand. The patient expends considerable energy in performing these activities uneconomically, which impairs the patient's tolerance and contributes to excessive fatigue. Conserving energy by performing these activities more economically from an energetic perspective will provide more energy to perform more of these or other activities.

Patients with generalized neuromuscular weakness require prophylactic management because of their high risk of developing life-threatening respiratory infections and complications. Prophylaxis should include flu shots, avoidance of polluted, smoky environments, smoking reduction and cessation, control of the types of food eaten and chewing well to avoid choking, and regular deep breathing, frequent movement, and change in body positions (even just shifting and taking some deeper breaths while seated in a wheelchair) to promote mucociliary transport. An optimal time to take deep breaths and to cough is during transfers, which usually are physically exerting and stimulate hyperpnea.

Individuals with Parkinson's Syndrome

Pathophysiology and Medical Management

Parkinson's syndrome is associated with reduced dopamine in the basal ganglia, resulting in the loss of normal reciprocal inhibitory and facilitatory neuronal input in the execution of smooth coordinated movement (Wilson et al, 1991). The clinical manifestations of the disease include stooped posture; stiffness and slowed motion; a fixed, mask-like expression; and tremor of the limbs. Patients with Parkinson's syndrome are hypertonic, rigid, and inflexible. Movement initiation is impaired and, once initiated, movement is not fluid. The patient walks with a quick, shuffling gait. These factors contribute to an increased energy cost of movement. Physical activity is restricted and function is compromised, contributing to impaired aerobic capacity, reduced movement efficiency, and hence reduced movement economy.

Although chest wall rigidity and respiratory muscle weakness are associated with a restrictive pattern of lung disease in the patient with Parkinson's syndrome (Mehta et al, 1978), obstructive type of respiratory dysfunction has been reported (e.g., reduced mid-tidal flow rates, increase airway resistance, impaired distribution of ventilation, and an increase in functional residual capacity) (Neu et al, 1966). This obstructive defect may reflect parasympathetic hyperactivity, which has been associated with the disease. The degree to which these cardiopulmonary manifestations of the disease are offset with anticholinergic drugs (used to treat rest tremor and reverse dystonia) has not been reported.

The upper extremities are rigid and held slightly abducted from the chest wall during locomotion. The rigidity and dyskinesia associated with Parkinson's syndrome lead to restricted movement and body positioning. The patient becomes deconditioned from disuse. Although the rigid, immobile chest coupled with reduced body position changes can contribute to restrictive cardiopulmonary pathology in this syndrome, chemoreceptor dysfunction has been documented (Serebrovskaya et al, 1998).

Principles of Physical Therapy Management

The goals of long-term management for the patient with Parkinson's syndrome include the following.

- Maximize the patient's quality of life, general health, and well-being through maximizing physiological reserve capacity
- Educate regarding cardiopulmonary manifestations of Parkinson's disease, self-management, smoking reduction and cessation, nutrition, weight control, airway protection, medications, infection control, and the role of a rehabilitation program
- Optimize alveolar ventilation
- Optimize lung volumes and capacities
- Optimize ventilation and perfusion matching and gas exchange
- Reduce the work of breathing
- Reduce the work of the heart
- Protect the airways from aspiration
- Facilitate mucociliary transport
- Maximize aerobic capacity and efficiency of oxygen transport
- Optimize physical endurance and exercise capacity
- Optimize general muscle strength and thereby peripheral oxygen extraction
- Design lifelong health and rehabilitation programs with the patient

Patient monitoring includes dyspnea, respiratory distress, breathing pattern (depth and frequency), arterial saturation, heart rate, blood pressure, and rate pressure product. Patients with cardiac dysfunction require ECG monitoring, particularly during exercise. Subjectively, breathlessness is assessed using a modified version of the Borg scale of perceived exertion.

Medication that is needed to maximize treatment response is administered before treatment (e.g., L-dopa). Knowledge of the type of medication, its administration route, and time to and duration of peak efficacy is essential if treatment is to be maximally efficacious. In addition, patients with Parkinson's syndrome may be on a beta-blocker to suppress action tremor. Because such medication reduces the heart rate and blood pressure, these patients are prone to orthostatic intolerance. In addition, heart rate and blood pressure responses to treatment and exercises will be less valid.

The primary interventions for maximizing cardiopulmonary function and oxygen transport in patients with Parkinson's syndrome include some combination of education, aerobic exercise, strengthening exercises, postural correction exercises, gait reeducation, chest wall mobility exercises, range of motion exercises, body positioning, breathing control and coughing maneuvers, activity pacing, and energy conservation. An ergonomic assessment of the patient's work and home environments may be indicated to minimize oxygen demand and energy expenditure in these settings. For optimal functional outcomes, prescriptive parameters focus on cross training rather than a single aerobic type exercise, and frequent, longer, less intense physical activity rather than less frequent, short, intense exercise. Flexibility exercise is prescribed to facilitate participation in regular physical activity and exercise.

Education is a principal focus of the long-term management of the patient with Parkinson's syndrome. Education includes the reinforcement of preventative health practices (e.g., infection control, airway protection, smoking reduction or cessation, cold and flu prevention, flu shots, aerobic exercise, strengthening exercise, nutrition, weight control, hydration, pacing of activities, and energy conservation).

Aerobic exercise is an essential component of the long-term management of the patient with Parkinson's syndrome to optimize the efficiency of oxygen transport overall, including maximizing alveolar ventilation and mobilizing secretions, as well as for its musculoskeletal benefits. Maximizing ventilation with mobilization is limited by the degree of hypertonicity and rigidity. Chest wall exercises include all planes of movement with a rotational component. Breathing control and coughing maneuvers are essential and should be coupled with body movement and positioning.

Individuals with Multiple Sclerosis

Pathophysiology and Medical Management

Multiple sclerosis is a demyelinating disease of the central nervous system. The focal or patchy destruction of myelin sheaths is accompanied by an inflammatory response (McFarlin & McFarland, 1982). The course of the disease consists of a variable number of exacerbations and remissions over the years from early adulthood. Exacerbations are also variable with respect to severity. The neurological deficits include visual disturbance, paresis of one or more limbs, spasticity, discoordination, ataxia, dysarthria, weak, ineffective cough, reduced perception of vibration and position sense, bowel and bladder dysfunction, and sexual dysfunction (Kasper et al, 2004). Breathing disturbances, including diaphragmatic paresis, may occur (Cooper et al, 1985). Autonomic disturbance in the form of impaired cardiovascular reflex function at rest and attenuated heart rate and blood pressure responses during exercise are relatively common in patients with multiple sclerosis (Neubauer & Gundersen, 1978; Pentland & Ewing, 1987; Senaratne et al, 1984).

Principles of Physical Therapy Management

The goals of long-term management for the patient with multiple sclerosis include the following.

- Maximize the patient's quality of life, general health, and well-being through maximizing physiological reserve capacity
- Educate regarding cardiopulmonary manifestations of multiple sclerosis, self-management, smoking reduction and cessation, nutrition, weight control, relaxation and stress management, sleep and rest, medications, infection control, and the role of a rehabilitation program
- Prescribe aids and devices as necessary to optimize function and activity
- Optimize alveolar ventilation
- Optimize lung volumes and capacities and flow rates
- Optimize ventilation and perfusion matching and gas exchange
- Reduce the work of breathing
- Reduce the work of the heart
- Protect the airways from aspiration
- Facilitate mucociliary transport
- Optimize secretion clearance
- Maximize aerobic capacity and efficiency of oxygen transport
- Optimize physical endurance and exercise capacity
- Optimize general muscle strength and thereby peripheral oxygen extraction
- Design lifelong health and rehabilitation programs with the patient

Patient monitoring includes dyspnea, respiratory distress, breathing pattern (depth and frequency), arterial saturation, cyanosis (delayed sign of desaturation), heart rate, blood pressure, and rate pressure product. Patients with cardiac dysfunction require ECG monitoring, particularly during exercise. Subjectively, fatigue can be assessed using a modified version of the Borg scale. Perceived exertion is assessed using the Borg scale.

Medication that is needed to maximize treatment response is administered before treatment (e.g., antispasticity medications). Knowledge of the type of medication, its administration route, and time to and duration of peak efficacy is essential if treatment is to be maximally efficacious. In addition, knowledge of the cardiopulmonary side effects of other medications is needed.

The primary interventions for maximizing cardiopulmonary function and oxygen transport in patients with multiple sclerosis include some combination of education, aerobic exercise, strengthening exercises (to maintain or reduce rate of decline), reduction of abnormal muscle tone, postural correction exercises, gait reeducation, chest wall mobility exercises, range of motion exercises, body positioning, breathing control and coughing maneuvers, airway clearance interventions, fatigue management, activity pacing, and energy conservation. An ergonomic assessment of the patient's work and home environments may be indicated to minimize oxygen demand and energy expenditure in these settings.

Prescriptive parameters are comparable to those for individuals with increased muscle tone; that is, frequent, less intense exercise, rather than less frequent, intense exercise that might be appropriate for someone without such a condition.

Education is a principal focus of the long-term management of the patient with multiple sclerosis. Education includes the reinforcement of preventative health practices (e.g., infection control, cold and flu prevention, flu shots, smoking reduction and cessation, nutrition, weight control, hydration, fatigue management, modified aerobic exercise, modified strengthening exercises, pacing of activities, and energy conservation). Multiple sclerosis is associated with significant fatigue. Thus activity and sleep patterns need to be assessed to ensure sleep is maximally restorative and not contributing to the patient's symptoms. By maintaining a log of activity and rest, the patient can observe relationships between these factors and identify the optimal time to rest.

Aerobic exercise is an essential component of the long-term management of the patient with multiple sclerosis to optimize the efficiency of oxygen transport overall. In mild-to-moderate cases the goals of aerobic exercise are to optimize cardiopulmonary conditioning and enhance movement economy. Optimizing cadence of walking or cycling is important to minimize discoordination, energy expenditure, and fatigue and to maximize safety. In more severe cases the goal is to maximize ventilation and gas exchange in the patient who has severe generalized muscular weakness, spasm, and excessive fatigue. Subjective parameters (i.e., fatigue and exertion) provide the basis for the intensity of the exercise program in conjunction with objective measures. Parameters, such as intensity and duration, may vary from session to session depending on the patient's general status, which tends to be variable. Aquatic exercise may be an alternative for patients whose discoordination precludes ambulation and cycling or who are troubled by heat. The use of a fan may also enhance the patient's work output.

Chest wall exercises include all planes of movement with a rotational component. Body positioning to optimize lung volumes and airflow rates is a priority. Breathing control and coughing maneuvers are coupled with body movement and positioning. If mucociliary clearance is impaired leading to secretion retention, postural drainage may need to be instituted coupled with deep breathing and coughing maneuvers.

Methods of facilitating effective coughing in patients with neuromuscular diseases are extremely important because they constitute life-preserving measures. Supported and unsupported coughing methods are described in detail in Chapters 21 and 22. Whenever possible, deep breathing and coughing are coordinated with chest wall movement to facilitate maximal inflation of the lungs before coughing and maximal exhalation of the lungs during coughing. Body positions are varied and changed frequently to simulate as much as possible shifts in alveolar volume and ventilation and perfusion that occur with normal movement and body position changes (Ray et al, 1974). In addition, body positioning is used to maximize the patient's coughing efforts.

Patients with generalized neuromuscular weakness require prophylactic management given their high risk of developing life-threatening respiratory infections and complications. Prophylaxis should include flu shots, avoiding polluted, smoky environments, smoking reduction and cessation, controlling the types of food eaten and chewing well to avoid choking, and regular deep breathing, frequent movement, and change in body positions (even just shifting and taking some deeper breaths while seated in a wheelchair) to promote mucociliary transport. An optimal time to take deep breaths and to cough is during transfers, which usually are physically exerting and stimulate hyperpnea.

Patients with multiple sclerosis often have remissions and exacerbations of their symptoms. Physical therapy focuses on all phases, with more intense treatment during stable periods. In this way it is hoped that periods between remissions are increased and exacerbations are less severe and shorter.

Individuals with Cerebral Palsy

Pathophysiology and Medical Management

Cerebral palsy results from insult to the central nervous system that usually occurs before birth (e.g., substance abuse and underoxygenation perinatally) (Kasper et al, 2004). The clinical presentation includes spasticity and residual deformity from severe muscle imbalance, hyperreflexia, and mental retardation. Although there are varying degrees of cerebral palsy severity, patients most frequently seen by the physical therapist have significant functional deficits and require long-term care. The loss of motor control and hypertonicity of peripheral muscles often restrict the mobility of patients such that they are wheelchair dependent. Loss of motor function limits physical activity and the exercise stimulus needed to maintain an aerobic stimulus and optimal aerobic capacity. Often coupled with motor deficits are cognitive deficits and mental retardation. These afflictions limit the degree to which the patient can follow instructions, perform treatments, and participate actively in a long-term rehabilitation program. Patients with cerebral palsy who are able to ambulate do so at exceptional energy expenditure both with and without walking aids (Campbell & Ball, 1978; Mossberg et al, 1990). Central neurological deficits, generalized hypertonicity, and musculoskeletal deformity contribute to increased metabolic demand for oxygen and oxygen transport.

Principles of Physical Therapy Management

The goals of long-term management for the patient with cerebral palsy include the following.

- Maximize the patient's quality of life, general health, and well-being through maximizing physiological reserve capacity

- Educate patient and/or family or care giver regarding cardiopulmonary manifestations of cerebral palsy, spasticity control, self-management, medications, nutrition, weight control, airway protection, infection control, and the role of a rehabilitation program
- Reduce spasticity to minimize undue energy cost
- Optimize alveolar ventilation
- Optimize lung volumes and capacities and flow rates
- Optimize ventilation and perfusion matching and gas exchange
- Reduce the work of breathing
- Reduce the work of the heart
- Protect the airways from aspiration
- Facilitate mucociliary transport
- Optimize secretion clearance
- Maximize aerobic capacity and efficiency of oxygen transport
- Optimize physical endurance and exercise capacity
- Optimize general muscle strength and thereby peripheral oxygen extraction
- Design lifelong health and rehabilitation programs with the patient or the family

Maximizing aerobic capacity and efficiency of oxygen transport and optimizing general muscle strength pertain to the patient with cerebral palsy that is mild in severity. Many patients seen by physical therapists have poorly controlled spasticity and marked intellectual limitations, which preclude full participation in aerobic and strengthening exercise programs. These patients are at risk for the sequelae of restricted mobility and recumbency.

Patient monitoring includes dyspnea, respiratory distress, breathing pattern (depth and frequency), arterial saturation, cyanosis (delayed sign of desaturation), heart rate, blood pressure, and rate pressure product. Unless mildly affected and not mentally incapacitated, patients with cerebral palsy are less able to provide subjective ratings of treatment response; thus the physical therapist relies particularly on clinical judgment in conjunction with the patient's objective responses to treatment.

Medication that is needed to maximize treatment response is administered before treatment (e.g., antispasticity medications). Knowledge of the type of medication, its administration route, and time to and duration of peak efficacy is essential if treatment is to be maximally efficacious.

The primary interventions for maximizing cardiopulmonary function and oxygen transport in patients with cerebral palsy include some combination of education, mobilization and coordinated activity (aerobic stimulation), strengthening exercises (strength is often difficult to assess and treat because of overwhelming spasticity), chest wall mobility exercises, range of motion exercises, body positioning, breathing control and coughing maneuvers, and airway clearance interventions.

Education is a principal focus of the long-term management of the patient with cerebral palsy. Whenever possible education is directed at the patient, but it more likely is directed at the parents and care providers. Education includes the reinforcement of preventative health practices (e.g., infection control, cold and flu prevention, flu shots, mobilization, coordinated activity, strengthening exercise, nutrition, weight control, and hydration). Individuals with cerebral palsy can be expected to have abnormal sleep patterns. First, central cerebral involvement may affect the periodicity of breathing. During sleep, the effects of such dysfunction are accentuated. Loss of normal periodic breathing and interspersed sighs impairs mucociliary transport. Secretions may accumulate and contribute to airway obstruction and areas of atelectasis. Second, individuals with cerebral palsy are unable to reposition themselves during the night in response to both cardiopulmonary and musculoskeletal stimuli. Third, patients often have poor swallowing and saliva control and thus are prone to aspiration and microatelectasis, particularly when recumbent at night. Inability to reposition themselves at night further increases the risk of aspiration and its sequelae.

Mobilization is an essential component of the long-term management of the patient with cerebral palsy in order to stimulate aerobic metabolism and optimize the efficiency of oxygen transport overall, including maximizing alveolar ventilation and mobilizing and removing secretions (Wolff et al, 1977). Maximizing ventilation with mobilization is limited if the patient has generalized spasticity. Furthermore, mobilization stimuli are selected specifically to minimize eliciting further muscle spasm. Prescriptive hydrotherapy and equinotherapy (horseback riding) can provide effective stimulation to the cardiopulmonary system in the multiply-handicapped individual and minimize the effects of spasticity. With training, coordination of ambulatory patients can be improved and aerobic energy expenditure reduced (Dresen et al, 1985). In addition, energy is conserved for performing more activity. Chest wall exercises include all planes of movement with rotation. Body positioning to optimize lung volumes and airflow rates is a priority. Breathing control and coughing maneuvers are essential and should be coupled with body movement and positioning. If mucociliary transport is impaired and leads to secretion retention, postural drainage and manual techniques may need to be instituted with appropriate monitoring to ensure they do not have a detrimental effect (Kirilloff et al, 1985).

In this patient population, clearing oral secretions and coughing maneuvers require special attention. Ventilatory strategies for facilitating effective coughing in patients with neuromuscular diseases are extremely important because they constitute life-preserving measures. Supported and unsupported coughing methods are described in detail in Chapters 23 and 24. Whenever possible, deep breathing and coughing is coupled with chest wall movement to facilitate maximal inflation of the lungs before coughing and maximal exhalation of the lungs during coughing. Body positions are varied and changed frequently to simulate as much as possible shifts in alveolar volume and ventilation and perfusion that occur with normal movement and body position changes. Microaspirations are likely a common occurrence in this patient population,

particularly at night. Nighttime positioning must be prescribed for a given patient to minimize aspiration.

Individuals with generalized neuromuscular weakness require prophylactic management given their high risk of developing life-threatening respiratory infections and complications. Prophylaxis should include flu shots, avoidance of polluted, smoky environments, control of the types of food eaten and chewing well to avoid choking, stimulation of deep breathing, airway clearance, and frequent movement and change in body positions (even just shifting and eliciting deeper breaths while seated in a wheelchair) to promote mucociliary transport. Wheelchair design and seating are also important areas of concern in which the physical therapist is actively involved.

Individuals with Spinal Cord Injury

Pathophysiology and Medical Management

The cardiopulmonary manifestations and complications of spinal cord injury are directly related to the level of the lesion (Murray & Nadel, 2000). Cardiopulmonary impairment results from the loss of supraspinal control of the respiratory muscles and the heart below the spinal cord lesion. Loss of diaphragmatic innervation results in ventilator dependency. Loss of abdominal and intercostal innervation reduces the ability to cough, mucociliary transport, and the ability to clear the airways. Denervation of the heart and orthostatism are less problematic in that the heart's autonomous function and increased responsiveness of the heart and blood vessels to circulating cathecolamines adequately compensate. The cough mechanism of people with quadriplegia is ineffective in clearing the airways (Estenne & Gorino, 1992).

Patients with quadriplegia are particularly prone to the effects of restricted mobility given the extent of their functional motor loss and sensory deficits, particularly on cardiopulmonary function (Bach, 1991). Mobilization and physical activity are essential for the patient with a spinal cord injury to maintain optimal cardiopulmonary function and oxygen transport efficiency and the optimal strength and endurance of the respiratory muscles. Patients with partial cord lesions will have a greater probability of ambulation with or without aids. Walking with aids is enormously costly in terms of energy cost (Smith et al, 1997), however, and may not be practical in daily life.

Because of the complexity and multisystem involvement of spinal cord lesions, the team works closely together. Even though the nurse may be primarily responsible for teaching and monitoring bowel and bladder routines, the physical therapist keeps informed of these because genitourinary and gastrointestinal problems can jeopardize physical therapy goals.

Principles of Physical Therapy Management

The goals of long-term management for the patient with spinal cord injury include the following.

- Maximize the patient's quality of life, general health, and well-being through maximizing physiological reserve capacity
- Educate regarding cardiopulmonary manifestations of spinal cord injury, self-management, medications, smoking reduction and cessation, nutrition, weight control, infection control, and the role of a rehabilitation program
- Ensure walking aids or wheelchair is optimal for the patient's needs to minimize energy cost, maintain optimal posture, and for safety
- Optimize alveolar ventilation
- Optimize lung volumes and capacities and flow rates
- Optimize ventilation and perfusion matching and gas exchange
- Reduce the work of breathing
- Reduce the work of the heart
- Protect the airways from aspiration
- Facilitate mucociliary transport
- Optimize secretion clearance
- Maximize aerobic capacity and efficiency of oxygen transport
- Optimize physical endurance and exercise capacity
- Optimize general muscle strength and thereby peripheral oxygen extraction
- Design lifelong health and rehabilitation programs with the patient

Patient monitoring includes dyspnea, respiratory distress, breathing pattern (depth and frequency), arterial saturation, cyanosis (delayed sign of desaturation), heart rate, blood pressure, and rate pressure product. Patients with high spinal cord injuries are somewhat more hemodynamically unstable and have more ECG irregularities than age-matched control individuals; thus their cardiopulmonary status should be monitored during treatment. Subjectively, perceived exertion is monitored using the Borg scale.

Medication that is needed to maximize treatment response is administered before treatment (e.g., antispasticity agents). Knowledge of the type of medication, its administration route, and time to and duration of peak efficacy is essential if treatment is to be maximally efficacious.

The primary interventions for maximizing cardiopulmonary function and oxygen transport in patients with spinal cord injury include some combination of education, aerobic exercise, strengthening exercises (to maintain or reduce rate of decline), postural correction exercises, chest wall mobility exercises, range of motion exercises, body positioning, breathing control and coughing maneuvers, airway clearance interventions, activity pacing, and energy conservation. An ergonomic assessment of the patient's work and home environments may be indicated to minimize oxygen demand and energy expenditure in these settings.

Education is a principal focus of the long-term management of the patient with spinal cord injury. Education includes the reinforcement of preventative health practices (e.g., infection control, cold and flu prevention, flu shots, aerobic exercise,

strengthening exercise, nutrition, weight control, hydration, pacing of activities, and energy conservation).

Aerobic exercise is an essential component of the long-term management of the patient with spinal cord injury in order to optimize the efficiency of oxygen transport overall, including maximizing alveolar ventilation and mobilizing and removing secretions. With higher lesions, exercise is usually confined to upper-extremity work in the form of wheelchair ambulation. Preservation of upper-extremity muscle function and minimization of overuse are primary goals from the outset. Patients can maintain adequate cardiopulmonary conditioning with wheelchair exercise; however, exercise prescription should be conservative to maximize the benefit-to-risk ratio of cardiopulmonary conditioning relying of upper-extremity work. Patients who are able to walk with leg braces and crutches expend considerable energy doing so. A decision must be made regarding the benefits of walking at high energy demand versus conserving energy for other activities. Chest wall exercises can be used and should include all planes of movement with a rotational component. Body positioning to optimize lung volumes and airflow rates is a priority. Breathing control and coughing maneuvers are essential and should be coupled with body movement and positioning. Coordination of respiration with aerobic activity and wheeling is taught to maximize work output.

Ventilatory muscle training has a role in the long-term rehabilitation of some patients with high spinal cord lesions. Such muscle training has long been known to increase the strength and endurance of the respiratory muscles (Gross, 1980) and may improve the functional capacity of some patients. A stronger, endurance-trained diaphragm will not fatigue as readily as an untrained diaphragm. Standardizing the resistance of the training stimulus alone, however, is not sufficient to produce a training effect. It is essential that flow rate is controlled using a gauge.

Methods of facilitating effective coughing in patients with neuromuscular diseases are extremely important because they constitute life-preserving measures. Supported and unsupported coughing methods are described in detail in Chapters 21 and 22. Whenever possible, deep breathing and coughing is coupled with chest wall movement to facilitate maximal inflation of the lungs before coughing and maximal exhalation of the lungs during coughing. Body positions are varied and changed frequently to simulate as much as possible shifts in alveolar volume and ventilation and perfusion that occur with normal movement and body position changes (Braun et al, 1984).

A comprehensive program includes stretching of the chest wall and passive range of motion exercises of the shoulder girdle. Maximal insufflations are encouraged in optimal body positions. Glossopharyngeal breathing can enable high quadriplegic patients to be freed from mechanical ventilation for hours at a time. Assisted or unassisted coughing is coordinated with deep breathing and rhythmic rocking motion. Manual assisted coughing and mechanical coughing aids, including functional electrical stimulation and insufflation-exsufflation devices, can be useful (Bach, 1991; Linder, 1993).

The pneumobelt is a device that can facilitate ventilation without a tracheostomy (Miller et al, 1988). This device counters loss of abdominal tone and helps preserve normal thoracoabdominal interaction during respiration, which is lost because of reduced ribcage compliance and increased abdominal compliance.

Patients with spinal cord injuries, particularly those with high lesions, require prophylactic management given their risk of developing life-threatening respiratory infections and complications. Prophylaxis should include flu shots, avoiding polluted, smoky environments, smoking reduction and cessation, controlling the types of food eaten and chewing well to avoid choking, regular deep breathing, airway clearance, and frequent movement and change in body positions (even just shifting and taking some deeper breaths while seated in a wheelchair is beneficial). An optimal time to take deep breaths and cough is during transfers, which usually are physically exerting and stimulate hyperpnea.

Individuals with the Chronic Effects of Poliomyelitis

Pathophysiology and Medical Management

The chronic effects of poliomyelitis affect a high proportion of survivors of poliomyelitis who contracted the disease during the epidemic of the 1950s. Three types of poliomyelitis were prevalent during the epidemic in the middle of this century, namely, spinal (the majority of cases), bulbar, and encephalitic. Half of survivors report new symptoms consistent with post polio syndrome (PPS) (see Chapter 6). New delayed symptoms include disproportionate fatigue, increased weakness, deformity, pain, reduced endurance, breathing and swallowing problems (Dean, 1991; Howard et al, 1988), and respiratory insufficiency (Lane et al, 1974). Although cardiopulmonary complications were not associated with the spinal form of poliomyelitis at onset, late-onset breathing and swallowing complications can appear as a late effect of the disease (Dean et al, 1991). In addition, these patients may be deconditioned and have poor movement economy (i.e., expend excessive energy because of postural deformities) (Dean & Ross, 1993). Thus delayed-onset cardiopulmonary complications, coupled with the effects of overuse and general deconditioning, increase the risk of cardiopulmonary compromise, reduce the ability to recover from these, and increase surgical and anesthetic risk.

Because of the nonspecific symptoms associated with PPS, it is a diagnosis of exclusion based on a detailed history.

Principles of Physical Therapy Management

The goals of long-term management for the patient with the chronic effects of poliomyelitis with or without PPS include the following.

- Maximize the patient's quality of life, general health, and well-being through maximizing physiological reserve capacity

- Educate regarding cardiopulmonary manifestations of the late sequelae of poliomyelitis, self-management, medications, smoking reduction or cessation, relaxation and stress management, rest and sleep, nutrition, weight control, infection control, orthoses, mobility and activities of daily living aids and devices, and the role of a rehabilitation program
- Ensure aids and devices provide an optimal level of support for a specific muscle or extremity, or whole body
- Optimize alveolar ventilation
- Optimize lung volumes and capacities and flow rates
- Optimize ventilation and perfusion matching and gas exchange
- Reduce the work of breathing
- Reduce the work of the heart
- Protect the airways from aspiration
- Maximize aerobic capacity and efficiency of oxygen transport
- Optimize movement economy
- Optimize physical endurance and exercise capacity
- Optimize general muscle strength and thereby peripheral oxygen extraction
- Design lifelong health and rehabilitation programs, including fall prevention strategies, with the patient,

Although there are commonalities between the management of individuals with a history of poliomyelitis with and without PPS, injudicious management of the individual with PPS can lead to further deterioration. Thus special attention is given to balancing rest with physical activity and developing modified exercise programs if they are indicated. Such programs are not indicated if an individual is exploiting maximal physiologic reserve capacity to meet the needs of each day. This individual has little reserve capacity and thus can lose functional capacity by increasing metabolic demands. With appropriate self-management and adherence to judicious recommendations, the prognosis for an individual with PPS can be favorable (Peach & Olejnik, 1991).

Patient monitoring includes dyspnea, respiratory distress, breathing pattern (depth and frequency), arterial saturation, cyanosis (delayed sign of desaturation), heart rate, blood pressure, and rate pressure product. Pain, a feature of PPS, can be subjectively assessed using an analog scale, perceived exertion is assessed using the Borg scale, and fatigue and breathlessness can also be assessed using modified versions of this scale.

Medication that is needed to maximize treatment response is administered before treatment (e.g., analgesia). Knowledge of the type of medication, its administration route, and time to and duration of peak efficacy is essential if treatment is to be maximally efficacious.

The primary interventions for maximizing cardiopulmonary function and oxygen transport in patients with PPS include some combination of education, aerobic exercise, strengthening exercises, postural correction exercises, chest wall mobility exercises, range of motion exercises, body positioning, breathing control and coughing maneuvers, activity pacing, and energy conservation. An ergonomic assessment of the patient's work and home environments may be indicated to minimize oxygen demand and energy expenditure in these settings. Aids and devices are reviewed to optimize energy expenditure (e.g., electric wheelchair or scooter versus manual wheelchair) and to reduce cardiopulmonary distress (e.g., home mechanical ventilation).

Education is a principal focus of the long-term management of the patient with the late sequelae of poliomyelitis. Education includes the reinforcement of preventative health practices (e.g., infection control, cold and flu prevention, flu shots, aerobic exercise, strengthening exercises, nutrition, weight control, hydration, pacing of activities, and energy conservation). Activity and sleep patterns must be assessed to ensure sleep is maximally restorative and not contributing to the patient's symptoms. Functional work capacity and activity tolerance may be increased by balancing activity with rest and maintaining fatigue below the patient's critical fatigue threshold (i.e., threshold requiring prolonged recovery time).

Aerobic exercise is an essential component of the long-term management of the patient with the late sequelae of poliomyelitis to optimize the efficiency of oxygen transport overall. The two principal goals of exercise are to optimize cardiopulmonary conditioning and movement economy. Maximizing ventilation with exercise is limited if the patient has severe generalized muscular weakness and increased fatigue. Disproportionate fatigue and other symptoms experienced by patients with the late sequelae of poliomyelitis have been attributed to overwork of affected and unaffected muscles, terminal axon degeneration, and impaired impulse transmission (Dean, 1991). Exercise is therefore prescribed judiciously to provide an optimal aerobic training effect without contributing to further other use abuse (i.e., prescriptive parameters based on subjective responses using semi-quantitative scales in conjunction with objective responses). Walking is the most functional type of aerobic exercise; however, aquatic exercise provides a useful medium for individuals with lower-extremity paresis, who require crutches to walk or are confined to a wheelchair. Reducing physical activity and exercise is indicated in some patients to optimize aerobic and muscle power. The effect of resting affected and unaffected muscles enhances functional capacity.

Individuals with PPS are likely to experience greater functional decline over time compared with survivors of poliomyelitis without the syndrome. The need for aids, devices, manual wheelchairs, and electric wheelchairs and scooters should be anticipated for some people. These, however, can be introduced with their intermittent use to provide rest to overused muscles and joints, minimize local and general fatigue, and preserve remaining muscle function to the greatest degree. Excessive use as well as under-use of such aids can contribute to rapid deterioration and decline. Thus the rehabilitation program includes recommendations about the appropriate use of aids and devices to optimize function, and these recommendations require periodic review.

Ventilatory strategies for facilitating effective coughing in patients with neuromuscular diseases are extremely important because they constitute a life-preserving measure. Supported and unsupported coughing methods are described in detail in Chapters 21 and 22. Whenever possible, deep breathing and coughing is coupled with chest wall movement to facilitate maximal inflation of the lungs before coughing and maximal exhalation of the lungs during coughing. Body positions are varied and changed frequently to simulate as much as possible shifts in alveolar volume and ventilation and perfusion that occur with normal movement and body position changes.

Progressive loss of pulmonary function in patients with ventilatory compromise at onset can lead to respiratory insufficiency. Comparable with other neuromuscular conditions, invasive mechanical ventilation is avoided. Promising alternatives are nasal and oral methods of noninvasive assisted mechanical ventilation (Bach et al, 1989). In addition, airway clearance can be further assisted with manual assisted coughing, glossopharyngeal breathing, mechanical exsufflation, and mechanical insufflation-exsufflation (Bach et al, 1993).

Survivors of poliomyelitis with ventilatory compromise are comparable with other patients with generalized muscle weakness. Of particular concern in this population is the necessity to establish the role of mobilization and exercise as a first line of defense in the management and prevention of cardiopulmonary dysfunction. For those patients with PPS and overuse abuse, however, additional exercise may be detrimental, though modified mobilization and exercise may be prescribed in an interval schedule (McArdle et al, 2001) (Chapter 18). The patient exercises for a period of time and then rests or reduces to a lower intensity of exercise to allow the muscles to rest. In addition to the multitude of benefits of mobilization and exercise on oxygen transport overall, these interventions also optimize respiratory muscle strength and endurance. If the patient does not recover within a few hours, the mobilization or exercise stimuli is excessive and should be modified. Chest wall mobility exercises to facilitate breathing and coughing may have a role.

Patients with generalized neuromuscular weakness require respiratory prophylactic management given their high risk of developing life-threatening respiratory infections and complications. Prophylaxis should include flu shots, avoiding polluted, smoky environments, controlling the types of food eaten and chewing well to avoid choking, regular deep breathing, airway clearance, and frequent movement and change in body positions (even just shifting and taking some deeper breaths while seated in a wheelchair is beneficial). An optimal time to take deep breaths and cough is during transfers, which usually are physically exerting and stimulate hyperpnea.

Individuals with Muscular Dystrophy

Pathophysiology and Medical Management

Individuals with muscular dystrophy and other types of degenerative neurological and muscular diseases have increased life expectancy and thus can expect prolonged morbidity. Prevention of complications as an individual becomes weaker and more limited in terms of participation in life is a priority. In addition to peripheral weakness, these conditions can lead to respiratory muscle weakness and alveolar hypoventilation (Black & Hyatt, 1971; Braun et al, 1983; Inkley et al, 1974). Vital capacity, forced expiratory volume, airflow rates, and maximum inspiratory and expiratory pressures are reduced. These patients are at risk for the development of atelectasis, impaired mucociliary transport, and pneumonia. In addition, long-term generalized muscular weakness, particularly of the thoracic cavity and abdomen, as well as restricted mobility and confinement to a wheelchair, predispose the patient to thoracic deformities (e.g., scoliosis and dropping of the ribs, and further muscle disuse). Patients with Duchenne's muscular dystrophy are susceptible to dysphagia and upper airway obstruction secondary to gag reflex depression and hypotonia of the pharyngeal structures (Murray & Nadel, 2000). These factors further compromise or threaten cardiopulmonary function and oxygen transport.

Cardiac dysfunction has also been reported in progressive muscular dystrophy (Moorman et al, 1985; Perloff et al, 1966). Although the majority of patients have no clinical evidence of cardiac dysfunction, a high proportion have abnormal ECGs at rest or during exercise and abnormal echo-cardiography and radionuclide ventriculography showing reduced left ventricular ejection fraction and abnormal ventricular wall motion. Fatty and fibrous tissue infiltrate the myocardium and conduction system, and electrical conduction is slowed. Thus subclinical cardiac involvement is prevalent in patients with muscular dystrophy and may explain sudden death in this patient population.

Chronic respiratory muscle weakness is characteristic of muscular dystrophy and other neuromuscular disorders. Because the cardiopulmonary system is seldom stressed due to musculoskeletal dysfunction in these patients, respiratory muscle weakness is seldom detected. Such weakness is significant, however, in that it contributes to several other serious problems, including thoracic mechanical abnormalities, diffuse microatelectasis, reduced lung compliance, a weak cough with impaired mucociliary transport and secretion accumulation, ventilation and perfusion imbalance, and nocturnal hypoxemia (Smith et al, 1987; Smith et al, 1989). Progressive respiratory muscle weakness increases the risk of respiratory muscle fatigue and failure (Macklem & Roussos, 1977).

The severity of disease is not consistently correlated with compromised pulmonary function; thus cardiopulmonary function must be assessed individually in each patient (Hapke et al, 1972). Patients with mild-to-moderate involvement of peripheral muscles may exhibit disproportionate respiratory compromise (Kilburn et al, 1959). This may be explained by differential changes in the degree of involvement of the diaphragm and the abdominal and intercostal muscles (Nakano et al, 1976). Over time, musculoskeletal changes of the chest wall lead to spinal deformity and stiffness with loss of its elastic recoil. Chronic alveolar hypoventilation leads

to respiratory insufficiency and the need for ventilatory assistance. With progressive respiratory insufficiency, nocturnal hypoventilation with hypercapnia and hypoxemia develop (Bach et al, 1987). Nocturnal respiratory support should be considered early to postpone the need for intubation and mechanical ventilation, which is associated with a poor prognostic outcome in patients who have chronically reduced vital capacities and weak cough.

Clinically, patients with muscular dystrophy present with low functional capacity commensurate with the extent of muscle weakness and impaired cardiopulmonary function, including alveolar hypoventilation, orthopnea (shortness of breath on reclining), impaired mucociliary transport, difficulty clearing secretions, and increased work of breathing. Abdominal muscle strength provides an index of pulmonary function in that it is correlated with vital capacity and expiratory flow rates (Hapke et al, 1972). The significant progressive functional loss associated with Duchenne's muscular dystrophy increases the patient's susceptibility to the sequelae of restricted mobility, including cardiopulmonary deconditioning and reduced efficiency of oxygen transport, circulatory stasis, muscular weakness, and bone loss.

Improved medical management of the complications of myopathies has significantly increased the life expectancy of patients, such as those with Duchenne's muscular dystrophy, over the past 20 years. With advancing age, further complications will arise from age-related changes in cardiopulmonary function (Dean, 1993; Leblanc et al, 1970). Thus in the years ahead an increasing number of patients with myopathies will be requiring cardiopulmonary management and prophylaxis.

Principles of Physical Therapy Management

The goals of long-term management for the patient with muscular dystrophy are to reduce the impact of progressive debility and prolonged morbidity throughout their longer life spans. Respiratory complications may advance from mild respiratory distress to the need for nocturnal noninvasive mechanical ventilation. Respiratory failure is the primary cause of death.

The long-term goals include the following.

- Maximize the patient's quality of life, general health, and well-being through maximizing physiological reserve capacity
- Educate about cardiopulmonary manifestations of muscle dystrophy, self-management, medications, nutrition, weight control, smoking reduction and cessation, airway protection, infection control, the role of a rehabilitation program, and the eventual need for mechanical ventilatory support
- Optimize aerobic capacity with a balance of judicious exercise, energy conservation, and rest
- Optimize capacity with judiciously prescribed and appropriately introduced aids and devices consistent with the patient's changing needs (e.g., walking aids, wheelchair design, and dressing and activities of daily living aids)

- Optimize alveolar ventilation
- Optimize lung volumes and capacities and flow rates
- Optimize ventilation and perfusion matching and gas exchange
- Protect the airways from aspiration
- Facilitate mucociliary transport
- Reduce the work of breathing
- Reduce the work of the heart
- Maximize aerobic capacity and efficiency of oxygen transport
- Optimize physical endurance and exercise capacity
- Optimize general muscle strength and thereby peripheral oxygen extraction
- Design lifelong health and rehabilitation programs with the patient that are in accordance with the anticipated loss of physical function

Patient monitoring includes dyspnea, respiratory distress, breathing pattern (depth and frequency), arterial saturation, cyanosis (delayed sign of desaturation), heart rate, blood pressure, and rate pressure product. Patients with cardiac dysfunction need to be cleared by a cardiologist before starting a rehabilitation program, particularly when it involves a mobilization or exercise program, to refine the prescriptive parameters of the program. If supplemental oxygen is used, the fraction of inspired oxygen (FIO_2) administered is recorded. Subjectively, breathlessness is assessed using a modified version of the Borg scale of perceived exertion. Assessment of nighttime and daytime cardiopulmonary function is needed because respiratory insufficiency often begins with nocturnal hypoxemia in patients with Duchenne's muscular dystrophy.

Medication that is needed to maximize treatment response is administered before treatment. Knowledge of the type of medication, its administration route, and time to and duration of peak efficacy is essential if treatment is to be maximally efficacious.

The primary interventions for maximizing cardiopulmonary function and oxygen transport in patients with muscular dystrophy include some combination of education; mobilization, primarily in the form of functional activities; strengthening exercises, primarily in the form of functional activities (to maintain strength or reduce rate of decline); ventilatory muscle training; postural correction exercises; chest wall mobility exercises; range of motion exercises; deformity prevention; body positioning; breathing control and coughing maneuvers; airway clearance interventions; activity pacing; and energy conservation. An ergonomic assessment of the patient's work and home environments may be indicated to minimize oxygen demand and energy expenditure in these settings. Such an assessment includes review of aids and devices (e.g., wheelchair type, weight, and size and noninvasive mechanical ventilation). Aids and devices are selected to minimize energy demand such that energy is conserved for other activities and undue fatigue is reduced.

The use of supplemental oxygen depends on the severity of the disease. Some patients have no need for supplemental oxygen, some need it only during exercise, and some patients require continuous oxygen with proportionately more delivered during activity and exercise compared with rest.

Education is a principal focus of the long-term management of the patient with muscular dystrophy. Education includes the reinforcement of preventative health practices (e.g., infection control, cold and flu prevention, flu shots, aerobic exercise, strengthening exercises, nutrition, weight control, hydration, pacing of activities, and energy conservation). Weight control is an important goal in patients with chronic neuromuscular diseases because they have the least capacity to compensate for the cardiopulmonary sequelae of obesity (Alexander, 1985). Obstructive sleep apnea is related to hypotonia of the upper airway musculature and obesity. Thus activity and sleep patterns must be assessed to ensure sleep is maximally restorative and not contributing to the patient's symptoms.

Mobilization is an essential component of long-term management of the patient with muscular dystrophy in order to optimize the efficiency of oxygen transport overall and minimize the sequelae of restricted mobility. Maximizing ventilation with mobilization is limited if the patient has severe generalized muscular weakness and increased fatigue. Functional activities provide the basis for the mobilization prescription. Although heavy resistive strengthening exercise has been advocated for these patients (Vignos & Watkins, 1966), a conservative approach including an exercise program based on functional goals and energy conservation is more justifiable physiologically. Chest wall mobility exercises include all planes of movement combined with a rotational component. Body positioning to optimize lung volumes and airflow rates is a priority. Breathing control and coughing maneuvers are coupled with body movement and positioning. If mucociliary transport is impaired and leads to secretion accumulation, which is refractory to mobilization and body positioning, it may be necessary to institute postural drainage coupled with deep breathing and coughing maneuvers.

Although the primary factor contributing to respiratory compromise is respiratory muscle weakness, the capacity of the respiratory muscles to respond to resistive loading is limited. Ventilatory muscle training may have some role in selected patients, however, particularly children (Adams & Chandler, 1974; Pardy & Leith, 1984). Improved respiratory muscle endurance and strength may have a generalized effect on functional capacity (Reid & Warren, 1984). The effect of walking alone, however, may be superior to the effect of ventilatory muscle training on ventilatory muscle strength and endurance. Thus ventilatory muscle training should be used selectively to elicit effects over and above those resulting from functional activities such as walking, given the multisystem and functional benefits of walking.

Patients with signs of ventilatory muscle fatigue, as opposed to weakness, benefit from ventilatory support at night. Rest of the respiratory muscles at night with continuous positive airway pressure or bi-level positive airway pressure optimizes their function during the daytime.

Methods of facilitating effective coughing in individuals with neuromuscular diseases are extremely important because they constitute life-preserving measures. Supported and unsupported coughing methods are described in detail in Chapters 21 and 22. Patients on noninvasive ventilatory support who are unable to generate adequate peak cough expiratory flow rates can benefit from manual assisted coughing and mechanical insufflation-exsufflation, thereby minimizing the need for endotracheal suctioning (Bach, 1993; Barrach et al, 1952). Tracheostomy is delayed as long as possible. Significantly reduced maximal insufflation capacity, however, is an indication for tracheostomy.

Whenever possible, deep breathing and coughing are coupled with chest wall movement. This facilitates maximal inflation of the lungs before coughing by increasing pulmonary compliance (Ferris & Pollard, 1960) and maximal exhalation of the lungs during coughing. Body positions are varied and changed frequently to simulate shifts in alveolar volume and ventilation and perfusion that occur with normal movement and body position changes. Glossopharyngeal breathing is a nonmechanical method of assisting ventilation. The patient is taught to use the tongue and pharyngeal muscles to swallow boluses of air past the vocal cords and into the trachea (Bach et al, 1987). The efficiency of training is monitored with spirometry to ensure the patient is able to achieve acceptable vital capacities. Some patients are able to support their ventilation, ventilator-free, for several hours in a day.

One intervention that is prolonging the life of patients with muscular dystrophy, as well as of patients with other progressive neuromuscular diseases, is the use of mechanical ventilatory support (Bach, 1992; Curran, 1981). Home mechanical ventilation provides a noninvasive method of providing positive airway pressure through an oral or nasal mask. This provides considerable advantage over invasive, full body or tracheostomy ventilatory support. Used in conjunction with an insufflation-exsufflation device, pulmonary complications can be minimized and life expectancy increased. Other forms of noninvasive mechanical ventilation include intermittent abdominal pressure ventilation, rocking bed, negative pressure tank ventilator, and chest shell ventilator. The type of ventilation is determined individually based on the indications for ventilation and the patient's status. The use of ventilatory aids as a component of a comprehensive rehabilitation program maintains pulmonary compliance and cough efficacy. Introduction of these devices early will facilitate increased use as the respiratory muscles progressively weaken. These aids are introduced to meet the individual's needs, and changed over time. Excessive use or dependence can contribute to deterioration.

Patients with generalized neuromuscular weakness require prophylactic management because of their high risk of developing life-threatening respiratory infections and complications. Prophylaxis should include flu shots, avoiding polluted, smoky environments, smoking reduction and cessation, controlling the types of food eaten and chewing well to avoid choking, and regular deep breathing, frequent movement, and change in body positions (even just shifting and taking some deep breaths while seated in a wheelchair) to promote mucociliary transport. An optimal time to take deep breaths and to cough is during transfers, which usually are physically exerting and stimulate hyperpnea. Wheelchair design is important for comfort, biomechanical and metabolic efficiency, and reducing unnecessary energy expenditure.

INDIVIDUALS WITH MUSCULOSKELETAL CONDITIONS

Individuals with Thoracic Deformities

Pathophysiology and Medical Management

Respiratory insufficiency can result from abnormalities of the chest wall secondary to congenital deformity, acquired neuromuscular disease, and trauma (Bates, 1989; Murray & Nadel, 2000). Congenital deformity of the chest wall reduces the mobility of the bony thorax, thereby increasing the work of breathing. Shallow, rapid breathing often results. Minute ventilation is increased at the expense of alveolar ventilation. Severe deformity leads to compression of the mediastinal structures. The heart can be displaced and rotated, impeding its mechanical function. Examples of chronic deformities that impinge on pulmonary function are kyphoscoliosis secondary to poliomyelitis, tuberculous osteomyelitis, and other causes and ankylosing spondylitis. Other examples of deformity include traumatic injury of the vertebral column, ribs, and sternum. Routine cardiopulmonary assessment should include a musculoskeletal examination of the spinal column and thoracic cavity.

Normal pulmonary function and gas exchange depend on symmetry of cardiopulmonary anatomy and physiological function. Asymmetry of the chest wall interferes with normal lung mechanics, regional gradients of ventilation and perfusion in the lungs, and the distribution of inspired gas (Bake et al, 1976; Sinha & Bergofsky, 1972). Significant decrease in lung compliance and increase in work performed against the elastic resistance of the lung are characteristic of kyphoscoliosis. Altered pressure gradients and uneven lung movement during the respiratory cycle may contribute to altered lung water balance and impaired lymphatic drainage. The effects of physiological dead space and shunt may be magnified, producing hypoxemia and hypercapnia. With severe chest deformity, a cycle of respiratory acidosis, pulmonary hypertension, and right heart failure can result in a life-threatening situation.

Principles of Physical Therapy Management

The goals of long-term management for the patient with thoracic deformity include the following.

- Maximize the patient's quality of life, general health, and well-being through maximizing physiological reserve capacity
- Educate regarding cardiopulmonary manifestations of thoracic deformity, self-management, medications, nutrition, weight control, infection control, smoking reduction and cessation, and the role of a rehabilitation program

- Optimize alveolar ventilation
- Optimize lung volumes and capacities and flow rates
- Optimize ventilation and perfusion matching and gas exchange
- Reduce the work of breathing
- Reduce the work of the heart
- Protect the airways from aspiration
- Facilitate mucociliary transport
- Optimize secretion clearance
- Maximize aerobic capacity and efficiency of oxygen transport
- Optimize movement economy
- Optimize physical endurance and exercise capacity
- Optimize general muscle strength and thereby peripheral oxygen extraction
- Design lifelong health and rehabilitation programs with the patient

Treatment is directed at the underlying problem contributing to threatened or impaired oxygen transport. In addition, these underlying problems that limit the individual's activities and participation are addressed primarily, with the exception of life-threatening impairments.

Patient monitoring includes dyspnea, respiratory distress, breathing pattern (depth and frequency), arterial saturation, cyanosis (delayed sign of desaturation), heart rate, blood pressure, and rate pressure product. Patients with cardiac dysfunction require ECG monitoring particularly during exercise. Subjectively, perceived exertion is assessed using the Borg scale, and breathlessness is assessed using a modified version of this scale.

The primary interventions for maximizing cardiopulmonary function and oxygen transport in patients with thoracic deformity include some combination of education, aerobic exercise, strengthening exercises, postural correction exercises, gait reeducation, chest wall mobility exercises, range of motion exercises, body positioning, breathing control and coughing maneuvers, airway clearance interventions, activity pacing, and energy conservation. An ergonomic assessment of the patient's work and home environments may be indicated to minimize oxygen demand and energy expenditure in these settings.

Education is a principal focus of the long-term management of the patient with thoracic deformity. Education includes the reinforcement of preventative health practices (e.g., infection control, cold and flu prevention, flu shots, smoking reduction or cessation, aerobic exercise, strengthening exercises, nutrition, weight control, and hydration).

Aerobic exercise is an essential component of the long-term management of the patient with thoracic deformity in order to optimize the efficiency of oxygen transport overall. Abnormal postural alignment may contribute to excessive energy cost and reduced movement economy. Improving alignment will help offset this effect. In severe cases, surgical correction is indicated.

Maximizing ventilation with exercise in patients with severe deformity may be limited. Optimizing alignment to minimize the cardiopulmonary limitations of the deformity during physical activity, exercise, and rest is a priority. Chest wall exercises include all planes of movement with a rotational component. Body positioning to optimize lung volumes and airflow rates is a priority. Breathing control and coughing maneuvers are essential and should be coupled with body movement and positioning. If mucociliary transport is impaired leading to secretion retention, postural drainage may need to be instituted, coupled with deep breathing and coughing maneuvers.

Ventilatory muscle training may have a role in the management of patients with reduced inspiratory pressures and associated decreases in total lung capacity and hypoxemia.

Methods of facilitating effective coughing in patients with musculoskeletal deformity are extremely important because they constitute life-preserving measures. Supported and unsupported coughing methods are described in detail in Chapters 21 and 22. Whenever possible, deep breathing and coughing is coupled with chest wall movement to facilitate maximal inflation of the lungs before and maximal exhalation during coughing. Body positions are varied and changed frequently to simulate as much as possible shifts in alveolar volume and ventilation and perfusion that occur with normal movement and body position changes.

Patients with chest wall deformities secondary to neuromuscular conditions require prophylactic management because of their high risk of developing life-threatening respiratory infections and complications. Prophylaxis should include flu shots, avoidance of polluted, smoky environments, smoking reduction and cessation, control of the types of food eaten and chewing well to avoid choking, regular deep breathing, airway clearance, and frequent movement and change in body positions (even just shifting and taking some deep breaths while seated in a wheelchair is beneficial). An optimal time to take deep breaths and cough is during transfers, which usually are physically exerting and stimulate hyperpnea.

Individuals with Osteoporosis

Pathophysiology and Medical Management

Osteoporosis is a condition associated with reduced bone mass per unit volume and appears to be on the increase (Smith et al, 1991) (see Chapter 1). Age-related bone loss begins earlier and accelerates faster in women, particularly after menopause, than men. Lifestyle factors, such as diet, exercise, and smoking, have a significant role in reducing bone mass. Caffeine has also been implicated as a contributing factor to bone loss secondary to increasing urinary calcium loss.

Osteoporosis is classified as idiopathic osteoporosis unassociated with other conditions, osteoporosis associated with other conditions (e.g., malabsorption, calcium deficiency, immobilization, or metabolic bone disease), osteoporosis as a feature of an inherited condition (e.g., osteogenica imperfecta or Marfan's syndrome), paralytic conditions prohibiting weight bearing and activity, and osteoporosis associated with other conditions but with a pathogenesis that is not understood (e.g., rheumatoid arthritis, alcoholism, diabetes mellitus, or chronic airflow limitation) (Kasper et al, 2004).

The most common clinical features are vertebral pain and spinal deformity resulting from vertebral compression and collapse. Vertebral bodies tend to collapse anteriorly, contributing to cervical lordosis, thoracic kyphosis, postural slumping, and loss of height. Acute episodes may be relieved by restricted mobility. Straining and sudden changes in position can exacerbate an acute episode. Cardiopulmonary complications of osteoporosis are secondary to spinal deformity, chest wall rigidity, and cardiopulmonary deconditioning resulting from restricted mobility. Vertebral compression fractures are also a feature of advanced osteoporosis. Collapse of the anterior surfaces of the vertebrae leads to kyphosis.

Osteoporosis is a condition associated with aging and older age groups. The pain of acute episodes leads to periods of restricted mobility and significant cardiopulmonary dysfunction in older persons (Dean, 1993; Dean, 2001). Exercise that is weight bearing and loads the muscles around bone maintains bone density and decelerates bone loss and thus has a central role in preserving bone health. Generally, the growth and remodeling of bone depends highly on the exercise prescription parameters (e.g., type of exercise, intensity, duration, and frequency). Bone mineral content is more closely related to cardiopulmonary conditioning than physical activity level. Furthermore, any detrimental effect of exercise on osteoporosis appears to relate more to malalignment and injury rather than activity itself.

The primary physiological mechanism underlying osteopenia and osteoporosis is negative calcium balance. Loss of calcium is associated with lack of exercise, smoking, alcohol consumption, consumption of caffeine, and meat consumption. Calcium supplementation is only part of the remedy as calcium loss may be the greater concern.

Principles of Physical Therapy Management

The etiology of osteoporosis is diverse; thus management must consider the underlying pathophysiology and that several factors may be contributing to the presentation of osteoporosis in the same patient.

The goals of long-term management for the patient with osteoporosis include the following.

- Maximize the patient's quality of life, general health, and well-being through maximizing physiological reserve capacity
- Educate regarding cardiopulmonary manifestations of osteoporosis, risk factors and preventive strategies, self-management, medications, nutrition, weight control, smoking reduction and cessation, infection control, and the role of a rehabilitation program
- Optimize alveolar ventilation
- Optimize lung volumes and capacities and flow rates
- Optimize ventilation and perfusion matching and gas exchange

- Facilitate mucociliary transport
- Maximize aerobic capacity and efficiency of oxygen transport
- Optimize physical endurance and exercise capacity
- Optimize general muscle strength and thereby peripheral oxygen extraction
- Reduce risk of falls, and teach fall prevention strategies
- Design lifelong health and rehabilitation programs with the patient

Patient monitoring includes heart rate, blood pressure, and rate pressure product. Patients with cardiac dysfunction require ECG monitoring, particularly during exercise. Subjectively, pain and discomfort are assessed with an analog scale or modified Borg scale, and perceived exertion is assessed using the Borg scale. These patients also require serial bone density assessments conducted over time. It is essential to obtain a bone density assessment early for reference over time.

Medication that is needed to maximize treatment response is administered before treatment (e.g., analgesics). Knowledge of the type of medication, its administration route, and time to and duration of peak efficacy is essential if treatment is to be maximally efficacious.

The primary interventions for maximizing cardiopulmonary function and oxygen transport in patients with osteoporosis include some combination of education, aerobic weight-bearing exercise, strengthening exercises, chest wall mobility exercises, range of motion exercises, activity pacing, and energy conservation. An ergonomic assessment of the patient's work and home environments may be indicated to minimize oxygen demand and energy expenditure in these settings.

Education is a principal focus of the long-term management of the patient with osteoporosis. Education includes the reinforcement of preventative health practices (e.g., infection control, cold and flu prevention, flu shots, smoking reduction and cessation, weight-bearing aerobic exercise, strengthening exercises, range of motion exercises, nutrition, weight control, hydration, pacing of activities, and energy conservation).

Aerobic and strength training are essential components of the long-term management of the individual with osteoporosis to optimize the efficiency of oxygen transport overall. Upright, weight-bearing aerobic exercise is essential to maintain bone density or reduce the rate of bone loss. Maximizing ventilation with exercise is limited if the patient has severe generalized muscular weakness and increased fatigue. Balance problems have also been identified in patients with osteoporosis, and these need to be addressed to minimize the risk of falling and its severe complications.

Chest wall exercises may have a role and include all planes of movement with a rotational component. Breathing control and coughing maneuvers are essential and should be coupled with body movement and positioning. Straining, Valsalva maneuvers, and jarring activity and exercise are contraindicated.

Methods of facilitating effective coughing in patients with osteoporosis are extremely important because they constitute life-preserving measures. Some patients fracture ribs and vertebrae during coughing. Patients at risk should rely on huffing maneuvers that do not require closing the glottis and do not generate high intrathoracic pressures (Hietpas et al, 1979).

INDIVIDUALS WITH COLLAGEN VASCULAR/CONNECTIVE TISSUE DISEASES

Individuals with Systemic Lupus Erythematosus

Pathophysiology and Medical Management

Systemic lupus erythematosus (SLE) is a condition characterized by the presence of multiple antibodies that contribute to immunologically mediated tissue inflammation and damage (Segal et al, 1985). The condition affects the major organ systems, including the central nervous, musculoskeletal, pulmonary, vascular, and renal systems. Symptoms include arthralgic and myalgic stiffness, pain, and fatigue.

The cardiopulmonary manifestations of SLE include atelectasis, which results from inflammation of the alveolar walls and perivascular and peribronchial connective tissue, effusions secondary to lung infarction, reduced surface tension, and splinting secondary to pleuritic pain. Other manifestations include pleuritis with or without effusion, pneumonitis, interstitial fibrosis, pulmonary hypertension, diaphragmatic dysfunction, pulmonary hemorrhage, systemic hypertension, myocarditis, constrictive pericarditis, dysrhythmias, tamponade, pericardial pain, arteritis, and defects of the mitral and aortic valves (Dickey & Myers, 1997). Other manifestations that affect cardiopulmonary function include anemia, leukopenia, thrombocytopenia, thrombosis, splenomegaly, ascitis, gastrointestinal bleeding, nephritis, and renal insufficiency (Kasper et al, 2004).

Principles of Physical Therapy Management

The goals of long-term management for the patient with SLE include the following.

- Maximize the patient's quality of life, general health, and well-being through maximizing physiological reserve capacity
- Educate regarding cardiopulmonary manifestations of SLE, self-management, nutrition, weight control, smoking reduction and cessation, medications, infection control, stress management, and the role of a rehabilitation program
- Optimize alveolar ventilation
- Optimize lung volumes and capacities and flow rates
- Optimize ventilation and perfusion matching and gas exchange
- Reduce the work of breathing
- Reduce the work of the heart
- Protect the airways from aspiration
- Facilitate mucociliary transport
- Optimize secretion clearance
- Maximize aerobic capacity and efficiency of oxygen transport
- Optimize physical endurance and exercise capacity

- Optimize general muscle strength and thereby peripheral oxygen extraction
- Design lifelong health and rehabilitation programs with the patient

Patient monitoring includes dyspnea, respiratory distress, breathing pattern (depth and frequency), arterial saturation, cyanosis (delayed sign of desaturation), heart rate, blood pressure, and rate pressure product. Patients with cardiac dysfunction should be cleared by a cardiologist before being prescribed an exercise program. Subjectively, discomfort, pain, fatigue, and breathlessness are assessed using analog scales or modified versions of the Borg scale, and perceived exertion is assessed using the Borg scale.

Medication that is needed to maximize treatment response is administered before treatment (e.g., analgesic and anti-inflammatory agents). Knowledge of the type of medication, its administration route, and time to and duration of peak efficacy is essential if treatment is to be maximally efficacious.

The primary interventions for maximizing cardiopulmonary function and oxygen transport in patients with SLE include some combination of education, aerobic exercise, strengthening exercises, postural correction exercises, chest wall mobility exercises, range of motion exercises, body positioning, breathing control and coughing maneuvers, airway clearance interventions, activity pacing, and energy conservation. An ergonomic assessment of the patient's work and home environments may be indicated to minimize oxygen demand and energy expenditure in these settings.

Education is a principal focus of the long-term management of the patient with SLE. Education includes the reinforcement of preventative health practices (e.g., infection control, cold and flu prevention, flu shots, smoking reduction or cessation, aerobic exercise, strengthening exercises, nutrition, weight control, hydration, pacing of activities, and energy conservation). An ergonomic assessment of the patient's work and home environments may be indicated to minimize oxygen demand and energy expenditure in these settings.

Aerobic exercise is an essential component of the long-term management of the patient with SLE in order to optimize the efficiency of oxygen transport overall, including maximizing alveolar ventilation and mobilizing and removing secretions. Parameters of the exercise prescription are based on subjective responses (e.g., discomfort, pain, breathlessness, and perceived exertion in conjunction with objective responses). Optimal types of aerobic exercise include walking and cycling. Aquatic exercise may be preferable for patients with musculoskeletal involvement that precludes walking and cycling. Chest wall exercises can be used and should include all planes of movement with a rotational component. Body positioning to optimize lung volumes and airflow rates is a priority. Breathing control and coughing maneuvers are essential and should be coupled with body movement and positioning. If mucociliary transport is impaired, leading to secretion retention, it may be necessary to institute postural drainage coupled with deep breathing and coughing maneuvers.

Individuals with Scleroderma

Pathophysiology and Medical Management

Scleroderma is characterized by the overproduction of collagen and progressive fibrosis of cutaneous and subcutaneous tissues (Gray, 1996). The cardiopulmonary manifestations of this condition result in interstitial pulmonary fibrosis with significantly reduced vital capacity, diffusing capacity, and arterial oxygen tension (Bates, 1989; Kasper et al, 2004). Reduced static compliance is the primary mechanical deficit. Pulmonary hypertension may be a complicating factor. Broncoalveolar lavage is consistent with an acute inflammatory process. Cardiomyopathy is associated with ischemia, areas of infarction, and myocardial fibrosis (Gray, 1996). Fibrosis of the conduction system predisposes the patient to conduction defects and dysrhythmias. Other cardiopulmonary manifestations include pericarditis with or without effusion and pulmonary and systemic hypertension from renal involvement. Half of patients with scleroderma have renal involvement including intimal hyperphasia, fibrinous necrosis of the afferent arterioles, and thickening of the glomerular basement membrane. Fibrotic changes and stenoses occur in the small arteries and arterioles systemically. Similar changes in the lymphatic vessels may obliterate lymph flow.

Esophageal involvement contributes to regurgitation of gastric contents, which is exacerbated when the patient is recumbent or bends over. Bloating and abdominal discomfort may reflect paralytic ileus and intestinal obstruction. Ascites and fluid accumulation in the gut increases abdominal pressure and encroaches on diaphragmatic motion.

Principles of Physical Therapy Management

The goals of long-term management for the patient with scleroderma include the following.

- Maximize the patient's quality of life, general health, and well-being through maximizing physiological reserve capacity
- Educate regarding cardiopulmonary manifestations of scleroderma, self-management, nutrition, weight control, smoking reduction or cessation, medications, infection control, stress management, and the role of a rehabilitation program
- Optimize alveolar ventilation
- Optimize lung volumes and capacities and flow rates
- Optimize ventilation and perfusion matching and gas exchange
- Reduce the work of breathing
- Reduce the work of the heart
- Protect the airways from aspiration
- Facilitate mucociliary transport
- Optimize secretion clearance
- Maximize aerobic capacity and efficiency of oxygen transport
- Optimize physical endurance and exercise capacity

- Optimize general muscle strength and thereby peripheral oxygen extraction
- Design lifelong health and rehabilitation programs with the patient

Patient monitoring includes dyspnea, respiratory distress, breathing pattern (depth and frequency), arterial saturation, cyanosis (delayed sign of desaturation), heart rate, blood pressure, and rate pressure product. Patients with cardiac dysfunction require ECG monitoring, particularly during exercise. If supplemental oxygen is used, the FIO_2 administered is recorded. Subjectively, breathlessness is assessed using a modified version of the Borg scale of perceived exertion, and perceived exertion is assessed using the Borg scale.

Medication that is needed to maximize treatment response is administered before treatment (e.g., immunosuppressive agents and antiplatelet therapy). Knowledge of the type of medication, its administration route, and time to and duration of peak efficacy is essential if treatment is to be maximally efficacious.

The primary interventions for maximizing cardiopulmonary function and oxygen transport in patients with scleroderma include some combination of education, aerobic exercise, strengthening exercises, postural correction exercises, chest wall mobility exercises, range of motion exercises, body positioning, breathing control and coughing maneuvers, airway clearance interventions, activity pacing, and energy conservation. An ergonomic assessment of the patient's work and home environments may be indicated to minimize oxygen demand and energy expenditure in these settings.

Patients with esophageal involvement are not treated or exercised immediately after a meal. These patients have frequent, small meals, antacids between meals, and do not lie down for a few hours after eating. When recumbent, these patients have the head of bed elevated to minimize the risk of aspiration of gastric contents.

Education is a principal focus of the long-term management of the patient with scleroderma. Education includes the reinforcement of preventive health practices (e.g., infection control, cold and influenza prevention, influenza shots, smoking reduction and cessation, aerobic exercise, strengthening exercise, range-of-motion exercises, nutrition, weight control, hydration, pacing of activities, and energy conservation). An ergonomic assessment of the patient's work and home environments may be indicated to minimize oxygen demand and energy expenditure in these settings.

Aerobic exercise is an essential component of the long-term management of the patient with scleroderma to optimize the efficiency of oxygen transport overall. The exercise program is modified according to the signs and symptoms (see Chapter 25). Chest wall exercises can be used and should include all planes of movement with a rotational component. Body positioning to optimize lung volumes and airflow rates is a priority. Breathing control and coughing maneuvers are essential and should be coupled with body movement and positioning. If mucociliary transport is impaired and leads to secretion retention, it may be necessary to institute postural drainage coupled with deep breathing and coughing maneuvers.

Individuals with Ankylosing Spondylitis

Pathophysiology and Medical Management

Ankylosing spondylitis results in reduced total lung capacity, vital capacity, and inspiratory muscle function (Lisboa et al, 1985; Rosenow et al, 1977). Ventilatory capacity is preserved given that the respiratory muscles are not involved. The condition can result in spinal and chest wall rigidity; thus there is greater reliance on diaphragmatic contribution to ventilation (84%) compared with healthy persons (68%) (Hoeppner et al, 1984). The patient with ankylosing spondylitis has an increased dependence on diaphragmatic function and therefore is at risk if administered respiratory depressant medications or if he or she undergoes thoracic or upper abdominal surgery (Grimby et al, 1974). These changes can lead to an increased respiratory rate during exercise to meet ventilatory demands. In combination with impaired respiratory mechanics, the work of breathing can increase.

During exercise, patients with ankylosing spondylitis show minimal chest wall expansion compared with healthy persons (Elliott et al, 1985). Although peak workload is reduced, diaphragmatic fatigue is more likely to be the limiting factor than ventilatory capacity, ventilation-perfusion mismatch, or abnormal blood gases.

Principles of Physical Therapy Management

The goals of long-term management for the patient with ankylosing spondylitis include the following.

- Maximize the patient's quality of life, general health, and well-being through maximizing physiological reserve capacity
- Educate regarding cardiopulmonary manifestations of ankylosing spondylitis, self-management, nutrition, weight control, infection control, smoking reduction and cessation, and the role of a rehabilitation program
- Optimize alveolar ventilation
- Optimize lung volumes and capacities and flow rates
- Optimize ventilation and perfusion matching and gas exchange
- Facilitate mucociliary transport
- Maximize aerobic capacity and efficiency of oxygen transport
- Optimize spinal mobility
- Optimize physical endurance and exercise capacity
- Optimize general muscle strength and thereby peripheral oxygen extraction
- Design lifelong health and rehabilitation programs with the patient

Patient monitoring includes dyspnea, respiratory distress, breathing pattern (depth and frequency), arterial saturation, cyanosis (delayed sign of desaturation), heart rate, blood pressure, and rate pressure product.

The primary interventions for maximizing cardiopulmonary function and oxygen transport in patients with ankylosing spondylitis include some combination of education, exercise, strengthening exercises, ventilatory muscle training, postural correction exercises, gait reeducation, chest wall mobility exercises, range of motion exercises, body positioning, breathing control and coughing maneuvers, pacing, and energy conservation. An ergonomic assessment of the patient's work and home environments may be indicated to minimize oxygen demand and energy expenditure in these settings.

Education is a principal focus of the long-term management of the patient with ankylosing spondylitis. Education includes the reinforcement of preventative health practices (e.g., smoking reduction or cessation, infection control, cold and flu prevention, flu shots, smoking reduction and cessation, aerobic exercise, strengthening exercises, nutrition, weight control, and hydration).

Aerobic exercise is an essential component of the long-term management of the patient with ankylosing spondylitis in order to optimize the efficiency of oxygen transport overall. Maximizing ventilation with mobilization is limited if the patient has extreme spinal rigidity. Chest wall exercises can be used and should include all planes of movement with a rotational component. Body positioning to optimize lung volumes and airflow rates is a priority. Breathing control and coughing maneuvers are essential and should be coupled with body movement and positioning. Ventilatory muscle training in conjunction with exercise may have some additional benefit in maximizing aerobic capacity.

Consistent with the physical activity/exercise pyramid recommendations of daily exercise, individuals with ankylosing spondylitis can benefit from frequent, prolonged, low-intensity cross training to offset the potential for loss of flexibility and range.

Individuals with Rheumatoid Arthritis

Pathophysiology and Medical Management

Rheumatoid arthritis (RA) is a multisystemic condition that is associated with well-documented cardiopulmonary and cardiovascular effects, including pleuritis with or without effusions, interstitial fibrosis, pulmonary vasculitis, an increased incidence of bronchitis and pneumonia myocarditis, epicarditis, endocarditis, dysrhythmias, neuritis, and vasculitis (Ekblom & Nordemar, 2003; Scott et al, 1987).

Individuals with RA have significant cardiovascular risk factors. Compared with individuals without RA, diastolic blood pressure and levels of thrombotic variables are elevated (McEntegart et al, 2001). Risk factor modification has an important role in the comprehensive management of individuals with RA.

Functional capacity is limited by pain and stiffness in the affected muscles and joints, weakness, the number of joints affected, fatigue, and whether the patient is having an acute episode. Self-limited physical activity and exercise contributes to cardiopulmonary deconditioning. Movement such as walking is often inefficient because of limping. Peak exercise tests are limited by musculoskeletal complaints; thus submaximal tests are more functional in this population. Tests of cardiovascular status must be non-weight–bearing to enable the patient to reach an acceptable stress level without confounding joint pain.

For patients with RA, 15 to 35 minutes of graded, low-intensity aerobic exercise performed three times a week can be sufficient to enhance aerobic capacity (Harkcom et al, 1985). In addition to improving aerobic capacity, such an exercise prescription results in increased exercise time, reduced affected joint count, improved activities of daily living, reduced joint pain, and general fatigue. Should a joint flare-up occur while the patient is on an exercise program, a few days or weeks of restricted mobility and abstinence from exercise frequently ameliorates the symptoms. Gentle mobilization (preferably weight bearing) coupled with range of motion exercises during this period will minimize the negative effects of reduced activity.

Prolonged use of steroids contributes to bone fragility. Thus physical activity and exercise prescriptions are modified accordingly.

RA is hallmarked by exacerbations and remissions. A lifelong health program helps to reduce the frequency and severity of exacerbations and enhance recovery from these. Further, such a program may help reduce the need for potent medication.

Principles of Physical Therapy Management

Traditionally the approach to the physical therapy management of RA has been largely from the orthopedic perspective. Exercise and stress of the oxygen transport system, however, are major components of overall management. Thus the secondary cardiovascular and pulmonary manifestations must be assessed to ensure that exercise prescription is safe as well as maximally therapeutic.

The goals of long-term management for the patient with RA include the following.

- Maximize the patient's quality of life, general health, and well-being through maximizing physiological reserve capacity
- Educate regarding cardiopulmonary manifestations of RA and associated cardiovascular risk factors, self-management, nutrition, weight control, smoking reduction or cessation, relaxation and stress management, medications, infection control, and the role of a rehabilitation program
- Optimize alveolar ventilation
- Optimize lung volumes and capacities and flow rates
- Optimize ventilation and perfusion matching and gas exchange
- Reduce the work of breathing
- Reduce the work of the heart

- Protect the airways from aspiration
- Facilitate mucociliary transport
- Optimize secretion clearance
- Maximize aerobic capacity and efficiency of oxygen transport
- Optimize physical endurance and exercise capacity
- Optimize general muscle strength and thereby peripheral oxygen extraction
- Design lifelong health and rehabilitation programs with the patient

Patient monitoring includes dyspnea, respiratory distress, breathing pattern (depth and frequency), arterial saturation, cyanosis (delayed sign of desaturation), heart rate, blood pressure, and rate pressure product. Subjectively, discomfort/pain and perceived exertion can be assessed using the Borg scale.

Medication that is needed to maximize treatment response is administered before treatment (e.g., steroids, nonsteroidal antiinflammatory drugs, and analgesics). Knowledge of the type of medication, its administration route, and time to and duration of peak efficacy is essential if treatment is to be maximally efficacious. Gentle, rhythmic, nonjarring exercise is prescribed, particularly for patients at risk of loss of bone mass secondary to long-term steroid use.

The primary interventions for maximizing cardiopulmonary function and oxygen transport in patients with RA include some combination of education, aerobic exercise, strengthening exercises, postural correction exercises, chest wall mobility exercises, range of motion exercises, body positioning, breathing control and coughing maneuvers, airway clearance interventions, activity pacing, and energy conservation. An ergonomic assessment of the patient's work and home environments may be indicated to minimize oxygen demand and energy expenditure in these settings. A review of mobility aids and devices is carried out to maximize the patient's function and exercise tolerance.

Education is a principal focus of the long-term management of the patient with RA. Education includes the reinforcement of preventative health practices (e.g., infection control, cold and flu prevention, flu shots, smoking reduction or cessation, aerobic exercise, strengthening exercises, range of motion exercises, nutrition, weight control, hydration, pacing of activities, and energy conservation).

Aerobic exercise is an essential component of the long-term management of the patient with RA in order to optimize the efficiency of oxygen transport overall both with respect to cardiopulmonary conditioning and improving movement economy. Mild-to-moderate exercise during subacute periods can be beneficial. Cycling efficiency of patients with RA is comparable with healthy persons. The efficiency of walking, however, is less in patients with RA because of limping and associated deformity and pain. Non-weight–bearing exercise is beneficial in patients with severe deformity and pain (e.g., aquatic exercise or water walking). Given the fluctuations in the patient's condition from day to day, exercise prescription is modified frequently to consider the patient's changing condition. Chest wall exercises include all planes of movement with a rotational component. Body positioning to optimize lung volumes and airflow rates is a priority. Breathing control and coughing maneuvers are essential and should be coupled with body movement and positioning.

Individuals with Chronic Renal Insufficiency

Pathophysiology and Medical Management

Patients with chronic renal disease have significant systemic complications. Cardiopulmonary manifestations include left ventricular hypertrophy and congestive heart failure secondary to chronic volume and pressure overload (American College of Sports Medicine, 2000). Patients have a high incidence of atherosclerosis, coronary artery disease, glucose intolerance, and diabetes. Also, generalized muscle weakness and fatigue compromises functional work capacity.

Chronically increased fluid volume, although regulated with dialysis, contributes to increased stroke work of the heart and cardiomegaly and hypertension. With respect to pulmonary function, increased fluid volume increases peribronchial fluid and airway closure. After dialysis, the reduction in body weight is related to a reduction in closing volume, increased vital capacity, and forced expiratory flow rates.

The pulmonary-renal syndromes reflect the close relationship between the lungs and kidneys. These syndromes are characterized by altered immunological status, alveolar hemorrhage, interstitial and alveolar inflammation, and pulmonary vascular involvement (Matthay et al, 1980).

The kidneys have a primary role in the production and regulation of certain humoral regulators of metabolism, hemodynamics, fluid balance, and oxygen transport (Rankin & Matthay, 1982). Thus pathology of the kidneys significantly affects those life-sustaining processes. Patients may be taking potent medications that are associated with severe side effects that can further compromise function.

Principles of Physical Therapy Management

The goals of long-term management for the patient with chronic renal insufficiency include the following.

- Maximize the patient's quality of life, general health, and well-being through maximizing physiological reserve capacity
- Educate regarding cardiopulmonary manifestations of renal insufficiency, self-management, medications, nutrition, weight control, relaxation and stress management, work simplification, stress management, infection control, and the role of a rehabilitation program
- Optimize alveolar ventilation
- Optimize lung volumes, capacities, and flow rates
- Optimize ventilation and perfusion matching and gas exchange
- Reduce the work of breathing
- Reduce the work of the heart

- Protect the airways from aspiration
- Facilitate mucociliary transport
- Optimize secretion clearance
- Maximize aerobic capacity and efficiency of oxygen transport
- Optimize physical endurance and exercise capacity
- Optimize general muscle strength and thereby peripheral oxygen extraction
- Design lifelong health and rehabilitation programs with the patient

Patient monitoring includes dyspnea, respiratory distress, breathing pattern (depth and frequency), arterial saturation, cyanosis (delayed sign of desaturation), heart rate, blood pressure, and rate pressure product. Subjectively, perceived exertion is assessed using the Borg scale.

Medication that is needed to maximize treatment response is administered before treatment. Knowledge of the type of medication, its administration route, and time to and duration of peak efficacy is essential if treatment is to be maximally efficacious. A lifelong health program has the potential of helping to reduce the need for potent medications for renal dysfunction.

The primary interventions for maximizing cardiopulmonary function and oxygen transport in patients with chronic renal insufficiency include some combination of education, aerobic exercise, strengthening exercise, chest wall mobility exercises, range of motion exercise, body positioning, breathing control and coughing maneuvers, airway clearance interventions, activity pacing, and energy conservation. An ergonomic assessment of the patient's work and home environments may be indicated to minimize oxygen demand and energy expenditure in these settings.

Education is a principal focus of the long-term management of the patient with chronic renal insufficiency. Education includes the reinforcement of preventative health practices (e.g., infection control, cold and flu prevention, flu shots, aerobic exercise, strengthening exercises, range of motion exercises, nutrition, weight control, hydration, pacing of activities, and energy conservation).

Aerobic exercise is an essential component of the long-term management of the patient with chronic renal insufficiency in order to optimize the efficiency of oxygen transport overall. Maximizing ventilation with exercise is limited if the patient has severe generalized muscular weakness and increased fatigue. Maximal oxygen uptake increases in hemodialysis patients along with improvement in other indices of cardiopulmonary conditioning (Painter et al, 1986). Patients may decrease or eliminate the need for anti-hypertension medications. Exercise carried out during hemodialysis treatment sessions is feasible and safe for appropriate patients. Because hemodialysis treatments require sessions of several hours multiple times weekly, aerobic training (e.g., cycle ergometry) can be effectively incorporated into treatment time (Shallom et al, 1984; Zabetakis et al, 1982). The exercise prescription of patients with blood glucose abnormalities and coronary artery disease is modified accordingly.

Chest wall exercises can be used and should include all planes of movement with a rotational component. Body positioning to optimize lung volumes and airflow rates is a priority. Breathing control and coughing maneuvers are essential and should be coupled with body movement and positioning.

Individuals who are Obese

Pathophysiology and Medical Management

Obesity and its multisystem sequelae are epidemic in industrialized countries; thus obesity must be managed by the physical therapist as a primary condition as well as secondary to other diagnoses. Any other pathology and problem is accentuated when compounded with obesity, and morbidity and mortality are increased for all health concerns (Desapriya, 2004; Orzano & Scott, 2004).

A detailed assessment is conducted to identify organ systems that are affected and may limit exercise. Central abdominal obesity (apple obesity) constitutes a greater cardiovascular risk than hip obesity (pear obesity) (Khan & Williamson, 1994; Flodmark et al, 1994). In younger people, low aerobic fitness in people who are obese appears to reflect deconditioning rather than a primary cardiac problem (Rowland et al, 2003). Individuals who are morbidly obese, however, may develop heart failure. Noninvasive approaches to weight control are superior to invasive approaches in terms of promoting lifelong change and multisystem benefit, health and well-being, and cost effectiveness.

Pharmacological approaches and surgery are extreme measures whose use is generally not restricted to those with morbid obesity. Vertical banded gastroplasy is increasingly being performed on patients with morbid obesity. One study that compared exercise responses before and six months after weight loss with surgery showed that cardiac diastolic function is improved along with $\dot{V}O_2$ and anaerobic threshold (Kanoupakis et al, 2001). The extent to which these and additional benefits would have occurred with conservative weight loss, however, and the long-term changes effected by both, were not studied.

Health risks associated with obesity are multisystemic (see Chapter 1). The cardiovascular and pulmonary risks are life threatening. In particular, the work of breathing, due to alveolar hypoventilation, and the work of the heart are increased with increasing body mass. The heart may enlarge to accommodate increased work load even at rest. Body mass over the chest wall can lead to alveolar hypoventilation and airway closure and reduced oxygenation. Individuals who are obese have problems when recumbent, particularly during sleep (e.g., obstructive sleep apnea, dysrhythmias, and shortness of breath). These problems are identified in the comprehensive assessment.

Principles of Physical Therapy Management

Obesity can be a primary referred problem or a secondary condition. Physical therapists are uniquely suited to counsel and coach patients with weight problems and promote physically active lifestyles, exercise programs, and provide basic knowledge on nutrition and diet commensurate with supporting this activity. Lessons learnt from tobacco control and smoking cessation have been extrapolated for use in the management of the obesity epidemic (Mercer et al, 2003).

Physical activity through the course of the day must be increased, and patients who are obese need to participate in a regular program of exercise.

The goals of long-term management for the individual who is obese include the following.

- Maximize the patient's quality of life, general health, and well-being through maximizing physiological reserve capacity
- Educate regarding cardiopulmonary manifestations of obesity, self-management, medications, nutrition, weight control, infection control, stress management, and the role of a rehabilitation program
- Maximize aerobic capacity and efficiency of oxygen transport
- Optimize physical endurance and exercise capacity
- Optimize general muscle strength and thereby peripheral oxygen extraction
- Design a lifelong health plan with the patient

Patient monitoring includes dyspnea, respiratory distress, breathing pattern (depth and frequency), arterial saturation (if indicated), heart rate, blood pressure, and rate pressure product. Subjectively, perceived exertion is assessed using the Borg scale.

Maintaining a healthy weight is a function of optimal nutrition and exercise (see recommendations in Chapter 1). The individual's readiness to change dietary and activity patterns must be assessed to determine the optimal time to introduce a structured program to maximize and sustain long-term outcomes (see Chapter 1).

A weight loss program is introduced concurrently with an increasing volume of regular physical activity and a structured exercise program. The parameters of the prescription, however, may require modification because of biomechanical stress and discomfort. As weight is lost, the prescriptive parameters are modified to increase the intensity and volume of exercise that is performed. Also, the individual's movement economy and efficiency will improve as the body's biomechanics normalize. Initially the hemodynamic responses to even low levels of exercise are likely to be excessive because of the weight that the individual carries during the performance of the activity. Before significant loss of weight, cycling may initially be preferable to walking if the person's biomechanics limit endurance. Physical activity must be comfortable both for sustainability and injury avoidance.

The role of the physical therapist as health coach is critically important in providing both support to the individual who is obese and long-term follow-up. The probability of success is increased with the involvement of a health care provider and follow-up. Facilitating weight loss and adopting healthy lifestyle behaviors long term can be life saving for a patient. Given the current epidemic of obesity, assisting an individual to attain a healthy lifestyle through optimal nutrition, exercise, and weight loss is a singularly important health outcome.

SUMMARY

This chapter reviews pathophysiology and medical management as they relate to the comprehensive physical therapy management of individuals with chronic, *secondary* cardiopulmonary pathology. Exercise testing and training is a major component of the comprehensive management of these conditions and is presented separately in Chapter 25.

This chapter specifically presents the comprehensive physical therapy management of chronic cardiopulmonary dysfunction *secondary* to neuromuscular, musculoskeletal, collagen vascular/connective tissue, and renal dysfunction. The neuromuscular conditions that are presented include stroke, Parkinson's syndrome, multiple sclerosis, cerebral palsy, spinal cord injury, chronic effects of poliomyelitis, and muscular dystrophy. The musculoskeletal conditions that are presented include thoracic deformity (kyphoscoliosis) and osteoporosis. The collagen vascular/connective tissue conditions that are presented include systemic lupus erythematosus, scleroderma, ankylosing spondylitis, and rheumatoid arthritis. Finally, management of the patient with chronic renal insufficiency and the person who is obese is presented.

The principles of patient management are presented rather than treatment prescriptions, which cannot be given without specific consideration of an individual patient. In this context, the goals of long-term management of patients with each condition are presented, followed by the essential monitoring required, and the primary interventions for maximizing cardiopulmonary function and oxygen transport. The selection of interventions for any given patient is based on the physiological hierarchy. The most physiological interventions are exploited followed by less physiological interventions and those whose efficacy is less well documented.

These principles must be considered if a patient has a chronic, *secondary* cardiopulmonary condition as a secondary diagnosis for which the patient is being treated by the physical therapist. These principles have implications for treatment prescription and monitoring in the management of the condition for which the patient is being primarily treated.

Review Questions

1. Analyze the limitations in participation and related activities that are associated with *chronic* cardiopulmonary pathophysiology that occurs secondary to stroke, Parkinson's syndrome, multiple sclerosis, cerebral palsy, spinal cord injury, late sequelae of poliomyelitis, muscular dystrophy, kyphoscoliosis, osteoporosis, systemic lupus erythematosus, scleroderma, ankylosing spondylitis, rheumatoid arthritis, chronic renal insufficiency, and obesity.

2. Relate cardiopulmonary physical therapy treatment interventions to the underlying pathophysiology of each of the above chronic conditions that a person may have, and provide the rationale for your choice.

REFERENCES

Adams, M.A., & Chandler, L.S. (1974). Effects of physical therapy program on vital capacity of patients with muscular dystrophy. Physical Therapy 54:494-496.

Alexander, J.K. (1985). The cardiomyopathy of obesity. Progress in Cardiovascular Diseases 28:325-334.

American College of Sports Medicine. (2000). Guidelines for exercise testing and prescription, ed 6. Philadelphia: Lippincott Williams & Wilkins.

Anonymous. (2002). National clinical guidelines for stroke: a concise update. Clinical Medicine 2:231-233.

Bach, J.R. (1991). New approaches in the rehabilitation of the traumatic high level quadriplegic. American Journal of Physical Medicine and Rehabilitation 70:13-19.

Bach, J.R. (1992). Pulmonary rehabilitation considerations for Duchenne muscular dystrophy: The prolongation of life by respiratory muscle aids. Critical Reviews in Physical and Rehabilitation Medicine 3:239-269.

Bach, J.R. (1993). Mechanical insufflation-exsufflation. Comparison of peak expiratory flows with manually assisted and unassisted coughing techniques. Chest 104:1553-1562.

Bach, J.R., Alba, A.S., Bodofsky, E., Curran, F.J., & Schultheiss, M. (1987). Glossopharyngeal breathing and noninvasive aids in the management of post-polio respiratory insufficiency. Birth Defects 23:99-113.

Bach, J.R., Alba, A.S., & Shin, D. (1989). Management alternatives for post-polio respiratory insufficiency. Assisted ventilation by nasal or oral-nasal interface. American Journal of Physical Medicine and Rehabilitation 68:264-271.

Bach, J.R., O'Brien, J., Krotenberg, R., & Alba, A.S. (1987). Management of end stage respiratory failure in Duchenne muscular dystrophy. Muscle and Nerve 10:177-182.

Bach, J.R., Smith, W.H., Michaels, J., Saporito, L., Alba, A.S., Dayal, R., & Pan, J. (1993). Airway secretion clearance by mechanical exsufflation for post-poliomyelitis ventilator-assisted individuals. Archives of Physical Medicine and Rehabilitation 74:170-174.

Bach-y-Rita, P., Wood, S., Leder, R., Paredes, O., Bahr, D., Wicab Back-y-Rita, E., & Murillo, N. (2002). Computer-assisted motivating rehabilitation (CAMR) for institutional, home, and educational late stroke programs. Topics in Stroke Rehabilitation 8:1-10.

Badics, E., Wittmann, A., Rupp, M., Stabauer, B., & Zifko, U.A. (2002). Systematic muscle building exercises in the rehabilitation of stroke patients. NeuroRehabilitation 17:211-214.

Bake, B., Dempsey, J., & Grimby, G. (1976). Effects of shape changes of the chest wall on distribution of inspired gas. American Review of Respiratory Disease 114:1113-1120.

Barrach, A.L., Beck, G.J., Bickerman, H.A., & Seanor, J.H. (1952). Physical methods of stimulating cough mechanisms. Use in poliomyelitis, bronchial asthma, pulmonary emphysema, and bronchiectasis. Journal of the American Medical Association 50:1380-1385.

Bastille, J.V., & Gill-Body, K.M. (2004). A yoga-based exercise program for people with chronic poststroke hemiparesis. Physical Therapy 84:33-48.

Bates, D.V. (1989). Respiratory function in disease, ed 3. Philadelphia: WB Saunders.

Black, L.F., & Hyatt, R.E. (1971). Maximal static respiratory pressures in generalized neuromuscular disease. American Review of Respiratory Diseases 103:641-650.

Braun, N.M.T., Arora, N.S., & Rochester, D.F. (1983). Respiratory muscle and pulmonary function in polymyositis and other proximal myopathies. Thorax 38:616-623.

Braun, S.R., Giovannoni, R., & O'Connor, M. (1984). Improving the cough in patients with spinal cord injury. American Journal of Physical Medicine 63:1-10.

Campbell, J., & Ball, J. (1978). Energetics of walking in cerebral palsy. Orthopedic Clinics of North America 9:374-377.

Cooper, C.B., Trend, P.S., & Wiles, C.M. (1985). Severe diaphragm weakness in multiple sclerosis. Thorax 40:631-632.

Curran, F.J. (1981). Night ventilation to body respirators for patients in chronic respiratory failure due to late stage muscular dystrophy. Archives of Physical Medicine and Rehabilitation 62:270-274.

Dean, E. (1991). Clinical decision making in the management of the late sequelae of poliomyelitis. Physical Therapy 71:752-761.

Dean, E. (1993). Advances in rehabilitation for older persons with cardiopulmonary dysfunction. In Katz, P.R., Kane, R.L., & Mezey, M.D. (Eds). Advances in long-term care, ed 2. New York: Springer Publishing.

Dean, E. (2001). Cardiopulmonary development. In Bonder, B.R., & Wagner, M.B. (Eds). Functional performance in older adults, ed 2. Philadelphia: F.A. Davis.

Dean, E. & Ross, J. (1992). Mobilization and exercise conditioning. In Zadai, C. (Ed). Pulmonary management in physical therapy. New York: Churchill Livingstone.

Dean, E., & Ross, J. (1993). Movement energetics of individuals with a history of poliomyelitis. Archives of Physical Medicine and Rehabilitation 74:478-483.

Dean, E., Ross, J., Road, J.D., Courtenay, L., & Madill, K. (1991). Pulmonary function in individuals with a history of poliomyelitis. Chest 100:118-123.

Desapriya, E. (2004). Obesity epidemic. Lancet 364:1488.

DeTroyer, A., De Beyl, T., & Thirion, M. (1981). Function of the respiratory muscles in acute hemiplegia. American Review of Respiratory Diseases 123:631-632.

Dickey, B.F., & Myers, A.R. (1997). Pulmonary manifestations of collagen-vascular diseases. In Fishman, A.P., Elias, J.A., Fishman, J.A., Grippi, M.A., Kaiser, L.R., & Senior, R.M. (Eds). Fishman's pulmonary diseases and disorders, ed 3. New York: McGraw Hill.

Dresen, M.H.W., de Groot, J.R., & Bouman, L.N. (1985). Aerobic energy expenditure of handicapped children after training. Archives of Physical Medicine and Rehabilitation 66:302-306.

Duncan, P., Studenski, S., Richards, L., Gollub, S., Lai, S.M., Reker, D., Perera, S., Yates, J., Koch, V., Rigler, S., & Johnson, D. (2003). Randomized clinical trial of therapeutic exercise in subacute stroke. Stroke 34:73-80.

Ekblom, B., & Nordemar, R. (2003). Rheumatoid arthritis. In Skinner, J. (Ed). Exercise testing and training for special cases, ed 3. Philadelphia: Lippincott Williams & Wilkins.

Elliott, C.G., Hill, T.R., Adams, T.E., Crapo, R.O., Nietrzeba, R.M., & Gardner, R.M. (1985). Exercise performance of subjects with ankylosing spondylitis and limited chest expansion. Bulletin of European Physiopathology and Respiration 21:363-368.

Estenne, M., & Gorino, M. (1992). Action of the diaphragm during cough in tetrapelgic subjects. Journal of Applied Physiology 72:1074-1080.

Ferris, B.G., & Pollard, D.S. (1960). Effect of deep and quiet breathing on pulmonary compliance in man. Journal of Clinical Investigations 39:143-149.

Flodmark, C.E., Sveger, T., & Nilssonehle, P. (1994). Waist measurement correlates to a potentially atherogenic lipoprotein profile in obese 12-14-year-old children. Acta Paediatrica 83:941-945.

Fluck, D.C. (1966). Chest movements in hemiplegia. Clinical Science 31:382-388.

Fugl-Meyer, A.R., & Grimby, G. (1984). Respiration in tetraplegia and in hemiplegia: A review. International Rehabilitation Medicine 6:186-190.

Gray, I.R. (1996). Cardiovascular manifestations of collagen vascular diseases. In Julian, D.G., Camm, A.J., Fox, K.M., Hall, R.J.C., & Poole-Wilson, P.A. (Eds). Diseases of the heart, ed 2. Philadelphia: W.B. Saunders.

Griggs, R.C., & Donohoe, K.M. (1982). Recognition and management of respiratory insufficiency in neuromuscular disease. Journal of Chronic Diseases 35:497-500.

Grimby, G., Fugl-Meyer, A.R., & Blomstrand, A. (1974). Partitioning of the contribution of rib cage and abdomen to ventilation in ankylosing spondylitis. Thorax 29:179-184.

Gross, D. (1980). The effect of training on strength and endurance on the diaphragm in quadriplegia. American Journal of Medicine 68:27-35.

Hapke, E.J., Meek, J.C., & Jacobs, J. (1972). Pulmonary function in progressive muscular dystrophy. Chest 61:41-47.

Harkcom, T.M., Lampman, R.M., Banwell, B.F., & Castor, C.W. (1985). Therapeutic value of graded aerobic exercise training in rheumatoid arthritis. Arthritis and Rheumatism 28:32-39.

Hoeppner, V.H., Cockcroft, D.W., Dosman, J.A., & Cotton, D.J. (1984). Nighttime ventilation improves respiratory failure in secondary kyphoscoliosis. American Review of Respiratory Diseases 129:240-243.

Howard, R.S., Wiles, C.M., & Spencer, G.T. (1988). The late sequelae of poliomyelitis. Quarterly Journal of Medicine 66:219-232.

Inkley, S.R., Alderberg, F.C., & Vignos, P.C. (1974). Pulmonary function in Duchenne muscular dystrophy related to stage of disease. American Journal of Medicine 56:297-306.

Kahn, H.S., & Williamson, D.F. (1994). Abdominal obesity and mortality risk among men in nineteenth-century North America. International Journal of Obesity 18:686-691.

Kanoupakis, E., Michaloudis, D., Fraidakis, O., Parthenakis, F., Vardas, P., & Melissas, J. (2001). Left ventricular function and cardiopulmonary performance following surgical treatment of morbid obesity. Obesity Surgery 11:552-528.

Kasper, D.L., Braunwald, E., Fauci, A., Hauser, S., Longo, D., Jameson, J.L., & Wilson, J.D. (Eds) (2004). Harrison's principles of internal medicine, ed 16. St. Louis: McGraw Hill.

Kilburn, K.H., Eagan, J.T., Sieker, H.O., & Heyman, A. (1959). Cardiopulmonary insufficiency in myotonic and progressive muscular dystrophy. New England Journal of Medicine 261:1089-1096.

Kirilloff, L.H., Owens, G.R., Rogers, R.M., & Mazacco, M.C. (1985). Does chest physical work? Chest 88:436-444.

Lane, D.J., Hazleman, B., & Nichols, P.J.R. (1974). Late onset respiratory failure in patients with previous poliomyelitis. Quarterly Journal of Medicine 43:551-568.

Leblanc, P., Ruff, F., & Milic-Emili, J. (1970). Effects of age and body position on "airway closure" in man. Journal of Applied Physiology 28:448-451.

Linder, S.H. (1993). Functional electrical stimulation to enhance cough in quadriplegia. Chest 103:166-169.

Lisboa, C., Moreno, R., Fava, M., Ferreti, R., & Cruz, E. (1985). Inspiratory muscle function in patients with severe kyphoscoliosis. American Review of Respiratory Diseases 132:48-52.

Macklem, P.T., & Roussos, C.S. (1977). Respiratory muscle fatigue: A cause of respiratory failure? Clinical Science and Molecular Medicine 53:419-422.

Maeshima, S., Ueyoshi, A., Osawa, A., Ishida, K., Kunimoto, K., Shimamoto, Y., Matsumoto, T., & Yoshida, M. (2003). Mobility and muscle strength contralateral to hemiplegia from stroke: benefit from self-training with family support. American Journal of Physical Medicine and Rehabilitation 82:456-462.

Malouin, F., Potvin, M., Prevost, J., Richards, C.L., & Wood-Dauphinee, S. (1992). Use of an intensive task-oriented gait training program in a series of patients with acute cerebrovascular accidents. Physical Therapy 72:781-793.

Matthay, R.A., Bromberg, S.I., & Putman, A.M. (1980). Pulmonary-renal syndromes-a review. Yale Journal of Biology and Medicine 53:497-523.

McArdle, W.D., Katch, F.I., & Katch, V.L. (2001). Exercise physiology, ed 5. Philadelphia: Lippincott Williams & Wilkins.

McEntegart, A., Capell, H.A., Creran, D., Rumley, A., Woodward, M., & Lowe, G.D. (2001). Cardiovascular risk factors, including thrombotic variables, in a population with rheumatoid arthritis. Rheumatology (Oxford) 40:640-644.

McFarlin, D.E., & McFarland, H.F. (1982). Multiple sclerosis. New England Journal of Medicine 307:1183-1188.

Mehta, A.D., Wright, W.B., & Kirby, B.J. (1978). Ventilatory function in Parkinson's disease. British Medical Journal 1:1456-1457.

Mercer, S.L., Green, L.W., Rosenthal, A.C., Husten, C.G., Khan, L.K., & Dietz, W.H. (2003). Possible lessons from the tobacco experience for obesity control. American Journal of Clinical Nutrition 77(Suppl 4):1073S-1082S.

Miller, H.J., Thomas, E., & Wilmot, C.B. (1988). Pneumobelt use among high quadriplegia population. Archive of Physical Medicine and Rehabilitation 69:369-372.

Moorman, J.R., Coleman, E., Packer, D.L., Kisslo, J.A., Bell, J., Hettlemna, B.D., Stajich, J., & Roses, A.D. (1985). Cardiac involvement in myotonic muscular dystrophy. Medicine 64:371-387.

Moseley, A.M., Stark, A., Cameron, I.D., & Pollock, A. (2003). Treadmill training and body weight support for walking after stroke. Cochrane Database and Systematic Review CD002840.

Mossberg, K.A., Linton, K.A., Friske, K. (1990). Ankle-foot orthoses: effect of energy expenditure of gait in spastic diplegic children. Archives of Physical Medicine and Rehabilitation 71:490-494.

Murray, J.F., & Nadel, J.A. (2000). Textbook of respiratory medicine, ed 3. Philadelphia: Elsevier.

Nakano, K.K., Bass, H., Tyler, H.R., & Carmel, R.J. (1976). Amyotrophic lateral sclerosis: A study of pulmonary function. Diseases of the Nervous System 37:32-35.

Neu, H.C., Connolly, J.J., Schwertley, F.W., Ladwig, H.A., & Brody, A.W. (1966). Obstructive respiratory dysfunction in Parkinsonian patients. American Review of Respiratory Diseases 95:33-47.

Neubauer, B., & Gundersen, H.J.G. (1978). Analysis of heart rate variations in patients with multiple sclerosis. Journal of Neurology, Neurosurgery, and Psychiatry 41:417-419.

Orzano, A.J., & Scott, J.G. (2004). Diagnosis and treatment of obesity in adults: an applied evidence-based review. Journal of the American Board of Family Practitioners 17:359-369.

Page, S.J., Gater, D.R., & Back-Y-Rita, P. (2004). Reconsidering the motor recovery plateau in stroke rehabilitation. Archives of Physical Medicine and Rehabilitation 85:1377-1381.

Painter, P.L., Nelson-Worel, J.N., Hill, M.M., Thornbery, D.R., Shelp, W.R., Harrington, A.R., & Weinstein, A.B. (1986). Effects of exercise training during hemodialysis. Nephron 43:87-92.

Pardy, R.L., & Leith, D.E. (1984). Ventilatory muscle training. Respiratory Care 29:278-284.

Peach, P.E., & Olejnik, S. (1991). Post-polio sequelae: effect of treatment and noncompliance on post-polio sequelae. Orthopedics 14:1199-1203.

Pentland, B., & Ewing, D.J. (1987). Cardiovascular reflexes in multiple sclerosis. European Neurology 26:46-50.

Perloff, J.K., de Leon, A.C., & O'Doherty, D. (1966). The cardiomyopathy of progressive muscular dystrophy. Circulation 33:625-648.

Rankin, J.A., & Matthay, R.A. (1982). Pulmonary renal syndromes. II. Etiology and pathogenesis. Yale Journal of Biology and Medicine 55:11-26.

Ray, J.F. 3rd, Yost, L., Moallem, S., Sanoudos, G.M., Villamena, P., Paredes, R.M., & Clauss, R.H. (1974). Immobility, hypoxemia, and pulmonary arteriovenous shunting. Archives of Surgery 109:537-541.

Reid, W.D., & Warren, C.P.W. (1984). Ventilatory muscle strength and endurance training in elderly subjects and patients with chronic airflow limitation: a pilot study. Physiotherapy Canada 36:305-311.

Rosenow, E.C., Strimlan, C.V., Muhm, J.R., & Ferguson, R.H. (1977). Pleuropulmonary manifestations of ankylosing spondylitis. Mayo Clinic Proceedings 52:641-649.

Ross, J., & Dean, E. (1992). Body positioning. In Zadai, C. (Ed). Clinics in physical therapy. Pulmonary management in physical therapy. New York: Churchill Livingstone.

Roth, E.J. (1994). Heart disease in patients with stroke. Part II. Impact and implications for rehabilitation. Archives of Physical Medicine and Rehabilitation 75:94-101.

Rowland, T., Bhargava, R., Parslow, D., & Heptulla, R.A. (2003). Cardiac response to progressive cycle exercise in moderately obese adolescent females. Journal of Adolescent Health 32:422-427.

Scott, T.E., Wise, R.A., Hochberg, M.C., & Wigley, F.M. (1987). HLA-DR4 and pulmonary dysfunction in rheumatoid arthritis. American Journal of Medicine 82:765-771.

Segal, A.M., Calabrese, L.H., Ahmad, M., Tubbs, R.R., & White, C.S. (1985). The pulmonary manifestations of systemic lupus erythematosus. Seminars in Arthritis and Rheumatism 14:202-224.

Senaratne, M.P.J., Carroll, D., Warren, K.G,. & Kappagoda, T. (1984). Evidence for cardiovascular autonomic nerve dysfunction in multiple sclerosis. Journal of Neurology, Neurosurgery, and Psychiatry 47:947-952.

Serebrovskaya, T., Karaban, I., Mankovskaya, I., Bernardi, L., Passino, C., & Appenzeller, O. (1998). Hypoxic ventilatory responses and gas exchange in patients with Parkinson's disease. Respiration 65:28-33.

Shallom, R., Blumenthal, J.A., Williams, R.S., McMurray, R.G., & Dennis, V.W. (1984). Feasibility and benefits of exercise training in patients on maintenance dialysis. Kidney International 25:958-963.

Sinha, R., & Bergofsky, E.H. (1972). Prolonged alteration of lung mechanics in kyphoscoliosis by positive pressure hyperinflation. American Review of Respiratory Disease 106:47-57.

Smith, W.E., Clark, P.F., MacArthur, D., Allatt, R.D., Hayes, K.C., & Cunningham, D.A. (1997). Oxygen costs using a reciprocating gait orthosis in a paraplegic (T9) patient with a bilateral below-knee amputation: case report. Spinal Cord 35:121-123.

Smith, P.E.M., Calverley, P.M.A., Edwards, R.H.T., Evans, G.A., & Campbell, E.J.M. (1987). Practical problems in the respiratory care of patients with muscular dystrophy. New England Journal of Medicine 316:1197-1205.

Smith, P.E.M., Edwards, R.H., & Calverley, P.M.A. (1989). Oxygen treatment of sleep hypoxaemia in Duchenne muscular dystrophy. Thorax 44:997-1001.

Smith, E.L., Smith, K.A., & Gilligan, C. (1991). Exercise, fitness, osteoarthritis, and osteoporosis. In Bouchard, C., Shephard, R.J., Sutton, J.R., & McPherson, B.D. (Eds). Exercise, fitness, and health. A consensus of current knowledge. Champaign: Human Kinetics Books.

Vignos, P.J., & Watkins, M.P. (1966). The effects of exercise in muscular dystrophy. Journal of the American Medical Association 197:843-848.

Wolff, R.K., Dolovich, M.B., Obminski, G., & Newhouse, M.T. (1977). Effects of exercise and eucapnic hyperventilation on bronchial clearance in man. Journal of Applied Physiology 43:46-50.

Zabetakis, P.M., Gleim, G.W., Pasternack, F.L., Saranitt, A., Nicholas, J.A., & Michelis, M.F. (1982). Long-duration submaximal exercise conditioning in hemodialysis patients. Clinical Nephrology 18:17-22.

Guidelines for the Delivery of Cardiovascular and Pulmonary Physical Therapy

Critical Care

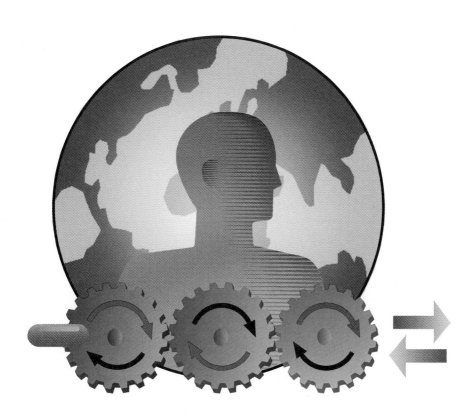

CHAPTER 33

Comprehensive Management of Individuals in the Intensive Care Unit

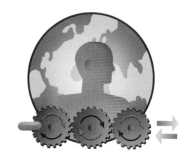

Elizabeth Dean and Christiane Perme

KEY TERMS

End-of-life issues
Evidence-based practice
Function optimization
Humanity
Management goals
Outcomes and measures

Physiological evidence
Prevention
Quality care
Scientific evidence
Treatment selection

Cardiopulmonary physical therapy in the intensive care unit (ICU) is a subspecialty within cardiopulmonary physical therapy. This chapter presents the principles of clinical and nonclinical aspects of patient management in this setting. An overview of the general goals of management and the rationale for prioritizing treatments according to a physiological hierarchy is described. End-of-life issues are also addressed.

The thrust toward evidence-based practice in health care and the development of conceptual bases for practice have had major implications for cardiopulmonary physical therapy practice in the ICU (Barlow et al, 1999; Dean, 1985; Dean, 1994a; Hislop, l975; Ross & Dean, l989; Shon, 1983). Superior knowledge of cardiopulmonary physiology, pathophysiology, pharmacology, multisystem dysfunction and its medical management, and ICU equipment and changing technology is essential. Clinical decision making in the ICU and rational management of patients is based on a tripod approach: knowledge of the underlying pathophysiology and basis for general care; knowledge of the physiological and scientific evidence for treatment interventions; and clinical reasoning and decision making in prioritizing treatments, prescribing their parameters, and performing serial evaluation to assess outcomes and further modify treatment (Figure 33-1). Quality

care is a function of these three areas of knowledge and expertise. Evidence-based practice and excellent problem solving ability will optimize outcomes (Thomas et al, 2002) and maximize the benefit-to-risk ratio of cardiopulmonary physical therapy interventions (Riegelman, 1991).

SPECIALIZED EXPERTISE OF THE ICU PHYSICAL THERAPIST

Effective clinical decision making and practice in the ICU demand specialized expertise and skill, including advanced, state-of-the-art knowledge in cardiopulmonary and multisystem physiology and pathophysiology, and in medical, surgical, nursing, and pharmacological management (Box 33-1). Physical therapists in the ICU need to be first-rate diagnosticians and observers. Given the multitude of factors that contribute to impaired oxygen transport (Dean, 1983; Dean, 1994b), the physical therapist needs to analyze these to define the patient's specific oxygen transport deficits and problems. Optimizing oxygen delivery in the patient who is critically ill (Kelly, 1996) by exploiting noninvasive interventions is the priority.

The role of the ICU physical therapist is to promote healing and recovery, and return the patient to the highest level of life

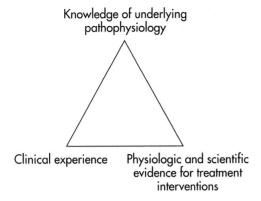

FIGURE 33-1 Tripod approach to patient management.

participation and satisfaction. Therefore the physical therapist must be capable of processing considerable amounts of objective information quickly, interpreting this information, and integrating it to provide the basis for a treatment prescription (i.e., the specific selection, prioritization, and implementation of treatment interventions) (Cutler, 1997). The integration and interpretation of the vast amount of multiorgan system data is perhaps the single most important skill in ICU practice and treatment prescription. With this data, the physical therapist identifies the indications for treatment, contraindications, and optimal timing of interventions. The condition of the patient in the ICU can change rapidly. The physical therapist works within narrow windows of opportunity to effect an optimal treatment response. Treatments are variable with respect to their intensity, duration, and frequency. Usually treatments are short and frequent. The maximally beneficial outcome with the least risk to the patient is the objective of every treatment. Although principles of management may be the same, specific knowledge requirements will differ depending on the type of critical care setting (e.g., burn, coronary care, neurosurgery, spinal cord injury, and trauma). Alternatively, a community hospital with a small general ICU will have a cross section of patients that the physical therapist will need to manage.

GOALS AND GENERAL BASIS FOR MANAGEMENT

The ultimate goals of cardiopulmonary physical therapy treatment in the ICU (Silver & Siebens, 1994) include the following:

1. return the patient to premorbid functional level to the greatest extent possible;
2. reduce patient morbidity, mortality, and length of hospital stay.

As a precursor to achieving these goals, the immediate goals relate initially to the attainment of optimal oxygen transport and hence cardiopulmonary function, and secondly to the attainment of optimal musculoskeletal and neurological function. In the ICU, the physical therapist must recognize the

BOX 33-1

Specialized Expertise and Skill of the ICU Physical Therapist

Detailed, comprehensive knowledge of cardiopulmonary physiology and pathophysiology, and pharmacology.
Thorough working knowledge of the monitoring systems routinely used in the ICU and an understanding of the interpretation of the output of these monitoring systems (e.g., ECG, arterial blood gases, fluid and electrolyte balance, hemodynamic monitoring, chest-tube drainage systems, intracranial pressure monitoring). This information is an integral component for assessing the underlying problems, and selecting, prioritizing, and progressing or modifying treatment.
Extensive expertise in cardiopulmonary assessment and treatment prescription; general experience in medicine and surgery is recommended.
Detailed understanding of multisystem physiology and pathophysiology and the cardiopulmonary manifestations of systemic disease.
Ability to practice effectively under pressure and in congested, suboptimal working conditions.
Knowledge regarding all emergency procedures, including those for respiratory and cardiac arrest, equipment, and power failure.
Knowledge regarding the paging system used in the unit for being contacted as well as for contacting other team members when they are out of the unit or out of the hospital.
On-call service, 24 hours a day, 7 days a week, is a common practice and should be considered in units without this service.
Knowledge regarding the roles of all team members.
Sensitivity toward each patient's psychosocial situation, culture, and values, and promotion of active involvement of the patient and family in clinical decision making, whenever feasible.
Superior communication skills (e.g., ability to work cooperatively with other members of the ICU team [see Figure 33-2] and give verbal presentations and discuss patients at rounds).

implications of cardiopulmonary insufficiency on neuromuscular status and that apparent impairment of neuromuscular status in not necessarily indicative of neurological dysfunction. Rather, reduced cardiac output and blood pressure, hypoxemia, hypercapnia, and increased intracranial pressure (ICP) may be indirectly responsible for these changes. Musculoskeletal and neurological complications can become life threatening and therefore need to be detected early and managed.

Key elements of the assessment of the patient in the ICU include risk factors for a suboptimal clinical outcome. In addition to age and comorbidity, risk factors include poor indices of PaO_2 with a high FIO_2, platelet count, cardiac index, blood urea nitrogen, creatinine, acute renal failure, peritoneal dialysis or hemodialysis, continuous infusion of antidysrhythmic agents, base deficit, reduced consciousness, pain, and cardiac arrest (Cullen et al, 1977). Thus patients with one or more of these conditions require close monitoring and management.

Many elements of the assessment of patients in the ICU are comparable to those for acute patients who are not critically ill but require respiratory support and mechanical ventilation (see Chapter 44). The primary difference is that, for patients in the ICU, the adequacy of the steps in the oxygen transport pathway are monitored closely, and the status and function of multiple organ systems are monitored in a serial (repeated at regular or judicious intervals) manner to observe trends over time so that treatment modifications can be titrated to the patient's responses. Serial vital signs including pain and distress are recorded along with arousal and cognitive status, neuromuscular status, musculoskeletal status, and functional mobility. Assessment of functional mobility ranges from the smallest movement to walking. Often it includes bed mobility, transfers to chair, and walking, which may require assistive devices. Related laboratory investigations are noted, including the results of electrocardiogram (ECG), x-rays, scans, blood work, blood sugar, and fluid and electrolyte balance, and are followed closely to quickly detect improvement or deterioration so that treatment can be correspondingly modified.

Mechanical ventilation and its modes and parameters are described in Chapter 44. The mode and settings and parameters of the mechanical ventilator are important indicators of changes in the patient's status and therefore must be included in the assessment and recorded at each treatment. In addition, the FIO_2 is recorded. Similarly, changes in FIO_2 are important outcomes and indicators of treatment response. This information is used collectively in clinical decision making before, during, and after weaning from mechanical ventilation.

Comparable to patients who are not critically ill, the assessment data are evaluated, problems and diagnoses made, and interventions prescribed based on the patient's needs and goals. With each treatment, the responses are reviewed and prescription parameters of the interventions are refined to progress the patient. One distinction in ICU patient management, compared with patients who are not critically ill, is that treatments are shorter, the intensity more moderate, and, if possible, treatments are more frequent.

Restricted Mobility and Recumbency

Hospitalization, particularly in the ICU, is associated with a considerable reduction in mobility (i.e., loss of exercise stimulus) and recumbency (i.e., loss of gravitational stimulus) (Dean, 2002) (see Chapters 18 and 19). These two factors are essential for normal oxygen transport; thus their removal has dire consequences for the patient with or without cardiopulmonary dysfunction.

In terms of a physiological hierarchy of treatment interventions (see Chapter 17), exploiting the physiological effects of acute mobilization, upright positioning, and their combination are the most physiologically justifiable primary interventions to maximize oxygen transport and prevent its impairment in patients who are critically ill.

Recumbency is nonphysiological; it is a position that, all too often, most patients are injudiciously confined. Changing

---

BOX 33-2

General Information Required Before Treating the Patient in the ICU

Sex and age
Premorbid status (e.g., lifestyle, ethnicity, culture, work situation, stress, cardiopulmonary conditioning, and oxygen transport reserve capacity)
Knowledge of patient's life roles and related activities for optimal return to daily life
Medical and surgical histories
General multisystem assessment findings
Pharmacological support
Smoking history
Hydration and nutritional status: deficiencies, obesity, or asthenia
Time of onset and course of present condition
Existing or potential medical instability
Indications or necessity for intubation and mechanical ventilation
Mode and parameters of mechanical ventilation
FIO_2
Invasive monitoring, lines, leads, and catheters
Existence of or potential for complications and multiorgan system failure
Coma
Elevated ICP and the need for ICP monitoring
Risk or presence and site(s) of infection
Quality of sleep and rest periods
Nutritional support during ICU stay
Pain control regimen

---

the position of the body from erect to supine positions results in significant physiological changes, which may jeopardize the patient's already compromised or threatened oxygen transport system (Box 33-2) (see Chapter 19).

The culmination of these deleterious effects offsets the increased homogeneity of ventilation and perfusion and their matching in the supine position. These effects compound the superimposed factors of restricted mobility, recumbency-induced central fluid shifts, prolonged lying without the normal stimulation or will to turn the body, and underlying pathophysiology or trauma that may contribute to impaired cardiopulmonary function and oxygen transport. Theoretically, the more compromised the patient, the greater the priority to maximize time spent in the upright position in conjunction with exploiting the benefits of acute mobilization.

Specificity of Cardiopulmonary Physical Therapy

Physical therapy interventions (see Chapter 17 and Part III) are specifically geared toward the status of each organ system, taking into consideration the pathophysiological basis for the patient's signs and symptoms, rationale for each intervention, and the physiological and scientific evidence supporting the efficacy of the intervention (Dean & Ross, 1992). Physical therapy provides both prophylactic and therapeutic interventions for the patient in the ICU. Conservative, noninvasive

---

BOX 33-3

Physiological Changes when Changing from the Upright to the Supine Position

Cephalad displacement of the visceral contents and diaphragm
Compression of the dependent lung fields
Cephalad fluid shift to the central circulation
↑ Stroke volume and cardiac output and over days a reduction due to renal compensation
↓ Total lung capacity
↓ Vital capacity
↓ Functional residual capacity
↓ Residual volume
↓ Forced expiratory volumes
↑ Airway resistance
↑ Closing volumes of small airways
↑ Restriction of chest wall and ↓ diaphragmatic excursion
↓ Pulmonary and chest wall compliance
↓ Arterial oxygen levels
↓ Cough effectiveness
↑ Preload, afterload, and myocardial work
↓ Myocardial efficiency
↓ Sympathetic stimulation and ↓ peripheral vascular resistance

---

BOX 33-4

General Physical Therapy Goals toward Function Optimization in the Patient in the ICU

Establish a detailed baseline of outcome measures and measures to be recorded serially to assess change
Maintain or restore adequate alveolar ventilation and perfusion and their matching in unaffected and affected lung fields and thereby optimize oxygen transport overall
Prolong spontaneous breathing (to the extent that is therapeutically indicated) and thereby avoid, postpone, or minimize need for mechanical ventilation
Minimize the work of breathing
Minimize the work of the heart
Design a positioning schedule to maintain comfort and postural alignment (distinct from therapeutic body positioning to optimize oxygen transport)
Maintain or restore general mobility, strength, endurance, and coordination within the limitations of the patient's condition and consistent with the patient's anticipated rehabilitation prognosis (distinct from therapeutic mobilization to optimize oxygen transport)
Maximally involve the patient in a daily routine including self-care, changing body position, standing, transferring, sitting in a chair, and ambulating in patients for whom these activities are indicated
Optimize treatment outcome by interfacing physical therapy with the goals and patient-related activities of other team members; coordinating treatments with medication schedules; and treating the patient specifically, on the basis of both results of objective monitoring available in the ICU and subjective findings

---

measures constitute initial treatments of choice to avert or delay the need for additional invasive monitoring and treatment, supplemental oxygen, pharmacological agents, and the need for intubation and mechanical ventilation. The physical therapist aims to avoid, reduce, or postpone for as long as possible the need for respiratory support. Even if the patient is mechanically ventilated, maintaining some level of spontaneous breathing, no matter how minimal, is associated with improved oxygenation and outcomes (Hedenstierna & Lattuada, 2002). In addition, the physical therapist helps to prevent the multitude of side effects of restricted mobility and recumbency during bed rest. A summary of general information required before treating the patient in the ICU is presented in Box 33-3.

Function Optimization

Function optimization refers to optimizing the capacity to participate in one's life roles and associated activities. This necessitates promotion of optimal physiological functioning at an organ system level, as well as promotion of optimal functioning of the patient as a whole. In critical care, primary goals related to function optimization are initially focused on cardiopulmonary function. With improvement in oxygen transport, increased attention is given to optimal functioning of the patient with respect to self-care, self-positioning, sitting up, and walking. General physical therapy goals related to function optimization are shown in Box 33-4. Outcomes can be tracked objectively by recording the length of time a patient sits over the edge of the bed, sits in a chair at bedside, stands, and walks. Also, the weight a patient lifts as well as

the number of repetitions and sets he or she performs can be readily quantified.

Consistent with being primarily a noninvasive practitioner, the physical therapist exploits noninvasive interventions to achieve therapeutic goals. Outcomes related to reduced reliance on invasive interventions are important physical therapy outcomes. These include reducing FIO_2; avoiding mechanical ventilation; minimizing mechanical ventilator support; increasing the amount of spontaneous breathing, even minimally, if the patient is mechanically ventilated; and reducing medication (e.g., bronchodilators, inotropes, chronotropes, sedation, narcotics, and analgesics).

Prophylaxis

General aspects of patient care related to physical therapy practice include the role of prophylaxis or prevention. The complications of restricted mobility and recumbency are described in Chapter 18 and relate primarily to the status of the cardiopulmonary, neuromuscular, and musculoskeletal systems, and overall functional capacity. In the ICU, the negative physiological effects of restricted mobility are amplified in patients who are severely ill and older. A primary objective of the physical therapist therefore is to avoid or reduce these untoward effects on the patient's recovery and

---

BOX 33-5

Specific Patient Information Required Before Treating the Patient in the ICU

Detailed knowledge of the patient's history, including the differential diagnosis on admission to the ICU, and relevant medical, surgical, and social histories

Knowledge of premorbid status related to the International Classification of Function (see Chapters 1 and 17) (i.e., limitations of structure and function [impairment], activities, and social participation [health-related quality of life])—these will provide a baseline of outcome measures on which clinical decisions about ICU discharge and hospital discharge will be made

Detailed understanding and knowledge of the medications administered to the patient, their indications, and side effects (especially those affecting response to physical therapy)

Knowledge regarding the stability of vital signs since admission, including heart rate and rhythm, respiration rate and rhythm, blood pressure, skin color, core temperature, and hemodynamic stability

Detailed knowledge of relevant findings of laboratory tests, procedures, and biopsies, including arterial blood gases, blood analysis, fluid and electrolyte balance, ECG, x-ray, thoracentesis, central venous pressure (CVP), left artrial

pressure (LAP), pulmonary artery wedge pressure (PAWP), microbiology and biochemistry reports, and urinalysis

Detailed understanding of the rationale for the ventilatory mode and parameters used if the patient is ventilated

With respect to establishing a patient database:

1. Conduct a thorough, detailed clinical assessment specific to the patient's condition(s), including inspection, palpation, percussion, and auscultation of the chest, as well as a neuromusculoskeletal assessment to rule out any secondary effects of cardiopulmonary dysfunction and to establish rehabilitation prognosis

2. Establish a physical diagnosis and problem list and prioritize the treatment goals and overall treatment plan

3. Determine the optimal assessment and treatment outcome measures and be knowledgeable about their interpretation

4. Conduct serial measurements to predict the patient's oxygen transport reserve capacity before treatment and stressing the oxygen transport system

As treatment progresses, record objective and relevant subjective treatment outcome measures and revise treatment goals as indicated by the patient's progress

---

the patient's length of stay in the ICU. Ventilator-associated pneumonia is a major complication of ICU care and warrants preventive measures from the outset (Cook, 2000).

Preventive physical therapy goals include reducing the deleterious effects of restricted mobility and pathology on cardiopulmonary and neuromuscular function and reducing the risk of musculoskeletal deformity, neurological dysfunction, and decubiti over pressure areas (back of the head, shoulders, elbows, sacrum, and heels). Special mattresses or a special bed may be indicated. The negative sequelae of recumbency and restricted mobility, which can be life threatening in people who are critically ill, are largely preventable. Particular care must be taken to avoid pressure sores because these significantly increase the risk of infection and deterioration, and can be life threatening. Physical therapists as well as nurses need to pay particular attention to individuals at risk, and to examine routinely for sites of redness, pressure, and potential skin lesions in every patient, regardless of expected length of stay in the ICU (Stillwell, 1992). The texture of bed covers, their smoothness, bunching of the bed gown, and irritation from lines and catheters to the patient must be routinely monitored. Prevention is key given the potentially reduced immunity and capacity to heal of patients in the ICU (Williams & Harding, 2003). Although pressure sores are largely preventable, the need to be vigilant remains given the deleterious consequences they may have for recovery. Unrelieved pressure and equipment failure have been identified as key causes of pressure sores in the patient after trauma (O'Sullivan et al, 1997). These causes of pressure sores are 100% avoidable with vigilance and monitoring. Physical therapists have a role for making recommendations about patient positioning between treatments in the interest of

preventing deleterious sequelae of recumbency and restricted mobility.

Preparation for Treating the Patient in the ICU

Patients in the ICU are generally characterized by some degree of life threatening medical instability or its risk. Before treating a given patient in the ICU, the physical therapist should be thoroughly familiar with the specific information shown in Box 33-5. Depending on the level of care in the ICU, nursing care is usually 1:1 or 1:2. Coordinating treatment with nursing interventions is efficient. It is helpful to have the nurse at hand to assist as required, particularly if the patient is beginning physical therapy. Alternatively, if the nursing care proved strenuous for the patient, physical therapy may be more beneficial if delayed.

GENERAL CLINICAL ASPECTS OF THE MANAGEMENT OF THE ICU PATIENT

Assessment

The fundamental assessment procedures for the cardiopulmonary system are described in detail in Part II. Laboratory reports, procedures, sputum culture, and x-rays supplement the findings of inspection, palpation, and auscultation of the chest. Of particular importance are the blood work, arterial blood gases (including SaO_2), ECG, fluid and electrolyte balance, hemodynamic monitoring, and intracranial pressure monitoring. These are the most commonly monitored parameters in the ICU in addition to vital signs, temperature, respiration rate, heart rate, blood pressure, respiratory distress, and pain.

Physical Therapy Uses of Monitoring Systems in the ICU

Establish the indications for and contraindications of cardiopulmonary physical therapy
Define treatment intensity, duration, and frequency for optimal treatment outcome
Determine the appropriateness of response to a specific intervention
Assess the need for supplemental oxygen before, during, and after treatment
Determine appropriate patient positioning between, during, and after treatments
Establish whether the patient is responding positively or negatively to treatment, or there is no change, and whether treatment should be modified or discontinued

Monitoring

Optimal physical therapy treatment depends on exploiting information from the monitoring systems available in the ICU. Monitoring systems can be used to establish the indications and contraindications for treatment as well as parameters of the treatment prescription and progression, and to assess the patient. These are summarized in Box 33-6. Physical therapists need to exploit the considerable amount of objective data available to them in patient management. A thorough knowledge and routine use of monitoring systems for each patient in the ICU cannot be overemphasized in terms of contributing to improved quality of care with less risk to the patient. Subjective responses of the patient are particularly important in the ICU, where the patient's power and self-responsibility are compromised. This can be achieved through a sign system, use of analog scales, and communication devices. The patient needs to be able to communicate basic needs if possible (e.g., discomfort/pain, anxiety, fear, and general distress).

The monitoring systems described in Chapter 16 provide essential information with respect to the management of the patient in the ICU. Information regarding acid-base imbalance and fluid and electrolyte balance helps to establish specific treatment goals. The Swan-Ganz catheter in situ gives the pressures for pulmonary artery pressure and wedge pressure, which provide an index of myocardial sufficiency and specifically left heart function. Central venous pressure gives an indication of fluid loading and the ability of the right side of the heart to cope with changes in circulating body fluids. Pressures related to heart function give the physical therapist an indication of pulmonary status and help to determine whether heart dysfunction is affecting lung function or lung dysfunction is affecting heart function, or both. Cardiopulmonary stress alerts the physical therapist to modify workloads or the physical demands of treatment to keep the patient medically stable and avoid undue fatigue and deterioration. The physical therapist conducts ongoing monitoring of the patient's responses to invasive care in the

ICU (e.g., responses to medication and fluid resuscitation, indications for intervention and refinement of its prescription) to ensure patient safety.

Changes in ECG may reflect heart disease, lung disease, altered acid base, and electrolyte and fluid balance. The physical therapist is responsible for identifying the patient's heart rhythm and ECG changes, which can be expected with improvement or deterioration in oxygen transport and secondary to medical management, drug intervention, changes in the course of the disease, and response to treatment generally.

Pharmacological Agents

The physical therapist needs a thorough knowledge of the common pharmacological agents used in intensive care (see Chapter 44). With this knowledge, the physical therapist can augment the effects of these agents and optimize physical therapy treatment response when treatments are coordinated with medication schedules. Most medications have optimal dosages for any given patient, optimal sensitivity, and peak-response time. Most medications have side effects. Side effects may cause deterioration in the patient's condition, create apparent signs and symptoms suggestive of other disorders, or alter response to treatment. The physical therapist therefore needs to identify the medications each patient is taking and their side effects. Medication that contributes to suboptimal therapeutic outcomes warrants discussion with the team in terms of finding an alternative. One physical therapy outcome is the minimization of medication with effective physical therapy.

Certain medications, such as bronchodilators, sedatives, mucolytic agents, antianginal medications, and analgesics, help the patient to cooperate and tolerate treatment. Special consideration must always be given to the different peak-response times of different medications. The patient can cooperate more actively in the treatment if pain and anxiety are reduced and breathing is easy. An enhanced treatment effect is therefore more likely. These advantages can result in shorter, more cost-effective, efficacious treatment, and more effective use of the physical therapist's time.

Some medication can attenuate a patient's response to mobilization/exercise and activity. Patients on beta-blocking agents, for example, may not show the normal changes in heart rate and blood pressure in response to exercise. In addition, beta-blockers contribute to fatigue. Caution must be observed when prescribing exercise for these patients. Another classification of drugs called vasopressor agents regulates blood pressure and heart rate. Patients on these agents may also exhibit abnormal mobilization/exercise responses. Monitoring is essential; however, vital signs to assess treatment response may be rather limited for patients on drugs acting on the cardiovascular system.

Narcotics are a commonly used classification of drug in the ICU and are often administered for their analgesic effects jointly with sedatives and tranquilizers. Despite pain relief, narcotics, particularly in combination with other sedative type drugs, interfere with physical therapy treatments because of the patient's reduced arousal, monotonous ventilation, and inability to cooperate with treatment. Further, narcotics tend to have multisystem effects rather than localized effects. Because physical therapy is the most physiological and noninvasive intervention available to the patient in the ICU, it behooves the physical therapist to ensure that pharmacological agents that are effective and more selective than narcotics in achieving the desired effect have been considered. Thus, as a team member, the physical therapist has a major role during rounds to ensure an integrative management program for each patient.

TREATMENT PRESCRIPTION IN THE ICU

Physical therapy treatments in the ICU are judiciously selected in a goal-specific manner. As a general guideline, treatments descend in a physiological hierarchy (Chapter 17). Mobilization, exercise, and body positioning are exploited first with respect to their direct and potent effects on oxygen transport overall. At the other end of the hierarchy (i.e., least physiological interventions that have a more limited effect on the steps in the oxygen transport pathway overall) are conventional interventions such as airway clearance techniques and suctioning. Assessment of the oxygen uptake and delivery relationship is essential given the high metabolic demands of patients in the ICU (Weissman & Kemper, 1993) and the documented associated exercise and stress responses associated with physical therapy (Horiuchi et al, 1997).

Supplemental Oxygen

Supplemental oxygen is usually administered continuously, whether the patient is ventilated or not, to maintain PaO_2 level within an optimal range (Dantzker et al, 1997). Oxygen concentrations can be increased before treatment to help compensate for associated stress. Oxygen, however, should always be increased to 100% and inspired for at least three minutes before and after suctioning. Should arterial desaturation be apparent during treatment, oxygen may need to be increased. If the patient is spontaneously breathing without oxygen, supplemental oxygen may also be indicated during treatment to avoid desaturation. Oxygen administration is regulated by the ICU team based on arterial blood gas including arterial saturation and subjective distress. Severe hypoxemia is known to result in irreversible tissue damage within minutes, but hyperoxia can also produce harmful effects within hours. By maximizing alveolar ventilation, gas exchange, and ventilation and perfusion matching, supplemental oxygen can be optimally used and the effects of acidemia minimized.

Treatment for respiratory acidosis in individuals with chronic pulmonary disease is aimed at increasing alveolar ventilation to improve the exchange of carbon dioxide and oxygen. Because the respiratory center is depressed by increased amounts of carbon dioxide (carbon dioxide narcosis), the lowered oxygen tension of the blood becomes the stimulus for respiration. If the patient inhales high concentrations of oxygen, the stimulation for respiration may be removed. For this reason, oxygen is never given to patients with carbon dioxide narcosis.

Low flow oxygen (one to three L/min) is given to a patient with chronic pulmonary disease who maintains a chronically elevated arterial PCO_2 in the presence of arterial hypoxemia. If intermittent positive pressure breathing is indicated, compressed or room air is used instead of oxygen.

Severe hypoxemia usually suppresses cardiac output to some degree. Cardiac output may be further compromised immediately after a patient is placed on a mechanical ventilator because of impaired venous return by the elevated transpulmonary pressure (Jardin et al, 1981). An attempt is made to carefully balance ventilation with an optimal or adequate cardiac output by shortening inspiratory time and minimizing transpulmonary pressures by using lower tidal volumes.

Breathing and Coughing Maneuvers

If the patient is nonventilated or recently extubated, breathing and coughing maneuvers in conjunction with moving and body positioning are emphasized to promote ventilation, flow rates, and secretion clearance (Bennett et al, 1990), decrease minute ventilation and respiratory rate, increase tidal volume, and improve arterial blood gases (Barach, 1974; Casciari et al, 1981). Breathing exercises for individual who breathe with long-time constants (e.g., patients with chronic pulmonary disease) are believed to be most effective if pursed-lips breathing is performed in conjunction with mechanical pressure applied over the abdomen (Irwin & Tecklin, 2004; Mueller et al, 1970). To derive the maximum benefits, breathing and coughing maneuvers should be performed in body positions that are most mechanically and physiologically optimal. In addition, they can be performed in the postural drainage positions to augment mucociliary clearance. To avoid airway closure, patients should not breathe below the end of normal tidal ventilation.

Mucociliary Transport and Secretion Clearance

The patient in the ICU needs special attention regarding fluid balance to carefully regulate hydration and fluid volume. Inhaled humidified air is a significant additional source of body fluid. Normally the alveolar gas is saturated with water vapor. The lining of the tracheobronchial tree is therefore protected from erosion and potential infection. This is particularly important in the patient who requires frequent suctioning. The effect of humidification can be assessed by the consistency of the patient's secretions. Thick secretions suggest humidification may be inadequate, and the patient may be dehydrated.

If the effects of mobilization on mucociliary transport and secretion accumulation have been exploited and further secretion clearance is warranted, postural drainage may be indicated. Postural drainage may be contraindicated in patients with unstable vital signs and is usually contraindicated immediately after feedings and meals. In some institutions, however, patients on continuous 24-hour tube feedings are tipped after feeding has been discontinued for 15 minutes. The cuff in the artificial airway is inflated to avoid aspiration. The specific postural drainage positions to be used are determined on the basis of the pathology, x-ray, and clinical examination. The recommended positions for the broncho-pulmonary segments involved should be approximated as closely as possible (see Chapter 20) and only modified if there are indications to do so. Frequently, specific positioning in the ICU is compromised as a result of the patient's status, intolerance to lying flat or being tipped, or limitations imposed by the monitoring apparatus or ventilator.

The role of manual techniques has been increasingly questioned because they have been associated with desaturation, atelectasis, musculoskeletal trauma, discomfort, cardiac dysrhythmias, and arrest (Kirilloff et al, 1985). Thus these techniques must be applied rationally, with appropriate monitoring, and modified accordingly. The precise sequence, duration, intensity, and frequency of treatment are based on treatment outcome rather than time. Oxygen demand has been shown to increase with manual airway techniques, and the hemodynamic and metabolic responses have been reported to resemble the response to exercise (Weissman & Kemper, 1993). The increases in cardiac output and blood pressure are thought to reflect increased sympathetic activity from stress as well as the exercise-like response (Horiuchi et al, 1997). The stressful responses to ICU procedures as well as conventional airway clearance procedures have been reported to be effectively modulated with medication (Cohen et al, 1996). A recent study reported no significant changes in $\dot{V}O_2$ and mean arterial pressure with conventional airway clearance interventions compared with undisturbed side-lying (Berney & Denehy, 2003). These discrepant findings may reflect differences in the intervention and subjects studied (stable patients who are ventilated patients). The application of manual techniques in the head-down position is contra-indicated in patients with acute myocardial infarction and increased intracranial pressure. Relative contraindications include hemorrhage, bronchopulmonary fistula, acute chest trauma, lung abscess, and gastric reflux (Lynn-McHale & Carlson, 2000). Given the adverse effects of manual airway clearance interventions that have been reported, the physical therapist needs to ensure that more physiological alternatives associated with fewer risks have been exploited.

Bagging

Although not universally accepted, bagging patients is practiced to varying degrees in ICUs. The purpose of bagging is to provide extra-large breaths during treatment, to maintain some degree of positive end-expiratory pressure, to assess lung compliance, and to facilitate the effect of instillation of a small volume of saline solution into the tracheobronchial tree

to loosen secretions. A self-inflating breathing bag is temporarily connected to the airway. Bagging must be performed cautiously. Aggressive bagging can produce bronchospasm. The lungs are manually inflated for a few breaths. The use of bagging in conjunction with suctioning is controversial. Some clinicians prefer to bag the patient after suctioning to avoid the possibility of the positive pressure pushing the mucus distally. Others maintain that because of the adherent quality of the mucus to the walls of the airway and the dilatation of the airways in response to positive pressure, bagging does not propel the mucus distally. Rather, it is believed that bagging before suctioning promotes air entry distal to the mucous plugs and movement of plugs centrally on expiration.

Certain body positions present a particular problem when a pressure-cycled ventilator is being used. The efficiency of the ventilator is greatly reduced when the patient's head is positioned below the hips because of an increase in total pulmonary resistance caused by the pressure of the abdominal contents. Therefore the use of a self-inflating breathing bag may be required to maintain pressure when changing from one position to another and during some postural drainage positions. Adequate tidal volume can be maintained by an assistant while the physical therapist assists the patient with bronchial drainage. With the use of the self-inflating bag, the physical therapist needs to ensure the patient is adequately ventilated and takes a larger than tidal breath every minute or so.

As soon as possible, spontaneous breathing is encouraged in conjunction with postural drainage. The small airways dilate slightly on inspiration and cause mucus to peel away from the walls; thus, during expiration, mucus plugs are moved centrally toward the trachea. The degree to which chest wall percussion, shaking, and vibration facilitate this movement is equivocal in the literature (Kirilloff et al, 1985; Dean & Ross, 1992). Thus these less substantiated, less physiological conventional procedures (i.e., manual techniques) should be considered carefully and only after other more supported and physiological treatments have been exploited. Furthermore, because of their documented adverse effects, it is essential that the patient be continuously monitored for safety reasons and to establish a favorable treatment outcome. For the patient who is unconscious or paralyzed, the ventilator or self-inflating bag can be used to increase inflation volumes. Research is needed to examine the role of bagging in mucous removal.

Instillation

Instillation is another procedure that should be used selectively in patients. A mucolytic effect of saline has not been well established. Beneficial effects may be more apparent in neonates.

Weaning from the Mechanical Ventilator

Depending on the institution and country, the physical therapist, the respiratory therapist, or both are often responsible for weaning the patient from mechanical ventilation. Thus coordinating their goals and working together to ensure the

BOX 33-7

General Steps in Weaning a Patient from the Mechanical Ventilator

1. An individualized weaning schedule is designed for each patient in which periods of time are spent off the ventilator and on a T tube that delivers appropriate oxygen and humidity.
2. The initial time period off the ventilator is carefully selected; mornings are often good times.
3. (a) Physical activity should be at a minimum during this period (e.g., not during or after physical therapy, not after meals, tests, or procedures, and not during family visits). (b) Supplemental oxygen and humidity are given.
4. The physical therapist offers support and reassurance.
5. Vital signs and signs and symptoms of respiratory distress are monitored continuously during weaning.
6. The patient is not left unattended in the initial weaning sessions until periods off the ventilator are reliably tolerated well for several successive minutes.
7. (a) Deterioration of vital signs, blood gases, and evidence of distress indicate that the patient will have to return to ventilatory assistance imminently. (b) Rest periods of at least an hour are strategically interspersed in the weaning schedule.
8. Blood gases are performed at regular intervals (e.g., 15, 30, 60, 90, and 120 minutes, or more or less frequently as indicated).
9. If blood gases stabilize within acceptable limits during the weaning period and the patient is generally tolerating the procedure well, the time off the ventilator is increased.
10. Patients with underlying cardiopulmonary disease who are older, malnourished, obese, or smoke can be expected to take longer to be completely weaned from the ventilator.
11. Weaning is generally faster in patients who have required a shorter period of mechanical ventilation.
12. To hasten the weaning process, synchronized intermittent mandatory ventilation (SIMV) has been reported to be useful in some patients. Others, however, have observed that the use of SIMV tends to fatigue the patient and delay the patient's progress in weaning. Thus SIMV must be used cautiously, and individual variability must be considered in terms of its effectiveness. Assist control ventilation is a well tolerated alternative.

weaning process is carried out expediently and with the least risk of weaning complications (e.g., postextubation atelectasis, aspiration, and hypoxemia) is a priority (Marini, 1984; Shoemaker et al, 1999).

Weaning can increase cardiovascular and psychological stress, and in turn $\dot{V}O_2$. Patients at particular risk of weaning failure must be identified and monitored by the physical therapist during this process. One study reported that cardiovascular responses to weaning in patients after heart surgery depended on the type of surgery (De Backer et al, 2000). Cardiac index, for example, was greater after abdominal aortic surgery than bypass or transplantation surgery. Although the oxygen extraction ratio remained stable after aortic surgery, it increased somewhat after bypass surgery, and markedly after transplantation surgery. Weaning patients with cardiac dysfunction from mechanical ventilation can lead to pulmonary edema due to increased venous return and release of catecholamines, reduced left ventricular compliance, compression of the heart by the lungs, and increased left ventricular afterload.

Because of its profound effect on pulmonary function and gas exchange, body position must be optimized for weaning to maximize weaning success and avoid the need for reintubation because of weaning failure. Patients who are overweight warrant particular attention. Low tidal volume and high respiratory rates can jeopardize weaning success. In patients who are obese, a semi-recumbent position may favor weaning compared to a 90-degree upright position, which may cause the abdomen to encroach on the underside of the diaphragm and limit its excursion (Burns et al, 1994).

Blood gas analysis and pulmonary function provide the indications for weaning. Ideally the patient's spontaneous tidal volume should approximate that delivered by the ventilator. Forced vital capacity should be two to three times the patient's required tidal volume. Weaning is not usually indicated if the patient requires positive end-expiratory pressure greater than 5 cm H_2O or FIO_2 greater than 0.4. In addition, patients who are unable to generate a negative inspiratory pressure of −20 mm Hg or greater are unlikely to be able to generate sufficient intrathoracic pressures for deep breathing and airway clearance and thus are poor candidates for weaning. Minute ventilation and maximum voluntary ventilation can be measured at bedside and contribute to the decision whether to wean. Although weaning protocols differ depending on the patient and the ventilatory mode used, general guidelines for this common ICU procedure are outlined in Box 33-7.

Special Noninvasive ICU Priorities and Considerations

Intubation and mechanical ventilation are delayed as long as possible, particularly in individuals with chronic obstructive pulmonary disease (COPD). These individuals have poor blood gases in combination with poor CO_2 ventilatory drive. Once mechanically ventilated, the patient tends to deteriorate rapidly, and the risk of failure to wean is increased. Noninvasive mechanical ventilation (see Chapter 44) has been a more recent advance to provide low-risk ventilatory support as a means of avoiding ICU admission and associated risks of invasive ventilation. Noninvasive mechanical ventilation (e.g., continuous positive airway pressure) can be administered at home. In patients who are medically stable, invasive mechanical ventilation is titrated judiciously to ensure the patient is initiating breaths as much as possible, which facilitates weaning.

Depending on the patient's response to ventilation, however, sedation and neuromuscular blockade may be indicated, which prevents the patient from cooperating fully with treatment. Further, weaning patients with COPD and neuromuscular conditions is complicated by respiratory muscle weakness and fatigue (see Chapter 26), which may indicate respiratory muscle training or rest. Because of these challenges, weaning necessitates close cooperation and coordination within the team to maximize weaning success.

Discharge from the ICU

To be recommended for discharge from the ICU, the patient should not require frequent physical therapy. The patient should be breathing spontaneously and independently and elicit a cough with or without assistance. The patient should be moving purposefully and have achieved, minimally, a low level of functional independence (at least 2 to 3 METs where 1 MET equals 3.5 ml O_2/kg body/min or the metabolic demand at rest).

The physical therapist is responsible for documenting the physical therapy treatment priorities and frequent progress notes during the ICU stay so that the team responsible for the patient after discharge can continue management with reduced risk of disruption of care or regression of the patient's condition. The patient should be consulted, if possible, and informed continually of his or her progress and plans made by the team and family. The patient should be given as many choices as possible about his or her care and be actively involved in long-term management planning.

NONCLINICAL ASPECTS OF THE MANAGEMENT OF THE PATIENT IN THE ICU

Team Work

Comprehensive patient care in the ICU must include a multidisciplinary team. Team work is the essence of optimal patient care and must include the patient and family as much as possible, particularly in the ICU (Imbus & Zawacki, 1986; Karlawish 1996). The physical therapist interacts frequently with other team members, particularly the medical staff, nurses, and respiratory therapists if in the ICU, regarding observations and changes in the patient's condition, treatment goals, and treatment response (Figure 33-2). In addition to providing therapy for patients and planning for discharge, the physical therapist is often consulted regarding ambulation, body positioning, lifting, transferring, chair sitting, and self-care.

Nutrition

Patients who are critically ill are hypermetabolic. Metabolic demand and oxygen consumption are increased after surgery and secondary to healing and repair, increased temperature, and altered thermoregulation. Patients with chronic cardiopulmonary limitation who are admitted to the ICU are often undernourished because of the effort required to purchase,

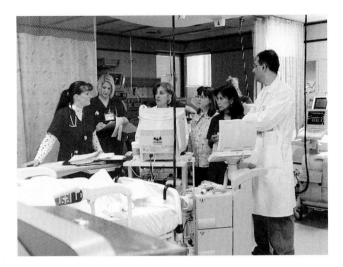

FIGURE 33-2 Multidisciplinary rounds in the ICU. Team work in the ICU is essential to facilitate communication and patient outcome. Note the presence of the nurse, respiratory therapist, pharmacist, social worker, physical therapist, and physician.

prepare, and consume food. Furthermore, these patients have increased $\dot{V}O_2$ and energy expenditure secondary to the increased work of breathing (Petty, 1985; Rochester & Esau, 1984). Without adequate nutrition, patients incur the effects of deconditioning faster, are debilitated, less capable of responding optimally to therapy, and more susceptible to infection. Intravenous hyperalimentation or external hyperalimentation is typically instituted early to maintain optimal nutritional status and avoid excessive physical wasting and deterioration. If a tracheostomy has been performed, the patient is able to eat normally provided risk of aspiration is minimal.

Regardless of the means by which nutritional support is provided, carbohydrate may be limited because of the increased CO_2 production resulting from its metabolism.

Infection Control

Infection control has become an even greater concern in hospitals and particularly ICUs now that superbugs have become prevalent. Superbugs are microorganisms that are resistant to broad spectrum antibiotics. The prevalence of these microorganisms has been attributed to the fact that many people today, over the course of their lives, have been on antibiotics, which has made them more susceptible to certain microorganisms and less sensitive to antibiotics. In addition, more patients with critical illness are surviving due to advances in management. Personal hygiene and good hygienic practice on the part of the physical therapist are mandatory because of the inherently high rate of infection in the ICU and compromised immunity of the patients. Patients in the ICU are prone to infection. Meticulous hand washing with an antiseptic detergent between patients is essential. Soaping for 30 seconds or more with a thorough scrubbing motion followed by thorough rinsing should be carried out. After contact with infected wounds, saliva, wounds, blood, pus, vomit, urine, or stool, the physical therapist must be particularly conscientious about washing immediately. Physical protection, including gowning, gloving, capping, and masking, is often required given the concerns regarding infection, and has in fact become common, routine practice in many ICUs.

There are several levels of infection control and there may be differences across ICUs in different hospitals. Some patients need to be protected from infection transmitted across patients in the ICU by health care staff, thus the need for meticulous hand washing. Some patients have types of infections from which the health care staff need protection. Often a combination of both types of precautions is indicated. The physical therapist needs to know the different level of infection control and precautions for each patient. In respiratory isolation, the patient remains in an isolated room for treatment. Masking and gloving will be required, and possibly gowning. Depending of the patient's diagnoses, eye protection may also be required. Contact isolation requires maximal infection control by those who come into contact with the patient; however, the patient can leave the room or restricted area.

The Patient as a Person

Although constraints do exist in the high technology environment of the ICU, the patient's dignity is observed as much as possible regardless of the reason for admission, the level of consciousness, or combative behavior directed toward the ICU staff. Gestures, such as using the patient's preferred name, explaining aspects of the patient's care, continually orienting the patient regarding person, place, time, and day, and having an interpreter available, if necessary, are widely practiced. A supportive caring atmosphere is created in which the patient is free to make choices and ask questions as much as possible. With endotracheal intubation, patients are unable to talk. Communication strategies are assessed to ensure the patient is maximally able to communicate his or her needs and maintain a sense of perceived control. Some strategies include mouthing (silent speech), use of a spelling board, writing, pointing to pictures, and responding with yes and no signs.

Other considerations that must be observed are related to disrobing, modesty, and privacy. These may reflect sex, age, physical image, culture, and individual differences. The patient needs to be asked about his or her comfort level with these, and also whether he or she is more comfortable with family present during treatment. Accommodating these individual differences is extremely important if the patient is to be maximally motivated to participate in treatment and adhere to recommendations between treatment sessions.

Patients may be in varying stages of cognitive awareness, from completely comatose to semi-comatose to reduced arousal. Patients who are comatose have been reported to have some awareness of their environment, and later can recall being talked about or wanting to communicate and having

BOX 33-8

Characteristics of the Patient who is at the End of Life

Failure of the peripheral circulation and profuse sweating, causing body cooling
Loss of strength, motion, and reflexes in the legs and then in the arms
Decreased sensitivity to touch and deep pressure and pain tends to remain
May experience pain, acute loneliness, and fear
May increase spiritual needs, particularly at night
An interval of quiescence just before death
Can be conscious until death

From Kinney, M.R., & Packa, D.R. (1995). Andreoli's comprehensive cardiac care (ed 7). Philadelphia: Elsevier.

been unable to do so. In addition, mechanical ventilation is a barrier to communication; thus methods of communicating need to be identified. Patients on neuromuscular blockade are unable to communicate but are aware (depending on the level of sedation) and do experience pain.

ICU as a Healing Environment

The physical environment of the ICU has a profound effect on the patient's recovery independent of the level of care received. Outside windows with daylight and pleasant views, for example, orient the patient to day and night and the passage of time. Other benefits include reduced number and types of complications and reduced length of stay in the ICU and in hospital overall. Minimizing the sense of social isolation is important, so family is encouraged to be present as much as feasible. In the absence of these supports, ICU neurosis and paranoia can emerge. Physical therapists who are involved in the designing of ICUs should consider psychosocial, environmental, technological, and clinical factors. Pet therapy may have some role in the ICU as it has been shown to have benefits in other care settings.

Circadian rhythms are associated with fluctuations in physiological and hormonal functions important to the patient's healing, recovery, and well being, and these are compromised with bed rest deconditioning. Normalizing circadian rhythms can be achieved by optimizing a sleep schedule with more wakeful periods during the day and reduction of noise at night (Shiraishi et al, 2003). If the patient is eating normally, meals need to be regularized.

END-OF-LIFE ISSUES

Anticipation of dying and death are traumatic for the patient, family and friends, and the health-care team. The phases of dying (Kinney & Packa, 1995) that can be anticipated when caring for the patient who is at the end of life are presented in Box 33-8.

The psychosocial issues in conjunction with support of the patient's physical status and comfort are priorities (Kuhl, 2002). Communicating effectively and being responsive to an individual's dignity and need is important. Each individual differs with respect to his or her needs, and time must be taken to identify these in an open and honest environment. Touching has a particularly important role in providing support and comfort as the end of life nears.

As the goal shifts from the provision of active treatment to supportive palliative care, the physical therapist needs to adjust treatment accordingly. Comfort and symptom management are the primary goals toward the end of an individuals life. If the patient is able to participate, modified active treatment in conjunction with a high level of support and attention to comfort can be of benefit. As the goals are revised, and if appropriate for the patient, he or she may remain actively engaged in planning and scheduling treatments.

If the patient is unable to cooperate actively with treatment, physical and psychological comfort and symptom management are maximized from a noninvasive perspective to support pharmacological support. Treatments may include relaxation, provision of comfort and human contact, noninvasive pain control strategies, breathing control and coughing maneuvers, and range of motion.

Principles of Physical Therapy Management

The family and friends of the patient who is dying have special needs that must be considered, and in fact constitute an integral part of the patient's overall care. In general the physical comfort and personal hygiene of the patient, as well as the quality of the immediate psychosocial environment, are paramount concerns. Optimal functional capacity is maintained as much as possible (Santiago-Palma & Payne, 2001) and has been shown to improve even in patients whose course is unstable (Sliwa & Marciniak, 1999). Nonetheless, the individual's priorities and needs may change quickly. The physical therapist needs to be flexible to accommodate these fluctuations, and sensitive to indications for no intervention. This may be a time for providing support and touching, if the patient wishes. Compassion, understanding, and respect for the patient and the family must be forthcoming from the ICU team as a whole. The ability to be attentive, comforting, and compassionate is an invaluable personal quality that needs to be developed to a high degree in the critical care area. The team needs to attend to how the patient, if sufficiently alert, is dealing with the possibility of dying and take their cues from the patient with respect to the role they need to play. If requested by the patient or family, spiritual care leaders are summoned.

If life support systems are being continued, the physical therapist may provide treatment to keep the patient as comfortable as possible. Conservative prophylactic cardiopulmonary physical therapy may be provided to reduce the work of breathing (body positioning and stress reduction, both of which can minimize oxygen cost). Treatments are kept to a minimum in terms of number and duration if death is inevitable. Range of motion exercises and skin care may help to reduce the discomfort of restricted mobility, facilitate nursing management and the basic care of the patient, and prevent complications. Analgesics may be continued along with other medications to reduce pain and suffering and maximize comfort. If so, these are prudently coordinated with treatments, if appropriate. In the presence of life supports the patient's needs may have to be anticipated somewhat more than without life supports because they severely limit communication. The dignity and modesty of the patient continue to be observed even after death.

The patient who has had life supports removed receives the same level of palliative care as the patient with supports. Weakness and wasting may contribute to the fatigue induced by treatment and coughing. Facilitated and supported coughing may help reduce the effort required to cough productively.

One's humanity is one of the most important attributes a health care provider can bring to the care of patients, and this is particularly true in palliative care. The use of human touch and talking (or being silent) may be the single most important means of communicating with and providing support to the patient who is dying and may be unable or disinterested in communicating. Supportive touching and handholding may be even more important to the patient on life support systems where the supports may be experienced as a physical barrier between the patient and those around him or her.

SUMMARY

Cardiopulmonary physical therapy in the ICU is a unique specialty. Despite the high-tech environment and severity of illness, most people are discharged after their ICU stays, which are variable in duration. Management focuses on returning the patient to a premorbid level of function or higher and, in the process, minimizing morbidity, mortality, and length of hospital stay. The general goals of critical care are function optimization (consistent with the International Classification of Function) and prophylaxis. Specific primary goals are defined by the underlying cardiopulmonary pathophysiology and multisystem dysfunction and its sequelae. Specific secondary goals are defined by the presence of or the potential for complications including musculoskeletal and neuromuscular dysfunction. This chapter elaborated on some general aspects of managing patients in the ICU. The knowledge base and experience of physical therapists working in the area were presented. A broad overview of the objectives of treatment and the rationale for prioritizing treatments according to a physiological hierarchy were described. General clinical and nonclinical aspects of patient management were discussed. Finally, end-of-life issues were presented.

Review Questions

1. Describe the elements of evidence-based practice in cardiopulmonary physical therapy.
2. Describe the general goals and principles of cardiopulmonary physical therapy in the ICU.
3. How do these goals reflect the International Classification of Function (i.e., limitations in participation, activity, as well as structure and function)?
4. Describe the role of monitoring in cardiopulmonary physical therapy care of the patient who is critically-ill.
5. Describe what is meant by "bringing one's humanity" to the management of people who are critically ill.
6. End-of-life issues are not only a concern in the intensive care unit. What attributes of the physical therapist are especially important in managing an individual at the end of life, irrespective of setting?

REFERENCES

Barach, A.L. (1974). Chronic obstructive lung disease: postural relief of dyspnea. Archives of Physical Medicine and Rehabilitation 55:494-504.

Barlow, D.H., Hayes, S.C., & Nelson, R.O. (1999). The scientist practitioner: research and accountability in the age of managed care. Boston: Allyn & Bacon.

Bennett, W.D., Foster, W.M., & Chapman, W.F. (1990). Cough-enhanced mucus clearance in the normal lung. Journal of Applied Physiology 69:1670-1675.

Berney, S., & Denehy, L. (2003). The effect of physiotherapy treatment on oxygen consumption and haemodynamics in patients who are critically ill. Australian Journal of Physiotherapy 49:99-105.

Burns, S.M., Egloff, M.B., Ryan, B., Carpenter, R., & Burns, J.E. (1994). Effect of body position on spontaneous respiratory rate and tidal volume in patients with obesity, abdominal distension and ascites. American Journal of Critical Care 3:102-106.

Casciari, R.J., Fairshter, R.D., Harrison, A., Morrison, J.T., Blackburn, C., & Wilson, A.F. (1981). Effects of breathing retraining in patients with chronic obstructive pulmonary disease. Chest 79:393-398.

Cohen, D., Horiuchi, K., Kemper, M., & Weissman, C. (1996). Modulating effects of propofol on metabolic and cardio-pulmonary responses to stressful intensive care unit procedures. Critical Care Medicine 24:612-617.

Cook, D. (2000). Ventilator associated pneumonia: perspectives on the burden of illness. Intensive Care Medicine 26(Suppl):S31-S37.

Cullen, D.J., Ferrara, L.C., Gilbert, J., Briggs, B.A., & Walker, P.F. (1977). Indicators of intensive care in critically ill patients. Critical Care Medicine 5:173-179.

Cutler, P. (1997). Problem solving in clinical medicine, from data to diagnosis, ed 3. Baltimore: Lippincott Williams & Wilkins.

Dantzker, D.R., Schay, S.M., & Fletcher, J. (1997). Cardiopulmonary critical care, ed 3. Philadelphia: Elsevier.

Dean, E. (1983). Research. The right way. Clinical Management 3:29-33.

Dean, E. (1985). Psychobiological adaptation model for physical therapy practice. Physical Therapy 65:1061-1068.

Dean, E. (1994a). Oxygen transport: a physiologically-based conceptual framework for the practice of cardiopulmonary physiotherapy. Physiotherapy 80:347-355.

Dean, E. (1994b). Invited commentary to "Are incentive spirometry, intermittent positive pressure breathing, and deep breathing exercises effective in the prevention of postoperative pulmonary complications after upper abdominal surgery? A systematic overview and meta-analysis." Physical Therapy 74:10-15.

Dean, E. (2002). Physiotherapy skills: positioning and mobilization of the patient. In Pryor, J.A., Ammani Prasad, S., & Webber, B.A. (Eds). Physiotherapy for respiratory and cardiac problems: adults and paediatrics, ed 3. St. Louis: Harcourt Health Sciences Group.

Dean, E., & Ross, J. (1992). Discordance between cardiopulmonary physiology and physical therapy. Chest 101:1694-1698.

De Backer, D., El Haddad, P., Preiser, J.C., & Vincent, J.L. (2000). Hemodynamic responses to successful weaning from mechanical ventilation after cardiovascular surgery. Intensive Care Medicine 26:1201-1206.

Hedenstierna, G., & Lattuada, M. (2002). Gas exchange in ventilated patients. Current Opinions in Critical Care 8:39-44.

Hislop, J.H. (1975). Tenth Mary McMillain lecture. The not-so-impossible dream. Physical Therapy 55:1069-1080.

Horiuchi, K., Jordan, D., Cohen, D., Kemper, M.C., & Weissman, C. (1997). Insights into the increased oxygen demand during chest physiotherapy. Critical Care Medicine 25:1347-1351.

Imbus, S.H., & Zawacki, B.E. (1986). Encouraging dialogue and autonomy in the burn intensive care unit. Critical Care Clinics 2:53-60.

Irwin, S., & Tecklin, J.S. (Eds). (2004). Cardiopulmonary physical therapy, ed 4. Philadelphia: Elsevier.

Jardin, F., Farcot, J.C., Boisante, L., Curien, N., Margairaz, A., & Bourdarias, J.P. (1981). Influence of positive end-expiratory pressure on left ventricular performance. New England Journal of Medicine 304:387-392.

Karlawish, J.H. (1996). Shared decision making in critical care: a clinical reality and an ethical issue. American Journal of Critical Care 5:391-396.

Kelly, K.M. (1996). Does increasing oxygen delivery improve outcome? Yes. Critical Care Clinics 12:635-644.

Kinney, M.R., & Packa, D.R. (1995). Andreoli's comprehensive cardiac care, ed 7. Philadelphia: Elsevier.

Kirilloff, L.H., Owens, G.R., Rogers, R.M., & Mazzocco, M.C. (1985). Does chest physical therapy work? Chest 88:436-444.

Kuhl, D. (2002). What dying patients want: practical wisdom for the end of life. Toronto: Random House of Canada Ltd.

Lynn-McHale, D.J., & Carlson, K.K. (2000). AACN procedure manual for critical care, ed 4. Philadelphia: Elsevier.

Marini, J.J. (1984). Postoperative atelectasis: pathophysiology, clinical importance, and principles of management. Respiratory Care 29:516-528.

Mueller, R.E., Petty, T.L., & Filley, G.F. (1970). Ventilation and arterial blood gas changes induced by pursed lips breathing. Journal of Applied Physiology 28:784-789.

O'Sullivan, K.L., Engrav, L.H., Maier, R.V., Pilcher, S.L., Isik, F.F., & Copass, M.K. (1997). Pressure sores in the acute trauma patient: incidence and causes. Journal of Trauma 42:276-278.

Petty, T.L. (1985). Chronic obstructive pulmonary disease, ed 2. New York: Marcel Dekker.

Riegelman, R.K. (1991). Minimizing medical mistakes. The art of medical decision making. Boston: Little, Brown and Company.

Rochester, D.F., & Esau, S.A. (1984). Malnutrition and the respiratory system. Chest 85:411-415.

Ross, J., & Dean, E. (1989). Integrating physiological principles into the comprehensive management of cardiopulmonary dysfunction. Physical Therapy 69:255-259.

Santiago-Palma, J., & Payne, R. (2001). Palliative care and rehabilitation. Cancer 92:1049-1052.

Schon, D.A. (1983). The reflective practitioner. How professionals think in action. New York: Basic Books.

Shiraishi, M., Kamo, T., Nemoto, S., Narita, M., Kamegai, M., Baevsky, R.M., & Funtova, H. (2003). Blood pressure variability during 120-day head-down bed rest in humans. Biomedical Pharmacotherapy 57(Suppl 1):35S-38S.

Shoemaker, W.C. (Ed). (1999). Textbook of critical care, ed 4. Philadelphia: Elsevier.

Silver, K.H., Siebens, A.A. (1994). Rehabilitation medicine. Surgical Clinics of North America 74:465-488.

Sliwa, J.A., & Marciniak, C. (1999). Physical rehabilitation of the cancer patient. Cancer Treatment Research 100:75-89.

Stillwell, S. (1992). Mosby's critical care nursing reference. St Louis: Mosby.

Thomas, D.C., Kreizman, I.J., Melchiorre, P., & Ragnarsson, K.T. (2002). Rehabilitation of the patient with chronic critical illness. Critical Care Clinics 18:695-715.

Weissman, C., & Kemper, M. (1993). Stressing the critically ill patient: the cardiopulmonary and metabolic responses to an acute increase in oxygen consumption. Journal of Critical Care 8:100-108.

Williams, D.T., & Harding, K. (2003). Healing responses of skin and muscle in critical illness. Critical Care Medicine 31:S547-S557.

CHAPTER 34

Intensive Care Unit Management of Individuals with Primary Cardiopulmonary Dysfunction

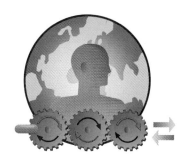

Elizabeth Dean and Christiane Perme

KEY TERMS

Cardiopulmonary failure
Coronary artery disease
Obstructive lung disease

Primary cardiopulmonary dysfunction
Restrictive lung disease
Status asthmaticus

This chapter presents the principles of cardiopulmonary physical therapy in the management of patients who are critically ill with *primary* cardiopulmonary dysfunction that can lead to cardiopulmonary failure. The categories of conditions presented are obstructive lung disease, status asthmaticus, restrictive lung disease, and coronary artery disease (medical and surgical conditions). Each category of condition is presented in two parts. The related pathophysiology and pertinent aspects of the medical management of each condition are presented as a basis for and in relation to the principles of physical therapy management. These are not mutually exclusive for each category because considerable overlap may exist when conditions coexist. Invasive care and noninvasive care have common goals and thus are complementary. Special considerations for the physical therapy management of patients in the ICU with examples of common conditions are highlighted.

These principles are not treatment prescriptions. Each patient must be assessed and treated individually, taking into consideration all factors that contribute to impaired oxygen transport (i.e., recumbency, restricted mobility, extrinsic factors related to the patient's care, intrinsic factors related to the patient, and the underlying pathophysiology) (see Chapter 2).

CARDIOPULMONARY FAILURE

Pathophysiology

The heart and lungs work interdependently; thus failure of one organ has significant implications for the function of the other organ (Vincent & Suter, 1987; Weber et al, 1983). Insufficiency or failure of the cardiopulmonary system refers to the inability of this system to maintain adequate oxygen and carbon dioxide homeostasis.

Pulmonary failure reflects a gas exchange defect or defect of the ventilatory pump. Table 34-1 shows the classification of pulmonary failure by specific causes and the mechanisms involved. Some common predisposing conditions include primary cardiopulmonary conditions (e.g., chronic lung disease, overwhelming pneumonia, and myocardial infarction) and secondary cardiopulmonary conditions (e.g., motor neuron diseases, spinal cord injury, stroke, and muscular dystrophy) (see Chapter 35). The oxygen and carbon dioxide tensions that have been used to define failure are variable because they depend on factors such as premorbid status, general health, age, prior blood gas profile, and the time frame for the development of failure. Arterial blood gases and pH are essential in the assessment of cardiopulmonary failure, which is usually diagnosed when the PaO_2 falls below 50 to 60 mm Hg and the $PaCO_2$ rises above 50 mm Hg (Shoemaker et al, 1999).

TABLE 34-1

Classification of Respiratory Failure by Cause and Mechanisms

ORIGIN	DRUGS	METABOLIC	NEOPLASMS	INFECTIONS	TRAUMA	OTHER

Brain	Narcotics
	Barbiturates
	Sedatives
	Poisons
	Anesthetics
		Hyponatremia
		Hypocalcemia
		Hypercapnia
		Alkalosis
		Hyperglycemia
		Myxedema
			Primary
			Metastatic
				Meningitis
				Encephalitis
				Abscess
				Bulbar polio
					Direct injury
					Increased
					   pressure
						Central alveolar
						   hypoventilation
						Obstructive sleep
						   apnea

Nerves and Muscles	Curariform drugs
	Arsenic
	Aminoglycosides
		Hypophosphatemia
		Hypomagnesemia
			Primary
			Metastatic
				Polio
				Tetanus
					Direct injury	Motor neuron
						   disease
						Myasthenia gravis
						Multiple sclerosis
						Muscular dystrophy
						Guillain-Barré
						   syndrome

Upper Airway			Tonsillar
			   adenoid
			   hyperplasia
			Goiter
			Polyps
			Malignant
			   tumors
				Epiglottitis
				Laryngotracheitis
					Vocal cord
					   paralysis
					Tracheomalacia
					Cricoarytenoid
					   arthritis
					Laryngeal
					   edema	

Chest Bellows					Flail chest
					Burn with
					   keloids
						Scleroderma
						Pleural interposition
						   (fibrosis, fluid,
						   tumor, air)
						Spondylitis
						Scoliosis
						Kyphosis

Contributing Factors						Massive obesity Ascites Ileus Pain Recumbency

Lower Airway and Parenchyma			Malignant
			Benign
				Viral
				   (bronchiolitis,
				   bronchopneumonia)
				Bacterial
				   (bronchitis,
				   pneumonia, abscess,
				   bronchiectasis)
				Fungal
				Mycoplasma
					Contused
					   lung
						Bronchospasm
						Heart failure
						   congestive
						   restrictive
						   obstructive
						COPD
						Respiratory distress
						   syndrome
						Interstitial lung
						   disease
						Atelectasis
						Cystic fibrosis
						Pulmonary emboli

From Civettia, J.M. Taylor, R.W. & Kirby, R.R (1988). Critical care, Philadelphia: JB Lippincott.

Primary cardiac failure reflects failure of the myocardium to pump blood to the pulmonary and systemic circulations and maintain adequate tissue perfusion (Austin & Greenfield, 1980). Significant dysfunction of the left ventricle can lead to pulmonary vascular congestion and cardiogenic pulmonary edema (i.e., congestive heart failure) (Matthay, 1985). Diseases of the heart that can lead to failure include significant myocardial damage as a result of infarction or myopathy, valvular heart disease, and congenital defects.

Both primary pulmonary and cardiac failure can be classified into acute and chronic stages. The compensation mechanisms that occur in the two stages are distinct. With adequate physiological compensation, patients can tolerate some degree of chronic failure. Patients with a mild degree of failure can live reasonably independent lives. Moderate failure is significantly more limiting, thus these patients may require home ventilatory support (e.g., supplemental oxygen and nighttime ventilation), and severe failure requires hospitalization and mechanical ventilatory support.

INDIVIDUALS WITH OBSTRUCTIVE LUNG DISEASE

Pathophysiology and Medical Management

Obstructive lung disease can result in ventilatory failure and admission of the patient to the intensive care unit (ICU), or it can complicate management if the patient is admitted for other reasons (Lynn-McHale & Carlson, 2000; Boggs & Wooldridge-King, 1993; Cheitlin, 2004). If conservative management fails or is unlikely to improve critically impaired oxygen transport and gas exchange and to adequately remove copious and tenacious secretions, intubation and mechanical ventilation are indicated (see Chapter 42). Complicating factors include impaired oxygen delivery, polycythemia, impaired respiratory mechanics secondary to lung damage and increased time constants impairing optimal inhalation and exhalation, flattened hemidiaphragms, rigid barrel-shaped chest wall, increased accessory muscle use and work of breathing, reduced diffusing capacity, impaired mucociliary transport, secretion accumulation, ineffective cough mechanism, increased oxygen consumption, increased work of the heart, and general debility and weakness.

The goal of intubation and mechanical ventilation is to support breathing by providing an airway and adequate alveolar ventilation, and is based on arterial blood gas analysis. A tidal volume and a respiratory rate that provide satisfactory blood gas and pH values are established and maintained unless the clinical condition changes. The precise regulation of mechanical ventilation helps to restore adequate blood gases and cardiopulmonary function, reduce the work of breathing, rest fatigued ventilatory muscles, and provide an optimal fraction of inspired oxygen (FIO_2) and humidification (Figure 34-1) (Wilson, 1992).

Minute ventilation can be seriously impaired with a leak in the mechanical ventilator circuitry. The tubes connecting sites are often the sites of air leakage. Complete disconnection at the endotracheal or tracheostomy connection may occur in

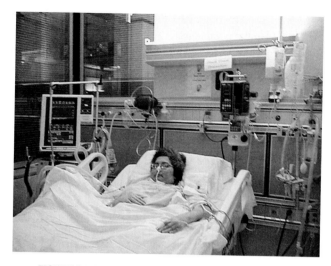

FIGURE 34-1 Patient receiving mechanical ventilation.

those patients with high pulmonary resistance. Close monitoring of the exhaled tidal volume and end tidal carbon dioxide will ensure the patient is receiving sufficient ventilation.

Positive end expiratory pressure (PEEP) is useful in promoting greater opportunity for gas exchange at end-expiration in mechanically ventilated patients. Venous return, myocardial perfusion, and cardiac output, however, may be impaired during positive pressure ventilation with PEEP administration (Jardin et al, 1981; Kumar et al, 1973). Excessive stimulation to cough in these ventilated patients should be avoided because this accentuates the cardiovascular side effects of PEEP. Continuous positive airway pressure (CPAP) can maintain airway patency during spontaneous ventilation. This mode of ventilation, however, seems to be preferred in children, whereas PEEP is used more commonly in adults.

Interference with the gag reflex in the patient with an endotracheal tube increases the risk of aspiration of the oropharyngeal and gastric contents and can result in pneumonitis and pneumonia. Risk of aspiration from the oropharyngeal cavity can be reduced by suctioning through the airway with the cuff of the airway inflated, in addition to suctioning the oropharynx after suctioning via the airway.

Suctioning can be performed frequently in a patient with an artificial airway and is less traumatic. Patients should be suctioned only as indicated because this procedure can produce significant desaturation (up to 60%), particularly in the ventilated patient (Walsh et al, 1989). Administration of 100% oxygen for three minutes before and after suctioning (i.e., hyperoxygenation) minimizes this desaturation effect. This can be accomplished by manually bagging the patient before treatment (i.e., manual hyperventilation) or by presetting the mechanical ventilator (Fell & Cheney, 1971). Risk of aspiration of gastric contents is reduced by the use of a nasogastric tube.

A common cause of acute respiratory failure is advanced chronic airflow limitation (Kirby et al, 1996). The pathophysiological deficits include significant loss of alveolar tissue, increased compliance of alveolar tissue, hyperinflated chest wall, impaired respiratory mechanics, flattened hemidiaphragms, impaired breathing efficiency, and reduced diffusing capacity. Proportional changes in lung volumes and capacities in patients with chronic airway limitation compared with healthy persons are presented in Figure 9-5. The primary abnormality is a significantly increased residual volume and inspiratory reserve volume and hence total lung capacity. Failure of oxygen transport ensues secondary to ventilation and perfusion mismatch, ventilatory muscle fatigue, reactive pulmonary hypertension, and right ventricular failure. Correcting the complications of respiratory failure, however, is often more problematic than treating the specific cause. Hypoxemia and hypercapnia are often present. Hypoxemia is usually improved with supplemental oxygen in the absence of significant diffusion defect or shunt.

Cardiovascular complications are among the most prevalent observed in ventilatory failure. Marked hypercapnia (increased arterial PCO_2) with acidemia (reduced pH) can produce extreme vasodilatation and hypotension resulting from the local action on blood vessels (Lynn-McHale & Carlson, 2000). Mild hypercapnia can produce reflex vasoconstriction and hypertension. Occasionally systemic hypertension is observed during weaning from the ventilator with the presence of a moderate degree of hypercapnia.

Right heart failure, cor pulmonale, is a well-known complication of chronic lung disease and congestive heart failure. Both hypoxia and reduced pH cause pulmonary vasoconstriction and an increase in pulmonary artery pressure. Consequently, reversing bronchospasm, hypoxemia, hypercapnia, and acidemia can often reduce pulmonary vasoconstriction, lower pulmonary artery pressure, and thereby improve hemodynamics.

End-stage respiratory failure results in a progressive increase in airway resistance, work of breathing, oxygen consumption, and carbon dioxide production. In areas of bronchial obstruction, marked alveolar hypoventilation results and ventilation and perfusion are severely mismatched. Hypoxemia and respiratory acidosis produce reactive pulmonary hypertension and further ventilatory failure. Profound carbon dioxide retention, refractory hypoxemia, and respiratory acidemia may terminate in a fatal dysrhythmia (Gibson et al, 1977; Macklem & Roussos, 1977; Rochester & Arora, 1983; Vincent & Suter, 1987; Weinstein & Skillman, 1980; Weissman et al, 1989).

Acidemia from respiratory causes with a pH of less than 7.25 is often harmful with respect to dysrhythmia production. Conversely, hypoventilation is equally harmful, and pH elevations greater than 7.5 may cause neurological and cardiovascular complications. In acute respiratory failure with profound acidemia, intravenous use of bicarbonate is used to buffer the hydrogen ion concentration until the underlying disorder is corrected. Bicarbonate infusion is guided by frequent pH measurements.

Transport of oxygen and carbon dioxide to and from the tissues depends on adequate pulmonary and systemic circulation. Frequently, blood volume has to be restored by fluids or blood replacement or both. Inotropic agents are used to maintain adequate circulation by augmenting myocardial contractility.

Of increasing interest in recent years has been the experience of illness and its contribution to disability (see Chapter 1). After their first episode of respiratory failure, patients with chronic obstructive pulmonary disease (COPD) report worse cognitive function and overall health status. After several months, however, these conditions may return to levels reported by individuals with similar disease severity who are being conservatively managed and have had no ICU admission (Ambrosino et al, 2002). The Nottingham Health Profile and Mini Mental Status can be useful tools for ongoing assessment of perceived health and cognition.

Principles of Physical Therapy Management

The principles of management of acute respiratory failure secondary to an exacerbation of COPD are based on interventions that will enhance oxygen transport (i.e., oxygen delivery, oxygen consumption, and oxygen extraction) and facilitate carbon dioxide removal (Gallagher & Civetta, 1980). Thus the steps of the oxygen transport pathway that have been identified as impaired or threatened by the patient's condition (i.e., immobility, recumbency, and extrinsic and intrinsic factors in addition to the underlying pathophysiology) (see Chapter 2) are the focus of treatment (Wong, 2000). On the basis of a detailed analysis of these factors, treatments are selected, prioritized, and applied to optimize the steps in the pathway that are affected. These may include treatments to maximize the patency of the airways, increase alveolar ventilation, facilitate mucociliary transport, facilitate airway clearance, optimize the mechanical position of the diaphragm, optimize ventilation and perfusion matching, optimize pH, eliminate carbon dioxide, optimize peripheral circulation and tissue perfusion, and reduce the work of breathing and of the heart. To optimize oxygen transport, the primary goals of physical therapy management include the following:

1. improve or maintain arterial oxygen tension (PaO_2) or prevent its deterioration;
2. improve or maintain arterial oxygen saturation (SaO_2) or prevent its deterioration;
3. improve or maintain arterial carbon dioxide levels ($PaCO_2$) and pH or prevent its deterioration;
4. optimize oxygen delivery and oxygen consumption relationship.

The means by which these goals are fulfilled depends on each patient's clinical presentation and the specific factors that contribute to cardiopulmonary dysfunction.

Mobilization: Special considerations

Mobilization and ambulation are requisite for normal physiological functioning of the human body (i.e., to stimulate exercise stress and gravitational stress and thereby optimize oxygen transport) (Dean & Ross, 1992). Although patients in the ICU are encouraged to move, exercise, sit up, stand, sit in chairs, take a few steps, and in some circumstances ambulate across the unit even if they are ventilated (Mackenzie et al, 1989), therapeutic mobilization is prescribed to exploit its acute effects, long-term cumulative effects, and preventive effects (see Chapter 18). These effects are physiologically distinct and need to be prescribed specifically to address each patient's problems. With the monitoring capability in the ICU, patients who are critically ill can move and be moved within safe therapeutic limits.

Given that cardiopulmonary physical therapy is among those activities that are the most metabolically demanding for patients in the ICU (Dean et al, 1995; Horiuchi et al, 1997; Weissman & Kemper, 1993; Weissman et al, 1984), the patient's capacity to meet a given increase in oxygen demand must be determined before treatment. Even though cardiopulmonary physical therapy stresses the oxygen transport system as a means of improving the function and efficiency of this system, unnecessary or excessive energy expenditure is undesirable and thus should be minimized. Interventions that can minimize oxygen demand include relaxation, judicious body positioning to facilitate oxygen transport, coordination of treatments with other interventions, scheduling treatments at appropriate times, timing treatments with medications so the maximal effect is achieved, pain control, and coordinating treatments with peak energy periods and around rest periods.

Mobilization and exercise are at the top of the hierarchy of physiological treatments; thus the potent and direct effects of these interventions are exploited first (see Chapter 17). Being moved to (passive) or moving into (active) the upright position promotes improved cardiopulmonary function and gas exchange. Chairs should be available at the side of every ICU bed to provide greater opportunity for the patient to be upright. The benefits of the upright sitting position are different to sitting propped up in bed. Stretcher chairs are particularly useful for patients who are unable to bear weight (Figure 34-2). Even minimal ability of the patient to assist with his or her bed mobility and transferring must be exploited, even if the maneuver takes several minutes and multiple assistants. These minimal efforts must be exploited. Without doing so, the patient's oxygen transport system deconditions further, which also reduces the patient's tolerance to be mobilized. What justifies this time and personnel cost is the greater therapeutic outcome that can be expected compared with passive interventions. The fundamental goal is enhanced recovery, reduced discomfort, reduced morbidity and mortality, and reduced ICU and hospital stay.

Significant benefit can be gained from standing the ventilated patient, provided there are no absolute contra-indications to being upright in terms of cardiopulmonary function, neuromuscular and musculoskeletal status, and skin integrity. Ambulating the patient who is ventilated is the priority whenever possible (Burns & Jones, 1975; Holton, 1972). The potential risks, however, must be recognized.

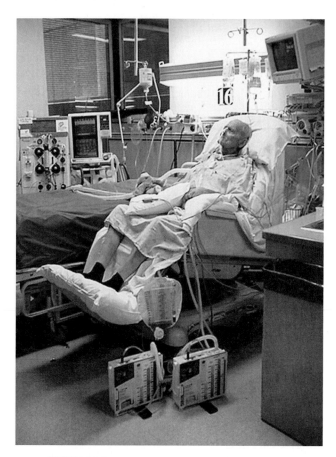

FIGURE 34-2 ICU patient sitting in a stretcher chair.

Mobilization and exercise must be prescribed specifically to ensure that the exercise stimulus is therapeutic (i.e., provides an adequate stressor to the oxygen transport pathway, yet is not hazardous).

Standing and walking even a few steps can be extremely strenuous for the patient in the ICU with respect to oxygen demand. Such activities need to be introduced gradually and with continuous monitoring to ensure the patient does not exceed the prescribed therapeutic intensity needed to maximize oxygen transport. Standing and walking are coordinated with other aspects of the patient's care and should be carried out in several stages (Figures 34-3, *A-E*). Monitoring of the electrocardiogram (ECG) and arterial saturation of the critically ill patient while he or she performs activities such as standing or walking cannot be overemphasized. By disconnecting these monitors, the physical therapist is working blindly and potentially dangerously because the leads do not reach or because of movement artifact. In anticipation of an increased workload, ventilatory parameters for ventilated patients may require adjusting. A greater concentration of oxygen should be delivered for at least three to five minutes before the activity and continued afterward for 10 minutes or so until the patient has recovered from the increased exertion and the heart rate and blood pressure have returned to within 5% to 10% of baseline values.

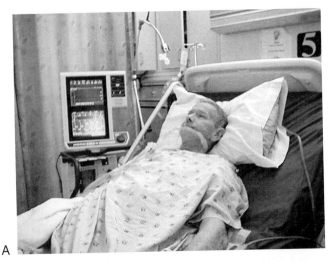

A

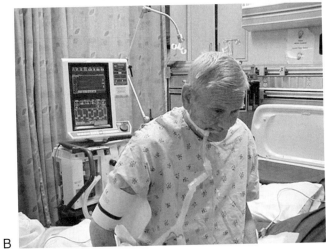

B

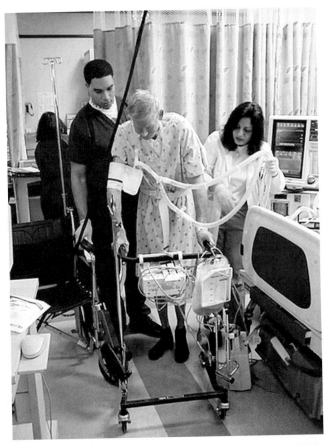

D

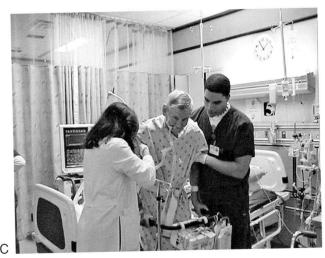

C

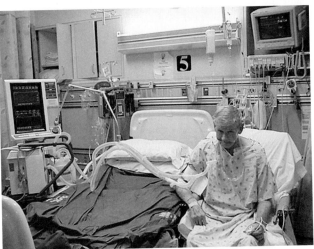

E

FIGURE 34-3 ICU patient receiving physical therapy treatment. **A,** Patient is on mechanical ventilation with an oral endotracheal tube. **B,** Patient sitting on the edge of the bed. **C,** Standing at the edge of bed with walker and assistance of two people. **D,** Walking around the bed. **E,** Patient sitting on a bedside chair after physical therapy treatment. Specific safety precautions must be followed at all times to safely mobilize the patient and to prevent accidental extubation.

Active movement has greater therapeutic effect on oxygen transport than assisted or passive movements; thus the benefits of active movements are exploited first. Movement recruiting large muscle groups minimizes the disproportionate hemodynamic stress associated with movement of small muscle groups or movements requiring excessive dynamic stabilization (Hanson & Nagel, 1987). If active movements cannot be performed or excessively stress the oxygen transport system, then active assisted movements are indicated. Passive movements have a role primarily when the patient is paralyzed or so hemodynamically unstable that the patient deteriorates with active movement. With respect to cardiopulmonary benefits, passive movement stimulates changes in ventilatory and circulatory patterns (West, 2004). These can be particularly beneficial in patients who have significant mobility restriction; however, they should not substitute for active and active-assisted movements, which are associated with even greater benefit because they are higher order activities on the physiologically based treatment hierarchy (see Chapter 17).

A recent study reported on the use of electrical stimulation in combination with active exercise of the limbs in patients with severe COPD who were mechanically ventilated (Zanotti et al, 2003). Muscle strength was improved and the number of days to transfer from bed to chair was reduced. The study's design precludes electrical stimulation as being superior to extended active exercise and progressive mobilization to the chair and ambulation.

Body Positioning: Special Considerations

Body positioning is a potent therapeutic intervention that promotes optimal oxygen transport and gas exchange in two ways; one, from the physiological benefits accrued from the specific positions themselves, and two, from the physiological benefits accrued from physically changing from one position to another (see Chapter 19). Body position can be used preferentially to augment alveolar volume, alveolar ventilation, ventilation and perfusion matching, respiratory mechanics, cough effectiveness, central and peripheral hemodynamics and fluid shifts, mucociliary transport, and secretion clearance (see Chapter 19). Both ventilation and perfusion are enhanced in the inferior lung fields. Thus in postural drainage positions the superior lung being treated is neither preferentially ventilated nor perfused. The less affected lung fields therefore may be contributing more substantially to improving arterial gases. Hence the physical therapist must consider the goals of treatment with respect to pulmonary function in both the involved and less-involved lung fields. During postural drainage, the length of time in a given position needs to be monitored to avoid drainage of secretions into the less involved, functional, inferior lung fields and to avoid the possibility of compression atelectasis in the inferior lung (Dean, 1985; Leblanc et al, 1970).

Although positions can be predicted that will optimize ventilation and perfusion matching, each patient will respond differently, depending on such factors as pathology, age,

weight, depth of breathing, and mechanical ventilation (Clauss et al, 1968; Ray et al, 1974). Therefore the patient's response to specific positioning must be observed, documented, and objectively monitored with respect to the effect on oxygen transport variables.

Another important goal of body positioning is to potentiate position-dependent fluid shifts to optimize cardiovascular function. For this reason the patient should be positioned upright as often as possible. There are other beneficial effects of the upright position on pulmonary function (e.g., maximize lung volumes and capacities, minimize alveolar collapse, decrease airway resistance, increase lung compliance and thereby reduce ventilator system pressure). To maximize the effect of gravity on promoting fluid shifts, the legs should be positioned dependently at frequent intervals. In a patient who is not self-supporting with or without assistance, fluid shifts can be stimulated with a high Fowler's position coupled with the use of the bed knee-break. Between sessions of therapeutic body positioning, a schedule of four-point turning (supine, left side, prone, right side) is ideal and should be attempted even in the ventilated patient if not strictly contraindicated (Dean, 2002).

Extreme 360-degree body position changes (i.e., randomized positioning in supine, prone, right and left side-lying) have been reported to have beneficial effects on oxygen transport in patients with acute respiratory failure (Kim et al, 2002). The head-down position has been shown to reduce respiratory distress in some patients with obstructive lung disease (Barach & Beck, 1954). The abdominal viscera are displaced cephalad, thereby elevating the typically flattened hemi-diaphragms and placing them in a mechanically advantageous position. This effect may be mimicked in other body positions by manual abdominal compression and abdominal binders. In some patients, however, the additional load imposed by the increased intraabdominal pressure on the underside of the diaphragm may inadvertently increase the work of breathing and increase respiratory distress. The prone position has been reported to be beneficial in patients with acute respiratory failure (Douglas et al, 1977; Piehl & Brown, 1976). A variant of the prone position, semi-prone, may be more beneficial in some patients by reducing intraabdominal pressure. In addition, the semi-prone position may be safer and more comfortable for the mechanically ventilated patient. The prescription of any body positioning must be based on its anticipated benefits on oxygen transport. The more extreme positions should be introduced in progressive stages and the patient's response monitored to ensure the response is favorable.

INDIVIDUALS WITH STATUS ASTHMATICUS

Pathophysiology and Medical Management

Status asthmaticus is a potentially life-threatening situation (Petty, 1982; Pryor et al, 2002). The pathophysiological features include marked airway resistance secondary to bronchospasm, edema, and mucous secretion and retention.

The work of breathing is markedly increased, resulting in respiratory distress. A cycle results in which the patient becomes more hypoxemic and hypercapnic secondary to alveolar hypoventilation, bronchospasm increases, and reactive pulmonary hypertension may ensue along with a further increase in the work of breathing and anxiety.

The classical signs and symptoms of a severe asthmatic attack that may progress to status asthmaticus include tachypnea, dyspnea, labored breathing, audible wheezing, tachycardia, cyanosis, anxiety, and panic. If the patient is able to cooperate with spirometric testing, the degree of reduced vital capacity, peak flow, and forced expiratory volume provide indices of the severity of airway obstruction (Brunner & Wolff, 1988).

Medical management is aimed at administering drugs and fluids to reduce hypoxemia with oxygen, decrease airway inflammation and resistance, and hence reduce the work of breathing and anxiety. Intravenous sodium bicarbonate helps to reverse respiratory acidosis and possibly metabolic acidosis (Kirby et al, 1996).

Principles of Physical Therapy Management

The prime objective of physical therapy is to optimize oxygen transport and avoid or delay the need for mechanical ventilation. Physical therapy can augment the medical management of the patient with status asthmaticus. In an attempt to avert intubation and mechanical ventilation the physical therapist coordinates treatment with the patient's medications (i.e., bronchodilators, muscle relaxants, steroids, and supplemental oxygen). The physical therapist promotes breathing control, enhances ventilation and perfusion matching, promotes mucociliary transport and secretion clearance, reduces hypoxemia, and teaches the patient to coordinate relaxed breathing with general body movement. Caution needs to be observed to avoid stimuli that potentiate bronchospasm and deterioration of the patient's condition (e.g., body positions that increase respiratory distress rather than relieve it, chest wall percussion, forced expiration maneuvers, aggressive bagging, and possibly instillation). Attention to relaxation and reduction of excessive oxygen demands is a priority, as was described for the patient with chronic airflow limitation. Certain body positions may have to be avoided (for example, because of the patient's intolerance and exacerbation of symptoms in those positions). Because of the relationship of altered pulmonary function in different positions, positioning (especially in patients in respiratory distress) must be applied cautiously within the patient's tolerance. Those body positions that reduce respiratory distress and the work of breathing and maximize alveolar ventilation, oxygen saturation, and blood gases are the positions of choice.

Major problems in status asthmaticus are alveolar hypoventilation, airway obstruction secondary to bronchospasm, mucosal edema, and secretions. Thus maximizing alveolar ventilation and facilitating mucociliary transport are priorities (Bates, 1989). Other problems include significantly increased

work of breathing because of an inefficient breathing pattern and an ineffective cough. Obtaining a productive cough without augmenting bronchospasm is a challenge. Deep breathing with pursed-lips expiration helps to prolong expiration and maintain the patency of the small airways. Deep, slow, and relaxed breathing is emphasized along with periodic effective, controlled huffing, and avoidance of forced expiratory maneuvers (Hietpas et al, 1979; Nunn et al, 1965).

Despite aggressive noninvasive management, blood gases may deteriorate and mechanical ventilation may be inevitable. Relaxation, maximizing alveolar ventilation, and reducing airway collapse and obstruction continue to be the primary goals; however, the means of achieving these goals differ when the patient is mechanically ventilated. Optimal prescriptive body positioning is the intervention of choice. Secretion clearance is achieved by judicious suctioning. Suctioning is performed as required because it can contribute to reduced oxygenation, airway collapse, atelectasis, increased arousal, increased work of breathing, and generally increased respiratory distress.

INDIVIDUALS WITH RESTRICTIVE LUNG DISEASE

Pathophysiology and Medical Management

Acute respiratory failure can be associated with primary restrictive lung disease (i.e., interstitial pulmonary fibrosis). This is distinct from restrictive defects secondary to neuromuscular and musculoskeletal diseases (e.g., Guillain-Barré syndrome, myasthenia gravis, and neuromuscular poisonings are common neuromuscular disorders that can precipitate respiratory failure in the absence of underlying primary lung disease) (Chapter 35). If paralyzed, the patient will likely be dependent on ventilatory assistance.

Restrictive lung dysfunction may complicate the management of patients admitted to the ICU for reasons other than cardiopulmonary disease. The lung parenchyma, the chest wall, or both may be involved. The underlying cause of respiratory failure may therefore reflect ventilatory pump failure, gas exchange failure, or both. The specific restrictions to cardiopulmonary function need to be identified and treated individually to optimize treatment. Obstructive and restrictive patterns of cardiopulmonary function frequently coexist; thus the contribution of both types of defects to a patient's oxygen transport must be determined. Typically, in restrictive lung disease, all lung volumes and capacities are reduced, although tidal volume can be relatively normal (see Figure 9-5). Patients with severe interstitial pulmonary fibrosis have increased pulmonary artery pressures with an associated increase in right ventricular work (Chung & Dean, 1989). These patients desaturate very readily.

Principles of Physical Therapy Management

Restrictive ventilatory dysfunction is commonly associated with both medical and surgical conditions. The principles of management of acute respiratory failure associated with these differ in that medical conditions are associated with underlying irreversible lung damage, whereas in the surgical patient the pulmonary restriction is reversible. The natural course of disease in the medical patient will be determined in part by the patient's premorbid status. The majority of surgical patients, however, will have had normal lung function before surgery and the development of cardiopulmonary complications (see Chapter 30). Regardless of whether mechanical ventilation is indicated, tissue oxygenation, carbon dioxide removal, regulation of blood pH, and an effective cardiac output are priorities. Supplemental oxygen is often effective in improving tissue oxygenation in conditions associated with restrictive lung disease in the absence of a right-to-left shunt. In the presence of shunt, supplemental oxygen does not reverse hypoxemia.

A judicious turning regimen can also be designed to optimize cardiopulmonary function (even if the patient is mechanically ventilated) reduce risks of cardiopulmonary complications, reduce musculoskeletal deformities and skin breakdown, and promote comfort. It is essential with body positioning for any purpose that the patient is not confined unnecessarily and does not assume any position for too long. Although lines, leads, monitoring devices, and catheters may be required, these are anchored as securely as possible with sufficient length to allow the patient to move spontaneously, be mobilized as much as possible, undergo as many positioning changes as possible, and facilitate routine patient care.

Mobilization and general body movement, particularly in upright positions, is always a priority in the ICU, as much and as often as possible given the patient's condition and safety considerations. Movements may be totally assisted but more often are likely to be active-assisted and active. No matter how weak the patient may be, active-assisted and active movements are the mainstay of the movement interventions performed by the physical therapist, particularly if these can be performed in near-upright positions. Assisted or passive movements should not be performed unless specifically indicated (i.e., the patient is unable to execute these movements completely alone). Even modest attempts at active-assisted movements, with perhaps only a minimal number of repetitions, benefit the patient considerably more both in terms of treatment goals related to cardiopulmonary and musculoskeletal function than assisted movements that do not contribute to muscle strength, endurance, and coordination. Injudicious application of totally assisted movements will contribute to the patient's deconditioning and physical deterioration. Regardless of the type of mobilization, the patient is observed closely for arterial desaturation, discomfort, respiratory distress, cyanosis, fatigue, and extent of cooperation if assisted-active and active movements are being performed.

Assisted movements are indicated to promote oxygen transport via their effects on ventilatory and circulatory patterns (West, 2004). Additionally, the goal is to maintain joint range of motion and prevent adaptive shortening of periarticular soft tissue in particular. Care must therefore be taken to perform these movements through the complete range of movement for each joint, with special attention to rotary components of joint movement. Lax joints can maintain range with one complete range of motion daily. Lax joints are unprotected and vulnerable to excessive strain. Protection may best be effected in these joints by moving the joint more slowly through the extremes of joint range and just short of complete range. In the presence of spasticity or limb splinting because of discomfort, the involved joints will benefit from two or more excursions through full range daily.

One approach that may be particularly beneficial in altering the distribution of ventilation and blood flow is general body and range of motion exercises, particularly of the upper limbs. If the patient is able to assist, however, greater cardiopulmonary stress occurs with upper limb exercise; thus heart rate, ECG, and blood pressure must be monitored. Lower-extremity movements, such as hip and knee flexion, may help to position the diaphragm for improved excursion. Lower-extremity movements will also increase venous return, which may or may not be desirable, depending on the patient. The goals of upper- or lower-extremity work must therefore be clearly defined. Possible benefits and untoward effects must be identified to ensure the patient benefits optimally from the prescribed exercise.

The treatment of choice in all patients is to simulate those conditions that maintain optimal oxygen transport in health or approximate those conditions as closely as possible. That is, the most physiological interventions are exploited first and the least physiological interventions are exploited last or when more physiological interventions are not possible. Physiological interventions such as mobilization may be contraindicated in patients whose oxygen delivery is too low. Without some reserve capacity in oxygen transport, the patient cannot sustain the additional metabolic load that mobilization imposes. Patients who are this critical are often put on neuromuscular blocking agents to reduce muscle tone and thereby reduce oxygen demand. Because these patients are in induced paralytic states, mobilization is not possible. In such cases, optimizing oxygen transport using body positioning and then nonphysiological interventions may be considered. Extreme caution must be observed when positioning these patients and moving their limbs because they are at risk of joint subluxation, strains, bruising, and pressure sores.

Interventions to promote mucociliary transport and secretion clearance are applicable to all situations in which secretions, mucosal edema, bronchospasm, or a combination of these factors occurs. If postural drainage is indicated to further facilitate mucociliary transport and secretion clearance, caution needs to be exercised to avoid inducing bronchospasm and hypoxemia; thus the use of percussion should be considered carefully.

INDIVIDUALS WITH MYOCARDIAL INFARCTION

Pathophysiology and Medical Management

The initial priority of management in the acute phase of myocardial infarction (MI) is the correction of the immediate problems including dysrhythmias, myocardial insufficiency, reduced cardiac output, hypoxemia, chest pain, and anxiety followed by implementation of a progressive rehabilitation program ranging from the acute medically stable phase to postdischarge rehabilitation phase (Kinney & Packa, 1995; Froelicher & Myers, 2000; Irwin & Tecklin, 2004). Before admission to the coronary care unit, continuous monitoring of the heart rate and rhythm is established. An intravenous line is routinely started for the administration of medications and fluids. An arterial line may be started for serial blood sampling for blood gases and enzyme measures. Initially pain medications, coronary vasodilators, and diuretics are frequently used to minimize the work of the heart, anginal pain, and discomfort. Drugs such as morphine serve to depress the respiratory drive; thus the physical therapist must be aware of corresponding changes in vital signs. Less potent sedatives and tranquilizers are more routinely prescribed. Increased pain and anxiety potentially worsen the patient's cardiac status by increasing myocardial oxygen demand and altering normal breathing pattern and gas exchange.

The primary purpose of oxygen administration to the cardiac patient is to reduce hypoxemia, myocardial work, and angina. Dyspnea, however, is commonly observed in the initial phases of myocardial infarction and can be effectively controlled by supplemental oxygen administered by nasal cannulae or mask. Oxygen may also correct potential ventilation-perfusion mismatching and hypoxemia. Oxygen is always administered with humidity to avoid drying the airways.

Blood gas analysis is performed within an hour of initiating oxygen therapy to establish a baseline of arterial saturation. In this way the oxygen dose can be altered to regulate blood gases and acid base balance.

INDIVIDUALS WITH MYOCARDIAL INFARCTION CONSERVATIVELY MANAGED

Principles of Physical Therapy Management

A primary principle of the management of the patient after myocardial infarction is to reduce myocardial oxygen demand and workload. The myocardium needs rest to promote optimal healing. Judicious rest of the myocardium is a priority that can often be balanced with gentle rhythmic, nonstatic movements. Box 34-1 illustrates several ways of reducing myocardial workload in patients with cardiopulmonary disease.

The physical therapist should be watchful at all times for signs of impending or silent infarction, including generalized or localized pain anywhere over the thorax, upper limbs, and neck, palpitations, dyspnea, lightheadedness, syncope, sensation of indigestion, hiccups, and nausea.

Depending on the degree of myocardial infarction and damage, varying lengths of modified mobility may be recommended (Kinney & Packa, 1995). Shorter initial periods of restricted mobility are safe and promote faster functional recovery (Herkner et al, 2003). During this period, the physical

---

BOX 34-1

Means of Reducing Myocardial Work Load in Patients with Cardiopulmonary Dysfunction

1. Provide a quiet environment without excessive noise and stimulation.
2. Prescribe low-intensity activity until medical stability has been maintained and patient shows signs of physical improvement.
3. Begin progressive mobilization in conjunction with patient's medical status, ECG stability, and unchanging or resolving enzyme levels.
4. Reduce patient's anxiety about his or her condition, self-care activities, and family and work responsibilities.
5. In general, begin gentle mobilization exercises, deep breathing, and coughing immediately as a prophylactic measure, unless, as frequently occurs in coronary patients, creptitations are audible in the bases of the lungs; treatments need to minimize pulmonary congestion and cardiac stress.
6. Promote relaxation with low-intensity activity. All levels of activity, including breathing exercises, are to be performed in a coordinated, rhythmic manner. Breath holding, Valsalva maneuvers, and isometric muscle contractions, (i.e., isometric exercise and exercise involving significant muscle or postural stabilization) are absolutely contraindicated during all activities in patients with coronary artery disease and should not be performed in any stage of a rehabilitation program.

---

therapist concentrates on rhythmic breathing exercises, gentle coughing exercises or huffing, and modified positioning with the bed head elevated at least 15 degrees to facilitate the gravity-dependent mechanical action of the heart and thereby reduce myocardial oxygen demand. Intermittent exposure to orthostatic stress by imposing the upright position is recommended for patients after acute myocardial infarction (Convertino, 2003). The patient is encouraged to perform deep breathing and coughing every hour during the day. Bed exercises including rhythmic, unresisted, hip, knee, foot and ankle exercises are usually performed as frequently as possible by the patient, or when the patient turns in bed. The patient is cautioned to exercise one leg at a time, sliding one heel up and down the bed and guarding against lifting the leg off the bed. These exercises, when performed correctly and coordinated with inspiration and expiration, require relatively little effort from and induce little additional physical stress on the individual with MI. Comparable with the management of the postoperative patient, these exercises are performed prophylactically to reduce the risk of venous stasis and formation of thromboemboli. In addition, they may help to regulate more coordinated breathing, encourage deep breaths and mucociliary transport, and reduce atelectasis. The patient is cautioned against performing the Valsalva maneuver and straining because these activities increase intrathoracic pressure and reduce cardiac output.

ECG monitoring of the patient with cardiac disease is the responsibility of all members of the health care team involved

Signs of Imminent Congestive Heart Failure

Development of tachydysrhythmias
Development of a ventricular gallop
Pulmonary crackles and other persistent adventitiae
Development of dyspnea
Development of increased jugular venous pressure and
    distention

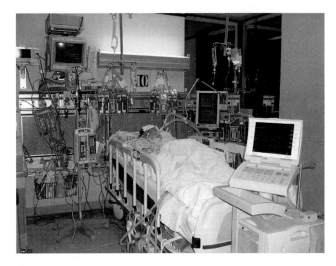

FIGURE 34-4 Patient after open heart surgery. Note mechanical ventilator, mediastinal drains and chest tubes, intraaortic balloon pump, and multiple intravenous drips.

in the patient's care. The physical therapist has a special responsibility to be proficient in ECG interpretation in the coronary care unit because physical therapy is one of the most metabolically demanding interventions for patients (Dean et al, 1995; Weissman et al, 1984). The physical therapist often has the responsibility of initiating new activities with the cardiac patient, which might include sitting over the edge of the bed, engaging in self-care (particularly involving the arms being maintained in a raised position), getting in and out of bed, sitting in a chair, going to the bathroom, walking around the room or in the hallways, and eventually exercising on the treadmill or ergometer. Changes in the ECG must be watched for, particularly when introducing new activities and increasing the intensity of workload in activities. Careful attention to ECG changes and serum enzyme levels will contribute to enhanced physical therapy care of the acute MI patient by optimizing the treatments prescribed and the margin of safety with which activities are performed.

Congestive heart failure may be unavoidable in cases of severe infarction or even milder infarction coupled with lung disease. Fluid intake and output and daily weight measurements promote early detection of congestive heart failure. Routine fluid intake by an intravenous line should not exceed 20 to 30 ml per hour. Signs of imminent and established congestive heart failure appear in Box 34-2. The work of the heart can be significantly reduced in the upright position (Levine & Lown, 1952).

Patients with cardiac conditions are prone to anxiety about their conditions and prognoses. The patient is given realistic guidelines at each stage of recovery with respect to the level of activity that can be safely performed, which can potentially avert deterioration and promote recovery. Involving the patient in rehabilitation planning from the onset facilitates the patient's planning realistically for the future and may help to reduce the depression often experienced by the acute MI patient.

The initial rehabilitation program is planned with the long-range rehabilitation goals in mind. The program designed for the cardiac patient is progressive in terms of types of activities, usually beginning with activities of daily living and with respect to the intensity, duration, and frequency of these activities (Bjore, 1972; Froelicher & Myers, 2000). The patient's tolerance and changes in ECG and vital signs are used as indicators for establishing and modifying the treatment

program. These physiological parameters must be observed carefully as the patient progresses to optimize the potential benefits of the therapeutic regimens as early as possible without endangering the patient.

Patient education and prevention of infarction are particularly important for the cardiac patient. As soon as the patient is alert and able to cooperate, information about his or her condition with guidelines about activity, diet, and stress management is reinforced. The more involved and informed the patient is in self-management, the greater the likelihood of receptivity and adherence to a rehabilitation regimen after discharge.

INDIVIDUALS AFTER OPEN HEART SURGERY

Principles of Physical Therapy Management

Patients scheduled for open heart surgery are considered moderately risky surgical candidates because of the nature and invasiveness of this type of surgery (Figure 34-4), regardless of their general level of health before surgery (Trekova et al, 1994). Whenever possible, patients prepare for surgery in advance by decreasing or stopping smoking, by avoiding exposure to respiratory tract infections, by avoiding stress, by eating a balanced diet, and by getting adequate sleep. Patients can benefit from a modified, prescriptive exercise program before surgery to maximize their aerobic capacity and thereby improve their perioperative course.

Preoperative teaching coupled with a conditioning program before hospitalization has a role in reducing hospital stay and complications (see Chapters 18, 30, and 31). During the preoperative period the physical therapist may spend additional time with patients scheduled for open heart surgery to provide teaching of the basic anatomy and physiology related to the surgery to be performed; the effect of anesthesia; the role of

---

BOX 34-3

Guidelines to Stages of Physical Therapy for the Patient after Open Heart Surgery

Stage 1

Post anaesthesia and recovery is where the patient is hemodynamicly stabilized. The patient may be seen in the post anesthesia and recovery room for a physical therapy assessment; the patient is usually extubated within 24 hours after surgery. Although the patient must be permitted to rest as much as possible in the initial 24-hour period, judicious body positioning is instituted to stimulate physiological "stir-up." Usually, once extubated, the patient is positioned side to side for deep breathing and coughing at least four times in the first 24 hours, and low-intensity mobilization is initiated. Medications are administered before treatment to ensure optimal effect during treatment. Depending on the findings of x-ray, physical examination, and arterial blood gases, the patient may require vibrations and possibly percussion. Postural drainage positions are modified to avoid tipping the patient head-down and causing increased myocardial strain. A sputum sample for culture and sensitivity testing may be taken at this time. The patient can usually tolerate being dangled over the edge of the bed for a few minutes. Special care is taken for all heart patients to avoid the Valsalva maneuver, forced coughing, and huffing, and to maintain a semi-recumbent or upright position for treatment. Blood pressure is checked before, during, and after treatment. Mobilization is progressed.

Stage 2

Deep breathing and coughing maneuvers coupled with mobilization are continued. Positioning for enhanced alveolar ventilation and ventilation and perfusion matching may be indicated. If secretion accumulation is a problem and the patient is too unstable to be optimally mobilized or positioned, postural drainage and possibly percussion and/or vibration may be indicated. Upper limb and neck exercises are introduced. Neck exercises are withheld if central venous pressure lines are still in place in the neck veins. The patient can sit in a chair at bedside as tolerated. The patient is encouraged to stand erect for a minute or so on transferring back and forth to the chair.

Stage 3

The patient can take short walks as tolerated. Ambulation is not begun until arterial lines and the Swan-Ganz catheter have been capped or removed. Vital signs are monitored before and after

standing and walking. Deep breathing and coughing maneuvers are continued even if the chest is clear, until the patient is up and about within reasonable limits as tolerated. The patient is encouraged in grooming and self-care.

Stage 4

Deep breathing and coughing should be done by the patient without supervision. The presence of atelectasis on x-ray or from assessment findings, however, would indicate the need for continuation of mobilization and body positioning with breathing exercises. Ambulation is increased as tolerated.

Stage 5

The patient can participate in individual or class activities, concentrating on trunk mobility, range of motion, coordinated breathing activities, posture, biomechanics, and gradually increasing endurance.

Stage 6

The patient can attempt six to eight stairs if progress has been satisfactory and as indicated. Aortic repairs in the first week or so are prone to rupture. Elevation of the blood pressure is therefore avoided to reduce the risk of breakdown of the aortic suture line. Vital signs are always monitored.

Stage 7

The patient depends primarily on ambulation for maintaining optimal alveolar ventilation and mucociliary transport rather than breathing and coughing exercises. The patient is cautioned to balance a period of exertion with a period of rest. The patient may be discharged. The physical therapist ensures that the patient fully understands the specific details of the home exercise program. The emphasis of exercise for cardiac patients continues to be on rhythmic, coordinated dynamic movements on discharge, avoiding isometric, static exercise. Precautions are reinforced with respect to avoiding stress to the incision, and this includes postponing driving for several weeks. If possible, the patient is invited to participate in a reconditioning and health promotion program as an outpatient in a physical therapy department. Follow-up medical and physical therapy visits are arranged before discharge around four to six weeks after surgery.

*The physical therapist must guard against excessively intense treatment of post open heart surgery patients as well as other patients who are receiving prophylactic anticoagulants.

---

intubation and mechanical ventilation; the incision lines to be expected over the chest, and the legs if veins are to be removed for bypass surgery; the lines, leads, chest tubes, and catheters that will be in place after surgery; interventions beginning postanesthesia and recovery (breathing control and coughing maneuvers, body positioning, foot and ankle exercises, and early mobilization); and the course of recovery the patient might expect barring complications (Chapter 17). The emphasis on patient education in most open heart surgery units may contribute to the generally low incidence of complications and mortality.

Some special considerations in physical therapy management of the patient after open heart surgery appear in Box 34-3, and

these expand on the concurrent medical course of patients in phase I cardiac rehabilitation (see Chapter 30). Patients are extubated early and rehabilitation is commenced as soon as possible (Cheng et al, 1996). These guidelines are to be applied thoughtfully and cautiously with regard to each specific patient's condition and observed recovery. Intermittent orthostatic stress and exercise stress are encouraged (Convertino, 2003). These guidelines suggest the upper limit of intensity of physical therapy, which should be applied if all is progressing well initially and reduced if warranted by the patient's condition. Progression from one stage to the next is based on an optimal and reliable treatment response at each level before proceeding. Different institutions may advocate different practices, depending on their facilities, the experience of the surgical and ICU team, and the incidence of post-operative complications and survival for that institution.

The physical therapist must guard against excessively intense treatment of both patients post open heart surgery and those patients for whom periods of relatively restricted mobility are anticipated. In addition to the fact that these patients may be hemodynamically unstable initially, they may be susceptible to soft tissue bruising from being on a prophylactic course of anticoagulants.

Patients are monitored for complications (see Chapters 17 and 36) and to guide treatment progression and detect untoward responses to treatment. After cardiac surgery, $\dot{V}O_2$ tends to increase due to increased cardiac output and oxygen delivery (Routsi et al, 1993). The oxygen extraction ratio may increase and SVO_2 decrease if cardiac function deteriorates.

Depression has been reported in patients in the ICU, particularly in those admitted for coronary care who are experiencing a physiological loss (Johnson & Roberts, 1996). Signs and symptoms of depression warrant monitoring and reporting to the team to maximize clinical and psychosocial outcomes.

Complications do occur in high risk ICU settings. Risk assessment is a fundamental component of the assessment (see Chapter 17). Common complications often related to premorbid status include restricted mobility, inability to wean from mechanical ventilation, deep vein thrombosis, pulmonary emboli, and stroke. Other complications are related to surgery (e.g., internal bleeding, overwhelming pneumonia, and lung collapse) or medication reaction. Complications are better managed if anticipated and detected early. Depending on the nature of the complication, physical therapy interventions may be stepped up in terms of intensity, duration, and frequency, modified, or discontinued until the patient is cleared with respect to stability.

Physical therapy follow-up should continue several months beyond discharge, at which point the patient should be well integrated into a cardiac rehabilitation program. Continuity and continuation of physical therapy throughout the entire rehabilitation period, from acute- to long-term, cannot be overemphasized given that achieving a maximal recovery from surgery is the priority.

SUMMARY

This chapter described the principles of cardiopulmonary physical therapy in the management of critically ill patients with primary cardiopulmonary dysfunction. Cardiopulmonary failure secondary to chronic lung disease and heart disease were described. Cardiopulmonary physical therapy management is based on the specific underlying pathophysiological mechanisms of these various disorders. These principles, however, cannot be interpreted to be guidelines for specific treatment in that each patient is an individual whose condition reflects multiple factors contributing to impaired cardio-pulmonary function or threatening it (i.e., the effects of recumbency, restricted mobility, extrinsic factors related to the patient's care, and intrinsic factors related to the patient in addition to the underlying pathophysiology).

Review Questions

1. With respect to patients who are critically ill with the following conditions, describe the pathophysiology of *primary* cardiopulmonary dysfunction, cardio-pulmonary failure, obstructive lung disease, status asthmaticus, restrictive lung disease, and coronary artery disease, and how the limitations related to structure and function threaten life.

2. Relate cardiopulmonary physical therapy treatment interventions to the underlying pathophysiology of *each* of the above conditions in the individual who is critically ill and provide the rationale for your choice.

REFERENCES

Ambrosino, N., Bruletti, G., Scala, V., Porta, R., & Vitacca, M. (2002). Cognitive and perceived health status in patients with chronic obstructive pulmonary disease surviving acute on chronic respiratory failure: a controlled study. Intensive Care Medicine 28:170-177.

Austin, G.L., & Greenfield L.J. (1980). Respiratory care in cardiac failure and pulmonary edema. Surgical Clinics in North America 60:1565-1575.

Barach, A.L., & Beck, G.J. (1954). Ventilatory effects of head-down position in pulmonary emphysema. American Journal of Medicine 16:55-60.

Bates, D.V. (1989). Respiratory function in disease, ed 3. Philadelphia: WB Saunders.

Bjore, D. (1972). Postmyocardial infarction: a program of graduated exercises. Journal of the Canadian Physiotherapy Association 24:22-25.

Brunner, J.X., & Wolff, G. (1988). Pulmonary function indices in critical care patients. New York: Springer-Verlag.

Cheng, D.C., Karski, J., Peniston, C., Asokumar, B., Raveendran, G., Carroll, J., Nierenberg, H., Roger, S., Mickle, D., Tong, J., Zelovitsky, J., David, T., & Sandle, A. (1996). Morbidity outcome in early versus conventional tracheal extubation after coronary artery bypass grafting: a prospective randomized controlled trial. Journal of Cardiovascular and Thoracic Surgery 112:755-764.

Chung, F., & Dean, E. (1989). Pathophysiology and cardiorespiratory consequences of interstitial lung disease-review and clinical implications. Physical Therapy 69:956-966.

Clauss, R.H., Scalabrini, B.Y., Ray, J.F. III, & Reed, G.E. (1968). Effects of changing body position upon improved ventilation-perfusion relationships. Circulation 37(Suppl 4):214-217.

Convertino, V.A. (2003). Value of orthostatic stress in maintaining functional status soon after myocardial infarction or cardiac artery bypass grafting. Journal of Cardiovascular Nursing 26:105-116.

Dean, E. (1985). Effect of body position on pulmonary function. Physical Therapy 65:613-618.

Dean, E. (2002). Physiotherapy skills: positioning and mobilization of the patient. In Pryor, J.A., Prasad, S.A., & Webber, B.A. (Eds). Physiotherapy for respiratory and cardiac problems: adults and paediatrics. St. Louis: Harcourt.

Dean, E., Murphy, S., Parrent, L., & Rousseau, M. (1995). Metabolic consequences of physical therapy in critically-ill patients. Proceedings of the world confederation of physical therapy congress, Washington, DC.

Dean, E., & Ross, J. (1992). Mobilization and body conditioning. In Zadai, C. (Ed). Pulmonary management in physical therapy. New York: Churchill Livingstone.

Douglas, W.W., Rehder, K., Beynen, F.M., Sessler, A.D., & Marsh, H.M. (1977). Improved oxygenation in patients with acute respiratory failure: the prone position. American Review of Respiratory Disease 115:559-566.

Fell, T., & Cheney, F.W. (1971). Prevention of hypoxia during endotracheal suction. Annals of Surgery 174:24-28.

Froelicher, V.F., & Myers, J.N. (2000). Exercise and the heart, clinical concepts, ed 4. Philadelphia: WB Saunders.

Gallagher, T.J., & Civetta, J.M. (1980). Goal-directed therapy of acute respiratory failure. Anesthesia and Analgesia 59:831-834.

Gibson, G.J., Pride, N.B., Davis, J.N., & Loh, L.C. (1977). Pulmonary mechanics in patients with respiratory muscle weakness. American Review of Respiratory Disease 115:389-395.

Herkner, H., Thoennissen, J., Nikfardjam, M., Koreny, M., Laggner, A.N., & Mullner, M. (2003). Short versus prolonged bed rest after uncomplicated acute myocardial infarction: a systematic review and meta-analysis. Journal of Clinical Epidemiology 56:775-781.

Hietpas, B.G., Roth, R.D., & Jensen, W.M. (1979). Huff coughing and airway patency. Respiratory Care 24:710.

Holten, K. (1972). Training effect in patients with severe ventilatory failure. Scandinavian Journal of Respiratory Diseases 53:65-76.

Irwin, S., & Tecklin, J.S. (Eds). (2004). Cardiopulmonary physical therapy, ed 4. Philadelphia: Elsevier.

Jardin, F., Farcot, J.C., Boisante, L., Curien, N., Margairaz, A., & Bourdarias, J.P. (1981). Influence of positive end-expiratory pressure on left ventricular performance. New England Journal of Medicine 304:387-392.

Johnson, L.H., & Roberts, S.L. (1996). A cognitive model for assessing depression and providing nursing intervention in cardiac intensive care. Intensive Critical Care Nursing 12:138-146.

Kim, M.J., Hwang, H.J., & Song, H.H. (2002). A randomized trial on the effects of body positions on lung function with acute respiratory failure patients. International Journal of Nursing Studies 39:549-555.

Kinney, M.R., & Packa, D.R. (1995). Andreoli's comprehensive cardiac care, ed 7. Philadelphia: Elsevier.

Kirby, R.R., Taylor, R.W., & Civetta, J.M. (1996). Critical care, ed 2. Philadelphia: Lippincott Williams & Wilkins.

Kumar, A., Pontoppiaan, H., Falke, K.J., Wilson, R.S. & Laver, M.B. (1973). Pulmonary barotrauma during mechanical ventilation. Critical Care Medicine 1:181-186.

Levine, S.A., & Lown, B. (1952). "Armchair" treatment of acute coronary thrombosis. Journal of American Medical Association 148:1365-1368.

Lynn-McHale, D.J., & Carlson, K.K. (2000). AACN procedure manual for critical care, ed 4. Philadelphia: Elsevier.

Mackenzie, C.F., Imle, P.C., & Ciesla, N. (1989). Chest physiotherapy in the intensive care unit, ed 2. Baltimore: Williams & Wilkins.

Macklem, P.T., & Roussos, C.S. (1977). Respiratory muscle fatigue: a cause of respiratory failure? Clinical Science and Molecular Medicine 53:419-422.

Matthay, M.A. (Ed). (1985). Pathophysiology of pulmonary edema. Clinics in Chest Medicine 6:301-314.

Nunn, J.F., Coleman, A.J., Sachithanandan, T., Bergman, N.A., & Laws, J.W. (1965). Hypoxemia and atelectasis produced by forced expiration. British Journal of Anesthesia 37:3-12.

Petty, T.L. (1985). Chronic obstructive pulmonary disease, ed 2. New York: Marcel Dekker.

Piehl, M.A., & Brown, R.S. (1976). Use of extreme position changes in acute respiratory failure. Critical Care Medicine 4:13-14.

Pryor, J.A., Prasad, S.A., & Webber, B.A. (2002). Physiotherapy for respiratory and cardiac problems: adults and paediatrics. St. Louis: Harcourt Health Sciences Group.

Ray, J.F. III, Yost, L., Moallem, S., Sanoudos, G.M., Villamena, P., Paredes, R.M., & Clauss, R.H. (1974). Immobility, hypoxemia, and pulmonary arteriovenous shunting. Archives of Surgery 109:537-541.

Rochester, D.F., & Arora, N.S. (1983). Respiratory muscle failure. Medical Clinics of North America 67:573-597.

Rochester, D.F., & Esau, S.A. (1984). Malnutrition and the respiratory system. Chest 85:411-415.

Routsi, C., Vincent, J.L., Bakker, J., De Backer, D., Lejeune P., d'Hollander, A., Le Clere, J.L., & Kahn, R.J. (1993). Relation between oxygen consumption and oxygen delivery in patients after cardac surgetry. Anesthesia Analgesia 77:1104-1110.

Shoemaker, W.C. (Ed). (1999). Textbook of critical care, ed 4. Philadelphia: Elsevier.

Trekova, N.A., Dementyeva, I.I., Dzemeshkevich, S.L., & Asmangulyan, Y.T. (1994). Blood oxygen transport function in cardiopulmonary bypass surgery for acquired valvular diseases. Intensive Surgery 79:60-64.

Vincent, J.L., & Suter, P.M. (1987). Cardiopulmonary interactions in acute respiratory failure. New York: Springer-Verlag.

Walsh, J.M., Vanderwarf, C., Hoscheit, D., & Fahey, P.J. (1989). Unsuspected hemodynamic alterations during endotracheal suctioning. Chest 95:162-165.

Weber, K.T., Janicki, J.S., Shroff, S.C., & Likoff, M.J. (1983). The cardiopulmonary unit: the body's gas exchange system. Clinics in Chest Medicine 4:101-110.

Weinstein, M.E., & Skillman, J.J. (1980). Management of severe respiratory failure. Surgical Clinics of North America 60:1403-1412.

Weissman, C., & Kemper, M. (1993). Stressing the critically ill patient: the cardiopulmonary and metabolic responses to an acute increase in oxygen consumption. Journal of Critical Care 8:100-108.

Weissman, C., Kemper, M., Damask, M.C., Askanazi, J., Hyman, A.I., & Kinney, J.M. (1984). Effect of routine intensive care interactions on metabolic rate. Chest 86:815-818.

Weissman, C., Kemper, M., Elwyn, D.H., Askanazi, J., Hyman, A.I., & Kinney, J.M. (1989). The energy expenditure of the mechanically ventilated critically ill patient. Chest 2:254-259.

West, J.B. (2004). Respiratory physiology-the essentials, ed 7. Baltimore: Lippincott Williams & Wilkins.

Wilson, R.F. (1992). Critical care manual, ed 2. Philadelphia: F.A. Davis.

Wong, W.P. (2000). Physical therapy for a patient in acute respiratory failure. Physical Therapy 80:662-670.

Woods, S.L. (2004). Cardiac nursing, ed 5. Philadelphia: Lippincott Williams & Wilkins.

Zanotti, E., Felicetti, G., Maini, M., & Fracchia, C. (2003). Peripheral muscle strength training in bed-bound patients with COPD receiving mechanical ventilation: effect of electrical stimulation. Chest 124:292-296.

Intensive Care Unit Management of Individuals with Secondary Cardiopulmonary Dysfunction

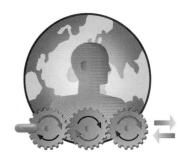

Elizabeth Dean and Christiane Perme

KEY TERMS

Burns
Head injury
Morbid obesity

Musculoskeletal trauma
Neuromuscular dysfunction
Spinal cord injury

This chapter describes the principles and practice of cardiopulmonary physical therapy in the management of *secondary* cardiopulmonary dysfunction that can lead to cardiopulmonary failure. Some common categories of conditions described include neuromuscular disease, morbid obesity, musculoskeletal trauma, head injury, spinal cord injury, and burns. Each category of condition is presented in two parts. The related pathophysiology and pertinent aspects of the medical management of the condition are presented in relation to the principles of physical therapy management. Invasive care and noninvasive care have common goals and thus are complementary. The principles presented are not treatment prescriptions. Each patient must be assessed and treated individually, taking into consideration the contribution of recumbency, restricted mobility, extrinsic factors related to the patient's care, and intrinsic factors related to the individual patient (see Chapter 17) in addition to the underlying pathophysiology.

INDIVIDUALS WITH NEUROMUSCULAR DISEASE

Pathophysiology and Medical Management

Amyolateral sclerosis, Guillain-Barré syndrome, myasthenia gravis, muscular dystrophy, multiple sclerosis, stroke, polio-myelitis, and neuromuscular poisonings are common neuro-muscular disorders that can precipitate respiratory failure in the absence of underlying *primary* lung disease (Cooper et al, 1985; Curran & Colbert, 1989; Dean et al, 1991; Fugl-Meyer & Grimby, 1984; Griggs & Donohoe, 1982; Lane et al, 1974). If paralyzed, the patient will likely be dependent on ventilatory assistance. Noninvasive mechanical ventilation has been an important advance in prolonging the lives of individuals with these serious progressive conditions. As cardiorespiratory failure becomes immanent, however, invasive mechanical ventilation is warranted.

Cardiopulmonary physical therapy has a central role in minimizing the need for mechanical ventilation in these patients because their prognosis for weaning is poor. Progressive respiratory insufficiency is best addressed early with the institution of nighttime ventilation at home (Curran, 1981) before the development of failure and necessity for hospitalization. Patients with progressive neuromuscular diseases (e.g., muscular dystrophy) are living longer; thus cardiopulmonary insufficiency will be compounded by age-related changes of the cardiopulmonary system (Dean, 1994a; Leblanc et al, 1970).

Neuromuscular conditions contribute to cardiopulmonary dysfunction in numerous ways (see Chapters 22 and 23). With progressive deterioration of inspiratory and expiratory muscle strength and endurance, respiratory insufficiency and failure can ensue (Black & Hyatt, 1971). Depending on the specific pathology, such deficits include reduced lung volumes and flow rates, reduced alveolar ventilation, increased airway resistance, ventilation and perfusion mismatch, impaired mucociliary transport, mucous accumulation, reduced cough and gag reflexes, relatively unprotected airway secondary to impaired glottic closure and weakness of the pharyngeal and laryngeal structures, and increased work of breathing.

Iatrogenic effects of medications can confound muscle weakness. Muscle relaxants and corticosteroids are used commonly in the intensive care unit (ICU). Myopathies related to these drugs have been reported in patients with stroke (Moukas et al, 2002). Ultrasonography can be used to assess muscle mass.

Principles of Physical Therapy Management

A patient with restrictive pulmonary disease secondary to neuromuscular conditions is at considerable risk of succumbing to the negative cardiopulmonary and cardiovascular sequelae of reduced mobility and recumbency, in addition to the pathophysiological consequences of respiratory failure. Provided the patient has some residual muscle power, the balance between oxygen demand and supply will determine the degree to which mobilization can be exploited to maximize oxygen transport. The treatment goals for these patients are to maximize oxygen delivery, enhance the efficiency of oxygen uptake and utilization, and thereby reduce the work of breathing. In these patients, minimizing oxygen demand overall (i.e., during mobilization as well as at rest) is a priority. Mobilization needs to be prescribed in body positions that enhance oxygen transport and its efficiency so that the benefits of mobilization can be exploited more fully without worsening arterial oxygenation (Dean, 1985). The patient requires continuous monitoring of oxygen transport and hemodynamic monitoring to ensure the exercise stimulus is optimally therapeutic and not excessive.

Although the mechanisms are different, patients with neuromuscular dysfunction can benefit from body positioning to reduce respiratory distress much like a patient with chronic airflow limitation (Barach, 1974). Upright and lean-forward positions will reduce distress to the greatest extent.

The patient's body position and length of time in any one position must be carefully monitored and recorded to minimize the risks of positions that are deleterious to oxygenation and ensure that a beneficial position is not assumed for too long because of the diminishing benefits over time. This is particularly important for the patient who is incapable of positioning himself or herself, who is incapable of communicating a need to turn, and in whom muscle wasting, bony prominences, and thinning of the skin may predispose the patient to skin breakdown.

Patients who are hypotonic and generally weak and debilitated fail to adapt normally to position-dependent fluid shifts and thus are more prone to orthostatic intolerance (Marini & Wheeler, 1997). Gravitational stimulation is essential to maintain the volume regulating mechanisms. Tilt tables

should be used judiciously given the potential risks in these patients, which are compounded by the loss of the lower-extremity muscle pump mechanism. Stretcher chairs may be preferable. Because of potential adverse reactions to fluid shifts and the potential for desaturation, falling PaO_2 levels and dysrhythmias, the patient's hemodynamic status must be monitored closely during gravitational challenges.

The importance of chest wall mobility to optimize three-dimensional chest wall excursion in individuals with chronic neurological conditions is emphasized in Chapters 22 and 23. This goal is particularly challenging if complicated by acute respiratory insufficiency. The goal is to promote alveolar ventilation, reduce areas of atelectasis, and optimize ventilation and perfusion matching and breathing efficiency to augment and minimize reliance on respiratory support (i.e., supplemental oxygen and mechanical ventilation) while minimizing respiratory distress. This is especially important because patients with neuromuscular conditions are poor candidates for being weaned off mechanical ventilation (Petty, 1982). In addition, these patients are prone to microaspirations. Promotion of mucociliary transport is therefore essential to facilitate clearing of aspirate and minimize bacterial colonization and risk of infection.

Another major problem for patients with restrictive lung disease secondary to generalized weakness and neuromuscular disease is an ineffective cough. Cough facilitation techniques (e.g., body positioning, abdominal counter pressure, and tracheal tickle; see Chapters 22 and 23) can be used to increase intraabdominal and intrathoracic pressures and cough effectiveness. A natural cough, even when facilitated, is preferable and more effective in dislodging mucus from the sixth or seventh generation of bronchi than repeated suctioning. Even a weak, facilitated cough may be effective in dislodging secretions to the central airways for removal by suctioning or for redistributing peripheral secretions (Hasani et al, 1991). Huffing, a modified cough performed with the glottis open and with abdominal support, may help mobilize secretions in patients with generalized weakness (Hietpas et al, 1979). In some cases suctioning may be the only means of eliciting a cough and clearing secretions simultaneously. Coughing attempts are usually exhausting for these patients. Thus ample rest periods must be interspersed during treatment, particularly for the ventilated patient. Coughing maneuvers must be strategically planned. Even though the patient may only be able to effect a series of a few weak coughs, it is essential that these attempts are maximized (i.e., the patient, optimally rested and medicated [e.g., bronchodilators, analgesia, reduced sedation and narcotics], is physically positioned to optimize length-tension relationship of the diaphragm and abdominal muscles, positioned vertically to optimize inspiratory lung volumes, expiratory flows, and avoid aspiration, and is provided thoracic and abdominal support during expiration to maximize intrathoracic and intraabdominal pressures) (see Chapter 22). These supportive measures will ensure that the benefits of the normal physiological cough mechanism, which is the single best secretion clearance technique, is maximized (i.e., the most productive cough with the least energy expenditure) (Bennett et al, 1990; Hasani et al, 1991; Kirilloff et al, 1985; Zinman, 1984). Forced chest wall compression or forced expiratory maneuvers are contraindicated because of airway closure and impairment of gas exchange (Nunn et al, 1965).

Impaired mobility, inability to cough effectively, decreased airway diameter, and bronchospasm contribute to impaired mucociliary transport and secretion accumulation. In addition, impaired glottic closure and increased risk of reflux in this patient population exposes the airway to risk of aspiration. Prophylacticly, multiple body positions and frequent position changes will minimize the risk of secretion accumulation and stasis. If mechanically ventilated, these patients are suctioned as indicated. If pulmonary secretions become a significant problem despite these preventative measures, postural drainage positions are selected to achieve the optimal effect (i.e., secretion mobilization and optimal gas exchange). Given the treatment response, manual techniques, of which manual vibration would have the greatest physiological justification, may yield some benefit.

Patients with chronic neuromuscular dysfunction and residual musculoskeletal deformity pose an additional challenge to the cardiopulmonary physical therapist in that cardiopulmonary function is less predictable because of altered lung mechanics (Bake et al, 1976) and possibly cardiac dynamics. Thus clinical decision making is more experiential in these patients and they require close monitoring.

INDIVIDUALS WHO ARE OBESE

Pathophysiology and Medical Management

Restriction of cardiopulmonary function secondary to morbid obesity is called the alveolar hypoventilation syndrome. In this syndrome the weight of excess adipose tissue over the thoracic cage and abdominal cavity restricts chest wall movement and movement of the diaphragm and abdominal contents, respectively, during respiration. In very heavy individuals, cardiopulmonary function can be significantly impaired, resulting in hypoxemia and cardiopulmonary failure. The major pathophysiological mechanisms include significant alveolar hypoventilation, reactive hypoxic pulmonary vaso-constriction, increased pulmonary vascular resistance, myocardial hypertrophy, increased right ventricular work, altered position of the thoracic structures, abnormal compression of the heart, lungs, and mediastinal structures, abnormal position of the heart, cardiomegaly, increased intraabdominal pressure, elevated hemidiaphragms with resulting pressure on the underside of the diaphragm, impaired cough effectiveness, impaired mucociliary transport, mucous obstruction of airways, airway narrowing, bronchospasm, impaired mechanical efficiency of diaphragmatic excursion, and impaired respiratory mechanics and breathing efficiency (Bates, 1989). In addition, such patients are likely to have poor cardiopulmonary reserve capacity secondary to increased metabolic rate and minute ventilation at submaximal work rates, increased metabolic cost of breathing, and increased work of breathing. Moderately heavy patients whose pulmonary function is normally not compromised may exhibit cardiopulmonary dysfunction when their oxygen transport systems are stressed because of illness.

Mechanical ventilation can be a challenge in that the system pressure required to inflate the lungs may predispose the patient to barotrauma. Furthermore, high system pressures contribute to reduced stroke volume and cardiac output. Adequate circulation is essential to fulfill the goals of medical management (i.e., to optimize tissue oxygenation and carbon dioxide removal). Thus a delicate balance between adequate alveolar ventilation, cardiac output, and peripheral circulation is maintained.

Principles of Physical Therapy Management

The patient who is obese can be treated aggressively provided there are no contraindications and he or she is being fully monitored. Treatments must be intense, to the limits of the patient's tolerance, provided this is not contraindicated. An aggressive approach is essential given that the obese patient is at greater risk of deteriorating between treatments than a nonobese patient. Recumbency is tolerated poorly by an individual who is obese. Positional decrements in PaO_2 and SaO_2 can induce dysrhythmias. The weight of the abdominal viscera limits diaphragmatic descent and elevates the resting position of the diaphragm, impeding its mechanical efficiency.

These patients need to be aggressively mobilized; both whole body exercise stress and range of motion exercises between mobilization sessions. Active and active assisted upper-extremity range of motion exercises are associated with increased hemodynamic stress; thus the patient must be monitored closely. Lower-extremity exercise, such as pedaling and hip and knee flexion and extension exercises may help position and improve the excursion of the diaphragm. Lower-extremity movement will augment venous return. Depending on the patient and the work of the heart, the effect of lower-extremity movement will require monitoring to ensure that myocardial work is not increased excessively.

The erect upright position is optimal to augment ventilation and reduce the work of the mechanical ventilator and the risk of barotrauma. The upright position, coupled with leaning forward, displaces the abdominal contents forward, thereby reducing intraabdominal pressure and facilitating diaphragmatic descent. The posterior lung fields, particularly of the bases, are at risk for dynamic airway closure and atelectasis. Numerous positions and position changes ensure that the dependent alveoli remain open. The time spent in the supine position should be minimized. In fact, greater emphasis should be placed on nursing these patients in the upright position (i.e., the position of least risk and its variants). In addition to its pulmonary benefits, the upright position can reduce compression of the heart and mediastinal structures and there is a potential decrease in stroke volume and cardiac output. The weight of the chest wall, in addition to the weight of internal fat deposits in and around the cardiopulmonary unit, can compromise cardiac output and contribute to dysrhythmias. Thus during all body position changes the patient should be monitored hemodynamically to ensure the position is being tolerated well. People who are obese often slump after being positioned in the upright position. It is crucial that the position of these patients is checked frequently and corrected. The slumped position can be counterproductive in that the benefits of the upright position are significantly reduced and can lead to deterioration.

Although patients who are obese do not tolerate the prone position well, the semi-prone position can be beneficial by simulating the benefits of the upright lean-forward position on the displacement of the abdominal viscera (Ross & Dean, 1992). This position also simulates the prone abdomen-free position, which is associated with even greater benefit than the prone abdomen-restricted position (Dean, 1985). The benefits of the prone position for the obese individual include increased lung compliance and enhanced gas exchange and oxygenation. The full prone abdomen restricted position is contraindicated in the obese individual with cardiopulmonary failure, however, because this position can compromise diaphragmatic descent and contribute to further cardiopulmonary distress and failure and possibly cardiac arrest.

Mucociliary transport is slowed and ineffective in individuals who are obese with cardiopulmonary failure. Frequent body positioning will facilitate mucociliary transport and lymphatic drainage. The postural drainage positions can be effective in mobilizing secretions should accumulation become a problem. Manual techniques are not likely to add much benefit, particularly in the person who is morbidly obese. Suctioning is essential to clear pulmonary secretions from the central airways.

A person who is obese is at risk for postextubation atelectasis. Thus aggressive mobilization and numerous positions and frequent position changes must be continued.

The spontaneously breathing obese patient has a weak ineffective cough, which will be even less effective after a period of intubation and mechanical ventilation. These patients are taught deep breathing and coughing maneuvers comparable with those described for the patient with neuromuscular disease. Body positioning to facilitate coughing and supported coughing must be instituted to maximize cough effectiveness. These maneuvers should be carried out in conjunction with hourly extreme position shifts.

People who are morbidly obese have a high incidence of upper airway obstruction and sleep apnea secondary to floppy compliant pharyngeal tissue. Thus the quality of their sleep and rest is suboptimal, and they are apt to desaturate significantly while sleeping. These patients are also at high risk for esophageal reflux and aspiration. The optimal resting position is with the head of the bed up.

Individuals who are obese must be positioned upright and mobilized particularly aggressively because of their cardiopulmonary risks. Positioning and mobilizing can be facilitated with hinged beds, heavy-duty lifts, and reinforced stretcher chairs and walking frames. These items are essential to ensure that the patients are physiologically perturbed as much as possible, and to minimize biomechanical injury to staff. The physical therapist has to ensure that the optimal devices are selected such that the individual is actively involved as much as possible, and optimal but not excessive support is provided. The care of the individual who is morbidity obese is a particular challenge in the ICU and places increased demand on coordinated team work in the unit.

INDIVIDUALS WITH MUSCULOSKELETAL TRAUMA

Pathophysiology and Medical Management

Crush and penetrating injuries of the chest are commonly seen in the ICU (Moylan, 1988). Damage to the chest wall, lung parenchyma, and heart contribute to the risk of cardiopulmonary failure (Box 35-1). Associated injuries of the head,

---

BOX 35-1

Factors Contributing to Cardiopulmonary Failure after Trauma and their Diagnostic Signs

Airway Obstruction

Respiratory insufficiency
Respiratory distress
Impaired blood gases

Inadequate Ventilation

Reduced thoracic movement
Paradoxical thoracoabdominal movement

Tension Pneumothorax

Cyanosis
Unilaterally absent breath sounds
Distended neck veins
Subcutaneous emphysema

Cardiac Tamponade

Distended neck veins
Muffled heart sounds
Narrowed pulse pressure
Paradoxical pulse

Open Pneumothorax

Decreased breath sounds
Penetration of thoracic wall

Myocardial Contusion

Dysrhythmia

Flail Chest

Loose segment
Multiple palpable fractured ribs
Decreased or moist breath sounds
Hemoptysis

Modified from Moylan, J.A. (Ed). (1988). Trauma surgery. Philadelphia: JB Lippincott.

spinal cord, and abdomen may also contribute. Fractures of long bones and the pelvis are associated with fat emboli, which pose the threat of pulmonary embolism. In addition, fluid loss in multiple trauma contributes to loss of blood volume, hypovolemia, and hemodynamic instability. The more extensive the injuries, the greater the pain and requirement for analgesia. Pain contributes significantly to reduced alveolar ventilation, airway closure, and inefficient breathing patterns.

Paradoxical motion of the chest wall associated with flail chest and rib fractures results from instability of portions of the rib cage after trauma to the chest. If severe, patients may require surgical stabilization of the ribs or stabilization by continuous ventilatory management. Chest wall injuries and rib fractures are particularly painful.

The presence of blood or air in the chest cavity and in the potential spaces of the pericardial sac and intrapleural cavity impairs cardiac distension and contraction, impairs ventilation, promotes retention of secretions, interferes with effective clearance, and impairs lymphatic drainage (Marini & Wheeler, 1989).

The presence of a pneumothorax or hemothorax can severely compromise lung expansion. A tension pneumothorax results when air collects under tension in the pleural cavity. The tension pneumothorax promotes lung collapse on both the ipsilateral and contralateral sides, which further threatens respiratory failure. Phrenic nerve injuries inhibit diaphragmatic function (Dureuil et al, 1986). The position of the affected hemidiaphragm rests higher in the thoracic cavity, which may restrict ventilation to the lung base and contribute to airway closure and basal atelectasis. Diaphragmatic injuries directly affect ventilation in two ways. First, the bellows action of the lungs is compromised. Second, the lung is displaced by herniation of the abdominal contents into the thoracic cavity.

Analysis of blood gases in the patient with posttraumatic injuries of the chest often shows severe hypoxemia and moderate elevations of arterial PCO_2. The presence of acidemia is common, which may have both respiratory and metabolic components. Patients with severe injuries have improved outcomes if hemodynamic status can be optimized (Velmahos et al, 2000). Being less than 40 years of age is the best predictor of achieving optimal levels. Increasing DO_2 and maintaining normal SVO_2 are particularly relevant goals (Kremzar et al, 1997).

Principles of Physical Therapy Management

Severe restlessness and dyspnea in a patient with chest injury are classic indications of respiratory failure. Auscultation and percussion can usually reveal an underlying pneumothorax or hemothorax. Tension pneumothorax is confirmed by chest x-ray or aspiration of the chest with a needle and syringe.

Flail chest refers to the asynchronous movement of the chest wall with two or more fractured ribs at two or more sites. This results in instability of the chest wall. The so-called flail segment is usually apparent on physical examination. Paradoxical movement of the flail segment can often be

observed. The chest is depressed rather than elevated over the site during inspiration. Rib fractures are indicated by tenderness and crepitations on physical examination and from x-ray findings. Nonventilatory management of chest injuries in the absence of severe hypoxemia is preferred in these patients.

Analgesia is timed such that peak effect is achieved at the time of treatment to maximize comfort, minimize distress, and maximize cooperation, motivation, and tolerance for as well as duration of treatment.

Rib Fractures

Simple uncomplicated rib fractures often receive no specific treatment. Pain from complicated fractures may be treated with intercostal nerve blocks and transcutaneous electrical nerve stimulation and analgesia. Optimizing alveolar ventilation and mucociliary transport and avoiding pulmonary complications are primary goals. Strapping the chest is avoided because this further restricts and compromises chest wall expansion.

The current method of therapy for flail chest is internal stabilization of the chest and use of a mechanical ventilator. Slight hyperventilation will usually reduce the respiratory drive of most patients to allow the ventilator to take over the full work of breathing. The flail segment is then stabilized by internal expansion of the lungs. The treatment ensures adequate ventilation with the least pain possible. After two weeks the flail segment is usually stable.

When the patient can maintain a reasonable tidal volume and normal blood gases, weaning is begun. As soon as tidal volume and forced vital capacity are within acceptable limits, oxygen can be administered through an endotracheal tube with a T tube assembly. Arterial blood gases are monitored closely after the ventilator has been discontinued. Once the blood gases are in acceptable ranges over a reasonable period of time (i.e., 12 to 24 hours), the endotracheal tube is removed.

Pneumothorax and Hemothorax

Air or blood in the pleural cavity after chest trauma must be removed through a chest tube. For a pneumothorax, the chest tube is positioned in the second or third intercostal space in the midclavicular line. For a hemothorax, the chest tube is positioned in the sixth intercostal space in the posterior axillary line. Usually the chest tubes are sutured and taped into position and therefore are not easily dislodged. If the tubes are pulled out, subcutaneous emphysema or a pneumothorax results. A pneumothorax will also result if the tube is disconnected from the underwater seal. This is the reason for securing the collecting reservoirs of a chest tube drainage system to the floor with tape. Mobilizing and frequently repositioning the patient facilitates chest tube drainage and re-expansion of collapsed alveoli. Care must be taken to avoid kinking or straining chest tubes during patient treatment.

A bronchopulmonary fistula can be responsible for a major loss of the tidal volume delivered by the ventilator. Small leaks can be tolerated and are usually compensated for by an increase in tidal or minute ventilation.

Multiple Trauma

The management of multiple trauma is a major challenge for the ICU team. Multisystem involvement and complications often present a precarious situation in which priorities have to be defined for each individual situation. Multiple trauma can include head injury, chest wall injuries, fractures, lung contusions, diaphragm injury, pleural space disorders, internal injuries, thromboemboli, fat emboli, and cardiac contusions. Deep vein thrombosis occurs in 20% to 40% of patients in the absence of prophylaxis (Piotrowski et al, 1996). Shock and acute respiratory distress syndrome (ARDS) may ensue (see Chapter 36). Early intervention with body positioning significantly lowers the incidence of ARDS compared with later intervention in patients with multiple trauma (Pape et al, 1998). The clinical picture of the patient with multiple trauma is compounded by the mobilization and positioning restrictions imposed (Ray et al, 1974). Positive end-expiratory pressure (PEEP) is frequently used to reduce the effects of lung congestion secondary to shock or ARDS (McAslan & Cowley, 1979). Arterial blood gases are assessed to evaluate the effectiveness of PEEP in effecting improved oxygen transfer.

Multiple Fractures

Multiple trauma patients are assumed to have spinal involvement, particularly of the cervical spine, until ruled out with appropriate scans and x-rays. Meanwhile the physical therapist performs repeated assessments to establish a baseline position for the patient and recommend positions that will maximize oxygen transport. Treatment to enhance oxygen transport and mucociliary transport is primarily restricted to body positioning using log rolling maneuvers and a selected range of motion exercises (i.e., not of the head and neck, and possibly shoulders).

Fixation, traction, and casting of fractures and dislocations of the limbs complicate the management of the trauma patient. Restrictions to mobilization and body positioning are primary concerns of the physical therapist (Mackenzie, 1989). Mobilization in the upright position provides both a gravitational stimulus and an exercise stimulus, both of which are essential to optimize oxygen transport. This is preferable to mobilization exercises in the recumbent position. In some cases, traction can be transferred from over the end of the bed to over a chair. A strict routine of body positioning is maintained, although severe limitations often exist with respect to the specific positions and the degree of turning permitted. Lower limb traction can be maintained when the patient is positioned in a modified side-lying position. Coordinating treatments with analgesia schedules reduces the patient's pain and fatigue, thereby improving tolerance to treatment and prolonging the treatment. These patients usually tolerate the head-down position well, provided head injury does not complicate the clinical picture.

The acute effects of mobilization that will benefit the patient with musculoskeletal trauma include augmentation of ventilation, perfusion, ventilation and perfusion matching,

and promotion of mucociliary transport and cough effectiveness. General mobilization exercises and proprioceptive neuromuscular facilitation (PNF) can be used to promote a mobilization stimulus. Cycle pedals can be attached to a chair or the end of the bed to provide a low-intensity exercise challenge for some patients. Maximal work output can be achieved within the patient's capacity using an interval training type schedule (i.e., schedule of work to rest periods). A mobilization program that promotes the long-term effects of exercise can be prescribed that involves as many large muscle groups as possible in rhythmic, dynamic exercise.

Frequent deep breathing and coughing is continued during and between treatments, depending on whether the patient requires mechanical ventilation. Body positioning is carried out within the limits of the patient's traction and casts. Impaired mucociliary transport is treated with body positioning and frequent position changes. Secretion accumulation may require postural drainage. Modified positions may be indicated because of the positioning restrictions imposed by the fractures, traction, and fixation devices. If indicated, manual techniques may be coupled with postural drainage (Mackenzie et al, 1980). Care must be taken to ensure the addition of manual techniques is beneficial and is tolerated by the patient.

Relaxation interventions, both active and passive, should be integrated into the treatment regimen for the trauma patient to reduce excessive oxygen consumption and promote comfort (Malamed, 2002). Active relaxation refers to relaxing the patient through participation of the patient in relaxation procedures. Passive relaxation refers to relaxing the patient using passive procedures (e.g., body positioning, physical supports, talking slowly and calmly, and taking adequate time for conducting treatments). Taking time to implement mobilization is essential. First, mechanically moving and having patients who have multiple injuries move requires a prolonged period of time. In addition, however, the cardiovascular and cardiopulmonary systems of the critically ill need time to adapt to new positions physiologically and to control discomfort. Prolonged periods of time may be required to turn a patient, dangle him or her over the bed, or transfer him or her to a chair with continuous monitoring. Every effort is made to maintain the patient's spirits, reduce stress, and encourage a positive attitude toward active participation early in the rehabilitation program that begins in the ICU.

Care must be taken to avoid under-treating or over-treating individuals with traumatic injury. A clear chest can rapidly regress because of general immobility and limitations to body positioning imposed by traction and pain. Treatments should always be coordinated with the patient's analgesics to optimize treatment response and for the patient's comfort. Whenever possible, the patient should be equipped with slings and pulleys and weights at bedside and a monkey bar overhead for bed mobility and upper-extremity exercise. In addition to their cardiopulmonary benefits, PNF patterns are useful in preparation for slings and pulleys. The use of PNF patterns for trauma and postoperative patients can be well tolerated by these patients. All activities are taught in conjunction with breathing control exercises and coordination with the respiratory cycle.

INDIVIDUALS WITH HEAD INJURY

Pathophysiology and Medical Management

Hypoxemia is observed in many patients with injury to the central nervous system (Demling, 1980). This may reflect primary damage to the cardiopulmonary centers of the brain or secondary effects of associated trauma. Arterial blood gases are therefore closely monitored in these patients.

Acute cerebral edema with sudden increase in intracranial pressure (ICP) and reduction in cerebral perfusion pressure rapidly affects central control of respiration (Borozny, 1987). Advancing cerebral edema is evidenced by deterioration in level of consciousness, pupillary reflexes, ocular reflexes, pattern of respiration, and exaggerated muscle tone and posture. The sequence of these clinical signs corresponds to progressively increasing ICP from the cortex toward the medullopontine region. With involvement of the brain stem, respiration becomes variable and uncoordinated. With loss of central control and imminent cessation of breathing, respiration is shallow and ataxic. The appearance of the jaw and laryngeal jerk with each inspiratory effort suggests a poor prognosis.

Physical therapy and the patient's normal routine may have a dramatic effect on the ICP. ICP can be elevated indirectly by an increase in intrathoracic pressure as a result of physical therapy or suctioning. Turning and positioning may produce obstruction to cerebral venous outflow. Noxious stimuli, such as arterial and venous punctures or cleansing wounds, can elevate ICP and relatively innocuous stimuli, such as noise or pupil checks. Whether these factors elevate ICP depend on cerebral blood volume and intracranial compliance. On cerebral stimulation, a chain reaction is initiated. Cerebral activity is increased, which in turn elevates metabolic rate, blood flow, and hence volume and ICP. Alternatively, increased cerebral blood volume secondary to gravitational effects increases ICP and reduces cerebral perfusion pressure.

The head of the bed is usually maintained between 30 and 40 degrees to promote venous drainage and thereby reduce ICP. The patient's head and neck can be fixed in a neutral position by halo traction or by sand bags positioned on either side (Figure 35-1). Mechanical hyperventilation is used to maintain PCO_2 below normal limits but above 20 mm Hg. Arterial blood gases are checked during or immediately after hyperventilation. Prolonged hyperventilation is avoided.

Barbiturate coma may be induced to decrease the cerebral metabolic rate for oxygen and hence cerebral blood flow. The reduction in cerebral metabolic rate exceeds the reduction in blood flow and thus oxygen supply exceeds demand, which is a desirable treatment outcome. Invasive hemodynamic monitoring is instituted in conjunction with barbiturate coma because barbiturates contribute to hemodynamic instability.

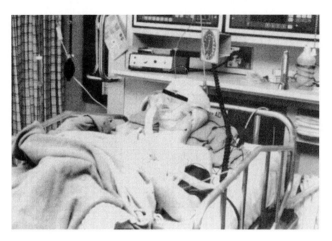

FIGURE 35-1 Patient after neurosurgery procedure; head of bed elevated 20 degrees to help reduce intracranial pressure.

A complication of head injuries is acute lung injury, specifically neurogenic pulmonary edema (see Chapter 36). Antonomical nervous system dysfunction contributes to hypertension and neurogenic pulmonary edema. The endothelial tight junctions in the pulmonary capillaries leak protein into the interstitium along with fluid. Constriction of the lymphatic vessels may also contribute to fluid accumulation by impeding the removal of lung water. Increased fluid accumulation in the interstitium may progress to the alveoli, contributing further to impaired gas exchange and reduced lung compliance.

Principles of Physical Therapy Management

Physical therapy priorities in the management of the patient with cardiopulmonary dysfunction secondary to head injury appear in Box 35-2. Body positioning, a mainstay of treatment for the patient with reduced consciousness, is based on a detailed assessment, consideration of multisystem status, and serial monitoring of the patient's response (Sullivan, 2000).

Intracranial pressure may increase with treatment and in particular with turning or suctioning. An ICP of up to 30 mm Hg may be acceptable provided the pressure returns to normal immediately after the removal of the pressure-potentiating stimulus. Prolonged elevation of ICP suggests low cerebral compliance and the possibility of potential brain damage unless pressure is reduced. Thus all interventions must be performed guardedly with due consideration being given to corresponding changes in ICP. Typically, management of patients with central nervous system trauma includes judicious tracheal suctioning, a stringent turning regimen, lung hyperinflation with the manual breathing bag in the nonventilated patient, or deep breathing with occasionally increased tidal volumes or sighs in the ventilated patients.

If the ICP is unstable and a risk of brain damage exists, physical therapy should follow sedation. Ideally treatments should be performed when the ICP is low and intracranial compliance is satisfactory. Patients whose cerebral compliance

---

BOX 35-2

Physical Therapy Priorities in the Management of the Patient with Cardiopulmonary Dysfunction Secondary to Head Injury

1. Prevent cerebral hypoxia by maintaining a patent airway
2. Reduce intracranial pressure and optimal cerebral perfusion pressure
3. Position the patient within the limits of fracture stabilization and elevated intracranial pressure to promote alveolar ventilation and ventilation and perfusion matching
4. Position the patient to reduce pathological patterns of muscle synergy and thereby promote ventilation and reduce oxygen consumption
5. Position the patient to reduce myocardial stress
6. Avoid activities and stimuli that increase ICP
7. Reduce atelectasis and its risk
8. Shift lung fluid accumulations and areas of atelectasis
9. Promote lymphatic drainage
10. Promote mucociliary transport and reduce pooling of secretions and risk of chest infection
11. Reduce the work of breathing and improve the efficiency of the muscles of respiration, particularly if long-term disability is a risk
12. Perform active, active-assisted, or passive movements as soon as possible to enhance cardiopulmonary function and secondarily to preserve musculoskeletal and neuromuscular function and reduce the risk of thromboemboli

---

is compromised need monitoring during position changes (Mavrocordatos et al, 2000). The head-down position is contraindicated. Noise and noxious stimulation that increases ICP should be kept to a minimum.

If the ICP is elevated, all noxious stimuli should be removed. In severe conditions a decision may have to be made by the team to limit or withdraw interventions that lead to an excessive ICP increase that does not remit instantly (e.g., physical therapy, positioning, suctioning, or neurological assessment).

Movement of the limbs is performed gently and in a relaxed manner. Patients in a comatose state may experience passive limb movement noxiously. Intracranial pressure may be elevated as a result. Passive movements, however, may have the added benefit of promoting improved tidal ventilation in the nonventilated patient by providing afferent stimulation to the respiratory center via peripheral muscle and joint receptors.

Severe head injury may produce flexor or extensor posturing. These synergies may be inhibited by appropriately positioning the patient. Judicious body positioning, in turn, reduces oxygen consumption and the patient's overall energy requirements.

Although arousing the patient and increasing oxygen consumption occurs with cardiopulmonary physical therapy, arousal and oxygen consumption are generally minimized to

reduce hemodynamic and metabolic demands in the patient with a head injury.

INDIVIDUALS WITH SPINAL CORD INJURY

Pathophysiology and Medical Management

The principal cause of death in the early stages of acute spinal cord injury, particularly for the high lesions, is cardiopulmonary complications. Lung volumes are reduced with the exception of residual volume, which increases. Vital capacity increases in the supine compared with the sitting position in quadriplegic patients. This does not, however, counter the negative effects of reduced functional residual capacity (FRC) and increased airway closure in this position and reduced flow rates.

Spinal cord injuries above C3 result in loss of phrenic nerve innervation, necessitating a tracheostomy and mechanical ventilation. The lower the level of the spinal cord lesion, the lower is the cardiopulmonary risk. All patients with spinal cord injuries are at risk for developing atelectasis and pneumonia. The coughing mechanics of patients with quadriplegia are abnormal and contribute to ineffective airway clearance (Estenne & Gorino, 1992). In addition the quadriplegic patient is at risk for developing pulmonary emboli. Prophylactic low-dose heparin is used routinely unless the presence of pulmonary emboli is suspected and higher dosages are indicated.

Patients with suspected spinal cord injuries usually undergo immediate spinal fixation on admission. Depending on the level of injury determined by clinical signs and x-rays, traction and fixation may be localized to the head and neck or spinal support and casting may be required in the thoracic or lumbar regions.

Principles of Physical Therapy Management

Because of the need to maintain relative immobility in the acute stabilization period of suspected spinal cord injury, therapeutic body positioning rather than mobilization is a primary intervention for optimizing oxygen transport. Although modified body positioning can be achieved, the provision of optimal care under these restricted conditions is a singularly important challenge to the physical therapist, particularly with respect to the management of adequate oxygen transport while the patient is in the ICU. Patients with high spinal cord lesions can be positioned in all positions within the limits of the cervical traction device being used, barring head injury. Both head and foot-tipped positions, however, are introduced cautiously and with hemodynamic monitoring because both positions can have significant cardiopulmonary and hemodynamic consequences secondary to spinal nerve loss and hence sympathetic nerve loss to the peripheral blood vessels. Turning frames such as the Stryker frame facilitate turning and tipping these hemodynamically labile patients in the supine and prone positions (Douglas et al, 1977).

Effective body positioning, despite the need in some cases for extensive modification, may be sufficient to optimize oxygen transport secondary to improved regional ventilation and perfusion to all lung fields. In the spontaneously breathing patient, deep breathing and coughing maneuvers need to be coupled with position changes to optimize mucociliary transport (Alverez et al, 1981; Braun et al, 1984). Some patients may not tolerate numerous positions and position changes and thus have impaired mucociliary transport. If secretion accumulation and stasis develop, postural drainage can be instituted; however, tipping must be attempted very cautiously. Patients should be monitored closely during and after treatment. Because of the hemodynamic lability of acute quadriplegic patients and the well-documented side effects of percussion and vibration (Kirilloff et al, 1985), these procedures must be applied cautiously, should they be indicated, depending on the severity of any complicating fracture-dislocation(s), the stability of fixation, the condition of the lungs, the presence of chest wall injuries, and hemodynamic lability.

The high-frequency oscillating ventilator may have some benefit in the management of multiple trauma patients with spinal injuries who require ventilation. The advantages of the high-frequency oscillating ventilator include improved spontaneous mucociliary clearance and reduced incidence of atelectasis (Gross & King, 1984). Weaning patients with high spinal cord lesions off the ventilator requires special skill because of the impaired function of the respiratory muscles. For these patients, weaning can be particularly fatiguing, frightening, and frustrating. Patients are weaned lying supine when they are alert and able to cooperate. Short periods off the ventilator on the T-piece are used initially. Use of the accessory muscles of respiration and any other muscular reserves are encouraged to compensate for the loss of function of the respiratory muscles. In some centers, patients are started in the weaning period on respiratory muscle training. The physical therapist must be well versed and practiced in this procedure before using it in conjunction with weaning the quadriplegic patient off the ventilator. Because of the potential risk of inappropriate application and of danger to the patient, respiratory muscle training must be effected knowledgeably to optimize its benefits for each individual patient.

Respiratory muscle weakness and fatigue, two physiologically distinct entities, are probably much more common in patients in the ICU than appreciated. These states need to be recognized and detected early because both can cause respiratory muscle failure (Macklem & Roussos, 1977). The distinction between the two conditions is that weakened muscles respond to resistive muscle training, whereas fatigued muscles do not. Exposing fatigued respiratory muscles to resistive loads can accentuate respiratory failure. The indication for respiratory muscle training, therefore, is weak rather than fatigued respiratory muscles. Rest is indicated for fatigued respiratory muscles. Whether the respiratory muscles are weak or fatigued must be established before prescribing respiratory muscle training. For further detail on respiratory muscle training refer to Chapter 26.

The combination of immobilization and cardiopulmonary involvement secondary to multiple trauma may result in disuse atrophy and weakness of the diaphragm similar to that observed in other skeletal muscles. Respiratory muscle weakness and fatigue can be a component of both obstructive and restrictive patterns of lung disease. Patients with spinal cord injuries do not have the same advantage of performing coordinated general body activity and relaxation maneuvers to help reduce the work of breathing. This contributes to a marked decrease in respiratory muscle strength and endurance resulting in reduced vital capacity, rib cage mobility, and the ability to cough. For these reasons, patients with paralysis and demonstrated respiratory muscle weakness are particularly well suited for respiratory muscle training. The quadriplegic patient has lost the function of the intercostal muscles, which are important muscles of inspiration and responsible for thoracic cage expansion. In addition, the absence of the abdominal muscles, which are the primary expiratory muscles, drastically reduces the ability to cough effectively and perform a forced expiration. The diaphragm and the accessory muscles of inspiration, namely the scaleni and sternocleidomastoid muscles, then become the quadriplegic patient's respiratory muscles. These factors as well as the effects of heat, humidity, and the vertical position, all predispose the individual with quadriplegia to the development of respiratory muscle weakness and failure. The physical therapist can help avert the effects of respiratory muscle weakness with respiratory muscle training (see Chapter 26).

Maximum inspiratory mouth pressure and vital capacity can be measured routinely to monitor change in diaphragmatic function. The level of inspiratory resistance and the duration for which the patient can use each resistor are indications of the endurance of the inspiratory muscles. Measurement of vital capacity and maximum inspiratory and expiratory mouth pressures provide an index of the strength of the inspiratory muscles.

Certain precautions must be observed with respiratory muscle training. Each time a new resistance is tried, the physical therapist should be with the patient. The patient selects his or her own rate and pattern of breathing. The inspiratory rate is usually constant. Breathing that is too shallow is inefficient, and breathing that is too slow and deep may result in accumulation of carbon dioxide. The patient is cautioned about avoiding hyperventilation. The physical therapist, or the patient when he or she is capable, should check the valving system on the respiratory muscle trainer before each training session to ensure it is functioning properly.

INDIVIDUALS WITH BURNS

Pathophysiology and Medical Management

Cardiopulmonary complications are common in patients with smoke inhalation with or without severe burns and are a major cause of death (Marini & Wheeler, 1989). Smoke and chemical inhalation produce edema, bronchospasm, cough, mucosal sloughing, hemorrhage, hoarseness, stridor, and profuse carbonaceous secretions. Irritation of the alveoli and acute pulmonary edema can result in a condition resembling adult respiratory distress syndrome (see Chapter 36).

On admission of the patient with burns to hospital, the patency of the airway is assessed immediately. Inhalation injuries are common in burn patients, resulting from smoke inhalation, heat trauma, and chemical and gas inhalation. Oxygen and humidification are usually administered immediately. Heat may cause laryngeal and bronchial edema. If airway occlusion from impending edema threatens, intubation is performed. If indicated early, intubation may avoid respiratory distress within the critical 24-hour period after admission. Particular care is given to children and older adults with inhalation injury because these patients have a higher risk of developing secondary cardiopulmonary complications.

Carbon monoxide poisoning may complicate the clinical picture further and seriously threaten tissue oxygenation (Cahalane & Deming, 1984; Cane et al, 1990). Hemoglobin has a higher affinity for binding with carbon monoxide than oxygen. A carboxyhemoglobin level greater than 20% denotes carbon monoxide poisoning. Levels in excess of 50% may produce irreversible neurological damage. The principal danger of carbon monoxide poisoning is that arterial PaO_2 can be adequate and tissue oxygen tension inadequate. Administration of high levels of oxygen is an initial priority to reduce the half-life of carbon monoxide from several hours to one hour.

Depending on the severity and extent of the burns, treatment ranges from conservative medical interventions to multiple surgeries related to progressive debridement and skin grafting. Both second and third degree burns can result in severe disfigurement and disability. Second-degree burns are partial thickness burns and tend to be painful. Third-degree burns are full thickness burns; these tend to be anesthetic in that the nerves themselves have been destroyed.

Treatment is directed at improving arterial saturation, maintaining fluid balance, and preventing infection. Hypoxemia is effectively treated with the administration of oxygen and maintenance of clear airways. If the patient is breathing spontaneously, oxygen is given via nasal cannulae or mask at flows of one to five L/min, depending on the arterial oxygen saturation. Moisture can be administered through a face tent with a heated nebulizer. Fluid balance is particularly challenging in the patient with burns because of the loss of skin, which is essential to the retention and compartmentalization of body fluids and in the regulation of fluid and electrolyte loss from the body. In addition, these patients may lose blood because of injury at the time of the accident. There is also a period without fluid replacement from before the injury to the time medical attention is available and IV fluid resuscitation commenced. Because of the nature of burns, even when fluid resuscitation has begun, fluid and electrolyte balance remains a challenge until considerable healing and repair have occurred. Fluid and electrolyte imbalances have considerable implications for hemodynamics and cardiopulmonary function

(see Chapter 16) and contribute to hemodynamic instability, which necessitates modification of the physical therapy management.

An airway may be inserted initially with burns to the face, airway, and lungs in anticipation of progressive edema, which would make the insertion of airway considerably more difficult hours or days later. Ventilatory assistance is indicated with evidence of respiratory insufficiency secondary to smoke inhalation, and burns of the nose, face, throat, airway, lungs, and chest wall. A nasotracheal tube is preferred to a tracheostomy tube because complications with a tracheostomy tube are greater in burn patients.

Cardiopulmonary complications are generally related to sepsis or fluid overload in the initial stage. Acute pulmonary edema and congestion are largely preventable with careful fluid therapy. Central venous pressure can be misleading in the burn patient because of severe fluid loss and may remain at low values despite pulmonary edema. Pulmonary artery pressure more accurately reflects the status of the pulmonary circulation in these patients. Treatment of pulmonary edema consists typically of digitalis, diuretics, and mechanical ventilation. Positive end expiratory pressure is usually indicated in the ventilated burn patient. Mist or aerosol inhalation is also used to reduce the thickness of pulmonary secretions.

Complications must be anticipated and prevented in the burn patient (Deming, 1985). These include impaired thermoregulation, hypermetabolism and increased energy expenditure, ileus and gastric distension, pain, and infection. Eschar formation associated with circumferential burns of the chest wall mechanically restricts chest wall movement and can lead to respiratory failure. Tissue edema that can continue for a few days after the burn contributes to increased tissue pressure and impaired tissue perfusion potentiating tissue ischemia and necrosis. Late complications include gastrointestinal bleeding secondary to stress ulceration and the continued high risk of infection.

Principles of Physical Therapy Management

Cardiopulmonary physical therapy is often required immediately for the patient with inhalation damage to maintain the patency of the airways, prevent atelectasis and retention of secretions, and improve or maintain gas exchange. Pulmonary function may be severely impaired as the net result of inhalation damage, burns and trauma to the chest wall, pain, and fluid imbalance.

Cardiopulmonary physical therapy often has to be modified in the patient with burns (Wright, 1984). Mobilization to enhance oxygen transport is exploited as much as possible; however, because of blood volume and hemodynamic problems, orthostatic intolerance may limit mobilization and positioning alternatives. With more severe burns and more extensive burn distribution, body positioning is the primary intervention. Positioning to effect an optimal therapeutic effect on oxygen transport is challenging because of the significant physical limitations that may exist. Given that body positioning profoundly influences ventilation and perfusion matching (Clauss et al, 1968), the reduced number of positioning alternatives will contribute to shunt, ventilation and perfusion mismatch, and hypoxemia. This effect will be accentuated if the patient is mechanically ventilated (see Chapter 33).

Body positioning to optimize oxygen transport is life-preserving; however, positioning and limb splinting must also be considered from the outset to minimize deformity and restore optimal neuromuscular and musculoskeletal status. Positioning priorities in burn patients must address both these aspects of management.

Patients who have skin grafts require particular care when moving or positioning because of the danger of sheering forces on the graft, which can disrupt the circulation, nutrition, and healing of the new skin. Sterile procedures must be observed at all times. The physical therapist is usually required to cap, gown, mask, and glove before treating the patient with extensive exposed areas and to cover the chest with a sterile drape. Facilitating mucociliary transport is a priority if the patient has significant mobility and positioning restrictions because of the burn severity. Wherever possible, mobilization in conjunction with multiple body positions and position changes is attempted to maximize mucociliary clearance (Wolff et al, 1977). If secretions have accumulated, positioning for postural drainage requires the same consideration as positioning for improved alveolar ventilation and ventilation and perfusion matching. In the spontaneously breathing patient, postural drainage positions can be used selectively to increase alveolar volume in the superior lung fields and alveolar ventilation to inferior lung fields, in addition to purposes of drainage of the superior bronchopulmonary segments. If the patient is mechanically ventilated, however, the superior lung fields are preferentially ventilated (see Chapter 33). Should the addition of manual techniques be indicated, percussion may not be comfortably tolerated in the presence of first and second degree burns. Manual vibration may substitute. Manual techniques are contraindicated over freshly grafted skin; however, manual vibration may be transmitted from a more distal site to a lung field that cannot be vibrated directly.

Risk of aspiration is increased if tube feedings are not discontinued for at least one hour before treatment. A nasogastric tube is often used and should be correctly positioned, particularly during treatment.

Stimulating exercise and gravitational stress may initially consist of being in the upright position, preferably with the legs dependent, performing selected limb movements and dangling over the edge of the bed for a few minutes if this can be tolerated. In patients with severe burns and significant fluid imbalance, however, active and active-assisted movements in an upright position that can be tolerated may substitute. As the patient's tolerance increases, free, unsupported sitting can progress to standing and walking. Ambulation during ventilator-assisted breathing should always be considered for any patient for whom this activity is not contraindicated. The upright position and physical activity in the upright position are likely to markedly enhance the patient's cardiopulmonary and neuromuscular function, and improve the patient's strength and endurance in preparation for long-term rehabilitation. If sitting up and ambulation are not imminent, appropriate limb movements, preferably active, can help provide an exercise stimulus that can enhance oxygen transport. Passive full range of motion exercises, in addition, are required to maximize joint range (a distinct goal from that to enhance oxygen transport) wherever possible.

Positioning to minimize deformity is a priority given the potential consequences for cardiopulmonary function and oxygen transport, as well as musculoskeletal and biomechanical reasons. Positioning a burn patient, regardless of the goal, should take into consideration alignment, pressure points, muscle balance, and effect on healing and grafted skin.

Certain precautions have to be observed in the management of the burn patient. First, skin loss contributes to substantial fluid loss, often resulting in labile fluid and electrolyte imbalance. This situation enhances myocardial irritability and the risk of dysrhythmia. Hemodynamic and electrocardiogram monitoring is performed routinely during physical therapy treatment. Second, large areas of skin loss increase the risk of infection; therefore the physical therapist must be familiar with sterile technique.

INIDIVIDUALS AFTER ORGAN TRANSPLANTATION

Organ transplantation has increased over the past decade, and survival rates are improving. Liver transplantation has become an accepted therapy for end stage liver disease. In addition to its metabolic consequences, liver disease has a marked effect on musculoskeletal complications including cachexia and osteoporosis, both of which can worsen postoperatively. Optimal nutrition and exercise have been advocated as means of improving outcomes before and after transplantation (Vintro et al, 2002).

SUMMARY

This chapter describes the principles and practice of physical therapy in the management of people with cardiopulmonary dysfunction *secondary* to neuromuscular and musculoskeletal conditions that can lead to cardiopulmonary failure. Categories of conditions included were neuromuscular conditions, musculoskeletal conditions, morbid obesity, head injury, spinal cord injury, and burns. A detailed understanding of the underlying pathophysiology of these conditions and their medical management provides a basis for defining the physical therapy goals and prescribing treatment. The principles described in this chapter cannot be interpreted as complete treatment prescriptions because each patient is an individual whose condition reflects multiple factors contributing to impaired oxygen transport or threat to it (i.e., the effects of recumbency, restricted mobility, extrinsic factors related to the patient's care, and intrinsic factors related to the patient in addition to the underlying pathophysiology).

Review Questions

1. With respect to patients who are critically ill, describe the pathophysiology of cardiopulmonary dysfunction *secondary to* the following conditions: neuromuscular dysfunction, morbid obesity, musculoskeletal trauma, head injury, spinal cord injury, and burns.

2. Relate cardiopulmonary physical therapy treatment interventions to the underlying pathophysiology of each of the above conditions in the patient who is critically ill and provide the rationale for your choice.

REFERENCES

Alvarez, S.E., Peterson, M., & Lunsford, B.R. (1981). Respiratory treatment of the adult patient with spinal cord injury. Physical Therapy 61:1737-1745.

Bake, B., Dempsey, J., & Grimby, G. (1976). Effects of shape changes of the chest wall on distribution of inspired gas. American Review of Respiratory Disease 114:1113-1120.

Barach, A.L. (1974). Chronic obstructive lung disease: Postural relief of dyspnea. Archives of Physical Medicine and Rehabilitation 55:495-504.

Bates, D.V. (1989). Respiratory function in disease, ed 3. Philadelphia: W.B. Saunders.

Bennett, W.D., Foster, W.M., & Chapman, W.F. (1990). Cough-enhanced mucus clearance in the normal lung. Journal of Applied Physiology 69:1670-1675.

Black, L.F., & Hyatt, R.E. (1971). Maximal static respiratory pressures in generalized neuromuscular disease. American Review of Respiratory Diseases 103:641-650.

Borozny, M.L. (1987). Intracranial hypertension: Implications for the physiotherapist. Physiotherapy Canada 39:360-366.

Braun, S.R., Giovannoni, R., & O'Connor, M. (1984). Improving the cough in patients with spinal cord injury. American Journal of Physical Medicine 63:1-10.

Cahalane, M., & Deming, R.H. (1984). Early respiratory abnormalities from smoke inhalation. Journal of the American Medical Association 25:771-773.

Cane, R.D., Davison, R., & Shapiro, B.A. (1990). Case studies in critical care medicine, ed 2. Philadelphia: Elsevier.

Clauss, R.H., Scalabrini, B.Y., Ray, J.F. III, & Reed, G.E. (1968). Effects of changing body position upon improved ventilation-perfusion relationships. Circulation 37(Suppl 4):214-217.

Cooper, C.B., Trend, P.S., & Wiles, C.M. (1985). Severe diaphragm weakness in multiple sclerosis. Thorax 40:631-632.

Curran, F.J. (1981). Night ventilation to body respirators for patients in chronic respiratory failure due to late stage muscular dystrophy. Archives of Physical Medicine and Rehabilitation 62:270-274.

Curran, F.J., & Colbert, A.P. (1989). Ventilator management in Duchenne muscular dystrophy and postpoliomyelitis syndrome: twelve years' experience. Archives of Physical Medicine and Rehabilitation 70:180-185.

Dean, E. (1985). Effect of body position on pulmonary function. Physical Therapy 65:613-618.

Dean, E. (1997). Oxygen transport deficits in systemic disease and implications for physical therapy. Physical Therapy 79:476-487.

Dean, E., Ross, J., Road, J.D., Courtenay, L., & Madill, K. (1991). Pulmonary function in individuals with a history of poliomyelitis. Chest 100:118-123.

Demling, R.H. (1980). The pathogenesis of respiratory failure after trauma and sepsis. Surgical Clinics of North America 60:1373-1390.

Demling, R.H. (1985). Burns. New England Journal of Medicine 31:1389-1398.

Douglas, W.W., Rehder, K., Beynen, F.M., Sessler, A.D., & Marsh, H.M. (1977). Improved oxygenation in patients with acute respiratory failure: The prone position. American Review of Respiratory Disease 115:559-566.

Dureuil, B., Viires, N., & Cantineau, J.P. (1986). Diaphragmatic contractility after upper abdominal surgery. Journal of Applied Physiology 61:1775-1780.

Estenne, M., & Gorino, M. (1992). Action of the diaphragm during cough in tetrapelgic subjects. Journal of Applied Physiology 72:1074-1080.

Fugl-Meyer, A.R., & Grimby, G. (1984). Respiration in tetraplegia and in hemiplegia: A review. International Rehabilitation Medicine 6:186-190.

Griggs, R.C., & Donohoe, K.M. (1982). Recognition and management of respiratory insufficiency in neuromuscular disease. Journal of Chronic Diseases 35:497-500.

Gross, D., & King, M. (1984). High frequency chest wall compression: A new non-invasive method of chest physiotherapy for mucociliary clearance. Physiotherapy Canada 36:137-139.

Hasani, A., Pavia, D., Agnew, J.E., & Clarke, S.W. (1991). The effect of unproductive coughing/FET on regional mucus movement in the human lungs. Respiratory Medicine 85(Suppl A):23-26.

Hietpas, B.G., Roth, R.D., & Jensen, W.M. (1979). Huff coughing and airway patency. Respiratory Care 24:710.

Kirilloff, L.H., Owens, G.R., Rogers, R.M., & Mazzacco, M. (1985). Chest 88:436-444.

Kremzar, B., Spec-Marn, A., Kompan, L., & Cerovic, O. (1997). Normal values of SVO_2 as therapeutic goal in patients with multiple injuries. Intensive Care Medicine 23:65-70.

Lane, D.J., Hazleman, B., & Nichols, P.J.R. (1974). Late onset respiratory failure in patients with previous poliomyelitis. Quarterly Journal of Medicine 43:551-568.

Leblanc, P., Ruff, F., & Milic-Emili, J. (1970). Effects of age and body position on "airway closure" in man. Journal of Applied Physiology 28:448-451.

Mackenzie, C.F. (Ed.). (1989). Chest physiotherapy in the intensive care unit, ed 2. Baltimore: Lippincott Williams & Wilkins.

Mackenzie, C.F., Shin, B., Hadi, F., & Imle, P.C. (1980). Changes in total lung/thorax compliance following chest physiotherapy. Anesthesia and Analgesia 59:207-210.

Macklem, P.T., & Roussos, C.S. (1977). Respiratory muscle fatigue: A cause of respiratory failure? Clinical Science and Molecular Medicine 53:419-422.

Malamed, S.F. (2002). Sedation: A guide to patient management, ed 4. Philadelphia: Elsevier.

Marini, J.J., & Wheeler, A.P. (1997). Critical care medicine—The essentials, ed 2. Baltimore: Lippincott Williams & Wilkins.

Mavrocordatos, P., Bissonnette, B., & Ravussin, P. (2000). Effects of neck position and head elevation on intracranial pressure in anaesthetized neurosurgical patients: preliminary results. Journal of Neurosurgery and Anesthesiology 12:10-14.

McAslan, T.C., & Cowley, R.A. (1979). The preventive use of PEEP in major trauma. American Surgeon 45:159-167.

Moukas, M., Vassiliou, M.P., Amygdalou, A., Mandragos, C., Takis, F., & Behrakis, P.K. (2002). Muscular mass assessed by ultrasonography after adminstration of low-dose corticosteroids and muscle relaxants in critically ill hemiplegic patients. Clinical Nutrition 21:297-302.

Moylan, J.A. (Ed). (1988). Trauma surgery. Philadelphia: J.B. Lippincott.

Nunn, J.F., Coleman, A.J., Sachithanandan, T., Bergman, N.A., & Laws, J.W. (1965). Hypoxaemia and atelectasis produced by forced expiration. British Journal of Anesthesia 37:3-12.

Pape, H.C., Remmers, D., Weinberg, A., Graf, B., Reilmann, H., Evans, S., Regel, G., & Tscherne, H. (1998). Is early kinetic positioning beneficial for pulmonary function in multiple trauma patients? Injury 29:219-225.

Piotrowski, J.J., Alexander, J.J., Brandt, C.P., McHenry, C.R., Yuhas, J.P., & Jacobs, D. (1996). Is deep vein thrombosis surveillance warranted in high-risk trauma patients? American Journal of Surgery 172:210-213.

Ray, J.F. III, Yost, L., Moallem, S., Sanoudos, G.M., Villamena, P., Paredes, R.M., & Clauss, R.H. (1974). Immobility, hypoxemia, and pulmonary arteriovenous shunting. Archives of Surgery 109:537-541.

Ross, J., & Dean, E. (1992). Body positioning. In Zadai, C. (Ed). Clinics in physical therapy, pulmonary management in physical therapy. New York: Churchill Livingstone.

Sullivan, J. (2000). Positioning of patients with severe traumatic brain injury: research-based practice. Journal of Neuroscience Nursing 32:204-209.

Velmahos, G.C., Demetriades, D., Shoemaker, W.C., Chan, L.S., Tatevossian, R., Wo, C.C., Vassiliu, P., Cornwell, E.E., 3rd, Murray, J.A., Roth, B., Belzberg, H., Asensio, J.A., & Berne, T.V. (2000). Endpoints of resuscitation of critically injured patients: normal or supranormal? A prospective randomized trial. Annals of Surgery 232:409-418.

Vintro, A.Q., Krasnoff, J.B., & Painter, P. (2002). Roles of nutrition and physical activity in musculoskeletal complications before and after liver transplantation. AACN Clinical Issues 13:333-347.

Wolff, R.K., Dolovich, M.B., Obminski, G., & Newhouse, M.T. (1977). Effects of exercise and eucapnic hyperventilation on bronchial clearance in man. Journal of Applied Physiology 43:46-50.

Wright, P.C. (1984). Fundamentals of acute burn care and physical therapy management. Physical Therapy 64:1217-1231.

Zinman, R. (1984). Cough versus chest physiotherapy. American Review of Respiratory Diseases 129:182-184.

C H A P T E R   3 6

Complications, Adult Respiratory Distress Syndrome, Shock, Sepsis, and Multiorgan System Failure

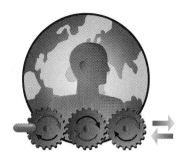

Elizabeth Dean and Christiane Perme

KEY TERMS

Acute lung injury
Acute respiratory distress syndrome
Multiorgan system failure
Perioperative complications

Respiratory failure
Sepsis
Shock

The purpose of this chapter is to describe some common complications seen in patients who are critically ill. Complications arising from the following conditions are included: respiratory failure, surgery, acute lung injury and acute respiratory distress syndrome, shock, sepsis, and multiorgan system failure. Furthermore, the implications for cardiopulmonary physical therapy are presented. Complications add further complexity to the diagnosis of the multiple factors contributing to impaired oxygen transport and to the challenge of prescribing effective treatment. Understanding the pathophysiological deficits in these complex conditions is the basis for efficacious management, reducing the risk of an untoward treatment response, and preventing worsening of the patient's condition. In addition, risks such as age, co-morbidity, severity of trauma, extent of surgery, obesity, deconditioning, smoking, and FIO_2 greater than 0.05 have been reported (Marx et al, 1998). Compared with nonsurvivors, survivors of these conditions have increased right ventricular ejection fraction, PaO_2, FIO_2, and oxygen consumption ($\dot{V}O_2$) (Boldt et al, 1995). With respect to vasoactive substances, atrial natriuretic peptide, catecholamines, renin, and vasopressin are lower in survivors. Cardiac index was not different between survivors and nonsurvivors, and there was no correlation between hemodynamics and circulating vasoactive substances.

Impending life threat is associated with global energetic failure secondary to cellular oxygen deficits.

COMPLICATIONS: MEDICAL AND SURGICAL

Complications that arise in the intensive care unit (ICU) either directly or indirectly relate to threat or dysfunction of oxygen transport. Medical and surgical complications often coexist. Medical complications include metabolic dysfunction, pulmonary dysfunction related largely to mechanical ventilation, acid base abnormalities, fluid and electrolyte disturbance, cardiac dysrhythmias, thromboembolism, myocardial dysfunction, gastrointestinal dysfunction, neurological dysfunction, and renal dysfunction. Surgical complications include hypoxemia, pain, deep vein thrombosis, and pulmonary embolism. The implications of these complications for physical therapy assessment and management are presented.

Metabolic Dysfunction

Complications associated with respiratory failure that can further impair tissue oxygenation are described in Box 36-1. The metabolic consequences of these complications and impairment of oxygen transport are life threatening for the

---

Complications of Respiratory Failure

Life-threatening impairment of oxygen transport and tissue oxygenation
Fluid and electrolyte imbalances
Cardiac dysrhythmias and hemodynamic instability
Myocardial dysfunction
Metabolic dysfunction
Thromboembolism
Neurological dysfunction
Gastrointestinal dysfunction
Renal dysfunction
Metabolic and blood sugar irregularities
Infection
Nutritional deficits
Complications of intubation and mechanical ventilation, including increased risk of infection
Complications of oxygen therapy

---

patient. Thus prevention of their development is a priority. Should complications develop, however, early detection and definitive management becomes the priority if the patient is to survive.

A hallmark of these complications is the impairment of multiple steps in the oxygen transport pathway, which adds to the complexity of management (Dantzker et al, 1997). The three major components of oxygen transport can be affected individually or in combination (i.e., oxygen delivery, consumption, and extraction) (Pallares & Evans, 1992; Wysocki et al, 1992).

In healthy individuals, the ratio of oxygen consumption to delivery is low (i.e., 23%, which ensures an over-supply of oxygen as a safety margin) (see Chapter 2). This safety margin also ensures that most patients are able to recover from insults to the oxygen transport system. If the insult is extreme, however, such as that resulting from complications of respiratory failure, surgery, acute lung injury and adult respiratory distress syndrome, shock, sepsis, and multiorgan system failure, significant metabolic dysfunction secondary to tissue hypoxia can result (Guiterrez, 1991).

The relationship between oxygen consumption and delivery has elucidated our understanding of hemodynamic and metabolic changes observed in critical illness (Vincent, 1991). The phenomenon of oxygen-delivery dependence of oxygen consumption occurs when a patient's oxygen transport system is unable to supply sufficient oxygen to meet basal oxygen demand (Phang & Russell, 1993). Oxygen delivery below 300 ml O_2/min/M^2 limits the oxygen diffusion gradient and reduces oxygen extraction and utilization at the cellular level. This is termed the *critical level of oxygen delivery.* When oxygen delivery exceeds 300 ml/min/M^2, $\dot{V}O_2$ does not depend on delivery. Thus the greater the delivery in relation to $\dot{V}O_2$, the greater the safety margin. When oxygen transport is so severely compromised that oxygen delivery falls below the critical level, anaerobic metabolism is triggered. Anaerobic

metabolism, however, may also be triggered at levels of oxygen delivery that exceed the normal critical threshold for anaerobic metabolism (Fenwick et al, 1990). This so-called pathological dependence of oxygen consumption on oxygen delivery occurs when the cells are inadequately extracting and using oxygen even in the presence of supranormal oxygen delivery levels. This phenomenon is observed in patients with adult respiratory distress syndrome and shock (discussed later this chapter).

Given that physical therapy is one of the most metabolically demanding ICU interventions (Dean et al, 1995; Weissman & Kemper, 1993), the physical therapist needs to be able to calculate this safety margin to prescribe the type of treatment and its parameters (i.e., intensity, duration, and frequency) such that treatment is maximally beneficial and associated with the least risk to the patient.

The ultimate treatment outcome measures are markers of oxygen tissue metabolism (Dantzker, 1993; Nightingale, 1993; Pallares & Evans, 1992). In addition, hourly assessment of oxygen delivery, consumption, and extraction provide the basis for directing management of oxygen transport deficits.

Pulmonary Dysfunction

Complications of the cardiopulmonary system can lead to respiratory failure (see Box 36-1) (Lynn-McHale & Carlson, 2002; Kirby et al, 1996). Some of these relate to being mechanically ventilated, such as ventilator-associated pneumonia. Certain technical problems related to the cuffs used in conjunction with artificial airways may occur (e.g., over-inflation, distortion, and herniation of the orifice of the tube). Mucous plugs can occlude the endotracheal tube or tracheostomy and impede ventilation. The common complications can be reduced if the tube is changed frequently and if minimal amounts of air are used for cuff inflation.

Prolonged endotracheal intubation can result in laryngeal edema, ulceration, and fibrosis. Mechanical ventilation may also rupture a bleb on the surface of the lung and produce a pneumothorax with rapid tension development. Chest tubes are inserted immediately to relieve the tension. Blebs occur when alveoli rupture, causing air to track to subpleural sites.

Mechanical ventilators can be a source of infection. The physical therapist can help minimize this risk by not directly handling the ventilator attachments that communicate with the air flow channels. Condensation from the hose should not be drained toward the ventilator or toward the patient. The physical therapist should be masked and gloved when connecting and disconnecting the patient to and from the ventilator.

Oxygen toxicity is a significant clinical complication of mechanical ventilation. Mechanical ventilators have precise oxygen controls to deliver the lowest possible inspired oxygen concentration needed to maintain arterial oxygen tensions. Because of the iatrogenic complications of high FIO_2 levels (i.e., denitrogen atelectasis and oxygen toxicity), oxygen above the patient's needs is never indicated other than short periods of hyperoxygenation before suctioning or in preparation for, during, and immediately after mobilization (Fell & Cheney, 1971; Shoemaker, 1984).

Flow-directed pulmonary artery catheters (i.e., Swan-Ganz catheters), commonly used in the intensive care unit (ICU) for monitoring patients who develop hemodynamic complications, are also associated with some complications (see Chapter 16). Infection may lead to bacteremia and septicemia. Judicious selection and application of any invasive procedure is warranted to minimize undue hazard. The presence of these catheters limits head and neck positions and requires mobilization be carried out cautiously within the patient's hemodynamic tolerance.

Acid-Base Abnormalities

Any combination of acid-base imbalance may occur either acutely or chronically during respiratory failure. Severe alkalemia associated with potassium and chloride losses may occur after mechanical ventilation and can precipitate serious cardiovascular and neurological complications (see Chapter 16) (Petty, 1982). Significantly impaired oxygen delivery to peripheral tissue may contribute to increased anaerobic metabolism and metabolic acidosis (Fenwick et al, 1990).

Fluid and Electrolyte Abnormalities

Fluid retention can occur with prolonged mechanical ventilation in a patient with no evidence of cardiac failure. Pulmonary edema, weight gain, decreased pulmonary compliance, and reduced oxygen transport are common signs. Fluid overload is a common cause of this fluid retention. Individuals who are mechanically ventilated are therefore usually maintained under-hydrated. Because of a tendency for sodium retention and hence fluid retention, intravenous saline solution is kept to a minimum. Humidifiers attached to mechanical ventilators are responsible for adding a considerable amount of water by absorption through the lungs.

Cardiac Dysrhythmias

Cardiac dysrhythmias are a common complication of respiratory failure. In addition, patients in respiratory failure tend to be older adults who as a group have a greater incidence of dysrhythmias secondary to cardiac disease. Electrocardiographic monitoring is therefore essential for all patients requiring ventilatory assistance in addition to patients with overt or suspected heart disease. Both atrial and ventricular tachydysrhythmias are seen in acute respiratory failure. Sinus tachycardia and premature ventricular contractions, however, are particularly common. Ventricular fibrillation or death may occur with rapid lowering of arterial PCO_2.

In the presence of respiratory failure and absence of cardiac disease, the management of cardiac dysrhythmias lies predominantly in the correction of blood-gas abnormalities. Effective supportive management can usually be achieved with pharmaceutical agents. Intravenous injection of lidocaine followed by continuous infusion is useful in managing premature ventricular contractions, which may be the precursor of potentially fatal tachydysrhythmias and cardiac arrest. Electrolyte replacement may also be required.

A thorough understanding of the clinical presentation, electrocardiographic diagnosis, and correct management of cardiac dysrhythmias is fundamental to the optimization of physical therapy treatments in the ICU and minimization of any risk to the patient. Cardiac dysrhythmias resulting from any cause necessarily require ongoing evaluation and therapy.

The physical therapist must be able to treat the patient optimally and safely within the restrictions of any dysrhythmia in addition to other medical or surgical conditions. The implications of the dysrhythmia on the patient's clinical presentation and for treatment selection and response must be recognized by the physical therapist and considered when designing the treatment plan.

Thromboembolism

A high incidence of pulmonary thrombosis or embolism exists in patients in acute respiratory failure. Early diagnosis and management of pulmonary thromboembolism have been greatly facilitated by the use of serial ultrasound procedures and scans. Physical therapy has a key role in preventing the development of thromboemboli by promoting frequent changes in position, specific bed exercises, particularly of the lower limbs, and passive range of motion exercises if indicated. It is essential that movement and repositioning are performed regularly to maximize their cardiopulmonary protective benefits. Pneumatic extremity cuffs apply pressure intermittently over the lower legs to minimize venous pooling and assist venous return (see Chapter 33). Compression stockings also may be applied over the feet and legs to increase circulatory transit time in the dependent areas and reduce circulatory stasis.

Myocardial Dysfunction

As in any clinical situation, acute myocardial infarction can occur during the management of acute respiratory failure. The risks are increased because patients in respiratory failure tend to be older and more susceptible to positional hypoxemia. The probability of heart failure and associated dysrhythmias is increased and significantly compounds the problems of the patient in respiratory failure.

Gastrointestinal Dysfunction

Stress ulceration leading to peptic ulcers is commonly associated with chronic airway obstruction. The stress of respiratory failure predisposes the patient to peptic ulceration. Profound hemorrhage may occur and blood replacement is necessitated.

Gastric dilation may occur in patients who are receiving mechanical ventilation. Gastric dilation is best managed by a nasogastric tube and intermittent suction. Care must be exercised to avoid hypokalemia and hypochloremia caused by excessive gastric suctioning. Special care is also taken to avoid fecal impaction, particularly in the patient who is paralyzed. This risk can be reduced with suitable fluid balance, mobilization, and frequent turning in conjunction with appropriate trunk and lower limb movements.

Muscular and Neurological Dysfunction

A close correlation exists between state of consciousness and arterial PO_2 and PCO_2. In addition, alteration in blood gases causes changes in alertness, personality, memory, and orientation. Motor changes include generalized or localized weakness, tremors, twitching, myoclonic jerks, gross clonic movements, convulsions, and flaccidity. Neurological complications of respiratory failure must be differentiated from those of nonpulmonary origin. The physical therapist must be aware of the spectrum of neurological complications that can result from respiratory failure and recognize that apparent improvement of neurological signs may reflect improved cardiopulmonary status.

Critical illness neuropathy is a serious complication of critical illness and is associated with metabolic disturbance during illness, paralysis, neuromuscular blockade, recumbency, and restricted mobility (Goellter et al, 2002). Prevention is a primary goal and includes early detection. Periodic ulnar nerve electrical stimulation has been one means of establishing nerve conduction integrity during an assault of critical illness requiring neuromuscular blockade and sedation. Medical management is focused on addressing its causes and reversing them. Rehabilitation potential is threatened in the presence of critical illness neuropathy.

Renal Dysfunction

The development of renal failure greatly compromises the chances of the patient's survival. Renal failure can result from gastrointestinal bleeding, sepsis associated with shock, drug-induced nephrotoxicity, and hypotension. Urinary outputs are maintained with adequate fluid and diuretics, with care not to induce pulmonary edema. Dialysis may need to be instituted if more conservative management fails (Phipps et al, 2002). If dialysis is anticipated, the physical therapist should review existing treatment goals to modify treatment accordingly.

POSTOPERATIVE COMPLICATIONS

Pathophysiology and Medical Management

Respiratory failure in a patient postoperatively is usually associated with a low PaO_2 and a high $PaCO_2$. This situation is likely to be more common than generally appreciated. If the patient is in good general health and is free from underlying cardiopulmonary disease, recovery is usually rapid. Otherwise, more severe complications and cardiopulmonary failure may

---

BOX 36-2

Common Postoperative Complications

Hypoxemia
Hypercapnia
Increased work of breathing
Increased work of the heart
Fluid shifts and third spacing
Fluid and electrolyte imbalances
Metabolic and blood sugar abnormalities
Reduced blood volume
Cardiac dysrhythmias
Reduced cardiac output
Reduced tissue perfusion and oxygenation
Anemia
Pain
Alveolar hypoventilation
Airway collapse
Atelectasis
Physiological shunting
Ventilation and perfusion mismatching
Impaired mucociliary transport
Mucus accumulation and stasis
Pneumonia
Thromboemboli
Pulmonary embolus
Coagulopathies
Sepsis
Shock
Multiorgan system failure

---

result and progress to a life-threatening situation. The effects of surgery on oxygen transport and on the various organ systems are described in Chapter 29. Common postoperative complications and their causes appear in Boxes 36-2 and 36-3. With severely reduced arterial oxygen content, hence oxygen delivery, oxygen extraction increases (Polonen et al, 1997).

Hypoxemia

The most common postoperative complication is hypoxemia secondary to alveolar hypoventilation, reduced functional residual capacity (FRC), airway closure, and postsurgical atelectasis (Leblanc et al, 1970; Marini, 1984; Ray et al, 1974). Adequate oxygenation, however, can be present despite hypoventilation when oxygen is being administered. The presence or absence of cyanosis may be an unreliable sign because peripheral cyanosis can occur despite adequate arterial PO_2. Morbidity and mortality has been reported to be reduced in patients with severe respiratory failure and system involvement when supranormal levels of oxygen delivery are achieved (Hayes et al, 1993; Waxman & Shoemaker, 1980; Yu et al, 1993).

Pain

Pain, in addition to the effects of anesthesia, frequently contributes to alveolar hypoventilation and atelectasis after

Factors Contributing to Postoperative Complications that Affect Oxygen Transport

Premorbid cardiopulmonary status
Premorbid oxygen transport (aerobic) capacity
Premorbid systemic disease
Premorbid general health and immune status
Smoking history
Age and sex
Lifestyle factors: nutritional status, stress, work situation, family situation, psychosocial support system, and substance abuse
Obesity
Pregnancy
Perioperative pain and anxiety
Perioperative reduced arousal
Perioperative reduced mobility
Perioperative recumbency
Perioperative medications (e.g., narcotics)
Perioperative nutritional deprivation
Perioperative reduction in normal sleep quality and quantity
Type of surgery
Extent of physical manipulation and compression of lung parenchyma, phrenic nerves, diaphragm, and the heart
Perioperative fever and increased oxygen consumptions
Duration of surgery
Position assumed during surgery
Duration of static positioning during surgery
Type, depth, and duration of anesthesia and sedation
Use of an airway
Use of mechanical ventilation
Oxygen therapy
Neuromuscular blockade
Fluid loss and chest tube drainage
Fluid accumulation and third spacing
Infusion of blood products
Site, number, and extent of incisions
Dressings and binders
Traction and splinting devices
Placement of lines, leads, catheters, and monitoring devices
Invasive monitoring equipment (e.g., Swan-Ganz catheter, Foley catheter, intracranial pressure monitor, central venous line, arterial lines, intravenous lines, and intraaortic balloon counter pulsation pump)
Need for cardiopulmonary bypass machine
Duration on cardiopulmonary bypass machine
Infection

abdominal or thoracic surgery. Rapid, shallow, and monotonous breathing may be spontaneously adopted by the patient to avoid pain and coughing. Although minute ventilation is favored, alveolar ventilation is compromised by the increased ratio of dead space to tidal volume. Furthermore, in the absence of deep breaths, coughs, and sighs, atelectasis may develop in the under-ventilated portions of the lungs. The ventilation-perfusion ratio is disturbed because blood flow to under-ventilated lung segments is ineffective, physiological shunting occurs, and arterial PO_2 tends to drop

although PCO_2 may be unchanged. An abnormally high transpulmonary pressure is then needed to reinflate these atelectatic alveoli. The physical therapist ensures good pain control before intervention, including mobilization. Patient controlled analgesia is used if the patient is able to cooperate sufficiently, as well as conventionally administered analgesia, as required.

Pulmonary Embolism and Deep Vein Thrombosis

Pulmonary embolism is a potentially life-threatening complication. Pulmonary embolism usually results from a thrombus forming in the veins of the lower limbs, pelvis, in the right atrium, or in the right ventricle. Patients may be at risk if they have varicose veins, chronic heart failure, or if they are obese, pregnant, or taking oral contraceptives.

The patient with a pulmonary thromboembolism usually has a sudden onset of tachypnea, radiating chest pain, and apparent anxiety. Occasionally, right heart failure follows. Enzymes are often elevated. Right heart strain may be evidenced on an echocardiogram or electrocardiogram (ECG). Right bundle branch block, peaked P waves, and inverted T waves may be seen. There may be no abnormality noted on chest x-ray.

Treatment consists of primary ventilatory and circulatory support, with adequate oxygenation of peripheral tissues. Anticoagulants, such as heparin, are infused intravenously to minimize further formation of thromboembolic substrates.

Principles of Physical Therapy Management

Significant impairment of lung volume, mechanics, and gas exchange uniformly occur after anesthesia and tissue dissection. The extent and duration of these changes increase with the magnitude of the operative procedure, degree of anesthesia required, and the patient's premorbid risk factors. These abnormalities observed in the postoperative period are characterized by gradual and progressive alveolar collapse. Total lung capacity, FRC, and residual volume are significantly decreased in patients who develop complications. Because of the significant decrease in FRC (30% or more), compliance is decreased, and therefore the work of breathing is increased. Hypoxemia secondary to transpulmonary shunting usually becomes maximal within 72 hours after surgery and often is completely resolved with conservative management within seven days. The FIO_2 will depend on the mode of 100% oxygen administration. Low oxygen flows and low amounts of FIO_2 tend to be delivered via nasal cannulae. Higher flows can deliver higher amounts of FIO_2 via oxygen masks and masks with reservoir bags. The FIO_2 must always be taken into account when interpreting arterial blood gases. The FIO_2 is selected to provide adequate oxygenation with the lowest oxygen concentration possible.

On the basis of patient assessment, arterial blood gases, fluid and electrolyte balance, hemodynamic status, and x-ray, a decision is made as to which treatments on the physiological hierarchy will optimize oxygen transport and what parameters will be used for each treatment. Positioning these patients upright and mobilizing them wherever possible will maximize FRC and reduce closing volumes and hence enhance gas exchange and oxygenation. What precludes mobilizing these patients even minimally is their lack of alertness, which must be explained. If the patient is unable to respond to treatment because of narcotics, for example, this can be discussed at rounds and other medications should be considered so that the patient is able to cooperate more. Thus even extreme body positioning will achieve more favorable results (Barlett et al, 1973; Clauss et al, 1968; Douglas et al, 1977; Piehl & Brown, 1976).

Endotracheal intubation and mechanical ventilation may be indicated if blood gases fail to improve with conservative management. The treatment priorities for the ventilated patient before and during weaning are presented in Chapter 33. Special attention in the postoperative patient is given to the pulmonary complications associated with diminished ability to move spontaneously, surgical pain, restrictions imposed by dressings and binders, and diminished ability to cooperate and to periodically hyperventilate the lungs.

Facilitating mucociliary transport is a primary goal in these patients. Impaired mucociliary transport can be precipitated by alveolar hypoventilation, perhaps the most common cause of postoperative complications. Sufficient impairment can lead to mucous stasis, airway obstruction, atelectasis, and infection. Multiple positions, including upright positions and 360-degree axial turns, and multiple position changes facilitate mucociliary transport. In the event of mucous accumulation and difficulty in removing pulmonary secretions, specific body positions are selected to optimize postural drainage of the affected bronchopulmonary segments and to maximize alveolar volume and ventilation. The addition of manual techniques can be detrimental in severely ill patients (Mackenzie, 1989; Poelaert et al, 1991), thus their use needs to be considered carefully.

Suctioning may be most effective immediately before and after position changes. The appropriate oxygen transport variables are monitored to assess treatment outcome and minimally to ensure the patient who may be unstable is not deteriorating. If the patient begins to deteriorate, treatment is discontinued until the patient stabilizes. Why the patient deteriorated is determined so that a decision can be made as to whether treatment can be reintroduced, and if so, what modifications are indicated.

Pain management is integral to the management of the surgical patient. Noninvasive and nonpharmacological pain control strategies need to be exploited for all surgical patients to augment or reduce the need for potent analgesics, especially narcotics. Chapter 30 described some physical therapy pain control strategies for surgical patients that can be applied with modification to the patient with surgical complications. Of these, use of electrotherapy modalities, such as transcutaneous electrical nerve stimulation, may be limited in the ICU because of electrical interference with monitoring devices.

Rest is prescribed as judiciously as treatment interventions to enable the patient to physiologically restore between and within treatments. This is particularly important for ICU patients who are hypermetabolic and have increased oxygen demands. Particular care must be observed in prescribing treatment threshold parameters for these patients. Suprathreshold states can be associated with an inappropriate balance between oxygen delivery and oxygen consumption such that the patient becomes compromised (e.g., hemodynamically unstable, cardiopulmonary distress is precipitated, or both). A greater volume of a mobilization stimulus, however, may be delivered to these patients with an intermittent mobilization regimen than with a single prolonged course of mobilization. Thus the benefits that would be accrued would be correspondingly increased.

Prevention of thromboemboli is a major treatment objective and is best achieved with mobilization, body positioning, passive movements, and physical devices, such as pneumatic cuff devices and stockings, to augment low-dose anticoagulants in patients at risk. Patients who develop pulmonary emboli are treated medically and physical therapy must be correspondingly modified to minimize oxygen consumption until the embolus resolves and the patient is in no imminent danger.

ACUTE LUNG INJURY AND ACUTE RESPIRATORY DISTRESS SYNDROME

Acute lung injury results from damage to the alveolar epithelium (Gattinoni et al, 1994). The extent of the damage reflects damage to the type I and type II alveolar cells. Damage to the type I cells results in alveolar edema, atelectasis, and loss of lung compliance secondary to loss of structural integrity of the alveoli provided by the type I alveolar cells. Damage to the type II cells also contributes to atelectasis and loss of lung compliance, but the mechanism relates to impairment of the production of surfactant and pulmonary fluid that covers the alveolar epithelium.

Pulmonary edema refers to the accumulation of vascular fluid in the interstitial spaces and alveoli. In acute lung injury the mechanism of pulmonary edema involves increased water movement across the pulmonary endothelial cells and increased permeability of the endothelium to protein. This type of pulmonary edema is referred to as noncardiogenic pulmonary edema. Pulmonary edema that is cardiogenic in origin results from left ventricular failure. An increase in hydrostatic pressure damages the interstitial tight spaces, which normally provide an effective barrier between the pulmonary circulation and alveoli. The critical distinction between the two types of pulmonary edema is that cardiogenic pulmonary edema primarily involves the movement of water across the alveolar capillary membrane, whereas noncardiogenic pulmonary edema involves the movement of protein and water into the interstitial and alveolar spaces. The clinical consequences reflect the location of the edema (i.e., interstitial, alveolar, or both) and the amount of fluid accumulation.

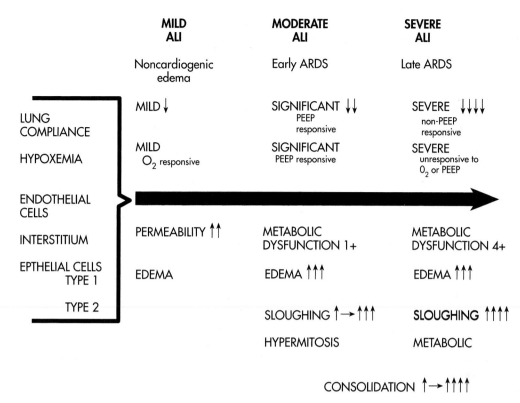

FIGURE 36-1 Major pathophysiological manifestations comprising the spectrum of acute lung injury from mild to severe disease. *(From Shapiro B.A., Peruzzi W.T. [1991]. Changing practices inventilatator management: a review of the literature and suggest clinical correlates. Surgery 117:121-133.)*

Acute lung injury is characterized as a clinical spectrum of parenchymal cell dysfunction. Mild injury reflects predominantly endothelial cell dysfunction and noncardiogenic edema. Severe injury reflects a progression to both endothelial and epithelial cell dysfunction and acute respiratory distress syndrome (ARDS). The clinical spectrum of acute lung injury and the clinical manifestations of mild and severe injury are shown in Figure 36-1. The clinical presentation of moderate injury falls between these two extremes.

ARDS results from major insult to the lung and injury to the alveolar-capillary membrane. Some of the causes of ARDS include shock, severe trauma or infection, overwhelming pneumonia, and inhaled toxins. Increased vascular permeability resembling that of the inflammatory response is a common feature. Fluid seeps into the interstitial spaces and overwhelms the alveoli, leading to pulmonary edema. Lung compliance and gas exchange are severely compromised. Thus the patient presents with severe dyspnea and hypoxemia. Diffuse pulmonary infiltrates appear on x-ray. Arterial hypoxemia results primarily from under-ventilated but perfused lung units and right to left shunt. In this situation, hypoxemia is relatively refractory to increases in FIO_2.

Fibrinogen in the fluids leaking into the alveoli contributes to fibrosis and reduction of lung compliance associated with ARDS. Increased lung surface tension and alveolar collapse tend to result from an inactivation of surfactant with the accumulation of fluid in the alveolar spaces. Thus reduced lung compliance produces a significant decrease in FRC in the patient with ARDS.

The signs and symptoms of ARDS may take up to 48 hours to fully manifest. Survival rate has increased significantly over the past decade from 50% to some 80% (Ullrich et al, 1999). The explanation for this improvement is unclear; however, the shift to an integrated management approach may be responsible (Houston, 2000; Stocker et al, 1997). Hypoxemia is a principal feature of the syndrome resulting from ventilation perfusion mismatch, and from a right to left shunt, whereby fluid-filled alveoli are ineffectively ventilated (Sinclair & Albert, 1997). Hyperventilation and labored respiration can be expected in conjunction with hypoxemia. Oxygen therapy has little effect in the presence of shunting. Hypercapnia is not usually a major problem in the patient with ARDS.

The metabolic perturbations that can result include problems with oxygen delivery, consumption, and extraction, as discussed previously. When oxygen delivery falls below the critical level, anaerobic metabolism is triggered, resulting in increased lactate production. Elevated serum lactates are associated with a poor prognosis. Changes in oxygenation may not be reflected in SVO_2 because of the abnormal dependence of oxygen consumption and delivery (Lorente et al, 1991). Positive end-expiratory pressure can worsen DO_2 in patients with ARDS who are mechanically ventilated and sedated (Spec-Marn et al, 1993). In turn, $\dot{V}O_2$ may become oxygen-supply dependent, thus peripheral-extraction may be increased. Recent advances in the medical management of ARDS include the use of partial liquid ventilation. Although not widely adopted, this form of ventilation may be more effective in recruiting dependent alveoli than conventional mechanical ventilation, and may augment the benefits of exogenous surfactant replacement, inhaled nitric oxide, and prone positioning (Wiedemann, 2000). In addition to improving oxygenation and respiratory mechanics, partial liquid ventilation may reduce ventilator-induced lung damage (Suh et al, 2000).

Principles of Physical Therapy Management

Intubation and ventilatory support are implemented if arterial blood gases are severely affected and respiratory distress worsened. An endotracheal tube can be placed through the nose or mouth or a tracheostomy can be performed in cases where prolonged ventilatory support is anticipated. The tidal volume is set at about 10 ml/kg of the patient's body weight. The patient usually establishes the respiratory rate, although it may be rapid. A positive end expiratory pressure (PEEP) of around 12 cm H_2O maintains the alveoli open and thereby optimizes gas transfer at end-expiration. Arterial oxygenation is usually improved with PEEP because the effect of shunting is reduced and a given FIO_2 tends to be more effective. Although the FIO_2 may be reduced, which reduces the possibility of oxygen toxicity, supranormal oxygen delivery can be beneficial in these patients (Bishop et al, 1993). Survival may be improved and frequency of multiorgan system failure reduced.

Further monitoring of respiratory status in conjunction with arterial blood gases is essential for following the progress of the syndrome. In addition to the oxygen transport variables, the principal parameters monitored in ARDS are reduced lung compliance, tachypnea, and the concentration of inspired oxygen needed to maintain acceptable levels of the arterial blood gases.

ARDS is characterized by a major pathophysiological restrictive component. Hence the principles of management of restrictive lung disease are applied. Changes in lung compliance and FIO_2 requirements provide guidelines to treatment required, treatment response, and course of the syndrome. Patients with ARDS require close monitoring and often frequent treatments aimed at promoting optimal gas exchange because of the severity of the syndrome and high incidence of mortality associated with it.

In severe ARDS, the patient may be heavily mechanically ventilated, on a high FIO_2, sedated, and thus require regular monitoring. Body positioning is initiated as much as tolerated without significant desaturation. Special attention is given to body positioning to promote ventilation and perfusion matching and mucociliary transport and to minimize the effect of restriction of diaphragmatic and chest wall excursion. Some patients, for example, benefit from side-lying in which excursion of the inferior hemidiaphragm is favored. Other patients, however, seem to deteriorate from apparent restriction of the inferior lung in side-lying. The underlying pathophysiology associated with ARDS is primarily related to respiratory mechanics, which could explain why improvements in oxygenation have not been associated with secretion clearance (Gillart et al, 2000). Each patient's condition and specific areas of lung involvement must be taken into consideration when prescribing a turning regimen. The effect of the patient's body position on blood gases helps to establish a suitable regimen on a rational basis. Optimal positioning can result in reduced supplemental oxygen needs (Swanlund, 1996).

With improvement (e.g., less heavily mechanically ventilated, reduced FIO_2, and satisfactory gases), the patient may be able to be mobilized with monitoring of vital signs, ECG, saturation, and subjective tolerance. The sitting position optimizes lung capacity even when a patient is intubated and mechanically ventilated. The airway can dislodge, however, so caution must be observed. The patient is carefully monitored and airway pressure recorded. Initially, if the patient is sedated, body positioning is exploited to maintain blood gases, and optimal range of motion and skin care are the focus of management. With improvement, the patient is mobilized. The use of a reclining chair at the bedside should be considered in the management of patients with acute lung injury. Theoretically, the potential function of all lung fields will be benefited with the lungs in a more upright position. Patients who are too unstable to tolerate upright positions and whose oxygenation is compromised in this position (Bittner et al, 1996) may respond favorably to extreme body positions and the prone position (Albert et al, 1987; Langer et al, 1988). The clinical benefits of the prone position in the management of the majority of patient with ARDS have been well documented over the past 20 years, thus physical therapists need to consider positioning these patients in prone as a common practice barring contraindications.

Improvements in oxygenation in patients with acute lung injury and ARDS with the prone position, including prone abdomen free, have been well documented for adult and pediatric populations (Curley, 1999; Curley et al, 2000; Lim et al, 2001; Tobin & Kelly, 1999; Ullrich et al, 1999). The benefits can persist when the patient is returned to the supine position, and further, the prone position does not adversely affect hemodynamics (Jolliet et al, 1998). The use of the prone position in the management of ARDS has been reported to be independently associated with survival (Venet et al, 2003). The literature is inconsistent, however, regarding whether patients respond differently depending on the underlying ARDS pathophysiology (pulmonary or nonpulmonary). Some investigators report no differences (Rialp et al, 2001), whereas others have reported marked differences with respect to radiographic changes, respiratory mechanics, and time course of oxygenation (Lim et al, 2001). These differences may be explained by pathophysiological differences of the primary disease insult responsible for ARDS, stage and severity, and co-morbidity. The mechanisms for improved gas exchange in prone in these severely ill patients have been the subject of much interest. Hypotheses have included improved alveolar recruitment and lung volumes, and homogeneous distributions of ventilation and perfusion (Breilburg et al, 2000), increased static lung compliance (Servillo et al, 1997), and reduced compressive forces compared to the supine position (Albert, 2000; Albert & Hubmayr, 2000). In the posterior lung fields in the prone position, in the areas where atelectasis, shunt, and ventilation to perfusion mismatch are most prevalent, transpulmonary pressure exceeds airway opening pressure without apparently compromising anterior lung fields (Lamm et al, 1996). A decrease on $PaCO_2$ with prone predicts survival (Gattinoni et al, 2003).

Problems with positioning patients in prone have been reported to be rare. Studies have been focusing on the differences between patients who respond favorably and those who do not (i.e., responders versus nonresponders). Patients may respond better in the early stages in which pulmonary edema is present versus the later stages in the presence of pulmonary fibrosis (Nakos et al, 2000). Alveolar recruitment procedures are more effective in improving PaO_2 in the prone position, and lower PEEP levels are needed to sustain improved PaO_2 compared with the supine position (Kacmarek, 2001). In addition, positive inspiratory pressure, hence barotrauma, and FIO_2 can be reduced (Breilburg et al, 2000). The effects of mechanical ventilation including PEEP (Lim et al, 1999), airway pressure release ventilation (Varpula et al, 2001), and certain pharmacological agents (inhaled nitric oxide) may be augmented in prone (Johannigman et al, 2001). Other studies have reported an even more significant effect of prone. One study reported that the prone position rather than PEEP improved oxygenation (Gainnier et al, 2003). Another study reported prone improves oxygenation significantly more than inhaled nitric oxide in patients with severe ARDS (Dupont et al, 2000).

Severely affected patients may require neuromuscular blockade to reduce their oxygen demand and enable them to respond to ventilatory assistance more effectively. Handling and positioning patients on neuromuscular blockade requires particular care because these patients lack muscle tone to protect their muscles and joints. Rotating beds can be extremely beneficial for these patients who are either too hemo-dynamically unstable or difficult to turn manually. These mechanical beds slowly rotate side to side through an arc, thus changing the patient's body position continuously (Gentilello et al, 1988; Pape et al, 1994). When the effects of continuous axial rotation on a kinetic bed are compared with prone, the effects have been shown to be comparable (Staudinger et al, 2001). The prescriptive parameters of the prone position in patients with ARDS, however, need to be based on a careful analysis of the pros and cons for each patient, and no single position will be maximally beneficial all the time. There are other physiological benefits to shifting the patient's position rather than maintaining a single position (see Chapter 19), provided that oxygenation is not compromised.

Although considerable evidence supports the clinical efficacy of the prone position to improve oxygenation, this position should be considered for the management of hypoxemia associated with other conditions as a means of simulating the normal effects of gravity of cardiopulmonary function. Favorable results have been reported in the management of hypoxemia associated with acute respiratory failure in acute myeloid leukemia (Schmidt et al, 2003), pulmonary hemorrage (Hayes-Bradley, 2004), and subarachnoid hemorrhage (Reinprecht et al, 2003).

Few complications have been reported with the use of body positioning, and in particular, the prone position. Normal precautions are taken to ensure that ventilator tubing and lines and leads are not compromised. Despite beneficial effects of oxygenation in patients with ARDS related to trauma (Fridrich et al, 1996), complications associated with prone positioning have been reported for such patients, including facial and chest wall skin necrosis, wound dehiscence, and cardiac arrest (Offner et al, 2000). Special precautions are necessary in this subgroup. Brachial plexopathy has also been reported when positioning patients prone in the ICU (Goettler et al, 2002). In addition to frequent body position changes, the semi-prone position may help to avoid the adverse effects of prone in some patients (Schmitz, 1991).

SHOCK

Common causes of shock include hypovolemia, septicemia, heart failure, and direct insult to the central nervous system. Some of the classical features of shock are hypotension, reduced cardiac output, tachycardia, hyperventilation, diaphoresis, pallor, confusion, nausea, and incontinence. Inadequate tissue perfusion results in extracellular acidemia and loss of potassium ions from the cells. The pulmonary blood vessels constrict in response to hypoxemia, which tends to increase pulmonary artery pressures.

Failure of cellular function secondary to shock can result from a deficiency of substrate for energy production, a reduced ability to use the nutrients for energy production, or both. The pathophysiological mechanisms responsible include hypoperfusion of the tissues, hormonal and metabolic cellular changes, and the toxic effects of the metabolic changes. Collectively, these produce cellular damage. With hypoperfusion and decreased oxygen delivery and other nutrients, the production of adenosine triphosphate is reduced. The maintenance and repair of cell membranes is disrupted, resulting in swelling of the endoplasmic reticular and eventually the mitochondria. Persisting cellular hypoxia contributes to rupture of the lysosomes, which releases enzymes that contribute to intracellular digestion and calcium deposition. Once the lysosomes have ruptured and intracellular digestion is triggered, irreversible cell damage ensues, impairing oxygen extraction and uptake (Wysocki et al, 1992).

The dependence between oxygen consumption and delivery is a marker for septic shock and thus provides justification for increasing oxygen delivery (see Chapter 2) (Friedman et al, 1998). More recently, the relationship of oxygen consumption and delivery has been used to evaluate patients who are critically ill with systemic inflammatory response syndrome and predict metabolic stress on this basis (Moriyama et al, 1999).

The pathology of shock and the effect on the respiratory membranes of the mitochondria follow a similar course regardless of cause. Swelling of the interstitial tissue disrupts the perfusion of the pulmonary capillaries. Congestive atelectasis and pulmonary edema ensue. In the advanced stages, hyaline membrane changes and pneumonitis may occur.

When shock is associated with heart failure, ventricular assist devices or intra aortic balloon pump may be indicated. These devices reduce the degree to which the patient can be positioned and moved; therefore, consultation with the team is essential in progressing such a patient.

Principles of Physical Therapy Management

Foremost, the physical therapist must be knowledgeable about the relationship of oxygen delivery and consumption in patients with shock, as well as the implications of the pathophysiological processes on oxygen extraction. The type of treatments and their parameters are based on a careful analysis of oxygen transport variables. Treatments are prescribed within the patient's safety margin. Physical therapists in the ICU must also be knowledgeable about the signs and symptoms associated with impending and frank shock. By recognizing and understanding the components of the different types of shock and the effect on the cardiopulmonary system, the physical therapist can better prescribe a rational treatment plan for the short- and long-term management of the patient.

Although physical therapy may be limited in reversing the signs and symptoms of shock, physical therapy can help to restore and maintain optimal cardiopulmonary function, reduce the risk of complications associated with restricted mobility and recumbency, and maintain physical status at an optimal level during the episode and in anticipation of the patient's recovery. The primary objective, however, is to minimize oxygen demand. A minimal objective is not to worsen the patient's condition by imposing excessive metabolic demand. This is the case in patients whose oxygen delivery is approaching the critical level with respect to oxygen consumption dependence. Excessive demands in these patients can be life threatening.

Patients in shock are usually unresponsive. The course of the shock episode is often complicated with the sequelae of immobility and recumbency. The specific goals related to optimization of cardiopulmonary and musculoskeletal function and prevention of further complications associated with cardiopulmonary function in particular are priorities.

Specific concerns for the patient in shock include the need for short, efficacious treatments and avoidance of unnecessarily fatiguing the patient. Treatment goals are therefore critically appraised and prioritized throughout each day to target physical therapy treatment only to the very immediate and essential needs of the patient. Prudent patient positioning is a priority because of the relative immobility and reduced spontaneous movement observed in these patients, and recumbency. Approximations to the upright position (i.e., head of bed up and foot of bed down) can augment sympathetic stimulation and improve hemodynamic status and reduce sympathomimetic medications. In addition, this position simulates the upright sitting position (although not perfectly) with respect to its beneficial effects on pulmonary and cardiac function.

Late stages of refractory shock leading to renal failure may necessitate dialysis. In peritoneal dialysis, a liter of fluid with a high osmotic fluid content is injected into the patient's abdomen to draw fluid out. The fluid is drained after about 30 minutes. Cardiopulmonary physical therapy is most effective if performed after the fluid has been completely drained from the peritoneum. After drainage of the fluid, the diaphragm is at a more optimal functional length for respiration, which potentially can improve treatment response. If hemodialysis is indicated, the patient is connected to a unit that dialyzes the blood externally. This process takes several hours and is usually repeated every few days.

Comparable to the management of other patients who are unstable and severely ill, physical therapy may constitute primarily supportive care and comprehensive monitoring in the patient with severe effects of shock regardless of whether he or she is in an acute or chronic stage.

SEPSIS AND MULTIORGAN SYSTEM FAILURE

Sepsis is the response to bacteremia or other byproducts of bacteria in the blood. The clinical features of sepsis include fever, tachycardia, tachypnea, and respiratory alkalemia. Metabolic abnormalities are also a common feature of sepsis. Sepsis is the most common predisposing factor contributing to multiorgan system failure (MOSF), which typically involves failure of more than two organ systems (Carrico et al, 1993; Vincent, 1993). Table 36-1 shows the major organs affected and their clinical manifestations (i.e., pulmonary, gastrointestinal, hepatic, renal, cardiovascular, hematological, and central nervous systems). The cascade of pathophysiological features of this MOSF is precipitated by multiple mediator systems. The release of these mediators impairs oxygen delivery and utilization of oxygen by the cells. Inadequate tissue oxygenation appears to be an important mechanism underlying MOSF (Bihara et al, 1987). Thus the supply of the major energy source to the cell, adenosine triphosphate, is reduced, which leads to structural and functional damage of the various organ systems. The mortality rate ranges from 60% to 80%.

Conditions that predispose a patient to MOSF include sepsis, overwhelming infection, multiple trauma and tissue injury, inflammation, and tissue perfusion deficits. Patients

TABLE 36-1		
Presentation of Multiorgan System Failure		
ORGAN	**CLINICAL PRESENTATION**	**SYNDROME**
Lungs	Hypoxemia, lung compliance, diffuse infiltrates	Acute lung injury/ARDS
Kidneys	Creatine >2 mg/dl	
	Urine output <500 ml/24 h	Oliguric ARF
	Urine output >500 ml/24 h	Nonoliguric ARF
Liver	Bilirubin 2 mg/dl, SGOT and LDH	Jaundice
	Intractible hyperglycemia or hypoglycemia	Hepatocyte failure
	Cholecystitis	Acalculous cholecystitis
Gut	Upper gastrointestinal bleed	Stress ulceration
Coagulation	Thrombocytopenia, prolonged PT and PTT	Hypofibrinogenemia, DIC
Heart	Hypotension, CI	Heart failure
CNS	Response only to painful stimuli	Obtundation

ARF, Acute renal failure; *SGOT,* serum glutamic oxaloacetic transaminase; *LDH,* lactate, dehydrogenase; *DIC,* disseminating intravascular coagulation; *PT,* prothrombin time; *PTT,* partial prothrombin time; *CI,* cardiac index.
Modified from Kirby, R.R., Taylor, R.W., & Civetta, J.M. (1996). Critical care, ed 2. Philadelphia: Lippincott.Williams & Wilkins.

who are older, have chronic diseases, are immunosuppressed, or have a severe initial presentation have an increased risk of failure and mortality.

Sepsis causes damage to peripheral nerves and muscles as well as organs and is termed critical illness polyneuropathy (CIP) (Hund, 2001). Although the pathogenesis is not understood, these effects must be detected early and addressed to avoid clinical manifestations including muscle weakness, prolonged recovery, and delayed weaning. The systemic inflammatory response and MOSF have been implicated, and neuromuscular blockers and steroids can exacerbate these manifestations. The use of steroids and muscle relaxants should be minimized. Stabilizing the underlying critical condition and avoiding sepsis are of major importance in preventing CIP.

General guidelines for current medical strategies for sepsis and septic shock have been recently documented (Dellinger et al, 2004). These include life support measures (i.e., fluid resuscitation), blood product administration, vasopressor and inotropic support, bicarbonate therapy, and hemodynamic stabilization. To control the sepsis process requires identification and management of the source or sepsis, as well as antibiotic and steroid administration. Sedation, analgesia, neuromuscular blockade, and glucose control are instituted to reduce excess metabolic demand. In the event of renal dysfunction, hemofiltration may be required along with intermittent hemodialysis. Preventive strategies are implemented to avoid the sequelae of recumbency and restricted mobility, of which deep vein thrombosis and embolism are risks. Comparable to other patients who are critically ill, those with extreme illness are at risk for stress ulceration, and therefore, stress ulceration prophylaxis is a component of routine medical management.

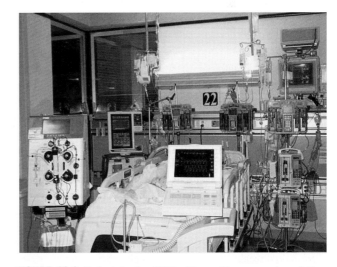

FIGURE 36-2 Patient in the ICU with multiorgan system failure. Note the ventilator, continuous dialysis, intra-aortic balloon pump and multiple intravenous drips.

Principles of Physical Therapy Management

The patient with sepsis and MOSF, like the patient in shock, is gravely ill and unlikely to be able to cooperate with treatment (Figure 36-2). The principles for management are comparable with those for managing the patient in shock; however; oxygen delivery is likely to be consistently compromised in these patients. If oxygen delivery is critically low, $\dot{V}O_2$ depends on oxygen delivery and the patient is in a state of metabolic acidosis (see Chapter 2). In this situation, where oxygen delivery is compromised to the point of not meeting tissue oxygen demands, the goal of treatment is to maximize oxygen delivery (Bishop et al, 1993; Roukonen et al, 1991; Yu et al, 1993) and minimize oxygen demand so that oxygenation of vital organs is threatened to the least extent. Thus the physical therapist must estimate the oxygen reserve capacity (i.e., the balance between oxygen demand and oxygen supply) in every assessment to select optimal treatment that is associated with the least risk. Treatments are selected to improve the efficiency of oxygen transport and utilization and thereby reduce the work of the heart and of breathing. Above all, treatment should not worsen the patient's oxygen transport status. Selective body positioning can augment oxygen transport and maximize the effective FIO_2. Even though the patient will likely benefit more from some positions than others, frequent body position changes, preferably a 360-degree turning regimen, are still necessary to avoid the sequelae of static body positioning. Semi-prone positions can substitute well for full prone positions if the patient is too hemodynamically unstable. Semi-prone positions may be tolerated better by the patient and may be safer. Even though hourly position changes may not be feasible in these severely ill patients, prolonged periods in a static position (more than two hours) are deleterious. Thus a balance between these two concerns must be achieved.

Promoting optimal mucociliary transport remains a priority even in the absence of secretion accumulation. Frequent position changes and numerous positions ensure pulmonary secretions are continually being redistributed to prevent accumulation and enhance removal. Should postural drainage be indicated, these positions may need to be modified. Head-down positions in particular may not be tolerated well. The relative benefits of superimposing manual techniques must be established on the basis of careful assessment because these procedures are associated with an increased metabolic demand to which the patient is not readily able to adapt. Increasing the oxygen demand of these patients may worsen their condition.

The assessment of neuromuscular function is challenging and inaccurate in patients who are severely ill. Patients may have marked weakness related to critical illness polyneuropathy and from interventions themselves (e.g., resting of the respiratory muscles with mechanical ventilation, and pharmacological agents including glucocorticoids, some antibiotics, and neuromuscular blockers) (Figure 36-3). Thus these interventions may be risk factors and their use needs to be assessed.

SUMMARY

This chapter presents several major complications that can develop in a patient *secondary* to various conditions in the ICU. Complications add significantly to the complexity of the physical therapy diagnoses of the patient's underlying problems with respect to oxygen transport and cardiopulmonary management. The complications highlighted in this chapter include those that impair multiple steps in the oxygen transport pathway and hence jeopardize metabolism at the cellular

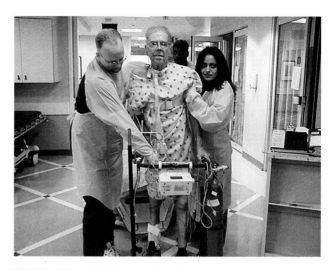

FIGURE 36-3 Mobilizing a patient in the ICU with critical illness polyneuropathy. Note the presence of marked muscle atrophy on both lower extremities.

level. This sequence of events is most frequently associated with the complications of respiratory failure, surgery, adult respiratory distress syndrome, shock, sepsis, and multiorgan system failure.

Physical therapy treatments in critical care areas are typically short, frequent, and should always be efficacious. Patients with complications, however, are usually severely compromised and often unable to cooperate with treatment, which necessitates particularly short and frequent sessions. Because of the severity of illness, patients with the complications described often require treatments that are more passive (i.e., stress to the oxygen transport system must be minimal, thus the treatments are lower on the physiological treatment hierarchy). These patients require frequent and comprehensive monitoring (often several times daily) of their oxygen transport capacity (i.e., the relationship between oxygen delivery and consumption, and oxygen extraction, to establish if and when treatment is indicated and the specific parameters of treatment). If a patient is thought to be too unstable for treatment at a given time, continued monitoring of her or his status is essential so that small windows of opportunity can be exploited during stable periods. During periods of monitoring (as opposed to periods of active treatment intervention), the physical therapist continues to have an important role in recommending body positions and frequency of body position changes so that these can yield the greatest benefit to oxygen transport. Treatment continues to progress in preparation for discharge to the ward. Ongoing physical therapy care is imperative throughout a patient's stay in the ICU because patients remain at risk of turns for the worse, which can occur suddenly while in the ICU. Prevention remains the overriding goal until the patient is discharged from the unit.

Review Questions

1. Describe the complications associated with respiratory failure.
2. Describe the implications for cardiopulmonary physical therapy (assessment and management) of respiratory failure, surgical complications, acute lung injury, adult respiratory distress syndrome, shock, sepsis, and multiorgan system failure.
3. Few longitudinal studies have examined the long-term prognosis for survivors of complications in the ICU. Identify some research questions related to long-term physical therapy outcomes (consistent with the International Classification of Function), and design some studies to address these.
4. Describe some methodological challenges related to physical therapy research in the ICU and how these might be addressed.

REFERENCES

Albert, R.K. (2000). Prone ventilation. Clinics in Chest Medicine 21:511-517.

Albert, R.K., & Hubmayr, R.D. (2000). The prone position eliminates compression of the lungs by the heart. American Journal of Respiratory and Critical Care Medicine 161:1660-1665.

Albert, R.K., Leasa, D., Sanderson, M., Robertson, H.T., & Hlastala, M.P. (1987). The prone position improves arterial oxygenation and reduces shunt in oleic-acid-induced acute lung injury. American Review of Respiratory Diseases 135:626-633.

Bartlett, R.H., Gazzaniga, A.B., & Geraghty, T.R. (1973). Respiratory maneuvers to prevent postoperative pulmonary complications. A critical review. Journal of the American Medical Association 224:1017-1021.

Bihara, D., Smithies, M., Gimson, A., & Tinker, J. (1987). The effects of vasodilation with prostacyclin on oxygen delivery and uptake in critically ill patients. New England Journal of Medicine 31:397-403.

Bishop, M.H., Shoemaker, W.C., Appel, P.L., Wo, C.-J., Zwick, C., Kram, H.B., Meade, P., Kennedy, F., & Fleming, A.W. (1993). Relationship between supranormal circulatory values, time delays, and outcome in severely traumatized patients. Critical Care Medicine 21:56-63.

Bittner, E., Chendrasekhar, A., Pillai, S., & Timberlake, G.A. (1996). Changes in oxygenation and compliance as related to body position in acute lung injury. The American Surgeon 62:1038-1041.

Boldt, J., Menges, T., Kuhn, D., Diridis, C., & Hempelmann, G. (1995). Alterations in circulating vasoactive substances in the critically-ill: a comparison between survivors and non-survivors. Intensive Care Medicine 21:1836-1849.

Breilburg, A.N., Aitken, L., Reaby, L., Clancy, R.L., & Pierce, J.D. (2000). Efficacy and safety of prone positioning for patients with acute respiratory distress syndrome. Journal of Advanced Nursing 32:922-929.

Carrico, C.J., Meakins, J.L., & Marshall, J.C. (1993). Multiple organ failure syndrome. The gastrointestinal tract: the motor of MOF. Archives of Surgery 121:197-208.

Clauss, R.H., Scalabrini, B.Y., Ray, J.F. III, & Reed, G.E. (1968). Effects of changing body position upon improved ventilation-perfusion relationships. Circulation 37(Suppl 4):214-217.

Curley, M.A. (1999). Prone positioning of patients with acute respiratory distress syndrome: a systematic review. American Journal of Critical Care 8:397-405.

Curley, M.A., Thompson, J.E., & Arnold, J.H. (2000). The effects of early and repeated prone positioning in pediatric patients with acute lung injury. Chest 118:156-163.

Dean, E., Murphy, S., Parrent, L., & Rousseau, M. (1995). Metabolic consequences of physical therapy in critically-ill patients. Proceedings of the World Confederation of Physical Therapy Congress. Washington, DC.

Dantzker, D.R., Schay, S.M., & Fletcher, J. (1997). Cardiopulmonary Critical Care, ed 3. Philadelphia: Elsevier.

Dantzker, D.R. (1993). Adequacy of tissue oxygenation. Critical Care Medicine 21:S40-S43.

Dellinger, R.P., Carlet, J.M., Masur, H., Gerlach, H., Calandra, T., Cohen, J., Gea-Banacloche, J., Keh, D., Marshall, J.C., Parker, M.M., Ramsay, G., Zimmerman, J.L., Vincent, J.L., & Levy, M.M. (2004). Surviving Sepsis Campaign guidelines for management of severe sepsis and septic shock. Critical Care Medicine 32:858-873.

Douglas, W.W., Rehder, K., Beynen, F.M., Sessler, A.D., & Marsh, H.M. (1977). Improved oxygenation in patients with acute respiratory failure: the prone position. American Review of Respiratory Disease 115:559-566.

Dupont, H., Mentec, H., Cheval, C., Moine, P., Fierobe, L., & Timsit, J.F. (2000). Short-term effect of inhaled nitric oxide and prone positioning on gas exchange in patients with severe acute respirtory distress syndrome. Critical Care Medicine 28:304-308.

Fell, T., & Cheney, F.W. (1971). Prevention of hypoxia during endotracheal suction. Annals of Surgery 174:24-28.

Fenwick, J.C., Dodek, P.M., Ronco, J.J., Phang, P.T., Wiggs, B., & Russell, J.A. (1990). Increased concentrations of plasma lactate predict pathologic dependence of oxygen consumption on oxygen delivery in patients with adult respiratory distress syndrome. Journal of Critical Care 5:81-86.

Fridrich, P., Krafft, P., Hochleuthner, H., & Mauritz, W. (1996). The effects of long-term prone positioning in patients with trauma-induced adult respiratory distress syndrome. Anesthesia and Analgesia 83:1139-1140.

Friedman, G., de Backer, D., Shahla, M., & Vincent, J.L. (1998). Oxygen supply dependency can characterize septic shock. Intensive Care Medicine 14:118-123.

Gainnier, M., Michelet, P., Thirion, X., Arnal, J.M., Sainty, J.M., & Papazian, L. (2003). Prone position and positive-end expiratory pressure in acute respiratory distress syndrome. Critical Care Medicine 31:2719-2726.

Gattinoni, L., Bombino, M., Pelosi, P., Lissoni, A., Pensenti, A., Fumagalli, R., & Tagliabue, M. (1994). Lung structure and function in different stages of severe adult respiratory distress syndrome. Journal of the American Medical Association 271:1772-1779.

Gattinoni, L., Vagginelli, F., Cariesso, E., Taccone, P., Conte, V., Chiumello, D., Valenza, F., Caironi, P., & Pesenti, A. (2003). Decrease in Paco2 with prone position is predictive of improved outcome in acute respiratory distress syndrome. Critical Care Medicine 31:2727-2733.

Gentilello, L., Thompson, D.A., Tonnesen, A.S., Hernandez, D., Kapadia, A.S., Allen, S.J., Houtchens, B.A., & Miner, M.E. (1988). Effect of a rotating bed on the incidence of pulmonary complications in critically ill patients. Critical Care Medicine 16:783-786.

Gillart, T., Bazin, J.E., Guelon, D., Constanin, J.M., Mansoor, O., Conio, N., & Schoeffler, P. (2000). Effect of bronchial drainage on the improvement in gas exchange observed in vertical decubitus in ARDS [English abstract]. Annales Francaises d'Anesthesie et de Reanimation 19:156-163.

Goettler, C.E., Pryor, J.P., & Reilly, P.M. (2002). Brachial plexopathy after prone positioning. Critical Care 6:540-542.

Gutierrez, G. (1991). Cellular energy metabolism during hypoxia. Critical Care Medicine 19:619-626.

Hayes, M.A., Yau, E.H.S., Timmins, A.C., Hinds, C.J., & Watson, D. (1993). Response of critically-ill patients to treatment aimed at achieving supranormal oxygen delivery and consumption. Chest 103:886-895.

Hayes-Bradley, C. (2004). Hypoxia from vasculitis pulmonary haemorrhage improved by prone position ventilation. British Journal of Anaesthesia 92:754-757.

Houston, P. (2000). An approach to ventilation in acute respiratory distress syndrome. Canadian Journal of Surgery 43:263-268.

Hund, E.F., Fogel, W., Krieger, D., DeGeorgia, M., & Hacke, W. (1996). Critical illness polyneuropathy: clinical findings and outcomes of a frequent cause of neuromuscular weaning failure. Critical Care Medicine 24:1328-1333.

Johannigman, J.A., Davis, K. Jr., Miller, S.L., Campbell, R.S., Luchette, F.A., Frame, S.B., & Branson, R.D. (2001). Prone positioning and inhaled nitric oxide: synergistic therapies for acute respiratory distress syndrome. Journal of Trauma 50:589-595.

Jolliet, P., Bulpa, P., & Chevrolet, J.C. (1998). Effects of the prone position on gas exchange and hemodynamics in severe acute respiratory distress syndrome. Critical Care Medicine 26:1934-1935.

Kacmarek, R.M. (2001). Strategies to optimize alveolar recruitment. Current Opinions in Critical Care 7:15-20.

Kariman, K., & Burns, S.R. (1985). Regulation of tissue oxygen extraction is disturbed in adult respiratory distress syndrome. American Review of Respiratory Diseases 132:109-114.

Kirby, R.R., Taylor, R.W., & Civetta, J.M. (1996). Critical care, ed 2. Philadelphia: Lippincott.Williams & Wilkins.

Lamm, W.J., Graham, M.M., & Albert, R.K. (1994). Mechanism by which the prone position improves oxygenation in acute lung injury. American Journal of Respiratory and Critical Care Medicine 150:184-193.

Langer, M., Mascheroni, D., Marcolin, R., & Cattinoni, L. (1988). The prone position in ARDS patients. A clinical study. Chest 94:103-107.

Leblanc, P., Ruff, F., & Milic-Emili, J. (1970). Effects of age and body position on "airway closure" in man. Journal of Applied Physiology 28:448-451.

Lim, C.M., Kim, E.K., Lee, J.S., Shim., T.S., Lee, S.D., Koh, Y., Kim, W.S., & Kim, W.D. (2001). Comparison of the response to the prone position between pulmonary and extrapulmonary acute respiratory distress syndrome. Intensive Care Medicine 27:477-485.

Lim, C.M., Koh, Y., Chin, J.Y., Lee, J.S., Lee, S.D., Kim, W.S., Kim, D.S., & Kim W.D. (1999). Respiratory and haemodynamic effects of the prone position at two different levels of PEEP in a canine lung injury model. European Respiratory Journal 13:163-168.

Lorente, J.A., Renes, E., Gomez-Aguinaga, M.A., Landin, L., de la Morena, J., & Liste, D. (1991). Oxygen delivery-dependent oxygen consumption in acute respiratory failure. Critical Care Medicine 19:770-775.

Lynn-McHale, D.J., & Carlson, K.K. (2000). AACN procedure manual for critical care, ed 4. Philadelphia: Elsevier.

Mackenzie, C.F. (Ed). (1989). Chest physiotherapy in the intensive care unit, ed 2. Baltimore: Lippincott Williams & Wilkins.

Marini, J.J. (1984). Postoperative atelectasis: pathophysiology, clinical importance, and principles of management. Respiratory Care 29:516-528.

Marx, G., Vangerow, B., Hecker, H., Leuwer, M., Jankowski, M., Piepenbrock, S., & Rueckoldt, H. (1998). Predictors of respiratory function deterioration after transfer of critically ill patients. Intensive Care Medicine 24:1157-1162.

Moriyama, S., Okamoto, K., Tabira, Y., Kikuta, K., Kikuta, I., & Hamaguchi, M. (1999). Evaluation of oxygen consumption and resting energy expenditure in critically ill patients with systemic inflammatory response syndrome. Critical Care Medicine 27:2133-2136.

Nakos, G., Tsangaris, I., Kostanti, E., Nathanail, C., Lachana, A., Koulouras, V., & Kastani, D. (2000). Effect of the prone position on patients with hydrostatic pulmonary edema compared with patients with acute respiratory distress syndrome and pulmonary fibrosis. American Journal of Respiratory and Critical Care Medicine 161:360-368.

Nightingale, P. (1993). Optimization of oxygen transport to the tissues. Acta Anaesthesiologica Scandinavica 98:32-36.

Offner, P.J., Haenel, J.B., Moore, E.E., Biffl, W.L., Franciose, R.J., & Burch, J.M. (2000). Complications of prone ventilation in patients with multisystem trauma with fulminant acute respiratory distress syndrome. Journal of Trauma 48:224-228.

Pallares, L.C.M., & Evans, T.W. (1992). Oxygen transport in the critically ill. Respiratory Medicine 86:289-295.

Pape, H.C., Regel, G., Borgman, W., Sturm, J.A., & Tacherne, H. (1994). The effect of kinetic positioning on lung function and pulmonary haemodynamics in posttraumatic ARDS: a clinical study. International Journal of the Care of the Injured 25:51-57.

Petty, T.L. (1982). Intensive and rehabilitative respiratory care, ed 3. Philadelphia: Lea & Febiger.

Phang, P.T., & Russell, J.A. (1993). When does VO_2 depend on DO_2? Respiratory Care 38:618-630.

Phipps, W.J., Monahan, F.D., & Sands, J. (Eds). (2002). Medical-surgical nursing: concepts and clinical practice, ed 7. Philadelphia: Elsevier.

Piehl, M.A., & Brown, R.S. (1976). Use of extreme position changes in acute respiratory failure. Critical Care Medicine 4:13-14.

Poelaert, J., Lannoy, B., Vogelaers, D., Everaert, J., Decruyenaere, J., Capiau, P., & Colardyn, F. (1991). Influence of chest physiotherapy on arterial oxygen saturation. Acta Anaesthesiologica Belgica 42:165-170.

Polonen, P., Hippelainen, M., Takala, R., Ruokonen, E., & Takala, J. (1997). Relationship between intra- and postoperative oxygen transport and prolonged intensive care after cardiac surgery: a prospective study. Acta Anaesthesidogica Scandinavica 41:810-817.

Ray, J.F. III, Yost, L., Moallem, S., Sanoudos, G.M., Villamena, P., Paredes, R.M., & Clauss, R.H. (1974). Immobility, hypoxemia, and pulmonary arteriovenous shunting. Archives of Surgery 109:537-541.

Reinprecht, A., Greher, M., Wolfsberger, S., Dietrich, W., Illievich, U.M., & Gruber, A. (2003). Prone position in subarachnoid hemorrhage patients with acute respiratory distress syndrome: effects on cerebral tissue oxygenation and intracranial pressure. Critical Care Medicine 31:1831-1838.

Rialp, G., Betbese, A.J., Perez-Marquez, M., & Mancebo, J. (2001). Short-term effects of inhaled nitric oxide and prone position in pulmonary and extrapulmonary acute respiratory distress syndrome. American Journal of Critical Care Medicine 164:243-249.

Roukonen, E., Takala, J., & Kari, A. (1991). Septic shock and multiple organ failure. Critical Care Medicine 19:1146-1151.

Schmidt, J.E., Tamburro, R.F., Sillos, E.M., Hill, D.A., Ribeiro, R.C., & Razzouk, B.I. (2003). Pathophysiology-directed therapy for acute hypoxemic respiratory failure in acute myeloid leukemia with hyperleukocytosis. Journal of Pediatric Hematology and Oncology 25:569-571.

Schmitz, T.M. (1991). The semi-prone position in ARDS: five case studies. Critical Care Nursing 11:22-30.

Servillo, G., Roupie, E., De Robertis, E., Rossano, F., Brochard, L., Lemaire, F., & Tufano, R. (1997). Effects of ventilation in ventral decubitus position on respiratory mechanics in adult respiratory distress syndrome. Intensive Care Medicine 23:1219-1224.

Shapiro, B.A., & Peruzzi, W.T. (1995). Changing practices in ventilator management: A review of the literature and suggested clinical correlates. Surgery 117:121-133.

Shoemaker, W.C. (Ed). (1984). Critical care: state of the art. Fullerton, Calif: Society of Critical Care Medicine.

Sinclair, S.E., & Albert, R.K. (1997). Altering ventilation-perfusion relationships in ventilated patients with acute lung injury. Intensive Care Medicine 23:942-950.

Spec-Marn, A., Tos, L., Kremzar, B., Milic-Emili, J., & Ranieri, V.M. (1993). Oxygen delivery-consumption relationship in adult respiratory distress syndrome patients: the effects of sepsis. Journal of Critical Care 8:43-50.

Staudinger, T., Kofler, J., Mullner, M., Locker, G.J., Laczika, K., Knapp, S., Losert, H., & Frass, M. (2001). Comparison of prone positioning and continuous rotation of patients with adult respiratory distress syndrome: results of a pilot study. Critical Care Medicine 29:51-56.

Stocker, R., Neff, T., Stein, S., Ecknauer, E., Trentz, O., & Russi, E. (1997). Prone positioning and low-volume pressure-limited ventilation improves survival in patients with severe ARDS. Chest 111:1008-1017.

Suh, G.Y., Chung, M.P., Park, S.J., Koh, Y., Kang, K.W., Kim, H., Han, J., Rhee, C.H., & Kwon, O.J. (2000). Partial liquid ventilation shows dose-dependent increase in oxygenation with PEEP and decreases lung injury associated with mechanical ventilation. Journal of Critical Care 15:103-112.

Swanlund, S.L. (1996). Body positioning and the elderly with adult respiratory distress syndrome: implications for nursing care. Journal of Gerontological Nursing 22:46-50.

Tobin, A., & Kelly, W. (1999). Prone ventilation-it's time. Anaesthesia and Intensive Care 27:194-201.

Ullrich, R., Lorber, C., Roder, G., Urak, G., Faryniak, B., Sladen, R.N., & Germann, P. (1999). Controlled airway pressure therapy, nitric oxide inhalation, prone position, and extracorporeal membrane oxygenation (ECMO) as components of an integrated approach to ARDS. Anesthesiology 91:1577-1586.

Varpula, T., Pettila, V., Nieminen H., & Takkunen, O. (2001). Airway pressure release ventilation and prone positioning in severe acute respiratory distress syndrome. Acta Anaesthesiologica Scandinavica 45:340-344.

Venet, C., Guyomarc'h, S., Pingat, J., Michard, C., Laporte, S., Bertrand, M., Gery, P., Page, D., Vermesch, R., Bertrand, J.C., & Zeni, F. (2003). Prognostic factors in acute respiratory distress syndrome: a restrospective multivariate analysis including prone positioning in management strategy. Intensive Care Medicine 29:1435-1441.

Vincent, J.L. (1991). Advances in the concepts of intensive care. American Heart Journal 121:1859-1865.

Vincent, J.L. (1993). Oxygen transport in severe sepsis. Acta Anaesthesiology Scandinavica 37(Suppl 98):29-31.

Waxman, K., & Shoemaker, W.C. (1980). Management of post-operative and posttraumatic respiratory failure in the intensive care unit. Surgical Clinics of North America 60:1413-1428.

Weissman, C., & Kemper, M. (1993). Stressing the critically ill patient: the cardiopulmonary and metabolic resposnes to an acute increase in oxygen consumption. Journal of Critical Care 8:100-108.

Wiedemann, P. (2000). Partial liquid ventilation for acute respiratory distress syndrome. Clinics in Chest Medicine 21:543-554.

Wysocki, M., Besbes, M., Roupie, E., & Brun-Buisson, C. (1992). Modification of oxygen extraction ratio by change in oxygen transport in septic shock. Chest 102:221-226.

Yu, M., Levy, M.M., Smith, P., Takiguchi, S.A., Miyasaki, A., & Myers, S.A. (1993). Effect of maximizing oxygen delivery on morbidity and mortality rates in critically ill patients: A prospective, randomized, controlled study. Critical Care Medicine 21:830-838.

Guidelines for the Delivery of Cardiovascular and Pulmonary Physical Therapy

Special Cases

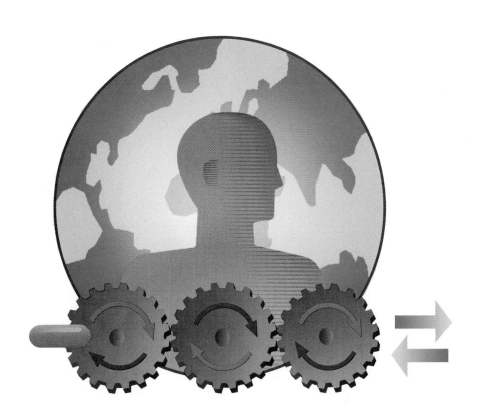

C H A P T E R 3 7

The Neonatal and Pediatric Patient

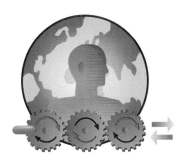

Victoria A. Moerchen and Linda D. Crane

KEY TERMS

Bronchopulmonary dysplasia
Cerebral palsy
Chest physical therapy with infants/children
Childhood asthma
Cystic fibrosis
Down syndrome
Endocardial cushion defect
Exercise
Handling for ventilation

Hyaline membrane disease
Muscular dystrophy
Obesity
Patent ductus arteriosus
Pediatric cardiac rehabilitation
Pediatric pulmonary rehabilitation
Pulmonary development
Transitional circulation
Trunk-ventilation interaction

Pediatrics entails a special application of cardiopulmonary physical therapy. This chapter stresses that cardiopulmonary development and its related vulnerabilities form the basis for cardiopulmonary practice with neonatal and pediatric patients.

The objectives of this chapter are to review cardiopulmonary development and related vulnerabilities; relate developmental pathologies to issues of adequate ventilation and oxygen transport; identify cardiopulmonary co-morbidities associated with reduced physical activity and obesity; present principles and precautions of direct respiratory care; and incorporate these principles into suggestions for practice.

This chapter begins with a brief description of critical events and important characteristics of cardiac and pulmonary development. Relevant diagnoses are then presented to build onto this developmental perspective and stress that cardiopulmonary pathology and ventilatory compromise are often related to developmental vulnerabilities. Obesity is presented as a complicating factor in the cardiopulmonary health of children with and without clinical diagnoses. Finally, treatment approaches are described, including pediatric cardiac rehabilitation, pulmonary care for neonatal and pediatric patients, pediatric pulmonary rehabilitation, and developmental motor approaches for trunk and ventilatory muscle function.

Knowledge of cardiopulmonary development, congenital and developmental cardiopulmonary pathology, and pediatric cardiopulmonary treatment is essential for any therapist serving children. Most pediatric patients require ongoing attention to respiratory function, whether as a primary focus of physical therapy or as an inherent aspect of motor development. This chapter is relevant to therapists who perform direct cardiopulmonary care and to therapists who incorporate a cardiopulmonary awareness into developmental motor therapy and the promotion of wellness in children.

657

CARDIOPULMONARY DEVELOPMENT

The application of cardiopulmonary physical therapy to infants and children requires a special understanding of developmental cardiopulmonary anatomy and physiology. Knowledge of normal development and its inherent points of vulnerability will help the reader understand some of what is known about cardiopulmonary pathology in pediatric patients.

Cardiac Development

Differences in fetal and neonatal gas exchange account for differences in the anatomy and physiology of fetal and neonatal circulation. A basic review of developmental circulation is essential for discussion of congenital heart defects and the role of pediatric cardiopulmonary physical therapy.

Fetal circulation

Placental oxygenation is a major characteristic of fetal circulation. Additionally, in fetal circulation, blood flow through the right and left sides of the heart occurs in parallel, such that cardiac output is actually combined ventricular output (CVO) (Heyman & Hanley, 1994). This is possible as a result of shunts in fetal circulation (Park, 1988).

Two points of shunting during fetal circulation are at the foramen ovale and the ductus arteriosus. The foramen ovale allows right-to-left blood flow through the atria, bypassing the lungs (Yao, 1983). Left ventricular output (LVO) is well-oxygenated blood that then enters the ascending aorta and flows to the brain and upper body. The ductus arteriosus similarly allows the lungs to be bypassed, as most of the right ventricular output (less well-oxygenated than the LVO) flows to the descending aorta and from there to the lower body.

Fetal blood flow to the lungs is minimal, secondary to high pulmonary vascular resistance during fetal circulation. Only 10% to 12% of CVO goes to the lungs (Koff, 1993; Phelan et al, 1994), and its function is to nourish the developing lung tissue rather than provide gas exchange.

Neonatal Circulation

Adult-like circulation occurs at or shortly after birth, with separation from the placenta and ventilation of the lungs resulting in closure of the ductus venous, foramen ovale, and ductus arteriosus. This process, referred to as transitional circulation, occurs early in neonatal life and increases the efficiency of oxygen uptake and transport (Heyman & Hanley, 1994; Rudolph, 1970).

The initiation of breathing and removal of lung fluid increase pulmonary blood flow. Whereas fetal circulation is characterized by high pulmonary vascular resistance and low systemic resistance, separation from the placenta causes a rise in systemic resistance and a decrease in pulmonary vascular resistance. As this shift in relative pulmonary and systemic resistances occurs, sites of intercommunication (shunts) close and the ventricles shift from working in parallel to working in series (Heyman & Hanley, 1994).

Closure of Foramen Ovale. The increased left atrial pressure that occurs during transitional circulation results in apposition of the valve of foramen ovale against the interatrial septum, functionally closing this site of fetal circulatory shunting (Rudolph, 1970). In most infants, anatomical closure occurs two to three months later (Emmanouilides & Baylen, 1988; Yao, 1983).

Closure of Ductus Arteriosus. Functional closure or constriction of the ductus arteriosus occurs postnatally within the first 15 to 72 hours in response to increased arterial oxygen saturation (Daniels et al, 1982). Anatomical closure of ductus arteriosus occurs by two to three weeks in most term neonates (Rudolph, 1970). The responsiveness of the ductal smooth muscle to arterial oxygen tension and to endogenous prostaglandins is impacted by gestational age (Park, 1988; Yao, 1983).

Pulmonary Development

Structural and functional characteristics of pulmonary development in infants and children are significant because they may contribute to aspects of respiratory vulnerability (Muller & Bryan, 1979).

Newborn Respiration

The pulmonary anatomy of the term infant is markedly different from the adult but also different from the child. An infant's airways are narrower from the nares to the terminal bronchioles. This presents a point of pulmonary vulnerability because a smaller diameter airway is more easily obstructed by mucus, edema, foreign objects, and enlarged lymphatic tissue. The infant also has a high larynx (Laitman & Crelin, 1980). Although this position of the larynx enables the newborn to breathe and swallow simultaneously, it may also contribute to predominant patterns of infant nasal breathing, which can result in increased work to breathe during any compromise of the nasal airway.

Even without airway compromise, the work of breathing is increased during the neonatal period. The initial low compliance of the newborn's lungs requires increased effort for ventilation, which results in a high rate of respiration and increased oxygen consumption.

Although the process of transitional circulation allows more efficient oxygen transport in the neonate than in the fetus, gas exchange in the newborn is still somewhat inefficient because of immature alveolar structure and function. The surface area for gas exchange in a newborn is one-twentieth that of an adult (Johnson et al, 1978), and the diffusion distance across the alveoli-capillary membrane is increased as a result of thick alveolar walls (Blackburn, 1992).

Functional characteristics of infant pulmonary development are also significant in terms of understanding possible contributions to pulmonary distress in infants. The diaphragm of a newborn has fewer type I (high oxidative) muscle fibers (25% compared with 50% in an adult) (Muller & Bryan, 1979). This difference predisposes an infant to earlier diaphragmatic fatigue when stressed.

TABLE 37-1	
Factors Contributing to Cardiopulmonary Dysfunction in the Premature Infant	
ANATOMICAL	**PHYSIOLOGICAL**
Capillary beds not well developed before 26 weeks' gestation	Increased pulmonary vascular resistance leading to right-to-left shunting
Type II alveolar cells and surfactant production not mature until 35 weeks' gestation; elastic properties of lung not well developed; lung space decreased by relative size of the heart and abdominal distention	Decreased lung compliance
Decreased responsiveness of the ductus arteriosus to oxygen tensions; delayed ductal closure	Left-to-right shunting
Type I, high-oxidative fibers compose only 10% to 20% of diaphragm muscle	Diaphragmatic fatigue: respiratory failure
Highly vascular subependymal germinal matrix not resorbed until 35 weeks' gestation, increasing the vulnerability of the infant to hemorrhage	Decreased or absent cough and gag reflexes; apnea
Lack of fatty insulation and high surface area to body/weight ratio	Hypothermia and increased oxygen consumption

Modified from Crane, L.D. (1995). Physical therapy for the neonate with respiratory disease. In Irwin, S., & Tecklin, J.S. (Eds). Cardiopulmonary physical therapy. St. Louis: Mosby

A biomechanical difference between the infant and child is the circular and horizontal alignment of the ribs and the concomitant horizontal angle at which the diaphragm inserts on the ribs during newborn and early infant chest development (Massery, 1991; Muller & Bryan, 1979). This, along with the more cartilaginous nature of the ribcage, results in less efficient chest wall mechanics. The result, again, is increased work to breathe (see Chapter 39 for a more complete discussion of chest development).

Respiration in the Child

Two residual structural differences exist beyond the newborn period and have potential implications for pulmonary vulnerability in the child. First, the somewhat horizontal angulation of the ribs persists until approximately seven years of age and results in less efficient chest wall mechanics (Muller & Bryan, 1979). Second, lymphatic tissue (especially adenoids) grows rapidly until about six years of age (Sinclair, 1978) and can continue to be a potential source of upper airway obstruction.

As infants and children grow and develop, however, most structural and functional disadvantages disappear. An aspect of growth and development that can be protective for infants and younger children is alveolar multiplication. This begins in the first year of life and continues until approximately eight years of age (Blackburn, 1992; Thurlbeck, 1975).

Cardiopulmonary Considerations in the Preterm Infant

All of the cardiopulmonary structural and functional characteristics of neonates that have been previously discussed apply to the premature infant. Additionally, there are significant gestational characteristics and aspects of cardiopulmonary vulnerability that are more pronounced and create more problems in premature infants (Table 37-1).

Recall that the transitional circulation of a term newborn includes a decrease in pulmonary vascular resistance over the first day. In preterm infants, however, lung immaturity and abnormal surfactant function (Jobe, 1988) may result in retained high pulmonary resistance (poor lung compliance), hypoperfusion, and respiratory distress syndrome (Walther et al, 1992). Persistent pulmonary hypertension will reinforce persistent right-to-left shunting through the ductus arteriosus (Nudel & Gootman, 1983; Rudolph, 1980). Respiratory distress syndrome (RDS) has been identified as the best predictor of prolonged patency of ductus arteriosus (Milne et al, 1989).

As the respiratory distress of the premature infant improves with neonatal intensive care, cardiopulmonary vulnerabilities can then occur in the opposite circulatory direction. Given the gestationally related responsiveness of ductus arteriosus to oxygen, some preterm infants retain patency of the ductus even when pulmonary vascular resistance falls (Archer, 1993). The result is left-to-right shunting that may lead to congestive heart failure (Nudel & Grootman, 1983; Park, 1988).

Most significantly, the immature status of cardiopulmonary anatomy in preterm infants predisposes them to hypoxia under any conditions that require increased oxygen (Blackburn, 1992). Cardiopulmonary pathophysiology and/or the stressors inherent to medical care often present challenges beyond the adaptive capacities of these fragile little systems.

COMMON PEDIATRIC DIAGNOSES

The sections that follow present and discuss specific cardiac and pulmonary diagnoses. Common neuromuscular or developmental diagnoses that have inherent to them the risk of compromised respiration or associated cardiopulmonary disease are also discussed. The diagnoses presented are not all inclusive but merely represent an attempt to give the reader

TABLE 37-2

Common Pediatric Diagnoses and Associated Heart Defects

DIAGNOSIS	HEART DEFECTS
Duchenne's muscular dystrophy	Cardiomyopathy (adolescence)
Fetal alcohol syndrome	Ventricular septal defect
	Tetralogy of Fallot
	Pulmonary value stenosis
	Patent ductus arteriosus
Friedreich's ataxia	Ventricular hypertrophy
	Congestive heart failure
HIV-1 infection	Myocarditis
	Ventricular dysfunction
Juvenile rheumatoid arthritis	Pericarditis
Marfan syndrome	Aortic aneurysm
	Aortic/mitral insufficiency
Noonan's syndrome	Dystrophic pulmonary valve (pulmonary stenosis)
Prematurity	Patent ductus arteriosus
Trisomy 13 (Patau's syndrome)	Ventricular septal defect
	Atrial septal defect
	Patent ductus arteriosus
Trisomy 18 (Edwards' syndrome)	Ventricular septal defect
	Patent ductus arteriosus (large)
Trisomy 21 (Down syndrome)	Endocardial cushion defect
	Ventricular septal defect
	Atrial septal defect
	Tetralogy of Fallot
Turner's syndrome	Coarctation of the aorta
Williams syndrome	Supravalvular aortic stenosis
	Supravalvular pulmonary stenosis

a preliminary knowledge of underlying pathologies and medical management of diagnoses commonly encountered in the practice of pediatric cardiopulmonary physical therapy.

Cardiac Diagnoses

Patent ductus arteriosus, endocardial cushion defects, and tetralogy of Fallot are the cardiac defects discussed within the limits of this chapter. Additionally, Table 37-2 provides a summary of common developmental diagnoses and their associated cardiac defects.

Patent Ductus Arteriosus

Patent ductus arteriosus (PDA), already introduced as a cardiopulmonary complication in preterm infants, is the most common heart defect during the neonatal period (Musewe & Olley, 1994). In term newborns, however, PDA accounts for 10% of congenital heart disease (Mitchell et al, 1971).

Gestational age, the presence of lung disease, the size of the ductus, and the direction of the shunt mediate the clinical features of PDA (Greene et al, 1994; Musewe & Olley, 1994). The preterm infant with very low birth weight will have the most extreme clinical picture. An infant or child with a large ductus will also have an obvious clinical presentation.

Tachycardia, an ejection systolic murmur, bounding peripheral pulses, increased respiratory distress, and poor feeding or poor weight gain are the classical signs of PDA (Archer, 1993; Greene et al, 1994; Musewe & Olley, 1994). In the term infant, PDA may be more clinically silent, especially when the ductus is small (Park, 1988).

Depending on the extent of the PDA, medical management includes nonsurgical (intravenous) use of indomethacin or direct, minimally invasive surgical closure (Georgeson & Robertson, 2004; Moore et al, 2005; Musewe & Olley, 1992; Smyth et al, 2004; Vanderkerckhove et al, 2005).

Endocardial Cushion Defects and Artrioventricular Defects

Endocardial cushion defects (ECD) represent a spectrum of defects characterized by malformation of the atrial septum, the mitral and tricuspid valves, and/or the ventricular septum (Emmanouilides & Baylen, 1988). Combinations of these defects are categorized as complete, transitional/intermediate, and partial, depending on degree of ventricular septal deficiency (Merrill et al, 1994; Spicer, 1984). In the complete form of ECD, all of the structures are deficient. In the partial form, only an atrial septal defect with a cleft mitral valve is present (Emmanouilides & Baylen, 1988; Merrill et al, 1994; Park, 1988).

There is marked variation in the underlying anatomy of this class of cardiac defects, such that clinical features are equally varied and difficult to inclusively summarize. In neonates with a complete defect, heart failure may manifest in infancy. Neonates with milder forms of this defect, however, may not be symptomatic until much later in development (Park, 1988). Additionally, endocardial cushion defects are frequently associated with other cardiac defects (Emmanouilides & Baylen, 1988).

Although the total incidence of endocardial cushion defects in infancy is 1% to 4%, the incidence in infants and children with Down syndrome is 40% (Freedom & Smallhorn, 1992). In these children, a complete ECD is the most common cardiac malformation (Spicer, 1984).

Operative management of infants and children with ECD depends on the morphology of the defect, the degree of pulmonary hypertension, and the extent of mitral valve regurgitation (Merrill et al, 1994). For infants with complete ECD, early surgical repairs are indicated (Bender et al, 1982; Graham & Bender, 1980).

Tetralogy of Fallot

Tetralogy of Fallot (TOF) is named for its tetrad of defects: ventricular septal defects, right ventricular outflow obstruction, right ventricular hypertrophy, and aortic override (Bove & Lupinetti, 1994; Pinsky & Arciniegas, 1990). A neonate with TOF will have symptoms dependent on the extent of right ventricular tract obstruction, which results in decreased pulmonary blood flow and the presence of right-to-left shunting (Bove & Luppinetti, 1994). The classical picture is one of cyanosis, especially with crying (Emmanouilides & Baylen, 1988; Pinsky & Arciniegas, 1990).

In neonates, initial medical management may include treatment of hypoxemia by pharmacologically maintaining patency or reopening the ductus arteriosus for additional pulmonary blood flow (Driscoll, 1990; Freedom & Benson, 1992). The elimination of conditions that produce hypoxemia may also include pharmacological agents to increase systemic vascular resistance and decrease myocardial contractility (Bove & Lupinetti, 1994). Surgical repairs are generally performed within the first year (Bove & Lupinetti, 1994; Starnes et al, 1994).

Pulmonary Diagnoses

The section that follows provides a brief discussion of common pulmonary disorders for which chest physical therapy is indicated. Additional physical therapy treatment and interactions of select diagnoses with obesity are described later in this chapter.

Hyaline Membrane Disease

The most common respiratory disorder in premature infants is hyaline membrane disease (HMD) or infant respiratory distress syndrome (IRDS or RDS). Occurring almost exclusively in preterm infants younger than 37 weeks' gestation, HMD results from lung immaturity and an inadequate amount and regeneration of surfactant (Phelan et al, 1994). Surfactant decreases alveolar surface tension and thus enables the neonate to stabilize terminal air spaces (Wallis & Harvey, 1979). Surfactant deficiency results in alveolar collapse and increased effort to breathe. Antenatal corticosteroids and surfactant replacement are standard care for very low birth weight, premature infants to reduce symptoms and sequelae of RDS.

Clinical signs of respiratory distress resulting from HMD occur early (usually within one to two hours) and persist for at least 48 to 72 hours (Farrell & Avery, 1975). Respiratory failure is common in these infants and necessitates oxygen therapy and assisted ventilation.

Chest physical therapy (CPT) is commonly indicated in the management of infants with HMD. There is usually a marked increase in airway secretions in the "recovery" state of the syndrome (after approximately two to three days), which is exacerbated by oxygen therapy and endotracheal intubation (Crane, 1981; Finer & Boyd, 1978).

Bronchopulmonary Dysplasia

As more preterm newborns survive neonatal respiratory distress, the prevalence of chronic lung disease, or broncho-pulmonary dysplasia (BPD), has increased (D'Angelo & Maniscalco, 2004; Parker et al, 1992). Although controversial, the etiology of BPD is usually linked with positive pressure ventilation and oxygen therapy in the treatment of respiratory distress during the neonatal period. The risk of BPD is highest in younger, low birth weight, premature infants (Abman & Groothius, 1994).

Northway, Rosan, and Porter's (1967) classical description of BPD includes four pathological stages. The first stage involves symptoms similar to HMD/RDS, but by the fourth stage, BPD has progressed to include characteristics of chronic lung disease (Voyles, 1981).

Clinically, infants with BPD often present with rales, wheezing, cyanosis, hypoxemia, increased incidence of lower respiratory tract infections, and abnormal chest radiographs by one month postnatal (Abman & Groothius, 1994). Medical management of BPD is primarily supportive. Long-term oxygen therapy is often necessary for infants who exhibit persistent severe hypoxemia.

The cardiopulmonary outcome of BPD is variable, ranging from near normal pulmonary function by age three to five in children with milder forms of BPD to continued poor cardiopulmonary function, chronic distress, and ongoing oxygen dependence in children with severe BPD (Berman et al, 1986; Gerhardt et al, 1987). Right-sided heart failure (cor pulmonale) is a common sequelae of this disease, especially in the first few years. Additionally, BPD survivors demonstrate an increased incidence of neurodevelopmental sequelae, including cerebral palsy and general development delay (Northway, 1979; Vohr et al, 1982).

Chest physical therapy is an important component of the management of an infant with BPD. Airway clearance problems are common due to submucosal and peribronchial smooth muscle hyperplasia, increased mucous secretions, oxygen therapy, and frequent lower respiratory tract infections. Infants with BPD also frequently have poor growth, which may be a consequence of a higher resting volume of oxygen utilization (VO_2), such that caloric needs are greater (Weinstein & Oh, 1981).

Transient Tachypnea of the Newborn

Transient tachypnea (TTNB) is another neonatal problem considered in the differential diagnosis of HMD/RDS. It is associated with delayed clearance of amniotic fluid from the lungs, results in early presentation of respiratory distress, and is most common in full-term and postterm neonates (especially if delivered by cesarean) (Avery et al, 1966; Emmanouilides & Baylen, 1988). CPT is occasionally indicated for infants with this problem, but TTNB is usually self-limited.

Meconium Aspiration Syndrome

Meconium is the content of fetal and newborn bowels. Although the cause of meconium passage is highly debated (Bacsik, 1977), once meconium is present in the uterine environment, the risk for aspiration is significant. It is generally accepted that meconium aspiration most frequently occurs with the first postnatal breaths of term or postterm infants (Gregory, 1977), but it may also occur with gasping in utero just before delivery (Katz & Bowes, 1992; Wiswell & Bent, 1993). Research has supported the contention that meconium aspiration syndrome (MAS) is often preventable if the upper and lower airways are suctioned immediately after birth (Wiswell et al, 1990). The lower airways especially should be suctioned in infants delivered through thick, particulate ("pea soup") meconium in amniotic material (Gregory, 1977).

Aspiration of meconium can result in serious and devastating pathophysiology. Most commonly the meconium will partially or completely block the peripheral airways (Wiswell & Bent, 1993). Atelectasis is the classical finding, but with partial obstruction, hyperexpanded areas will also be observed as a result of air that was inspired but then trapped in distal, small airways. Common complications of MAS include tension pneumothorax, persistent pulmonary hypertension, and bronchiolitis and pneumonitis secondary to chemical irritation from the components of the meconium (Wiswell & Bent, 1993). Additionally, long-term pulmonary sequelae have been reported (MacFarlane & Heaf, 1988; Swaminathan et al, 1989).

Medical management of MAS is supportive, with supplemental oxygen and, if necessary, mechanical ventilation. Chest physical therapy is especially advocated during the first eight hours of life, although it may be necessary for a longer period of time if the infant requires assisted ventilation.

Pneumonia

Neonatal Pneumonia. The most common organisms producing neonatal septicemia associated with pneumonia in neonates are group B *streptococcus* and *Hemophilis influenzae* (Emmanouilides & Baylen, 1988). Neonatal pneumonia mimics HMD/RDS in clinical presentation and chest radiographs.

Aspiration Pneumonia. Aspiration is an unfortunate result of small children's "indiscreet curiosity" (Waring, 1975) in exploring their environment and relying on their mouths for sensory learning. Aspiration can also result from gastroesophageal reflux and decreased upper airway neuromuscular control (Orenstein & Orenstein, 1988).

Bronchial drainage techniques are often indicated as part of the medical management of infants and children after aspiration to aid with airway clearance and reduce the possibility of bacterial superinfection.

Pneumocystis Carnii Pneumonia/HIV-Infected Children. Pulmonary involvement is often the leading cause of symptoms in children with HIV (Marolda et al, 1991). In infants with perinatally acquired HIV, *pneumocystis carnii pneumonia* (PCP) frequently occurs within the first 15 months of life (Connor et al, 1991). The risk of mortality during the infant's first episode of PCP is high (Bagarazzi et al, 1990; Bernstein et al, 1989; Scott et al, 1989).

The clinical presentation of PCP includes failure to thrive, cough, dyspnea, tachypnea, fever, hypoxemia, and chest radiograph evidence of prominent air bronchograms and multiple cysts or bullae (Bagarazzi et al, 1990; Berdon et al, 1993; Bernstein et al, 1989). PCP is most often diagnosed after bronchoalveolar lavage studies (Phelan et al, 1994).

Treatment is supportive and includes antibiotic therapy, antiretroviral therapy, nutritional support, and mechanical ventilation as needed (Bagarazzi et al, 1990; Phelen et al, 1994).

Asthma

Although asthma is discussed in detail in Chapter 5, a discussion of pediatric pulmonary problems would not be complete without some discussion of this common cause of childhood lung disease. An estimated 8% to 10% of children in the United States have asthma, with asthma accounting for the most lost time from school and 33% of pediatrician visits per year (Magee, 1991).

Childhood asthma can begin at any age, and its clinical etiology and clinical course are variable. Children with early medical histories that include very low birth weight, bronchopulmonary dysplasia, and respiratory syncytial virus infection may be at increased risk for developing asthma (Pullen & Hey, 1982; Rickards et al, 1987; Smyth et al, 1981).

Medical management usually includes avoidance of known precipitants, adrenergic drugs, and corticosteroids (in chronic, severe cases). CPT for this disease includes patient and family education in breathing control, relaxation, effective coughing, and exercise. Older children in particular may benefit from CPT, especially when they are responding slowly to pharmacological treatment alone (Asher et al, 1990). Exercise is also highly effective in the treatment and management of asthma and is discussed in a later section of this chapter.

Asthma is under-diagnosed and under-tracked among minorities and children from families with low socioeconomic status (SES) (Galant et al, 2004). Some studies suggest that detection and treatment in schools may be part of the solution (Galant et al, 2004; Knorr et al, 2004). Similarly, education regarding asthma management of children from minority or low SES families may be effectively implemented in schools by positioning the school nurse as the case manager (Galant et al, 2004; Homer, 2004; Knorr et al, 2004; Taras et al, 2004). For a child attending school in a district that does not have a full-time nurse in each school, the physical therapist may need to track and be aware of asthma in the child before he or she engages in physical exertion.

Cystic Fibrosis

Cystic fibrosis (CF) is a complex, autosomal-recessive disorder that occurs at a frequency of one in 3400 live births (Kosorok et al, 1996). A defect in a single gene, the CF regulator, leads to pathological changes in exocrine glands including airways, sweat glands, pancreas, bilary tract, and gut (Staab, 2004).

The disease progression is one of chronic lung infection that results in fibrosis and bronchiectasis that lead to respiratory insufficiency, the primary factor in morbidity by the second or third decade of life (Staab, 2004). Definitive diagnosis of CF includes positive family history, obstructive pulmonary disease, recurrent pulmonary infection, intestinal malabsorption, poor growth, the presence of *Staphylococcus aureus* or *Pseudomonas aeruginosa* in the respiratory tract, and, most importantly, a positive sweat chloride test (Cystic Fibrosis Foundation, 1990). As the disease progresses, chronic nocturnal hypoxia becomes a stimulus for the development of pulmonary hypertension and right ventricular failure and is associated with poor prognosis (Milross et al, 2004).

The chronic pulmonary disease in CF is related to increased secretion of abnormally viscous mucus, impaired mucociliary transport, airway obstruction, bronchiectasis, overinflation, and infection. Radiographic changes are most pronounced in the upper lobes, especially the right (Wood et al, 1976). Early detection and early treatment are key to the management of CF, with prevention being the yet unattained goal. The major marker of pulmonary disease in this population is forced expiratory volume in one second (FEV_1) (McColley, 2004). A recent study, however, that used high resolution computed tomography (HRCT) to examine the lungs of children six through 10 years of age who had no abnormality of FEV_1, revealed air trapping and bronchiectasis (Brody et al, 2004). Similarly, when $FEV_{0.5}$ was used as a marker, airway function was noted to be diminished soon after diagnosis in infants with CF (Ranganathan et al, 2004). These results support the belief that early intervention in children for whom detection occurs during infancy may be more critical than previously appreciated (McColley, 2004). The future of genetic diagnostics and gene therapy may address both early identification and effective, if not preventative, early treatment (Greisehnbach et al, 2004).

The early institution of prophylactic pulmonary physical therapy, including postural drainage and the judicious use of antibiotics, provides effective measures for controlling or slowing the effects of bronchiolar and bronchial obstruction. Involvement of the child and family in pulmonary care is particularly important. Family understanding of the nature of the disease and the purpose of each therapeutic measure promotes successful management of the child. A home program of CPT should be established for each child, taking into consideration the child's ongoing pulmonary needs and the family's unique contributions and constraints.

Bronchial drainage is an aspect of conventional treatment for CF with several options that allow both efficacy and patient independence (Davis, 1994). Airway clearance techniques are described in detail in Chapter 21, but alternatives to traditional percussion and postural drainage warrant mention within the context of CPT for children with CF. Specifically, the forced-expiration technique (FET) as part of the active cycle of breathing (ACB) technique, use of a positive expiratory pressure (PEP) mask, autogenic drainage (AD), and use of the flutter device have been shown to be effective in assisting sputum expectoration, often in greater amounts and in less time per treatment compared with other treatments (Konstan et al, 1994; Mahlmeister et al, 1991; Pryor, 1991; Pryor & Webber, 1979; Shoni, 1989). The efficacy of PEP in this population remains equivocal (Elkins et al, 2004; Darbee et al, 2004).

Although postural drainage, percussion, and vibration remain the treatment of choice for infants and children who are unable to be instructed in techniques that use patterns of voluntary breathing, other techniques are available for children who can follow specific breathing instructions and who can perform a reliable pulmonary function test. Children as young as two to three years of age can be taught to "huff" as part of FET (Pryor, 1991), the PEP mask has been used with children as young as three years (Mahlmeister et al, 1991), and AD can reportedly be taught to children at four to six years of age (DeCesare & Graybill, 1990; Shoni, 1989). The benefits of each technique should be carefully considered relative to each child's cognitive, respiratory, and motor planning abilities when choosing or modifying the child's program for airway clearance. Additionally, there is some debate about whether standard postural drainage techniques may exacerbate gastro-esophageal reflux and impact oxygen saturation in infants with CF who also have gastroesophagial reflux disorder (Button, 1999; Button et al, 1998; Button et al, 2004; Phillips et al, 1998). Clearly, each child's response to any technique must be carefully monitored.

Ventilatory muscle training is an important aspect of pulmonary treatment in older children with CF. Studies have demonstrated that training to improve the endurance of ventilatory muscles decreases dyspnea and increases general exercise tolerance in patients with CF (Keens et al, 1977; Reid & Loveridge, 1983).

The role of general exercise in the cardiopulmonary management of children with CF is specifically discussed within the context of pulmonary rehabilitation later in this chapter. It is important to realize, however, that some debate exists as to whether exercise can replace more traditional airway clearance techniques. Pryor (1991) has suggested that exercise should be an additional component rather than a substitute for breathing techniques. Cerney (1989) in contrast, reported that some children with mild disease may be able to use regular exercise in place of bronchial drainage treatments. The severity of the disease process and the child's condition at any particular point in time will clearly mediate the appropriateness and effectiveness of exercise as either a component or primary means of airway clearance.

Special Respiratory Problems Associated with Intubation and Tracheostomy

Once an infant or child develops respiratory failure, intubation and mechanical ventilation are usually required. The goals of medical management are then to treat the cause of the respiratory failure as aggressively as possible and to wean the child from mechanical ventilation as quickly as possible.

If a child's condition necessitates long-term mechanical ventilation, or if an artificial airway is needed to bypass an upper airway obstruction, a tracheostomy is usually performed (Scott & Koff, 1993).

Infants and children who have a tracheostomy and are intubated for long periods of time require vigorous prophylactic airway management, such as bronchial drainage and airway suctioning. CPT, including postural drainage and vibration emphasizing right upper lobe segments, has been shown to significantly decrease the incidence of postextubation

TABLE 37-3

Functional Relationship of Trunk Control and Respiration

BIOMECHANICAL COMPONENT	POSTURAL/TRUNK CONTROL CONSEQUENCES	RESPIRATORY CONSEQUENCES
Weak abdominal obliques	Passive lumbar lordosis Protruding tummy Lower rib flaring Decreased trunk rotation Unable to weight shift Dependence on rectus abdominis	Ineffective cough High chest Retained horizontal rib alignment Tight rectus abdominis may lead to pectus excavatum Child may use diaphragm for trunk control, limiting its function as a primary muscle of respiration Decreased support of abdominal contents under diaphragm
Tight pectoralis minor	Forward shoulders Scapula pulled laterally and anteriorly, away from the thoracic wall Upper thoracic flexion	Anterior upper chest cannot adequately expand
Weak serratus anterior	Weak upper fibers—medial edge of scapula leaves the thoracic wall	Decreased structural reinforcement of the posterior chest wall Interdigitation of the lower fibers of serratus anterior with the external abdominal oblique will interact to affect the dynamic stability of the ribcage
Decreased active upper thoracic extension	Kyphotic upper trunk Passive overlengthening of the scapular retractors	Approximation of upper ribs → decreased upper chest mobility → decreased oxygenation of the upper lobe → abdominal breathing
Decreased ribcage stability	Serratus anterior will elevate the ribs rather than stabilize the scapula against the thoracic wall	Decreased structural support for the respiratory muscles to work from

Modified from Moerchen VA. (1994). Respiration and motor development: a system perspective. Neurology Report 18:8-10. Reprinted from the Neurology Report with the permission of the Neurology Section, APTA.

atelectasis in infants intubated for more than 24 hours (Finer et al, 1979).

Pulmonary Considerations in Neuromuscular and Motor Diagnoses

Although cardiopulmonary symptoms may not be the primary reason for referral to physical therapy in children with neuromuscular and general motor developmental diagnoses, these children do have motor involvement that can result in respiratory and postural muscle weakness, immobile chests, and hypoventilation. Furthermore, many of these children have had medical histories remarkable for cardiopulmonary complications or have diagnoses that entail progressive processes that will result in cardiopulmonary compromise.

Table 37-3 provides an extensive summary of the interactions between trunk musculature and ventilation in children with atypical development. Although the biomechanical deviations noted are frequently seen in children with atypical tonal presentations, they are also common in children with scoliosis, sternal deformity, or general immobility of the thorax. These deviations and other aspects of ventilatory

compromise are discussed with regard to motor diagnoses common to pediatric practice.

Cerebral Palsy

Children with cerebral palsy generally have weak trunk and postural muscles, which, when combined with atypical neural mechanisms, produce atypical movement patterns and functional alignment deviations. The trunk and respiration relationships described in Table 37-3 are consistent with the clinical picture of external pulmonary development in children with cerebral palsy.

Although the extent of mobility impairment is variable among children with cerebral palsy, hypoventilation, increased work to breathe, inefficient cough, increased risk for aspiration, and poor breath support for vocalization can occur (Alexander, 1993). Limited active mobility and the use of habitual patterns that show little deviation from the center of gravity beyond the base of support contribute to thoracic stiffness. A high chest, flattened anteriorly, with excessive rib flaring is common in these children (Figure 37-1).

Therapeutic attention to respiration should first identify possible aspiration and suggest modifications for positioning

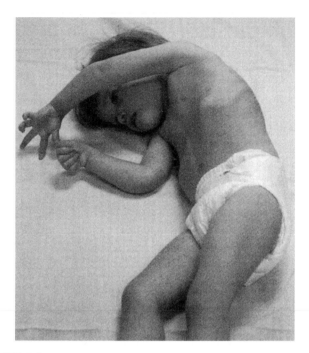

FIGURE 37-1 Flattened anterior chest with marked rib flaring in a child with cerebral palsy.

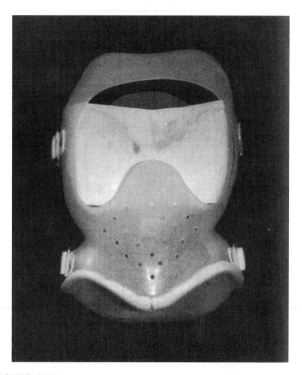

FIGURE 37-2 An anterior cut-out and elastic support in a body jacket/spinal orthosis aids diaphragm function.

during feeding. Additionally, certain postures for sleep and play may be less restrictive for chest excursion and should be incorporated into a home program. Mobilization of the ribs and thoracic spine are important precursors to improving chest excursion during ventilation.

CPT may be indicated if the child develops a primary pulmonary complication. Prophylactic postural drainage can also be integrated into many sensory stimulation programs for more severely involved children. Additional "handling" to address ventilatory function will be discussed in a subsequent section on motor approaches to respiratory treatment.

Myelomeningocele

Myelomeningocele, or spina bifida, is a diagnosis that physical therapists generally equate with issues of ambulation and mobility; however, central ventilatory dysfunction is prevalent in infants, children, and adolescents who also have an associated Arnold-Chiari type II malformation (Hays et al, 1989; Swaminathan et al, 1989; Ward et al, 1986).

The Arnold-Chiari type II malformation, which occurs in 90% of infants with myelomeningocele, is a hindbrain malformation consisting of a caudal herniation of the cerebellum and brain stem into the cervical canal (Charney et al, 1987). Ventilatory problems associated with a symptomatic Arnold-Chiari type II malformation include inspiratory stridor (vocal cord paralysis), central apnea, and respiratory distress (Hays et al, 1989; Hesz & Wolraich, 1985; Oren et al, 1986). Abnormal ventilatory patterns, however, have also been observed in asymptomatic infants (Ward et al, 1986) and adolescents (Swaminathan et al, 1989).

Ventriculoperitoneal shunting (management of hydro-cephalus) and, if necessary, cervical decompression are the surgical approaches to treatment of life-threatening ventilatory complications in this population.

Other pulmonary issues in children with myelomeningocele warrant discussion. Trunk weakness and hypotonia are observed early in the motor development of infants and toddlers who have shunted hydrocephalus. Additionally, in children with thoracic and high lumbar level lesions, abdominal muscle support for diaphragm function may be insufficient. The use of abdominal binders and spinal orthoses/body jackets with (anterior) diaphragm cut-outs and an elastic insert are indicated to aid in diaphragm function (Figure 37-2). Although progressive scoliosis is not the natural history of children with spina bifida, it is a symptom of unstable neurology (tethered cord), and attention to ventilatory ability is necessary both for general monitoring and for possible preoperative evaluation.

Down Syndrome

Impaired pulmonary function in children with Down syndrome is clearly related to generalized weakness of trunk musculature (Dichter et al, 1993). The postural deviations common in these children reflect (Figure 37-3) inefficient muscle function for both ventilation and movement (Moerchen, 1994). The trunk-ventilation relationships delineated in Table 37-3 summarize the subtle but significant clinical presentation of external pulmonary development in these children. Too often only motor development is addressed by physical therapists who are treating children with Down

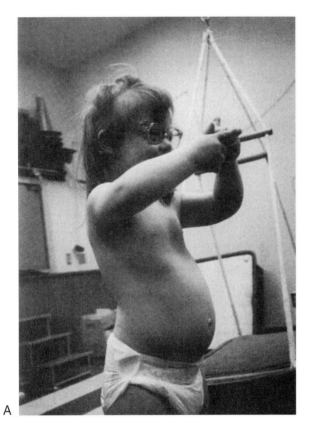
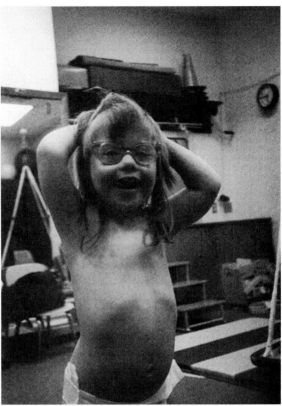

A   B

FIGURE 37-3 A, Characteristic posture of a child with Down syndrome/hypotonia. Note the abdominal protrusion and sternal retraction. **B,** Rib flaring with upper extremity movement; the abdominal obliques are not stabilizing the lower ribs. *(Photos from Moerchen, V.A. [1994]. Respiration and motor development: a systems perspective. Neurology Report 18:8-10. Reprinted with the permission of the Neurology Section, APTA.)*

syndrome. Respiration needs to be considered if therapy goals include increased vocalizations or improved tolerance for exercise.

Pulmonary hypoplasia may also challenge the respiratory function of these children. Cooney and Thurlbeck (1982) observed a consistent combination of decreased numbers of alveoli and larger alveolar ducts in individuals with Down syndrome, not related to age or incidence of heart disease. Although these researchers had a small sample size, their results do suggest that trisomy 21 may result in lung vulnerability.

Muscular Dystrophy

Duchenne's muscular dystrophy (DMD) is an example of a diagnosis in which the neuromotor and chest wall impairments together lead to ventilatory failure. End-stage respiratory failure in this disease results from progressive respiratory muscle weakness, thoracic deformity, reduced lung compliance, retained secretions, ventilation-perfusion imbalance, and hypoxemia (Bach et al, 1987; Smith et al, 1987). In 70% to 90% of these patients, death is directly related to restrictive respiratory complications (Bach et al, 1987;

Smith et al, 1987). In addition to ventilatory failure, cardiac function also deteriorates in DMD. Dilated cardiomyopathy or congestive heart failure develops during or after puberty (Cox & Kunkel, 1997).

Physical therapists are typically involved in treatment of these patients for preservation of motor function. Early attention to ventilation, however, is warranted. Prophylactic spinal fusion to prevent scoliosis-related compromise of ventilation in these patients considers both the progression of the spinal curvature and vital capacity (VC) (Rideau et al, 1984).

CPT should be a component of the overall physical therapy management of children with muscular dystrophy. Deep breathing, coughing, and activities to address endurance are recommended but will require ongoing modification as the disease progresses. Inspiratory muscle training in these children remains controversial. Although some researchers have demonstrated improved endurance of ventilatory muscles (DiMarco et al, 1985; Martin et al, 1986; Stern et al, 1991), other researchers have suggested that inspiratory resistance may over-tax respiratory muscles that are already near fatigue from working against incompliant structures (lungs, thorax) (Smith et al, 1988).

Respiratory dependence does occur as the disease progresses. Protocols for point of initiation and type of mechanical ventilation are continuously evolving. Close monitoring of VC and nocturnal hypoventilation can allow respiratory support to be implemented before the onset of acute respiratory failure (Bach et al, 1981; Bach et al, 1998; Bach et al, 1987; Curran, 1981). The speed of progression of the disease is significant to the timing of noninvasive positive pressure ventilation (NPPV). Symptoms of nocturnal hypoventilation may be treated initially with continuous positive airway pressure (CPAP), especially if obstructive sleep apnea is noted (Hukins & Hillman, 2000; Vianello et al, 1994). Transitioning to NPPV is typically required when diurnal hypercapnia is noted (Raphael et al, 1994), unless severe bulbar weakness is present (Shneerson & Simonds, 2002). Further, when NPPV in combination with insufflation/ exsufflation is used to treat adolescents with end-stage DMD, pulmonary complications requiring hospitalization have been reduced (Bach et al, 1998). Peak cough flow is greater with in-exsufflation than with manual cough techniques (Bach, 2003). Progressing to tracheostomy (invasive) ventilation is elective and may be avoidable with combined noninvasive methods initiated earlier in the disease process.

Miscellaneous Conditions

Multiple other pediatric diagnoses and musculoskeletal conditions include clinical presentations (strength, alignment, and limited mobility) that should cue the therapist's attention to pulmonary function. Syndromes that involve sternal deformity, such as Marfan syndrome or Poland's syndrome, will clearly entail possible ventilatory compromise. Children with juvenile rheumatoid arthritis (JRA) may have inflammation of thoracic joints or may splint through their trunks when they try to move painful extremities. With these children, breathing exercises will have a role both in pulmonary care and in pain management.

Put simply, children who make compensations in their movement patterns to accommodate pain, weakness, or deformity may limit the mechanics of their thoraces. Conversely, children who cannot adequately oxygenate may make compensations in their movement patterns to support ventilation. Clearly, attention to ventilation should be an inherent aspect of observing motor development and quality of movement in all children.

Obesity as a Cardiopulmonary Co-morbidity

The childhood obesity epidemic that is occurring across cultures in most Western countries (Stubbs & Lee, 2004) cannot go unmentioned as a co-morbity associated with cardiopulmonary diagnoses. Clearly overeating and immobility (either elective or secondary to motor impairments) super-imposed on cardiopulmonary diagnoses create an additional set of risk-factors about which physical therapists need to be appraised. A brief review of these co-morbidities is provided.

Obesity and Asthma

Asthma and obesity present an interaction of factors that are somewhat cyclical in their effects. Children with asthma may be less active, especially if their asthma is exercise induced and they have not been instructed in how to prepare for physical activity. Inactivity superimposed on excessive energy intake (overeating) leads to overweight status. Among children with asthma, obese children wheeze more, use their inhalers more frequently, and have higher bronchial hyper-reactivity, than nonobese children (Bibi et al, 2004). There is debate about whether high body mass index (BMI) is a risk factor for asthma or chest symptoms related to obesity mimic asthma (Bibi et al, 2004; Chinn, 2003; Chinn & Rona, 2004).

Obesity and Obstructive Sleep Apnea

The incidence of obstructive sleep apnea (OSA) related to obesity in clinical as well as nonclinical populations of children is alarming. In typically developing children, the severity of OSA is positively related to degree of obesity (Arens & Marcus, 2004; Marcus et al, 1996; Ng et al, 2004). Additionally, obese children have elevated blood pressures (Ng et al, 2004). Further, obesity obscures the normal anatomical landmarks used for emergency airway management, complicating emergency care (Ray & Senders, 2001).

Obesity and Low Muscle Tone

In clinical populations with known low neuromotor tone of the upper airways, such as Down syndrome and Prader Willi syndrome, obesity is associated with higher incidence of obstructive sleep apnea (Dearlove et al, 1998; Dyken et al, 2003; Harris & Allen, 1996; Ng & Chan, 2003; Schrander-Stumpel et al, 2004).

PHYSICAL THERAPY TREATMENT APPROACHES

Postoperative Pediatric Cardiac Rehabilitation

Postoperative physical therapy consists largely of techniques to increase respiration, mobilize secretions, and progress physical mobility. Positional rotation for pulmonary care is possible if the child has a stabilized sternum. Breathing exercises and coughing will need to be modified based on the child's age and cognitive level. Huckabay and Daderian (1990) reported improved postoperative cooperation in children three to 10 years of age when choice making was incorporated into a breathing program.

Immobilization after cardiac surgery is to be avoided as much as medically possible. Passive range of motion may be initiated immediately, taking care to avoid compromising arterial lines. Ambulation is generally initiated once the child is extubated and has had atrial and groin lines removed (Johnson, 1991).

Child and family education as part of pediatric cardiac rehabilitation has been observed to reduce parent and child anxiety related to safe levels of physical activity (Balfour et al, 1991; Calzolari et al, 1990; Mathews et al, 1983). Although studies of pediatric cardiac rehabilitation have been focused on children older than six years, monitored exercise has been shown to safely produce an increase in peak oxygen consumption and a decrease in resting heart rate (Balfour et al, 1991; Calzolari et al, 1990; Mathews et al, 1983).

Exercise prescription for cardiopulmonary rehabilitation of older children who have undergone cardiac repairs at an early age will require careful monitoring. Lower exercise VO_2 values, lower cardiac output, and lower values of diffusion capacity of the lung for carbon monoxide have been observed in response to exercise in children who have undergone cardiac surgery compared with the responses of age-matched controls (Gildein et al, 1994; Tomassoni et al, 1991). Exercise recommendations include submaximal performance (Tommassoni et al, 1991) and technique training to increase the biomechanical efficiency of movement while decreasing the associated metabolic costs (Gildein et al, 1994).

CPT for Neonates and Infants

The primary goal of CPT for neonates and infants is to improve airway clearance. If techniques of bronchial drainage can increase the diameter of the airways through secretion mobilization, then ventilation may also be improved and the work of breathing reduced. These techniques should be judiciously applied for prophylaxis and treatment in infants who have or are at risk for developing airway clearance problems. Applying bronchial drainage techniques to infants requires a thorough understanding of each infant's condition and the precautions and considerations inherent to any technique or combination of techniques.

Positional Rotation

Frequent changing of position will prevent prolonged dependency of any one portion of the lung so that pooling of secretions can be limited or avoided and improved ventilation can be achieved (Menkes & Britt, 1980; Ross & Dean, 1989). Whereas positional rotation programs for adults emphasize the lower lobes, positional programs for infants must emphasize all lung areas (Figures 37-4 to 37-6). The upper lobes and right middle lobe are common sites of airway collapse and atelectasis in infants, and the right middle lobe bronchus is surrounded by a collar of lymph nodes, making it vulnerable to extrinsic compression. Important considerations and essentials of a positional rotation program for infants are outlined in Box 37-1.

Premature infants do tolerate and benefit from prone positioning. Studies have demonstrated improved oxygenation, tidal volume, dynamic lung compliance, and synchrony of chest wall movement when preterm infants are put in prone positions (Hutchinson et al, 1979; Lioy & Manginello, 1988; Martin et al, 1979).

Positional rotation is generally performed manually every two hours, and although this provides pulmonary benefit, it may also contribute to the disruption of homeostasis that has been documented to occur in the course of neonatal intensive care (Long et al, 1980; Yeh et al, 1984). Use of nursery beds that provide continuous positional oscillation (from right side to supine to left side, and so forth) might provide an option that allows the benefits of position change while also minimizing the homeostatic disruption. Murai and Grant (1994) demonstrated that continuous positional oscillation as part of a total chest physical therapy program decreased the duration of oxygen supplementation without adversely affecting the cardiopulmonary status of the neonates.

Postural Drainage

Postural drainage positions to promote gravity-assisted drainage of specific segmental airways can be safely applied to infants and children. In the acute care setting, however, many of the head-down positions are modified according to tolerance and precautions or contraindications (Table 37-4). The rule for modification of any position for postural drainage is that the position used should be as close to the classical (anatomically correct) position for that segment as safely possible. Examples of the classical postural drainage positions for each bronchopulmonary segment are pictured in Figure 37-7.

Tiny infants (especially premature infants weighing less than 800 grams) usually require and benefit from modification of the head-down position. Horizontal to slightly elevated positioning of the head may be best (Thoresan et al, 1988). This modification is primarily due to the high incidence of intraventricular hemorrhage in premature infants (Crane et al, 1978; Emery & Peabody, 1983). Other precautions for Trendelenburg positioning of infants include but are not limited to abdominal distention, congestive heart failure, dysrhythmias, hydrocephalus, frequent episodes of apnea and bradycardia, and acute respiratory distress.

Chest Percussion and Vibration

Percussion and vibration are used in conjunction with postural drainage to augment the effect of gravity in the removal of secretions. There are several ways to perform percussion on infants. For a larger infant, it is possible to use a cupped hand in a manner similar to percussing an adult's chest. For a smaller infant, some modification of this technique is needed. Chest percussion for a smaller infant is accomplished by the use of tenting three fingers, four fingers, or using any of the commercially available percussion devices made for neonates (Figure 37-8). A small anesthesia mask or "palm cup" can also be used effectively.

Precautions for chest percussion in the infant include but are not limited to unstable cardiovascular or oxygenation status (although percussion may be provided safely if continuous transcutaneous monitoring is available), coagulopathy, subcutaneous emphysema, or intraventricular hemorrhage. Additionally, percussion is generally contraindicated over a healing thoracotomy incision or if the child displays irritability and signs of respiratory distress with the treatment.

Vibration is accomplished either through manual vibratory motion of the therapist's fingers on the infant's chest wall

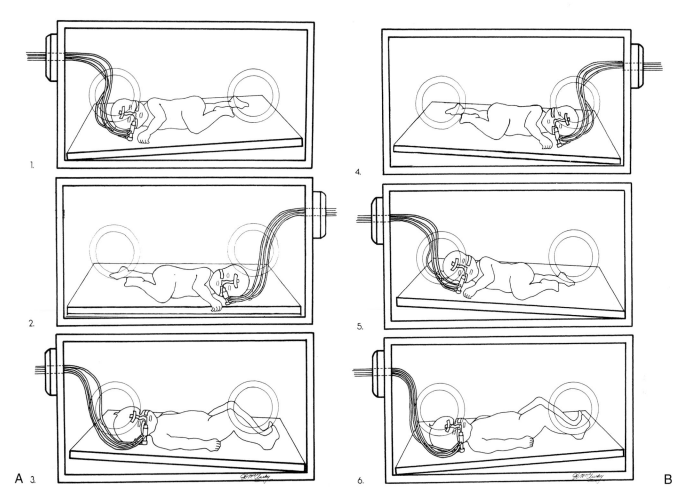

FIGURE 37-4 *Sequence for positional rotation. Position 1.* Segments that come off the left lower bronchus posteriorly are drained by positioning the infant on his or her right side, three-fourths prone with a head-down angle. *Position 2.* The posterior segment of the right upper lobe is drained by positioning on the left side, three-fourths prone with the bed flat. *Position 3.* The anterior segments of the upper lobes are drained by positioning supine with the head of the bed elevated or flat. *Position 4.* Segments that come off the right lower lobe bronchus posteriorly are drained by positioning on the left side, three-fourths prone with a head-down angle. *Position 5.* The posterior segment of the left upper lobe is drained by positioning on the right side, three-fourths prone with the head of the bed elevated. *Position 6.* Segments that come off the tracheobronchial tree anteriorly are drained by positioning supine with a head-down angle. *Positions 7 and 8.* Segments such as the right middle lobe or lingula that come off the tracheobronchial tree anterolaterally will be drained in a three-fourths spine position, slightly head down (see Figure 37-5). Babies on ventilators may also be positioned prone. This is usually done by the therapist rather than in a routine positional rotation (see Figure 37-6).

(Figure 37-9) or through the use of a mechanical vibrator. An electric toothbrush can be adapted by padding the bristle portion with foam (Curran & Kachoyeanos, 1979). Vibration has been observed to occasionally increase irritability and may be less well tolerated than percussion. The most common precaution for vibration is increased irritability with the development of bradycardia and respiratory distress.

The decision to use chest percussion and vibration will depend on the reviewed principles and precautions, the medical condition of the infant, and the infant's tolerance to handling. Continuation of percussion and vibration will depend on the day-to-day medical status of the infant and the infant's response to treatment.

Airway Suctioning

Sterile airway suctioning is discussed in detail in Chapter 44; however, some special considerations for suctioning the airway of an infant must be highlighted (Durand et al, 1989; McFadden, 1981; Perlman & Volpe, 1983).

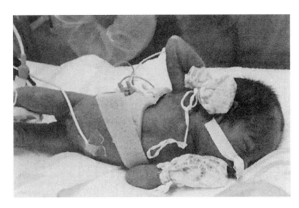

FIGURE 37-5 Three-fourths supine position for right middle lobe. Lingula is the same three-fourths supine position with the patient lying on his or her right side.

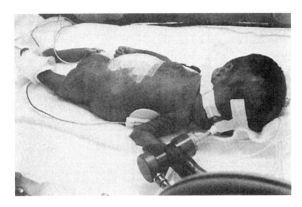

FIGURE 37-6 Premature infants (even those on ventilators with numerous catheters) may be placed prone when care is taken.

1. If possible, suction with a transcutaneous oxygen monitor in place. These monitors give continuous feedback regarding the infant's oxygenation status.
2. Bagging should be done only with a bag attached to a pressure manometer to ensure that sufficient pressures are being used without exceeding the maximum safe levels (these limits should be similar to the ventilator settings).

BOX 37-1

Essentials of a Positional Rotation Program

1. Care should be taken to coordinate any change in the infant's position with other nursing procedures to avoid unnecessary stimulation.
2. Infants should never be left unattended when in a head-down position.
3. Vital signs should be monitored closely by respiration and heart rate monitors. The alarms should be turned on.
4. The infant's chest should be auscultated for adventitious breath sounds after positioning.
5. While the infant is in a drainage position, secretions will be more easily mobilized. The infant's trachea or endotracheal tube should be suctioned as needed.
6. Avoid placing the infant in a head-down position for approximately one hour after eating to avoid aspiration of regurgitated food.
7. Any change in the infant's position should be done slowly to minimize stress on the cardiovascular system.
8. Infants with umbilical arterial lines can be placed on their abdomens; however, one should always check that the line has not been kinked.
9. Some infants might require modified drainage positions. Infants with severe cardiovascular instability or suspected intracranial bleeding should not be placed in a head-down position.

TABLE 37-4

Precautions and Contraindications for Postural Drainage in a Neonate*

POSITION	PRECAUTION	CONTRAINDICATION
Prone	Umbilical arterial catheter Continuous positive airway pressure in nose Excessive abdominal distention Abdominal incision Anterior chest tube	Untreated tension pneumothorax
Tendelenburg position (head down)	Distended abdomen SEH/IVH* (grades I and II) Chronic congestive heart failure or cor pulmonale Persistent fetal circulation Cardiac dysrhythmias Apnea and bradycardia Infant exhibiting signs of acute respiratory distress Hydrocephalus Less than 28 weeks' gestational age	Untreated tension pneumothorax Recent tracheoesophageal fistula repair Recent eye or intracranial surgery Intraventricular hemorrhage (grades III and IV) Acute congestive heart failure or cor pulmonale

*Subependymal hemorrhage/intraventricular hemorrhage.
From Crane, L.D. (1995). Physical therapy for the neonate with respiratory disease. In Irwon, S., Tecklin, J.S. (Eds). Cardiopulmonary physical therapy. St. Louis: Mosby.

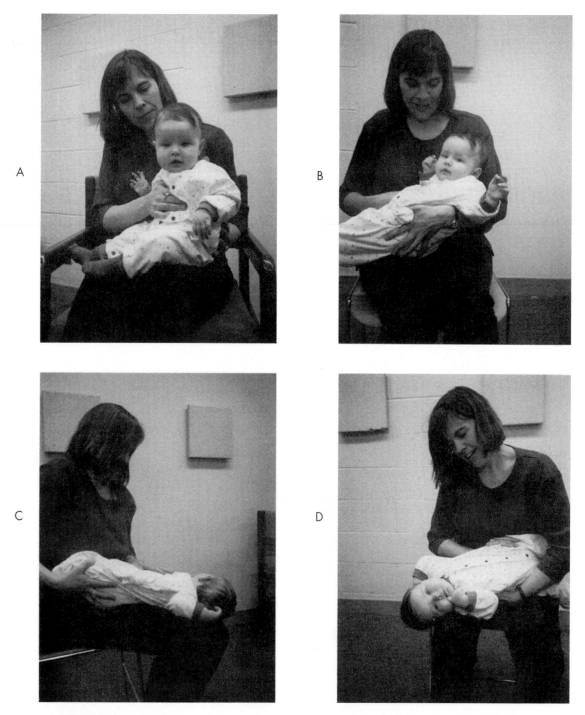

FIGURE 37-7 Postural drainage with an infant. **A,** Both upper lobes—apical segments. **B,** Left upper lobe—anterior segment. **C,** Right upper lobe—anterior segment. **D,** Lingula.

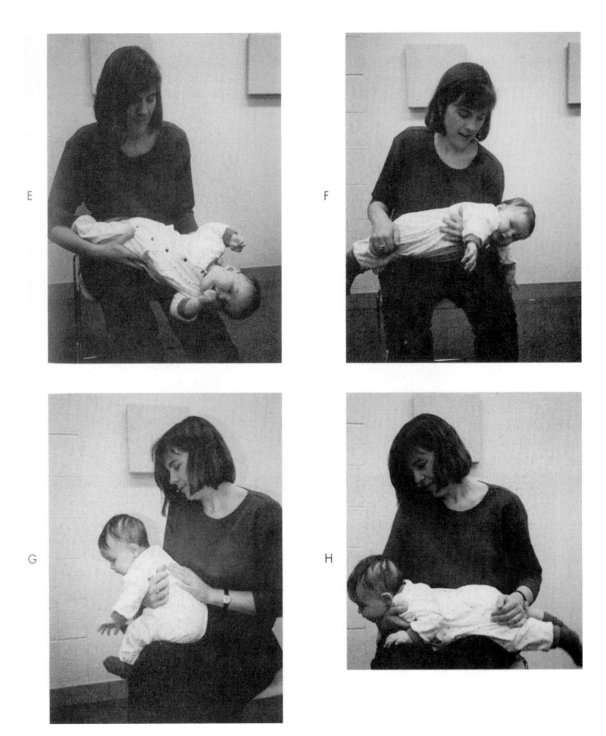

FIGURE 37-7 Cont'd E, Right middle lobe. **F,** Right upper lobe—posterior segment. **G,** Left upper lobe—posterior segment. **H,** Both lower lobes—apical (superior) segments.

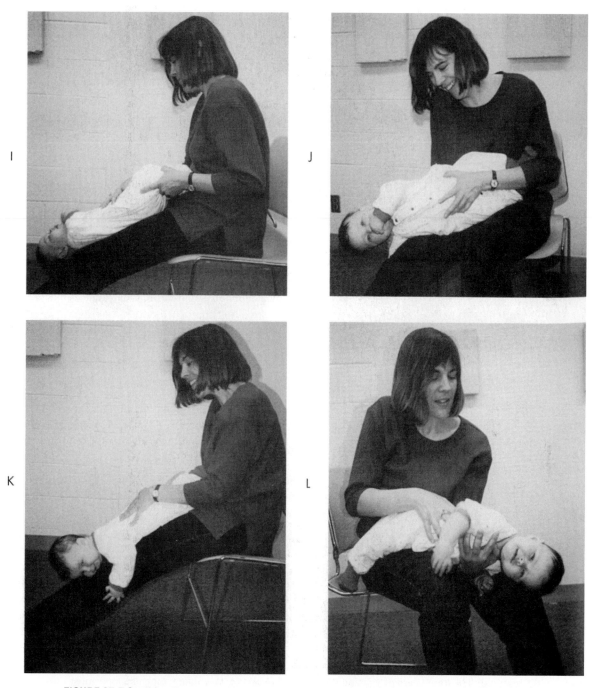

FIGURE 37-7 Cont'd I, Both lower lobes—anterior basal segments. **J,** Left lower lobe—lateral basal segment; right lower lobe—carduac (medial) segment. **K,** Both lower lobes—posterior basal segments. **L,** Right lower lobe—lateral basal segment.

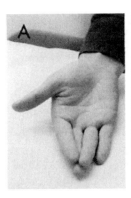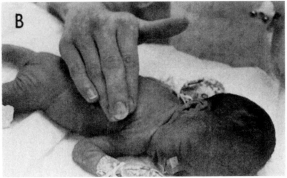

FIGURE 37-8 "Tenting" of the finger for percussion of premature infants or small children.

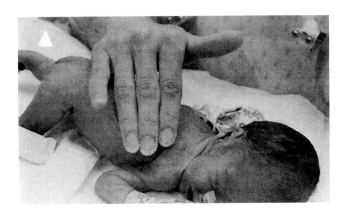

FIGURE 37-9 Manual chest wall vibration of a premature infant.

3. Suction for no more than five seconds with each catheter withdrawal.
4. Infants should be carefully hyperoxygenated when hyperventilated so as to minimize hyperoxia and hypoxia. Bagging usually does not need to continue for more than five to 10 seconds to maintain adequate oxygen levels.

Monitor the blood pressure of preterm infants before, during, and after suctioning. Change in blood pressure may indicate increased intracranial pressure and risk for intracranial hemorrhage.

CPT for Children

The goals for CPT with children (two years of age and older) include more than improving airway clearance. Children are capable of following directions and imitating a therapist's demonstration of deep breathing, coughing, and active exercise. CPT in children is focused on improving ventilation, improving the efficiency of breathing, increasing general strength and endurance with an emphasis on muscles of respiration, improving posture, and addressing relaxation, breathing control, and pacing.

The application of CPT with children often requires patience and creative adaptation (Figure 37-10). The challenge is to make it seem less like a treatment and more like a game. It is important, however, to be honest in your explanations and to speak to the child with respect and at a level appropriate to the child's age and development.

Involving the family in CPT treatment of a child can be invaluable. In some cases the parent may do most of the "hands-on" and repeat instructions to the child under the direct guidance of the therapist. This arrangement will also help reinforce parent and family education for carry-over of home therapy.

Positional Rotation

The goal of positional rotation and postural drainage is to prevent the accumulation of secretions and to aid in their removal. Any child who is immobile, receiving artificial ventilation, or not expanding his or her chest adequately should have his or her position changed at least every two hours. Recall that positional changes will enhance oxygen transport and promote pulmonary drainage (Ross & Dean, 1989). If the child is reluctant to have his or her position changed, changing the location of the television may be helpful. Be creative!

Young Children. In younger children (18 months to three years of age), deep breathing is usually encouraged by blowing bubbles, tissue paper, mobiles, or simple horns. To achieve maximal chest expansion, the child should be positioned on each side while playing blowing games or singing. The theory behind the side lying position is that the downside lung ventilates more effectively (see Chapter 19). Additionally, if the poorly ventilated lung is uppermost, stretch techniques can facilitate deeper breathing (see Chapter 23).

Spontaneous coughing in younger children often occurs with a change in position or with crying. For the child who does not cough spontaneously or whose cough is inadequate to clear secretions, nasopharyngeal suctioning may be necessary.

Older Children. School-age children can be more specifically instructed in various breathing exercises, such as diaphragmatic breathing, pursed-lip breathing, and segmental

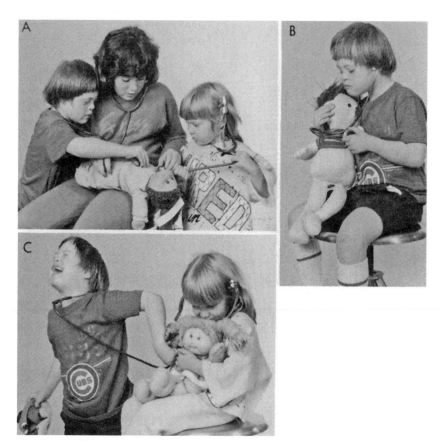

FIGURE 37-10 A-C, Few areas of health care delivery require creative adaptation and problem solving to the extent that pediatrics does.

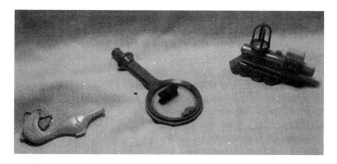

FIGURE 37-11 Whistles such as these encourage increased inspiration and controlled, sustained expiration to make the whistle components move. *Left*, a fish with a wheel that moves at its back fin; *middle*, a race car that drives around a track and makes whirling sounds; *right*, a ball that moves up and down in a train.

lateral costal breathing. They may also be candidates for using relaxed deep breathing for control and pacing of activity. Cooperation with this age group, however, still remains higher if some aspect of therapy is fun. Elaborate whistles are available that encourage deep breathing; they make therapy fun by challenging the patient to make the whistle components move (Figure 37-11). Additionally, pediatric incentive spirometers are available with cheerful, "cool" pictures to make respiration exercises more like a game (Figure 37-12).

Older children (not infants) can be stimulated to cough by applying a firm pressure over the trachea in the suprasternal notch. Be aware that coughing, whether spontaneous or stimulated, may elicit gagging and vomiting, especially if airway clearance is scheduled too soon after a child has eaten.

Preoperative and Postoperative Care

The efficacy of postoperative CPT is highly related to preoperative care. The appropriate application of preoperative assessment, instruction, and treatment by therapists helps to decrease the incidence of postoperative complications.

Preoperative teaching is extremely important for both the child and the family. Parents can often be more anxious than the child, so patient and family education is important. The level of preoperative training with the child will depend on the child's age.

If the child is very young (under two years of age), the therapist needs to meet with the parents and explain the purpose of bronchial drainage treatments, potential airway clearance problems, and possible complications. The preventative nature of these treatments should be stressed, and

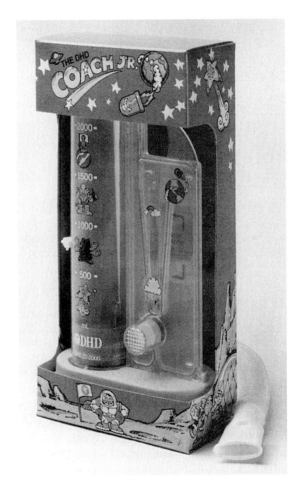

FIGURE 37-12 A pediatric incentive spirometer. *(Photo provided courtesy of DHD Medical Products.)*

procedures that might be done with the child after surgery should be demonstrated and discussed. These might include positioning, chest percussion, vibration, and airway suctioning. In addition, always allow time for the parents to ask questions.

If the child is able to understand simple concepts, the therapist can, in addition to parent orientation, instruct the child in various breathing games, use of an incentive spirometer, coughing, and general upper and lower extremity exercises.

In older children (eight years of age or older), postoperative procedures can be explained and demonstrated. The importance of bronchial hygiene should be stressed during demonstration of deep breathing and coughing. The child can be shown how to splint the incision using a pillow or stuffed animal to assist with comfort while coughing. Do not tell the child that coughing will not hurt; be honest but reinforce that splinting will help. Teach the child diaphragmatic and pursed-lip breathing with an inspiratory-hold maneuver, and, if appropriate, teach the child how to use an incentive spirometer.

Postoperative pulmonary complications may not be as prevalent in the pediatric age group as in adults, but they still occur. The most common complications are atelectasis,

infection secondary to pooling of secretions, and airway obstruction. Infants and children with the following characteristics will be at risk for developing postoperative pulmonary complications: preexisting lung disease, thoracic or upper abdominal location of incision, prolonged postoperative bed rest or restricted mobility, and neuromuscular involvement that affects the ability to be mobile, cough, and breathe deeply.

Postoperative treatments generally focus on increasing ventilation, coughing, and active mobility. Specific bronchial drainage is used only if the child is unable to clear his or her airways or is at risk due to chronic lung disease.

After high abdominal or thoracic surgery, there may be a tendency for the child to splint on the side of his or her incision. Arm, shoulder, and trunk movement should be encouraged to prevent any postoperative complications. For the younger child, chest mobility can be encouraged by clapping the hands overhead or by dramatizing songs such as *The Itsy Bitsy Spider.* More conventional exercises may be taught to the older child.

Children tend to mobilize very quickly (unless their movement is limited secondary to motor involvement or to a specific surgical procedure). Once the child is out of bed and moving about, with clear lungs and an effective cough, postoperative CPT treatments can generally be discontinued.

Pediatric Pulmonary Rehabilitation

Rehabilitation programs for pediatric patients with chronic lung disease include the same components and have essentially the same goals as adult pulmonary rehabilitation. The major difference is related to different diagnoses being most prevalent in the children versus adult age groups. Asthma and CF are the most common diagnoses of children who are candidates for pulmonary rehabilitation.

Exercise and Asthma

Exercise and conditioning are very important components of the treatment of the child with asthma. Improved chest and trunk mobility, control of breathing, strength, posture, and an increased tolerance to exercise are all goals that can be addressed in the design of exercise programs for these children (Magee, 1991; Nixon, 1996; Seligman et al, 1970).

The transient airflow obstruction associated with physical exertion may render children (and their parents) wary of exercise. Several approaches may be beneficial at promoting and maintaining exercise in this population. First, aerobic conditioning will reduce the ventilation requirement for activity, thus reducing the increased rate of ventilation with exertion. This prolongs the time period that the nose and trachea remain in the location at which air is warmed and humidified before moving to the intrathoracic region, thus raising the threshold for exercise-induced symptoms (de Bisschop et al, 1999; Milgrom & Taussig, 1999). Second, because many younger children perform bursts of activity at unpredictable times of day and often are not allowed to carry their inhalers with them in school or during sports activity, the physical therapist may be influential in communicating with the child's physician to identify longer acting medications that might be given at home (Milgrom & Taussig, 1999). Third, postexercise deep bronchoconstriction in some children may be reduced with warm-up exercise that consists of repeated activity that varies in intensity and includes burst periods of high intensity (de Bisschop et al, 1999).

Part of a pulmonary rehabilitation program may involve providing recommendations for the child's participation in physical education (PE). Certain aspects of exercise relative to pulmonary function in children with asthma need to be communicated to the PE teacher. Running is the form of exercise most likely to aggravate exercise-induced asthma, especially if performed in a cool, dry environment. Swimming, by contrast, is an excellent activity. Continuous or high burst exercise might induce bronchospasm, whereas short periods of exercise (less than six continuous minutes) may be beneficial for conditioning without bronchial aggravation (Magee, 1991). PE teachers should also be aware that the child may need to use a pre-exercise inhaler to participate in PE without pulmonary consequence (Magee, 1991).

Exercise and CF

Physical activity designed to improve exercise tolerance helps children with CF to mobilize secretions and improve body image. In terms of preventing opportunistic infections in these children, exercise is also associated with an increased immune responsiveness (Boas et al, 2000). Further, quality of life measures also increase when exercise is part of the overall management program of children with CF (Klign et al, 2004; Selvadurai et al, 2002).

The development of an exercise program for children with CF should be done on an individualized basis and a pre-exercise assessment should include but not be limited to the following:

1. Assessment of range of motion, strength, and posture.
2. Complete chest evaluation.
3. Evaluation of ADL tolerance and limitations.
4. Inspiratory muscle strength (maximal inspiratory negative pressure at the mouth) and endurance testing. This inspiratory endurance testing can be done with an inspiratory muscle training device by having the child breathe for a predetermined length of time at progressively increased resistances until tolerance is reached.
5. Exercise tolerance testing, performed with electrocardiogram, blood pressure, and oxygen monitoring.

A basic exercise program for children with CF should include activities to strengthen the back and shoulder extensors, elongate the trunk flexors, and address overall endurance. Vigorous exercise and fitness training in these children requires careful monitoring of pulmonary response. Considerable research exists to support aerobic and anaerobic training in these children (Klign et al, 2004; Selvadurai et al, 2002).

Among hospitalized children with CF, children who received either aerobic or resistance training protocols had better aerobic and strength outcomes, respectively, than children in a standard CPT program, with no significant differences between the exercise and nonexercise groups in disease severity or length of hospital stay (Selvadurai et al, 2002). Attention to nutritional status in these children is paramount to both prevent decreased activity and promote exercise tolerance and quality of life (Boucher et al, 1997; Marin et al, 2004; Moorcroft et al, 1997). The evidence base suggests that the benefits of exercise will likely outweigh the risks in this population when other aspects of health are optimized.

Motor Approaches to Maximize Trunk and Ventilatory Function

Attention to pulmonary function is easily accomplished within any "handling" approach to motor therapy for children with trunk weakness, tightness, alterations in tone, or general immobility. Most "handling" consistent with a neurodevelopmental technique (NDT) approach lends itself readily to a dual focus on movement quality and ventilation. Extrinsic pulmonary development is clearly interrelated with musculoskeletal and motor development of the trunk.

Treatment should begin with assessment and initial handling for functional range of motion through the trunk. This will typically require elongation of the pectoral, sternocleidomastoid, upper trapezius, and rectus abdominis muscles. Manual lowering of the ribcage will also be necessary to work toward maximizing chest mobility (Figure 37-13).

Passive elongation of muscles must always be followed by active elongation. Controlled prone extension off a large inflated ball is both fun for the child and effective for the therapist (Figure 37-14). Manual guidance for upper extremity abduction and external rotation will facilitate active elongation of the pectoral muscles via active firing of the scapular retractors. The ball can be used to impart movement and support the lower ribcage. This elongates the anterior trunk (rectus abdominis), lengthens intercostal muscles, and facilitates increased upper chest expansion.

Handling to achieve proprioceptive input of the scapulae on the posterior thorax will help reinforce active thoracic extension and anterior chest expansion. The therapist's hands can stabilize the ribcage to reinforce abdominal oblique function during movement (Figure 37-15).

Activities requiring alternating extension-rotation and flexion-rotation will recruit control of the abdominal obliques and maintain active upper trunk extension. Bubble blowing, whistle toys, and singing are excellent means of monitoring the ventilatory changes that occur with active use of increased upper chest expansion. As tidal volume increases, vocalizations should increase in frequency, sound higher, and become louder.

The concept of functional carryover is central to the treatment approach presented here. Addressing ventilation and trunk control simultaneously has intuitive appeal based

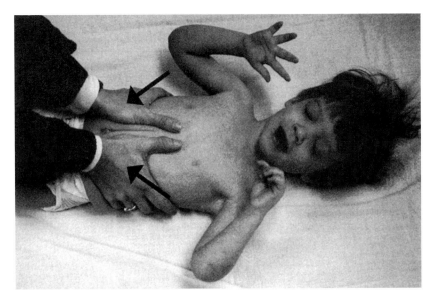

FIGURE 37-13 Manual lowering of the rib cage. *Arrows* indicate direction of therapist's hand movement (caudal and medial).

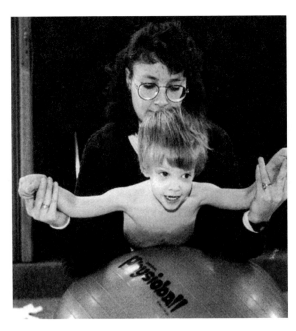

FIGURE 37-14 Handling to facilitate active upper thoracic extension as a means of actively opening the anterior chest and lengthening the rectus abdominis while supporting the lower ribcage on the ball.

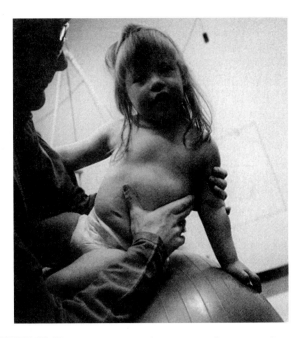

FIGURE 37-15 Handling to reinforce upper chest expansion and abdominal oblique stabilization of the lower ribs.

not only on shared musculoskeletal relationships but also on the necessity of pulmonary tolerance for motor activity.

SUMMARY

Cardiopulmonary physical therapy with infants and children begins with an understanding of the issues related to development and developmental vulnerabilities. Specific cardio-

pulmonary diagnoses in pediatrics have been described and treatment recommendations provided. Cardiopulmonary development and function are the basis for indications and precautions for treatment of neonatal and pediatric patients.

The link between pulmonary and motor function is also important. Many children with motor involvement are at risk for or have medical histories remarkable for cardiopulmonary dysfunction. Motor approaches that maximize ventilatory function are critical because efficient oxygenation is a priority not only for children with primary cardiopulmonary diagnoses but also for children with motor compromise.

Review Questions

1. Discuss the importance of changes in pulmonary blood flow during transitional circulation, and relate these changes to closure of foramen ovale and ductus arteriosus.

2. Describe six characteristics of an infant's pulmonary anatomy that contribute to the increased work of breathing and potential for pulmonary distress in this age group.

3. Identify and discuss two aspects of cardiopulmonary vulnerability in the preterm infant.

4. Compare the goals of chest physical therapy for infants and older children. What are the similarities and differences?

5. When treating infants to improve airway clearance, what are the precautions/considerations of:
   - positional rotation?
   - postural drainage?
   - percussion?
   - vibration?
   - airway suctioning?

6. How might neuromotor (neuromuscular) dysfunction affect pulmonary development?

7. Identify two cardiopulmonary complications of obesity in typically developing children. How are these complications exaggerated in children with low muscle tone?

8. Describe goals, precautions, and suggested monitoring for exercise in children who have the following:
   - a history of cardiac surgery.
   - asthma.
   - cystic fibrosis.

REFERENCES

Abel, E.L. (1984). Fetal alcohol syndrome and fetal alcohol effects. New York: Plenum Press.

Abman, S.H., & Groothius, J.R. (1994). Pathophysiology and treatment of bronchopulmonary dysplasia. Pediatric Clinics of North America 41:277-315.

Alexander, R. (1993). Respiratory and oral-motor functioning. In Connolly, B.H., & Montgomery, P.C. (Eds). Therapeutic exercise in developmental disabilities, ed 2. Hixson, Tenn: Chattanooga Group.

Archer, N. (1993). Patent ductus arteriosus in the newborn. Archives of Disease in Childhood 69:529-532.

Arens, R., & Marcus, C.L. (2004). Pathophysiology of upper airway obstruction: a developmental perspective [review]. Sleep 27: 997-1019.

Asher, M.I., Douglas, C., Airy, M., Andrews, D., & Trenholme, A. (1990). Effects of chest physical therapy on lung function in children recovering from acute severe asthma. Pediatric Pulmonology 9:146-151.

Avery, M.E., Gatewood, O.B., & Brumley, G. (1966). Transient tachypnea of newborn. American Journal of Disease in Children 111:380-385.

Bach, J.R. (2003). Mechanical insufflation/exsufflation: has it come of age? [commentary]. European Respiratory Journal 21: 385-386.

Bach, J.R., Alba, A., Pilkington, L.A., & Lee, M. (1981). Long-term rehabilitation in advanced stage of childhood onset, rapidly progressive muscular dystrophy. Archives of Physical Medicine and Rehabilitation 62:328-331.

Bach, J.R., Isikawa, Y., & Kim, H. (1998). Prevention of pulmonary morbidity for patients with Duchene muscular dystrophy. Chest 112:1024-1028.

Bach, J.R., O'Brien, J., Krptenberg, R., & Alba, A.S. (1987). Management of end stage respiratory failure in Duchene muscular dystrophy. Muscle and Nerve 10:177-182.

Bacsik, R.D. (1977). Meconium aspiration syndrome. Pediatric Clinics of North America 24:463-479.

Bagarazzi, M.L., Connor, E.M., McSherry, G.D., & Oleske, J.M. (1990). *Pneumocystis carnii pneumonia* (PCP) among human immunodeficiency virus (HIV) infected children: ten years experience. Pediatric Research 27:166.

Balfour, I.C., Drimmer, A.M., Nouri, S., Pennington, D.G., Hemkins, C.L., & Harvey, L.L. (1991). Pediatric cardiac rehabilitation. American Journal of Disease in Childhood 145:627-630.

Bender, H.W., Hammon, J.W., Hubbard, S.G., Muirhead, J., & Graham, T.P. (1982). Repair of atrioventricular canal malformation in the first year of life. Journal of Thoracic and Cardiovascular Surgery 84:515-522.

Berdon, W.E., Mellins, R.B., Abramson, S.J., & Ruzal-Shapiro, C. (1993). Pediatric HIV infection in its second decade-the changing pattern of lung involvement. Radiologic Clinics of North America 31:453-463.

Berman, W., Katz, R., Yabek, S.M., Dillon, T., Fripp, R.R., & Papile, L. (1986). Long-term follow-up of bronchopulmonary dysplasia. Journal of Pediatrics 109:45-50.

Bernstein, L.J., Bye, M.R., & Rubinstein, A. (1989). Prognostic factors and life expectancy in children with acquired immuno-deficiency syndrome and *pneuomocystitis carnii pneumonia*. American Journal of Disease in Childhood 143:775-778.

Bibi, H., Shoseyov, D., Feigenbaum, D., Genis, M., Friger, M., Peled, R., & Sharff, S. (2004). The relationship between asthma and obesity in children: is it real or a cause of overdiagnosis? Journal of Asthma 41:403-410.

Blackburn, S. (1992). Alterations of the respiratory system in the neonate: implications for clinical practice. Journal of Perinatal Nursing 6:46-58.

Boas, S.R., Danduran, M.J., McBride, A.L., McColley, S.A., & O'Gorman, M.R. (2000). Postexercise immune correlates in children with and without cystic fibrosis. Medicine and Science in Sports and Exercise 32:1997-2004.

Boehme, R. (1991). How do I get scapular stability in my patients? Team Talk 1:1-3.

Boehme, R. (1992). Assessment and treatment of the respiratory system for breathing, sound production, and trunk control. Team Talk 2:2-8.

Boucher, G.P., Lands, L.C., Hay, J.A., & Hornby, L. (1997). Activity levels and the relationship to lung function in children with cystic fibrosis. American Journal of Physical Medicine and Rehabilitation 76:311-315.

Bove, E.L., & Lupinetti, F.M. (1994). Tetralogy of Fallot. In Mavroudis, C., & Backer, C.L. (Eds). Pediatric cardiac surgery, ed 2. St. Louis: Mosby.

Bozynski, M.A., Naglie, R.A., Nicks, J.J., Burpee, B., & Johnson, R.V. (1988). Lateral positioning of the stable ventilated very-low-birth-weight infant: effect on transcutaneous oxygen and carbon dioxide. American Journal of Disease in Childhood 142:200-202.

Button, B.M. (1999). Postural drainage techniques and gastro-oesphageal reflux in infants with cystic fibrosis. European Respiratory Journal 14:1456.

Button, B.M., Heine, R.M., Catto-Smith, A.G., & Phelan, P.D. (1998). Postural drainage in cystic fibrosis: is there a link with gastro-oesophageal reflux? Journal of Paediatrics and Child Health 34:330-334.

Button, B.M., Heine, R.M., Catto-Smith, A.G., Phelan, P.D., & Olinsky, A. (2004). Chest physiotherapy, gastro-oesophageal reflux, and arousal in infants with cystic fibrosis. Archives of Disease in Childhood 89:435-439.

Calzolari, A., Turchetta, A., Biondi, G., Drago, F., De Ranieri, C., Gagliardi, G., Giambini, I., Giannico, S., Kofler, A.M., Perrotta, F., Santilli, A., Vezzoli, P., Ragonese, P., & Maecelletti, C. (1990). Rehabilitation of children after total correction of tetralogy of Fallot. International Journal of Cardiology 28:151-158.

Cerney, F.J. (1989). Relative effects of bronchial drainage and exercise for hospital care of patients with cystic fibrosis. Physical Therapy 69:633-639.

Charney, E.B., Rorke, L.B., Sutton, L.N., & Schut, L. (1987). Management of Chiari II complications in infants with myelomeningocele. Journal of Pediatrics 11:364-371.

Chinn, S. (2003). Obesity and asthma: evidence for and against a causal relation. Journal of Asthma 40:1-16.

Chinn, S., & Rona, R.J. (2004). Obesity and asthma in children (comment). American Journal of Respiratory and Critical Care Medicine 170:95.

Coates, A.L. (1992). Oxygen therapy, exercise, and cystic fibrosis. Chest 101:2-4.

Connor, E., Bagarazzi, M., McSherry, G., Holland, B., Boland, M., Denny, T., & Oleske, J. (1991). Clinical and laboratory correlates of *Pneumocystis carnii pneumonia* in children infected with HIV. Journal of the American Medical Association 265:1693-1697.

Cooney, T.P., & Thurlbeck, W.M. (1982). Pulmonary hypoplasia in Down's syndrome. New England Journal of Medicine 307:1170-1173.

Cox, G.F., & Kunkel, L.M. (1997). Dystrophies and heart disease. Current Opinion in Cardiology 12:329-343.

Crane, L. (1981). Physical therapy for neonates with respiratory dysfunction. Physical Therapy 61:1764-1773.

Crane, L.D., Zombek, M., Krauss, A.N., & Auld, P.A.M. (1978). Comparison of chest physiotherapy in infants with HMD. Pediatric Research 12:559.

Curran, F.J. (1981). Night ventilation by body respirators for patients in chronic respiratory failure due to late stage Duchenne muscular dystrophy. Archives of Physical Medicine and Rehabilitation 62:270-273.

Cystic Fibrosis Foundation Center Committee and Guidelines Sub-committee. (1990). Cystic fibrosis foundation guidelines for patient services, evaluation, and monitoring in cystic fibrosis centers. American Journal of Disease in Childhood 144: 1311-1312.

D'Angelo, C.T., & Maniscalco, W.M. (2004). Bronchopulmonary dysplasia in preterm infants: pathophysiology and management strategies. Paediatric Drugs 6:303-330.

Daniels, O., Hopman, J.C.W., Stoelinga, G.B.A., Busch, H.J., & Peer, P.G.M. (1982). Doppler flow characteristics in the main pulmonary artery and the Lratio before and after ductal closure in healthy newborns. Pediatric Cardiology 3:99-104.

Darbee, J.C., Ohtake, P.J., Grant, B.J., & Cerny, F.J. (2004). Physicologic evidence for the efficacy of positive expiratory pressure as an airway clearance technique in patients with cystic fibrosis. Physical Therapy 84:524-537.

Davis, P.B. (1994). Evolution of therapy for cystic fibrosis. New England Journal of Medicine 331:672-673.

de Bisschop, C., Guenard, H., Desnot, P., & Vergeret, J. (1999). Reduction of exercise-induced asthma in children by short, repeated warm ups. British Journal of Sports Medicine 33: 100-104.

Dearlove, O.R., Dobson, A., & Super, M. (1998). Anaesthesia and Prader-Willi syndrome. Paediatric Anaesthesia 8:267-271.

Dichter, C.G., Darbee, J.C., Effgen, S.K., & Palisano, R.J. (1993). Assessment of pulmonary function and physical fitness in children with Down syndrome. Pediatric Physical Therapy 5:3-8.

DiMarco, A.F., Kelling, J.S., DiMarco, M.S., Jacobs, I., Shields, R., & Altose, M.D. (1985). The effects of inspiratory resistive training on respiratory function in patients with muscular dystrophy. Muscle and Nerve 8:284-290.

Driscoll, D.J. (1990). The cyanotic newborn. Pediatric Clinics of North America 37:1-23.

Durand, M., Sangha, B., Cabal, L.A., Hoppenbrowers, T., & Hodgman, J.E. (1989). Cardiopulmonary and intracranial pressure changes related to endotracheal suctioning in preterm infants. Critical Care Medicine 17:506-510.

Dyken, M.E., Lin-Dyken, D.C., Poulton, S., Zimmerman, M.B., & Sedars, E. (2003). Prospective polysomnographic analysis of obstructive sleep apnea in down syndrome. Archives of Pediatrics and Adolescent Medicine 157:655-660.

Elkins, M.R., Jones, A., & van der Schans, C. (2004). Positive expiratory pressure physiotherapy for airway clearance in people with cystic fibrosis [review]. The Cochrane Database of Systematic Reviews 4.

Emery, J.R., & Peabody, J.L. (1983). Head position affects intracranial pressure in newborn infants. Journal of Pediatrics 103:950-953.

Emmanouilides, G.C., & Baylen, B.G. (1988). Neonatal cardio-pulmonary distress. St. Louis: Mosby.

Farrel, P.M., & Avery, M.E. (1975). Hyaline membrane disease. American Review of Respiratory Disease 111:657-688.

Finer, N.N., & Boyd, J. (1978). Chest physiotherapy in the neonate: a controlled study. Pediatrics 61:282-285.

Finer, N.N., Moriartey, R.R., Boyd, J., Phillips, H.J., Stewart, A.R., & Ulan, O. (1979). Postextubation atelectasis: a retrospective review and a prospective controlled study. Journal of Pediatrics 94:110-113.

Freedom, R.M., & Benson, L.N. (1992). Tetralogy of Fallot. In Freedom, R.M., Benson, L.N., & Smallhorn, J.F. (Eds). Neonatal heart disease. London: Springer-Verlag.

Freedom, R.M., & Smallhorn, J.F. (1992). Atrioventricular septal defect. In Freedom, R.M., Benson, L.N., & Smallhorn, J.F. (Eds). Neonatal heart disease. London: Springer-Verlag.

Galant, S.P., Crawford, L.J., Morphew, T., Jones, C.A., & Bassin, S. (2004). Predictive value of a cross-cultural asthma case-detection tool in an elementary school population. Pediatrics 114: 307-316.

Georgeson, K.E., & Robertson, D.J. (2004). Minimally invasive surgery in the neonate: review of current evidence. Seminars in Perinatology 28:212-220.

Gerhardt, T., Hehre, D., Feller, R., Reifenberg, L., & Bancalari, E. (1987). Serial determination of pulmonary function in infants with chronic lung disease. Journal of Pediatrics 110:448-456.

Gildein, P., Mocellin, R., & Kaufmehl, K. (1994). Oxygen uptake transient kinetics during constant-load exercise in children after operations of ventricular septal defect, tetralogy of Fallot, transposition of the great arteries, or tricuspid valve atresia. American Journal Cardiology 74:166-169.

Graham, T.P., & Bender, H.W. (1980). Preoperative diagnosis and management of infants with critical congenital heart disease. Annals of Thoracic Surgery 29:272-288.

Greene, M.A., Mavroudis, C., & Backer, C.L. (1994) Patent ductus arteriosus. In Mavroudis, C., & Backer, C.L. (Eds). Pediatric cardiac surgery. St Louis: Mosby.

Gregory, G.A., Gooding, C.A., Phibbs, R.H., & Tooley, W.H. (1974). Meconium aspiration in infants-a prospective study. Journal of Pediatrics 85:848-852.

Griesenbach, U., Geddes, D.M., & Alton, E.W. (2004). Gene therapy for cystic fibrosis: an example for lung gene therapy. Gene Therapy 11(Suppl 1):S43-S50.

Harris, J.C., & Allen, R.P. (1996). Is excessive daytime sleepiness characteristic of Prader-Willi syndrome? The effects of weight change. Archives of Pediatrics and Adolescent Medicine 150:1288-1293.

Hays, R.M., Jordan, R.A., McLaughlin, J.F., Nickel, R.E., & Fisher, L.D. (1989). Central ventilatory dysfunction in myelodysplasia: an independent determinant of survival. Developmental Medicine and Child Neurology 31:366-370.

Hesz, N., & Wolraich, M. (1985). Vocal-cord paralysis and brainstem dysfunction in children with spina bifida. Developmental Medicine and Child Neurology 27:522-531.

Heymann, M.A., & Hanley, F.L. (1994). Physiology of circulation. In Mavroudis, C., & Backer, C.L. (Eds). Pediatric cardiac surgery. St Louis: Mosby.

Homer, S.D. (2004). Effect of education on school-age children's and parent's asthma management. Journal for Specialists in Pediatric Nursing 9:95-102.

Huckabay, L., & Daderian, A.D. (1990). Effect of choices on breathing exercises post-open heart surgery. Dimensions of Critical Care Nursing 9:190-201.

Hukins, C.A., & Hillman, D.R. (2000). Daytime predictors of sleep hypoventilation in Duchene muscular dystrophy. American Journal of Respiratory Critical Care Medicine 161:166-170.

Hutchinson, A.A., Ross, K.R., & Russell, G. (1979). The effects of posture on ventilation and lung mechanics in preterm and light-for-date infants. Pediatrics 64:429-432.

Jobe, A. (1988). The role of surfactant in neonatal adaptation. Seminars in Perinatology 12:113-123.

Johnson, B. (1991). Postoperative physical therapy in the pediatric cardiac surgery patient. Pediatric Physical Therapy 3:14-22.

Johnson, T.R., Moore, W.M., & Jeffries, J.E. (1978). Children are different: developmental physiology, ed 2. Columbus, Ohio: Ross Laboratories.

Kapandji, I.A. (1982). The physiology of the joints, ed 1. New York: Churchill Livingstone.

Katz, V.L., & Bowes, W.A. (1992). Meconium aspiration syndrome: reflections on a murky subject. American Journal of Obstetrics and Gynecology 166:171-183.

Keens, T.G., Krastins, I.R.S., Wannamaker, E.M., Levison, H., Crozier, D.N., & Bryan, A.C. (1977). Ventilatory muscle training in normal subjects and patients with cystic fibrosis. American Review of Respiratory Disease 116:853-860.

Klign, P.H., Oudshoorn, A., van der Ent, C.K., van der Net, J., Kimpen, J.L., & Helders, P.J. (2004). Effects of anaerobic training in children with cystic fibrosis: a randomized controlled study. Chest 125:1299-1305.

Knorr, R.S., Condon, S.K., Dwyer, F.M., & Hoffman, D.F. (2004). Tracking pediatric asthma: the Massachusetts experience using school health records. Environmental Health Perspectives 112:1424-1427.

Koff, P.B. (1993). Development of the cardiopulmonary system. In Koff, P.B., Eitzman, D., & Neu, J. (Eds). Neonatal and pediatric respiratory care. St Louis: Mosby.

Konstan, M.W., Stern, R.C., & Doershuk, C.F. (1994). Efficacy of the Flutter device for airway mucus clearance in patients with cystic fibrosis. Journal of Pediatrics 124:689-693.

Kosorok, M.R., Wei, W.H., & Farrell, P.N. (1996). The incidence of cysteic fibrosis. State Medicine 15:449-462.

Laitman, J.T., & Crelin, E.S. (1980). Developmental change in the upper respiratory system of human infants. Perinatology and Neonatalogy 4:15-21.

Lioy, J., & Manginello, F.P. (1988). A comparison of prone and supine positioning in the immediate postextubation period of neonates. Journal of Pediatrics 112:982-984.

Long, J.G., Phillip, A.G.S., & Lucey, J.F. (1980). Excessive handling as a cause of hypoxemia. Pediatrics 65:203-207.

MacFarlane, P.I., & Heaf, D.P. (1988). Pulmonary function in children after neonatal meconium aspiration syndrome. Archives of Disease in Childhood 63:368-372.

Magee, C.L. (1991). Physical therapy for the child with asthma. Pediatric Physical Therapy 3:23-28.

Mahlmeister, M.J., Fink, J.B., Hoffman, G.L., & Fifer, L.F. (1991). Positive-expiratory-pressure mask therapy: theoretical and practical considerations and a review of the literature. Respiratory Care 36:1218-1229.

Marcus, C.L., Curtis, S., Koerner, C.B., Joffe, A., Serwint, J.R., & Loughlin, G.M. (1996). Evaluation of pulmonary function and polysomnography in obese children and adolescents. Pediatric Pulmonology 21:176-83.

Marin, V.B., Velandia, S., Hunter, B., Gattas, V., Fielbaum, O., Herrera, O., & Diaz, E. (2004). Energy expenditure, nutrition status, and body composition in children with cystic fibrosis. Nutrition 20:181-186.

Marolda, J., Pace, B., Bonforte, R.J., Kotin, N.M., Rabinowitz, J., & Kattan, M. (1991). Pulmonary manifestations of HIV infection in children. Pediatric Pulmonology 10:231-235.

Martin, A.J., Stern, L., Yeates, J., Lepp, D., & Little, J. (1986). Respiratory muscle training in muscular dystrophy. Developmental Medicine and Child Neurology 28:314-318.

Martin, R.J., Herrell, N., Rubin, D., & Fanaroff, A. (1979). Effects of supine and prone positions on arterial oxygen tension in the preterm infant. Pediatrics 63:528-531.

Massery, M. (1991). Chest development as a component of motor development: implications for pediatric physical therapists. Pediatric Physical Therapy 3:3-8.

Mathews, R.A., Nixon, P.A., Stephenson, R.J., Robertson, R.J., Donovan, E.F., Dean, F., Fricker, F.J., Beerman, L.B., & Fischer, D.R. (1983). An exercise program for pediatric patients with congenital heart disease: organizational and physiologic aspects. Journal of Cardiac Rehabilitation 3:467-475.

McColley, S.A. (2004) Cystic fibrosis lung disease: when does it start, and how can it be prevented? The Journal of Pediatrics 145:6-7.

McFadden, R. (1981). Decreasing respiratory compromise during infant suctioning. American Journal of Nursing 81:2158-2161.

Mellins, R.B., & Berdon, W.E. (1994). The lung in human immunodeficiency virus infection. In Phelan, P.D., Olinsky, A., & Robertson, C.F. (Eds). Respiratory illness in children, ed 4. Boston: Blackwell-Scientific Publications.

Merrill, W.H., Hoff, S.J., & Bender, H.W. (1994). Surgical treatment of atrioventricular septal defects. In Mavroudis, C., & Backer, C.L. (Eds). Pediatric cardiac surgery. St. Louis: Mosby.

Milgrom, H., & Taussig, L.M. (1999). Keeping children with exercise-induced asthma active. Pediatrics 104:38-42.

Milne, M.J., Sung, R.Y.T., Fok, T.F., & Crozier, I.G. (1989). Doppler echocardiographic assessment of shunting via the ductus arteriosus in newborn infants. American Journal of Cardiology 64:102-105.

Milross, M.A., Piper, A.J., Dobbin, C.J., Bye, P.T., & Grunstein, R.R. (2004). Sleep disordered breathing in cystic fibrosis. Sleep Medicine Reviews 8:253-255.

Mitchell, S.C., Korones, S.B., & Berendes, H.W. (1971). Congenital heart disease in 56,109 births: incidence and natural history. Circulation 43:323-331.

Moerchen, V.A. (1994) Respiration and motor development: a systems perspective. Neurology Report 18:8-10.

Moorcroft, A.J., Dodd, M.E., & Webb, A.K. (1997). Long-term change in exercise capacity, body mass, and pulmonary function in adults with cystic fibrosis. Chest 111:338-343.

Moore, J.W., Levi, D.S., Moore, S.D., Schneider, D.J., & Berdis, F. (2005). Interventional treatment of patent ductus arteriosus in 2004. Catheter Cardiovascular Intervention 64:91-101.

Muller, N.L., & Bryan, A.C. (1979). Chest wall mechanics and respiratory muscle in infants. Pediatric Clinics of North America 26:503-516.

Murai, D.T., & Grant, J.W. (1994). Continuous oscillation therapy improves pulmonary outcome of incubated newborns: results of a prospective, randomized, controlled trial. Critical Care Medicine 22:1147-1154.

Musewe, N.N., & Olley, P.M. (1994). Patent ductus arteriosus. In Freedom, R.M., Benson, L.N., & Smallhorn, J.F. (Eds). Neonatal heart disease. London: Springer-Verlag.

Ng, D.K., & Chan, C-H. (2004). Obesity is an important risk factor for sleep disordered breathing in children with down syndrome [comment]. Sleep 27:1023-1024.

Ng, D.K., Lam, Y.Y., Kwok, K.L., & Chow, P.Y. (2004). Obstructive sleep apnea in children. Hong Kong Medical Journal 10:44-48.

Nixon, P.A. (1996). Role of exercise in the evaluation and management of pulmonary disease in children and youth [review]. Medicine and Science in Sports and Exercise 28:414-420.

Northway, W.H., Rosan, R.C., & Porter, D.Y. (1967). Pulmonary disease following respirator therapy of hyaline membrane disease: bronchopulmonary dysplasia. New England Journal of Medicine 276:357-368.

Northway, W.H. (1979). Observations on bronchopulmonary dysplasia. Journal of Pediatrics 95:815-818.

Nudel, D.B., & Gootman, N. (1983). Clinical aspects of neonatal circulation. In Gootman, N., & Gootman, P.M. (Eds). Perinatal cardiovascular function. New York: Marcel Dekker.

Oren, J., Kelly, D.H., Todres, D., & Shannon, D.C. (1986). Respiratory complications in patients with myelodysplasia and Arnold-Chiari malformation. American Journal of Disease in Childhood 140:221-224.

Orenstein, S.R., & Orenstein, D.M. (1988). Gastoesophageal reflux and respiratory disease in children. Journal of Pediatrics 112:847-858.

Parker, R.A., Lindstrom, D.P., & Cotton, R.B. (1992). Improved survival accounts for most, but not all, of the increase in bronchopulmonary dysplasia. Pediatrics 90:663-668.

Park, M.K. (1988). Pediatric cardiology for practitioners. St. Louis: Mosby.

Perlman, J.M., & Volpe, J.J. (1983). Suctioning in the preterm infant: effects on cerebral blood flow velocity, intracranial pressure, and arterial blood pressure. Pediatrics 72:329-334.

Phelan, P.D., Olinsky, A., & Robertson, C.F. (Eds). (1994). Respiratory illness in children. Boston: Blackwell-Scientific Publications.

Phillips, G.E., Pike, S.E., Rosenthal, M., & Bush, A. (1998). Holding the baby: head downwards positioning for physiotherapy does not cause gastro-oesophageal reflux. European Respiratory Journal 12:954-957.

Pinsky, W.W., & Arciniegas, E. (1990). Tetralogy of Fallot. Pediatric Clinics of North America 37:179-192.

Pullan, C.R., & Hey, E.N. (1982). Wheezing, asthma, and pulmonary dysfunction 10 years after infection with respiratory syncytial virus in infancy. British Medical Journal 284:1665-1669.

Pryor, J.A. (1991). The forced expiration technique. In Pryor, J.A. (Ed). Respiratory care. London: Churchill-Livingstone.

Pryor, J.A., & Webber, B.A. (1979). An evaluation of the forced expiration technique as an adjunct to postural drainage. Physiotherapy 65:304-307.

Ranganathan, S.C., Stocks, J., Dezateux, C., Bush, A., Wade, A., Carr, S., Castle, R., Dinwiddie, R., Hoo, A.F., Lum, S., Price, J., Stoobant, J., & Wallis, C. (2004). The evolution of airway function in early childhood following clinical diagnosis of cystic fibrosis. American Journal of Respiratory and Critical Care Medicine 169:928-933.

Raphael, J-C., Chevret, S., Chastang, C., & Bouvet, F. (1994). Randomised trial of preventative nasal ventilation in Duchene muscular dystrophy. Lancet 343:1600-1604.

Ray, R.M., & Senders, C.W. (2001). Airway management in the obese child. Pediatric Clinics of North America 48:1055-1063.

Reid, W.D., & Loveridge, B.M. (1983). Ventilatory muscle endurance training in patients with chronic obstructive airway disease. Physiotherapy Canada 35:197-205.

Rickards, A.L., Ford, G.W., Kitchen, W.H., Doyle, L.W., Lissenden, J.V., & Keith, C.G. (1987). Extremely-low-birth-weight infants: neurological, psychological, growth and health status beyond five years of age. Medical Journal of Australia 147:476-481.

Rideau, Y., Glorion, B., Delaubier, A., Tarle, O., & Bach, J. (1984). The treatment of scoliosis in Duchene muscular dystrophy. Muscle and Nerve 7:281-286.

Ross, J., & Dean, E. (1989). Integrating physiological principles into the comprehensive management of cardiopulmonary dysfunction. Physical Therapy 69:255-259.

Rudolph, A.M. (1970). The changes in the circulation after birth: their importance in congenital heart disease. Circulation 41:343-359.

Rudolph, A.M. (1980). High pulmonary vascular resistance after birth: physiologic considerations and etiologic classification. Clinical Pediatrics 19:585-590.

Schrander-Stumpel, C.T., Curfs, L.M., Sastrowijoto, P., Cassidy, S.B., Schrander, J.J., & Fryns, J.P. (2004). Prader-Willi syndrome: causes of death in an international series of 27 cases. American Journal of Medical Genetics 124:333-338.

Scott, G.B., Hutto, C., Makuch, R.H., Mastrucci, M.T., O'Connor, T., Mitchell, C.D., Trapido, E.J., & Parks, W.P. (1989). Survival in children with perinatally acquired human immunodeficiency virus type 1 infection. New England Journal of Medicine 321:1791-1796.

Scott, A.A., & Koff, P.B. (1993). Airway care and chest physiotherapy. In Koff, P.B., Eitzman, D., & Neu, J. (Eds). Neonatal and pediatric respiratory care. St. Louis: Mosby.

Seligman, T., Randel, H.O., & Stevens, J.J. (1970). Conditioning program for children with asthma. Physical Therapy 50:641-647.

Selvadurai, H.C., Blimkie, C.J., Meyers, N., Mellis, C.M., Cooper, P.J., & Van Asperen, P.P. (2002). Randomized controlled study of in-hospital exercise training programs in children with cystic fibrosis. Pediatric Pulmonology 33:194-200.

Shneerson, J.M. & Simonds, A.K. (2002). Noninvasive ventilation for chest wall and neuromuscular disorders. European Respiratory Journal 20:480-487.

Shoni, M.H. (1989). Autogenic drainage: a modern approach to physiotherapy in cystic fibrosis. Journal of the Royal Society of Medicine 82(Suppl 16):32-37.

Sinclair, D. (1978). Human growth after birth. London: Oxford University Press.

Smith, P.E.M, Calverley, P.M.A, Edwards, R.H.T., Evans, G.A., & Campbell, E.J.M. (1987). Practical problems in the respiratory care of patients with muscular dystrophy. New England Journal of Medicine 316:1197-1205.

Smith, P.E.M., Coakley, J.H., & Edwards, R.H.T. (1988). Respiratory muscle training in Duchene muscular dystrophy. Muscle and Nerve 11:784-785.

Smyth, J.A., Tabachnik, E., Duncan, W.J., Reilly, B.J., & Levison, H. (1981). Pulmonary function and bronchial hyperreactivity in long-term survivors of bronchopulmonary dysplasia. Pediatrics 68:336-340.

Smyth, J.M., Collier, P.S., Darwish, M., Millership, J.S., Halliday, H.L., Peterson, S., & McElnay, J.C. (2004). Intravenous indometacin in preterm infants with symptomatic patent ductus arteriosus. A population pharmacokinetic study. British Journal of Clinical Pharmacology 58:249-258.

Spicer, R.L. (1984). Cardiovascular disease in Down syndrome. Pediatric Clinics of North America 31:1331-1343.

Staab, D. (2004). Cystic fibrosis—therapeutic challenge in cystic fibrosis children. European Journal of Endocrinology 151 (Suppl 1):S77-S80.

Starnes, V.A., Luciani, G.B., Latter, D.A., & Griffin, M.L. (1994). Current surgical management of tetralogy of Fallot. Annals of Thoracic Surgery 58:211-215.

Stern, L.M., Martin, A.J., Jones, N., Garrett, R., & Yeates, J. (1991). Respiratory training in Duchene dystrophy. Developmental Medicine and Child Neurology 33:649.

Stubbs, C.O., & Lee, A.J. (2004). The obesity epidemic: both energy intake and physical activity contribute. Medical Journal of Australia 181:489-491.

Swaminathan, S., Paton, J.Y., Ward, S.L.D., Jacobs, R.A., Sargent, C.W., & Keens, T.G. (1989). Abnormal control of ventilation in adolescents with myelodysplasia. Journal of Pediatrics 115:898-903.

Swaminathan, S., Quinn, J., Stabile, M.W., Bader, D., Platzker, A.C.G., & Keens, T.G. (1989). Long-term pulmonary sequelae of meconium aspiration syndrome. Journal of Pediatrics 114:356-361.

Taras, H., Wright, S., Brennan, J., Campana, J., & Lofgren, R. (2004). Impact of school nurse case management on students with asthma. Journal of School Health 74:213-219.

Thoresen, M., Cowan, F., & Whitelaw, A. (1988). Effect of tilting on oxygenation in newborn infants. Archives of Disease in Childhood 63:315-317.

Thurlbeck, W.M. (1975). Postnatal growth and development of the lung. American Review of Respiratory Disease 111:803-844.

Tomassoni, T.L., Galioto, F.M., & Vaccaro, P. (1991). Cardiopulmonary exercise testing in children following surgery for tetralogy of Fallot. American Journal of Disease in Childhood 145:1290-1293.

Vandekercckhove, K, Macrae, D. & Slavik, Z. (2005). Nonsurgical treatment of patent arterial duct in term neonates with congenital heart disease: The role of intravenous indomethacin. Pediatric Cardiology January 27 [ePub ahead of print].

Vianello, A., Bevilacqua, M., Salvador, V., Cardaioli, C., & Vincenti, E. (1994). Long-term nasal intermittent positive pressure ventilation in advanced Duchene's Muscular Dystrophy. Chest 105:445-448.

Vohr, B.R., Bell, E.F., & Oh, W. (1982). Infants with bronchopulmonary dysplasia: growth pattern and neurologic and developmental outcome. American Journal of Disease in Childhood 136:443-447.

Voyles, J.B. (1981). Bronchopulmonary dysplasia. American Journal of Nursing 81:510-514.

Wallis, S., & Harvey, D. (1979). Respiratory distress: its cause and management. Nursing Times 75:1264-1272.

Walther, F.J., Benders, M.J., & Leighton, J.O. (1992). Persistent pulmonary hypertension in premature neonates with severe respiratory distress syndrome. Pediatrics 90:899-903.

Ward, S.L.D., Jacobs, R.A., Gates, E.P., Hart, L.D., & Keens, T.G. (1986). Abnormal ventilatory patterns during sleep in infants with myelomeningocele. Journal of Pediatrics 4:631-634.

Waring, W.W. (1975). Respiratory diseases in children—an overview. Respiratory Care 20:1138-1145.

Weinstein, M.R., & Oh, W. (1981). Oxygen consumption in infants with bronchopulmonary dysplasia. Journal of Pediatrics 99:958-961.

Wiswell, T.E., & Bent, R.C. (1993). Meconium staining and the meconium aspiration syndrome. Pediatric Clinics of North America 40:955-981.

Wiswell, T.E., Tuggle, J.M., & Turner, B.S. (1990). Meconium aspiration syndrome: have we made a difference? Pediatrics 85:715-721.

Wood, R.E., Boat, T.F., & Doershuk, C.F. (1976). Cystic Fibrosis. American Review of Respiratory Disease 113:833-878.

Yao, A.C. (1983). Cardiovascular changes during the transition from fetal to neonatal life. In Gootman, N., & Gootman, P.M. (Eds). Perinatal cardiovascular function. New York: Marcel Dekker.

Yeh, T.F., Lilien, L.D., Leu, S.T. & Pildes, R.S. (1984). Increased O_2 consumption and energy loss in premature infants following medical care procedures. Biology of the Neonate 46:157-162.

CHAPTER 38

The Aging Patient

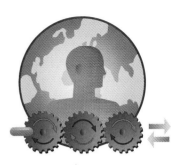

Elizabeth J. Protas

KEY TERMS   Aging
                 Autonomic
                 Cardiovascular changes

Exercise changes
Pulmonary changes

Cardiopulmonary and autonomic nervous system functions are dynamic and undergo changes as people age. It is important for physical therapists to be aware of changes that occur with normal aging in order to better understand the impact of disease and impairment on these systems' functions. In addition, a clear understanding of how these systems respond to exercise training will assist the clinician in prescribing and evaluating exercise interventions in elders.

Understanding aging is more complicated than simply taking into account chronological age. As people age, greater variability occurs between individuals, making predications about any one individual difficult. The trends of some changes are probably not linear but curvilinear, with changes accelerating after age 65. Thus many of the physiological studies that have been done with 60-year-olds may not apply to individuals who are 80, 90, or 100 years of age. Most of the studies that are available on exercise in older individuals have been conducted with subjects who are under 65 years of age. The vast majority of these studies only used men as subjects or had a small number of women in the sample. Sex may be an important variable in relation to exercise and aging, but the data available on this issue are limited. Another consideration is the composition of study populations. With increasing age there is a greater incidence of disease. Latent cardiovascular disease and histories of chronic illnesses are common in older populations. Comorbidities are frequently encountered in

elders. It may be more common for a person over 75 years of age to have health problems than be healthy. As a physical therapist, I may be more interested in the responses of a frail 85- or 90-year-old woman who has a history of hypertension, coronary artery disease, and diabetes than someone who is healthy at this age because this reflects the population who is referred to physical therapy. The occurrence of disease states in study populations may impact the cardiopulmonary responses to exercise. Furthermore, the study of the physiological aspects of exercise and aging is still evolving. The literature can be confusing and contradictory, making conclusions and generalizations difficult. An attempt is made in this chapter to provide some direction in this confusing maze of information.

An additional issue is a model of aging that might sort out some of the determinants of aging (Figure 38-1). The model identifies biological factors, disuse, disease, and psychosocial concerns as determinants of aging. Biological factors address genetics, sex, cellular mechanisms, and metabolic and physiological responses that influence aging. Disuse is implicated in the more sedentary lifestyle led by many elders, which results in loss of exercise capacity (Bortz, 1993). With exercise training, it should be possible to reverse or attenuate capacities that decline as a result of disuse. The emphasis in this chapter is on the biological and disuse characteristics of aging. The impact of various diseases is discussed in other chapters. Psychosocial issues related to exercise and aging are not discussed.

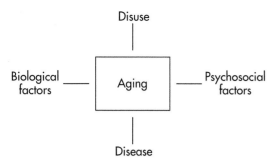

FIGURE 38-1 A model of aging that identifies the major determinants underlying the aging process.

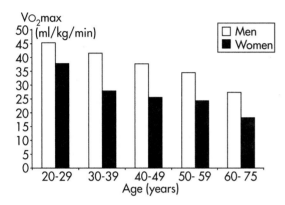

FIGURE 38-2 Decline in VO_{2max} from 20 to 75 years of age in both men and women. *(From Hossack, K.F., & Bruce, R.A. [1982]. Maximal cardiac function in sedentary normal men and women: comparison of age-related changes Journal of Applied Physiology 53:799-804.)*

CARDIAC CHANGES WITH AGING

Aerobic Capacity

Aerobic capacity is the maximum ability to perform exercise with large muscle groups. This ability is produced by interaction of the lungs, heart, and peripheral tissues. The most common indirect measure of aerobic capacity is maximum oxygen consumption (VO_{2max}), or the maximum amount of oxygen used during exercise. VO_{2max} is directly related to cardiac output (the amount of blood pumped by the heart) and the arteriovenous oxygen difference (the amount of oxygen extracted in the periphery). Cardiac output is the product of heart rate times stroke volume. Aerobic capacity reflects the central cardiac function and the efficiency of the peripheral tissues to extract and use oxygen.

VO_{2max} declines with age (McGuire et al, 2001; Beere et al, 1999) at a rate of between 0.40 to 0.50 ml/kg/min per year in men and between 0.20 to 0.35 ml/kg/min per year in women (Figure 38-2) (Buskirk & Hodgson, 1987). The reduction is approximately 10% per decade. The decline is faster and greater in men than in women; however, men have a larger capacity than women (Cunningham et al, 1999; Hossack &

Bruce, 1982). VO_{2max} is related to body size, which tends to be smaller in women than men. Increases in body weight along with aging result in reduced VO_{2max}, even if aerobic capacity remains the same, because relative oxygen consumption is related to body weight. Reduced physical activity with aging also contributes to a loss of VO_{2max}.

Considerable disagreement exists regarding the mechanisms that contribute to the decline in VO_{2max} with age. Both cardiac and peripheral changes contribute to the loss. A reduction in maximum cardiac output was proposed to account for 50% to 100% of the total reduction in VO_{2max} (Dempsey & Seals, 1995; Ogawa et al, 1992; Saltin, 1986). McGuire et al (2001), however, suggested that reductions in peripheral oxygen withdrawal were the dominant mechanism responsible for reduced VO_{2max} with age. A major component to the decline in maximum cardiac output is a decreased maximum heart rate (Beere et al, 1999; Ogawa et al, 1992; Hagberg, 1987). The decline in heart rate is linearly related to age and occurs in both sedentary and active persons (Cunningham et al, 1999; Sidney & Shephard, 1977). Discrepancies in the age-related response of maximum stroke volume also exist; observations have found reduced, preserved, and increased maximum stroke volume with age (Lakatta, 2002; McGuire et al, 2001; Beere et al, 1999; Ogawa et al, 1992). The decline in VO_{2max} associated with aging is most likely attributable to a decrease in maximum heart rate, stroke volume, and arteriovenous oxygen difference, although each component's contribution varies (Dempsey & Seals, 1995; Lakatta, 1993).

Cardiac Mechanics

Age-related changes in cardiac structure occur in the form of left ventricular wall thickness (Gates et al, 2003; Lakatta, 2002) and are attributed to an increase in size of cardiac myocytes (Olivetti et al, 1991) and increased collagen (Lakatta, 2002). Additional cardiac structural changes include increases in vascular intimal thickness, vascular stiffness, and left arterial dimension (Lakatta, 2003; Lakatta, 2002).

The diastolic properties (cardiac filling) of the heart alter with age. Diastole requires relaxation of the myocardial fibers, sufficient venous return to rapidly fill the heart, and timing of the atrial contraction to contribute to the end diastolic volume. Relaxation is possibly hampered by an increase in ventricular stiffness, although there is limited evidence of this in humans (Lakatta, 1993). The period of the isovolumic myocardial relaxation (the time between aortic valve closing and mitral valve opening) is prolonged (Gates et al., 2003). Likewise, the peak rate of left ventricular filling during early diastole is progressively reduced so that between the ages of 20 and 80 years, the average rate can be reduced up to 50% (Lakatta, 2002). Despite the changes in early diastole, the resting left ventricular end-diastolic volume remains the same because of an enhanced left atrial contribution to ventricular filling (Lakatta, 2002). This is accompanied by an enlarged left atrium and an audible fourth heart sound in most older adults (Lakatta, 2002; Fleg et al, 1988).

Considerable disagreement exists regarding what happens to diastolic function during exercise. End-diastolic volume index (end-diastolic volume normalized for body surface) increases similarly in both young and older men during submaximal exercise; however, only older men remain at these elevated levels during exhaustive exercise (Lakatta, 2002). Filling pressures during exercise in men increase with age (Ehrsam et al, 1983). In addition, peak left ventricular diastolic filling rate during submaximal and maximal exercise decreases with aging (Levy et al, 1993; Schulman et al, 1992). Decreased filling rate is associated with increased ventricular stiffness and prolonged relaxation times (Ehsani, 1989).

Resting measures of systolic and cardiac pump function do not change with aging. The resting end-systolic volume and stroke volume do not change with age. Likewise, ejection fraction at rest (end-diastolic volume – [end-systolic volume/end-diastolic volume]) is similar in healthy older and younger individuals (Lakatta, 2002).

Unlike resting systolic function, the pumping function of the heart changes considerably in response to exercise. Myocardial contractility as measured by the ratio of end-systolic volume to systolic arterial pressure declines during exercise as people age (Lakatta, 1993). The end-systolic volume index increases, whereas the ejection fraction decreases during exercise (Lakatta, 2002). Reduced contractile performance is related to a decrease in the response to beta-adrenergic stimulation, changes in the myocardium, increased systolic blood pressure, and ventricular wall abnormalities (Dempsey & Seals, 1995).

Impact of Exercise Training on Aerobic Capacity and Cardiac Mechanics

Older persons who remain active reduce the rate of decline in VO_{2max} to 5% per decade, compared with an anticipated decline of 10% per decade in sedentary adults (Hagberg, 1987). A metaanalysis of 29 studies on endurance training, which included 1030 men and 466 women between the ages of 61 and 78 years, concluded that endurance training significantly increases functional capacity in young elders (Green & Crouse, 1995). Less improvement was seen with increasing age, a shorter length of training, low VO_{2max} before training, and short duration of exercise sessions. The analysis suggests that a healthy 68-year-old individual who exercises for 30 minutes three times per week for four to six months can improve VO_{2max} by 14% (Green & Crouse, 1995). Similar improvements occur in both men and women (Kohrt et al, 1991; Warren et al, 1993).

The mechanisms underlying improvements in VO_{2max} in elderly persons who engage in endurance training are not clear. One consistent finding is greater extraction of oxygen in the exercising skeletal muscle, which produces a wider arteriovenous oxygen difference in both older men and women (Wilmore et al, 2001; Ogawa et al, 1992; Ehsani, 1989). This implies that adaptations in the peripheral skeletal muscles

account for some of the increase in VO_{2max} in elders. The impact of exercise training on maximum cardiac output is uncertain (Ehsani, 1989). Maximum cardiac output can either remain the same or increase after exercise training, depending on the effect of training on maximum stroke volume and maximum heart rate. Maximum heart rate remains the same in older men regardless of activity level, suggesting that the decline in maximal heart rate depends on factors other than exercise and physical fitness (Seals et al, 1985). A decrease in response to circulating catecholamines is most often cited as the reason for changes in maximum heart rate with aging (Rodeheffer et al, 1984). Relatively intense endurance training for a year or more can increase peak stroke volume in men (Coudert & Praagh, 2000; Ehsani et al, 1991; Seals et al, 1994). Adaptations to exercise training in older women have been attributed predominantly to peripheral changes in arteriovenous oxygen difference rather than central changes in cardiac function (Spina, 1999; Spina et al, 1993). This apparently occurs despite intensive endurance training over a year-long period. In contrast, a relatively recent study that compared men and women who were masters athletes with healthy sedentary seniors, healthy young persons, and sedentary controls reported that stroke volume for any given filling pressure was greater for masters athletes compared to age-matched sedentary elders (Arbab-Zadeh et al, 2004). Further studies examining the outcomes of prolonged, sustained endurance training in older men and women are needed to determine what adaptations occur in women.

The diastolic changes that occur with aging can be reversed by exercise training (Levy et al, 1993). Levy et al intensively endurance trained 13 rigorously screened older men aged 60 to 82 years (mean age 68 years) and 11 younger men in their twenties for six months. The training produced increased resting, submaximal, and peak filling rates for the older group comparable to the changes seen in the younger group (Levy et al, 1993). End-diastolic peak volume at rest and exercise also increase after lengthy endurance training (Ehsani et al, 1991). Thus training reduces the age-associated diastolic changes. The mechanisms of this response are uncertain in humans. Studies in rats have shown that exercise training increases calcium uptake in cardiac sarcoplasmic reticulum, decreases relaxation time, reduces the decline of left ventricular pressure, enhances fatty acid oxidation, and increases cytochrome c oxidase levels (Levy et al, 1993; Tate et al, 1990; Starnes et al, 1983). All of these changes have been associated with reduced diastolic function with aging.

Exercise training can also improve systolic performance in older men as reflected by the increase in exercise stroke volume. Increased peak stroke volume occurs with an increased exercise ejection fraction, a decrease in end-systolic volume, and greater left ventricular wall mass (Beere et al, 1999; Ehsani et al, 1991; Seals et al, 1994). These changes apparently do not occur in older, estrogen-deficient women (Spina et al, 1993). Table 38-1 contains a summary of these changes.

TABLE 38-1

Cardiac Changes with Aging

	BECAUSE OF AGING	AFTER EXERCISE TRAINING
Maximum Exercise		
Oxygen consumption	↓	↑
Heart rate	↓	↔
Stroke volume	↓	↑, ↔
Arteriovenous oxygen difference	↓	↑
Cardiac output	↓	↑, ↔
Cardiac function		
Diastolic		
Left ventricular wall thickness	↑, ↓ after 80	↑
Left ventricular filling rate	↓	↑
End-diastolic volume	↔	↑
Systolic		
Myocardial contractility	↓	↑, ↔*
End-systolic volume	↑	↓, ↔*
Ejection fraction	↓	↑, ↔*

↑, Increase; ↓, decrease; ↔, no change.
*In women.

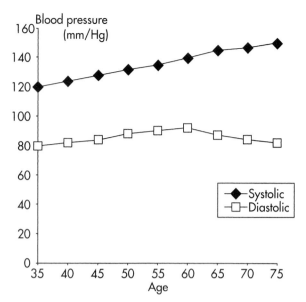

FIGURE 38-3 Changes in systolic and diastolic blood pressures as people age. *(From Timiras, P.S. [Ed] [1988]. Cardiovascular alterations with age: atherosclerosis, coronary heart disease and hypertension. In Physiological basis of aging and geriatrics. Boca Raton, Fla: CRC.)*

Vascular and Autonomic Changes with Aging

Aging results in an increase in arterial stiffness because of a loss of elastin, elastin fractures, and an increase in collagen and calcification (Lakatta, 2003; Roach & Burton, 1959). Arterial wall thickness and diameter and resting systolic pressure also increase (Figure 38-3) (Lakatta, 2003; Lakatta, 1993). It is unclear whether peripheral vascular resistance increases in normotensive older adults. Changes in the structure, size, and reactivity of the arteries increase the work of the left ventricle and have been directly implicated in the increase in cardiac myocyte size.

Complaints of dizziness when an older patient moves from supine to standing are frequently encountered by the physical therapist. Postural hypotension, or orthostatic intolerance, generally does not occur in healthy community dwelling elders but is common in debilitated, institutionalized individuals over the age of 70 years (Tsutsui et al, 2002; Lipsitz, 1989). Orthostatic intolerance is associated with decreased resting diastolic function, possibly decreased stroke volume, extreme inactivity, and, in individuals with hypertension, high levels of systolic blood pressure (Harris et al, 1991).

There are decreases in baroreceptor and cardiopulmonary reflexes with aging (Lakatta, 1993; Cleroux et al, 1989). Arterial and venous dilation are reduced, but vasoconstriction is relatively spared. The heart demonstrates an overall decrease in responsiveness to autonomic stimulation. Older individuals experience higher central venous and mean arterial pressures, but lower forearm blood flow and forearm vascular resistance in response to passive leg raising (Cleroux et al, 1989). During submaximal and maximal exercise, arterial blood

pressure is either unchanged or increased when younger subjects are compared with older subjects (Seals, 1993). There also appears to be impaired peripheral vasodilation in skeletal muscle in response to exercise (Ogawa et al, 1992). Redistribution of blood flow during exercise normally involves the shunting of blood from inactive limbs and viscera. There seems to be an enhanced vasoconstriction in inactive muscles during dynamic exercise in healthy older men (Taylor et al, 1992).

Effect of Exercise Training on Vascular and Autonomic Function in Aging

Exercise training improves peripheral blood flow in skeletal muscle in 60-year-old men and women (Beere et al, 1999; Martin et al, 1991). Exercise training, specifically aerobic training, has been shown to decrease blood pressure (ACSM, 2004). Meta-analysis revealed that four or more weeks of aerobic training could decrease systolic and diastolic blood pressure (Halbert et al, 1997) and mean arterial blood pressure responses when compared with sedentary individuals (Martin et al, 1991). Aerobic training also reduces the age-related decline in cardiovagal baroreflex sensitivity and partially restores diminished cardiovagal baroreflex sensitivity in older men (Monahand et al, 2000). Aerobic training alters the autonomic nervous system and its control over resting heart rate by enhancing parasympathetic activity and attenuating sympathetic activity (Carter et al, 2003). During vigorous exercise, the predominant activity of the autonomic nervous system is to increase sympathetic nerve activity, producing an

TABLE 38-2		
Vascular and Autonomic Changes with Aging*		
	BECAUSE OF AGING	AFTER EXERCISE TRAINING
Arterial wall thickness	↑	?
Systolic blood pressure	↑	↓
Diastolic blood pressure	↑ and ↔	↓
Orthostatic tolerance	↔	?
Arterial and venous dilation	↓	?
Vasoconstriction	↔	↔
Central venous pressure	↑	?

*↑, Increases; ↓, decreases; ↔, unchanged; ?, insufficient data on older adult subjects.

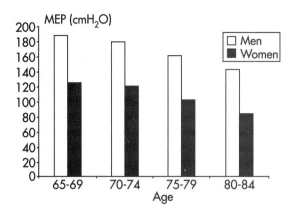

FIGURE 38-4 Decrease in maximum expiratory pressures between 65 and 84 years of age for both men and women. This is a measure of respiratory muscle strength. *(From Enright, P.L., Kronmal, R.A., Monlio, T.A., Schenker, M.B., & Hyatt, R.E. [1994]. Respiratory muscle strength in the elderly. American Journal of Respiratory Critical Care Medicine 149:430-438.)*

increase in norepinephrine concentrations and increasing blood flow via dilation of the large arteries and constriction of the veins (Lakatta, 2002; Ng et al, 1994) (Table 38-2). Long-term aerobic training, however, reduces sympathetic nerve activity for a given work rate, thereby lowering the exercise heart rate at a given work rate (Carter et al, 2003).

PULMONARY FUNCTION

Structural and Functional Changes with Aging

Two major changes to the pulmonary system associated with aging are decreased elastic recoil and stiffening of the chest wall (Zaugg & Lucchinetti, 2000; Dempsey & Seals, 1995). Elastic recoil of the lungs depends on the composition of the connective tissue, the structure of the connective tissue, and alveolar surface tension produced by surfactant (Dempsey & Seals, 1995). Very limited evidence suggests that the structure of the connective tissue may be the primary mechanism for age-associated change in elastic recoil. Chest wall stiffness is accompanied by an increase in chest anterioposterior diameter, costal cartilage calcification, narrowing of the intervertebral disks, and changes in the rib to vertebrae articulations (Zaugg & Lucchinetti, 2000; Crapo, 1993).

Decreases occur with the alveolar-capillary surface area, the alveolar septal surface area, and the total surface area of lung parenchyma (Brody and Thurlbeck, 1985). This reduces the alveolar surface area available for gas exchange and increases the amount of physiological dead space (Zaugg & Lucchinetti, 2000).

Loss of elastic recoil with aging is directly associated with reduced forced expiratory flow (Babb & Rodarte, 2000). Limitations in exhalation are caused by airway narrowing and closure at all lung volumes; thus reducing forced expiratory volume in one second (FEV_1) (Dempsey & Seals, 1995). Additionally, early airway closure also produces an early closing volume and a relative increase in the total residual volume. The combination of reduced elastic recoil and increased chest wall stiffness further increases residual volume and

leads to a decrease in forced vital capacity in older individuals (Mahler et al, 2003; Janssens et al, 1999). Flow rates are also significantly lower in women and African-Americans than in white men at any age (Dempsey & Seals, 1995).

Respiratory muscle strength, as reflected by the ability to create pressure over a range of lung volumes and flow rates, is similar when comparing healthy 30- and 70-year-olds (Johnson & Dempsey, 1991). This suggests that respiratory muscle strength does not change with aging; however, maximal inspiratory and expiratory pressures have been reported to decrease 15% between the sixth and eighth decades (Figure 38-4) (Enright et al, 1994). Perhaps these observed differences are similar to the differences observed with submaximal and maximal cardiac responses with the dynamic pressure measures over different volumes and flows considered submaximal.

Changes in the surface area result in a decrease in the diffusion capacity of the lung (Mahler et al, 2003; Murray, 1986). Both the loss of surface area and a decrease in pulmonary capillary blood volume contribute to reduced and uneven ventilation-to-perfusion matching in elders. The resting partial arterial pressure of oxygen declines five to 10 mm Hg between the ages 25 and 75 years (Dempsey & Seals, 1995). These changes do not affect the arterial oxymyoglobin saturation or oxygen content. Parallel changes in the peripheral vasculature, pulmonary vascular resistance, and pulmonary arterial pressure at rest increase (Table 38-3).

Changes in Pulmonary Responses to Exercise with Aging

In addition to the structural and functional changes at rest, a number of significant changes occur in breathing during acute exercise. Expiratory flow limitations occur at lower exercise intensities as people age. A normal, healthy 69–year-old will begin to experience flow limitations even in response to moderate exercise (Dempsey & Seals, 1995). Practically, the

TABLE 38-3

Pulmonary Function Changes with Aging

Structure and Function	BECAUSE OF AGING	AFTER EXERCISE TRAINING
Elastic recoil	↓	
Chest wall stiffness	↑	
Alveolar-capilary surface area	↓	
Forced expiratory flow	↓	
Total residual volume	↑	
Forced vital capacity	↓	
Maximum inspiratory and expiratory pressure	↓	
Ventilation-perfusion matching	↓	
Partial arterial pressure oxygen	↓	
Oxygen saturation	↔	
Pulmonary vascular resistance	↑	
Exercise response		
Expiratory flow limitation	↑	↔
Minute ventilation	↑	↓*, ↑†
Work of breathing	↑	↓
Respiratory muscle oxygen consumption	↑	↓
Arterial hypoxemia	↔, ↑	↑
Pulmonary artery pressure	↑	↔
Pulmonary wedge pressure	↑	↔

↑, Increases; ↓, decreases; ↔, unchanged.
*Submaximal.
†Maximal.

individual may experience this by having greater difficulty catching his or her breath during exercise.

Normally as people exercise, the tidal volume increases directly with increasing exercise intensity up to about 50% to 60% of the vital capacity. This remains unchanged as people age, although the vital capacity for elders is reduced (McClaran et al, 1995). Likewise, as exercise and the tidal volume increase there is a slight drop in the ratio of dead space to tidal volume. This drop is not affected by aging, although the older person will breathe more (have a higher minute ventilation) in response to submaximal exercise (Dempsey et al, 2003).

The work of breathing is increased during exercise as people age as a result of a number of factors. Older adults require an increased ventilatory response to exercise in order to attain the same alveolar ventilation and $PaCO_2$ (Dempsey et al, 2003). Combined with the loss of elastic recoil, which causes airway closure at higher lung volumes, expiratory flow limitation occurs at moderate exercise intensities (an expiratory volume of 70 to 100 L·min^{-1}), producing a hyperinflation, a noticeable increase in elastic and flow resistive work of breathing, and shortness of breath (Dempsey et al, 2003). In addition, an increase in the end-expiratory lung volume with increasing exercise results in breathing that occurs at a stiffer

point in the lung-volume relationship. The increased stiffness imposes a higher elastic recoil on the ventilatory muscles, requiring greater pressure development by the inspiratory muscles. The increase in expiratory flow resistance likewise requires greater pressure development by the expiratory muscles. Both the inspiratory and expiratory changes increase the work of breathing. The increase in the work of breathing increases the respiratory muscle oxygen consumption so that the respiratory muscles alone can require 10% to 12% of the total body oxygen consumption during maximal exercise in a sedentary 70-year-old man (Dempsey & Seals, 1995).

What is also apparent is that the reserves used to respond to exercise represent a greater percent of the available capacity. An older individual can exceed 50% of inspiratory muscle capacity even during moderate exercise. This is in contrast to the younger individual who rarely exceeds 50% of the inspiratory muscle capacity with exercise (Dempsey & Seals, 1995). Thus the reserve capacity to generate pleural pressure is reduced in elders by virtue of the fact that greater capacity is needed for even moderate exercise.

The variability characteristic of exercise responses in older individuals is particularly evident when considering gas exchange and pulmonary-vascular hemodynamics. In general, most individuals demonstrate only slight changes in arterial blood-gas homeostasis, but a small number of individuals demonstrate arterial hypoxemia with exercise (Dempsey & Seals, 1995). Some studies suggest that this response may be a factor of fitness level. More fit older individuals showed progressive arterial hypoxemia and carbon dioxide retention during mild-to-moderate exercise (Prefaut et al, 1994; Anselme et al, 1994).

Pulmonary artery pressure increases with age at any oxygen consumption or cardiac output during exercise (Reeves et al, 1989). In addition, the maximum pulmonary artery pressure at maximal exercise is reached at substantially lower oxygen consumption and cardiac output levels in older individuals compared with younger persons. Pulmonary wedge pressure also increases with age and can exceed 25 mm Hg during peak supine exercise (Dempsey & Seals, 1995). Limited data suggest that these high pressures may in turn induce pulmonary edema during intense exercise in elders. Pulmonary edema would limit diffusion and may contribute to ventilation perfusion maldistribution (Dempsey & Seals, 1995).

Effects of Exercise Training on Pulmonary Function

Aerobic training in elders can reduce some of the changes that have been described. Studies that address some of the changes, such as chest wall compliance or pulmonary artery pressure, are limited or nonexistent. The studies that are available deal with relatively young subjects who are 60 to 70 years of age, which does not provide insights into what exercise might do for the those in their seventies and eighties, or beyond.

Aerobic training can significantly decrease submaximal minute ventilation (Makrides et al, 1986; Warren et al, 1993).

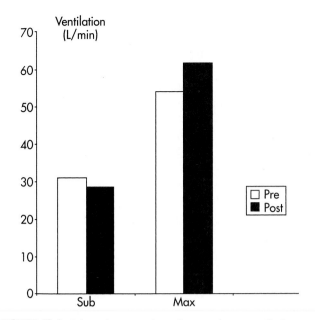

FIGURE 38-5 Submaximum and maximum minute ventilation preexercise and postexercise training with a 12-week walking program in women whose mean age was 72.5 years. *(From Warren, B.J., Nieman, D.C., Dotson, R.G., Adkins, C.H., O'Donnell, K.A., Haddock, B.L., & Butterworth, D.E. [1993]. Cardiorespiratory responses to exercise training in septuagenarian women. International Journal of Sports Medicine 14:60-65.)*

One study used a walking program with 70-year-old women over a 12-week period and demonstrated a 7.7% drop in submaximal minute ventilation (Figure 38-5) (Warren et al, 1993). Decreased minute ventilation is accompanied by a decrease in carbon dioxide production, respiratory exchange ratio (carbon dioxide production/oxygen consumption), and blood lactate level for any given level of submaximal exercise (Makrides et al, 1986; Warren et al, 1993). Thus the improved ventilatory efficiency after training may have more to do with improved efficiency in the periphery rather than an impact on the pulmonary system directly. Improved peripheral metabolic efficiency results in the production of less carbon dioxide; therefore the lungs do not have to work as hard to eliminate carbon dioxide. The important functional results of these changes are that the older adults who engage in exercise training will experience less breathlessness, a lower perceived exertion, and will use a lower percentage of their maximal ventilatory capacity during exercise (Jones, 1986).

Exercise training also increases maximum ventilatory responses during maximal exercise (Warren et al, 1993; Jones, 1986). The 12-week walking program referred to above increased maximum minute ventilation by 14% in 70-year-old women (see Figure 38-5) (Jones, 1986). These women walked five days per week at an intensity of 78% of the maximal treadmill heart rate, or 118 beats per minute on average, so even though the program was not very strenuous it produced substantial changes in maximum ventilation. Exercise training can improve submaximal ventilatory

efficiency and increase maximum ventilation in elders. Table 38-3 summarizes the pulmonary changes seen with aging and exercise.

SUMMARY

As people age, profound changes occur at rest and in response to submaximal and maximal exercise. Many of these changes are reduced or reversed as a result of exercise training. The implication is that many of these changes may have more to do with disuse than aging per se. Sedentary individuals tend to show these changes to a greater extent than more active seniors. Prevailing evidence suggests that elders at any age can derive benefits from exercise training. Even very modest, short-term interventions have proven efficacious. Older individuals should be encouraged to engage in regular physical activity to improve their exercise capacity.

Review Questions

1. What are the major changes that occur with aging in the cardiovascular system?
2. What outcomes will exercise training produce in an older adult's cardiovascular system?
3. What are the major changes that occur with aging in the autonomic nervous system in response to exercise, and which of these changes can be influenced by exercise training?
4. What are the major changes that occur in the pulmonary system with aging and in response to exercise?
5. Describe the possible impact of exercise training on the aging pulmonary system.

REFERENCES

American College of Sports Medicine. (2004). Position stand on exercise and hypertension. Medicine and Science in Sports and Exercise 36:533-553.

Anselme, F., Caillaud, C., Couret, I., Rossi, M., & Prefaut, C. (1994). Histamine and exercise-induced hypoxemia in highly trained athletes. Journal of Applied Physiology 76:127-132.

Arbab-Zadeh, A., Dijk, E., Prasad, A., Fu, Q., Torres, P., Zhang, R., Thomas, J.D., Palmer, D., & Levine, B. (2004). Effect of aging and physical activity on left ventricular compliance. Circulation 110:1799-1805.

Babb, T.G. & Rodarte, J.R. (2000). Mechanism of reduced maximal expiratory flow with aging. Journal of Applied Physiology 89:505-511.

Beere, P.A., Russell, S.D., Morey, M.C., Kitzman, D.W., & Higginbotham, M.B. (1999). Aerobic exercise training can reserve age-related peripheral circulatory changes in healthy older men. Circulation 100:1085-1094.

Bortz, W.M. (1993). The physics of frailty. Journal American Geriatric Society 41:1004-1008.

Brody, J.S., & Thurlbeck, W.M. (1985). Development, growth, and aging of the lung. In Fishman, A.P. (Ed). Handbook of physiology, ed 3.

Brown, C.M., Hetch, M.J., Weih, A. Neundorfer, B. & Hilz, M.J. (2003). Effects of age on the cardiac and vascular limbs of the arterial baroreflex. European Journal of Clinical Investigations 33:10-16.

Buskirk, E.R., & Hodgson, J.L. (1987). Age and aerobic power: the rate of changes in men and women. Federation Proceedings 46:1824-1829.

Carter, J.B., Banister, E.W. & Blaber, A.P. (2003). Effect of endurance exercise on autonomic control of the heart. Sports Medicine 33:33-46.

Cleroux, J., Giannattasio, C., Bolla, G., Cuspidi, C., Grassi, G., Mazzola, C., Sampieri, L., Seravalle, G., Valsecchi, M., & Mancia, G. (1989). Decreased cardiorespiratory reflexes with aging in normotensive humans. American Journal of Physiology 257:H961-H968.

Coudert, J., & Praagh, E.V. (2000). Endurance exercise training in the elderly: effects on cardiovascular function. Current Opinion in Clinical Nutrition and Metabolic Care 3:479-483.

Crapo, R.O. (1993). The aging lung. In Mahler, D.A. (Ed). Pulmonary disease in the elderly. New York: Marcel Dekker.

Cunningham, D.A., Paterson, D.H., Koval, J.J. & St. Croix, C.M. (1999). A model of oxygen transport capacity changes for independently living older men and women. Canadian Journal of Applied Physiology 22:439-453.

Davy, K.P., & Seals, D.R. (1994). Total blood volume in healthy young and older men. Journal of Applied Physiology 76: 2059-2062.

Dempsey, J.A., Sheel, A.W., Haverkamp, H.C., Babcock, M.A. & Harms, C.A. (2003). The John Sutton lecture CSEP, 2002: pulmonary system limitations to exercise in health. Canadian Journal of Applied Physiology 28(Suppl):S3-S24.

Dempsey, J.A., & Seals, D.R. (1995). Aging, exercise, and cardio-pulmonary function. In Holloszy, J. (Ed.). Perspectives in exercise science. New York: Williams & Wilkins.

Ehrsam, R.E., Perruchoud, A., Oberholzer, M., Burkhart, F., & Herzog, H. (1983). Influence of age on pulmonary hemo-dynamics at rest and during supine exercise. Clinical Science 65:653-660.

Ehsani, A.A. (1989). Cardiovascular adaptations to exercise training in the elderly. Federation Proceedings 46:1840-1843.

Ehsani, A.A., Ogawa, T., Miller, T.R., Spira, R.J., & Jilka, S.M. (1991). Exercise training improves left ventricular systolic function in older men. Circulation 83:96-103.

Enright, P.L., Kronmal, R.A., Manolio, T.A., Shenker, M.B., & Hyatt, R.E. (1994). Respiratory muscle strength in the elderly. American Journal Respiratory Critical Care Medicine 149: 430-438.

Fleg, J.L., Gerstenbleth, G., & Lakatta, E.G. (1988). Pathophysiology of the aging heart and circulation. In Messerli, F.H. (Ed). Cardiovascular disease in the elderly, ed 2. Boston: Martinus Nihoff.

Gates, P.E., Tanaka, H., Graves, J., & Seals, D.R. (2003). Left ventricular structure and diastolic function with human aging. European Heart Journal 24:2213-2220.

Green, J.S., & Crouse, S.F. (1995). The effects of endurance training on functional capacity in the elderly: a meta-analysis. Medical Science of Sport Exercise 27:920-926.

Hagberg, J.M. (1987). Effect of training on the decline of VO_{2max} with aging. Federation Proceedings 46:1830-1833.

Halbert, J.A., Silagy, C.A., Finucane, P., Withers, R.T., Hamdorf, P.A., & Andrews, G.R. (1997). The effectiveness of exercise training in lowering blood pressure a meta-analysis of randomised controlled trials of 4 weeks or longer. Journal of Hypertension 11:641-649.

Harris, T., Lipsitz, L.A., Kleinman, J.C., & Cornoni-Huntley, J. (1991). Postural change in blood pressure associated with age and systolic blood pressure. Journal Gerontology Medicine Science 46:M159-M163.

Hossack K.F., & Bruce, R.A. (1982). Maximal cardiac function in sedentary normal men and women: comparison of age-related changes. Journal of Applied Physiology 53:799-804.

Janssens, J.P., Pache, J.C., & Nicod, L.P. (1999). Physiological changes in respiratory function associated with aging. European Respiratory Journal 13:197-205.

Johnson, B.D., & Dempsey, J.A. (1991). Demand vs. capacity in the aging pulmonary system. In Holloszy, J. (Ed). Exercise and sport sciences review, ed 19. Baltimore: Williams & Wilkins.

Jones, N.L. (1986). The lung of the Master's athlete. In Sutton, J.R., & Beck, R.M. (Eds). Sports medicine for the mature athlete. Indianapolis: Benchmark Press.

Kohrt, W.M., Malley, M.T., Coggan, A.R., Spina, R.J., Ogawa, T., Ehsani, A.A., Bourey, R.E., Martin, W.H. 3rd, & Holloszy, J.O. (1991). Effects of gender, age, and fitness level on response of VO_{2max} to training in 60-71 yr olds. Journal of Applied Physiology 71:2004-2011.

Lakatta, E.G. (2003). Arterial and cardiac aging: major shareholders in cardiovascular disease enterprises. Part 1: Aging arteries: a "set up" for vascular disease. Circulation 107:139-146.

Lakatta, E.G. (2002). Age-associated cardiovascular changes in health: impact on cardiovascular disease in older persons. Heart Failure Review 7:29-49.

Lakatta, E.G. (1993). Cardiovascular regulatory mechanisms in advanced age. Physiology Review 73:413-467.

Levy, W.C., Cerqueira, M.D., Abrass, I.B., Schwartz, R.S., & Stratton, J.R. (1993). Endurance exercise training augments diastolic filling at rest and during exercise in healthy young and older men. Circulation 88:116-126.

Lipsitz, L.A. (1989). Orthostatic hypotension in the elderly. New England Journal Medicine 321:952-957.

Mahler, D.A., Fierro-Carrion, G. & Baird, J.C. (2003). Evaluation of dyspnea in the elderly. Clinic in Geriatric Medicine 19:19-33.

Makrides, L., Heigenhauser, G.J., & Jones, N.L. (1986). Physical training in young and older healthy subjects. In Sutton, J.R., Brock, R.M. (Eds). Sports medicine for the mature athlete. Indianapolis: Benchmark Press.

Martin, W.H. 3rd, Ogawa, T., Kohrt, W.M., Malley, M.T., Korte, E., & Stolz, S. (1991). Effects of aging, gender, and physical training on peripheral vascular function. Circulation 84:654-664.

McClaran, S.R., Babcock, M.A., Pegelow, D.F., Reddan, W.G., & Dempsey, J.A. (1995). Longitudinal effects of aging on lung function at rest and exercise in healthy active fit elderly adults. Journal of Applied Physiology 78:1957-1968.

McGuire, D.K., Levine, B.D., Williamson, J.W., Snell, P.G., Blomqvist, C.G., Saltin, B., & Mitchell, J.H. (2001). A 30-year follow-up of the Dallas bed rest and training study. Circulation 104:1350-1357.

Monahand, K.D., Dinenno, F.A., Tanaka, H., Clevenger, C.M., DeSouza, C.A., & Seals, D.R. (2000). Regular aerobic exercise modulates age-associated declines in cardiovagal baroreflex sensitivity in healthy men. Journal of Physiology 529:263-271.

Murray, J.F. (1986) Aging in the normal lung, ed 2. Philadelphia: WB Saunders.

Ng, A.V., Callister, R., Johnson, D.G., & Seals, D.R. (1994). Endurance exercise training is associated with elevated basal sympathetic nerve activity in healthy older humans. Journal of Applied Physiology 77:1366-1374.

Ogawa, T., Spina, R.J., Martin, W.H. 3rd, Kohrt, W.M., Schechtman, K.B., Holloszy, J.O., & Ehsani, A.A. (1992). Effects of aging, sex, and physical training on cardiovascular responses to exercise. Circulation 86:494-503.

Prefaut, C., Anselme, F., Caillaud, C., & Masse-Biron, J. (1994). Exercise-induced hypoxemia in older athletes. Journal of Applied Physiology 76:120-126.

Reeves, J.T., Dempsey, J.A., & Grover, R.F. (1989). Pulmonary circulation during exercise. In Weir, E.K., & Reeves, J.T. (Eds). Pulmonary vascular physiology and pathophysiology. New York: Marcel Dekker.

Roach, M.R., & Burton, A.C. (1959). The effect of aging on the elasticity of human iliac arteries. Canadian Journal Biochemistry Physiology 37:557-570.

Rodeheffer, R.J., Gerstenblith, G., Becker, J.L., Fleg, J.L., Weisfield, M.L., & Lakatta, E.G. (1984). Exercise cardiac output is maintained with advancing ages in healthy human subjects: cardiac dilatation and increased stroke volume compensate for diminished heart rate. Circulation 69:203-213.

Saltin, B. (1986). The aging endurance athlete. In Sutton, J.R., & Brock, R.M. (Eds). Sports medicine for the mature athlete. Indianapolis: Benchmark Press.

Schulman, D.D., Lakatta, E.G., & Fleg, J.L., Lakatta, L., Beder, L.C., & Gerslenblith, G. (1992). Age-related decline in left ventricular filling at rest and exercise. American Journal of Physiology 263:H1932-H1938.

Seals, D.R. (1993). Influence of aging on autonomic-circulatory control in humans at rest and during exercise. In Gisolfi, C.V., Lamb, D.R., & Nadel, E.R. (Eds). Perspectives in exercise science and sports medicine, ed 6. Exercise, heat, and thermoregulation. Dubuque: Brown & Benchmark.

Seals, D.R., Hagberg, J.M., Hurley, B.F., Ehsani, A.A., & Holloszy, J.O. (1985) Endurance training in older men and women. I. Cardiovascular response to exercise. Journal of Applied Physiology 57:1024-1029.

Seals, D.R., Hagberg, J.M., Spina, R.J., Rogers, M.A., Schechtman, K.B., & Ehsani, A.A. (1994). Enhanced left ventricular performance in endurance trained older men. Circulation 89:198-205.

Sidney, K.H., & Shephard, R.J. (1977). Maximum and submaximum exercise tests and men and women in the seventh, eighth, and ninth decades of life. Journal of Applied Physiology 43:280-287.

Spina, R.J. (1999). Cardiovascular adaptations to endurance exercise training in older men and women. Exercise and Sports Science Review 27:317-332.

Spina, R.J., Ogawa, T., Kohrt, W.M., Martin W.H. 3rd, Holloszy, J.O., & Ehsani, A.A. (1993). Differences in cardiovascular adaptations to endurance exercise training between older men and women. Journal of Applied Physiology 75:849-855.

Starnes, J.W., Beyer, R.E., & Edington, D.W. (1983). Myocardial adaptations to endurance exercise in aged rats. American Journal of Physiology 245:H560-H566.

Stevenson, E.T., Davy, K.P., Reiling, M.J., & Seals, D.R. (1995). Maximal aerobic capacity and total blood volume in highly trained middle-aged and older female endurance athletes. Journal of Applied Physiology 77:1691-1696.

Tate, C.A., Taffet, G.E., Hudson, E.K., Blaylock, S.L., McBride, S.P., & Michael, L.H. (1990). Enhanced calcium uptake of cardiac sarcoplasmic reticulum in exercise-trained old rats. American Journal of Physiology 27:H431-H435.

Taylor, J.A., Hand, G.A., Johnson, D.G., & Seals, D.R. (1992). Augmented forearm vasoconstriction during dynamic exercise in healthy older men. Circulation 86:1789-1799.

Timiras, P.S. (1988). Cardiovascular alterations with age: atherosclerosis, coronary heart disease and hypertension. In Timiras, P.S. (Ed). Physiological basis of aging and geriatrics. Boca Raton, Fla: CRC.

Tsutsui, Y., Sagawa, S., Yamauchi, K., Endo, Y., Yamazaki, F., & Shiraki, K. (2002). Cardiovascular responses to lower negative pressure in the elderly: role of reduced leg compliance. Gerontology 48:133-139.

Warren, B.J., Nieman, D.C., Dotson, R.G., Adkins, C.H., O'Donnell, K.A., Haddock, B.L., & Butterworth, D.E. (1993). Cardiorespiratory responses to exercise training in septuagenarian women. International Journal of Sports Medicine 14:60-65.

Wilmore, J.H., Stanforth, P.R., Gagnon, J., Rice, T., Mandel, S., Leon, A.S., Rao, D.C., Skinner, J.S. & Bouchard, C. (2001). Cardiac output and stroke volume changes with endurance training: the heritage family study. Medicine and Science in Sports and Exercise 33:99-106.

Zaugg, M., & Lucchinetti, E. (2000). Respiratory function in the elderly. Anesthesiology Clinics of North America 18:47-58.

C H A P T E R   3 9

Multisystem Consequences of Impaired Breathing Mechanics and/or Postural Control

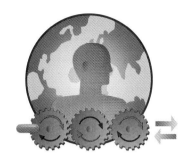

Mary Massery

KEY TERMS

Abnormal or compensatory breathing patterns
Abdominal binder
Breathing mechanics
Gastrointestinal impairments
Gravity's influence on development
Integumentary impairments
Internal organs
Multisystem interactions
Musculoskeletal impairments
Neuromuscular impairments

Normal and abnormal development of chest wall
Paradoxical breathing
Pelvic floor
Postural control
Reflux
Sandifer's syndrome
Scoliosis
Soda-pop can model of respiratory and postural control
Spinal cord injury
Vocal folds

The cardiovascular/pulmonary (CP) system is unique in that it provides both physiological support (oxygen delivery) as well as a mechanical support (respiratory/trunk muscle control) for movement. The physiological components have been covered extensively in other sections of this book. This chapter focuses on the mechanical aspect of ventilation and its interactions with other body systems in both health and dysfunction and includes three major points of focus:

1. Breathing is a three-dimensional motor task that is influenced by gravity in all planes of motion.
2. Breathing is an integral part of multisystem interactions and consequences that simultaneously support respiration and postural control for all motor tasks.
3. The mechanics of breathing influence both health and motor performance outcomes related to participation.

The four motor impairment categories identified in the *Guide to Physical Therapist Practice*, second edition, will be

incorporated into this chapter (APTA, 2001). An additional fifth category, the internal organ (IO) system, is added by this author (Box 39-1). In addition to addressing the impact of these impairment categories on health and motor performance from a ventilatory viewpoint, this author also presents a method to cross-check impairment-based findings with functional limitations. Six everyday functional tasks that require the integration of breathing and movement are presented (Box 39-2).

BREATHING: A THREE-DIMENSIONAL ACTIVITY WITHIN GRAVITY'S INFLUENCE

Planes of Ventilation and Gravity's Influence

Ventilation does not take place in a one-dimensional plane but rather as a three-dimensional activity. During every breath, the chest has the potential to expand in an anterior-posterior

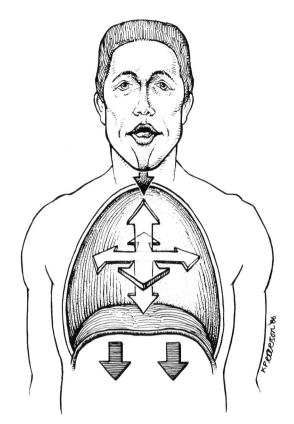

FIGURE 39-1 Planes of respiration: anterior-posterior, inferior-superior, and lateral.

plane, an inferior-superior plane, and a lateral plane (Figure 39-1). This means that the muscles that support breathing are resisted by gravity in one direction, assisted by gravity in another direction, and relatively unaffected in other directions. For example, in an upright position, superior expansion of the chest is resisted by gravity while inferior expansion is assisted, and other movements of the chest (lateral, anterior, and posterior expansion) are relatively unaffected by gravity. The adverse effects of gravity are counteracted by muscles that can function even with the resistance of gravity. If the respiratory muscles become dysfunctional through weakness, paralysis, fatigue, or some other condition, the patient may no longer be able to breathe effectively within gravity's influence. Therefore, positioning of patients with impaired breathing mechanics must take into consideration how gravity will affect the muscles that support breathing in any particular posture.

Effects of Gravity on Normal and Abnormal Chest Wall Development

Gravity also plays an extremely crucial role in the skeletal development of the chest in the newborn. Normally-developing infants move freely in and out of postures, such as prone, hands-knees, and standing, as they progress developmentally, allowing gravity to alternately assist or resist the movements. Moving through these postures, the infant strengthens and develops muscle groups and learns to interact with the gravitational force in his or her environment (Bly, 1994). The combination of normal movement patterns experienced within a gravitational field and genetic predisposition influences the normal development of the bones, muscles, and joints that comprise the thoracic cage (ribcage) and thoracic spine. Infants with limited ability to move within their environment and limited ability to counteract the force of gravity develop atypical joint alignment and atypical muscle support that may lead to impaired breathing mechanics or vice versa (Bach, 2003; Lissoni et al, 1998; Papastamelos, 1996). Severe neuromuscular (NM) deficits such as cerebral palsy, spinal muscle atrophy, cerebral vascular accidents, head traumas, and spinal cord injuries are examples of conditions that can cause such a muscle imbalance in children. Muscle weakness or fatigue of the trunk muscles can also be caused by conditions arising outside of the NM system, such as oxygen transport deficits from bronchopulmonary dysplagia (BPD), congenital heart defects, etc., or from nutritional deficits such as gastroesophygeal reflux, absorption problems, etc. Therefore, a variety of reasons may account for an infant's inability to change his or her own positions in space. Impairments to breathing mechanics may be caused by muscle weakness, muscle tone problems such as hypertonicity or hypotonicity, motor planning deficits, motor learning deficits, and/or medical fragility (Toder, 2000).

Children with breathing mechanics impairment typically spend significantly more time in a supine posture than in any

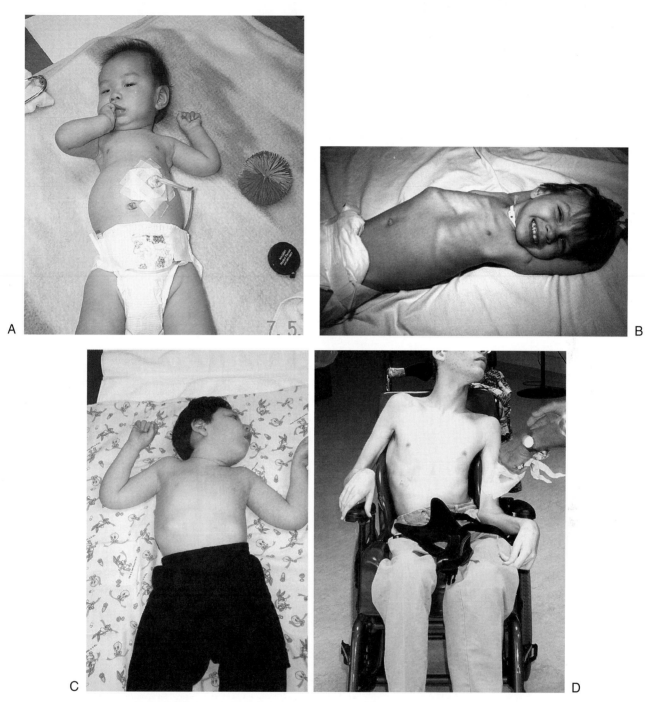

FIGURE 39-2 A, Caitlin, six months of age. Caitlin has spinal muscle atrophy, type I. Note persistent immature triangular shaping of chest wall secondary to pronounced muscle weakness and an inability to counteract gravity effectively. **B,** Melissa, three-and-a-half years of age. Melissa has a C5 complete spinal cord injury due to birth trauma. Melissa's chest wall has become more deformed than Caitlin's chest due to the prolonged exposure to the severe muscle imbalance of the respiratory muscles within gravity's constant influence. Note the marked pectus excavatum and anteriorly flared ribs in supine. **C,** Carlos, 5 years of age and **D,** Kevin, 17 years of age. Both have spastic cerebral palsy. Note the lateral flaring of the lower ribcage, the asymmetry of the trunk, and the flattening of the entire anterior ribcage, all of which are more noticeable in the older child.

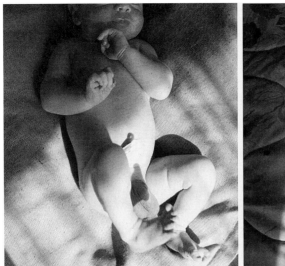
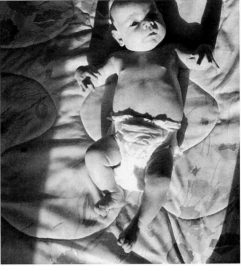

FIGURE 39-3 **A** and **B,** Newborn chest. Note triangular shape, short neck, narrow and flat upper chest, round barreled lower chest. Muscle tone is primarily flexion and breathing is primarily diaphragmatic and on one plane: inferior.

other posture, which can lead to unbalanced gravitational influence and undesirable changes in the thorax. These deformities may include retaining the more primitive triangular shape of the newborn chest (Figure 39-2, *A*). In some cases, the child's diaphragm remains functional yet unbalanced by weak or paralyzed abdominal and intercostal muscles, and this has a significant affect on the developing skeleton (Figure 39-2, *B*). Pronounced muscle imbalance of the trunk can result in such severe chest wall deformities that it impairs the child's ability to meet his or her ventilatory needs. Common musculoskeletal (MS) abnormalities are anteriorly flared lower ribs; a dynamic cavus deformity, likely a pectus excavatum or less often a pectus carinatum; laterally flared ribs and/or asymmetry (Figure 39-2, *B, C, D*) (Bach, 2003; Papastamelos, 1996; Massery, 1991). These deformities may be more devastating in one posture than another because of the child's unequal inability to counteract gravity's force.

Understanding normal chest wall development is essential for accurately assessing abnormal chest deformities seen in children (Massery, 1991). Initially the newborn's chest is triangular: narrow and flat in the upper portion and wider and more rounded in the lower portion (Figure 39-3). The infant's short neck renders the upper accessory muscles nonfunctional as ventilatory muscles. The infant's arms are held in flexion and adduction across the chest, significantly hampering lateral or anterior movement of the chest wall. The infant, forced to be a diaphragmatic breather, shows greater development of the lower chest and this leads to the triangular shaping of the ribcage. Newborns breathe primarily on a single plane of motion, inferior, rather than the three dimensions of the adult.

From three to six months of age the infant begins to develop more trunk extension tone and spends more time in a prone position on his or her elbows. The baby begins to reach

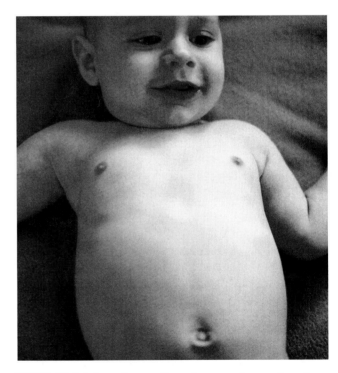

FIGURE 39-4 Infant chest wall at three to six months of age. Increased upper chest width. More convex shaping of entire chest as antigravity movements are becoming possible. Still has a short neck and two functionally separate chambers: thorax and abdomen.

out into the environment with his or her upper extremities. This facilitates development of the anterior upper chest. Constant stretching and upper extremity weight bearing helps to expand the anterior upper chest both anteriorly and laterally, while increasing posterior stabilization (Bly, 1994).

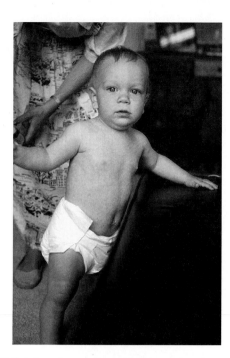

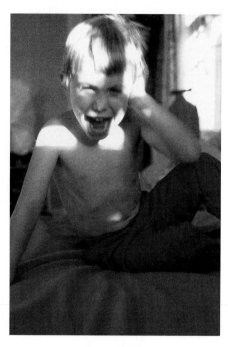

FIGURE 39-5 Infant chest wall at six to 12 months of age. The infant spends more time in upright. The activation of abdominal muscles, gravity's influence, and increased postural demands result in a more elongated chest wall, wider rib spacing, and increased intercostal muscle activation, as well as a functional interface of the ribcage onto the abdomen with the abdominal and intercostal muscles. This improves both the respiratory dynamics by giving more external support to the diaphragm at the mid chest level, and the postural stabilization potential needed for more complex motor tasks. Note that the base of the ribcage is no longer barrel shaped like it is in the newborn.

FIGURE 39-6 A four-year-old boy. Note the elongated chest, which occupies more than half of the trunk space, the wide intercostal spacing, the effective muscle stabilization of the lower ribcage with the abdominal muscles, the rectangular shaping of the chest from a frontal view, and the elliptical shaping of the chest from a transverse view.

An increase in intercostal and pectoralis muscle strength improves the infant's ability to counteract the force of gravity on the anterior upper chest in the supine position, leading to the development of a slight convex configuration of the area and a more rectangular shaping of the thorax from a frontal plane (Figure 39-4). The baby begins to breathe in more than one plane of motion.

The next significant development occurs when the child begins to independently assume erect postures (e.g., sitting, kneeling, or standing). Until this time, the ribs are aligned relatively horizontally, with narrow intercostal spacing (see Figure 39-3). The newborn's chest only comprises approximately one third of the total trunk cavity. As the child begins to consistently move up against the pull of gravity, the ribs, with the aid of the abdominal muscles and gravity, rotate downward (more so in the longer lower ribs), creating the sharper angle of the ribs (Figure 39-5). This markedly elongates the ribcage until it eventually occupies more than half of the trunk cavity (Figure 39-6). A comparison of chest x-rays of newborns and adults, as well as pictures of infants, clearly shows these developmental trends (Figure 39-7, *A, B*), which are summarized in Table 39-1.

Optimum respiratory function cannot be expected from a severely underdeveloped or deformed chest and/or spine. As long as the condition that caused the trunk muscle imbalance persists, regardless of whether that deficit was a true NM disorder or an impairment in another motor impairment category (see Box 39-1), the chest wall and spine will likely develop abnormally. Frequent position changes, management of adverse NM tone, facilitation of weakened chest muscles, promotion of optimal breathing patterns, incorporation of ventilatory strategies with movement, as well as integration of physical therapy goals within the child's overall development and medical program, will stimulate the optimal chest and trunk development.

MULTISYSTEM INTERACTIONS AND THEIR INFLUENCE ON HEALTH AND MOTOR PERFORMANCE: THE RELATIONSHIP BETWEEN RESPIRATION AND POSTURAL CONTROL

A single body system acting in isolation does not produce normal movement. Every person is composed of multiple body systems that interact and overlap in duty: the summed interaction results in normal movement. If these interactions are not normal or adequately compensatory in nature, then motor impairments may result. Because of this, this author suggests that every physical therapy examination and evaluation should include a multisystem screening of all five impairment categories (see Box 39-1) in order to determine

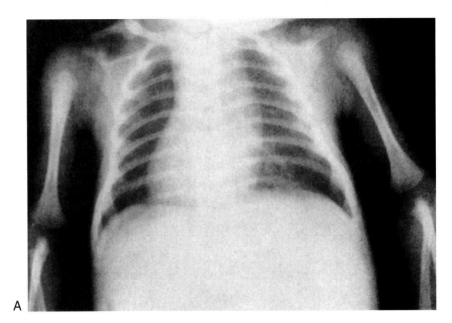

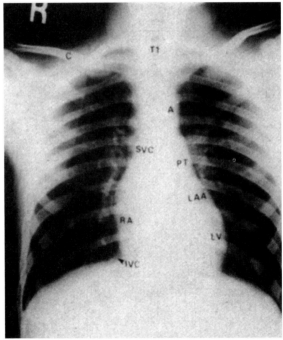

FIGURE 39-7 A, Newborn chest x-ray. Note triangular shaping of ribcage and narrow intercostal spacing. **B,** Normal adult chest x-ray. Chest shape is rectangular, ribs angled downward, upper and lower chest equally developed.

TABLE 39-1		
Trends of Normal Chest Wall Development from Infant to Adulthood		
CHEST	**INFANT**	**ADULT**
Size	Thorax occupies one third trunk cavity	Thorax occupies more than half trunk cavity
Shape	Triangular frontal plane, circular A-P plane	Rectangular frontal plane, elliptical A-P plane
Upper chest	Narrow, flat apex	Wide, convex apex
Lower chest	Circular, flared lower ribs	Elliptical, lower ribs integrated with abdominals
Ribs	Evenly horizontal	Rotated downward, especially inferiorly
Intercostal spacing	Narrow, limits movement of thoracic spine and trunk	Wide, allows for individual movement of ribs and spine
Diaphragm	Adequate, minimal dome shape	Adequate, large dome shape
Accessory muscles	Nonfunctional	Functional

the impact of each body system on total motor performance. The following Soda-Pop Can model of respiratory and postural control was developed by this author to aide the reader in understanding the multisystem interactions between the mechanics of breathing and the simultaneous needs of postural control in both pediatric and adult populations.

Soda-Pop Can Model of Respiratory and Postural Control

Muscles of respiration are also muscles of postural support, and vice versa. Every muscle that originates or inserts onto the trunk is both a respiratory and postural muscle. This duality of function means that respiration and postural control can never be evaluated as isolated responses. External and internal forces that affect the function of the respiratory muscles will also affect postural responses. The Soda-Pop Can model seeks to illustrate this dual purpose.

Structurally Weak, Yet Functionally Strong

The shell of a soda-pop can is made out of a thin, flimsy aluminum casing that is easily smashed when empty. However, this same can, when it is full and unopened, is almost impossible to compress or deform without puncturing the exterior shell. The strength of the can is derived from the positive pressure it exerts against atmospheric pressure and gravity through its closed (unopened) system (Figure 39-8, A). As soon as the closed system is compromised, however, by flipping open the pop-top or inadvertently puncturing the side of the can, it loses its functional strength. It is no longer capable of counteracting the positive pressure forces that act upon it. Once opened, it is possible to completely smash the can into a tiny fragment of its original shape (Figure 39-8, B).

The trunk of the body uses a concept similar to the soda-pop can to prevent being "smashed" by external forces. The skeletal support of the trunk is not inherently strong. The spine and ribcage alone are not capable of maintaining their alignment against gravity without the muscular support that gives them the capability of generating pressures that can withstand the compressive forces of gravity. This is demonstrated daily by patients in intensive care unit (ICU)

settings. Weakened from prolonged illnesses and/or medical procedures, patients in the ICU typically slump into a forwarded, flexed posture when they sit up for the first time, showing impaired ability to generate adequate pressure support through muscle activation to support an ideal alignment of the spine and ribcage in an upright posture. In pediatrics, the results can be even more alarming. Melissa, who suffered a C5 spinal cord injury during a vaginal birth injury, shows a complete collapse of the ribcage and spine in upright. Melissa was incapable of taking a single effective inspiratory effort in this posture, which explains why she had no tolerance for upright activities. Her soda-pop can was crushed, and with it her breathing mechanics (Figure 39-8, C).

Positive Pressure Support Instead of More Skeletal Support

The aluminum can is a chamber. Once the chamber is filled with carbonated fluid and sealed, carbonated gases are released inside, resulting in positive pressure pushing outwardly upon the can, thus providing dynamic support to the metal. Likewise, the trunk of the body is composed of thoracic and abdominal chambers that are dynamically supported by muscle contractions to provide positive pressure in both chambers for respiratory and postural support.

The thoracic and abdominal chambers are completely separated by the diaphragm (Figure 39-9). The chambers are "sealed" at the top by the vocal folds, at the bottom by the pelvic floor, and circumferentially by the trunk muscles. Muscle support allows these chambers to match or exceed the positive pressure exerted upon them by outside forces in order to support the "flimsy" skeletal shell. The primary muscles involved in this support are the intercostal muscles, which generate and maintain pressure for the thoracic chamber; the abdominal muscles, which generate and maintain pressure for the abdominal chamber, especially the transverse abdominus; the diaphragm, which regulates and uses the pressure in both chambers; and the back extensors, which provide stabilizing forces for the alignment of the spine and articulation with the

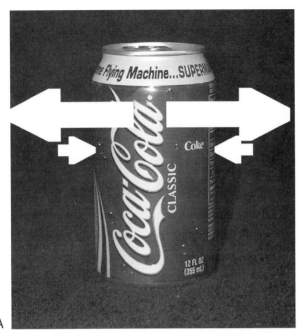

A

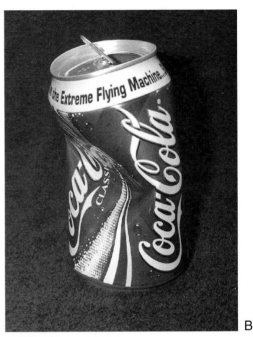

B

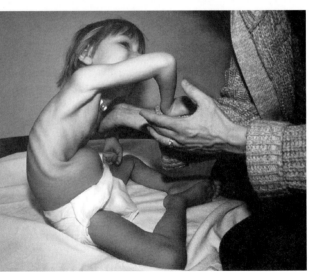

C

FIGURE 39-8 Soda-Pop Can model of respiratory and postural control. **A,** A soda-pop can derives its functional strength because the internal pressure of the carbonated drink is higher than the atmospheric pressure acting upon it, not because of its thin aluminum shell. **B,** Without the internal pressure support, the aluminum can is easily deformed and compressed. **C,** Melissa, age three-and-a-half years: C5 complete spinal cord injury due to birth trauma. Clinical example of a crushed trunk resulting in severely compromised respiratory mechanics in spite of the fact that her lungs are normal. Melissa was incapable of generating adequate positive pressures to counteract the constant force of gravity and atmospheric pressure upon her developing skeletal frame.

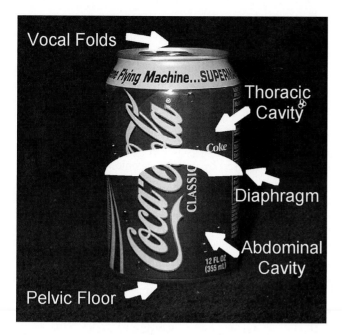

FIGURE 39-9 A soda-pop can as a three-dimensional model for trunk muscle support for breathing and postural control. Note that the control of pressure begins at the level of the vocal folds and extends all the way down to the pelvic floor. A breach in pressure anywhere along the cylinder will impair the total function of the can, and likewise for the patient's trunk.

ribcage. These muscles work synergistically to adjust the pressure in both chambers so that the demands of ventilation and posture are simultaneously met (Primiano, 1982; McGill, Sharratt & Seguin, 1995; Bouisset & Duchene, 1994; Rimmer et al, 1995; Bach, 2002; Faminiano & Celli, 2001).

A quick synopsis of the biomechanics of breathing will illustrate the normal interaction among the diaphragm, intercostals, and abdominals within the construct of a positive pressure chamber (Flaminiano & Celli, 2001; Cala, 1993; Nava et al, 1993; Rimmer & Whitelaw, 1993). The diaphragm is well known as the primary respiratory muscle, but this author asks the reader to see the diaphragm instead as a pressure regulating muscle. The diaphragm completely separates the thoracic cavity from the abdominal cavity and as such is capable of creating and utilizing pressure differences in the chambers to support the simultaneous needs of respiration and trunk stabilization. It is the interactions among the diaphragm, intercostals, and abdominal muscles, in addition to support from other trunk muscles, that work together to generate, regulate, and maintain thoracic and abdominal chamber pressures necessary for the ongoing, concurrent needs of breathing and motor control of the trunk (Hodges et al, 2001). The support works both ways: the diaphragm is dependent on the support of the intercostal and abdominal muscles for effective and efficient breathing, and likewise the trunk is dependent on the diaphragm to increase its muscular support and for increased pressure support during motor tasks with higher postural demands (Hodges et al, 2001; Grimstone

& Hodges, 2003; Hodges et al, 2002; Gandevia et al, 2002). One cannot be considered separate from the other.

When the diaphragm contracts to initiate inhalation, the central tendon descends inferiorly, creating negative pressure in the thoracic cavity and causing air to be drawn into the lungs due to the pressure differential with atmospheric pressure. Simultaneously, the intercostal muscles are activated to avoid being drawn inward toward the negative pressure (Lissoni et al, 1998; Rimmer et al, 1995; Wilson et al, 2001; De Troyer et al, 2003). Inadequate intercostal muscle support would cause the chest to collapse inward, eventual development of a MS deformity such as a pectus excavatum, and a secondary loss of chest wall compliance (see Figure 39-2, *B*) (Lissoni et al, 1998; Rimmer & Whitelaw, 1993; Skjodt et al, 2001; Han, et al 1993; Sumarez, 1986). While the diaphragm is descending, it creates positive pressure in the abdominal cavity due to the support of abdominal muscles, particularly the deepest muscle, the transverse abdominus (Hodges & Gandevia, 2000). The positive pressure created is equal to the negative pressure created in the thorax according to Newton's Law, which states that for every action, there is an equal and opposite reaction (Serway & Faughn, 1992). The diaphragm uses positive abdominal pressure like a fulcrum to stabilize the central tendon. This central stability then mechanically supports the effective contractions of the lateral (peripheral) fibers up and over the abdominal viscera (lateral and superior chest wall expansion) (Flaminiano, 2001).

The abdominal cavity has relatively higher pressure at rest than the thoracic cavity, as reflected by the natural positioning of the diaphragm within the trunk. Its dome is convex superiorly because the higher pressure from the abdominal cavity pushes it upward. During lung disease, this relationship of pressure may reverse and severely compromise the mechanics of breathing. For example, patients who have obstructive lung disease such as emphysema trap air distally in the diseased lung segments (Cherniack & Cherniack, 1983). Eventually the build up of air, as well as other aspects of the disease cause the thoracic cavity to become the higher pressure chamber at rest, pushing the diaphragm inferiorly until the dome of the diaphragm becomes flat. At that point, the diaphragm's mechanical support is so compromised that it can no longer function as an inspiratory muscle. To compensate, patients with end stage emphysema often lean forward on extended arms, flex their trunks, and activate their abdominal muscles to increase abdominal pressures and hopefully restore the correct pressure relationship with the thoracic chamber. If successful, they can temporarily push the dome of the diaphragm upward to give it a chance to function as an inspiratory muscle again and gain some relief from their constant dyspnea. This is an example of pathologic positive pressure support.

Top and Bottom of the "Soda-Pop Can": The Vocal Folds and Pelvic Floor

Vocal Folds and Vocal Apparatus. Normal positive thoracic pressure is needed for both postural support of the upper trunk and for many expiratory maneuvers such as talking, coughing, and bowel and bladder evacuation (Pierce & Worsnop, 1999; Wood et al, 1986; Deem & Miller, 2000). The vocal folds and vocal apparatus provide the superior valve or pressure regulation of the thoracic chamber. If the vocal folds are compromised due to an impairment of the upper airway or because they are bypassed altogether with a tracheostomy or endotracheal tube, the patient becomes incapable of generating positive thoracic pressure support. Once the patient has inhaled maximally and reached pressure in the lungs equal to the pressure outside the lungs, the air will simply "fall out." There is no valve at the top to hold the pressure inside the chest. Activities of the trunk that require positive pressure in the thorax will then be compromised. For example, without the vocal folds to regulate the controlled release of thoracic pressure during exhalation, there is no way for the patient to slowly, or eccentrically, release the air such as needed for talking or eccentric trunk or extremity activities. Thus, the therapist may notice speech and/or eccentric motor impairments. The same is true for concentric contractions. Without the vocal folds as the pressure valve, the patient can not build up adequate intrathoracic pressure to produce an effective cough (Bach & Saporito, 1996). Similarly, if the patient can not close the glottis and direct thoracic positive pressure downward toward the pelvic floor, then bowel and bladder evacuation may be compromised (Borowitz & Borowitz, 1997; Borowitz & Sutphen, 2004). For example, in the clinical setting, patients with tracheostomies are noted to often experience constipation, which improves as soon as they are decanulated and the vocal folds have been restored as an active component of trunk pressure regulation.

The patient with compromised vocal folds can generate a brief moment of positive expiratory pressures for activities such as coughing or yelling by learning to recruit a quick and forceful concentric contraction of the trunk flexors, primarily the abdominals, pectoralis and/or latissimus dorsi muscles immediately at peak inspiratory lung volume. This positive thoracic expiratory pressure, however, cannot be sustained because the expiratory pathway (e.g., tracheostomy tube or paralyzed vocal folds) is wider than the normal opening of the vocal folds, and this causes a larger volume of air to be expelled per second. Unlike patients with obstructive lung disease who have an abnormally prolonged expiratory phase, patients with impairment to the pressure regulator at the top of the chamber have no natural mechanism to prolong exhalation either for eccentric or concentric motor tasks.

In addition to regulating the airflow out of the lungs, the vocal folds play an important role in generating the increased thoracic pressures needed for trunk stabilization associated with lifting, pushing, upper extremity weight bearing activity, etc (Hayama et al, 2002). This response is called the glottal effort closure reflex (Deem & Miller, 2000). The entire length of the vocal folds adducts and prevents any air leakage while the chest wall muscles and the abdominals contract to increase abdominal and thoracic pressures. This increased pressure stabilizes the shoulder complex to allow for greater force production from the upper extremities. For example, a tennis player with a strong serve often uses a functional glottal effort closure reflex. The server throws the ball up while taking a deep breath in, then he or she closes the glottis at the peak of inspiration using the trapped air and the activation of the chest and abdominal muscles to increase thoracic pressure. Then, when the tennis racket makes contact with the ball, the server explosively expels the air (usually with a grunt) to maximize the force production of the serve. This concept is used by ordinary people on a daily basis to perform tasks such as pushing a heavy door open, lifting a heavy box, or leaning on a table with one arm and reaching across the table to pick something up with the other arm, and when an infant bears weight on his or her arms while crawling, etc. All these activities require the full or partial glottal effort closure response in order to increase the functional strength of the arms. This concept is consistent with the Soda-Pop Can model's concept of pressure regulation for functional strength and control.

In pediatrics, the importance of the vocal folds as the superior pressure regulator may be observed in a child with a tracheostomy due to an airway impairment, or a child with poor vocal control for other reasons, without a NM diagnosis. The therapist may see that the infant crawls with elbow flexion rather than on extended arms, even though there is no muscle weakness in the arms. In this author's clinical assessment, it may be the inability of the vocal folds to keep adequate positive pressure in the chest during weight bearing (glottal effort closure reflex) that causes the elbows to flex, rather than weak triceps. In this case, strengthening the vocal folds, or adding a Passy Muir valve (speaking valve) to a tracheostomy tube if it is present, will improve the child's potential to meet the positive thoracic pressures necessary for higher level postural activities. In other words, working on restoring the trunk's pressure support system (the soda-pop can) may result in greater functional gains than working on upper extremity exercises.

Other types of vocal fold interactions occur within this pressurized system to optomize speech, breathing, and/or postural control. For example, the vocal folds will have improved function as a speech valve if abdominal pressure is restored via an abdominal binder in patients with spinal cord injury (Hoit et al, 2002). Similarly, for children with laryngeal malacia or other types of upper airway obstructions, excessive inspiratory flow rates, which create excessive negative pressure in the upper airway, may result in decreased voicing or the appearance of exercise induced asthma (Mandell & Arjmand, 2003).

Pelvic Floor. The pelvic floor muscles provide support at the other end of the cylinder, at the base of the abdominal cavity. If there is dysfunction of these muscles, the abdominal cavity's positive pressure potential will be adversely affected (Hodges & Gandevia, 2000). For example, when abdominal pressure is intended to be directed upward toward the vocal folds for coughing, sneezing, yelling, laughing, etc., insufficient pelvic floor musculature will result in a loss of positive

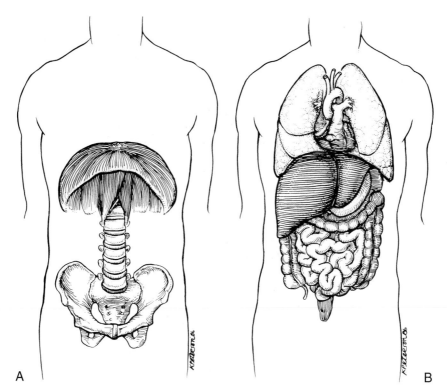

A

B

FIGURE 39-10 A, Note the diaphragm's position as the pressure regulator between the thoracic and abdominal cavities. **B,** Note the amount and alignment of the IOs within the trunk that are affected by the changes in the diaphragm's position during respiration.

pressure through the pelvic opening. This is often expressed as urinary stress incontinence, rendering the intended respiratory or postural maneuver less effective (Sapsford et al, 2001). There are numerous conditions that compromise the integrity of the pelvic floor, but the most obvious example is women who are postpartum. The overstretched pelvic floor muscles from childbirth cause them to inadvertently release positive pressure through the pelvic floor during demanding activities such as sneezing, coughing, and running. Women in this state learn to cross their legs or perform other pressure supporting compensatory behaviors to reduce urinary incontinence stresses while their pelvic floor heals. Other conditions, such as adult females with cystic fibrosis, experience a high incidence of urinary stress incontinence secondary to repetitive stress on the pelvic floor from the positive pressure associated with their chronic coughs (Langman et al, 2004; Dodd, 2004). Incontinence is not restricted to patients with primary pulmonary disease. Women with low back pain and impaired postural responses have also been noted to have a higher incidence of incontinence (Saspsford et al, 2001).

IOs. The organs in the trunk generate and/or use pressure changes in the thorax and abdomen to augment their own function. For example, the neuromuscular system creates the pressure changes in the thorax and abdomen. The lungs and esophagus use this pressure change in the thorax to create

efficient breathing and improved upper gastrointestinal motility. The cardiac system causes small changes in thoracic pressures. Using these changes and the changes from the respiratory mechanics, the heart and circulatory system can optimize blood circulation or blood pressure. The abdomen also uses pressure changes for its IOs. It uses the rhythmic pressures through the intestines for lumbar stabilization, improved lower gastrointestinal motility, optimal hemodynamic flow of body fluids, and optimal lymphatic drainage (Figure 39-10) (De Looze et al, 1998).

Without normal pressure support, which includes the rhythmic change in the thorax from negative to positive pressure and the rhythmic change in the abdomen from neutral to positive pressure (making the abdomen the relatively higher pressure system), the function of the IOs may be compromised. The dysfunction may be expressed as a drop in blood pressure (hypotension), inefficient respirations, gastroesophygeal reflux, poor bladder emptying (increasing risk for urinary tract infections), or constipation, to name a few, during acute spinal cord injury where the ability to generate and use pressure support is immediately lost after the injury (De Looze et al, 1998; Noreau et al, 2000; Winslow & Rozovsky, 2003). These dysfunctions may not be caused solely by the lack of normal pressure support, but the lack of pressure support is a major cause of the dysfunction.

BOX 39-3

Compensatory Breathing Patterns Associated with Insufficient Muscular Support

1. Paradoxical breathing
   a. Functioning diaphragm with paralyzed or weak intercostals and abdominal muscles
   b. Paralyzed or weak diaphragm with functional accessory muscles; may or may not have functioning abdominal muscles
2. Diaphragm and upper accessory breathing
   a. Paralyzed or weak intercostals
3. Upper accessory muscles breathing
   a. Paralyzed or weak diaphragm and intercostals; abdominal muscles may or may not be functional
4. Asymmetrical breathing
   a. Paralyzed or weak trunk muscles on one side
   b. Often associated with hemiparesis or scoliosis
5. Lateral or "gravity-eliminated" breathing
   a. Generalized weakness, no paralysis
   b. Breathing takes place in the plane with the least resistance to gravity
   c. Often associated with weakness due to prolonged illness
6. Shallow breathing
   a. Small tidal volumes
   b. Often associated with high NM tone or painful conditions

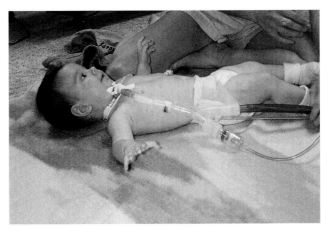

FIGURE 39-11 Nicholas, one year of age. Nicholas was born with both hemi-diaphragms paralyzed and requires full-time mechanical ventilation. When he is off the ventilator for brief periods of time to assess his independent breathing pattern, he demonstrates the second type of paradoxical breathing: a rising upper chest and falling abdomen during inhalation.

Summary

The Soda-Pop Can model of respiratory and postural control provides a three-dimensional, dynamic illustration of how the trunk meets its concurrent needs for breathing, postural control, and IO function. When the patient has lost the ability to generate, regulate, and/or maintain appropriate internal pressures in both the thoracic and abdominal chambers, the mechanics of breathing, as well as numerous other body functions, may be impaired. Inadequate pressure support may start as an impairment to the mechanics of breathing, such as in a NM or MS disorder, or it may start as an impairment to another body system such as cardiovascular, pulmonary, airway, integumentary (INT), or the IOs but result in impaired breathing mechanics none the less. The overlapping of function precludes trunk motor performance from being accurately assessed in isolation of all other body systems, especially respiratory mechanics.

COMPENSATORY BREATHING PATTERNS ASSOCIATED WITH INSUFFICIENT MUSCULAR SUPPORT

As illustrated in the Soda-Pop Can model, the trunk muscles are needed to provide the necessary pressure changes for normal breathing. What happens if the muscles are weak, paralyzed, fatigued, or otherwise nonsupportive? What kinds of compensatory breathing patterns may develop? Six different compensatory breathing patterns are described herein (Box 39-3).

Paradoxical Breathing

Paradoxical breathing is named for the paradoxical movements of the chest noted during inspiration. It is sometimes clinically referred to as belly breathing, see-saw breathing, or reverse breathing. The first type of paradoxical breathing is caused by a strong contraction of the diaphragm in the absence of adequate muscular support from the two other triad muscles: the intercostal muscles and abdominal muscles. The diaphragm contracts, the abdomen rises excessively because inadequate abdominal muscle function does not stop the descent of the diaphragm with positive pressure, and the upper chest collapses because of a lack of the stabilizing contraction of the intercostal muscles (see Figure 39-2, *A*). This is the more common form of paradoxical breathing, and although it is not efficient, it is usually sufficient for breathing without mechanical ventilator support (Lissoni et al, 1998).

The second type of paradoxical breathing occurs when the diaphragm is weak or paralyzed while the upper accessory muscles are still intact. The abdominal muscles may or may not be functional. The inspiratory action now is opposite of the motion that was described for the first type (Figure 39-11). The abdomen is drawn inward toward the negative pressure in the thorax created by the upper accessory muscle during inhalation. Thus the chest rises and the belly falls. Generally this second type of paradoxical breathing requires at least part-time mechanical ventilation support because the accessory muscles are not designed to meet the needs of long-term independent ventilation and are more likely to fatigue and cause respiratory distress. The loss of the diaphragm as

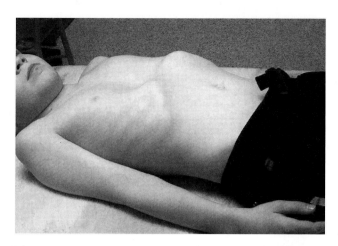

FIGURE 39-12 Justin, nine years of age. Justin has a congenital pectus excavatum. No neurological impairment. His breathing pattern is primarily diaphragm and upper accessory muscles. Note the persistent elevation of the ribcage and the inward collapse of the lower sternum (pectus excavatum). Justin's sternum moved paradoxically with every inspiratory effort, especially during high respiratory and postural demand.

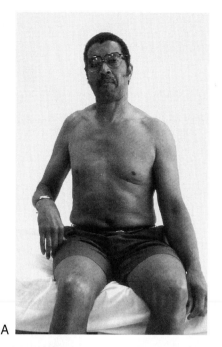

A

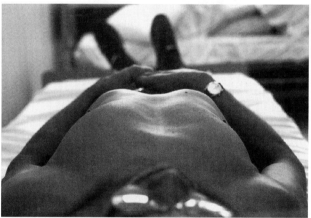

B

FIGURE 39-13 Charles. Right hemiparesis from a CVA. **A,** Note asymmetry of trunk in sitting during breathing and postural control. **B,** Note the weakness in the right upper chest. Charles' right upper chest moved less during inhalation than the left, which accentuated his asymmetrical trunk alignment and was probably a contributing factor to his impaired posture and upper extremity function in stance and during gait.

the primary respiratory muscle results in a much greater inspiratory volume loss than the loss of just the accessory-muscles support noted in the first paradoxical pattern. Loss of the diaphragm as the primary pressure regulator for the trunk also results in significant deficits in postural control.

Diaphragm and Upper Accessory Muscles Only (Paralyzed or Nonfunctional Intercostal Muscles)

Another type of compensatory breathing pattern occurs when the intercostal and abdominal muscles are paralyzed or weak but the diaphragm and upper accessory muscles still function (i.e., patients with tetraplegia, high paraplegia, some congenital pectus excavatum deformities, upper airway obstructions, or asthma). These patients learn to counterbalance the strength of the diaphragmatic inferior pull by using their sternocleidomastoid muscles and possibly their scalene, trapezius, and pectoralis muscles. Allowing for superior and possibly some anterior and lateral expansion of the chest, this compensatory breathing pattern prevents the collapse of the upper chest that is seen in paradoxical breathing. This must be cognitively coordinated with the inspiratory phase and is generally a more effective breathing pattern for patients with NM weakness but may not be an efficient choice for patients with asthma. On subjective breathing assessment, these patients often present with shortened neck muscles. Intercostal retractions, or the collapsing of the intercostal spaces on inspiration, may be seen here, especially at the level of the xiphoid. The paralyzed or weak intercostal muscle tissue will be sucked in toward the lungs during the creation of negative pressure within the chest, thus the observance of the intercostal retractions that in the long term can develop into a

pectus excavatum (Figure 39-12) (Bach & Bianchi, 2003; Massery, 2005).

Upper Accessory Muscles Only

If the patient lacks all of the "triad ventilatory muscles," independent breathing can only be attempted using the upper accessory muscles in a superior plane and possibly some anterior expansion as well. Generally these patients will need mechanical ventilation to augment their independent effort because the lung volumes they can generate will not be adequate to support the oxygen needs of the body.

A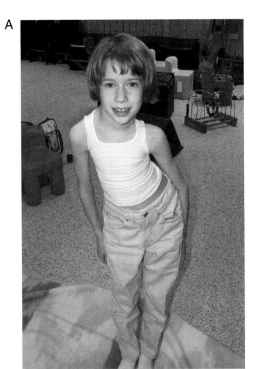

B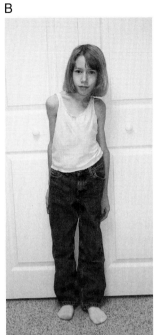

C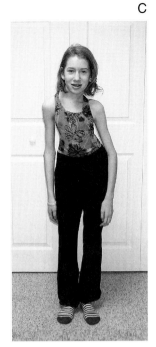

FIGURE 39-14 A, Katie nine years of age; diagnosis of infantile scoliosis. Presurgical workup showed her FVC at 33% of predicted value. **B,** Katie age 10 years, one year later. Her surgeon felt that the improvements in lung volumes and a slight reduction in the scoliosis would allow him to postpone the surgery in order to allow Katie more time to grow before the surgery fixed her adult height. Katie's loose shirt partially occludes the severity of the spinal deformity. **C,** Katie age 13 years, six months after back surgery. Scoliosis reduced as far as possible given her fused ribs (from surgery as a toddler) and other joint limitations.

Asymmetrical Breathing

Patients with asymmetrical movement of the chest due to a cerebral vascular accident (CVA), a scoliosis, or other types of asymmetric impairments may demonstrate an asymmetric breathing pattern. This is generally sufficient for breathing without a mechanical ventilator because the strong side compensates for the weak side (Lanini et al, 2003). This compensation, however, may lead to asymmetric alignment of the trunk that adversely affects postural control in upright postures. In addition, the adverse effects on posture can lead to undesired MS changes over a prolonged period of time, especially for the pediatric patient. Prevention of these secondary changes is of utmost importance (Sobus et al, 2000) (Figure 39-13).

Lateral or Gravity Eliminated Breathing

Patients with generalized weakness, such as with benign hypotonia, prolonged illness, an incomplete spinal cord injury, etc., may show a tendency to breathe wherever gravity provides the least resistance. For example, in a supine position, patients with weakened chest muscles cannot effectively oppose the force of gravity in the anterior plane, thus they alter their breathing pattern to expand primarily in the lateral plane

where gravity is eliminated. In sitting, these same patients would tend to breathe inferiorly where gravity would assist the movement. Likewise, in a side-lying position they would tend to breathe in an anterior plane. Overall these patients have the best prognosis for effective breathing retraining methods because they have weakness, not complete paralysis.

Shallow Breathing

Shallow breathing typically results from injuries to the central nervous system resulting in high tone, such as Parkinson, head injuries, cerebral palsy, etc. It can also occur secondary to painful conditions such as low back pain. The breathing patterns are altered not so much by muscle weakness as by the following: chest immobility because of abnormally high NM tone (spasticity, rigidity, tremors), which severely limits chest expansion in any plane; cerebellar discoordination; improper sequencing because of lesions in the brain, most commonly seen with medullary lesions; or painful conditions that cause the patient to limit changes in trunk pressures in order to limit changing pressures on the MS lesion. The breathing pattern is usually symmetrical, shallow, sometimes asynchronous, and frequently tachypneic (respiratory rates over 25 breaths/min). Initiation and follow-through of a volitional maximal

Identifying Katie's Motor Impairments from a Multisystem Model and Planning a Targeted Intervention Strategy

IMPAIRMENT CATEGORIES	MS	NM	CP	INT	IO
Identify primary pathology	Scoliosis				
Identify the progression of impairments	MS→	NM→	CP→	IO→	(INT)
List current impairment problems	**MS**: abnormal joint alignment, proximal worse than distal; abnormal length tension relationship of all muscles affected by joint malalignment resulting in weakness proximal > distal **NM**: trunk muscle weakness and malalignment resulting in the development of inadequate postural control strategies and a constant conflict between breathing and postural needs **CP**: severe restrictive lung condition resulting in significant endurance impairments; impaired breathing mechanics, including paradoxical breathing (weak intercostal muscles); RR 32/min (tachypneic); forced exhalations even at rest; weak cough; chronic nocturnal hypoventilation; inadequate respiratory reserves for inhalation or exhalation demands; 3–5 syllables/breath (normal 8-10); sustained phonation 2–3 sec (normal 10 seconds); no cardiac symptoms (yet) **INT**: none (yet) **IO**: malnutrition; dehydration; no reflux; no connective tissue limitations around scars from previous surgeries or around her shoulders or pelvis				
Functional limitations and impact on participation	Functional limitations were noted in all activities that required greater oxygen or caloric fuel than Katie's restricted body could provide or that required effective coordination of breathing with movement. This resulted in limitations from the most basic motor activity of breathing to limitations in coughing, sleeping, talking, eating, and moving, thus causing severe limitations in Katie's ability to participate in normal childhood activities such as running, walking, biking, etc.				
Prioritize the current problems by categories	IO→	MS→	NM→	CP→	(INT)
Diagnosis	Nine-year-old girl with congenital idiopathic progressive kyphoscoliosis with severe secondary restrictions to her breathing mechanics and lung growth, nutritional health, strength and alignment of the entire musculoskeletal frame, resulting in pain, endurance impairments, significant health risks, and overall limitations in the child's physical capabilities and participation.				
Prognosis	Marked compromises of the musculoskeletal and neuromuscular support for breathing and movement, combined with Katie's poor nutritional status, limit the pulmonary status she needs immediately for surgical clearance. I believe that Katie can improve the alignment, mobility, strength, and control of her rib cage and respiratory mechanics necessary to meet the pulmonary demands of surgery if given enough time to achieve a true change in the muscle function (minimum of 4–6 weeks of training). After surgery, Katie will need an aggressive physical therapy program to develop new neuromuscular strategies that effectively utilize her new musculoskeletal alignment to maximize breath support and postural control in order to reduce her long-term cardiopulmonary, nutritional, and musculoskeletal health risks, and to increase her potential to participate in normal childhood activities.				
Pre and post surgical goals	Pre surgery: Improve nutritional status, hydration, skeletal alignment of the trunk, and strength and control of the trunk musculature in order to improve Katie's breathing mechanics and cough effectiveness such that she can survive the scoliotic reduction surgery and the recovery phase. Post surgery: Use Katie's improved breathing mechanics to initiate an effective airway clearance program and to develop neuromuscular strategies to utilize and maintain her new spine alignment in order to reduce the risk of post surgical pulmonary complications and to maximize breath support and postural control long term in order to reduce her ongoing cardiopulmonary, nutritional, and musculoskeletal health risks and to increase her potential to participate in normal childhood activities.				
Interventions specific to Katie's short-term goal of surgical readiness	**MS**: rib mobilization to maximize inspiratory lung volumes; other ROM of joints as needed **NM**: NM reeducation to increase intercostal activation for inspiratory lung volumes and chest wall stabilization; NM reeducation to reduce recruitment of abdominal muscles for forced exhalation strategies; incorporation of new breathing pattern into postural demanding tasks starting with low level activities such as walking **CP**: endurance training—ventilator muscle training, including both resistive inspiratory and expiratory devices to increase respiratory endurance and low level power production; power training—using peak flow meter and incentive spirometers for visual feedback for maximal effort breathing; coughing strategies for improved airway clearance **INT**: no short term interventions needed **IO**: devised plan for increasing overall hydration and caloric intake through multiple small meals/snacks and constant sipping of water throughout the day, including school hours; school approval was critical to carryover				

inspiration is difficult or impossible for these patients. This will markedly curtail the ability to produce an effective cough, to maintain bronchial hygiene, or to yell (Grimstone & Hodges, 2003).

APPLICATION OF THE SODA-POP CAN MODEL TO A CLINICAL EXAMPLE

Implicit in the Soda-Pop Can model of respiratory and postural control is the concept that impaired pressure regulation of the trunk may have resulted from an impairment in any body system that generates or uses this pressure, and thus all systems must be screened for their potential role in the motor dysfunction of breathing or postural control. Five such impairment categories were identified at the beginning of this chapter (see Box 39-1) as well as six functional activities that require the effective coordination of the mechanics of breathing and the postural demand of motor tasks (see Box 39-2). These ideas will now be applied to a clinical case.

Multisystem Evaluation, Examination, and Intervention

Case History

Katie is a 9-year-old female (Figure 39-14, *A*) with a congenital idiopathic scoliosis (infantile scoliosis) that required surgical stabilization of two upper thoracic vertebrae at three years of age. Several ribs fused on the concave side of the scoliosis after surgery and contributed to a continued progressive kyphoscoliosis as Katie matured. Spinal fusion from T1 to S1 was planned at age nine-and-a-half when the scoliosis reached 97 to 98 degrees despite conservative bracing from three years of age and close monitoring by the orthopedic surgeon.

The presurgical work up revealed that Katie's lungs were so severely restricted by her MS impairment that the pulmonologist was unsure she would survive the surgery. In other words, Katie's can of soda-pop was crushed, resulting in multiple body system dysfunctions even though the original impairment was in a single system: the MS system. Katie was referred to physical therapy to attempt to improve her restrictive lung condition in order to become a viable surgical candidate. Katie had not been referred to physical therapy before this time for any other type of intervention.

Impairment Categories. Using a multisystem examination and evaluation from the Soda-Pop Can model point of view, Katie's pathology was no longer noted as a single system motor dysfunction. The progression of her impairments, starting with the original insult to the MS system, is identified in (Table 39-2).

1. Katie's pathology started in the MS system, specifically the spinal skeletal system. Her skeletal support, the "aluminum can," had collapsed. Katie's muscle support matured around those deformities and did not develop optimal length tension relationships for maximal force production (strength). Her muscle weakness was primarily in the trunk and proximal joints. Her distal extremity muscles showed less weakness. In particular, her chest intercostal muscles were so weak and underutilized that the negative pressure of inhalation caused her chest to be sucked inward (paradoxical breathing). She could not generate enough muscle force to counteract the internal negative pressures associated with normal inspiratory lung volumes. Fortunately, the paradoxical movement had not caused a pectus excavatum, but over time it was a real possibility. Her hips and shoulders matured around the malaligned spine, which resulted in additional joint dysfunction. Katie's mom reported that Katie was not a physically active girl, which was expected with her multiple joint limitations.

2. The MS weaknesses resulted in a secondary NM problem as her muscle recruitment and balance strategies developed around an atypical MS alignment that neither supported the symmetrical development of the body nor effectively supported the concurrent demands of pressure support in the trunk for respiratory and postural control. As a result, Katie's breathing pattern was atypical (paradoxical) and likely contributed to her reduced lung volumes.

3. Reduced lung volumes and limited physical activity led to significant endurance and mechanical impairments in the CP system. Katie's breathing mechanics were so compromised and her potential lung space so compressed that she developed a severe restrictive lung condition. No heart or vascular problems were noted per her physician at the time of her initial evaluation. Right-sided heart failure, cor pulmonale, however, which develops secondary to chronic pulmonary dysfunction, was a real risk for Katie as she matured.

4. The shape of the scoliosis severely impinged on the size of Katie's stomach, causing IO impairment that resulted in malnutrition and dehydration. Katie could only eat less than 200 calories per meal before feeling full. Fluids filled her up even quicker and made it hard for Katie to adequately hydrate herself and consume adequate calories. Fortunately Katie did not develop gastroesophageal reflux disease (GERD) from the abnormal pressures and malalignment.

5. Katie's INT system was functioning well and did not appear to cause any limitations in her motor performance. Her prior scars were well healed and not adhered to underlying surfaces. In spite of the severe spinal deformity, the connective tissue around her trunk and extremities was easily moved to allow the maximum mobility of the underlying skeletal structures. It would not have been a surprise, however, to have found connective tissue limitations preventing maximal MS movement.

Functional limitations. A functional assessment was also done to cross-check the evaluation from both perspectives: impairments and functional limitations. The functional findings confirmed the impairment findings: Katie had significant functional limitations due to impaired breathing mechanics that were impacting her quality of life.

1. Katie's breathing pattern at rest showed excessive diaphragmatic excursion, underutilization of intercostals (especially on the left, concave side of her chest), and paradoxical breathing. Her respiratory rate (RR) was 32 breaths per minute with forced exhalations (normal RR is 10 to 20 breaths/min). With minor increased physical workload, such as walking fast, she responded by breathing faster, but not deeper. Not surprisingly, she had very poor physical endurance compared with her peers. Her forced vital capacity (FVC) was 33% of predicted value for her age and height, indicating a severe restrictive lung status.

2. Her cough sequence was normal, but the small lung volume impaired her expiratory force because there was simply not enough air to force out. Her peak expiratory flow rate (PEFR) was 59% of predicted value. Clinically, less than 60% of predicted PEFR has been associated with ineffective cough and increased risk of secondary pulmonary complications.

3. Katie's teachers complained that Katie fell asleep almost every afternoon in school and often complained of headaches. Given her severe restrictive lung condition and weak trunk muscles, I suspected nocturnal hypoventilation even though a sleep study three years prior showed no abnormalities. Hypoventilation can contribute to overall poor lung function during the day due to fatigue and could therefore account for some of her poor growth patterns. Her pulmonologist concurred and ordered a new sleep study. The chronic hypoventilation was confirmed in the sleep study.

4. Katie has always been quiet according to her mother. The question was whether she was naturally quiet or conserving energy. Her speech was three to five syllables per breath. Normal speech is eight to 10 syllables per breath (Deem & Miller, 2000). Her sustained phonation was 2.4 to 3.1 seconds. Normal sustained phonation is 10 seconds (Deem & Miller, 2000). Katie yelled when asked to do so, but her mom reported that she rarely ever yelled. Her lack of breath support could explain her quiet speech, short answers, and apparent reserved style. It was impossible to know whether Katie was quiet naturally or became quiet due to poor breath support over her entire lifetime.

5. Katie's stomach was compromised by the kyphoscoliosis, which made her feel full with less than 200 calories. Katie not only had poor weight gain, but as she got older and needed more calories for vertical growth, she actually started to loss weight and was not achieving the conservative vertical height goals that her orthopedic surgeon was hoping for before the spinal fusion.

6. Not surprisingly, Katie had marked endurance limitations in normal, age appropriate physical activities. Specifically, Katie fatigued when walking more than one-and-a-half lengths of the grammar school gym or riding her bike more than two-and-a-half blocks. Katie's body was focused on surviving, not thriving. Her weak muscles and poor breathing mechanics combined with inadequate caloric, hydration, and oxygen fuel, meant that few reserves were left over from survival needs to support the thriving needs of gross motor activities such as running and jumping. Katie's body simply could not meet both the needs of breathing and higher level postural demands of normal childhood activities (Hodges et al, 2001; Gandevia et al, 2002). Katie preferred to engage in lower oxygen consuming activities such as playing the violin, reading, and playing quietly. The question was whether she really had a choice regarding her activities.

Priorities of Interventions. Understanding Katie's progression of impairments streamlined the screening process. Katie's pulmonary system was preventing her from having surgery. But pulmonary did not start out as her primary pathology. The questions this presented were how all five motor impairment categories contributed to her current pulmonary status and how to clinically prioritize the interventions to meet the short-term respiratory/surgical goals. In the short term, the evaluation directed me to prioritize the following interventions. Katie's long-term health and participation goals were developed after surgery.

1. Katie's poor nutritional status meant she had no caloric reserves to effectively engage in a conditioning program to strengthen her respiratory muscles in preparation for surgery. Likewise, her general state of dehydration would cause decreased mobility of pulmonary secretions, thus increasing her postsurgical risk of pneumonia and/or atelectasis. Thus, focusing on increasing Katie's nutritional and hydration needs was the first priority. Katie was instructed to eat at least six meals per day rather than three, and was given permission from her teachers to bring a water bottle to class. In school she was encouraged to drink at the start of every new subject. Katie's nutritional content was managed by her pediatrician.

2. Surgery was the recommended intervention to improve the long-term alignment of her spine and ribcage. In the short term, however, manual mobilization of her ribcage was a priority to gain any possible additional movement that could be used to increase lung volumes.

3. After Katie's ribcage mobility was increased and a position that gave her the best support for chest wall movement was identified (sitting), a NM program was initiated to improve the respiratory mechanics. The focus of the program was:

   a. to increase the recruitment, strength, and function of the intercostal muscles as inspiratory muscles (for increased lung volume) and as chest wall stabilizers (to stop the paradoxical breathing), while decreasing the use of forced abdominal muscle exhalations, thus reducing her overall energy cost of breathing by using her trunk pressures more effectively,

   b. to increase the power production of both inspiratory and expiratory muscles for increased lung volume and increased cough effectiveness through use of peak flow meters and incentive spirometers for visual feedback of specific targeted performance (large effort, low repetitions),

c. to increase endurance and overall fitness of the respiratory muscles through use of an aggressive daily ventilatory muscle training program involving both the inspiratory and expiratory muscles (low resistance, high repetitions); ventilatory muscle training resistance was used instead of a traditional fitness training program such as treadmill training because Katie's weakness, malalignments, and painful joints would have prevented her from exercising long enough to be effective and may have actually caused other joint problems,

d. to improve Katie's ability to meet the conflicting needs of respiration and postural control necessary for functional endurance and motor performance by prescribing low level activities (walking) to start, increasing the distance (endurance), and providing instruction on how to use the new breathing pattern within a functional task to challenge her balance and respiratory needs simultaneously.

4. By addressing the contributions that all body systems had on the efficiency and effectiveness of Katie's breathing mechanics, her lung volumes, cough effectiveness, endurance impairments, and postural conflicts were targeted through multiple interventions to address her most pressing problem: pulmonary clearance for orthopedic surgery.

5. Katie's INT system did not show any impairments and was not a significant contributor to her poor pulmonary status. However, after surgery, her dehydrated condition predisposed her to a potential skin breakdown and poor scar healing and therefore she had to be monitored for any emerging problems.

Diagnosis and Prognosis. Katie's MS pathology impaired the structural support of her trunk and respiratory mechanics. As a result of the innate interactions between the body systems, the MS restrictions resulted in dysfunction in numerous other systems. She was referred to physical therapy for one specific task: to improve her breathing mechanics such that she could undergo surgery to correct the initial pathology, the scoliosis. After the PT exam, the pulmonologist was contacted to discuss the findings and told that Katie's condition showed potential for improvement, but a minimum of four to six weeks was needed to achieve a true training effect that would hopefully sustain her through the long surgery. Surgery was put off for eight weeks to allow Katie the maximum benefit of the physical therapy intervention. For her long-term goals of improved health and participation in normal childhood related activities, it was obvious that improving her breathing mechanics was only one aspect that needed to be addressed. The other issues were to be addressed after surgery.

Outcomes. Katie and her mom understood the surgical risk and were very motivated to participate in an aggressive physical therapy program that relied heavily on their home participation. Katie and her mom were instructed regarding the necessity of a home exercise program five days a week for four to six weeks in order to effect a true change in the status of the muscle strength and endurance. Katie did the exercises seven days per week instead. Specific pulmonary function test improvements are noted below along with their influence on her surgical status.

1. Katie's pulmonary function test (PFT) baseline for FVC was .45 L, which is 33% of predicted value (1.36 L), and her PEFR was 1.64 L/s, or 59% of predicted value.

   a. Three weeks later, Katie's FVC improved to .57 L, or 42% of predicted value.
   b. Five months later, FVC had increased to .63 L, or 45% of predicted value, where it held steady.
   c. Three months after initating her program, PEFR improved to 2.31 L/s, making it 81% of predicted value, which is within a normal range for effective cough.
   d. Two years later, after a sleep study confirmed chronic hypoventilation and after successful initiation of bi-level positive airway pressure machine (Bi-PAP) nocturnal support, FVC improved to .71 L, but this value was now only 40% of predicted value for her age and height (1.78 L). The predicted values continue to climb with age in children, but Katie's lungs did not keep pace with expectations for a typically developing child. A predicted FVC value of 60% is often used as the clinical measurement of adequate lung volume necessary for normal pulmonary maneuvers such as coughing, sighing, sneezing, etc. At 40% she was still at long-term risk for secondary respiratory problems due to impaired lung volumes.

2. At four months, the orthopedic surgeon decided to put the surgery on hold because her scoliosis had reduced from 97 to 98 degrees to 90 to 92 degrees. He felt that her improved pulmonary status had a positive effect on her skeletal frame and that as long as she remained stable, it was worth holding off the surgery to give her every chance to grow and continue making respiratory gains before fusing her spine (see Figure 39-14, *B*).

   a. Katie's surgery was held off for three-and-a-quarter years until Katie was 12 years old, allowing her to establish more vertical growth before the spinal fusion. The orthopedic surgeon expressed his surprise that she did not require the surgery before 10 years of age.
   b. Katie continued to do her exercises three to four days a week for that entire time. She had no postoperative respiratory complications. Her scoliosis was markedly reduced but not eliminated (Figure 39-14, *C*). Katie may require additional surgeries later for her shoulders, hips, and fused ribs.

Numerous other aspects were involved in Katie's care, including an eventual gastric surgery for a gastrostomy-tube placement to foster more effective nutritional gains, the initiation of growth hormones, the use of bi-PAP nocturnal support to reverse chronic hypoventilation and its effects on her physical endurance and growth, as well as a more comprehensive physical therapy program to focus on her overall growth and maturation. This report focused on the initial physical therapy intervention to illustrate how a multi-system assessment could be used to develop a differential diagnosis regarding her physical and pulmonary limitations. In this case Katie's scoliosis and subsequent muscle development made her incapable of generating, maintaining, and regulating adequate pressures in her trunk to support normal respiration, postural control, and IO function. The Soda-Pop Can model helped to explain why the impairment to her MS system had such far reaching implications on her health and the function of her other systems.

Quality of Life. In additional to medical improvement, Katie's mom reported that the respiratory and multisystem approach to Katie's physical therapy program "absolutely saved her life." Katie's confidence in her ability to influence her own destiny was noted at the second physical therapy visit, during which she saw the positive results of her diligent adherence to the home program: her impairment level improved in terms of PFTs and she achieved functional gains in her 12-minute walk test. Within six months of the initiation of the physical therapy program, Katie's paradoxical breathing was gone, she no longer used forced abdominal exhalations, her chest wall expansion improved, and her sustained phonation improved 50% (from 3.1 seconds to 4.7 seconds), all of which contributed to her increased physical activity. She started swimming lessons, joined recreational softball, and generally reported that she "likes this new feeling. It's easier to move and breathe." Her mom reported that Katie smiled more often.

Interpretation of the Clinical Relevance of this Case to Impaired Respiratory Mechanics. The CP system is one of many systems that creates and utilizes pressure support in the trunk for optimal performance, and it should not be assessed or treated in isolation from the potential influence that other body systems have on its performance. The body always functions as a whole unit with all the individual systems interacting and supporting one another; it does not act as a single system. In particular, postural control and the mechanical support for breathing are interdependent; yet breathing needs will always take precedence over postural needs. Therefore, mechanical support for breathing should be assessed and treated within the context of the mechanical support for postural control because both activities utilize the same space and the same muscles.

A diagnosis that stems from the MS system, such as for Katie, cannot be assessed from a single system perspective. As we saw with Katie, although the initial pathology stemmed from the MS system, her current problems were more pressing in the NM system (motor planning and strength), the CP system (severely impaired respiratory mechanics, inadequate respiratory endurance, and the risk for cardiac

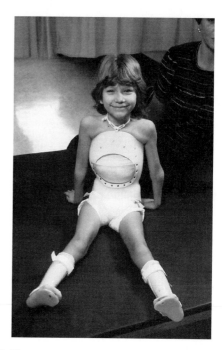

FIGURE 39-15 Melissa, six years of age. Note the use of the TLSO with an abdominal cutout supported by an abdominal binder. This provided support for her developing spine and trunk while still allowing for optimal support for breathing mechanics. Note that the TLSO provided an ideal alignment of the proximal extremity joints (shoulders and hips) as well as the ideal head alignment for normal functions such as talking and eating.

impairments), and the IOs (persistent malnutrition and dehydration). If Katie had been treated for a single system impairment, this author does not believe that she would have had the significant clinical and functional successes that allowed her surgeon to delay her impending surgery more than three years.

BROADER APPLICATION

Pathologies stemming from any motor impairment category may result in impaired breathing mechanics and/or a conflict in postural control and breathing that interferes with motor performance. For example, a patient with a NM insult such as a spinal cord injury, cerebral palsy, CVA, or head injury will show impaired breathing mechanics and impaired postural control due to paralysis, weakness, or impaired motor planning or execution associated with those NM disorders. The therapist would need to assess such a patient from the neuro-motor perspective as well as that system's interaction with the MS, CP, INT, and IO systems before feeling confident that the major limiting impairment to motor performance and health had been correctly identified and prioritized for intervention. Dramatic changes in chest wall and trunk alignment can be achieved long term from a multisystem approach. See Melissa's changes from three to 12 years of age after a SCI birth trauma (compare Figures 39-15 and 39-16 with Figures 39-2, *B* and

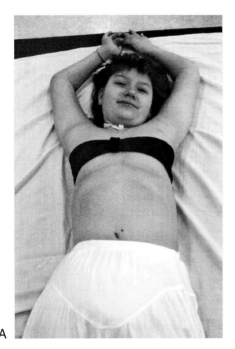

A

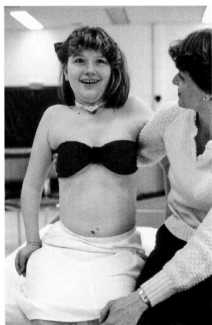

B

FIGURE 39-16 Melissa, 12 years of age, after orthopedic surgery to reduce scoliosis. **A,** Note that the chest wall deformities that were so prevalent at age three are almost completely absent. The only noticeable skeletal restriction is the slight reduction in mid chest expansion noted around ribs six through eight, which looks like a high "waistline" just under her bra strap line in supine. The intercostal muscles, which were paralyzed, are the only support for the ribcage at that level. Melissa used her upper accessory muscles to support breathing and chest wall alignment of the upper chest, and the diaphragm for the lower ribcage. **B,** Melissa continues to wear an abdominal binder in upright postures, but it was removed for this picture.

39-8, *C*). Melissa's chest wall and spinal deformities were almost completely reversed after years of interventions from a multidisciplined team approach to her multisystem impairments (Massery, 1991). Melissa was not seen by a physical therapist or any physical medicine discipline until she was three-and-a-half years old. A few key long-term interventions and outcomes follow.

1. Melissa used an abdominal binder whenever she was upright to provide the abdominal pressures needed for IO support and improved breathing mechanics and lumbar stabilization. This will be a lifelong intervention.

2. In addition, Melissa needed a body jacket, or thoracic-lumbar-sacral orthosis (TLSO), with an abdominal cutout and abdominal binder. An abdominal binder alone was not enough support for her developing spine and proximal joints. She still developed a scoliosis, but she did not develop a kyphosis or axial rotation of the curve. The orthopedic surgeon stated that this made the eventual surgical correction easier, safer, and faster.

3. An aggressive NM reeducation program was implemented to teach Melissa how to engage her upper accessory muscles, especially her pectoralis muscles, as substitute chest wall stabilizers and how to use them as long-term inspiratory muscles to balance the excessive inward pressure generated by the isolated contractions of the diaphragm. She was also instructed in how to use her breath support (ventilatory strategies) to improve her mobility skills, such as in rolling over and reaching.

4. A comprehensive airway clearance program was developed to minimize the family's reliance on suctioning. Melissa and her family learned multiple manual assistive cough techniques that effectively expectorated the mucus. They reduced her suctioning from 24 to 36 times per day to one to three times per day. She had multiple pneumonias in her first three-and-a-half years of life, but none from age three to 12.

5. Melissa's nutrition and hydration needs were attacked as a whole team to increase her caloric and hydration status. Her 12-year-old picture clearly shows that she learned to consume adequate calories for growth. (A gastrostomy tube was not used as it had not yet been invented when Melissa was a young girl.)

6. Melissa was initiated on nocturnal positive pressure ventilation support at approximately six years of age due to nocturnal hypoventilation and the conflict between the use of calories for growth or breathing. The positive pressure support obviously relieved her work of breathing and gave her muscles a daily rest, but it also provided pressure support to reverse the pectus forces.

The same concept can be applied for any other impairment category. For example, in Katie's case, if her INT system showed connective tissue restrictions secondary to the kyphoscoliosis, then her INT system would have been the primary limiting factor to improving her pulmonary status rather than her NM and IO systems. In other words, if her

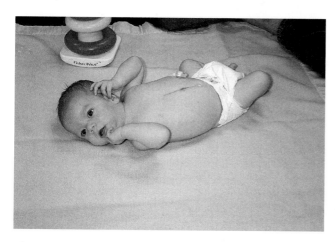

FIGURE 39-17 Jonathan, six months of age. His severe gastroesophygeal reflux required surgical support (gastrostomy tube and Nissen fundoplication procedures) at five months of age. His mother reports that his favorite posture when in supine is extreme trunk extension and right head rotation. This may have developed as a compensatory strategy against the noxious stimulus from reflux and a possible upper airway obstruction that was yet undiagnosed.

ribcage was capable of being mobilized but the overlying skin did not allow movement into the new range due to connective tissue shortening, then Katie would not have been capable of learning to use new breathing strategies to increase her lung volumes. This is noted dramatically in patients who have connective tissue disorders such as scleroderma or severe burns: the skin no longer has the mobility to allow the underlying muscles to move the chest wall adequately to inhale lung volumes necessary to meet the oxygen needs of motor tasks. How restrictive their breathing is depends on the severity of the condition and damage to the INT structures.

Conditions related to the IO system may have a more subtle influence on postural control and breathing. Infants with severe gastroesophygeal reflux may assume a posture of trunk extension and right head rotation in a supine position (Sandifer's syndrome) (Werlin et al, 1980; Senocak et al, 1993; Gorrotxategi et al, 1995; de Ybarrondo & Mazur, 2000; Demir et al, 2001) (Figure 39-17). This posturing may be mistaken initially for a true NM lesion. In fact, the infant may use this posturing to move away from the noxious stimulus of reflux experienced whenever he or she moves into a flexed trunk posture of head turning and lateral trunk bending to the left. If the child is not assessed from a multisystem perspective, the physical therapist may erroneously treat the excessive extension tone and asymmetry of the trunk rather than the underlying cause of the motor behavior, which stems from the IO system. If untreated, these infants tend to develop more trunk extension and upper chest breathing strategies to avoid exacerbating the reflux, which occurs when the diaphragm descends onto the irritable stomach, and to avoid

increasing intraabdominal pressure, which may also contribute to reflux. Over time, that child may develop impairments in all motor systems, and this could affect the child's overall health and participation potential. For example, children with cystic fibrosis are tipped downward for postural drainage to improve lung function, but it is now known that the treatment predisposes the children to reflux and a worsening of their pulmonary condition (Button et al, 2003; Button et al, 2004). The outline below describes how all motor systems could be affected by a pathology starting in the IO system.

1. IO system: The pathology started here.
2. NM system: Inadequate motor control of trunk flexors, necessary for balance, forced expiratory maneuvers, and lumbar stabilization, may develop. An IO pathology potentially predisposes the child to later low back dysfunction and pain because normal positive pressure stabilization motor strategies, especially from the diaphragm and abdominal muscles, are not developed in childhood.
3. MS system: A sequelae of connected events is possible, such as (a) excessive ligamentous shortening of lumbar vertebrae secondary to the chronic lordotic posture, and/or (b) elevated ribcage alignment, which results when the trunk flexors never actively engage in pulling the ribcage inferiorly and the over-recruitment of upper accessory muscles continues to promote this position, which can contribute to (c) increased risk for low back pain secondary to poor lumbar stabilization strategies, weak abdominal muscles, and atypical vertebral alignment.
4. CP system: Poorer overall endurance may result if the child develops an upper chest breathing pattern as his or her primary breathing pattern in response to the noxious feedback received in response to using the diaphragm as the primary respiratory muscle. This could also predispose the child to neck and/or shoulder dysfunction because the conflict between the respiratory recruitment of the upper accessory muscles and the dual role these same muscles play in upper quadrant movement may cause over-utilization and later complaints of pain, fatigue, headaches, etc.
5. INT system: This is generally not a major problem area, but the potential exists for inadequate connective tissue mobility that may restrict movement into flexion patterns of the trunk, shoulder, or hip.

The clinical examples are endless. Impaired breathing mechanics do not occur only because of a direct impairment of the lungs, airways, or chest wall muscles. Impaired breathing mechanics can occur from insults to any system that influences motor performance. The CP system should be seen as an integral part of all motor assessments in order to determine whether the mechanics of breathing are working for or against the patient's overall motor performance. In other words, breathing mechanics may be the cause or the consequence of motor dysfunction and a thorough multisystem evaluation should help the clinician determine the difference.

SUMMARY

In this chapter, the role of the respiratory mechanics as they relate to other body systems has been explored. Gravity was presented as a significant influence on both the potential movement of the chest and the normal development of the chest and trunk. The relationship of the dual role of the trunk in support of both respiration and postural control was introduced in the form of the Soda-Pop Can Model. These concepts were then applied to clinical cases from multiple motor impairment categories to illustrate how trunk control, breathing, and internal functions are dependent on the ability of the body to generate, maintain, and regulate pressure in the thoracic and abdominal chambers; the control of which extends from the vocal folds down to the pelvic floor. Using clinical examples, all five motor impairment categories—MS, NM, CP, INT, and IO systems—were screened for their potential role in motor performance and breathing mechanics because each system influences the performance of the other. This information was then used to design a treatment plan that effectively targeted the primary impairments and successfully achieved a desired motor outcome that involved the trunk and breathing.

Review Questions

1. Explain the role of gravity in normal chest wall development of infants.
2. Explain how the pressure in the thorax and abdomen helps to provide postural support for the trunk and the role of the diaphragm in that process.
3. Explain the role of the vocal folds and the pelvic floor in normal respiration and in high postural demanding activities.
4. Expalin the relationship between the gastrointestinal system and respiration.
5. Take one of your patients and apply the concept of a multisystem evaluation, examination, and intervention planning as was demonstrated in this chapter.

REFERENCES

APTA. (2001). Guide to Physical Therapist Practice, ed 2. Physical Therapy 81:.

Bach, J.R., Baird, J.S., Plosky, D., Navado, J., & Weaver, B. (2002). Spinal muscular atrophy type 1: management and outcomes. Pediatric Pulmonology 34:16-22.

Bach, J.R., & Bianchi, C. (2003). Prevention of pectus excavatum for children with spinal muscular atrophy type 1. American Journal of Physical Medicine and Rehabilitation 82:815-819.

Bach, J.R. & Saporito, L.R. (1996). Criteria for extubation and tracheostomy tube removal for patients with ventilatory failure. A different approach to weaning. Chest 110:1566-1571.

Bly, L. (1994). Motor skills acquisition in the first year. San Antonio, Tex: Therapy Skill Builder.

Borowitz, S.M., & Borowitz, K.C. (1997). Gastroesophageal reflux in babies: impact on growth and development. Infants and Young Children 10:14-26.

Borowitz, S.M., & Sutphen, J.L. (2004). Recurrent vomiting and persistent gastroesophageal reflux caused by unrecognized constipation. Clinical Pediatrics 43:461-466.

Bouisset, S., & Duchene, J.L. (1994). Is body balance more perturbed by respiration in seating than in standing posture? Neuroreport 5:957-960.

Button, B.M., Heine, R.G., et al. (2003). Chest physiotherapy in infants with cystic fibrosis: to tip or not? A five-year study. Pediatric Pulmonology 35:208–213.

Button, B.M., Heine, R.G., et al. (2004). Chest physiotherapy, gastro-esophageal reflux, and arousal in infants with cystic fibrosis. Archive of Diseases in Childhood 89:435–439.

Cala, S.J. (1993). Abdominal compliance, parasternal activation, and chest wall motion. Journal of Applied Physiology 74:1398-1405.

Cherniack, R.M. & Cherniack, L. (1983). Respiration in health and disease, ed 3. Philadelphia, Pa: W.B. Saunders Co.

De Looze, D., Van Laere, M., De Muynck, M., & Elewaut, A. (1998). Constipation and other chronic gastrointestinal problems in spinal cord injury patients. Spinal Cord 36:63-66.

De Troyer, A., Gorman, R.B., & Gandevia, S.C. (2003). Distribution of inspiratory drive to the external intercostal muscles in humans. Journal of Physiology 546:943-954.

de Ybarrondo, L., & Mazur, J.L. (2000). Sandifer's syndrome in a child with asthma and cerebral palsy. Southern Medical Journal 93:1019-1021.

Deem, J.F. & Miller, L. (2000). Manual of voice therapy, ed 2. Austin, Tex: PRO-ED, Inc.

Demir, E., Saka, E., et al. (2001). A case of Sandifer's syndrome with hand tremor. Turkish Journal of Pediatrics 43:348-350.

Dodd, M.E. (2004). Incontinence in cystic fibrosis. London: Presented at The Royal Society of Medicine Conference on Cystic Fibrosis.

Flaminiano, L.E. & Celli, BR. (2001). Respiratory muscle testing. Clinics in Chest Medicine 22:661-677.

Gandevia, S.C. Butler, J.E., Hodges, P.W., & Taylor, J.L. (2002). Balancing acts: respiratory sensations, motor control and human posture. Clinical and Experimental Pharmacology and Physiology 29:118-121.

Gorrotxategi, P., Reguilon, M.J, et al. (1995). Gastroesophageal reflux in association with the Sandifer syndrome. European Journal of Pediatric Surgery 5:203-205.

Grimstone, S.K. & Hodges, P.W. (2003). Impaired postural compensation for respiration in people with recurrent low back pain. Experimental Brain Research 151:218-224.

Han, J.N., Gayan-Ramirez, G., Dekhuijzen, R., & Decramer, M. (1993). Respiratory function of the rib cage muscles. European Respiratory Journal 6:722-728.

Hayama, S., Honda, K., et al. (2002). Air trapping and arboreal locomotor adaptation in primates: a review of experiments on humans. Zeitschrift fur Morphologie und Anthropologie 83:149-159.

Hodges, P.W. & Gandevia, S.C. (2000). Activation of the human diaphragm during a repetitive postural task. Journal of Physiology 522:165-175.

Hodges, P.W., & Gandevia, S.C. (2000). Changes in intra-abdominal pressure during postural and respiratory activation of the human diaphragm. Journal of Applied Physiology 89:967-976.

Hodges, P.W., Gurfinkel, V.S., Brumagne, S., Smith, T.C., & Cordo, P.C. (2002). Coexistence of stability and mobility in postural control: evidence from postural compensation for respiration. Experimental Brain Research 144:293-302.

Hodges, P.W., Heijnen, I., & Gandevia, S.C. (2001). Postural activity of the diaphragm is reduced in humans when respiratory demand increases. Journal of Physiology 537:999-1008.

Langman, H., Orr, A., et al. (2004). Urinary incontinence in CF: why does it happen? Eighteenth Annual North American Cystic Fibrosis Conference, St. Louis, Mo. Pediatric Pulmonology 27(Suppl):154-155.

Lanini, B., Bianchi, R., Romagnoli, I., Coli, C., Binazzi, B., Gigliotti, F., Pizzi, A., Grippo, A., & Scano, G. (2003). Chest wall kinematics in patients with hemiplegia. American Journal of Respiratory and Critical Care Medicine 168:109-113.

Lissoni, A., Aliverti, A., Tzeng, A.C., & Bach, J.R. (1998). Kinematic analysis of patients with spinal muscular atrophy during spontaneous breathing and mechanical ventilation. American Journal of Physical Medicine and Rehabilitation 77:188-192.

Massery, M. (2005). Asthma: multisystem implications. In Campbell, S., Palisano, R., & Vander Linden, D., (Eds). Physical therapy for children. Philadelphia, Pa: W.B. Saunders.

Massery, M.P. (1991). Chest development as a component of normal motor development: implications for pediatric physical therapists. Pediatric Physical Therapy 3:3-8.

McGill, S.M., Sharratt, M.T., & Seguin, J.P. (1995). Loads on spinal tissues during simultaneous lifting and ventilatory challenge. Ergonomics 38:1772-1792.

Nava, S., Ambrosino, N., Crotti, P., Fracchia, C., & Rampulla, C. (1993). Recruitment of some respiratory muscles during three maximal inspiratory manoeuvres. Thorax 48:702-707.

Noreau, L., Proulx, P., Gagnon, L., Drolet, M., & Laramee, M.T. (2000). Secondary impairments after spinal cord injury: a population-based study. American Journal of Physical Medicine and Rehabilitation 79:526-535.

Papastamelos, C., Panitch, H.B., & Allen, J.L. (1996). Chest wall compliance in infants and children with neuromuscular disease. American Journal Respiratory Critical Care Medicine 154: 1045-1048.

Pierce, R.J. & Worsnop, C.J. (1999). Upper airway function and dysfunction in respiration. Clinical and Experimental Pharmacology and Physiology 26:1-10.

Primiano, F.P. Jr. (1982). Theoretical analysis of chest wall mechanics. Journal of Biomechanics 15:919-931.

Rimmer, K.P., Ford, G.T., & Whitelaw, W.A. (1995). Interaction between postural and respiratory control of human intercostal muscles. Journal of Applied Physiology 79:1556-1561.

Rimmer, K.P. & Whitelaw, W.A. (1993). The respiratory muscles in multicore myopathy. American Review of Respiratory Disease 148:227-231.

Sapsford, R.R., Hodges, P.W., Richardson, C.A., Cooper, D.H., Markwell, S.J., & Jull, G.A. (2001). Co-activation of the abdominal and pelvic floor muscles during voluntary exercises. Neurourology and Urodynamics 20:31-42.

Senocak, M.E., Arda, I.S, et al. (1993). Torticollis with hiatus hernia in children. Sandifer syndrome. Turkish Journal of Pediatrics 35:209-213.

Serway, R., & Faughn, J. (1992). College physics. Orlando, Fla: Harcourt Brace Jovanovich.

Skjodt, N.M., Farran, R.P., Hawes, H.G., Kortbeek, J.B., & Easton, P.A. (2001). Simulation of acute spinal cord injury: effects on respiration. Respiratory Physiology 127:3-11.

Sobus, K.M.L., Horan, S.M., et al. (2000). Respiratory management of neuromuscular diseases in children. Physical Medicine and Rehabilitation: State of the Art Reviews 14:285-299.

Sumarez, R.C. (1986). An analysis of action of intercostal muscles in the human rig cage. Journal of Applied Physiology 60:690-701.

Toder, D.S. (2000). Respiratory problems in the adolescent with developmental delay. Adolescent Medicine 11:617-631.

Werlin, S.L., D'Souza, B.J., et al. (1980). Sandifer syndrome: an unappreciated clinical entity. Developmental Medicine and Child Neurology 22:374-378.

Wilson, T.A., Legrand, A., Gevenois, P.A., & De Troyer, A. (2001). Respiratory effects of the external and internal intercostal muscles in humans. Journal of Physiology 530:319-330.

Winslow, C., & Rozovsky, J. (2003). Effect of spinal cord injury on the respiratory system. American Journal of Physical Medical Rehabilitation 82:803-814.

Wood, R.P. 2nd, Jafek, B.W., & Cherniack, R.M. (1986). Laryngeal dysfunction and pulmonary disorder. Otolaryngology Head and Neck Surgery 94:374-378.

C H A P T E R 4 0

The Transplant Patient

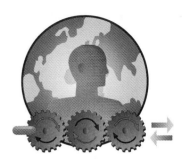

Susan A. Scherer

KEY TERMS   Cardiac rehabilitation   Organ donation
                Immunosuppression   Pulmonary rehabilitation

The ability to transplant an organ from one individual into another is a relatively new phenomenon. New advances in surgical techniques and immunosuppressive drugs, the ability to detect and treat rejection, and improved outcomes have made transplantation of solid organs a viable treatment option for patients with end-stage cardiac and pulmonary conditions. The increased life expectancy of transplant patients means that physical therapists have many opportunities for patient intervention both before and after transplantation in various settings. Trends in patient demographics indicate that a physical therapist may see a transplant patient not only in a regional medical center setting but also in outpatient and rural clinics. This chapter contains guidelines for managing patients who have undergone heart or lung transplantation.

BACKGROUND

Transplantation of tissues and organs has been of interest to physicians and surgeons since the 18th century. Advances in understanding of the immune system, development of immunosuppressive medications, and techniques such as cardiopulmonary bypass provided the opportunity for successful organ transplants. In 1954, the first kidney was successfully transplanted. Other first successful organ transplants include the heart in 1968, a combined heart-lung transplant in 1981, and a single lung transplant in 1983 (http://www.OPTN.org).

Organ transplantation has become a viable alternative to medical treatment of many conditions. Because of the success rates, many types of transplants are no longer considered experimental but appropriate treatment for organ failure. Due to improved survival, long-term outcomes are as important as short-term outcomes as a measure of successful transplantation. The number of Medicare-approved medical centers that perform lung and heart-lung transplants has grown to 45 in the United States, and there are 104 certified heart transplant centers (http://www.cms.hhs.gov). More than 2000 heart transplants and 1000 lung transplants have been performed annually since 2000. The five-year survival rates for heart transplant are reported as 70.6%, and for lung transplants as 45%. Other national data on median waiting time and survival rates as indicated by the Organ Procurement and Transplantation Network (OPTN) are shown in Table 40-1 (based on OPTN data as of June 25, 2004).

The number of organs available for transplant remains well below the need for donor organs. Currently there are over 85,000 individuals on the national waiting list for all organs (based on OPTN data as of August 27, 2004). Once an organ donor has been identified, a computer generated list of potential recipients is ranked according to the criteria established for each organ. A general list of criteria is provided in Box 40-1. Criteria may include blood or tissue type, size of organ, medical status of the patient, and the amount of time the patient has been on the waiting list. The organ procurement

Heart Lung Transplantation National Data

	HEART	LUNG
Number transplants, 1998-March 2004	35,056	11,480
Median waiting time (days), 2001-2002	Status IA, 40	Cystic fibrosis, 821
	Status IB, 73	COPD, 502
	Status II, 335	Pulmonary fibrosis, 570
1 year survival (all status)	85.8%	8.75%
5 year survival	70.6%	45.1%

Data from http://www.optn.org.

General Criteria for Transplant Waiting Lists

Age under 65 years (under 60 years in some centers)
Terminal illness (expected lifespan less than 1 year)
Nonsmoker
Adequate social support system
Disease free in other systems

coordinator confers with the transplant surgeons until a potential recipient is identified. Surgical teams then travel to the donor hospital while the recipient is concurrently prepared for surgery. Heart, lung, and liver transplantation success is optimized when the transplant occurs within six hours of removal of the donated organ. Surgical methods that allow for longer travel times or changes in management of the donor organ have increased the number of available organs; however, the number of available organs remains significantly below the need.

Organ Donation

The major limitation of organ transplantation is the limitation of supply in the face of an increasing demand. The number of patients who could benefit from transplant significantly exceeds the number of organs available. The OPTN is an organization whose primary goal is to increase the availability of donated organs available and improve organ sharing. OPTN was established by the National Organ Transplant Act of the United States Congress in 1984, and is administered by the private, non-profit organization United Network for Organ Sharing (UNOS), under contract with the US Department of Health and Human Services (http://www.optn.org).

ISSUES ASSOCIATED WITH TRANSPLANTATION

There are many ethical, psychological, and social concerns surrounding organ transplantation. Ethical issues relate to increasing potential donor sources and distributing available organs. Psychological issues include stress due to an unknown waiting time, the potential of moving from home to a location near a transplant center and possible employment

disruption. The transplant process affects not only the individual patient, but the social support systems as well. In addition, adequate social support is a factor in long-term transplant success and quality of life.

Ethical Considerations

The ethical considerations of organ transplantation relate to increasing potential donor sources and distributing available organs. The bioethical issues around appropriate organ donors continue to generate considerable debate. For example, one important issue is whether the donor's family should be compensated monetarily for the organ donation. Currently there is no monetary gain from organ donation in the United States.

Other bioethical considerations include how to allocate the available organs to individuals waiting for transplant. All patients are screened for medical and psychological conditions that would adversely affect the outcome of transplantation. The specific acceptance criteria are different for each organ; lung transplant criteria differ from heart transplantation criteria. In general, waiting list time remains the primary factor that determines who is next in line to receive an available organ; however, other matching factors are considered for each available organ. Patients who are current smokers are not candidates for lung transplantation, although most centers allow former smokers to qualify for a lung transplant. Patients with documented alcohol abuse are not candidates for transplantation. Criteria are used so that individual preferences of team members are not given priority. In addition, ethnicity, sex, religion and financial status are *not* part of the transplant criteria. The general criteria for being listed on a transplant waiting list are listed in Box 40-1.

Psychological and Social Considerations

There are many psychological issues associated with organ transplantation, such as feelings of uncertainty, upheaval associated with moving, and issues of psychological adjustment. The time spent waiting for a transplant can vary considerably. During the waiting period, patients struggle with the need to carry on with their lives, knowing that at any moment they may be called to the hospital for transplant. In addition, the patient is torn between wanting to remain hopeful that a transplant will provide new life and the reality of knowing they have a terminal condition. Anxiety and depression have been identified as prevalent psychological issues related to transplant (Brown et al, 2004; Limbos et al, 2000).

The number of transplant centers in the United States is limited. Because organs are viable for only hours after removal from the donor, patients waiting for transplant are frequently required to live within a several-hour radius of the transplant center in which the surgery will occur. Patients need information and logistical assistance to relocate to a city that has a transplant center. They may also require emotional and financial support for this transition (Monterosso, 2003). The demands of waiting and relocation put considerable stress on the patient and his or her significant other. Those patients who relocate to a city near a transplant centers may have the most difficult time psychologically, especially as they leave family and significant others behind. The psychological stresses are somewhat different on spouses. Spouses speak of the struggle to remain hopeful yet plan for a future that may not include their loved one. If the patient and spouse move to a new city to wait for transplant, they may find themselves with more time together than before. In this forced retirement, new stresses are added to relationships. Transplant teams usually include a psychologist or social worker to whom patients may be referred for individual or family counseling, if needed.

Other concerns include psychological adjustment and the effect of social supports on mediating coping skills. Feelings of being useless are common because patients waiting in a foreign city are outside of their own environment and must find some meaningful activities. Coping strategies appear to strengthen psychological outcomes (Dew et al, 2000). After transplant, patients are often emotionally overwhelmed with a feeling of gratefulness that they are alive and feelings of guilt that someone else's grief has given them a chance to rejoice. A strong support system is considered an essential component of a successful transplant and improves psychosocial outcomes after transplantation (Dew et al, 2000). Therapists can assist patients by listening to their feelings, being supportive, and encouraging participation in support groups. Support groups, which include patients who are waiting for and patients who have undergone a transplant, can offer significant psychosocial support. Spouses and significant others also benefit from group support.

PHYSICAL THERAPY CONSIDERATIONS

As important members of the transplant team, physical therapists need an understanding of the physiological components of both the pretransplant disease and posttransplant state, as well as knowledge of the influence of surgery, medications, and rejection on musculoskeletal structure and function. In addition, physical function may be decreased due to both the primary cardiopulmonary condition and overall deconditioning. Knowledge of medical management including medications,

ventilatory support, and hemodynamic monitoring assists the therapist in determining whether modifications to a plan of care are needed during rehabilitation.

Physical therapists have a role in the management of the transplant patient in all stages of transplant: before, in the acute postoperative phase, and in the rehabilitation phase. The purpose of physical therapy before transplant is to identify baseline function and to screen for impairments that may limit rehabilitation goals. Pretransplantation offers an opportunity to address limitations in strength, range of motion, or endurance and improve physical function. Because of the surgical intervention, bed mobility, ventilation, secretion management, range of motion, and pain control are important areas to address in the immediate postoperative phase. In the posttransplantation rehabilitation phase, physical therapy goals are to return the patient to the highest functional level. Upper and lower extremity muscle strength and range of motion are addressed, as well as posture, shoulder and trunk mobility, breathing pattern, breath sounds, and functional mobility.

Oxygen Transport

Cardiac and pulmonary conditions leading to transplant produce limitations in the oxygen transport pathway. An understanding of the limitations in the oxygen transport pathway assists the therapist in designing a plan of care specific for each individual. Oxygen transport may be affected by the primary disease process, the surgical or medical intervention, or the medications used posttransplant. Cardiac conditions lead to impairments in myocardial function, leading to decreased oxygen availability for daily activities. Peripheral muscle dysfunction often occurs concurrently with the myocardial condition.

Pulmonary conditions lead to impairments in the mechanics of the lungs and chest wall and diffusion abnormalities, producing a low blood oxygen content that is inadequate for daily activities. Myocardial function may be decreased secondary to increased vascular resistance in the lung. Likewise, peripheral utilization of oxygen may be decreased as a result of the pulmonary condition or inactivity.

Surgical and Medical Considerations

Physical therapists need to consider the effect of surgery, medication, and possible graft rejection on oxygen transport and functional ability. In patients who have undergone a surgical procedure, physical therapists must identify and manage problems related to anesthesia, pain control, hemodynamic instability, and alterations in muscle function affected by the site of surgical incisions. The medication regimen for patients after organ transplant is complex, and in many cases more cumbersome than the medical management of the underlying condition. Patients must take immuno-suppressant medications for the remainder of their lives. These medications, and others used to manage the symptoms related to the immune suppressants, have consequences for peripheral muscle function and energy production. Limitations in physical function may be due to the primary condition, lack of physical activity, side effects of medications, or all three. Specifics will be covered later in this chapter.

The principle limitation to survival is graft rejection. Although advances in immune suppression have been successful, long-term rejection remains a difficult medical problem. During the first year after transplant, the primary causes of morbidity and mortality relate to acute cellular rejection and infection. Long-term, chronic rejection is problematic. In heart transplant patients, cardiac allograft vasculopathy, an accelerated form of atherosclerosis, remains a primary limitation to long-term survival (Weis & von Scheidt, 1997).

REHABILITATION OF THE TRANSPLANT PATIENT

To assist in management of the patient with transplant, rehabilitation is categorized into the following four phases: pretransplant, surgery and the postoperative acute phase, postoperative outpatient phase, and community or home-based phase. Although the ultimate goal of transplant rehabilitation is to improve the patient's function and quality of life, each phase of rehabilitation has its own emphasis.

Pretransplant Rehabilitation

Heart Transplant and End-Stage Cardiac Disease

Patients are referred for heart transplantation for end-stage cardiac conditions. The primary diagnoses for adults requiring a heart transplant are severe coronary artery disease (44%) or end-stage cardiomyopathy/heart failure (44%). In children, the primary diagnoses requiring transplant are congenital cardiac abnormalities (Hosenpud et al, 2000).

Patients with heart failure report symptoms of fatigue, dyspnea, and orthopnea. Physical signs include the presence of a third heart sound, pulmonary rales that do not reverse with coughing, jugular venous distension, peripheral edema, and hepatomegaly. Compensatory mechanisms include increased sympathetic nervous system activity, increased resting heart rate, and activation of the rennin-angiotensin system, which increases blood pressure.

Patients with heart failure generally meet the heart transplant selection criteria if they have New York Heart Association (NYHA) class III or IV heart failure that is unresponsive to medical management. Specific criteria for recipient status vary somewhat from center to center, although the American Heart Association and the International Society for Heart and Lung Transplantation (ISHLT) have similar recommendations for defining status (Cupples & Spruill, 2000; Costanzo et al, 1995). Patients frequently have left ventricular ejection fraction (LVEF) of less than 20% and peak oxygen consumption (VO_{2peak}) of less than 14 ml/kg/min, but these are not considered absolute criteria for heart transplantation (Costanzo et al, 1995). Recipients waiting for heart transplantation are classified based on severity of disease. Patients

***

BOX 40-2

Heart Transplant Recipient Status

Status IA

Patient requires mechanical circulatory assistance

Mechanical circulatory support has been required for more than 30 days with concurrent device-related complications

Continuous infusion of high-dose inotropic medications with continuous hemodynamic monitoring

Life expectancy without transplant is less than 7 days

Status IB

Patient requires at least one of either of the following: (a) left or right ventricular assist device for more than 30 days, (b) continuous infusion of IV inotropic medications

Status II

Those patients not meeting Status IA or IB criteria

Source: UNOS

***

in the worst medical condition (Status IA) are higher on the transplant recipient list. Box 40-2 provides some definitions of heart transplant recipient status.

Pretransplant management of the patient with heart failure is designed to preserve cardiac output until the transplant can be completed. Outpatient medical management includes medications and supplemental oxygen. Hospitalization may be needed for inotropic medication support such as dobutamine. Left ventricular assist devices (LVADs) are devices designed to augment cardiac output and allow the patient a bridge to transplantation.

The main goal in the preoperative period is to prevent losses of function. Maintenance of range of motion, soft tissue extensibility, and muscle strength are suggested goals. While patients with severe disease may be unable to participate in therapy, cardiac rehabilitation is an effective treatment for improving functional status of patients with significant heart failure and those with LVADs, whether or not transplantation is anticipated (Stewart et al, 2003; Cahalin, 1998). Recent literature demonstrates that exercise training is both safe and effective at improving functional capacity in patients on LVAD devices awaiting heart transplantation (Arena et al, 2000).

Lung Transplant and End-Stage Pulmonary Disease

Patients are referred for lung transplantation for end-stage pulmonary conditions. The primary diagnoses for adults requiring a lung transplant are severe chronic obstructive pulmonary disease (COPD) (44%), idiopathic pulmonary fibrosis (IPF) (17%), and cystic fibrosis (CF) (15%). Other conditions include pulmonary hypertension (PH) (Hosenpud et al, 2000). Single-lung transplants are usually performed for patients with COPD or IPF, whereas double-lung transplants are preferred for patients with CF. A small number of living-donor transplants (1%) are performed each year (OPTN data).

TABLE 40-2		
Preoperative Pulmonary Rehabilitation		
ACTIVITY	**TIME**	**SPECIFIC ACTIVITIES**

Warm-up (group)	10 minutes
	   Upper body
	   Lower body
	   Trunk
		Active range of motion

Individualized Endurance Program	10 to 30 minutes, may be done as intervals	Cycle ergometer, 25 to 30 watts Treadmill, 0.8 to 1.5 mph 0% to 5% grade Arm ergometer, 0 to 25 watts (forward or backward)

Individualized Strength Program	15 to 20 minutes	1 set of 8-12 repetitions (pulleys, Theraband)
		Latissimus pull-downs
		Rhomboids
		Shoulder extension/rotation
		Shoulder flexion
		Pectoral muscles
		Triceps
		Lower Extremity
		   Quadriceps
		   Hip extensors
		   Hip abductors

Cool-down (group)	10 minutes	Stretching (full-body) Breathing retraining Relaxation

Patients with pulmonary conditions report symptoms of dyspnea, which limits daily activities. COPD is characterized by destruction of lung tissue, leading to overdistension of the lungs and increased work of breathing accompanied by carbon dioxide retention. Typically, to qualify for lung transplantation, patients with COPD should demonstrate a forced expiratory volume in one second (FEV_1) of less than 25% of the predicted value, and partial pressure of carbon dioxide ($PaCO_2$) must equal 55 mm Hg with elevated pulmonary artery pressures. Cigarette smoking is a concern for patients with COPD and emphysema. Patients who continue to smoke are not considered candidates for lung transplantation and must demonstrate a nonsmoking status for four to six months before being listed for transplant. Random nicotine samples are taken from patients with a recent smoking history.

Idiopathic pulmonary fibrosis (IPF) is characterized by scarring of lung parenchyma leading to decreased lung volumes and decreased diffusing capacity. Typically, patients with IPF qualify for a lung transplant if their vital capacity is less than 60% of the predicted value and diffusing capacity is less than 50% of the predicted value. Patients with IPF have the highest mortality while waiting for transplant, so early referral to the transplant center is recommended (Maurer et al, 1998).

Transplant recommendations for patients with pulmonary hypertension continue to be debated. Some patients may exhibit improvement in function with vasodilator therapy such as prostacyclin. In patients who require transplant, there is no consensus on whether single- or double-lung transplant is better, or whether a heart-lung block transplant is preferred.

Pulmonary rehabilitation is an essential component to the management of patients with chronic lung conditions even without transplant and is becoming an accepted requirement for patients awaiting lung transplantation. Clinical data from pulmonary rehabilitation programs suggest that patients with better physical function before transplant have improved posttransplantation outcomes (Kesten, 1997; Scherer, 1995; Manzetti et al, 1994; Resnikoff & Ries, 1998). Some centers use a six-minute walk test as baseline data and suggest that patients must be able to walk at least 450 feet in six minutes to be placed on the waiting list. Although there is no data to support a minimum walking distance necessary for a successful clinical outcome, clinical expertise reinforces the clinical data from pulmonary rehabilitation programs and suggests that patients with greater physical capacity before transplant will have higher levels of physical function posttransplant.

Using the pretransplant waiting time to maximize physical function may reduce the time needed posttransplant to return to functional activities. Reasonable goals for pretransplant rehabilitation include normal muscle strength in lower extremity musculature, functional upper extremity muscle strength and endurance, functional shoulder and chest wall range of motion, demonstration of coordinated diaphragmatic breathing with exercise and activities, and improved cardiovascular endurance. Due to the significant effect of the immunosuppressive medications on muscle strength, there is a greater emphasis on resistance training in a patient awaiting lung transplantation than in most typical pulmonary rehabilitation programs. An example of a preoperative pulmonary rehabilitation program is shown in Table 40-2.

In patients with primary pulmonary hypertension or Eisenmenger's syndrome, a moderate exercise program is frequently contraindicated. If cardiac output is monitored and the physician agrees, however, range of motion exercises may be taught and light strengthening exercises may be performed. For example, a 22-year-old woman with primary pulmonary hypertension on the lung transplant waiting list was referred for physical therapy for shoulder injury leading to decreased range of motion in a capsular pattern. In consultation with the physician, joint mobilization, range of motion activities and modalities were used with few precautions. Strengthening exercises were used cautiously to avoid breath-holding and Valsalva maneuvers.

Patient Education. The waiting period provides an ideal opportunity for patient education. Nurses generally provide the patient with much of the education regarding preoperative expectations and medication issues. Rehabilitation teaching includes breathing training, airway clearance techniques, and activity progression.

Other Transplants

Patients awaiting other organ transplants may also be referred to physical therapy for treatment of musculoskeletal problems. Because of the level of metabolic abnormality in patients awaiting liver and kidney transplants, endurance training is difficult to perform. Other physical therapy interventions, however, may be used as appropriate (i.e., muscle strengthening, range of motion).

Surgical Implications

Surgical procedures have implications for the physical therapist in the areas of pain, abnormal hemodynamic responses, and movement patterns. The surgical approach for transplant is chosen to provide the surgeon the optimal working area and visual field. The choice of incision may affect patient comfort and function after surgery. Patients may have pain in the area of the incision and may demonstrate decreased muscle function and joint pain related to the muscles that were incised during surgery. The physical therapist should be familiar with the surgical incisions and their impact on rehabilitation. Other physical therapy related complications include injury to the phrenic nerve, brachial plexus injury, and peroneal nerve injury secondary to prolonged positioning during surgery and recovery.

Heart transplants are usually performed through a median sternotomy incision and cardiopulmonary bypass is used. The native heart is excised, leaving a portion of the right atrium (atrial cuff) including the sinoatrial node. The left atrium of the donor heart is sutured to the recipient's atrial cuff and the major vessels are reattached, starting with the pulmonary arterial vessels and followed by the aorta. Drainage tubes are placed in the pleural and mediastinal spaces and an epicardial pacing wire is placed before closure of the sternum. Total heart ischemic time is minimized, with les than four hours recommended. Finally, the two halves of the sternum are wired together, the new heart defibrillated, cardiopulmonary bypass discontinued, and the patient awakened.

Lung transplantation surgical incisions depend on whether a single- or double-lung transplant is to be performed. It is technically easier to perform a single-lung transplant on the left side. Single-lung transplants are performed through a standard posterolateral thoracotomy incision, made through the fourth or fifth intercostal space. The latissimus dorsi and lower trapezius muscles may be incised, as are the intercostal muscles at this level. If the rib at the surgical level fractures, it can be resected so that the bone ends do not rub or puncture the lung. The serratus anterior muscle is preserved if at all possible, but the lateral portion of the rhomboid may be cut to allow more access for the surgeon. Postoperative pain and impaired upper quarter movement patterns may present significant problems for patients.

Double-lung transplants are performed as two single-lung transplants, in a technique referred to as bilateral sequential lung transplantation (Meyers et al, 1999). This technique uses an anterior thoracotomy in the fourth or fifth intercostal space and minimizes the need for cardiopulmonary bypass.

Acute Phase Rehabilitation

The acute phase of rehabilitation begins in the intensive care unit and continues throughout the patient's hospital stay. Interventions are focused on facilitating normal cardiovascular and pulmonary function and increasing functional abilities in self-care and ambulation.

Heart Transplant Acute Management

Postoperative management of the patient after heart transplantation is similar to that of other cardiac surgeries. Patients experience hemodynamic instability, dysrhythmias, pulmonary hypertension, bleeding, and acute rejection. Factors that may lead to a complicated postoperative course include length of ischemic time and reperfusion injury. Prolonged ischemic time is associated with graft dysfunction (Hosenpud et al, 2000). Reperfusion injury is also associated with poor short-term outcomes.

Patients are weaned from mechanical ventilation within 24 to 36 hours, and chest tubes and pacing wires removed after two days. Acute cellular rejection is characterized by lymphocytes and myocyte infiltration into the cardiac muscle, resulting in dyspnea, fatigue, and heart failure. The symptoms of acute cellular rejection are often mild; therefore, patients undergo cardiac biopsy at regular intervals to identify the presence of rejection. Biopsy specimens are obtained by inserting a catheter in the jugular or subclavian vein into the right atrium. Humoral rejection is observed in the first weeks or months after an organ transplant. Humoral rejection is considered an immune system response that results in inflammation and thickening of the endothelial lining of the cardiac vessels.

Exercise Guidelines. Goals of the acute phase of rehabilitation include the following: regain normal postural cardiovascular responses (no postural hypotension), and increase functional activities. The former is primarily focused

TABLE 40-3

University Hospital Cardiovascular Rehabilitation Supervised Exercise/Activity Plan/Surgical Patients

STEP	EXERCISE	ACTIVITY
1 (1.5 METS)	Active/passive ROM, in bed for 5 reps Turn, cough, deep breathe and use incentive spirometer, q2-4°	Partial self care Feed self Use of bedside commode
2 (1.5-2.0 METS)	Active ROM, sit on edge of bed for 5 reps Teach perceived rate of exertion	Partial/complete self care Sitting bed bath Up in chair for meals
3 (2 METS)	Walk 100 feet at slow pace Active ROM 10 reps	Complete self care Incentive spriometer independently
4 (2.5 METS)	Walk 150 feet at average pace Teach pulse counting Warm-ups, standing for 10 reps	Use of bathroom with assistance May take warm shower after pacer wire removed
5 (3-3.5 METS)	Walk 300 feet at average pace Walk down flight of stairs Instruct in home exercise	May stand at sink for activities of daily living Dressing independently
6 (4 METS)	Walk up flight of stairs Walk 500 feet at average pace Schedule submaximal exercise tolerance test Enroll in Phase II	All self care independent

ROM, Range of motion.
Guidelines for exercise:
Patient heart rate to be 50-120 beats/min; no significant arrhythmias.
Exercise heart rate not more than 20 beats above rest; systolic blood pressure <200, diastolic blood pressure <120 during exercise.
No worsening ST changes; <10-15 diastolic blood pressure drop during exercise.
Rate of perceived exertion <10; no angina or other symptoms.
Patient to complete entire step before advancing to next step.

on the patient being able to tolerate changes in position, increase time in upright sitting, and transfer independently. Upper and lower extremity range of motion and strength need to be adequate to perform activities of daily living. An example of a cardiac rehabilitation program is shown in Table 40-3.

Specific issues for physical therapists include abnormal electrocardiogram (ECG) and cardiovascular control. ECG readings may be normal because the donor heart has an intact conduction system, although the atrial cuff left from the native heart may cause the ECG to have two P waves. Control of cardiovascular responses is altered due to cardiac denervation that occurs with surgery. When the donor heart is removed, the extrinsic nervous supply, including vagus nerve and sympathetic trunk, is severed. Consequently, there is no direct innervation to the heart to control heart rate response during change in position or during exercise. Heart rate and stroke volume increase due to the effect of preload as demonstrated by the Frank-Starling law and through circulation of catecholamine compounds. For the physical therapist, this means that heart rate and blood pressure respond more slowly to changes in position and exercise, and require a longer time between position or activity changes. In addition, other complications of heart transplant include sternum instability, infection, and/or pain.

Lung Transplant Acute Management

Postoperative management of the patient after lung transplantation begins in the intensive care unit. After lung transplantation, patients are generally mechanically ventilated for 24 to 72 hours. Often, paralytic agents are used during this period so that ventilation can be optimized. Chest tubes are likely in place, and patients are medicated for pain. Infection control is imperative; isolation rooms with negative-pressure ventilation are used and respiratory isolation procedures are maintained.

Specific problems in the immediate lung transplantation period include ineffective airway clearance, poor gas exchange, and acute rejection. Hypotension and hypoxemia can lead to decreased blood flow at the site of anastamosis for the new lung, creating necrotic changes and impairment in airflow. Problems with airway clearance are related to the denervation of the transplanted lung, specifically the autonomic nervous system pathways. The lack of innervation leads to ineffective cough and decreased ciliary clearance. Problems with gas exchange occur as a result of postoperative edema. The patient is managed by being kept "dry" (i.e., decreasing plasma volume without compromising cardiac output).

Exercise Guidelines. In the immediate postoperative period, the major goals are to prevent lung infection, optimize ventilation-perfusion ratio, increase time out of bed, and

TABLE 40-4

Goals and Interventions for Acute Posttransplant Rehabilitation: Lung Transplant

PROBLEM	GOAL	ACTIVITY
Decreased secretion clearance	Independent secretion management (because the lungs are denervated, there is decreased sensation of secretions)	Incentive spirometer Airway clearance techniques Assisted cough Positioning (single-lung, operative side up while side-lying to facilitate drainage) Double-lung avoid supine
Incisional pain	Pain management (postoperative pain is related to the surgical incision and decreased movement of muscles)	Pain medication Active range of motion shoulder girdle Positioning Mild heat Massage/soft tissue techniques
Abnormal postural hemodynamic responses	Normalize hemodynamic response (i.e., no postural hypotension; normal heart rate, respiratory rate, and blood pressure response to exercise)	Progressive mobilization from supine to sitting, sit in chair, walking in room Monitor heart rate, blood pressure, respiratory rate, SaO_2
Increased oxygen/ventilatory requirements	Adequate oxygenation without supplementation (SaO_2 94%-96% on room air) Normal vital capacity Diaphragmatic breathing	Instruction of diaphragmatic breathing Facilitation of diaphragmatic breathing Lateral costal expansion techniques (surgery side) Incentive spirometry
Decreased functional mobility	Independent activities of daily living (dressing, hygiene, shower, toilet; need adequate shoulder range of motion to perform these activities)	Active and active-assisted range of motion for shoulder Wand exercises Encourage and assist with activities of daily living (hygiene, shower, toilet)
Decreased exercise tolerance	Independent transfers Independent ambulation of 500 feet Out of bed most of day	Daily schedule Assisted ambulation (room progressing to hallway) Bicycle in room, 2 minutes initially, progress to 10 minutes
Compromised nutrition	No supplemental feedings (IV)	Schedule rehabilitation around meals Medical management of nausea

increase active range of motion on the surgical side. The primary goal is to mobilize the patient out of bed and increase daily activity. Patients are encouraged to be out of bed, walk in the hallway, and in some cases a stationary bike is brought into the room to help the patient increase endurance. Therapeutic interventions vary greatly. In general an intervention may continue until an abnormal exercise response is reached. Abnormal responses include a decrease in heart rate or blood pressure with an increase in exercise, a decrease in oxygen saturation below recommended levels (88% to 90%), or symptoms of dizziness and diaphoresis.

Airway clearance techniques are an essential component of acute care management. Many techniques are considered appropriate. Breathing training that targets diaphragm function is also considered an essential component of acute management for the patient after lung transplantation. Suggested goals and interventions are shown in Table 40-4.

Posttransplant Outpatient Rehabilitation

Rejection

One of the most common complications of organ transplantation is organ rejection. Acute rejection occurs within the

first six months of transplantation, whereas chronic rejection remains a long-term problem. Rejection episodes are monitored closely, often with biopsy, and treated with a variety of immune-suppressant medications.

Acute rejection is mediated by T cells. These T cells infiltrate the new organ allograft, multiply, and expand, causing tissue destruction. Chronic rejection appears as hypertrophy of the intima in the transplanted organ, which progresses to fibrosis. In heart transplants, chronic rejection is seen as accelerated atherosclerosis. In lung transplants, chronic rejection appears in the airways as bronchiolitis obliterans. There is no effective treatment for chronic rejection, and chronic rejection is prevented by aggressively managing acute rejection episodes.

Heart Transplant

After heart transplant, patients continue to experience decreased aerobic capacity and endurance, muscle atrophy, and decreased physical function (Kavanagh et al, 1988; Brubaker et al, 1997). In addition, immune suppression increases the risk of infection and leads to loss of muscle and bone. Rejection remains a significant risk, and heart transplant patients are likely to acquire premature atherosclerosis. Despite these problems, aerobic capacity and physical function are

TABLE 40-5

Effect of Heart Transplant on Selected CV Variables Compared to Normal Age Predicted Values

	HEART RATE	STROKE VOLUME	BLOOD PRESSURE	VO$_2$
Rest	Lower than normal	Lower than normal with little change when changing positions	Higher than normal	NA
Exercise	Lower (approximately 15 beats less)	Decreased and late onset	Higher than normal	May approximate normal with appropriate exercise training program

VO$_2$, Oxygen consumption. *Adapted from Sadowsky, H.S. (1996). Cardiac transplantation: a review. Physical Therapy 76:498-515.*

amenable to rehabilitation. Common long-term impairments are chest wall soreness, abnormal upper quarter movement patterns, and low back and knee pain from overuse. Once the patient leaves the hospital, rehabilitation looks much like phase II cardiac rehabilitation. The overall objective is to increase functional activity to within normal limits.

Cardiac and Respiratory Physiology in Heart Transplant. Functional capacity (oxygen consumption) in patients after heart transplantation is approximately 50% that of control subjects, and heart rate, blood pressure, and ventilatory abnormalities exist as well. In posttransplant patients, peak heart rate is lower than that in controls (156 vs 168 beats/min), although heart rate kinetics are not different than controls (Borrelli et al, 2003; Tegtbur et al, 2003). In regard to long-term effects of heart transplantation on heart rate, some children who have received heart transplantation do acquire a normal heart rate response to exercise (Marconi et al, 2002). The ventilatory response to exercise is abnormal, as demonstrated by a decreased diffusing capacity (Ewert et al, 2000). In addition, there may be some peripheral limitations that contribute to decreased functional capacity; these include decreased capillary density in muscle (Lampert et al, 1998). A summary of how cardiac variables are affected by heart transplant is shown in Table 40-5.

Signs of Rejection. The primary signs and symptoms of rejection include flu-like symptoms including low-grade fever and muscle aches. Dysrhythmias and bradycardia below 60 or relative bradycardia (decreased compared with patient's normal resting heart rate) are significant and should be reported to the physician immediately. Rejection episodes are monitored by biopsy. Exercise can continue if the rejection episode is mild or moderate as determined by biopsy.

Exercise and the Heart Transplant Patient. Exercise training is important for reversing the physiologic abnormalities observed after heart transplant, returning patients to improved functional status, and preventing disability incurred from the immunosuppressant regimen. The outpatient phase of rehabilitation resembles phase II cardiac rehabilitation, which generally continues for a duration of 8 to 12 weeks, at which time the patient is encouraged to continue exercise on his or her own or at a fitness facility. Guidelines for exercise for the posttransplant cardiac patient are shown in Box 40-3.

BOX 40-3

Summary Guidelines for Posttransplant Cardiac Rehabilitation

Use cardiac phase II protocols
Heart rate is not best indicator of exercise intensity
Increase warm-up and cool-down to 10 to 15 minutes
Rate of perceived exertion 11 to 13 (20-point Borg scale)
No exercise when patient is in severe rejection (biopsy)
Continue exercise when patient is in mild rejection

As mentioned before, implications for exercise response are that heart rate increases can only be accomplished using circulating catecholamines. For the patient in phase II cardiac rehabilitation, this means that the warm-up and cool-down portions of exercise should be slowly increased to 10 to 15 minutes. Exercise intensity should not be determined by heart rate alone, due to the effects of denervation. In addition, rating of perceived exertion (RPE) scales remain an unreliable method for determining exercise intensity after heart transplant due to large interindividual variations in the relationship of RPE and maximal oxygen consumption (Shephard et al, 1996). While there is no strong clinical consensus about the optimal method for prescribing and monitoring exercise intensity for patients after heart transplant, rate-pressure product (RPP) or a combination of RPE and physiological monitoring is recommended. Endurance and strength exercise can be performed in this rehabilitation stage, although upper extremity strengthening should only be started after the sternum has healed. To protect the sternum, lifting should be limited to less than 10 pounds for six to eight weeks. Treadmill, bike, arm ergometry, and indoor cross-country ski equipment are all appropriate choices.

Cardiac rehabilitation provides substantial increases in aerobic capacity, with patients able to improve 20% to 50% over prerehabilitation levels (Kobashigawa et al, 1999; Kavanagh et al, 1988). The mechanisms that contribute to increased aerobic capacity include increased maximal heart rate, improved ventilatory capacity, improved oxygen extraction, and increased capillary density in the exercising muscle

(Richard et al, 1999; Kobashigawa et al, 1999; Keteyian et al, 1996; Lampert et al, 1998). Supervised exercise programs lead to greater increases in aerobic capacity than home exercise programs (49% vs 18% improvement) (Kobashigawa et al, 1999).

Resistance training has been used in patients after heart transplantation as an essential component of cardiac rehabilitation, to improve physical function and prevent losses of muscle strength associated with corticosteroid use. Resistance training does appear to increase bone mineral density close to pretransplant levels and to increase muscle strength (Braith et al, 1996; Braith et al, 1998; Braith et al, 2003).

Despite the evidence that cardiac rehabilitation is beneficial in increasing aerobic capacity and exercise capacity, there is no literature that suggests that exercise training prevents allograft arteriopathy atherosclerosis or improves quality of life.

Lung Transplant

Patients who have received a lung transplant may be referred to physical therapy as early as 10 to 14 days after transplantation occurs. In the early stages of this postoperative outpatient phase, patients are medically labile and need once- or twice-a-week monitoring of medical status. Rehabilitation should progress in this phase, but close communication with medical personnel is recommended because of the many medication changes. Blood levels of immunosuppressive drugs are monitored and metabolic function (fluid and electrolyte levels, kidney and liver function) are followed.

Cardiac and Respiratory Physiology in Lung Transplant. After lung transplant, patients continue to experience decreased aerobic capacity and endurance, muscle atrophy, and decreased physical function. In addition, immune suppression increases the risk of infection and leads to loss of muscle and bone. Rejection remains a significant risk. Despite these problems, aerobic capacity and physical function are amenable to rehabilitation. Patients in the outpatient phase of rehabilitation begin at low levels of function and progress to having few functional limitations. Therapists need to adapt and progress the rehabilitation program appropriately. Because of the debilitating side effects of immunosuppressive medications, rehabilitation needs to be aggressive and preventive in nature. Rehabilitation can occur in a group setting and/or on an

individual basis. General guidelines for posttransplant lung rehabilitation are shown in Box 40-4.

After transplantation, functional capacity remains between 40% and 60% of predicted oxygen uptake, whether the patient receives a single- or double-lung transplant (Williams et al, 1992). Although there are mild ventilatory abnormalities, the decreased VO_2 is not well explained by the decrease in ventilation, low oxygen saturation, or anemia (Evans et al, 1991). Instead, several articles suggest that the main cause of decreased aerobic capacity is a peripheral muscle limitation (Evans et al, 1997; McKenna et al, 2003). Problems in the periphery include decreased peripheral oxygen utilization, decreased mitochondrial capacity, and decreased type I fibers, as well as decreased muscle power (Tirdel et al, 1998; Wang et al, 1999; Lands et al, 1999).

Rejection. The primary symptoms of acute rejection are shortness of breath, exercise intolerance, and desaturation at rest or with exercise. Patients generally have a portable oximeter at home and may report episodes of desaturation. Rejection should be suspected and reported if a decrease in SaO_2 of 4% to 5% for the same amount of activity is seen. Monitoring of ventilatory status should be the primary consideration of the therapist. Respiratory rate and oxygen saturation should be followed closely during exercise sessions.

Exercise and the Lung Transplant Patient. Patients are generally excited about the improvement in shortness of breath and frequently surprised at the level of muscle weakness observed in the lower extremities. Once ventilation is no longer a limiting factor in function, other deficits emerge. In the initial stages of outpatient rehabilitation, patients may have multiple complaints about the side effects of medications and often generally do not feel well. Rehabilitation should continue through these periods of malaise. The overall objective of outpatient rehabilitation is to improve function to levels appropriate for the patient's age and interests. Generally, patients are closely followed-up by the medical staff for two to three months after transplant, and rehabilitation two to three times per week continues throughout this period. The most common impairments that limit function are decreased cardiopulmonary endurance, decreased muscle strength and endurance, range of motion limitations, and abnormal movement patterns of the shoulder or trunk. Impairments may be caused by the surgical procedure itself or may be the result of years of abnormal muscle mechanics, posture, and decreased activity.

Aerobic exercise training for patients with lung transplantation provides substantial benefits in aerobic capacity to 60% of prerehabilitation levels and 14% over baseline testing in a six-week training period. The mechanisms by which aerobic capacity increases include decreased resting minute ventilation, which suggests an increase in efficiency of oxygen utilization. In addition, this study demonstrated that heart rate and ventilation decreased for the same amount of submaximal exercise, indicating a training effect (Stiebellehner et al, 1998).

Peripheral muscle deconditioning contributes to decreased exercise ability and limited physical function (Wang et al,

---

BOX 40-4

Summary Guidelines for Posttransplant Lung Rehabilitation

Keep SaO_2 above 90%
Add supplemental oxygen if necessary during treated acute rejection episodes
Patient should wear mask when with people
Increase strength program during prednisone bursts
Evaluate for musculoskeletal dysfunction

TABLE 40-6

Outpatient Posttransplant Physical Therapy Management: Lung Transplant

PROBLEM	GOAL	ACTIVITY
Decreased aerobic capacity	Daily functional activities including leisure 30 minutes of aerobic exercise at moderate intensity (60%-70% Vo₂ max) at least 3 times a week Peak Vo₂ of 70%	Pulmonary rehabilitation Supervised aerobic exercise program with Sao₂ monitoring
Decreased lower extremity muscle strength due to deconditioning and effects of prednisone	Functional muscle strength for sit to stand and stairs Leg press 60% of body weight Manual muscle test lower extremity muscle groups 5/5	Strength training program (1 set 8-12 reps) leg press knee extension hamstring curls
Abnormal upper extremity (shoulder girdle) mechanics for single-lung transplant due to thoracotomy incision	Able to perform all upper extremity activities in a normal fashion Range of motion to within functional limits Muscle strength for function Muscle endurance for overhead activities	Strength training program (1 set 8-12 reps) Latissimus pull-down Shoulder retraction Fly Endurance training program (2- 3 sets of 10) Upper body ergometer
Abnormal coordination of breathing with activity or decreased diaphragm performance	Coordinate breathing with activity most of time Perform diaphragm breathing during exercise Demonstrate dyspnea recovery techniques	Breathing training Breathing facilitation techniques

1999; Pantoja et al, 1999). Although resistance training has been used in patients after heart transplantation, little knowledge is available as to the efficacy in patients after lung transplantation. Lower extremity strengthening can begin early, but upper extremity resistance training should be delayed until wound and tissue healing is complete (generally about six weeks because of the delays in wound healing secondary to prednisone). Other important aspects of rehabilitation include posture reeducation, range of motion, and upper extremity movement patterns. Guidelines for outpatient physical therapy are provided in Table 40-6.

To improve physical function after lung transplantation, a pulmonary rehabilitation protocol may be used, or the therapist may creatively design a rehabilitation program. Except for delaying upper extremity strengthening for six weeks after surgery, no therapeutic interventions are contraindicated. For endurance training, stationary bicycles, treadmills, arm ergometers, indoor ski machines, rowers, and stair climbers may be used. Pulleys, weight equipment, free weights, resistive elastic bands, or gymnastic balls all may be appropriate for strengthening and facilitation of normal movement patterns. Because of the effects of prednisone, proximal muscle function must be addressed and strengthening programs should be consistent with those designed to increase muscle force production: generally one set of eight to 12 repetitions at 60% of the patient's one-repetition maximum (1RM). Once a patient has achieved a satisfactory level of function (determined by the therapist and patient), formal rehabilitation may be discontinued and the patient should participate in a community based rehabilitation program.

Community or Home-Based Rehabilitation

Patients are generally followed-up at the transplant center until the medical staff is satisfied with patient progress. Return home can occur at this point in time, whether or not rehabilitation goals have been met. For patients who have left their home community to wait for transplant, the transition to home frequently occurs three months after transplant. The major goal of community-based rehabilitation is a return to normal function with minimal limitations. Therapists in rural settings and community hospitals may be involved with a transplant patient's plan of care in this phase. Therapists should be comfortable treating patients in many settings, addressing the common complications, and watching for signs of rejection. In the initial stages of posttransplant rehabilitation, a supervised program is recommended. Hospital-based phase III cardiac rehabilitation programs are appropriate, or patients may elect to independently exercise in a fitness facility. Some follow-up by the transplant center is important to encourage compliance in exercise programs. Once patients reach their desired level of fitness, a community-based program is appropriate for maintaining endurance, aerobic capacity, strength, and flexibility. Patients who participate in training can attain high levels of exercise performance with an appropriate training regimen (Kuehls, 2003).

Influence of Medications on Treatment

Rejection Issues

Although transplants are often successful, some health professionals believe that patients are merely exchanging one

TABLE 40-7

Side Effects of Immunosuppressive Medications

MEDICATION TYPE	TRADE NAME	ACTION	ADVERSE EFFECTS
Antilymphocytic	ATGAM OKT3 Zenapax (Daclizumab)	These are monoclonal or polyclonal antibodies that cause T-cell death or movement of T-cells out of vasculature	Flu-like symptoms Unstable vital signs
Antimetabolites	Azathioprine (Imuran) Mycophenolate mofetil (CellCept)	Inhibits enzymes and prevents lymphocytes from proliferating	Blood—leukopenia, bone marrow suppression GI—pancreatitis Hepatic—toxicity
Glucocorticoids	Prednisone	Block production of interleukins, stimulates protein breakdown	CNS—euphoria, insomnia Eyes—cataracts GI—hyperglycemia Skin—acne, delayed wound healing Muscle—weakness Bone—osteoporosis
Immune modulators	Cyclosporine (Neoral) Tacrolimus (FK 506)	Decrease production of interleukins and T-lymphocytes	Blood—leukopenia CNS—tremor, seizure Hepatic—toxicity Renal—toxicity

set of problems for another. For a transplant to be successful, a patient must remain on powerful immunosuppressive drugs for the remainder of his or her life. Some of these medications have crippling side effects. The effects of long-term prednisone are well known: osteoporosis, muscle weakness, and glucose intolerance. The long-term effects of cyclosporine and azathioprine affect the patient's ability to fight infection. Patients also need to manage medication side effects on a daily basis. It is these medications, however, that make for impressive survival rates.

Types of Medications

The drugs used to cause immune suppression are categorized as inhibitors. Each of these medications affects a different component of the immune system and they are used in various combinations.

Antilymphocytic Medications. The antilymphocytic class of medications includes the monoclonal or polyclonal antibodies to human lymphatic tissue. These antibodies have a powerful effect on decreasing T cell activity by causing cell death or movement of the T cells out of the vasculature. These drugs are most commonly used in treating acute rejection. ATGAM (polyclonal antibody antithymocyte gamma globulin), OKT3, and daclizumab (Zenapax) are included in this category. Given intravenously, these drugs lead to flu-like symptoms and potentially unstable vital signs due to a large increase in cytokine activity. Rehabilitation exercises should not be performed during administration of these medications.

Antimetabolites. The antimetabolite class of drugs is used for long-term immune suppression. These drugs inhibit various enzymes within the cell energy production pathways, preventing lymphocytes from proliferating. Azathioprine (Imuran) and mycophenolate mofetil (CellCept) are included in this category. Both of these drugs commonly cause gastrointestinal upset. Intestinal absorption is easily affected by food intake or drug interactions (e.g., antacids decrease absorption

of CellCept). These drugs also may cause significant bone marrow suppression and increase the risk of infection. Bone marrow suppression (leukopenia, anemia) is common, as are gastrointestinal symptoms of nausea, vomiting, and anorexia.

Glucocorticoids. Glucocorticoids such as prednisone are believed to block the production of interleukins and decrease the inflammatory response. They have been a mainstay of organ transplant management for many years. Common adverse effects of glucocorticoids include hypertension, diabetes, obesity, cataracts, delayed wound healing, muscle weakness, and osteoporosis. Steroid therapy may be delayed until primary wound closure is certain (1 to 2 weeks), at which time the patient is started on low-dose oral steroids. Acute rejection episodes are treated with oral or intravenous steroid pulses.

Immune Modulators. Immune modulators bind to proteins in the cells, decreasing the production of interleukin-2 or T-lymphocytes. Cyclosporine (Neoral, Sandimmune) and tacrolimus (FK-506) are the most common of these drugs and are a main component of immune suppressant therapy. The main complication is renal toxicity, which may be reversible if the dose is decreased. Cyclosporine is considered a nervous system irritant, leading to hand tremor and possible seizures. Therapists should be aware of these side effects. In addition, absorption of these drugs is affected by other medications and food intake. Serum concentrations of these drugs are increased with intake of grapefruit juice, as well as drugs such as erythromycin, diltiazem, and corticosteroids. Because of potential drug interactions, serum levels of these drugs are monitored closely. Table 40-7 summarizes the effects of common immunosuppressive medications.

Long-term Complications of Transplant Management

Osteoporosis

Osteoporosis remains a prevalent and disabling problem for patients after organ transplantation surgery. There is a high incidence of vertebral and other atraumatic fractures between 8% and 65% in the first year after transplant, which can significantly limit physical function and complicate the posttransplantation rehabilitation course (Spira et al, 2000). Physical therapists have a role in identifying physical limitations of osteoporosis and prescribing appropriate exercise programs (Scherer, 2001). Osteoporosis medications such as alendronate (Foxamax) are considered essential components of care, and the addition of resistance exercise to a medication regimen does improve bone mineral density (Mitchell et al, 2003).

Cardiac Allograft Vasculopathy

One of the most troubling long-term complications of heart transplantation is cardiac allograft vasculopathy, an accelerated form of coronary disease affecting cardiac arteries. Blockage of the arteries occurs and is thought to be due to epithelial injury and scarring of the coronary arteries (Waller et al, 2003). Physical therapists must continue to identify signs and symptoms of cardiac ischemia and refer patients for appropriate treatment. Patients may be on medications to lower cholesterol (statins) and manage hypertension as preventive measures, and they may be candidates for stenting or coronary artery bypass surgery as well (Weis, 2002).

Bronchiolitis Obliterans

Long-term chronic rejection of the transplanted lung results in a condition labeled bronchiolitis obliterans (BO). It is the main problem seen in long-term survivors of lung transplantation. Bronchiolitis obliterans results from lymphocyte infiltration into the basement membrane of the small airways, followed by migration through the intima into the respiratory mucosa. This process leads to epithelial damage and scarring, which may partially or fully occlude the small airways. As a complication of transplant, BO is usually irreversible. The primary pulmonary function that is affected is FEV_1, and thus BO is considered an obstructive lung condition. The diagnosis is made through transbronchial biopsy.

Physical therapists who are working with long-term survivors of lung transplant may find that the patients are demonstrating decreased lung function and symptoms of dyspnea with activity. The therapist, therefore, must continue to monitor ventilatory status and oxygen saturation in the lung transplant patient. Long-term complications of organ transplantation are summarized in Box 40-5.

Quality of Life

Although quality of life generally improves after heart and/or lung transplantation, many factors may influence quality of life (Gross et al, 1995). Patients report improved physical function, general health, and social functioning (Limbos et al, 2000; Bunzel, 1999). Although physical function is improved, some abnormalities exist. One study reports that at five years after lung transplantation, 74% of patients were active and working, 13% were active but not working, 10% had some

---

BOX 40-5

Long-Term Complications of Organ Transplant

Accelerated atherosclerosis/hypertension/hypercholesterolemia
Infections
Cancers
Osteoporosis
Steroid myopathy with muscle weakness
Glucose intolerance
Nephrotoxicity
Delayed wound healing

---

limitations, and 3% were disabled (Chaparro et al, 1997). Decreased emotional wellbeing, however, may occur after five years (Bunzel, 1999). It is unclear whether the declines in quality of life in long-term survivors are due to declines in physical condition or other factors. Patients with lung transplantation generally have increased quality of life until the onset of BO, which then causes a decline in quality of life. Quality of life is an important outcome of transplant rehabilitation and should be assessed regularly.

SUMMARY

Physical therapy plays an important role in maintaining and improving functional levels of patients both before and after organ transplant. Knowledge of cardiovascular and pulmonary physiology, along with the ability to analyze movement and function allow rehabilitation professionals to maximize a patient's quality of life. The field of organ transplantation is exciting and growing. New advances in long-term management of transplant recipients mean that rehabilitation professionals need to continue to develop and evaluate approaches to care.

Review Questions

1. What are the psychological and social implications of organ transplant?
2. What is the role of pretransplant pulmonary rehabilitation?
3. How does the surgical incision affect the musculoskeletal function of a posttransplant patient?
4. What are the signs of organ rejection in the cardiac transplant patient? The lung transplant patient?
5. How is the rehabilitation of the heart transplant patient similar to and different from traditional cardiac rehabilitation?
6. How is the rehabilitation of the lung transplant patient different from other forms of pulmonary rehabilitation?
7. How do immunosuppressive drugs affect a patient's neuromuscular function? Muscle strength? Cardiopulmonary endurance?
8. What are the long-term complications of heart or lung transplantation?

REFERENCES

Arena, R., Humphrey, R., & Peberdy, M.A. (2000). Safety and efficacy of exercise training in a patient awaiting heart transplantation while on positive intravenous inotropic support. Journal of Cardiopulmonary Rehabilitation 20:259-261.

Borrelli, E., Pogliaghi, S., Molinello, A., Diciolla, F., Maccherini, M., & Grassi, B. (2003). Serial assessment of peak VO_2 and VO_2 kinetics early after heart transplantation. Medicine and Science in Sports and Exercise 35:1798-1804.

Braith, R.W., Magyari, P.M., Fulton, M.N., Aranda, J., Walker, T., & Hill, J.A. (2003). Resistance exercise training and alendronate reverse glucocorticoid-induced osteoporosis in heart transplant recipients. Journal of Heart and Lung Transplantation 22: 1082-1090.

Braith, R.W., Mills, R.M., Welsch, M.A., Keller, J.W., & Pollock, M.L. (1996). Resistance exercise training restores bone mineral density in heart transplant recipients. Journal of the American College of Cardiology 28:1471-1477.

Braith, R.W., Welsch, M.A., Mills, R.M., Jr., Keller, J.W., & Pollock, M.L. (1998). Resistance exercise prevents glucocorticoid-induced and myopathy in heart transplant recipients. Medicine and Science in Sports and Exercise 30:483-489.

Brown, P.A., Launius, B.K., Mancini, M.C., & Cush, E.M. (2004). Depression and anxiety in the heart transplant patient: a case study. Critical Care Nursing Quarterly 27:92-95.

Brubaker, P.H., Brozena, S.C., Morley, D.L., Walter, J.D., & Berry, M.J. (1997). Exercise-induced ventilatory abnormalities in orthotopic heart transplant patients. Journal of Heart and Lung Transplantation 16:1011-1017.

Bunzel, B., & Laederach-Hofmann, K. (1999). Long-term effects of heart transplantation: the gap between physical performance and emotional well-being. Scandinavian Journal of Rehabilitative Medicine 31:214-222.

Cahalin, L.P. (1998). Exercise training in heart failure: inpatient and outpatient considerations. AACN Clinical Issues 9:225-243.

Chan, C.K., & Kesten, S. (2000) Psychological functioning and quality of life in lung transplant candidates and recipients. Chest 118:408-416.

Chaparro, C., Scavuzzo, M., Winton, T., Keshavjee, S., & Kesten, S. (1997). Status of lung transplant recipients surviving beyond five years. Journal of Heart and Lung Transplantation 16:511-516.

Costanzo, M.R., Augustine, S., Bourge, R., Bristow, M., O'Connell, J.B., Driscoll, D., & Rose, E. (1995). Selection and treatment of candidates for heart transplantation. A statement for health professionals from the Committee on Heart Failure and Cardiac Transplantation of the Council on Clinical Cardiology, American Heart Association. Circulation 92:3593-3612.

Cupples, S.A., & Spruill, L.C. (2000). Evaluation criteria for the pretransplant patient. Critical Care Nursing Clinics North America 12:35-47.

Dew, M.A., Switzer, G.E., DiMartini, A.F., Matukaitis, J., Fitzgerald, M.G., & Kormos, R.L. (2000). Psychosocial assessments and outcomes in organ transplantation. Progress in Transplant 10:239-259; quiz 260-1.

Evans, A.B., Al-Himyary, A.J., Hrovat, M.I., Pappagianopoulos, P., Wain, J.C., Ginns, L.C., & Systrom, D.M. (1997). Abnormal skeletal muscle oxidative capacity after lung transplantation by 31P-MRS. American Journal of Respiratory Critical Care Medicine 155:615-621.

Ewert, R., Wensel, R., Bruch, L., Mutze, S., Bauer, U., Plauth, M., & Kleber, F.X. (2000). Relationship between impaired pulmonary diffusion and cardiopulmonary exercise capacity after heart transplantation. Chest 117:968-975.

Gross, C., Savik, K., Bolman, R.M., & Hertz, M.I.(1995). Long-term health status and quality of life outcomes of lung transplant recipients. Chest 108:1587-1593.

Hosenpud, J.D., Bennett, L.E., Keck, B.M., Boucek, M.M., & Novick, R.J. (2000). The Registry of the International Society for Heart and Lung Transplantation: seventeenth official report—2000. Journal of Heart and Lung Transplantation 19:909-931.

Kavanagh, T., Yacoub, M.H., Mertens, D.J., Kennedy, J., Campbell, R.B., & Sawyer, P. (1998). Cardiorespiratory responses to exercise training after orthotopic cardiac transplantation. Circulation 77:162-171.

Kesten, S. (1997). Pulmonary rehabilitation and surgery for end-stage lung disease. Clinics in Chest Medicine 18:173-181.

Keteyian, S.J., Levine, A.B., Brawner, C.A., Kataoka, T., Rogers, F.J., & Schairer, J.R. (1996). Exercise training in patients with heart failure: a randomized, controlled trial. Annals of Internal Medicine 124:1051-1057.

Kobashigawa, J.A., Leaf, D.A., Lee, N., Gleeson, M.P., Liu, H., Hamilton, M.A., Moriguchi, J.D., Kawata, N., Einhorn, K., Herlihy, E., & Laks, H.. (1999). A controlled trial of exercise rehabilitation after heart transplantation. New England Journal of Medicine 340:272-277.

Kuehls, D. (2003). Truimph of the heart: each day is a precious gift for Greg Osterman, who runs marathons with another person's heart beating in his chest. Runner's World 38:72-77.

Lampert, E., Mettauer, B., Hoppeler, H., Charloux, A., Charpentier, A., & Lonsdorfer, J. (1998). Skeletal muscle response to short endurance training in heart transplant recipients. Journal of the American College of Cardiology 32:420-426.

Lands, L.C., Smountas, A.A., Mesiano, G., Brosseau, L., Shennib, H., Charbonneau, M., & Gauthier, R. (1999). Maximal exercise capacity and peripheral skeletal muscle function following lung transplantation. Journal of Heart and Lung Transplantation 18:113-120.

Limbos, M.M., Joyce, D.P., Chan, C.K., & Kesten, S. (2000). Psychological functioning and quality of life in lung transplant candidates and recipients. Chest 118:408-416.

Manzetti, J.D., Hoffman, L.A., Sereika, S.M., Sciurba, F.C., & Griffith, B.P. (1994). Exercise, education, and quality of life in lung transplant candidates. Journal of Heart and Lung Transplantation 13:297-305.

Marconi, C., Marzorati, M., Fiocchi, R., Mamprin, F., Ferrazzi, P., Ferretti, G., & Cerretelli, P. (2002). Age-related heart rate response to exercise in heart transplant recipients. Functional significance. Pflugers Archives 443:698-706.

Maurer, J.R., Frost, A.E., Estenne, M., Higenbottam, T., & Glanville, A.R. (1998). International guidelines for the selection of lung transplant candidates. The International Society for Heart and Lung Transplantation, the American Thoracic Society, the American Society of Transplant Physicians, the European Respiratory Society. Journal of Heart and Lung Transplantation 17:703-709.

McKenna, M.J., Fraser, S.F., Li, J.L., Wang, X.N., Carey, M.F., Side, E.A., Morton, J., Snell, G.I., Kjeldsen, K., & Williams, T.J. (2003). Impaired muscle Ca2+ and K+ regulation contribute to poor exercise performance post-lung transplantation. Journal of Applied Physiology 95:1606-1616.

Meyers, B.F., Sundaresan, R.S., Guthrie, T., Cooper, J.D., & Patterson, G.A. (1999). Bilateral sequential lung transplantation without sternal division eliminates posttransplantation sternal complications. Journal of Thoracic and Cardiovascular Surgery 117:358-364.

Mitchell, M.J., Baz, M.A., Fulton, M.N., Lisor, C.F., & Braith, R.W. (2003). Resistance training prevents vertebral osteoporosis in lung transplant recipients. Transplantation 76:557-562.

Monterosso, L. (2003). Relocation information needs of lung transplant recipients and careers. Transplant Nurses' Journal 12:16-22.

Pantoja, J.G., Andrade, F.H., Stoki, D.S., Frost, A.E., Eschenbacher, W.L., & Reid, M.B. (1999). Respiratory and limb muscle function in lung allograft recipients. American Journal of Respiratory Critical Care Medicine 160:1205-1211.

Resnikoff, P.M., & Ries, A.L. (1998). Maximizing functional capacity. Pulmonary rehabilitation and adjunctive measures. Respiratory Care Clinics North America 4:475-492.

Resnikoff, P.M., & Ries, A.L. (1998). Pulmonary rehabilitation for chronic lung disease. Journal of Heart and Lung Transplantation 17:643-650.

Richard, R., Verdier, J.C., Duvallet, A., Rosier, S.P., Leger, P., Nignan, A., & Rieu, M. (1999). Chronotropic competence in endurance trained heart transplant recipients: heart rate is not a limiting factor for exercise capacity. Journal of the American College of Cardiology 33:192-197.

Scherer, S.A. (2001). Clinical perspective: framework and rationale for physical therapy management of lung transplant patients with osteoporosis. Cardiopulmonary Physical Therapy 12:75-82.

Scherer, S.A. (1995). Pre-operative pulmonary rehabilitation reduces post-operative length of hospital stay after lung transplantation. International Conference on Pulmonary Rehabilitation and Home Ventilation, Denver, Colo.

Shephard, R.J., Kavanagh, T., Mertens, D.J., & Yacoub, M. (1996). The place of perceived exertion ratings in exercise prescription for cardiac transplant patients before and after training. British Journal of Sports Medicine 30:116-121.

Spira, A., Gutierrez, C., Chaparro, C., Hutcheon, M.A., & Chan, C.K. (2000). Osteoporosis and lung transplantation: a prospective study. Chest 117:476-481.

Stewart, K.J., Badenhop, D., Brubaker, P.H., Keteyian, S.J., & King, M. (2003). Cardiac rehabilitation following percutaneous revascularization, heart transplant, heart valve surgery, and for chronic heart failure. Chest 123:2104-2111.

Stiebellehner, L., Quittan, M., End, A., Wieselthaler, G., Klepetko, W., Haber, P., & Burghuber, O.C. (1998). Aerobic endurance training program improves exercise performance in lung transplant recipients. Chest 113:906-912.

Tegtbur, U., Pethig, K., Machold, H., Haverich, A., & Busse, M. (2003). Functional endurance capacity and exercise training in long-term treatment after heart transplantation. Cardiology 99:171-176.

Tirdel, G.B., Girgis, R., Fishman, R.S., & Theodore, J. (1998). Metabolic myopathy as a cause of the exercise limitation in lung transplant recipients. Journal of Heart and Lung Transplantation 17:1231-1237.

Waller, J., Brook, N.R., & Nicholson, M.L. (2003). Cardiac allograft vasculopathy: current concepts and treatment. Transplant International 16:367-375.

Wang, X.N., Williams, T.J., McKenna, M.J., Li, J.L., Fraser, S.F., Side, E.A., Snell, G.I., Walters, E.H., & Carey, M.F. (1999). Skeletal muscle oxidative capacity, fiber type, and metabolites after lung transplantation. American Journal of Respiratory Critical Care Medicine 160:57-63.

Weis, M. (2002). Cardiac allograft vasculopathy: prevention and treatment options. Transplant Procedures 34:1847-1849.

Weis, M., & von Scheidt, W. (1997). Cardiac allograft vasculopathy: a review. Circulation 96:2069-2077.

Williams, T.J., Patterson, G.A., McClean, P.A., Zamel, N., & Maurer, J.R. (1992). Maximal exercise testing in single and double lung transplant recipients. American Review of Respiratory Diseases 145:101-105.

C H A P T E R   4 1

The Patient in the Community

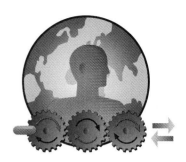

Donna Frownfelter and Ryan Hartley

KEY TERMS   Assisted living   Outpatient
                 Continuity of care   Subacute hospitals
                 Home care   Skilled nursing and rehabilitation facilities
                 Managed care   Transitional care units

Physical therapy in the community may take on a wide variety of forms. The practice has certainly changed dramatically over the last few years. Diagnostic related groupings (DRGs) during the 1980s began a trend that saw patients leaving the hospital earlier and often in a more acute stage of recovery. Subacute hospitals, Medicare skilled nursing, long-term acute care facilities, and rehabilitation facilities with transitional care units provide therapy and improved costs of care (Carson, 1999) and facilitate patient progression so that patients will be back home within a few short days or weeks, depending on their condition. Managed care has had a significant impact on the type of diagnosis given to patients and the number of therapy sessions authorized for given diagnoses or symptoms. This may be seen as decreased delivery of physical therapist service to the patient, but it also opens up opportunities for new paradigms of delivery of health care services and new models of care for people with chronic illnesses. There needs to be a movement toward more patient-centered health care delivery systems and more self-care and self-management. Studies have shown that by using concepts of self-management, people have improved quality of life and decreased hospitalizations (Epping-Jordan, 2004; Guinn, 2004; Hainsworth, 2005; Holman, 2004; Hughes, 2004; Jerant, 2005; Marks, 2005; Monninkhof, 2004; O'Donnell, 2004; Tanner, 2004). This chapter uses the case of people with

chronic obstructive pulmonary disease (COPD) to demonstrate how health care professionals may facilitate the management of chronic conditions.

Working with people in the community is different than working with patients in an acute care hospital. When people are in the community, their focus is on optimal health, not on disease or a surgical procedure or trauma, as it usually is in the acute care setting. People with COPD (or other chronic disease or dysfunction) and the health care team can work in a collaborative, self-advocacy and self-help model. It is not that collaboration, self-advocacy, and self-help are not part of acute care but that they should be available in other settings, as well. In the setting of skilled nursing, rehabilitation, or long-term care, if support and interventions are necessary, the patient should be given choices and allowed input into decisions regarding his or her care as much as the patient and his or her family or significant other are able. Dr. Thomas Petty, who devoted his life to people with COPD, called this "do it yourself rehab." This model is at times difficult for the health care team who, in the old models of rehabilitation, prescribes and tells a patient what to do and expects him or her to do it "as ordered," often with little collaboration. Today it is more our role to treat and educate people so that they can make better decisions about their health and proceed in positive directions toward improving their health. One person with COPD shared the following. "The health care team talks about 'wellness.' I will never be 'well' with moderate to severe COPD, so I am striving for 'optimal health.'"

This chapter focuses on attaining optimal health and function for patients who are receiving physical therapy in the home or long-term care setting. These concepts and ideas, however, can be applied in the nursing home, skilled nursing facility, senior housing, transitional or assisted living facilities, adult day care, and outpatient settings. The settings described in this chapter will be used only as examples on which to focus the discussion.

Continuity of care is an essential component of quality health care in light of the trend toward earlier hospital discharge either to a skilled nursing/rehabilitation facility or to the home with nursing and therapy support. A colleague in hospital practice recently commented that she feels more like a triage therapist than a physical therapist. At times the absolute basics of therapy (i.e., safety, transfers and ambulation with an assistive device) may be all that a patient is able to receive before leaving the hospital setting, and home exercises are not often implemented or strongly emphasized by hospital staff at discharge. Combined with a general decrease in endurance due to recent insult/injury and bed rest during hospitalization, the postdischarge patient is not likely to assume as active a lifestyle as is necessary to regain function and avoid further complications.

The types and diagnoses of people seen in the community vary; often they are the very young, the very old, and those with chronic illness. The medical community has improved its ability to quickly and more effectively handle complicated medical situations, from premature births to cancer to joint replacements. These patients are now returning home much faster than in the past, though often with unresolved cardiopulmonary impairments. Specialty hospitals have been developed to care for the medically fragile, ventilator-assisted or ventilator-dependent patient who is not stable enough or lacks the resources to be at home. These long-term acute care hospitals are able to provide quality care at improved cost of care (Senoff, 2000). Many patients, especially children on ventilators whose parents can provide some care and are assisted by nursing staff, are returning home successfully on ventilators. They integrate into the community in school and recreation, function well, and perceive a high quality of life. As with other children with a variety of disabilities, there is funding available for support through age 21 and very limited support after that age. Quality of long-term care and the continuity of care and service as children age into adulthood is an area of major concern.

In times of acute or long-term loss of independent function, the availability of able caregivers will often determine the level of function a patient can enjoy in the home and community. Although sons and daughters, friends, fellow churchgoers, or paid workers can provide this service, the caregiver may be an elderly spouse or friend who also has medical problems and a limited physical ability to assist the patient. Additionally, many potential caregivers (especially sons and daughters of

those needing care) have families and obligations of their own, and this "sandwich generation" is often torn between caring for their aging parents and their own immediate families (Guinn 2004). Many elderly patients will try valiantly to remain at home and independent, amazing the most seasoned clinician with their inventiveness and family/friend supports. Other patients will recognize that they are no longer able to care for themselves and that the caregiver, due to physical or time limitations, cannot continue in that role.

Nursing homes, long thought of as a place "to go to die," have become centers of skilled nursing and rehabilitation. Some have developed beautiful, hotel-like atmospheres with a range of services. The residents may live in independent apartments and, if a disease or trauma occurs, may return to the skilled nursing area to receive rehabilitation services. As their condition allows, they later step down to an assisted living area, then transfer back to their apartments or remain in a higher level of care.

Transitional care units are common discharge destinations for patients who are not quite ready to go home but no longer need the constant care and monitoring found in the hospital. Patients are admitted for up to one month and receive continued daily rehabilitation therapies to allow them to return home safely.

Even after an acute incident (e.g., a cerebral vascular accident [CVA]), a patient may not be able to return home in a month but may continue to make gains for up to a year or more as strength, balance, and endurance improve. Therapists can screen residents and continue to try to improve their physical status and enable them to live to their fullest capacity.

When considering these practice settings, it becomes obvious that cardiovascular and pulmonary concerns are highlighted. From the very young to the very old, primary and secondary cardiovascular and pulmonary issues are often the limiting factors in a patient's rehabilitation progress, and so should be addressed as part of standard physical therapy care.

The focus in home and long-term care settings is to help individuals achieve optimal health in the environment in which they live.

PHYSICAL THERAPY IN HOME AND LONG-TERM CARE

Treating patients in the home or long-term care facility is unique because the therapist is constantly adapting treatment to the patient's living quarters, observing and anticipating safety concerns, and finding new and creative ways to improve the patient's quality of life. Although there are many adaptations a physical therapist must make when treating patients in the home or long-term care facility, many of the physical therapy interventions performed in the home and long-term care facility are similar to those used in hospitals for patients of similar ages and conditions. Activities to improve safety, strength, endurance, transfers, ambulation, and activities of daily living (ADLs) are common, and often traditional methods such as supervised repetition of tasks (i.e., transfers and ADLs) are used as they would be elsewhere. Theraband and other basic therapy equipment may be indicated and prescribed according to the patient's needs and ability to pay for the equipment.

Education is especially important in home and long-term care, to prepare the patient, family, and caregivers to function safely and independently when the therapist is not present. Safety and medical issues may arise unexpectedly. Patients must be familiar with signs and symptoms indicating their condition is changing (such as shortness of breath, changes in secretions, increased fatigue, inability to perform usual ADLs, depression, loss of appetite, etc.). Knowing how to handle these issues—knowing when to call 911, call for an appointment with the physician, or when to just rest—requires a great deal of problem solving and awareness on the part of each person involved.

The following sections discuss ways in which the physical therapist can adapt his or her observations, examination, assessment, interventions, goals, and progression for people in the community.

SPECIFIC CARDIOVASCULAR AND PULMONARY CONCERNS IN THE COMMUNITY

Patients who move into nursing homes or alternative long-term care and independent living facilities or return home after an episode of care for disease or trauma often have several problems in common. They may have decreased strength, endurance, and balance, leading to decreased independence, mobility, and activity level. They often have poor posture, and are at risk for falls due to poor balance and weakness. They are frequently poorly nourished from lack of appetite or dysphagia. Returning home with a decrease in independent functioning can have negative emotional effects, which may further decrease appetite, activity level, motivation, and social/community interactions.

Many patients have preexisting cardiovascular and pulmonary impairments, such as asthma, hypertension, or congestive heart failure, or co-morbidities such as diabetes. They may have previously had hip fractures, joint replacements, CVAs, or myocardial infarctions. The cardiovascular and pulmonary impairments related to any of these may in fact be the limiting consideration to progress with therapy. These concerns need to be addressed so that the individual is able to reach his or her full rehabilitation potential.

CHRONIC ILLNESS AND SELF-MANAGEMENT

Many people at home or in long-term care have chronic diseases that may or may not be the reason they are receiving physical therapy. These chronic diseases can affect not only the person's physical capabilities, but his or her emotions, attitude, and motivation as well, in ways those of us without chronic conditions may not fully appreciate. Leading a full life with a chronic disease or a decline in function is quite possible; it often requires active effort on the part of the patient and the therapist, and often requires positive self-management. People will manage one way or the other. The choices they make about their health care, exercise, and how they are going to self-manage will lead to better or worse health-related quality of life.

Positive self-management involves a combination of positive emotional outlook, active involvement in decision making, and maintenance of a lifestyle that is as optimal as possible. The therapist, or any other person for that matter, cannot do this for the patient. The physical therapist needs to be caring and fully present with the patient, and though the therapist can provide the initial stimulus for the process, effective self-management comes only from within the patient. The therapist can continue to be a resource and provide interventions as the need may arise, but the goal is for the patient to be his or her own case manager and decision maker regarding health care and optimal function.

In the home or community setting, the person with a chronic illness needs to make several choices. How does he or she decide what will promote optimal function and health? In the case of the person with COPD, there may be a referral to an outpatient pulmonary rehabilitation program after an acute care stay. This is not always the case, however, and many people will be discharged without referral to home care or outpatient therapy. If they do go to a pulmonary rehab program, when it is over or if there are not third party payers or financial support for continued participation, the individual needs to decide how to continue moving toward optimal health. Do they go to a health club or YMCA or walk in the malls, practice yoga, continue to pay privately for a therapist, continue with a long-term pulmonary rehab program, or just exercise at home? The answers are as different as the people making the decision about what optimal health is in relationship to their personal circumstances. At times it may be a matter of trial and error; perhaps the person's choice is not the same as that of a physician or other health care professional, but it is their decision and choice. They need to have the right to try, to succeed or fail, and perhaps make other decisions. They need to know how to access the health care system if there are medical problems, and learning to do so must be an integral part of the patient education process.

Actively playing a role in decision-making (i.e. self-management) empowers patients, making them more motivated, positive, active, and successful than passive patients who only do what the therapist (and physician, etc.) tells them. And with the decrease in visits allowed by managed care, patient self-management and empowerment can be a valuable source of efficiency in treatment. This chapter will explore ways in which the therapist can help patients cultivate positive self-management strategies for themselves, for a more active, healthy lifestyle.

The therapist can help this process by providing a caring and supportive presence. This has been referred to as a "healing presence," which may lead to a more beneficial, therapeutic, positive experience for the patient (Authier, 2004; McDonough-Means, 2004). The American Physical Therapy

Association promoted this through the phrase "the science of healing, the art of caring."

IF YOU CANNOT BREATHE YOU CANNOT FUNCTION

Functioning depends on the ability to breathe and move. An example of this was seen in a patient who fell in the parking lot of a hospital while going to a pulmonary rehabilitation program. She was in a long leg cast at home and became very short of breath with sit-to-stand transfers. Limited by severe shortness of breath, she could barely ambulate across the room with her pick-up walker. When observed using her bronchodilator metered-dose inhaler (MDI), she was found to be using it improperly. After she was instructed on how to use it properly, she used the bronchodilator before transfer and her gait was like that of a different person. She was able to coordinate her breathing pattern with control to match her activity, and her endurance was remarkably improved.

With these principles in mind, we can look at some of the considerations in nursing home and home health settings.

LONG-TERM CARE FACILITIES AND NURSING HOMES

As mentioned previously, with the changes in health care, much rehabilitation is now taking place in transitional care units, Medicare skilled nursing homes, and assisted living facilities.

The following are special considerations for working in a long-term care setting.

- There are several layers of care, from aides and general floor nurses to head nurses, geriatric specialist nurse consultants, and on-call physicians.
- Most patient care is given by aides.
- Communication and cooperation are key to achieving patient goals and success.
- Input from and involvement of the patient and family or significant other is essential in developing goals.
- Clear and achievable goals must be developed and revisited as the patient progresses or regresses in therapy. Is the goal to transition to a more independent living facility (i.e., home or an assisted living facility), or to maximize function within the current living facility?
- Quality of life issues must be taken into consideration. How mobile is the patient? Is he or she independent? When is therapy going to be most efficient time-wise? Is he or she a morning person? Will therapy conflict with his or her other interests and activities? Will therapy provide moral support or act as a distracter? Will therapy provide real recreation?
- Nutritional concerns must be taken seriously. Is the patient losing or gaining weight? Is he or she aspirating? Poor denture fit and food allergies may also affect the patient's ability to eat. Gastroesophageal reflux (GERD) may be occurring. The patient may be depressed and have no appetite. The patient may not want to take fluids because he or she has a difficult time getting to the bathroom

independently. Patients with severe COPD become extremely short of breath just eating. Nurses and aides on the floor and in the dining area, as well as family and friends, may provide valuable insight into these areas.

- Is the patient sleeping? After surgery, trauma, or a CVA, many patients are left overnight in positions that they may not have slept in before, such as supine or side-lying. Nurses and care staff can often help in positioning patients so they can rest comfortably and safely. The patients should be asked what their previous positions were for sleeping. If the patient has difficulty waking in the morning, or has headaches or difficulty following directions, issues such as sleep apnea should be considered. Issues ranging from incontinence and chronic pain to emotions and a busy environment outside the patient's door can contribute to loss of sleep and should be addressed as much as possible.
- Excellent results are often seen when aspects of physical therapy are incorporated into the patient's everyday life with the help of nurses and aides. This can help with the patient's physical capabilities as well as the learning process. For example, if the patient is taught in therapy to use ventilatory strategies with movement, such as inspiring when extending the trunk (see Chapter 23), this should be communicated to other caregivers and consistently encouraged. If the goal is for the patient to walk to meals, the physical therapist and caretakers can have the patient transition from walking to one meal (or as far as he or she can toward the dining room) to walking to two meals, to more functional goals such as walking to activities, social settings, out to the car to meet the family, and so on.
- In-services for nurses and care staff that help reinforce therapy techniques should be done both individually and in formal classes. Classes are helpful to discuss and instruct several staff members on a particular topic; they can be repeated for new staff and as a refresher for some aides who have not used or practiced the techniques. Even more essential, though, are ongoing one-on-one therapist/aide education sessions. These can be patient- or condition-specific and occur during treatment sessions or times that are mutually convenient. The aides may at first feel they are too busy and unable to do the job, but it is to both their benefit and that of the patient because in the long run the patient will be able to do more and the aide will have less work. In addition, the family members will be pleased and regard the work of the aide more highly. This will also benefit the nursing home because it will be known for its individualized, excellent patient care, which will please the director of nursing and the administrator. Furthermore, most aides like to do the best for their patients and provide the best care they can render.
- Try to get other programs and nursing home activity groups to follow through with therapeutic goals. Talk with the activity department if patients need extra encouragement or help with oxygen to participate. If patients need to drink more water for increased hydration, ask the activity department to remind the patient and provide water.

- As a therapist, be willing to pitch in and help whenever you are able, even if it "isn't in your job description." Your willingness to be a team player will be noticed. If an aide is off sick and you are available at lunch and see there is a problem passing out trays, offer to help. The next time you ask an aide for help there will probably be more willingness. If there is a patient that is difficult to transfer, offer to help in getting the patient up for physical therapy. This will serve as both a teaching opportunity and as a help to the aide. Look for ways to blend your therapy with the needs of the nursing staff.
- Give recognition to aides who have been remarkable in their patient care follow through of therapy goals. Be on the lookout for ways to praise and thank them in a sincere manner. They will be more willing to help in the future.
- Sponsor open house times in the therapy department so that the staff can come in and see the therapists. You can provide educational material for the staff (and food). Welcome their input and suggestions for patients who may benefit from therapy but are not on the physical therapy caseload.
- Prepare a bulletin board to share the accomplishments of patients in pictures and writing. We all love success stories and being part of the success. Show pictures of aides, as well as therapists, helping the patients.
- In addition to chart reviews and talking about patients with the nurses, screen patients in the dining rooms, activity sessions, and halls. The aides will be a terrific source of patient referrals because they are with the patients more than anyone else.

MONITORING CARDIOVASCULAR AND PULMONARY STATUS IN THE LONG-TERM CARE FACILITY

Because of shorter hospital stays, patients in long-term care facilities may be less stable than in the past. With this increase in patient acuity, it is more important than ever to monitor the patient's response to activity. Many long-term care and subacute facilities provide pulse oximeters and portable electrocardiogram monitors because they have more unstable patients. In addition, all therapists should be competent in blood pressure monitoring and taking heart rates. Auscultation training is highly recommended (see Chapter 15).

During the initial evaluation, vital signs and oximetry should be taken with the patient at rest in a supine or semi-Fowler's position for baseline, and then in sitting and standing positions. It is helpful to take the blood pressure on both arms to see if there is a difference in the readings. The arm with the higher reading should be used for recording and monitoring.

Initially, vital signs and oximetry should be evaluated before each therapy session and after the intervention or ambulation to assess the physiological response to exercise. Blood pressure and pulse should increase in relation to the activity. An increase of 20% to 30% or 20 to 30 beats above resting heart rate would be within normal limits, with a recovery time of 5 to 10 minutes back to baseline.

Many patients without primary cardiovascular and pulmonary diagnoses have abnormal responses to exercise, either from a preexisting but undetected dysfunction or a more recent change. Each patient must be observed closely and measured objectively to be sure he or she is responding properly to exercise. An example of this was seen in a patient one month post-CVA in a home-care setting. The patient was very fatigued and complained that his knees felt like they were going to buckle. This patient had been doing quite well and was not being monitored. Once the patient expressed the feeling of weakness, however, the therapist took vital signs after the patient rested and walked again. The patient's blood pressure and heart rate dropped during the exercise. The doctor was informed and ordered a blood test that revealed the patient did not have an appropriate blood level of digitalis. Medication was increased and the patient improved. Had the therapist not checked the vital signs and continued to push the patient, there could have been serious consequences.

SPECIAL MONITORING CONSIDERATIONS FOR PATIENTS ON OXYGEN

Oxygen therapy is usually prescribed due to a patient being hypoxemic (low levels of oxygen in the arterial blood) or to relieve myocardial work, such as in cases of severe myocardial infarction or other cardiac dysfunction.

It is important to note that arterial blood gases are drawn at rest with no patient activity unless specifically noted otherwise (such as an exercise test blood gas). Generally, Medicare guidelines require that a patient with a PO_2 of 55 mm Hg (Torr) be placed on oxygen. This is on the steep part of the oxyhemoglobin dissociation curve. When the patient exercises, he or she consumes more oxygen than at rest. Consequently, if a patient is on oxygen at rest and the PO_2 is 55 or 60 mm Hg, he or she may desaturate during exercise as the red blood cells give up more oxygen to supply the exercising muscle. The patient will experience increased shortness of breath and the oximeter will note a drop below 90%. Blood pressure and heart rate may initially increase because of the stress, but later drop because the heart cannot continue to compensate for the decrease in oxygen level.

The pulse oximetry reading (oxygen saturation) of normal subjects is 97.5% or above at rest, and it is clinically acceptable to maintain oxygen saturation at 90% or above. This saturation corresponds with keeping the PO_2 generally above 55 mm Hg; below 55 mm Hg, a dramatic drop in oxygen saturation will occur for a small drop in PO_2.

If the facility or home care agency does not have an oximeter, the durable medical equipment company that supplies the oxygen may be called and will bring an oximeter when they check the oxygen set up. Best practice, however, delineates that there should be oximeters available.

Any patient on oxygen at rest should be tested for desaturation. If it hasn't been ordered already, the therapist can call the patient's doctor to request an increase in oxygen during exercise. For example, a patient can have a prescription written for one l/min at rest and three l/min during exercise. The increase in oxygen is usually no problem as long as the oxygen is decreased back to the resting amount as soon as the patient recovers to baseline. This is true even for people who retain carbon dioxide and whose oxygen is carefully titrated to prevent taking away the hypoxic drive to breathe.

DOCUMENTATION

Functional outcomes are key to documentation. As we evaluate patients and write care plans, we set goals for both the short and long term. Each goal should be linked to functional outcomes that enable the patient to be safe and as mobile, functional, and independent as possible in the care setting in which he or she lives.

Documentation needs to show progress toward the functional outcomes the therapist has developed with the patient. Goals should be attainable and realistic. If there is poor or slow progress to a goal, there needs to be documentation and explanation in the notes of what has occurred and how the treatment program will be modified or how the goals need to be changed.

When functional outcomes have been met, the patient is reassessed to see if he or she can accomplish more or if therapy should be replaced with a maintenance program. A screening date should be set to reevaluate for maintenance, improvement, or decline in condition. At times patients who have "plateaued" will improve and may be picked up on a screening to request a doctor's order to have additional therapy with specific increased goals defined. If a patient's condition has declined, the patient can be reevaluated to see whether therapy should be resumed to regain his or her former status or to set more realistic functional goals.

It is important to remember that third party payers read these notes to understand the examination, evaluation, plan of intervention for the patient, and the progress that has been made in meeting functional outcomes. Because the patient is receiving long-term therapy, the more therapy the patient needs, the more necessary accurate documentation becomes in order to communicate with the third-party payer or the managed care group. A good quote to remember is, "if it wasn't written, it wasn't done!"

Every patient in a long-term facility may have cardiovascular and pulmonary concerns. The cardiovascular and pulmonary system must be optimized for the patient to reach maximal outcomes. Cooperation with the nurses and aides, as well as with the special activities staff and family members, is essential for follow-through of treatment programs and patient success. Teamwork is the key, including the patient in decision making and goal planning. Communication and documentation are vital to provide information on the progress and continued needs of the patient.

CARDIOVASCULAR AND PULMONARY CONCERNS IN HOME CARE

Home care takes the practice setting one step further from the hospital. Managed care has had a major impact on this area of therapy and nursing care. Patients are home faster after surgery and spending less time in the hospital in general, so patients receiving physical therapy at home can be quite acute. Therapists unaccustomed to addressing cardiovascular and pulmonary issues must do so in the home because nearly every patient (e.g., post-op, recent decline in function) will experience difficulty with breathing or endurance upon returning home. Often these individuals will have difficulty returning to their previous level of function without the help of home-based physical therapy.

In the home-care setting, the therapist is alone, although support is available through the nursing and home-care agencies. The therapist must be prepared to evaluate patients and their progress with very little supervision or consultation, and know how to obtain necessary information and equipment for the patient. This area of practice demands that therapists have experience and the ability to function independently. They need to be creative in adapting equipment, and innovative if the patient cannot afford to purchase medical equipment. In addition, they must be able to handle emergencies and crisis situations. All home-care therapists must have a basic CPR certification renewed annually. A firm grasp on policies and procedures for handling emergencies, infection control, and safety are essential for any therapist in the home. Therapists need to be able to evaluate the need for referrals to other health care workers or social service. They need to be aware of possible abuse or neglect. If the patient's condition declines or the patient shares that he or she has been falling or a new condition has arisen, the therapist needs to be able to do a medical screening and decide whether further intervention or notification of the patient's physician needs to be made. This is not the setting for new graduates, but rather for the experienced therapist.

Patients at home, even though they are receiving physical therapy and often have a caregiver, must be able to monitor their cardiovascular and pulmonary status themselves, to prevent overexertion and accidents. Therapists should teach patients self-monitoring strategies, such as the Borg Rating of Perceived Exertion scale (see Chapter 18), and heart rate monitoring, and therapists should check the reliability and validity of patients' self-assessments. When the therapist is satisfied in the patient's ability to self-monitor properly and without cues, he or she can be more confident that the patient can make better decisions about his or her own activity level independently and safety. The patient should be confident of his or her self-management and empowered and encouraged to pursue further functional gains.

WORKING IN THE HOME SETTING

In the hospital or outpatient center, the patient comes to *your place of business*. They come where you work. With long-term care and home care, *you go to work where they live.* Etiquette is required when going into a patient's residence. Permission must be requested to enter the residence, alter the living space, put in grab bars, remove scatter rugs and telephone cords that are seen as a safety hazard, or rearrange rooms that you may consider too cluttered and unsafe. The therapist must remember that this is the patient's home and must be tactful in the way recommendations are made. The cluttered room may hold treasures that have been accumulated over a lifetime. Patients may surround themselves with items that are all they have left to remember of loved ones. It may be true that a path is needed for safe walker ambulation, but how this is communicated may make all the difference in developing a good relationship between the home-care therapist and the patient. Therapists should also remember that returning home can make a patient very proud as well as very intimidated. Indicating that you are sensitive to this situation and want to help can also assist in establishing rapport.

Initially an evaluation of the patient's home needs to be made. Safety is a primary consideration. Are there electrical or phone cords across the floor? Are scatter rugs loose or tacked down with carpet tape? Can the patient pick up his or her foot sufficiently to walk over the scatter rug without tripping? Are there pieces of kitchen linoleum that have come up and might trip the patient? Are the kitchen chairs on rollers and the patient's balance poor? If the patient is on oxygen, does he or she have a gas stove? Are the close relatives, friends, or caretakers smokers? Signs need to be posted to warn of the danger of smoking and flames around oxygen. Patients who are smokers need to have this reinforced very clearly.

If the patient lives alone, what provision is there for an accident or fall? Does the patient have an alert necklace device or a cell phone that he or she can carry in a pocket? What procedure will be followed? Does the patient know how and when to contact 911 for help? Are there neighbors or family that can regularly check on the patient?

Does the patient have stairs? Is the bedroom upstairs? Is there a first floor bathroom? If the bathroom is on the second floor, can the patient get up the stairs safely and in a timely manner or does a commode on the lower level seem more appropriate?

Does the patient have the proper adaptive equipment and assistive devices? Is it in working order, and does the patient know how to use it? Often a patient borrows "grandpa's cane" and does not realize that he or she is eight inches shorter than grandpa. Modifications may need to be made so that existing equipment fits properly and is safe and functional. Grab bars in bathrooms and toilet seat risers may need to be ordered.

Is there family support or a caretaker if the patient is not independent? Is the designated caregiver able to safely and consistently perform all the duties required for the patient's wellbeing? If the spouse needs to work or go out, how long can the patient be safely left alone? Does the patient know how to obtain a caretaker? Are they able to financially afford the support?

Is the bed the proper height? Are there handrails? Is it difficult for the patient to transfer into bed? Is a device needed to help the patient transfer independently?

The question of the bed arose with one home-care patient who had a fractured pelvis. During the initial examination she was asked how she had broken her pelvis and she replied, "Hopping into bed." The therapist questioned what she meant and she said, "I'll show you." In the bedroom it was quickly noted that this very short patient had a very tall bed. The mattress was between her iliac crest and waist when she backed up to the bed. She stated, "I used to have a stool that I climbed into bed on, but my son thought it wasn't safe and took it away. Now I have to hop up into bed!" She had returned home to do the same activity that had put her in the hospital with a fractured pelvis. Looking at the bed, it was noted that there were three-inch rolling casters and a caster pad under the bed. The son was called and the casters and pads removed. The patient was quite pleased that the bed was four inches lower and she could now transfer in easily.

Most home-care agencies have social worker support to help patients discover resources available to them. A physician's referral is needed and the service is generally covered under Medicare.

Cost effective yet excellent therapy with quality perceived by the patient is the goal of managed care. There is a great deal of creativity; deals can be made if a provider group can demonstrate that the patient will benefit at a cost savings to the managed care group. We are seeing coalitions form between contract-service therapy agencies, durable medical equipment companies, nursing agencies, and enteral feeding companies to provide "one-stop shopping" groups, so that the managed care companies can make one call for these services.

COMMUNICATION AND REFERRALS TO OTHER DISCIPLINES

It is essential that communication take place between the members of the home-care team. Communication is difficult because everyone is on the road and traveling to patients' homes. Generally, pager and cell phone numbers of therapists and nurses are exchanged and compliance with answering pages and calls is good; however, consideration needs to be given to the realization that we do not like to be interrupted frequently when seeing patients. Generally a system of timing the calls or pages is welcomed. A "911" can be placed after the page number to indicate that the call is urgent or that information needs to be given immediately.

Because the home patient is away from the constant monitoring of the hospital environment, the home-care nurses and therapists often are the most familiar with the patient's day-to-day condition. Also, in the chaos of discharging from the hospital, some referrals or orders for services such as occupational therapy or social work may have been made but not followed-up or filled. If the therapist notices that the patient may benefit from additional services, he or she should consider addressing the issue formally (a referral filed through the home-care agency or nurse case manager) or informally (a phone call to the appropriate health care professional).

If the patient needs additional physical therapy, a referral should be made by calling the home-care agency or the patient's nurse case manager. Identify the problem and why you feel the additional therapy is indicated. The physician will be called and the order generally obtained. It would then be helpful for the referring therapist to call the new therapist for an update on the patient and reason for the referral. This communication should be documented to show the necessary communication and coordination between the therapists and nurses.

At times it is helpful to combine treatment sessions with another discipline, such as a co-treatment between a physical therapist and an occupational therapist, or a physical therapist and a speech-language therapist. This can provide focus and continuity of goals between disciplines, as well as ease the strain on patients who initially lack the endurance to tolerate several treatment visits a day. For example, a physical therapist and a speech-language therapist may meet to focus on a patient with poor posture who lacks breath support for phonation or to address better positioning for swallowing during meals. A patient who is having difficulty feeding because of trunk weakness and who is sitting in flexion with a forward head and neck and is having difficulty swallowing may benefit from speech and occupational therapists who can help with seating systems and feeding. The interaction and communication between therapists facilitates ideas for both therapists, provides continuity and follow-through, and helps to optimize patient care.

MONITORING CARDIOVASCULAR AND PULMONARY STATUS AT HOME

Cardiovascular and pulmonary monitoring at home is similar to that in a long-term care facility. Blood pressure and heart rate monitoring should be done at rest on both arms, in sitting and standing, and before and after exercise as previously mentioned.

A portable pulse oximeter (Figure 41-1) must also be taken on visits to patients who have primary cardiovascular and

pulmonary diagnoses or functional limitations; desaturation is a major determinant of exercise intolerance and a potential medical concern for these patients. It is a good idea to have an oximeter handy for all other patients as a precaution. Several models of portable oximeters are available and many home therapy companies own at least one.

Self-monitoring (Borg Rating of Perceived Exertion scale, heart rate) should be incorporated with therapy and independent activities as the patient is able. Caregivers and family members may also be taught to monitor the patient's blood pressure (with a sphygmomanometer and stethoscope or an automated device) as well as heart rate. Caregivers and family members may also be able to observe changes such as increased shortness of breath, increase or decrease in amount and color of secretions, dizziness or light-headedness, color changes such as cyanosis or flushed skins, diaphoresis, unsteadiness with ambulation, and mental status changes, and report them promptly to the therapist or physician.

EXERCISE AND ACTIVITY AT HOME

Therapists must remember that the baseline activity level and exercise tolerance of patients seen at home can be very low, particularly in those with primary cardiovascular and pulmonary diagnoses. Establishing an exercise program with these patients may be difficult, especially when the patient is used to an inactive lifestyle or has attempted exercising before with unsuccessful or unpleasant results. Exercise in the traditional sense is less likely to be successful given this negative impression, and a different approach may be necessary to address the patient's need for increased activity for functional and health reasons.

The therapist may want to choose a more agreeable method of exercise in which activity is incorporated into other aspects of life that are enjoyable for the patient, such as playing with grandchildren, gardening, taking walks around the block, or visiting family and friends (which involves ambulating to and from the car as well as several transfers along the way).

The frequency and intensity of these activities can be minimal to start and increase as the patient becomes accustomed to (and hopefully partial to) the activity. Progress the patient as tolerated, with the input of the patient. Self-monitoring (heart rate, Borg Rating of Perceived Exertion scale) and input from the patient should be encouraged. Some patients have elected to purchase their own oximeter and use it as a self-monitoring tool as well (Figure 41-2).

As mentioned earlier, adding choices and patient participation in the establishment of an exercise scheme can help empower the patient and lead to increased compliance with as well as a more positive impression of an exercise program that continues even after therapy has ended.

The therapist must first be sure that the patient can perform the exercises and activities of daily living safely and independently (with the appropriate device or caregiver support) while properly and accurately monitoring his or her own

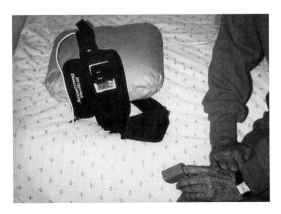

FIGURE 41-1 Pulse oximeter.

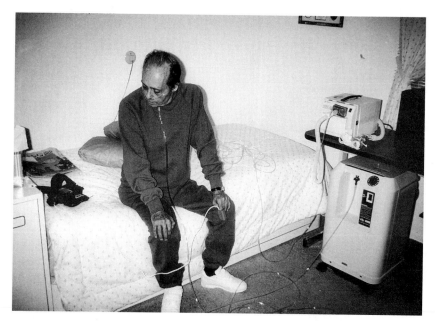

FIGURE 41-2 Patient monitoring oximeter with exercise.

condition and modifying the intensity or distance appropriately without cues. Once the patient can do this reliably, he or she can begin to pursue activities of his or her choice, which allows for faster progression of therapy goals and a patient who is more actively involved with his or her rehabilitation process.

HOME OXYGEN

Home oxygen may be supplied by an oxygen concentrator, tanks, or a liquid oxygen system (Figure 41-3 and Chapter 43). Often, several extensions of oxygen tubing are needed to allow patients mobility to go to the bathroom, the kitchen, and the living room (Figure 41-4). Although oxygen is a safety concern the home-care therapist must deal with, the long tubing still allows for proper oxygen delivery; compensated flow meters measure the amount of oxygen actually reaching the patient, and problems such as kinks will be indicated by a decreased flow reading. Still, some portable oxygen systems, particularly demand oxygen systems, will sometimes not deliver the exact amount expected (Figure 41-5). It is necessary to use oximetry to determine whether the patient has an appropriate oxygen saturation reading.

Patients need to be taught to coil the tubing or use a similar strategy to be sure that they do not trip over the tubing. Some patients have more than one tank or concentrator in the home in order to prevent having long lengths of tubing.

Patients with sleep apnea may use nocturnal nasal continuous positive airway pressure (CPAP) (Figure 41-6) or bi-phasic continuous positive airway pressure (Bi-PAP), which provide varying levels of assistance with ventilation during the night. A Bi-PAP unit allows the patient to rest and let the machine assist ventilation by providing pressure support on inspiration and exhalation. Therapists should encourage the

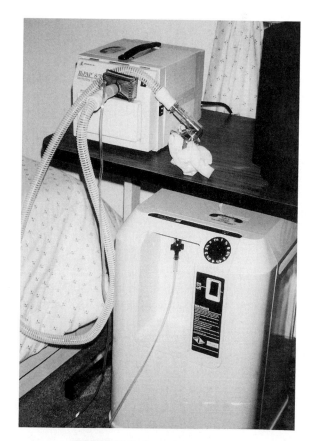

FIGURE 41-3 Oxygen concentrator.

patient to use this device every night because, although the patient may have difficulty adjusting to the nasal CPAP at first, the patient will adapt to the assistance in time and feel it is beneficial.

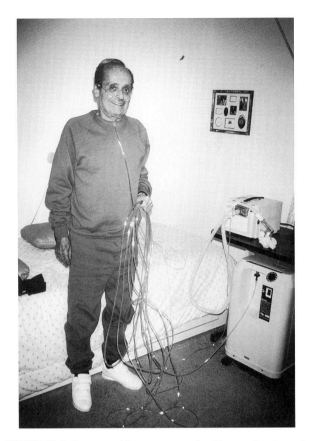

FIGURE 41-4 Oxygen tubing presents a significant safety hazard.

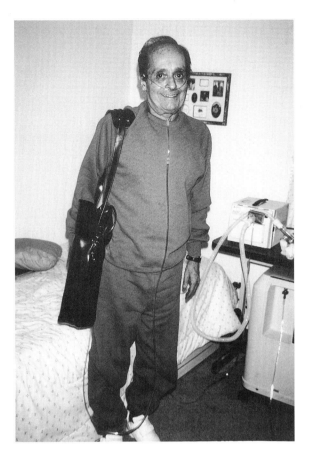

FIGURE 41-5 Portable demand oxygen system.

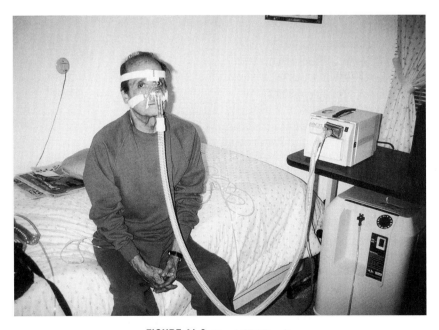

FIGURE 41-6 Nasal CPAP unit.

SUPPORT FOR PEOPLE IN THE HOME OR COMMUNITY

An important part of achieving optimal health upon returning home or settling into a new living facility is having the necessary social and emotional support. Remember, nobody does it alone. Family and friends help the patient feel like a real person, which hospital stays or new functional limitations can often prevent.

Support can also come in the form of groups of people with similar diagnoses or limitations formed in the community or over the Internet. These can be extremely important for patients, regardless of the amount of support they receive from family and friends. Peers in these groups may be the only people who understand what the patient is going through; support from these peers, as well as the opportunity for the patient to support those peers in return, may help inspire physical and personal gains impossible through therapy interventions alone.

Peer groups, in person or over the Internet, can also be valuable resources to help patients with chronic illness make choices concerning their health and life situations (Anhoj, 2004; Gunnarsdottir, 2004; Jamison, 2004; Lieberich, 2004; Nguyen, 2005; Wantland, 2004). Two good examples for people with COPD are the National Emphysema/COPD Association (NECA) Web site at www.NECACommunity.org and www.COPD-Alert.com. NECA's vision statement states that they are "a patient-centered, member-driven, and member-governed organization. Our mission is to empower people with emphysema/COPD and their families and caregivers to improve the quality of patient care and the quality of their lives." (NECA News, Fall/Winter, 2003). People with COPD are given free membership to this group, and health care professionals and supporters pay a nominal fee for the newsletters and information. They host grass roots efforts such as conferences and informational sessions on self-care management and patient empowerment. They have a newsletter that discusses research and provides tips from people living with COPD to help share information that has proven beneficial. The NECA lets people know they are not alone and that there are resources they can draw on for help and decision making as they live with COPD.

There are numerous other patient friendly Web sites for COPD (and other conditions), all of which are easily accessed through search engine Web sites and the links sections of related Web sites. Box 41-1 contains examples of Web sites that may be helpful for people with COPD and their families or caregivers. This is only a partial listing, and links to many other Web sites can be found by accessing those in Box 41-1.

THERAPEUTIC GOALS FOR HOME-CARE PATIENTS WITH CARDIOVASCULAR AND PULMONARY DYSFUNCTION

To be independent at home, it is necessary for patients with cardiovascular and pulmonary dysfunction to the following.

- Understand the dysfunction or disease and how it affects their functioning.

BOX 41-1

Patient Friendly COPD Web sites

www.NECACommunity.org — National Emphysema COPD Association
www.COPD-ALERT.org — self-care, sharing of information for people with COPD
www.chestnet.org — American College of Chest Physicians
www.lungsusa.org/diseases/ — American Lung Association
www.lung.ca/copd/ — Canadian Lung Association
www.lib.uiowa.edu/hardin/md/resp.html — library links to respiratory/lung disease
www.intellihealth.com — Harvard University Medical School, COPD and pulmonary disease
www.mdlinx.com/pulmonaologylinx/index.cfm — journal articles
www.medicinenet.com/lungs/focus.htm — medical information site geared to patients
www.nhlbi.nih.gov/health/public/lung/index.htm — National Heart, Lung and Blood Institute
www.alphaone.org — information on alpha-1-antitrypsin deficit

This is a partial listing of some Web sites for people with COPD and their families or caregivers. There are numerous other helpful informational sites. This is meant as a starting point. Many links to other Web sites will be found by accessing these Web sites.

- Acquire all necessary adaptive equipment and assistive devices for use in the home and community.
- Acknowledge their functional limitations (i.e., not try to push their limits without monitoring their responses) to ensure safety.
- Be compliant with medications and the direction of physicians and other health care professionals. Discuss what is working well and what is not and work collaboratively to find better solutions and interventions.
- Arrange for caregivers to safely and consistently provide assistance at the level needed.
- Learn preventative care (i.e., prevent pulmonary infections and do not increase salt/water intake if on cardiac precautions or taking steroids).
- Learn ventilatory strategies to increase comfort and function (see Chapter 23).
- Learn to monitor themselves for signs of impending trouble (i.e., increased shortness of breath, swelling in ankles, productive cough, change in mucus, decreased urine output, or rapid weight gain).
- Pace activity and use energy conservation techniques and rest periods to accomplish more with less stress.
- Optimize nutrition and hydration, notify health care professionals about increases or decreases in weight, and seek referral to a dietician for significant concerns.
- Develop a social support network to provide emotional support when needed, and to check on them occasionally.
- Engage in a walking program and increasing general exercise to continue functional gains.

SUMMARY

Education, self-monitoring, compliance to medication, reduction of risk factors, nutrition, and hydration are essential in the progress and maintenance of people living with chronic conditions at home. As health care practitioners, we offer helpful suggestions for modification of the patient's home environment and lifestyle. We cannot, however, force a patient to comply or accept what we have proposed. The patient in the home setting needs to be independent in his or her judgments and activities. We need to respect that and at the same time provide our experience and therapeutic judgment and expertise. This setting is often the most rewarding a therapist can have, although at times it also may be the most frustrating. One thing is certain, if you ask a patient where he or she wants to be, the answer sounds like "There's no place like home!"

Review Questions

1. What are some common problems patients in the community may experience?
2. What role does a preexisting cardiopulmonary condition play in a new diagnosis or trauma (e.g., CVA, hip fracture)?
3. What are some situations or concerns particular to patient care delivery in a nursing home, assisted living center, and home care?
4. What role can a physical therapist play in optimizing the patient's self-management in the above settings?
5. How can cardiovascular and pulmonary function be monitored outside in long-term care and home care?
6. What special patient instructions and considerations should be provided for a patient on oxygen?
7. How can caregivers and family members be incorporated into the management of patients with chronic illness in the home and long-term care setting?

REFERENCES

Anhoj, J., & Jensen, A.H. (2004). Using the Internet for life style changes in diet and physical activity: a feasibility study. Journal of Medical Internet Resources 6:33.

Authier, P. (2004). Being present—the choice that re-instills caring. Nursing Administration 28:276-279.

Emlet, C., Cragtree, J., Condon, V., & Tremel, L. (1995). In-home assessment of older adults, an interdisciplinary approach. Gaithersburg, Md: Aspen Publishers.

Epping-Jordan, J.E., Pruitt, S.D., Bengoa, R., & Wagner, E.H. (2004). Improving the quality of health care for chronic conditions. Quality Safe Heath Care 13:299-305.

Guinn, M.J. (2004). A daughter's journey promoting geriatric self-care: promoting positive health care interactions. Geriatric Nursing 2595:267-271.

Hainsworth, T. (2005). A new model of care for people who have long-term conditions. Nursing Times 101:L28-L29.

Harrington, J. (1983). The case for home health specialization. Clinical Management in Physical Therapy 3:17.

Holman, H., & Lorig, K. (2004). Patient self-management: a key to effectiveness and efficiency in care of chronic disease. Public Health Report 119:239-243.

Hughes, S. (2004). Promoting self-management and patient independence. Nursing Standard 19:L47-L52.

Jackson, B.N. (1984). Home health care and the elderly in the 1980's. American Journal of Occupational Therapy 38:717.

Jackson, D.E., & Wilhoire, M.J. (1985). Home health physical therapy, considerations for the provision of care. Clinical Management in Physical Therapy 5:10.

Jerant, A.F., et al. (2005). Walk a mile in my shoes: a chronic illness care workshop for first year students. Family Medicine 37:L21-L26.

Lorig, K., et al. (2000). Living a healthy life with chronic conditions, self-management of heart disease, arthritis, diabetes, asthma, bronchitis, emphysema and others, ed 2. Boulder, Colo: Bull Publishing Company.

Marks, R., Allegrante, J.P., & Lorig, K. (2005). A review and synthesis of research evidence for self-efficacy-enhancing interventions for reducing chronic disability: implications for health education practice (part I). Health Promotion Practice 6:37-43.

May, B.J. (1993). Home health and rehabilitation: concepts of care. Philadelphia: F.A. Davis.

May, B.J. (1990). Principles of exercise for the elderly. In Basmajian, J.V., & Wolf, S.L. (Eds). Therapeutic exercise, ed 5. Baltimore: Williams & Wilkins.

McDonough-Means, S.I., Kreitzer, M.J., & Bell, I.R. (2004). Fostering a healing presence and investigating its mediators. Journal of Alternative and Complementary Medicine 10(Suppl 1): S25-S41.

Monninkhof, E., van der Aa, M., van der Valk, P., van der Palen, J., Zielhuis, G., Koning, K., & Pieterse, M. (2004). A qualitative evaluation of a comprehensive self-management programme for COPD patients: effectiveness from the patients' perspective. Patient Education Counseling 55:177-184.

Nguyen, H.Q., Carrieri-Kohlman, V., Rankin, S.H., Slaughter, R., & Stulbarg, M.S. (2005). Is Internet-based support for dyspnea self-management in patients with chronic obstructive pulmonary disease possible? Results of a pilot study. Heat and Lung 34:51-62.

O'Donnell, D.E., Aaron, S., Bourbeau, J., Hernandez, P., Marciniuk, D., Balter, M., Ford, G., Gervais, A., Goldstein, R., Hodder, R., Maltais, F., & Road, J. (2004). State of the art compendium: Canadian Thoracic Society recommendations for the management of chronic obstructive pulmonary disease. Candian Respiratory Journal 11(Suppl B):7B-59B.

Pfau, J. (1989). Adult exercise instruction sheets: home exercise for rehabilitation. Tucson, Ariz: Therapy Skill Builders.

Polich, C. (1990). The provision of home health care services through health maintenance organizations: conflicting roles for HMOs. Home Health Care Quarterly 11:17.

Sallade, J. & Adam, L. (1986). Geriatric exercise booklet. Clinical Management in Physical Therapy 6:32.

Schaefer, K. & Lewis, C. (1986). Marketing geriatric programs—a home care example. Clinical Management in Physical Therapy 6:11-17.

Tanner, E.K. (2004). Chronic illness demands for self-management in older adults. Geriatric Nursing 25:313-317.

Vassif, J.A. (1985). The home health care solution. New York: Harper & Row.

Wentland, D.J., et al. (2003). The effectiveness of Web-based vs. non-Web based intervention on a meta-analysis of behavioral change outcomes. Journal of Medical Internet Resources 6:40.

Zola, I.K. (1990). Aging, disability and the home care revolution. Archives of Physical Medicine and Rehabilitation 71:93.

Related Aspects of Cardiovascular and Pulmonary Physical Therapy

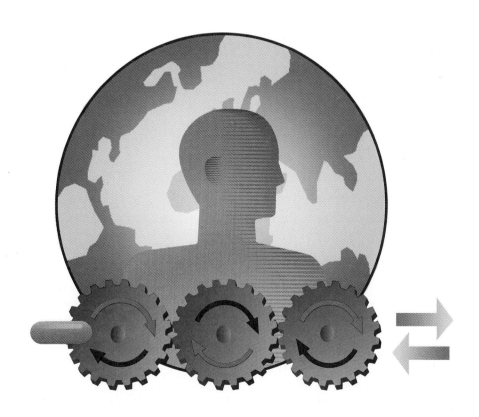

CHAPTER 42

Body Mechanics—The Art of Positioning and Moving Patients

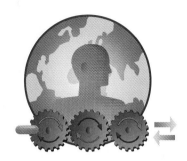

Donna Frownfelter and Mary Massery

KEY TERMS

Body mechanics
Dependent patients
Lifting and moving
"Positioning for success"

Ventilation related to:
    Neutral head and shoulder alignment
    Prone
    Side-lying
    Supine
    Upright

Body mechanics may be defined as the efficient use of one's body as a machine and locomotive entity. When working with critically ill or chronically dependent patients, it is essential to accomplish optimal body positioning to facilitate maximal ventilatory potential and improved patient outcomes. Therapists and nurses attempting to position or move dependent patients must understand and use proper body mechanics (McConnell, 2002; Hefti et al, 2003; Karahan & Bayraktar, 2004; Neil, 1959; Fuerst & Wolff, 1969) because they are necessary to reduce stress and trauma and promote success for both the patient and the health care team. Positioning and moving dependent patients is an art that is quite different than working with a patient who can move independently and assume any given position with ease. In this chapter, the principles of body positioning and moving dependent patients are discussed.

POSITIONING FOR OPTIMAL VENTILATION

Because of the three-dimensional nature of breathing, one of the therapist's most important goals is to facilitate chest excursion in all three planes of ventilation: anterior-posterior, superior-inferior, and lateral (Massery, 1994). This can be accomplished by improving the length-tension relationships of the muscles used in inspiration (Crosbie & Myles, 1985; Kendall et al, 1993). Massery reasons that the success of proper positioning to enhance inspiratory muscles will do the following.

1. Improve the length-tension relationship of the accessory ventilatory muscles involved in that posture.
2. Incorporate a passive stretch of the chest wall.
3. Use the natural coordination of the trunk-chest wall movement with inspiration and exhalation patterns to maximize movement.

The following are some common improvements that can be incorporated into normal positioning.

Supine Position

All activity is performed within the field of gravity. Patients in a supine position may find breathing difficult because they must overcome gravity to move the chest wall with each breath. Using towel rolls or pillows to facilitate a better position may significantly improve the patient's opportunity

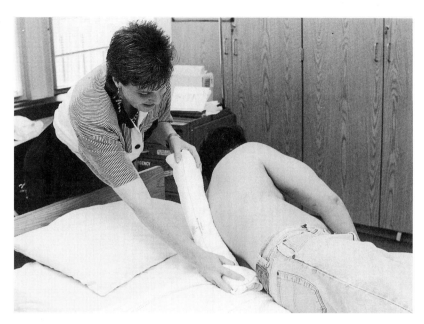

FIGURE 42-1 Placement of a vertical towel roll.

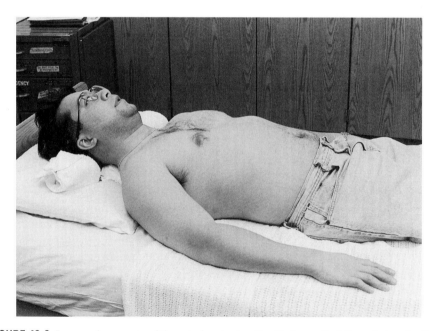

FIGURE 42-2 Increased openness of the anterior chest wall with the vertical thoracic towel roll and the occipital towel roll combined.

for improved ventilation. All positioning suggestions, however, need to be applied with the individual patient's comfort and tolerance in mind.

Upper chest expansion can be increased by removing pillows from under the patient's head to increase thoracic extension. This will increase the length-tension relationship of the neck accessory muscles (scalene and sternocleidomastoid muscles). Increased movement will be noted in the upper chest in a superior and anterior plane (Massery et al, 1997). Further anterior expansion can be achieved by using a towel roll placed longitudinally at the vertebral spine to open the anterior chest of a patient who tends toward excessive flexion of the trunk (Figure 42-1).

If the patient needs support under his or her head to achieve a neutral chin tuck to protect his or her swallowing ability, a thin pillow or horizontal towel roll under the occiput may be used (Figure 42-2).

External rotation of the shoulders with the scapula in a neutral or retracted position will place the pectoralis and intercostal muscles on stretch. This will improve lateral and

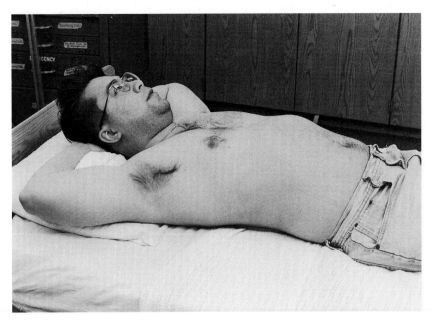

FIGURE 42-3 Butterfly position with a thoracic towel roll to open the anterior chest.

anterior chest wall movement (Ishii et al, 2004; Kendall et al, 1993). If a patient has full range of motion (ROM) and is comfortable with the arms placed overhead or in full flexion/ abduction/external rotation for maximal stretch, this is the optimal position for full excursion of the anterior chest wall (Figure 42-3). If there are significant shoulder limitations, moderate shoulder abduction with forearm supination may be the best position available to facilitate chest excursion. Whenever significant limitations are found, the therapist should try to modify the position to accommodate the patient and achieve optimal ventilation.

Side-lying Position

Side-lying is an optimal position that may improve breathing patterns. Gravity is eliminated for anterior expansion and the diaphragm moves freely. Preterm infants placed in a side-lying or prone position have been shown to have fewer stress behaviors, and this resulted in longer periods of sleep with less fussiness and crying (Grenier et al, 2003). It is important to consider the shunt effects if a patient has lung pathology. For example, if a patient has right lower lobe pneumonia or atelectasis, side-lying on the unaffected side will improve oxygenation. Conversely, side-lying with the affected side down will cause a decrease in oxygenation (differential shunt) because a patient with decreased ventilation receives more perfusion to the down lung and more shunting will occur. The patient's hip and knee joints should be flexed and supported for comfort. The upper extremities can be moved up and away from the body to allow for free movement of the upper chest wall. A pillow can be used to support the upper arm anteriorly, or the patient can be placed in a three quarter supine position

with a pillow behind the back to support the uppermost arm. If the patient has full ROM and is comfortable, a butterfly position of the arms can be used. This will automatically open the rib cage, put the pectoral muscles at a lengthened range, and facilitate inspiration.

Prone Position

Prone positioning has been found to improve oxygenation in a number of patient populations, including patients who are critically ill and medically fragile (such as those with acute respiratory distress syndrome [ARDS], hypoxemic acute respiratory failure, and preterm infants) (Oczenski et al, 2005; Vollman, 2004; Piedalue & Albert, 2003; Harcombe, 2004; Guerin et al, 2004; Gainnier et al, 2003; Grenier et al, 2003), with minimal untoward effects. There have been some cases where difficulties have been noted. One instance of severe hypotension was noted in a child that had scoliosis, pectus excavatum, and neurofibromatosis who presented for a spinal fusion. It is recommended that sternal pressure be avoided in patients with chest wall deformities (Alexianu et al, 2004). Early enteral nutrition is poorly tolerated in critically ill patients receiving invasive mechanical ventilation in the prone position. Medication can be given to enhance gastric emptying and prevent vomiting. Feeding the patient in the prone position presents a difficult situation in which both the nutrition and mechanical ventilation are extremely important (Reignier et al, 2004).

When a patient is mechanically ventilated and has numerous tubes and monitors, turning him or her to the prone position takes a good amount of planning and is staff intensive but can have significant impact on his or her outcome.

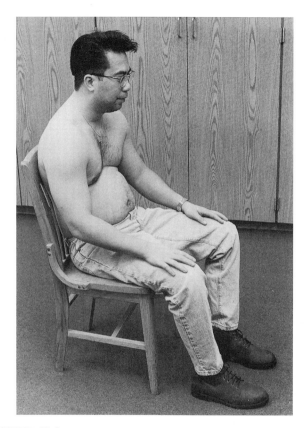

FIGURE 42-4 Unsupported upright position of a patient with T1 paraplegia. Note the posterior pelvic tilt and excessive thoracic khyphosis with resulting collapse of the anterior chest wall.

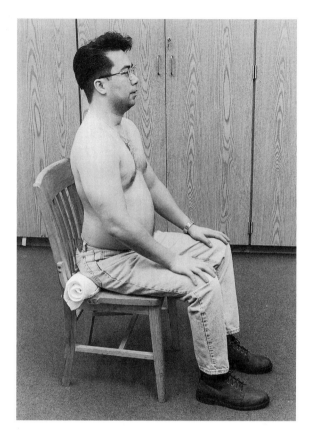

FIGURE 42-5 Ischial towel roll to support the pelvis in anterior tilt in a patient with T1 paraplegia. Note the changes in the thoracic spine and open anterior chest wall as well as improved head and neck alignment.

Upright Postures

Upright postures create new challenges to breathing by adding the components of balance and an unsupported spinal column. Many patients, however, spend prolonged periods of time in their wheelchairs or in other situations where they are sitting or standing. Many patients with poor trunk support tend to sit in a slumped position, which results in a decrease in tidal volume and minute ventilation. Improvement in sitting posture will improve pulmonary function and allow better breath support for function.

Pelvic alignment is a key component to optimal posture. A relatively anterior tilted pelvis in healthy, flexible adults will tend to do the following: reduce the kyphotic curve in the thoracic spine, adduct the scapula toward a neutral position, produce a more neutral or externally rotated upper-extremity position, and pull the head back into a neutral chin tuck (Woodhall-McNeal, 1992; Borello-France et al, 1988). The anterior tilt of the pelvis will improve upper-extremity ROM and ventilation potential. Attending to this one consideration may be all that is necessary to improve the breathing capacity in some patients, allowing them to continue to advance in their exercise programs or rehabilitation courses. This may be facilitated by the use of a lumbar roll.

Another simple means of attaining an anterior pelvic tilt in sitting is to have the patient lean forward over his or her legs, then slide a towel roll horizontally just behind the ischial tuberosities, which will prevent the pelvis from rolling back into a posterior tilt (Johnson, 1989) (Figures 42-4 and 42-5). This is well tolerated for many patients with intact sensation and a pelvis that is at least minimally mobile. For patients with neurological impairment who have impaired sensation or less pelvic mobility, a wedge may be substituted; however, caution must be used because some sliding may occur.

Neutral Alignment of the Head and Shoulders

A vertical or horizontal towel roll may also be used with wheelchair positioning to bring the shoulders and head back into a more neutral alignment. The anterior chest wall will also be more open with this technique.

A neutral head and neck position is important for patients with impaired speech volume or endurance and for patients with swallowing or aspiration impairments. A neutral chin tuck will optimize the length-tension relationship of the vocal folds, minimize vocal strain, and improve protective airway reflexes (Massery, 1994).

It is also vital to evaluate the patient's shoulder positioning. Internal rotation of the shoulders and scapular protraction tends to block the upper chest from reaching its full expansion potential. Alternately, external rotation of the shoulders will increase upper chest wall movement and thoracic extension (Ishii et al, 2004). Clinically, improved lung volumes will be noted when these positioning considerations are taken into consideration. Often these small, seemingly insignificant changes may position the patient for success with other therapeutic activities. If unattended, these small factors can impede patient outcomes. Positioning is vital to improving ventilation and functional skills.

LIFTING AND MOVING DEPENDENT PATIENTS

There have been changes in the concepts and principles of lifting. As discussed, the body has historically been thought of in terms of a machine. It was believed that improper mechanics of lifting would result in tremendous loads on the disks. The key components of lifting were to "keep it close," "bend the knees," and "lift with the legs." Spinal posture later became the center of attention during lifting (Physical Therapy Forum, 1985).

On the basis of observation, lifting seems to occur "naturally": the therapist begins with slightly bent knees and the patient rears backward as the therapist extends his or her knees and starts to lift the patient gluteal area first. Most injuries seem to occur with the back in flexion. The rationale for strengthening the core muscles is to promote safer lifting. Abdominal strength is necessary to support the pelvis during lifting. Many commercially available lumbar and abdominal elastic supports are now available and widely used. They provide additional abdominal wall support as well as a reminder to lift safely. Unfortunately they are at times worn loosely or not properly applied.

Another school of thought advocates maintaining the lordotic lumbar curve while lifting. This is the technique used by weight lifters. When these individuals are questioned about backaches, they usually deny any problems.

The lifting technique used may require modification because of other factors, such as limited space (i.e., small hospital rooms), clothing, or impairments of the health care team members (such as degenerative knee joints).

The first consideration in body mechanics is the need to maintain proper posture and balance (body stability). Consideration should be paid to the relationship between gravity, posture, and body stability (Figure 42-6). It is commonly known that gravitational force is always exerted in a vertical direction toward the center of the earth. In addition, that point in a patient or object at which all of its mass is centered is called the center of gravity (the point at which the patient's maximum weight is concentrated). When standing, the human body's center of gravity is located at a height of approximately 55% of the body's total height: in the pelvic cavity, slightly anterior to the upper part of the sacrum. The lower a person's center of gravity, the greater his or her body

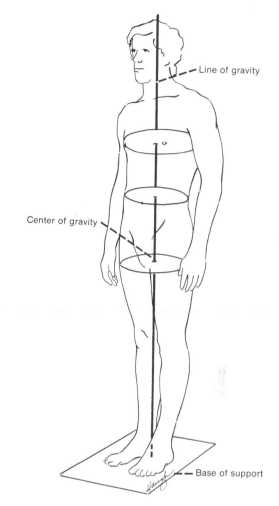

FIGURE 42-6 The line of gravity passes through the center of gravity and the base of support to maintain body stability.

stability. Consequently, when the human body is used as a machine to lift an object, increasing muscular effort great enough to maintain stability and to lift against the force of gravity is necessary as the lifter's center of gravity is further removed from the object. Therefore, one way for the therapist to conserve energy and maintain stability is to carry the weight of the patient (or object) as close to his or her own center of gravity as possible. This allows the lifter maximum concentration of energy toward movement of the patient and minimal stress or injury. To help accomplish this, the bed should be adjusted so the therapist or nurse can reach the patient comfortably. Usually, adjusting the bed to the lifter's hip level is adequate. This places the patient close to the therapist's center of gravity.

The majority of lifting should be done with the legs (knees) as opposed to straining to lift with the arms and back (Figure 42-7). Whenever there is a question about a single therapist's ability to lift a patient alone, it should not be done—assistance should be obtained (Rantz & Courtial, 1977).

Another point to consider is the base of support while lifting. The base of support is defined as the area between the

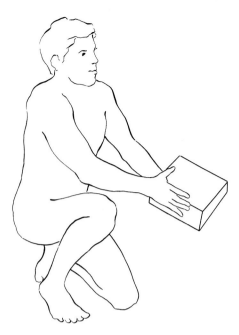

FIGURE 42-7 Reach work level by bending the knees and hips rather than the back. Lift with the legs! This can also be done with a full double knee squat similar to techniques by weightlifters.

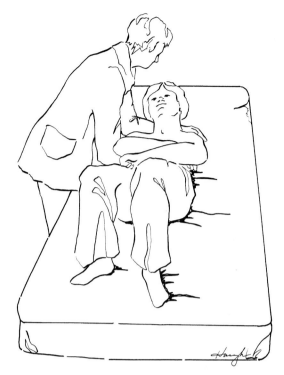

FIGURE 42-8 The patient should be prepared for a position change: knees bent, arms crossed over chest and head lifted up to reduce friction between the patient's body and the bed.

feet, which provides the body's stability. It is easily appreciated that the wider the base of support, the greater the body's stability. To enlarge on this concept, it is also necessary to define the line of gravity and its relationship to body stability. The line of gravity is an imaginary line passing through the center of gravity of an object and perpendicular to the surface on which the object (body) rests (see Figure 42-6). The closer the line of gravity passes to the center of the base of support, the greater the body's (object's) stability. Increasing muscular effort is exerted in proportion to the distance the line of gravity shifts away from the base of support (Rauch, 1971).

The following guidelines summarize and apply the concepts discussed above.

1. The lower your center of gravity, the wider your base of support, and the nearer the line of gravity falls to the center of your base of support, the greater your body's stability. When lifting, stand with your feet well apart, knees slightly flexed, and one foot forward. Keep your head and trunk in proper alignment.
2. When a body is used as a machine, the external weight on which it works displaces the body's center of gravity in the direction of the weight being lifted. To conserve energy and maintain stability, carry the weight as close to your own center of gravity as possible. Lower your hips to the level of the surface supporting the weight you plan to lift by flexing your hips and knees. Adjust the bed up as high or down as low as you need for comfortable and efficient work.
3. The effort required to perform a given activity depends on the weight of the object to be lifted. Know your limits. Do not attempt to lift alone if you have any doubts about your ability to do so. Don't be a hero in a back brace. Obtain assistance for the sake of both the patient and yourself.

4. Other general tips for lifting are as follows (see Figure 42-7):
   • Lift with your legs. Keep legs in a position that permits them to supply most of the force for shifting your trunk.
   • Do not attempt to lift with your arms and back.
   • When lifting, avoid rotation of the spine. Shift your feet into a position that supports the patient's weight shift when moving or lifting the patient.
   • Stabilize your body against a stationary object whenever possible.
   • For best efficiency, coordinate the move by a synchronized verbal expression understood by therapists and patient, such as "one, two, three, lift."

One additional consideration must be noted—moving against the resistance of friction. Friction is defined as a force that opposes the movement of one object over the surface of another. Friction is reduced as the amount of surface-area contact between two objects is reduced.

When moving a patient side to side or up and down in bed, the therapist or nurse attempts to reduce the contact between the patient's body surface and the bed. This can be accomplished by several maneuvers: use of a turning sheet (placed just above the patient's shoulders to just below the patient's hips), crossing the patient's arms over his or her chest or abdomen, having the patient flex his or her knees and hips, and asking the patient to flex his or her neck and raise his or her head as he or she is lifted (if the patient is unable to do this, the therapist or nurse will assist) (Figure 42-8).

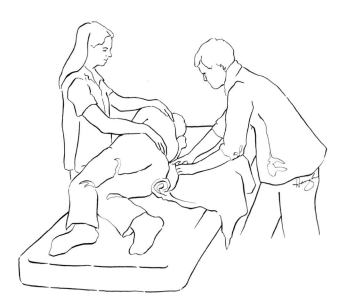

FIGURE 42-9 To insert the draw sheet, the patient is turned onto his or her side and the half-rolled draw sheet is tucked under the patient (from just above the shoulders to just below the hips). The patient rolls over the draw sheet and it is pulled out behind him or her.

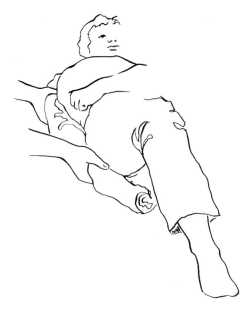

FIGURE 42-10 The draw sheet should be rolled close to the patient's body. A flexion hand grip at the patient's shoulders and hip is most efficient.

MOVING DEPENDENT PATIENTS

I. Moving the patient up or down (Roper, 1973; Lewis, 1976; Neil, 1976).
    A. Using a turning sheet (Figures 42-9 to 42-11).
        1. Sheet should cover the patient from shoulders to hips.
        2. Gather material as close to the patient's body as possible.

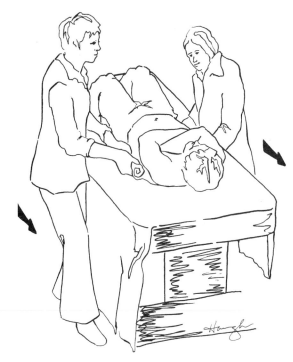

FIGURE 42-11 Moving the patient toward the head of the bed. The patient is prepared. The therapist is positioned to move toward the head of the bed in order to shift his or her body weight to move the patient.

        3. Hold at shoulders and hips, with a flexion pattern (see Figure 42-10).
        4. Cross patient's arms over his or her chest; flex knees and hips.
        5. Ask the patient to raise his or her head if possible.
        6. Synchronize action by counting "one, two, three, lift."
        7. Shift weight from one leg to the other rather than lifting up and pulling on back.
    B. Without a turning sheet (up or down), two people.
        1. Follow basic procedure: cross patient's arms, ask patient to lift head, flex knees and hips.
        2. The therapist places his or her hands and forearms under the patient's shoulders and hips.
        3. If patient is extremely heavy or tall, another person can bend knees and assist.
II. Moving the patient to the side of the bed.
    A. With turning sheet.
        1. Cross patient's arms, and other body parts, toward the side to which the patient is to be moved.
        2. Therapist places his or her hands at the patient's hips and shoulder on material close to the patient's body.
        3. One therapist pushes, the other pulls.
    B. Without turning sheet.
        1. Both therapists stand on the desired side.
        2. One therapist's forearms go under the patient's shoulder, the other's under the patient's hips.

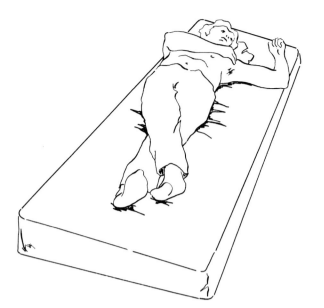

FIGURE 42-12 Preparation for the patient to turn onto his or her left side: move the patient to the right side of the bed, position his or her left arm up to the side at a 90-degree angle, cross the right leg and arm over his or her body and turn the patient's head to the left.

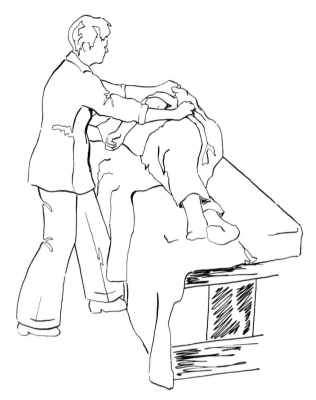

FIGURE 42-13 A one-person turn to the right side using a draw sheet. The patient's body position is the same as for the turn to the side. The therapist is positioned with one foot forward, the other back. The therapist pulls the sheet with his or her hands positioned at the hips and shoulders of the patient.

3. Synchronize action by counting "one, two, three, pull."

III. Turning the patient onto his or her side.
  A. With turning sheet (to right side) (Figures 42-12 and 42-13).
    1. Move the patient supine to the opposite side of the turn (e.g., if turning onto right side, move the patient to the left side of the bed).
    2. Bring the patient's right arm to the side at a 90-degree angle up and away from the body.
    3. Place the patient's left arm across the chest.
    4. Place the patient's left leg over the right leg.
    5. Pull the sheet at the patient's back to turn.
  B. Without turning sheet (to right side).
    1. Move patient to opposite side (therapist's hands and forearms under patient's shoulders and hips).
    2. Same steps as 2, 3, and 4 above.
    3. Roll patient to right side by pushing or pulling patient's left shoulder and left hip.
IV. Turning the patient prone (e.g., roll to right side) (Figure 42-14).
  A. With or without turning sheet.
    1. Move the patient to the opposite side of the bed from the side toward which he or she is turning.
    2. Cross the patient's left arm and left leg over the body.
    3. Tuck in patient's right hand and arm at the body side as close as possible.
    4. Push or pull on the patient's hips and shoulders to turn.

5. Free both arms; do not allow the patient to lie on the arm or hand.
6. A pillow may be placed under the patient's hips and lower legs to bend the knee and relieve back strain at the lumbar spine.

SUMMARY

Patient positioning and movement is a necessary and integral function of physical therapy. It is too often taken for granted and performed with little thought or planning. Therapists and nurses need to analyze their physical activities in relation to the principles of efficient movement and the proper application of body mechanics before they start to move a patient. A "tube index," counting and identifying each technical attachment (e.g., IV, Foley catheter, arterial blood gas stent, or chest tubes), should be taken before moving a patient. Extra care needs to be taken to prevent dislodging important medical equipment. This could prove life threatening if ventilator tubing is pulled and a patient is extubated. The practical application of body mechanics will not only conserve energy and preserve muscles and joints but will also allow the patient to be moved with a minimum amount of pain and discomfort, thereby providing greater safety for both the patient and health care team.

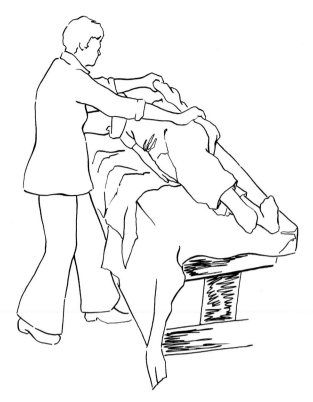

FIGURE 42-14 Positioning the patient prone (example: rolling to the right side). The patient's right arm is tucked in at his or her side with the left arm and leg crossed over.

Review Questions

1. How many staff will it take to position a patient who needs maximum assistance and is mechanically ventilated into a prone position? What are the determining factors?

2. How can changing a patient's position affect ventilation?

3. How can the therapist use towel rolls and easily accessible equipment to improve a patient's position and potential for improved ventilation?

4. What ventilation/perfusion changes occur when a patient is turned from the "affected" side down to the "unaffected" side down?

5. Can positioning alone be considered therapeutic (skilled) when it accomplishes the treatment goal?

6. How would positioning to reach a therapeutic goal be documented?

REFERENCES

Alexianu, D., et al. (2004). Severe hypotension in the prone position in a child with neurofibromatosis, scoliosis and pectus excavatum presention for posterior spinal fusion. Anesth Analg 98: 3334-3335.

Borello-France, D.P., Burdett, R.G., & Gee, Z.L. (1988). Modification of sitting posture of patients with hemiplegia using seat boards and backboards. Physical Therapy 68:68-71.

Crosbie, W.J., & Myles, S. (1985). An investigation into the effect of postural modification on some aspects of normal pulmonary function. Physiotherapy 7:311-314.

Fuerst, E., & Wolff, L. (1969). Fundamentals of nursing, ed 4. Philadelphia: J.B. Lippincott.

Gainnier, M., Michelet, P., Thirion, X., Arnal, J.M., Sainty, J.M., & Papazian, L. (2003). Prone position and positive end-expiratory pressure in acute respiratory distress syndrome. Critical Care Medicine 31:2719-2726.

Grenier, I.R., Bigsby, R., Vergara, E.R., & Lester, B.M. (2003). Comparison of motor self regulatory and stress behaviors of preterm infants across body positions. American Journal of Occupational Therapy 57:289-297.

Guerin, C., Gaillard, S., Lemasson, S., Ayzac, L., Girard, R., Beuret, P., Palmier, B., Le, Q.V., Sirodot, M., Rosselli, S., Cadiergue, V., Sainty, J.M., Barbe, P., Combourieu, E., Debatty, D., Rouffineau, J., Ezingeard, E., Millet, O., Guelon, D., Rodriguez, L., Martin, O., Renault, A., Sibille, J.P., & Kaidomar, M. (2004). Effects of systematic prone positioning in hypoxemic acute respiratory failure: a randomized controlled trial. Journal of the American Medical Association 292:2379-2387.

Harcombe, C.J. (2004). Nursing patients with ARDS in the prone position. Nursing Standard 18:33-39.

Hefti, K.S., Farnham, R.J., Docken, L., Bentaas, R., Bossman, S., & Schaefer, J. (2003). Back injury prevention: a lift team success story. AAOHN J 51:246-251.

Is there a right way to lift? (1985). Physical Therapy Forum 4:23.

Ishii, M., Matsuo, Y., et al. (2004). Optimizing forced vital capacity with shoulder positioning in a mechanically-ventilated patient with amyotrophic lateral sclerosis. Cardiopulmonary Physical Therapy Journal 15:12-16.

Johnson, G. (1989). Functional orthopedics I. San Ansellmo, Calif: Institute of Physical Art. Chicago: Course presentation June 8-11, 1989.

Karahan, A., & Bayraktar, N., (2004). Determination of the usage of body mechanics in clinical settings and the occurrence of low back pain in nurses. International Journal of Nursing Studies 41:67-74.

Kendall, F.P., McCreary, E.K., & Provance, P.G. (1993). Muscles testing and function. Baltimore: Williams & Wilkins.

Lewis, L. (1976). Fundamental skills in patient care. Philadelphia: J.B. Lippincott.

Massery, M., Dreyer, et al. (1997). Chest wall excursion and tidal volume change during passive positioning in cervical spinal cord injury [abstract]. Cardiopulmonary Physical Therapy 8:27.

Massery, M. (1994). What's positioning got to do with it? Neurology Report 18:11-14.

McConnell, E.A. (2002). Using proper body mechanics. Nursing 32:17.

Neil, C. (1959). Body management in nursing. Nursing Times 55:163.

Oczenski, W., Hormann, C., Keller, C., Lorenzl, N., Kepka, A., Schwarz, S. & Fitzgerald, R.D. (2005). Recruitment maneuvers during prone positioning in patients with acute respiratory distress syndrome. Critical Care Medicine 33:54-61.

Piedalue, F., Albert, R.K. (2003). Prone positioning in acute respiratory distress syndrome. Respiratory Care Clinics of North America 9:495-509.

Rantz, M., & Courtial, D. (1977). Lifting, moving and transferring patients: a manual. St. Louis, Mosby.

Rauch, B. (1971). Kinesiology and applied anatomy. Philadelphia: Lea & Febiger.

Reignier, J., Thenoz-Jost, N., Fiancette, M., Legendre, E., Lebert, C., Bontemps, F., Clementi, E., & Martin-Lefevre, L. (2004). Early enteral nutrition in mechanically ventilated patients in the prone position. Critical Care Medicine 32:94-99.

Roper, N. (1973). Principles of nursing, ed 2. New York: Churchill Livingstone.

Vollman, K.M. (2004). Prone positioning in the patient who has acute respiratory distress syndrome: the art and science. Critical Care Nursing Clinics of North America 16:319-336.

Woodhall-McNeal, A.P. (1992). Changes in posture and balance with age. Aging 4:219-225.

C H A P T E R 4 3

Respiratory Care Practice Review

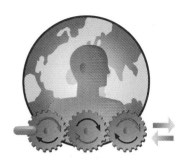

Donna Frownfelter and Michael Wade Baskin

KEY TERMS

Aerosol
Biphasic positive pressure ventilation
Continuous positive airway pressure
Humidity
Incentive spirometry

Mechanical ventilation
Noninvasive mechanical ventilation
Oxygen
Positive airway pressure

Proper care of the pulmonary patient involves a multidisciplinary approach, and all professionals involved should have a working knowledge of each individual profession's scope of care. As respiratory therapists, physical therapists, occupational therapists, and nurses apply their expertise in providing care for pulmonary patients, it becomes evident that coordinated teamwork is essential for optimal outcomes. The purpose of this chapter is to provide an overview of respiratory care principles and modalities frequently encountered in the various settings for other involved health care professionals. Interaction with the various modalities and pieces of equipment is also discussed. A knowledge and comfort level with respiratory therapy modalities and equipment will relieve anxiety and promote more effective interventions.

OXYGEN THERAPY

The atmosphere contains 20.95% oxygen, one of the most essential elements necessary to sustain human life. Oxygen exerts a partial pressure of 159.6 mm Hg at sea level (dry air) and approximately 97 mm Hg (Torr) in arterial blood. The normal range as measured by arterial blood gas analysis is 80 to 100 mm Hg (Torr). Under normal circumstances, this molecule travels from the atmosphere to the mitochondria at

the cellular level where it is used to produce ATP in a process called aerobic metabolism. The oxygen transport pathway involves the airways and lungs, heart and cardiovascular system, and the muscle tissue where the mitochondria reside. Any process that inhibits the transport of oxygen from the atmosphere to the cellular level can cause tissue hypoxemia, decreased function, and, ultimately, death.

When oxygen is prescribed it should be considered a drug. A particular dosage must be ordered by a set prescription. In general, a health care practitioner (i.e., a physical therapist) does not instruct a patient to increase or decrease a medication he or she is taking. In the same manner, an increase or decrease in oxygen intake must be discussed and orders changed by a physician. Some practices have standing orders that allow the health care team to change oxygen settings. For example, a prescription may be for one l/min of oxygen by nasal cannula at rest titrated up to four l/min to keep oxygen saturation above 90%.

Patients with cardiovascular and pulmonary impairments frequently need oxygen supplementation (AARC, 2002). Respiratory care practitioners and the nursing staff are generally responsible for administration of this drug under a physician's order. There are several different methods a therapist may choose to deliver oxygen in the most effective way, which will be discussed. Long-term oxygen therapy for patients with chronic obstructive pulmonary disease (COPD) who are hypoxemic has been found to improve quality of life and life expectancy (Web & Haas, 1998; Petty, 1999; Dunne, 2000; DesRosiers & Russo, 2000) .

The purpose of oxygen therapy is to treat and prevent hypoxemia, excessive work of breathing, and excessive myocardial work (Kacmarek et al, 1990). Although individual oxygen appliances offer suggested guidelines regarding oxygen administration, the only way to ensure effective delivery from a given device is by blood gas monitoring of PaO_2, partial pressure of oxygen in the arterial blood, or monitoring hemoglobin saturation by oximetry. Oxygen therapy is usually administered by one of two methods: low-flow or high-flow systems.

Low-Flow Systems

A low-flow oxygen system is one that is not intend to meet the total inspiratory requirements of the patient (does not deliver the entire inspired atmosphere to the patient). For example, using a normal minute ventilation (minute ventilation = tidal volume [TV] × respiratory rate [RR]) of eight l/min (500 CC × 16 breaths per minute) with a patient receiving one l/min of oxygen, the patient is breathing eight l/min but the device only provides one l/min. Thus seven l/min are coming from the room air and the device does not provide the entire inspired atmosphere to the patient. Every time the patient changes his or her breathing pattern, tidal volume and respiratory rate, the fraction of inspired oxygen (FIO_2) may change. Ideally, for efficient use of a nasal cannula, the patient should have a normal tidal volume, respiratory rate, and breathing pattern. This is often not the case, but the cannula is used as it is well tolerated by the patient. This method of oxygen delivery is not used when a specific concentration of oxygen is needed (Burton et al, 1991).

The nasal cannula (also called nasal prongs) is one of the most common low-flow devices encountered because of its low expense and high patient compliance (Figure 43-1). This device supplies approximately 24% and 40% oxygen with flow rates from one l/min to six l/min. Flow rates greater than six l/min can cause nasal mucosa irritation and drying. The approximate liter flow and resultant FIO_2 values are shown in Table 43-1.

Nasal cannulas deliver 100% oxygen; however, this percentage significantly lessens as the oxygen mixes with inspired air from the room. The amount of oxygen delivered depends on the flow rate and the ventilatory pattern of the patient. A larger minute volume (TV ∞ RR) would dilute the oxygen at any given flow rate and cause a greater decrease in the percentage delivered to the lungs. In other words, the faster and deeper a patient breathes, the more diluted the oxygen will become. On the other hand, if a patient has a low minute volume, the oxygen percentage delivered will increase (Kacmarek et al, 1990). If precise control of FIO_2 is needed, the nasal cannula should not be used (Bazuaye et al, 1992). In these cases a high-flow system (i.e., a venture mask) may be used.

Skin integrity, especially behind the ears, needs to be evaluated because the pressure of the cannula can cause skin breakdown.

Mouth breathing by patients on a nasal cannula typically causes concern from some of the health care team. This concern, however, may be unnecessary. If the nasal passages are unobstructed, then oxygen is able to collect in the oral and nasal cavity (anatomical reservoir). On inspiration, the oxygen collected in this area is drawn into the airways and lungs. If a patient with a nasal cannula is mouth breathing, the practitioner should ensure the nasal passages are unobstructed. If there is concern that the patient is not receiving adequate oxygen, a blood gas or oxygen saturation measurement should be obtained. If this is not feasible, or if the patient is unable to breathe through the nose, it may be appropriate to switch the patient to a mask.

The patient should be encouraged to breathe through the nose to receive maximum benefit from the nasal cannula; however, mouth breathing does not mean the patient will not receive appropriate oxygen (Dunlevy & Tyl, 1992). Clinically it is found that some patients who mouth breathe do so

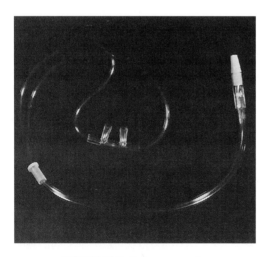

FIGURE 43-1 Oxygen cannula.

TABLE 43-1	
Approximate Liter Flow and Resultant FIO_2 Values	
FLOW (L/MIN)	**FIO_2 (%)**
1	24
2	28
3	32
4	36
5	40
6	44

Adapted from the American College of Sports Medicine. (2000). Guidelines for exercise testing and prescription, ed 6. Philadelphia: Lippincott, Williams & Wilkins.

because of nasal polyps, sinus congestion, deviated septum, or other physical issues. If the work of breathing is increased when the patient tries to breathe through the nose, it may be counterproductive.

The simple mask, or open-face mask, is another low-flow oxygen delivery device commonly used. It can deliver from 40% to 60% oxygen, depending on the flow rate and the patient's ventilatory pattern. This device requires a flow rate of five to six l/min to prevent rebreathing and excessive respiratory work (Jensen et al, 1991). As with the nasal cannula, this type of oxygen delivery method should not be used if precise control of oxygen concentration (FIO_2) is required.

The partial rebreathing mask is basically a mask with a reservoir bag attached. The oxygen source supplies the bag with 100% oxygen where it mixes with exhaled anatomical dead-space air that has not taken place in gas exchange. This exhaled air is rich in oxygen. The exhaled air that has taken place in gas exchange and contains CO_2 is vented through the open ports on each side of the mask. This mask can deliver oxygen concentrations from 70% to greater than 80%, and it requires flows between seven and 10 l/min to keep the bag from fully collapsing during inspiration (Kacmarek et al, 1990).

The nonrebreathing mask is another low-flow delivery device that also contains a bag reservoir, but it can deliver up to 100% oxygen. This mask contains valves at the reservoir bag and the side vents to prevent ambient air mixing on inspiration and exhaled air mixing on expiration. For this mask to operate effectively, a good seal between the patient's face and the mask must be achieved. The bag should partially deflate during inspiration (Figure 43-2).

Another form of low-flow oxygen delivery is the transtracheal oxygen catheter. This has been used in pediatric patients as well as the adult population (Christopher, 2003; Preciado, 2002). It is surgically placed into the trachea via a small incision between the second and third tracheal rings. Generally these devices are seen in home-oxygen patients. Transtracheal oxygen catheters are more efficient than nasal cannulas, and they have a high patient acceptance rate with low complications (Christopher et al, 1987). Because the oxygen is administered directly into the trachea, 50% less oxygen is needed (Kacmarek et al, 1990). For people who use portable oxygen systems and for those who require high oxygen flow rates, tracheal oxygen catheters may be beneficial (Jackson et al, 1992). The catheter can be covered by the patient's clothing and is therefore cosmetically appealing. Complications such as plugging of the catheter and subcutaneous emphysema have been reported (Veen et al, 1996; Rothe et al, 1996).

HIGH-FLOW SYSTEMS

A high-flow oxygen delivery system is that which delivers a specific oxygen concentration despite the patient's ventilatory pattern. It does deliver the entire inspired atmosphere to the patient. Everything the patient breathes comes from the device. If it is found that a patient requires oxygen delivered at an FIO_2 of 50% to keep the oxygen saturation at a safe level, then a high-flow system would be the method of choice. If a patient has CO_2 retention and a hypoxic drive to breathe, a high-flow system with an exact FIO_2 can be used. This is often the case when a patient with COPD who is a CO_2 retainer gets pneumonia and goes into respiratory failure. The physician wants to give adequate oxygen but hopefully will not have to place the patient on a mechanical ventilator. A high flow system in this acute care setting will be optimal. Patient tolerance of the ventimask is often less than optimal. A patient who is acutely ill and very dyspneic may tolerate the mask, but as the patient feels better, he or she may feel claustrophobic from the mask covering his or her face and the high flow of gas.

The Venturi mask is a common method of delivering high-flow oxygen concentrations from 24% to 50%. This mask operates via the Venturi principle, which provides for a mixing of 100% oxygen and entrained ambient air. The oxygen flows though a narrow orifice at a high velocity, causing a sub-atmospheric pressure. This drop in pressure is what causes the ambient air to be entrained through a port. The size of the port determines the amount of air that is entrained and thus the percentage of oxygen delivered. The Venturi mask has a rotating air entrainment port that allows the health care provider to "dial in" the desired FIO_2 (Figure 43-3). Flow rates of 40 to 80+ l/min provide minute ventilation at rates that are higher than those the patient could attain without the aid of the mask. Consequently, no matter what the respiratory rate, tidal volume, or breathing pattern, the oxygen delivery will be consistent.

Mechanical aerosol systems also operate via air entrainment, but the mask is connected to the aerosol unit by large-bore tubing to allow a specific FIO_2 to be delivered with high humidity (Figure 43-4). Although drainage bags are usually

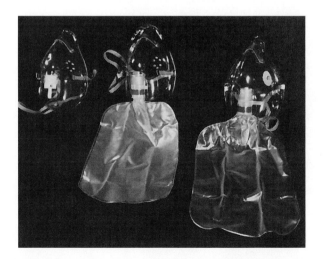

FIGURE 43-2 From left to right: mask without bag, partial rebreathing bag, nonbreathing bag. Note the valves on the mask and at the junction between the mask and bag.

attached to the tubing to collect condensation, the tubing must be monitored for possible pooling of water, which causes flow obstruction to the patient. If partial obstruction occurs, a mild back pressure results in the tubing, causing less air entrainment. This means that a higher concentration of oxygen will result, and a higher dosage of oxygen than desired may be delivered to the patient.

PORTABLE OXYGEN

As health care continues to move out of the hospital setting and into the home, more health care practitioners will be providing care to patients who require oxygen in their homes. Oxygen is most commonly delivered in the home for those

patients needing long-term oxygen, usually COPD patients who are hypoxemic. Generally one to two l/min is prescribed via nasal cannula, but the flow rate will depend on the patient's need.

Home oxygen-delivery systems can be divided into three categories: high-pressure oxygen cylinders, low-pressure liquid oxygen (Kampelmacher et al, 1998), and oxygen concentrators (Burton et al, 1991). Additional options include continuous flow versus demand or pulsed oxygen delivery (Tiep et al, 2002; Garrod et al, 1999; Johann et al, 2001). There are also a variety of oxygen conserving devices (McCoy, 2000). When a continuous system is changed to either a demand or pulsed system, or when a new oxygen conserving device is started, the patient must be monitored carefully. Clinical experience has shown that some patients may not tolerate the same liter flow with a pulsed system, and oximetry and perceived exertion must be evaluated when there is any change in oxygen delivery.

High-pressure oxygen tanks come in various sizes. The larger ones, such as the H and K sizes, are used as a base unit or reservoir. Long oxygen tubing connected to these tanks allows for patient mobility. Smaller tanks are used for portability and can provide up to three hours of use. They can be refilled by transferring gas from the larger reservoir tank.

Liquid oxygen is a low-pressure oxygen delivery method, and it tends to be more convenient than using the high-pressure tanks, especially for the active oxygen patient. The canisters are lightweight and allow patients to be away from the home reservoir for up to eight hours. The down side is that liquid oxygen costs more, and the reservoirs need to be filled up to twice a week with continuous use. If high flows are needed, these units are not recommended.

Oxygen concentrators are commonly seen in the home health setting, especially because Medicare offers coverage

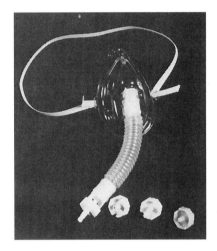

FIGURE 43-3 Venturi mask.

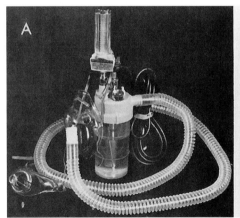
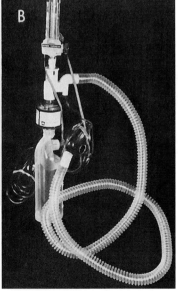

FIGURE 43-4 **A,** Heated aerosol. **B,** Nebulizers.

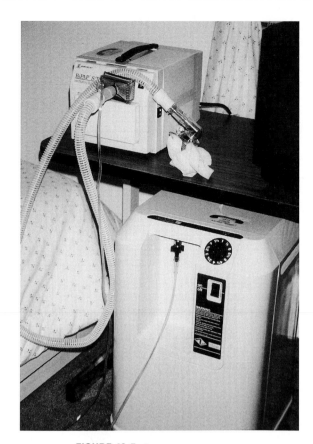

FIGURE 43-5 Oxygen concentrator.

for these devices (Figure 43-5). They generally tend to be expensive initially but are actually less expensive for long-term use. They are electrically powered and create oxygen by drawing ambient air across a semipermeable membrane, separating oxygen from nitrogen. They generally operate at two l/min and provide 90% oxygen. Long oxygen tubing, up to 50 feet, allows patients extra mobility. Patients using concentrators should have a back-up device, such as a portable tank, in case of a power outage.

CONTINUOUS (CONSTANT) POSITIVE PRESSURE BREATHING

Continuous positive airway pressure (CPAP) is oxygen delivered with pressure above atmospheric pressure. Whereas normally during the respiratory cycle there is a negative pressure during inspiration, the pressure curve in CPAP is always above atmospheric pressure (positive pressure) on the airways.

CPAP may be used to improve oxygenation (Squadrone, 2005; AARC, 2004) for patients in whom the usual means of oxygen delivery are not effective and patients with obstructive sleep apnea (Skinner et al, 2004), and it has been used to help the transition of weaning from mechanical ventilation (Halliday, 2004). An elevated head of the bed posture has also been shown to be a good second line treatment for obstructive sleep apnea (Skinner et al, 2004). In addition, CPAP has been

shown to help infants after cardiac surgery to more smoothly stabilize during weaning from a ventilator and resume a better spontaneous breathing pattern (Imanaka et al, 2004), and it has been useful in the management of respiratory distress in premature babies and decreases the need for invasive mechanical ventilation (Upadhyay, 2004). Early intervention using CPAP in elderly patients with cardiogenic pulmonary edema has also been effective (L'Her et al, 2004).

Quality of life predictors have been shown to be positive a year after initiation of CPAP: improvement was noted at three months after initiation of CPAP and continued at one year (Lloberes et al, 2004; Buttner & Ruhle, 2004).

A concern for compliance and effectiveness of CPAP is noted in patients who are mouth breathers. Those with moderate to severe sleep disordered breathing were found to be less adherent to CPAP therapy than those who are nose breathers. This is related to a leak that compromises the CPAP (Bachour et al, 2004).

USE OF OXYGEN TO IMPROVE EXERCISE

Oxygen has been shown to increase exercise performance in patients with COPD who have moderate to severe airflow obstruction and mild hypoxemia at rest (Fujimoto et al, 2002; Snider, 2002; Brusasco & Pellegrino, 2003). It has also been shown to benefit patients with COPD who are nonhypoxemic at rest (Emtner et al, 2003; Jolly et al, 2001). Breathlessness is the most common symptom that limits exercise tolerance. Oxygen supplementation often will give an increased driving pressure of oxygen, which allows the patient to decrease the work of breathing (AARC, 2001). Peripheral muscle weakness has been found in many patients with COPD. Improving exercise tolerance will result in improved muscle strength and endurance. Another consideration is that, if hyperoxia is not enough, the use of noninvasive positive pressure (NPPV) may be beneficial. This is still somewhat controversial and requires more study, but in this author's clinical opinion it can be very beneficial (Ambrosino & Strambi, 2004).

RESPIRATORY MODALITIES

Incentive Spirometry

Incentive spirometry (IS), also called sustained maximum inspiration (SMI), is simply a visual and/or audio feedback device that encourages slow, deep inspiration (Figure 43-6). Generally this treatment is performed frequently, up to every hour, and its purpose is to treat and prevent atelectasis and pneumonia, especially in postoperative patients who are considered a high risk for postoperative complications (AARC, 1991; Lezon, 1999; Pullen, 2003; Hall,1996; King, 2000). In many acute care settings, IS is done routinely. Several articles challenge the routine use of IS and have found that the addition of IS added no benefit to breathing exercise postoperatively (Weiner et al, 1997; Crowe & Bradley, 1997; Gosselink et al, 2000; Overend et al, 2001). In a study of

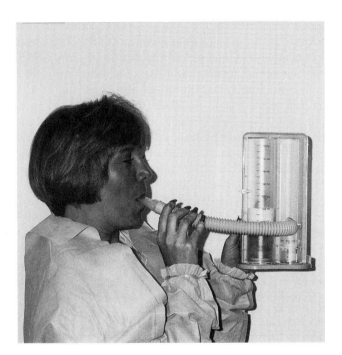

FIGURE 43-6 Incentive spirometry device in use.

patients pre-lung resection, when a combination of inspiratory muscle training and IS was performed before and after lung resection, there were significant lung function improvements in FEV1 that were higher postoperatively than preoperatively (Weiner et al, 1997).

There may be potential benefits to using IS with patients with neuromuscular and musculoskeletal impairments as well. They often demonstrate a decreased vital capacity and decreased chest wall mobility. IS devices encourages deep breathing and a sustained inspiration. During the sustained inspiration, collateral ventilation can occur as areas of the lung that are well ventilated equilibrate with areas that are poorly ventilated. This is an area for future research, perhaps combining inspiratory muscle training and IS.

There are many commercially available incentive spirometers. Some are focused on volume, others on flow rates. Regardless of the type, the importance of patients using them should be stressed. Patients with COPD may have these prescribed when they are undergoing surgical procedures. Care must be taken not to have them continue to use them when the acute episode is over. These patients have air trapping and should not continue IS long term.

HUMIDITY AND AEROSOL THERAPY

Humidity Therapy

Under normal circumstances, when inhalation takes place, air becomes 100% saturated with water vapor before entering the lower airway tracts below the carina. This humidification process is important to mucous production, ciliary activity, and a healthy respiratory tract. When this normal humidification

process is interfered with, such as in patients with endotracheal or tracheostomy tubes, other methods of adding moisture to the respiratory system must be employed.

Humidification is the addition of water vapor in its molecular form to a gas. When a dry gas is administered to a patient (e.g., via a nasal cannula), some type of humidification appliance is used to prevent unnecessary complications. Flows of two l/min or less may not require humidification when using a nasal cannula. Humidification therapy is also indicated in the presence of thick tenacious secretions and when an artificial airway is in place. Artificial airways, such as endotracheal and tracheostomy tubes, bypass the normal humidification system (the upper airway); therefore, supplementation is essential (Frownfelter, 1987).

There are basically two types of humidifiers. Bubble-through humidifiers are those that are generally used with simple oxygen appliances. The pass-over type of humidifier is usually found in conjunction with a mechanical ventilator. Both bubble-through and pass-over humidifiers are available for ventilators (AARC, 1992), and they are usually heated to warm the humidified air to body temperature before it enters the airway (Kacmarek et al, 1990).

Aerosol Therapy

An aerosol is created when a suspension of liquid or solid particles exists in a gas. Two common forms of medication aerosol delivery in the clinical setting are the small-volume nebulizer (SVN) and the metered-dose inhaler (MDI). A bland aerosol is administration of water or saline solution to the patient's lungs (AARC, 2003).

In general the goals of aerosol therapy are to hydrate dried retained secretions, to improve cough efficiency, to restore and maintain function of the mucociliary elevator, to deliver medications, and to humidify gases delivered through artificial airways. The MDI is strictly used for medication delivery (see Chapter 45).

Other forms of aerosol delivery are the spinning disk (such as in a room humidifier or mist tent) and the ultrasonic nebulizer. Both of these are electrically powered as opposed to the SVN, which is pneumatically powered (Figure 43-7) (Branson & Seger, 1988).

A key element in aerosol delivery is particle size. The size of the aerosol particle will determine its ability to penetrate the airway before depositing or raining out. The therapeutic range is considered one μ, with the smaller range of particles having the greatest penetrating ability. The larger particles deposit sooner. If they are greater than five μ then the chances of entry into the airway are less. The particles may deposit in the nose and proximal airway. The greatest amount of alveolar deposition (95% to 100%) occurs in the one to two μ range. On the other hand, aerosol particles smaller than one μ are so stable that they may not deposit at all (Kacmarek et al, 1990).

Although particle size is important in determining appropriate deposition, a patient's ventilatory pattern is probably more important in that it is the more variable and controllable of the two. Gravity also plays a factor, and it too can be used to benefit particle deposition. Patients should be sitting up as much as possible while taking slow, deep breaths with a short three- to four-second inspiratory hold. Mouth breathing is encouraged if aerosol therapy is delivered by mask. Nasal breathing may filter out particles of optimal size. Not all patients will be able to achieve this position and ventilatory pattern, and the therapist must modify accordingly.

Comparisons between the ability of SVNs and MDIs to deliver medications have found that the MDI is either equal in efficacy or outperforms nebulizers. Significant cost savings are also realized by those institutions that recognize MDI usage as an effective means of aerosol medication delivery over SVN (Orens et al, 1991).

To further enhance the efficacy of the MDI treatment, a spacer or holding chamber may be attached to trap the aerosol particles before inhalation. This device allows greater drug particle deposition to the airways and reduces oropharyngeal

deposition (Ashworth et al, 1991). Ventilator patients who are receiving drug aerosol therapy also receive greater benefit from an in-line MDI with a holding chamber compared with a jet nebulizer (Fuller et al, 1990).

Aerosol-Therapy Precautions

It should be mentioned that there are hazards associated with aerosol therapy. Bronchospasm may occur as the smooth muscles of the bronchial passages react to foreign particles entering the lung. Shortness of breath and respiratory distress may also occur as a result of dried retained secretions swelling and occluding portions of the lung. Cross contamination is a concern in that aerosol devices may harbor organisms that can be transmitted to patients. Frequent equipment changes and proper sterilization and cleaning techniques are key in preventing this occurrence.

Intermittent Positive Pressure Breathing

Intermittent positive pressure breathing (IPPB) continues to be used in some settings, but there is little evidence to supports its efficacy as a treatment modality (AARC, 2003).

This particular technology was developed during World War II to assist pilots breathing in unpressurized cabins at high altitudes. IPPB subsequently became a very popular respiratory therapy device in the 1960s and 1970s (Figure 43-8). Its use began to decline in the 1980s. In 1983 the National Heart, Lung, and Blood Institute reported that IPPB has limited therapeutic benefit. This clinical trial is only one of several studies that show IPPB is an outmoded medical technology. Research dating back to the 1950s questions the efficacy of this device (Duffy & Farley, 1992).

The purpose of the IPPB machine is to increase alveolar ventilation, improve the ventilation-perfusion ratio, mobilize and facilitate expectoration of thick secretions, decrease the work of breathing, and deliver aerosolized medications. It is a pressure-cycled ventilator that, when triggered by a patient's inhalation, delivers ambient air or oxygen to the patient until

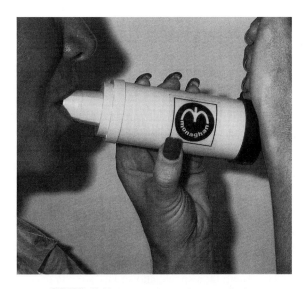

FIGURE 43-7 Commonly used spacer device.

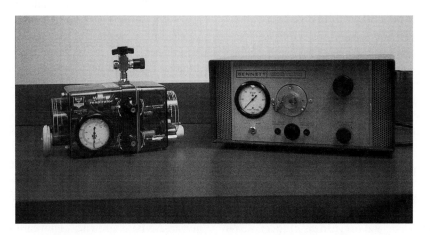

FIGURE 43-8 Left to right: Bird Mark machine, Bennett AP-5 IPPB machine.

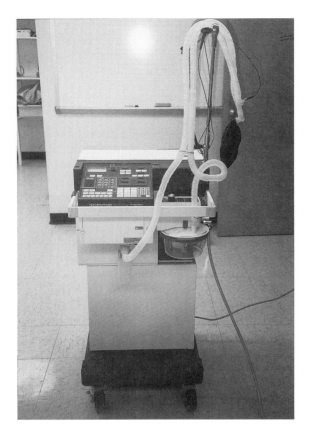

FIGURE 43-9 Puritan Bennett 7200a microprocessor driven ventilator.

a preset pressure is reached. It is basically a lung expansion device that helps deliver an increased tidal volume. IPPB is used for a variety of pulmonary conditions, and treatment sessions usually last 10 to 15 minutes.

The modality of IPPB comes into question in the clinical setting because it has not been shown to provide benefits over that of other simpler respiratory treatment methods. It also introduces potential complications and hazards that the other treatments do not. Typically IPPB has been used to treat asthma, COPD, and postoperative atelectasis; however, other therapies, such as IS, postural drainage, and aerosol therapy, tend to prevail as the treatment of choice over IPPB.

Although IPPB is questionable in regards to its clinical efficacy, it may be a beneficial form of treatment in acute asthma or COPD that is refractory to standard therapy, atelectasis that has not responded to simpler therapy, and the prevention of respiratory failure in patients with kyphoscoliosis and neuromuscular disorders (Handelsman, 1991).

MECHANICAL VENTILATION

Many disease states that lead to cardiac and/or respiratory failure will require mechanical ventilation to support the patient's effort to ventilate and oxygenate (Figure 43-9). Patients receiving mechanical ventilator support can be found in many settings, from the acute care hospital to skilled nursing facilities and home care. Children who live in the home and community need to be integrated into the school system and community recreational facilities. Acute exacerbations of disorders such as emphysema, COPD, and chronic bronchitis may require mechanical ventilation and are generally seen in hospital intensive care units. Disorders requiring long-term ventilation, such as spinal cord injury, brain injury, and certain neuromusculoskeletal diseases, may be found receiving mechanical ventilation in rehabilitation hospitals, the home, or a long-term care facility.

Mechanical ventilator assistance is provided primarily by machines that deliver preset volume and positive pressure breaths to the patient. Positive pressure ventilation is the opposite of normal physiological ventilation in that normal ventilation occurs when negative pressure, created by contraction of the diaphragm, causes air to enter the lungs. Whereas normal inspiration occurs by pulling air into the lungs, ventilators push air into the lungs (positive pressure). This is important because the thoracic cavity becomes an area of higher pressure, which may create adverse cardiovascular and hemodynamic events. Monitoring of heart rate and blood pressure is vital when patients are placed on a mechanical ventilator to make sure there is not cardiovascular compromise with increases in pressure.

Invasive Versus Noninvasive Mechanical Ventilation

Invasive mechanical ventilation involves the insertion of an artificial airway into the trachea that attaches to ventilator tubing. Noninvasive mechanical ventilation (NIV) is delivered by a nasal or facial mask that attaches to a positive airway pressure BIPAP machine. Noninvasive mechanical ventilation is growing in use. It has been used primarily for patients with acute hypercapnic ventilatory failure, especially for acute exacerbations of COPD. Benefits of NIV include a reduction in the need for intubation, a decrease in complication rate, and a reduced length of hospitalization. One factor in the success of NIV is the early delivery of ventilation in patients with respiratory failure (Brochard, 2003).

In a study involving medical-surgical intensive care units in North American, South America, Spain, and Portugal, 1,638 patients were studied who were receiving mechanical ventilation. The median age of the study patients was 61 years. Indications for mechanical ventilation were acute respiratory failure (66%), acute exacerbation of COPD (14%), coma (10%), and neuromuscular disorders (10%). Mechanical ventilation was administered via endotracheal tube in 75%, tracheostomy tube in 24%, and facial mask in 1% of patients. A total of 47% of patients were ventilated on an assist-control mode and 46% were ventilated with synchronized intermittent mandatory ventilation (SIMV), pressure support, or a combination of both modes (Esteban et al, 2000). In North America it seems that, clinically, the trend towards NIV is growing significantly (Antonelli et al, 2003; Wysocki & Antonelli, 2001; Abreu, 2000).

Patients with chest wall restriction such as severe kyphoscoliosis also benefit from NIV. Ventilation and oxygenation go hand in hand. If the chest wall is not moving, ventilation is decreased. Just giving oxygen to patients with severe thoracic restriction will not bring them to optimal respiratory function. The NIV provides improved ventilation that will improve patient function and endurance (Schonhofer et al, 2001).

BIPAP is a noninvasive form of ventilation that uses a tightly fitted nasal mask that delivers positive pressure at two different levels, one for inspiration and another for exhalation, both of which are above atmospheric pressure. It may also be referred to as pressure release ventilation. Indications for BIPAP include signs of respiratory failure or chronic respiratory failure in patients with severe COPD, increased work of breathing, patients with neuromusculoskeletal impairments that limit ventilation and thus oxygenation, and sleep disordered breathing. Use of BIPAP has improved outcomes in terms of less daytime fatigue and improved activity levels. In addition, it may be used as a bridge for patients such as those at the end stage of cystic fibrosis who need lung transplants (Padman et al, 1992; Hill et al, 1995).

It is important to assess skin integrity because the pressure from the strap on the face and around the head can cause skin breakdown. This is an important consideration to discuss with the patient.

Modes of Mechanical Ventilation

The physician and respiratory therapist have a wide variety of choices from which to select the most appropriate method of ventilation for a given patient. Terms defining properties of mechanical ventilation can be confusing. Choosing the appropriate mode of ventilation is at times considered more of an art than a science. There are basic fundamental starting points for mechanical ventilation, then the variable modes are adjusted to optimize each individual patient's needs. Before describing the modes of ventilation, the following terms are defined.

1. Trigger—Variable that causes a breath to be delivered by the ventilator. A patient may inhale, causing the ventilator circuit pressure to drop to a preset number (i.e., less than one or two cm H_2O). This is called a pressure trigger. Some ventilators are volume and flow triggered.
2. Flowrate—The speed at which the ventilator breath is delivered. This parameter is usually measured in liters per minute.
3. Frequency—Refers to the number of breaths delivered over time (e.g., 10 breaths per minute).
4. Spontaneous breath—Breathing through the ventilator circuit without assistance.

The following are descriptions of common current ventilator modes.

- Controlled mechanical ventilation (CMV)—The control mode is a lesser used method of ventilation and generally requires the patient to be sedated and paralyzed. The ventilator delivers all breaths at a preset frequency, volume or pressure, and flow rate. The patient cannot take spontaneous breaths or trigger the machine.
- Assist control (AC)—The patient receives a preset pressure or volume, frequency or number of breaths, and flow rate. In between machine-cycled breaths, the patient can trigger the machine to deliver another breath at the preset parameters. All breaths are machine delivered. No spontaneous breathing can occur.
- Assisted mechanical ventilation—This mode is similar to AC, however, there is no set frequency. The patient triggers the machine at will to deliver a set pressure or volume at a set flow rate.
- Intermittent mandatory ventilation (IMV)—As the ventilator delivers a set mandatory frequency and volume or pressure, the patient is allowed to take spontaneous breaths between cycles. This is a former popular mode.
- SIMV—This mode improves on that of IMV in that it synchronizes the machine-delivered breaths with the patient's spontaneous breaths. In IMV the machine may cycle a breath before the patient can completely exhale a spontaneous breath. If no inspiratory effort is present, the machine delivers the mandatory breaths.
- CPAP—The patient spontaneously breathes and a preset level of pressure is constantly maintained. This method of ventilation can also be achieved through use of commercially available pneumatically powered units that hook directly into the oxygen wall outlet. A tight fitting mask is secured around the patient's mouth and nose, and a preset pressure and oxygen percentage is delivered.
- BIPAP—A noninvasive form of mechanical ventilation usually delivered through a tight fitting nasal mask. There are different pressures for inspiration and exhalation, which are always above atmospheric levels.
- Airway pressure release ventilation (APRV)—This may also be called pressure release ventilation. The patient is allowed to spontaneously breathe with a set amount of CPAP. If additional ventilation is required, the CPAP will be dropped periodically, releasing the pressure, causing the patient to exhale. When the exhalation is complete, CPAP is restored. Proponents of this mode claim that by allowing the patient control, patient comfort and compliance are high.
- Pressure support ventilation (PSV)—When using pressure support the patient is allowed to breathe spontaneously and he or she receives a preset amount of inspiratory support until the flow rate reaches a minimal level. The patient controls the frequency, tidal volume, and inspiratory time. This mode is often used in conjunction with SIMV. This mode is also popular due to high patient compliance.
- Mandatory minute ventilation (MMV)—The patient is allowed to breathe spontaneously; however, a minimal level of minute ventilation will be achieved through ventilator-assisted breaths. This is usually accomplished by using PSV.
- Volume-assured pressure support (VAPS)—This is one of the newest modes of ventilation. It allows the patient to

breathe spontaneously in the PSV mode and monitors each breath's tidal volume. If the breath is not going to reach the set volume, the ventilator will hold the flow rate constant and increase the pressure until the desired volume is reached (Branson & Chatburn, 1992).

Alarm Management and Precautions

When working with patients on mechanical ventilators, it is inevitable that alarms will sound. Alarms are important indicators of a change in patient condition or a machine malfunction. All alarms should be recognized and valued as excellent sources of information. If alarms are silenced or ignored without interpretation, patient fatalities may result. Alarms should not be turned off. When therapy is being delivered, the alarms are a valuable tool. The therapist, however, needs to realize they are treating the patient, not the machine. If an alarm sounds during a therapy treatment, stop the intervention and wait a few seconds to see if the alarm stops. Evaluate which alarm went off and why before continuing therapy. If it is not clear why the alarm sounded, contact the respiratory care practitioner or the patient's nurse.

The most common alarms are those that monitor high and low pressure, FIO_2, apnea, disconnection, and volume. The high pressure alarm is the one that sounds most commonly when the patient is receiving physical therapy. Generally, if the high-pressure alarm continues to sound, the patient should be checked for secretions. Suctioning can remedy this problem. The ventilator tubing should also be checked for possible occlusion from compression or excessive water buildup (Figure 43-10). Other reasons for high pressure alarms to sound are bronchospasm or breath holding. Do not use strong resistance exercise with patients on mechanical ventilation because they may hold their breath and perform a Valsalva maneuver, which will cause increased circuit pressure to deliver the tidal volume to the patient. Low pressure may signify a leak in the ventilator circuitry or a disconnection from the machine. Before turning a patient or performing upper extremity exercise, make sure there is clearance and ease of movement in the ventilator circuit tubing to prevent it from coming off during the interventions. In one case (in an unnamed medical center's intensive care unit) a patient's low pressure alarm sounded and the patient was bagged while the cause was evaluated. The source was a disconnect that occurred when a housekeeping person had unplugged the ventilator to use the plug for a cleaning machine. When the low pressure alarm sounds, first consider that the patient is not being ventilated.

If you are unfamiliar with a particular ventilator and an alarm sounds that you are unable to identify and/or remedy, first ensure the patient is not in any extra distress. Assess the overall appearance of the patient and, most importantly, the rise and fall of the patient's chest as the ventilator cycles. If the patient does not appear to be receiving breaths, immediate action should be taken to remove the ventilator from the patient and begin manual ventilation with a self-inflating bag.

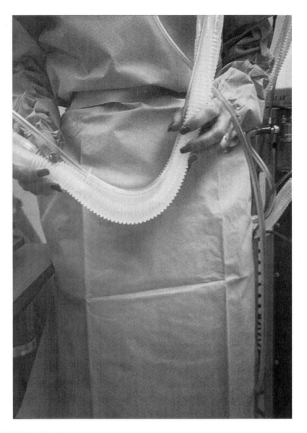

FIGURE 43-10 Condensation build-up in ventilator tubing—a potential hazard.

The respiratory care practitioner should be called to rectify the situation. When the problem is resolved, the patient should be returned to the mechanical ventilator.

Another significant precaution to take when working with a patient on a ventilator is to watch for condensation in the tubing that could accidentally be poured directly into the patient's lungs, especially during turning. When moving a ventilator patient, plan ahead by securing all lines, wires, and tubing. Follow the appropriate procedure for emptying any water from the ventilator tubing before moving the patient. Aspiration of water from ventilator tubing can be fatal.

Weaning from Mechanical Ventilation

Weaning is generally initiated when the reason for placing the patient on mechanical ventilation is reversed. Several factors need to be evaluated. Is there adequate oxygenation? During weaning the work required by the patient to breathe may increase and oxygen may need to be titrated appropriately. Hemodynamic stability must be monitored. Using CPAP during weaning may provide the bridge necessary to wean with less stress and decreased ventilatory demand. In general in patients who are receiving mechanical ventilation, the ventilator is discontinued and then the artificial airway is evaluated and removed. In some patients with neuromuscular and musculoskeletal issues, however, ventilator weaning by lung expansion with NIV and decannulation will be a better solution (Bach & Goncalves, 2004). Some patients with neuromusculoskeletal concerns may use other mechanical means of ventilation such as a pneumobelt (Ayoub, 2002). This is a noninvasive devices placed over the abdomen. There is a bladder that inflates and mechanically puts pressure on the abdomen thereby causing exhalation. When the bladder deflates the diaphragm descends and inspiration occurs. There are other negative pressure devices that also help patients with neurological deficits, such as a chest curaiss, which resembles a turtle shell placed over the chest wall. Negative pressure is applied to the chest wall, which elevates the thorax to provide inspiration, then releases to allow for exhalation. The benefits of these mechanical aids are that the patient does not need an artificial airway and he or she is provided with a more physiological means of ventilation. They are well received by many people with neurological impairments.

ROLE OF THE PHYSICAL THERAPIST

The physical therapist can have a significant role in keeping the patient who is mechanically ventilated from having decreased aerobic capacity by helping the patients perform aggressive mobilization (see Chapters 18 and 19), exercise, and breathing strategies and interventions (see Chapters 20, 21, 22, and 23). The physical therapist can also play a role in finding optimal positions to support the patient when being weaned. Therapists who have been working on breathing strategies can be a source of comfort and encouragement during the weaning periods. Active mobilization early on in the course of mechanical ventilation will result in more successful outcomes.

SUMMARY

Physical therapists need to understand the basic equipment and principles of respiratory care in order to optimize the functional outcomes of their patients. The team approach is vital in acutely ill patients. Working in collaboration with respiratory care practitioners and nurses will maximize interventions and improve patient outcomes.

Review Questions

1. Why does a high flow system provide the most accurate oxygen delivery?
2. What circumstances will drive the physician to order a low-flow system when a high-flow system would be optimal?
3. Why do low-flow oxygen masks require a certain minimum liter flow (i.e., five to 10 l/min for a simple mask)?
4. How does oxygen improve exercise performance?
5. Which ventilator monitor would alert the therapist that the patient has become disconnected from the machine?
6. Which circumstances would cause the high pressure alarm to sound on a patient who is mechanically ventilated?
7. What precautions should a physical therapist use when exercising a patient who is on a mechanical ventilator?
8. What is the role of the physical therapist in the health care team that case for patients who are mechanically ventilated?

REFERENCES

AARC Clinical Practice Guidelines. (1991). Incentive spirometry. Respiratory Care 36:1402-1403.

AARC Clinical Practice Guidelines. (1992). Humidification during mechanical ventilation. Respiratory Care 37:887-890.

AARC Clinical Practice Guidelines. (2001). Exercise testing for evaluation of hypoxemia and/or desaturation. Respiratory Care 46:514-522.

AARC Clinical Practice Guidelines. (2002). Oxygen therapy for adults in the acute care facility. Respiratory Care 46:717-720.

Ambrosino, N., Strambi, S., (2004). New strategies to improve exercise tolerance in chronic obstructive pulmonary disease. European Respiratory Journal 24:313-322.

Antonelli, M., Pennisi, M.A., & Conti, G. (2003). New advances in the use of noninvasive ventilation for acute hypoxaemic respiratory failure. European Respiratory Journal 22(Suppl 42):65s-71s.

Ashworth, H.L., Wilson, C.G., Sims, E.E., Wotton, P.K., & Hardy, J.G. (1991). Delivery of propellant soluble drug from a metered dose inhaler. Thorax 46:245-247.

Bach, J.R., & Goncalves, M. (2004). Ventilator weaning by lung expansion and decannulation. American Journal of Physical and Medical Rehabilitation 83:560-568.

Bachour, A., & Maasilta, P. (2004). Mouth breathing compromises adherence to nasal continuous positive airway pressure therapy. Chest 126:1248-1254.

Barbarash, R.A., Smith, L.A., Godwin, J.E., & Sahn, S.A. (1990). Mechanical ventilation. DICP, The Annals of Pharmacotherapy 24:959-970.

Bazuaye, E.A., Stone, T.N., Corris, P.A., & Gibson, G.J. (1992). Variability of inspired oxygen concentration with nasal cannulas. Thorax 47:609-611.

Branson, R.D., & Seger, S.M. (1988). Bronchial hygiene techniques. In Kacmarek, R.M., & Stoller, J.K. (Eds). Current respiratory care. Philadelphia: B.C. Decker.

Branson, R.D., & Chatburn, R.L. (1992). Technical description and classification of modes of ventilator operation. Respiratory Care 37:1026-1044.

Brochard, L. (2003). Mechanical ventilation: invasive versus noninvasive. European Respiratory Journal 47(Suppl):31S-37S.

Brusasco, V., Pellegrino, R., (2003). Oxygen in the rehabilitation of patients with chronic obstructive pulmonary disease: an old tool revisited. American Journal of Respiratory Critical Care Medicine 168:1021-1022.

Burns, S.M. (1990). Advances in ventilatory therapy: high-frequency, pressure support, and nocturnal nasal positive pressure ventilation. Focus on Critical Care 17:227-237.

Burton, G.G., Hodgkin, J.E., & Ward, J.J. (1991). Respiratory care a guide to clinical practice, ed 3. Philadelphia: J.B. Lippincott.

Buttner, A., Ruhle, K.H. (2004). Quality of life before an during CPAP. Pneumologie, 58:651-659.

Casanova, C., Celli, B.R., Tost, L., Soriano, E., Abreu, J., Velasco, V., & Santolaria, F. (2000). Long-term controlled trial of nocturnal nasal positive pressure ventilation in patients with severe COPD. Chest 118:1582-1590.

Christopher, K.L., Spofford, B.T., Petrun, M.D., McCarty, D.C., Goodman, J.R., & Petty, T.L. (1987). A program for transtracheal oxygen delivery: assessment of safety and efficacy. Annals of Internal Medicine 107:802-808.

Christopher, K.L. (2003). Transtrachel oxygen catheters. Clinical Chest Medicine 24:489-510.

Crowe, J.M., & Bradley, C.A. (1997). The effectiveness of incentive spirometry with physical therapy for high-risk patients after coronary artery bypass surgery. Physical Therapy 77:260-268.

DesRosiers, A., Russo, R. (2000). Long term oxygen therapy. Respiratory Care Clinic of North America 6:625-644.

Duffy, S.Q., & Farley, D.E. (1992). The protracted demise of medical technology: the case of intermittent positive pressure breathing. Medical Care 30:718-734.

Dunne, P.J., (2000). The demographics and economics of long term oxygen therapy. Respiratory Care 45:223-228.

Dunlevy, C.L., & Tyl, S.E. (1992). The effect of oral versus nasal breathing on oxygen concentrations received from nasal cannulas. Respiratory Care 37:357-360.

Emtner, M., Porszasz, J., Burns, M., Somfay, A., & Casaburi, R. (2003). Benefits of supplemental oxygen in exercise training in nonhypoxemic chronic obstructive pulmonary disease patients. American Journal of Respiratory Critical Care Medicine 168:1034-1042.

Esteban, A., Anzueto, A., Alia, I., Gordo, F., Apezteguia, C., Palizas, F., Cide, D., Goldwaser, R., Soto, L., Bugedo, G., Rodrigo, C., Pimentel, J., Raimondi., G., & Tobin, M.J. (2000). How is mechanical ventilation employed in the intensive care unit? An international utilization review. American Journal of Respiratory Critical Care Medicine 161:1450-1458.

Frownfelter, D.L. (1987). Chest physical therapy and pulmonary rehabilitation an interdisciplinary approach, ed 2. St Louis: Mosby.

Fujimoto, K., Matsuzawa, Y., Yamaguchi, S., Koizumi, T., & Kubo, K. (2002). Benefits of oxygen on exercise performance and pulmonary hemodynamics in patients with COPD with mild hypoxemia. Chest 122:457-463.

Fuller, H.D., Dolovich, M.B., Posmituck, G., Pack, W.W., & Newhouse, M.T. (1990). Pressurized aerosol versus jet aerosol delivery to mechanically ventilated patients: comparison of dose to the lungs. American Review of Respiratory Disease 141:440-444.

Garrod, R., Bestall, J.C., Paul, E., & Wedzicha, J.A. (1999). Evaluation of pulsed dose oxygen delivery during exercise in patients with severe chronic pulmonary disease. Thorax 54:242-244.

Gosselink, R., et al, (2000). Incentive spirometry does not enhance recovery after thoracic surgery. Critical Care Medicine 28: 679-683.

Jall, J.C., et al, (1996). Prevention of respiratory complications after abdominal surgery: a randomized clinical trial. British Medical Journal 312:148-152.

Halliday, H.L. (2004). What interventions facilitate weaning from the ventilator? A review of the evidence from systematic reviews. Paediatric Respiratory Review 5(Suppl A):S347-S352.

Handelsman, H. (1991). Intermittent positive pressure breathing (IPPB) therapy. Health Technology Assessment Reports 1:1-9.

Hill, A.T., et al, (1995). Nasal intermittent positive pressure ventilation in cystic fibrosis, more than a bridge to transplantation? Pediatric Pulmonology 285:259.

Hodgkin, J.E., Connors, G.L., & Bell, C.W. (1993). Pulmonary rehabilitation guidelines to success, ed 2. Philadelphia: J.B. Lippincott.

Imanaka, H., Takeuchi, M., Tachibana, K., Takauchi, Y., & Nishimura, M. (2004). Changes in respiratory pattern during continuous positive airway pressure in infants after cardiac surgery. Journal of Anesthesiology 18:241-249.

Jackson, M., King, M.A., Wells, F.C., & Shneerson, J.M. (1992). Clnical experience and physiologic results with an implantable intratracheal oxygen catheter. Chest 102:1413-1418.

Jensen, A.G., Johnson, A., & Sandstedt, S. (1991). Rebreathing during oxygen treatment with face mask: the effect of oxygen flow rates on ventilation. Acta Anaesthesiologica Scandinavica 35:289-292.

Johann, U., Fichter, J., & Sybrecht, G.W. (2001). Efficacy of demand oxygen delivery systems in patients with chronic obstructive lung disease. Pneumologie 55:306-310.

Jolly, E.C., Di Boscio, V., Aguirre, L., Luna, C.M., Berensztein, S., & Gene, R.J. (2001). Effects of supplemental oxygen during activity in patients with advanced COPD without severe resting hypoxemia. Chest 120:437-443.

Kacmarek, R.M., Mack, C.W., & Dimas, S. (1990). The essentials of respiratory care, ed 3. St. Louis: Mosby.

Kampelmacher, M.J., Cornelisse, P.B., Alsbach, G.P., van Kesteren, R.G., Melissant, C.F., Douze, J.M., & Lammers, J.W. (1998). Accuracy of oxygen delivery by liquid oxygen canisters. European Respiratory Journal 12:204-207.

King, M.S. (2000). Preoperative evaluation. American Family Physician 62:308-311.

Lezon, K. (1999). Teaching incentive spirometry. Nursing 29:60-61.

L'Her, E., Duquesne, F., Girou, E., de Rosiere, X.D., Le Conte, P., Renault, S., Allamy, J.P., & Boles, J.M. (2004). Noninvasive continuous positive airway pressure elderly cardiogenic pulmonary edema patients. Intensive Care Medicine 30:882-888.

Lloberes, P., et al, (2004). Predictive factors of quality of life improvements and continuous positive airway pressure use in patients with sleep apnea-hypopnea syndrome:study at 1 year. Chest 126:1241-1247.

McCoy, R. (2000). Oxygen-conserving techniques and devices. Respiratory Care 45:95-103.

Orens, K.D., Kester, L., Fergus L.C., & Stoller, J.K. (1991). Cost impact of metered dose inhalers vs small volume nebulizers in hospitalized patients: the Cleveland clinic experience. Respiratory Care 36:1099-1104.

Overend, T.J., Anderson, C.M., Lucy, S.D., Bhatia, C., Jonsson, B.I., & Timmermans, C. (2001). The effect of incentive spirometry on postoperative pulmonary complications: a systematic review. Chest 120:971-978.

Padman, R., et al, (1992). Noninvasive mechanical ventilation for cystic fibrosis patients at end stage disease. Pediatric Pulm A 232:297.

Petty, T.L. (1999). Controversial indications for long term respiratory care: long term oxygen therapy. Monaldi Archives of Chest Disease 54:58-60.

Pilbeam, S.P. (1992). Mechanical ventilation physiological and clinical applications. St. Louis: Mosby.

Preciado, D.A., Thatcher, G., Panitch, H.B., & Rimell, F.L. (2002). Transtracheal oxygen catheters in a pediatric population. Ann Otol Rhinol Laryngol 111:310-314.

Pullen, R.L. (2003). Teaching bedside incentive spirometry. Nursing 33:24.

Rothe, T.B., Frey, J.G., Ciobanu, T.D., & Karrer, W. (1996). Dangerous complication of transtracheal oxygen therapy with the SCOOP system. Pneumologie 50:700-702.

Schonhofer, B., Wallstein, S., Wiese, C., & Kohler, D. (2001). Non-invasive mechanical ventilation improves endurance performance in patients with chronic respiratory failure due to thoracic restriction. Chest 119:1371-1378.

Skinner, M.A., Kingshott, R.N., Jones, D.R., Homan, S.D., & Taylor, D.R. (2004). Elevated posture for the management of obstructive sleep apnea. Sleep Breath 8:193-200.

Snider, G. (2002). Enhancement of exercise performance in COPD patients by hyperoxia. Chest 122:1830-1837.

Squadrone, V., Coha. M., Cerutti, E., Schellino, M.M., Biolino, P., Occella, P., Belloni, G., Vilianis, G., Fiore, G., Cavallo, F., Ranieri, V.M., & Piedmont Intensive Care Units Network (PICUN). (2005). Continuous positive airway pressure for treatment of postoperative hypoxemia: a randomized controlled trial. Journal of the American Medical Association 293:589-595.

Tiep, B.L., Barnett, J., Schiffman, G., Sanchez, O., & Carter, R. (2002). Maintaining oxygenation via demand oxygen delivery during rest and exercise. Respiratory Care 47:887-892.

Upadhyay, A., & Deorari, A.K. (2002). Continuous positive airway pressure: a gentler approach to ventilation Indian Pediatrics 41:459-469.

Veen, J.C., Stolk, J., & Dijkman, J.H. (1996). Complications in the use of the subcutaneous tunnelled intratracheal oxygen catheter. Netherlands Journal of Medicine 48:8-10.

Web, J.G., & Haas, C.F. (1998). Long term oxygen therapy for COPD: improving longevity and quality of life in hypoxemic patients. Postgrad Medicine 103:143-144, 147-148, 153-155.

Weiner, P., Man, A., Weiner, M., Rabner, M., Waizman, J., Magadle, R., Zamir, D., & Greiff, Y. (1997). The effect of incentive spirometry and inspiratory muscle training on pulmonary function after lung resection. Journal of Thoracic Cardiovascular Surgery 113:552-557.

Wysocki, M., Antonelli, M. (2001). Noninvasive mechanical ventilation in acute hypoxaemic respiratory failure. European Respiratory Journal 18:209-220.

Zadai, C.C. (1992). Pulmonary management in physical therapy. New York: Churchill Livingstone.

C H A P T E R   4 4

Care of the Patient with an Artificial Airway

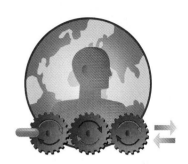

Donna Frownfelter and Lisa Sigg Mendelson

KEY TERMS Airway clearance Suctioning technique
Artificial airway Tracheostomy
Open and closed suctioning systems Tracheostomy tube/cuff

An artificial airway is a tube inserted in the trachea either through the mouth or nose or by a surgical incision. Artificial airways have been known to medical science for 3000 years. George Washington ultimately died of upper airway obstruction because his physicians could not agree on the use of tracheostomy. It was not until 1909, when Chevalier Jackson published his classic paper on tracheotomy, that this procedure gained some acceptance. The procedure did not become a highly specialized technique in patient care until the invention of modern tracheostomy tubes and the development of intermittent positive-pressure ventilators. In today's clinical practice, artificial airways have the following four basic purposes: to bypass upper airway obstruction, to assist or control respirations over prolonged periods, to facilitate the care of chronic respiratory tract infections, and to prevent aspiration of oral and gastric secretions. Multiple disease processes and traumatic problems can require an artificial airway, but each situation, simple or complex, can fit into one or several of these categories (Box 44-1).

INDICATIONS OF NEED—OBSERVATION

The respiratory care team can play a vital role in recognizing patient need for a tracheostomy by noting physiological changes that indicate respiratory distress (St. John & Malen, 2004). Cardinal signs of dangerous airway obstruction are stridor and chest wall retractions. Early clinical signs may include restlessness, agitation, tachycardia, confusion, motor dysfunction, and decreased oxygen saturation on pulse oximetry. These signs may be accompanied by headache, flapping tremor, audible wheezing and congestion and diaphoresis. Cyanosis from impaired oxygenation of the blood is a late, ominous sign.

In children, restlessness is due to the lack of oxygen unless another factor (e.g., thirst) is clearly evident. Extreme fatigue and an inability to sleep indicate impending danger. Apprehension, restlessness, and mental confusion at any age may be taken as early signs of hypoxemia.

Complications of Tracheostomy

Selection of the appropriate airway is made depending on the patient's impairment by the following factors: What is the best means of accomplishing the goal? Is it an emergency or a controlled, determined situation? Will the airway be needed for long-term care? In general, oral endotracheal tubes are inserted in emergencies. They are the quickest and easiest tubes to insert, even for relatively untrained personnel. A nasotracheal tube will generally replace the oral endotracheal tube for a long-term intubation. The nasal tube is more efficient in that it is better secured, allows the patient to eat, is easier to suction, and is generally more comfortable for the patient.

BOX 44-1

Disease Processes that Could Require an Artificial Airway Because of Respiratory Insufficiency

1. Primary lung disease (e.g., emphysema, chronic bronchitis, pulmonary fibrosis, cystic fibrosis, severe pneumonia, burned lung, and toxic inhalation)
2. Systemic disease with secondary lung involvement (e.g., cardiac failure, renal failure [fluid overload], and multi-organ system failure)
3. Neuromuscular disease (e.g., polio, Guillain-Barré syndrome, myasthenia gravis, use of muscle relaxants, and tetanus)
4. Central nervous system depression (e.g., drugs, post-anesthesia, metabolical coma, cerebrovascular accident, meningitis, and central nervous system tumors)
5. Trauma (e.g., head/neck/chest surgery or injuries)
6. Diseases complicated by extremes of age (e.g., premature infant or elderly)
7. Mechanical obstruction (e.g., upper airway infection, laryngeal paralysis, tumor, edema, bleeding, foreign body, and thyroid malignancy)
8. Recurrent aspiration (e.g., glottic incompetence, occlusive diseases of the esophagus, and swallowing disorders of various causes)

From Selecky, P.A. (1974). Tracheostomy-a review of present day indications, complications and care, Heart Lung 3:272-283.

There are certain complications with nasotracheal tubes. Among these are sinus blockage and pain, vocal cord damage, and pressure necrosis to the cartilaginous structure of the nose. To reduce these complications, the airway should be evaluated daily. The tube should be removed as quickly as possible when the indication for intubation is reversed. If there appears to be a need for a more long-term airway, however, a tracheostomy should be considered. The procedure should not be taken lightly because many additional complications may occur.

Complications of tracheostomy can be surgical, postoperative, or physiological. Complications that occur at the time of the operation are more frequently direct results of the surgical procedure itself. Delayed complications may result directly or indirectly from surgery, postoperative care, or the abrupt physiological changes resulting from tracheostomy. Objectives of caring for the patient after a tracheostomy are to maintain patency of the tube, cleanliness of the wound site, and good aeration of the lungs, as well as to observe any changes in the patient's vital signs and oxygenation by pulse oximetry.

In patients with artificial airways the normal physiological mechanism for adding moisture to the air via the nasal mucosa is bypassed. Therefore supplemental humidification is extremely important to protect the mucosa from drying and crusting, which results in obstruction.

The dressing under the tracheostomy tube and tracheostomy ties should be changed when they become soiled because dried blood and other secretions near the incision can encourage bacterial growth. The incision should be checked frequently for bleeding. The skin may be cleaned with half-strength hydrogen peroxide and sterile saline when a new dressing is applied. The dressing should be folded into place, never cut. This eliminates the possibility of lint or frayed threads being aspirated. Commercially prepared dressings best meet these criteria.

When changing the tapes that hold the tube in place, it is best to have one nurse hold the tube in place while another replaces the old tapes. An angle is cut at the end of the tape to facilitate its placement through the flange of one side of the tube. The tape is then threaded through the back of the tracheostomy tube and through the other flanged opening and tied securely with a square knot placed on one side of the patient's neck. One finger should be placed under the twill tape while tying to prevent the tape from being tied too tight.

Pneumothorax can occur immediately after tracheostomy because of laceration of the mediastinal pleura at the time of or within 24 hours of surgery (this arises often in children and patients with chronic obstructive lung disease). Other problems include air embolism, aspiration, and subcutaneous and mediastinal emphysema. Recurrent laryngeal nerve damage or posterior tracheal penetration may occur but is uncommon.

Postoperative Physiological Complications

Attentive nursing care is the single most essential factor in postoperative tracheostomy management. Vigilant monitoring and observation by the entire respiratory care team is of vital importance.

A patient with an artificial airway is understandably apprehensive and has special communication needs. He or she should also be reminded that the inability to phonate is only temporary. The patient must be reassured that he or she will be attended to frequently and can trust and depend fully on the health care team to attend to his or her needs. If alert, the patient must be equipped with a signal light or bell, paper and pencil, magic slate, or picture board for communication.

Airway obstruction is the foremost complication that exists postoperatively for the patient who has undergone tracheostomy. Tracheal secretions are the major source of obstruction, particularly if they are excessive or viscous. When using a cuffed tube, acute obstruction might occur from overinflating the cuff, which allows it to balloon over the end of the tube. Other causes of obstruction are dislodgement of the tube into a false tract anterior to the tube tracheal opening, and kinking of softened plastic cannula.

Tracheobronchitis, inflammation of the trachea and bronchus, is a complication resulting primarily from irritation due to incorrect suctioning technique and the presence of a foreign body in the trachea.

Crusting is a common and complex problem that may result from inadequate humidification of inspired air or patient dehydration. In many instances, ulceration of the tracheal mucosa results from irritation by the airway or incorrect suctioning. This ulcerated area becomes infected with various organisms and is virtually covered by crust. Further suctioning removes the crust, causing discharge of serum and bleeding. The discharge produces a wet eschar that is covered with mucus. Because of the drying effect of air passing over this mass, a hard crust can form. The development of this crust in the trachea might eventually produce a mass large enough to completely plug the tracheal cannula and almost completely obstruct the trachea. Cases have been cited in which an entire cast of the tracheobronchial tree has been removed.

Other physiological complications may be related to the following: hypoxemia developing before or during the procedure and resulting in an uncontrollable patient, cardiac arrest, and increased myocardial sensitivity to adrenalin; alkalosis developing from rapid carbon dioxide wash-out after establishment of the airway, resulting in myocardial fibrillation and apnea; cardiac failure, resulting in profuse bronchorrhea caused by pulmonary edema and shock.

Chronic complications cited by Dailey et al (1992) include the following: infection at the surgical site, aspiration, aerophagia, persistent stoma, and tracheal stenosis.

Postoperative Mechanical Complications

Dislocation of the tube may result from unsatisfactory nursing care, poor attention to the airway during positioning, or ventilator tubing pulling on the airway. If the tracheostomy tube tapes are not kept tight and tied with a square knot or if they become loose as a result of subcutaneous emphysema or edema, the tube may be coughed out of the trachea and become lodged in the tissues of the neck and obstruct the airway. In pediatric patients, stay sutures are frequently used to prevent dislodgement of the tracheostomy tube. These sutures are valuable during recannulization of the tube if it comes dislodged before a tract has been well established. Stay sutures will prevent entry into a false tract. Advantages of this technique include the following: blocked or displaced tubes can be rapidly replaced, exposure of the trachea at surgical intervention is improved, firm anchoring of the trachea at the moment of incision, decreased trauma associated with extubation, and uniform tracheostomy technique for all ages.

Dislodgement of the outer cannula or required removal before a tract has been well established (usually 5 to 10 days) again requires diligence and quick action by the nurse. No attempt at reinsertion should be made without adequate light, satisfactory tissue retraction, tracheal hook, and a Trousseau's dilator. A Trousseau's dilator and tracheal hook should be readily available. A spare tracheostomy tube of the correct size should be kept at the patient's bedside at all times. Should the tube be coughed out, the nurse uses the Trousseau's dilator to hold the wound apart while summoning the physician. Tragedies have occurred from inserting the tube into the soft tissues of the neck or mediastinum because of a dislodged cannula and the frantic efforts to replace it. Once the tracheostomy tract has been firmly established, the tube can be replaced by the nurse on written order of the physician.

TRACHEOSTOMY TUBES

Metal Tubes

Tracheostomy tubes are of two basic types: metal and polyvinyl chloride (hard and soft). Metal tubes are not commonly seen but some patients with long-standing tracheostomies may prefer not to switch to a polyvinyl choride tube. Metal tubes can be made of either stainless steel or sterling silver and are composed of the following three parts: an outer cannula that fits into the tracheal incision, an inner cannula that fits into the outer cannula, and an obturator that facilitates insertion of the tube. These three parts comprise a tracheostomy set and are not interchangeable with any other set. Before the outer cannula is inserted into the tracheal incision, the obturator is placed inside. The lower end of the obturator protrudes from the end of the outer cannula and facilitates its insertion into the trachea. This is the only purpose of the obturator. The protruding end of the obturator obstructs the lumen of the outer cannula. When the obturator is removed, it is immediately replaced with the inner cannula. If one part is lost or damaged, the entire set is useless. Therefore, each part, including obturator, must be accounted for carefully. Plastic tubes generally have interchangeable parts. Care should be exercised in handling sterling silver tubes because silver is easily dented.

The inner cannula should always be inspected to be sure it is clean and clear of secretions before it is reinserted. Mucus that has dried inside the inner cannula cannot be cleaned by merely rinsing it with water. The cannula should be soaked in hydrogen peroxide and scrubbed with a tracheostomy brush and rinsed with saline to be sure all secretions have been removed. If a silver inner cannula becomes discolored, it may be cleaned with silver polish.

To prevent dislodgement, lock the inner cannula into position after reinsertion. The locking mechanism is different with each tube and the therapist should become familiar with the types used. If the inner cannula is not locked it may come out if the patient has a forceful exhalation or position change. It is vital that the inner cannula be reinserted quickly if the patient is on mechanical ventilation, especially if the patient is on full support.

Polyvinyl Chloride (Plastic) Disposable Tubes and Cuff Inflation

The development of plastic tracheostomy tubes came about for the following three important reasons: application of silicone to the inner surface of the plastic tube minimizes crusting and adherence of secretions; there is greater ease in attaching a safe, dependable, permanent inflatable cuff to the plastic tube that cannot slip off and occlude the tracheal opening; and lower costs allow the tube to be disposable. Plastic tubes come with and without cuffs.

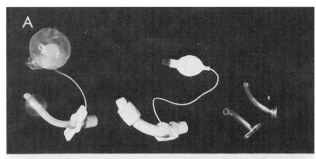

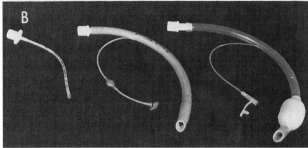

FIGURE 44-1 A, Cuffed adult tracheostomy tubes, uncuffed pediatric tracheostomy tube (far left). **B,** Cuffed adult endotracheal tubes, uncuffed pediatric endotracheal tube (far left).

The cuffed tracheostomy tube is primarily used in conjunction with a positive-pressure ventilator to form a closed system (Figure 44-1). It is also used to reduce the possibility of aspiration because of absent, protective laryngeal, and pharyngeal reflexes. The inflatable cuff is located around the lower portion of the tube and, when inflated, seals the trachea from most airflow except through the tube itself (see Figure 44-1). The cuff, usually made of pliable plastic, is inflated by injecting air into the fine-bore tubing. A small pilot balloon is located proximally in the tubing and indicates that the cuff is inflated. The inflation end of the cuff and the balloon must be checked before insertion of the tube into the trachea to be certain that there are no leaks. The Luer valve inflation port to the pilot balloon is self-sealing. Some Luer valves have a relief valve when pressure exceeds 25 mm Hg.

Cuff Inflation

There are two commonly used methods of cuff inflation: the minimal air leak, in which a small amount of air escapes on inspiration; and minimal occlusive volume, in which just enough air is placed in the cuff to stop air from escaping on inspiration. According to Crabtree Goodnough (1988), the minimal leak cuff technique may produce less injury than the minimal occlusive volume inflation technique. Regardless of which technique is used, the pressure of the cuff should be checked every four to eight hours and the pressures documented. With continued research and monitoring of tracheal cuff pressures, potential tracheal injury can be prevented.

Once the cuff is inflated, the only route for air exchange is through the patient's tracheostomy tube; therefore, careful observation of the patient is essential. If the patient is on mechanical ventilation, observation is essential. Alarms are always to be in the "on" position when a patient is being mechanically ventilated. Some means of resuscitation, such as a manual resuscitation bag with mask, must be available at the bedside to ventilate the patient in case the tracheostomy tube comes out or is dislodged.

Considerable emphasis has been given to the incidence of tracheal ischemia and resulting stenosis from the use of a cuffed tube. Tracheal ischemia results from the pressure of the cuffed tube against the tracheal wall, which heals with scar formation and thereby leads to subsequent stenosis. This complication can be reduced or eliminated by minimal air leak or minimal occlusive volume. For the minimal occlusive volume, the cuff must be inflated to eliminate any air leak on inspiration. Cuff pressures should be monitored and documented every four to eight hours to prevent tracheal injury. The recommended cuff pressure is 15 to 25 mm Hg. The cuff is inflated until there is no air leak between the wall of the trachea and the cuff, and then a small amount of air is released to allow only a slight air leak between the walls of the trachea and the cuff. This reduces the pressure of the cuff, still allows the ventilator to function properly, and reduces the likelihood of tracheal ischemia. Any difficulty in properly inflating the cuffed tracheostomy tube should be immediately reported to the physician.

If the tracheotomized patient is conscious, he or she may attempt to speak. If the cuff is properly inflated, he or she will be aphonic because no air can pass over the vocal cords. If he or she needs to speak, the cuff can be deflated, and the patient may be given a sterile dressing to hold over the tube. This will allow him or her to speak and also clear secretions by rapid exhalation (simulated cough).

To prevent the formation of crusts, inspired air must be continuously and adequately humidified by means of nebulizing equipment. The equipment used for this purpose can be a possible source of infection. Therefore the nebulizer and tubing should be changed every eight hours ideally, but at least once every 24 hours.

The Communitrache I is a tracheostomy tube that permits the removal of secretions above the inflation cuff without nasotracheal suctioning. The other benefit to this tracheostomy tube is the patient's ability to communicate, especially while on a ventilator. When the patient is weaned from the ventilator, a fenestrated tube may be used. Fenestrated comes from the French word *fenestre,* meaning window. There is a window (fenestration) in the outer cannula. When the tube is used for speaking, the cuff is deflated, the inner cannula removed, and an external plug is inserted to cap the tracheostomy tube to allow the patient to speak. The cuff must be deflated when the cap is in place. If the cuff is inflated, the patient is unable to breathe air into the lungs and will exhibit immediate distress. If a patient with a fenestrated tube needs to be suctioned, the inner cannula must be replaced so that the suction catheter does not enter the fenestration and cause injury to the tracheal wall mucosa.

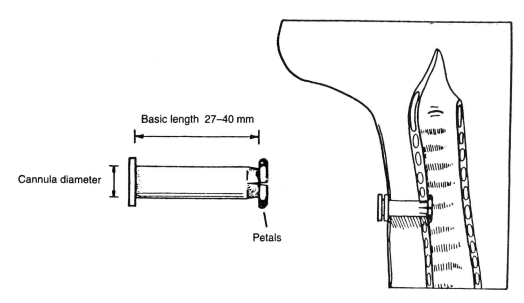

Basic length 27–40 mm

Cannula diameter

Petals

FIGURE 44-2 Dimensions and actual positioning of an Olympic tracheostomy button. *(From Pierson, D.J. & Kacmarek, R.M. [1992]. Foundations of respiratory care. Churchill Livingstone. Edinburgh. © David J. Pierson.)*

Other Airway Devices

The Olympic tracheostomy button is used as an interim airway after tracheostomy tube removal (Figure 44-2). This method is another example of weaning a patient from the tracheostomy tube but still maintaining the stoma should a tracheostomy be again needed. Patients that may benefit most from this device are people with chronic obstructive pulmonary disease (COPD). This is one method used to facilitate secretion removal after hospitalization when it becomes necessary because of the disease process. The Olympic tracheostomy button allows the tracheostomy patient the opportunity to reestablish an unobstructed airway and at the same time allows the patient to speak.

There are many other speaking tracheostomy tubes (Fitsimones, 2003). Airway clearance needs to be optimized before a speaking valve is used. If a patient has increased secretions, he or she may find it difficult to tolerate the procedure. A benefit of the valve, however, is that the patient may be able to simulate coughing and promote mobilization of upper airway secretions.

One common speaking valve is the Passy-Muir valve (Figure 44-3). The Passy-Muir is a one-way valve that allows inspiration only and forces exhalation through the upper airway. It is important to note that the cuff must be deflated when using the valve or a cuffless tracheostomy tube may be used. Breath stacking (taking a few breaths in without exhaling) can be used to get more air into the lungs before exhalation. Using the valve, the upper airway muscles gradually recover, allowing for transition to a fenestrated tube or a smaller size tracheostomy tube and thereby preparing the patient for eventual decannulation (Pierson & Kacmarek, 1992). Another

benefit may be improved ability to swallow. Also, some patients claim that they can taste their food again, which may promote improved nutrition and hydration, (Elpern, 1999, Lichtman et al, 1995).

The management of major airway obstruction by tracheal tumor, external compression, or tracheal disease below the thoracic inlet still presents difficult problems. The Montgomery T tube is a bifurcated silicone rubber stent designed to preserve patency of the airways in a patient with injury to the trachea or main stem bronchi (Figure 44-4). When the T tube is in place, the patient breathes normally through the nose and mouth and can speak. The T tube is helpful in long-term therapy to alleviate obstruction or during reconstructive surgery. This device does not cause any adverse tissue reaction on a long-term basis, according to Montgomery (Wahidi & Ernst, 2003).

Airway Care

Normally the mucociliary escalator and the cough reflex provide airway clearance. When these mechanisms fail, suctioning of the airways, manual cough assistance, or the cough machine is indicated. Suctioning does have potential hazards, but it should be a safe procedure with proper guidance and care (Dean, 1997). Health care professionals also need to protect themselves during open system suctioning. This procedure can cause dissemination of particle droplets in the immediate area. Ng et al studied 50 consecutive suctioning procedures with entubated patients using an open system (i.e., the mechanical ventilator tubing is removed from the tracheostomy or endotracheal tube to suction the patient).

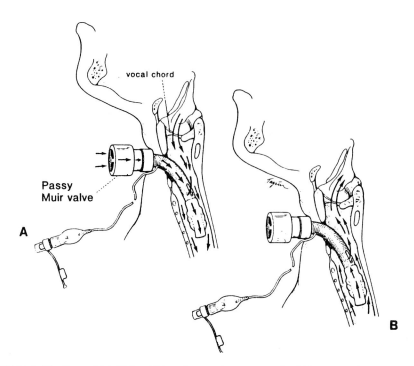

FIGURE 44-3 The Passy-Muir Valve. This valve attaches to a standard 15-mm tracheostomy adapter. It allows inspriration **A,** via the valve, but exhilation **B,** must occur via the upper airway. *(From Pierson, D.J. & Kacmarek, R.M. [1992]. Foundations of respiratory care. Churchill Livingstone. Edinburgh. © David J. Pierson.)*

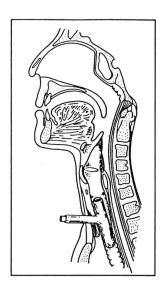

FIGURE 44-4 The Montgomery T-tube. *(From Montgomery, W.W. [1980]. Manual care of the Montgovery silicone tracheal T-tube. The Annals of Otology Rhinology & Laryngology 89 [Suppl 73]:3.)*

Visible droplets were scattered from 25 to 168 cm from the artificial airway. When they were cultured, the same bacteria aspirated grew on the agar plates. This highlights the importance of protective eyewear for and precautions to be taken by the person performing the suction procedure (Ng, 1999).

Suctioning

When preparing to suction, three phases should be considered: (1) Preparation before suctioning, (2) the actual suctioning procedure, and (3) postsuctioning (Day et al, 2002, AARC Clinical Practice Guideline, 2004).

Open versus Closed Suctioning Systems

Patients on mechanical ventilators may either be suctioned by disconnecting the ventilator tubing and suctioning (open system) or directly in line with the ventilator tubing (closed system). Studies have shown that a closed system maintains better physiologic stability, less oxygen desaturation and fewer dsyrhythmias (Kalyn et al, 2003; Lee et al, 2001; Johnson et al, 1994; Grossi, 1995,).

Before Suctioning

Patient assessment and preparation as well as hyper-oxygenation are essential. Proper catheter size will be discussed later in the chapter.

During Suctioning

There needs to be an awareness of the appropriate depth of insertion, and time limits for the procedure need to be observed. A decision will need to be made as to how many

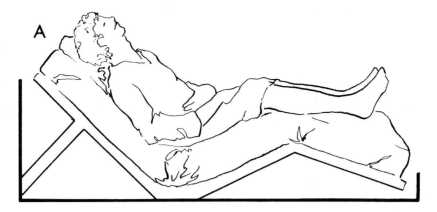

Fowler 60-70 degrees

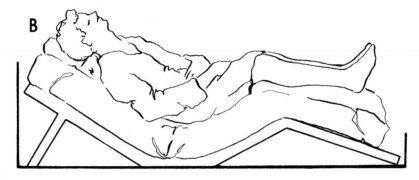

Semi-Fowler 10-12"

FIGURE 44-5 A, Fowler's and **B,** Semi-Fowler's positions.

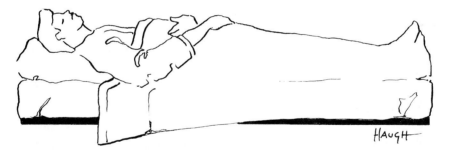

FIGURE 44-6 Supine position.

passes of the catheter will be needed. Monitoring of the patient by EKG monitor and pulse oximetry will demonstrate the patient's tolerance of the procedure.

Postsuctioning

The patient needs to be reassured and positioned comfortably. Reconnection to the ventilator or previous level of equipment must be completed in cases of open system suctioning.

Suction Procedure

Proper explanation of the suctioning technique to the patient helps allay apprehension and enhance cooperation.

Medicate the postoperative patient before suctioning to decrease the pain of coughing. Always maintain a calm and reassuring manner.

Maintain aseptic technique throughout the entire procedure. Use sterile gloves and a sterile, disposable catheter for each suctioning.

Position the patient properly unless contraindicated. Nasotracheal and/or pharyngeal suctioning should be done with the patient in Fowler position, 60 to 70 degrees, or semi-Fowler position, approximately 45 degrees, with the neck hyperextended (Figure 44-5). The supine position is best for the patient with tracheostomy or endotracheal tubes (Figure 44-6).

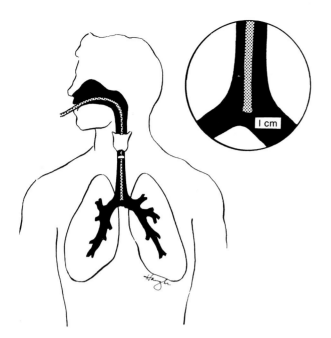

FIGURE 44-7 The catheter will simulate coughing when it contacts the carina (in a patient with cough reflex).

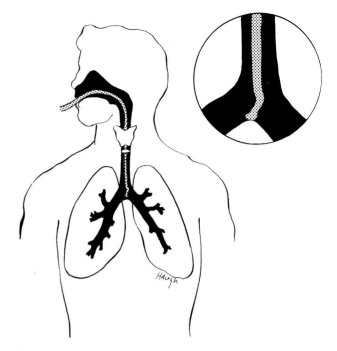

FIGURE 44-8 The catheter is withdrawn 1 cm after it reaches the carina, before applying suction.

Pharyngeal suctioning may be necessary before deflating the cuffed tracheostomy tube. The nurse should not suction the pharynx and then the trachea with the same catheter, but the trachea may be suctioned first and then the pharynx with the same catheter.

Duration of suctioning is very important. Each suctioning procedure should last no longer than five to 10 seconds to avoid hypoxia.

Prolonged suctioning may result in precipitating a dysrhythmia or cardiac arrest. A good way to judge the elapsed time is to hold one's own breath and be guided by the development of discomfort. This is most important for the patient who depends on ventilatory assistance.

Use the lowest possible vacuum settings (below 120 mm Hg) that will still support suctioning the tracheostomy tube. The higher the setting is raised, the greater the risk of trauma to the tracheal mucosa. Caution should be exercised to avoid kinking the suction tubing or catheter. When negative pressure is excessive and released suddenly, inadvertent removal of portions of tracheal mucosa may occur.

Insertion of the suction catheter should be done gently, using aseptic technique and sterile gloves. Goggles are used as part of universal precautions if there is any danger of coughed-out secretions. The catheter should first be moistened in sterile saline or with a water-soluble gel. Suction is not applied while the catheter is passed down into the trachea. Proper insertion of the catheter will stimulate coughing when it contacts the carina (Figure 44-7). It is then immediately withdrawn one cm before suction is applied (Figure 44-8). Do not force the catheter up and down while suctioning. Suction is applied only while the catheter is being withdrawn. Rotating the catheter during withdrawal results in suctioning a larger

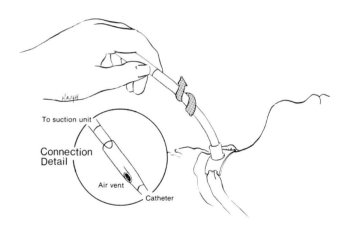

FIGURE 44-9 The catheter is rotated during withdrawal in order to suction a larger surface area.

area and increases the surface contact of the trachea and tracheostomy tube (Figure 44-9).

Left main-stem bronchus aspiration is more difficult because of the anatomical arrangement of the bronchus. It was formerly thought that left bronchial aspiration was facilitated by turning the patient's head to the right. Studies by Kirimli et al (1970) and Panacek et al (1989) indicate that left bronchial aspiration is best accomplished by using a Coudé tip catheter. After its insertion into the trachea, the curved tip should be positioned to point toward the left main-stem bronchus. Even so, insertion is difficult, and auscultation by stethoscope is necessary to thoroughly access the suctioning.

Right main-stem bronchus aspiration is the usual case because of the more direct alignment of this bronchus with the trachea. This can almost always be carried out with a straight tracheal catheter. The deeper suction would rarely be indicated; generally when the catheter hits the carina it is withdrawn before suctioning.

Excessive suctioning can be harmful. Use judgment to determine just how often a patient requires suctioning. It should not be routine, it should be based on the need of the patient (Wood, 1998; Gilbert, 1999). Assessment by auscultation and patient clinical observations should be used to determine the need for suctioning. Suction only when it is needed (Carroll, 1994). Allow the patient to rest and breathe between each insertion of the suction catheter and, if necessary, ventilate him or her for a few minutes before further suctioning. Remember that each suctioning attempt removes air as well as secretions. Hyperoxygenation with 100% oxygen has been suggested to provide better results and fewer complications. Hyperventilation was previously encouraged, but studies have shown that it is not necessary; hyperoxygenation is the important factor (Grapp, 1996, Pritchard et al, 2001).

Complications from tracheal suctioning include the following: hypoxemia, cardiac dysrhythmia, bronchospasm, and infection. Suctioning can lead to hypoxemia because oxygen is removed from the airways, and this could lead to tissue hypoxia. To minimize this problem, patients should receive preoxygenation with 100% oxygen for three to five breaths. This can be done on the ventilator without disconnection. Cardiac dysrhythmias, such as premature ventricular contractures, bradycardia, and tachycardia, can be diminished by hyperoxygenating the patient with 100% oxygen. If any dysrhythmias occur on the monitor, the suctioning procedure should be discontinued momentarily to allow the patient to stabilize and increase his or her oxygen level. Bronchospasm may be effectively prevented by administration of a bronchodilator, such as albuterol, before suctioning. Infection can be decreased by maintaining sterile techniques with sterile gloves and sterile catheters when suctioning.

Suctioning Artificial Airway

Nasotracheal, Endotracheal, and Tracheostomy

1. Check equipment; be sure that all necessary equipment is present and maintain a sterile field.
2. Check monitors.
3. Wash hands.
4. Inform the patient of the procedure.
5. Hyperoxygenate with 100% oxygen for three to five breaths with manual resuscitation bag.
6. Place the patient's neck in extension.
7. Put on sterile gloves and goggles.
8. Lubricate the catheter with sterile saline or water-soluble gel.
9. Place the catheter (without suction) upward and backward in short increments. Continue until an obstruction (the carina) is reached.

10. When the carina is stimulated, the patient will generally cough unless his or her reflexes are obtunded.
11. Pull the catheter back slightly from the carina, then apply suction with no more than 120 mm Hg pressure as the catheter is withdrawn in a rotating motion.
12. Aspiration time should be within 10 to 15 seconds total. (A good guideline is for the therapist to hold his or her breath during suctioning [because the patient is also not breathing]. This gives the therapist a better sensitivity for what the patient is experiencing.)
13. Allow the patient to rest for several seconds and preoxygenate him or her again.
14. Check the patient's breath sounds and repeat the procedure if necessary to remove more secretions.
15. Suction pharynx.
16. Observe the patient and monitor for any dysrhythmias.
17. Use pulse oximetry to monitor desaturation.
18. Discard used equipment and remove gloves and goggles.
19. Wash hands.

Nasopharyngeal Airways

When frequent, aggressive nasopharyngeal suctioning is indicated in a patient that is comatose, a nasopharyngeal airway (NPA) will lessen the trauma of frequent passage of the catheter. The NPA is a soft latex material that provides easy access to the trachea for nasopharyngeal suctioning. The nasal and pharyngeal mucosa are protected and the procedure thus becomes more comfortable to the patient. In addition, a fiberoptic bronchoscope may be passed through the airway if the procedure is indicated.

Endotracheal or Tracheostomy Suctioning

Sterile technique is followed for endotracheal and tracheostomy suctioning. Usually no lubrication is necessary, although it may be used if there is difficulty passing the catheter.

Sterile Suctioning

The technique for correct sterile suctioning of artificial airways is perhaps the most important and vital segment of care for the patient because it removes secretions that would otherwise obstruct the airway. If suctioning is not performed properly, it can cause physiological or psychological trauma to the patient.

The equipment necessary for proper sterile suctioning includes the proper mechanical apparatus, connecting tubing, sterile gloves, sterile saline, suction catheters, dressings, and goggles as indicated with universal precautions. It must be remembered that while suctioning the patient, his or her only air passage is being partially occluded. Thus the suction catheter should never be larger than one half the diameter of the tube opening; if it is larger, it may completely occlude the patient's air passage.

TABLE 44-1	
The Pediatric Tracheostomy Card	
TRACHEOSTOMY SIZE	**RECOMMENDED CATHETER SIZE**
Pediatric Tubes	
00 PT	6.5 F
0 PT	6.5 F
1 PT	8 F
2 PT	8 F
3 PT	10 F
4 PT	10 F
Neonatal Tubes	
00 NT	6.5 F
0 NT	6.5 F
1 NT	6.5 F
SCT-Single Cannula Tracheostomy Tubes	
5 SCT	10 F
6 SCT	12 F
7 SCT	14 F
8 SCT	14 F

From Warnoch, C., & Porpora, K. (1994). A pediatric trache card: transforming research into practice. Pediatric Nursing 20:186-188.

One method for determining the size of the catheter used for suctioning is to double the size of the tracheostomy tube in place and add two. For example, if the patient has a #6 tube, the calculation would be as follows: 6 + 6 = 12, 12 + 2 = 14. Therefore a 14-F catheter would be the largest catheter that could be used to suction the #6 tracheostomy. See Table 44-1 for a correlation of tracheostomy sizes to catheter sizes.

The catheter used for pharyngeal suctioning should never be used for subsequent suctioning of the artificial airway, but using an artificial airway suction catheter for pharyngeal suction is acceptable. Aseptic technique is absolutely necessary to minimize the risk of infection and, ideally, only disposable catheters should be used.

Suctioning may be necessary every few minutes when the patient initially returns from surgery because there is an increase in secretions, which is usually the result of irritation of the endotracheal tube plus a reflex mechanism initiated by the surgical trauma. Usually, by paying attention to the patient's color, respiratory rate, lung sounds, and oxygen saturation on pulse oximetry, the nurse or therapist can determine the amount of secretions present. Excessive mucus in the trachea or large bronchi is usually indicated by coarse, rattling sounds. Fine bubbling sounds usually suggest fluid located more peripherally (i.e., in the alveolar spaces). If accumulated secretions are not cleared, they can cause respiratory and cardiac rates to increase; effective oxygen and carbon dioxide transfer is impaired, causing cyanosis to appear and low-grade fever to develop.

Instillation of Saline

Saline instillation is not recommended. Studies have shown that it is ineffective and can cause reflex and uncomfortable airway responses (i.e. cough, bronchospasm). It is not a recommended practice (McKelvie, 1998, Akgul & Akylcu, 2002).

Extubation/Decannulation

Extubation or decannulation is the removal of the artificial airway. In general it is done when the reason for establishing the artificial airway no longer exists. In certain cases the artificial airway may be removed to facilitate airway clearance and aspiration. This can be prevented with thorough attention and care of the tracheostomy tube (Ross, 2003, Bach, 1995). The patient is aided in gradually relearning normal breathing through his or her upper respiratory tract before the tube is removed. This can be a time of considerable fear and anxiety for patients because they have learned they can breathe safely through their tracheostomy, and they may become apprehensive when asked to breathe in a normal manner. The relearning process can be accomplished under the physician's direction by reducing the lumen of the tube for a day or two or by partially obstructing the tube's outer opening for increasing lengths of time. Eventually the patient is able to tolerate the complete occlusion of the tracheostomy opening. This is sometimes difficult and similar to breathing through a straw.

When occluding the tracheostomy opening with a cuffed tube, the cuff must be deflated first. Failure to do this will result in total obstruction of the patient's airway as the tube opening is occluded.

Fenestrated tubes have also been excellent for weaning the patient from the tracheostomy tube. They do not actually increase the airway resistance as in the above method and are probably more effective. They also allow the patient to talk and attempt to cough to mobilize secretions. Other methods used in decannulation include the Olympic tracheostomy button and the Passy-Muir valve. The Olympic tracheostomy button allows the airway to remain patent for suctioning and reinsertion of a tracheostomy tube should it become necessary. The Passy-Muir valve allows for normal recovery of the upper airway muscle, making it possible to reduce the size of the tracheostomy tube, leading to eventual plugging and decannulation. Careful observation and documentation of the patient's ability to ventilate must be done when either of these devices is used in the decannulation process.

Close supervision should continue after extubation. After a tracheostomy tube is removed, the skin edges are usually taped together with butterfly strips for a few days until the wound heals. While healing, air will escape through the wound and reduce the effectiveness of the patient's cough. The patient should be instructed that the noise from the partially closed trachea is normal, and small secretions should be removed from this area. The patient should be taught and instructed to hold a sterile dressing firmly over the incision when coughing until the opening heals.

SUMMARY

Artificial airways are commonly used and the health care team needs to be proficient at using them and comfortable working with patients who have them. Precautions need to be observed and techniques need to be consistently applied to prevent respiratory tract infections and unplanned decannualtion. Training and orientation needs to be thorough so that suctioning procedures are safe for the patient and the health care team. Knowing the indications for the artificial airway will help identify when the airway is no longer needed. For patients who require life-long use of tracheostomy tubes, the patient, family, and care taker will need to be instructed in the airway clearance and cleaning procedures.

Review Questions

1. What physiological changes occur with surgical placement of a tracheostomy tube?
2. Discuss possible psychosocial concerns of patients with an artificial airway.
3. When would a speaking valve be indicated? What is the cuff position?
4. How does the patient-care team prepare the patient with a trachestomy for self care?
5. Compare emergency care, acute care, and long-term care for a patient with upper airway obstruction and tracheostomy placement.

REFERENCES

AARC Clinical Practice Guideline. (2004). Nasotracheal suctioning-revision and update. Irving, Tex: American Association for Respiratory Care.

Akgul, S., & Akyolcu, N. (2002). Effects of normal saline on endotracheal suctioning. Journal of Clinical Nursing 11:826-830.

Bach, JR. (1995). Indications for tracheostomy and decannulation of tracheotomized ventilator users. Monaldi Archives of Chest Disease 50:223-227.

Carroll, P. (1994). Safe suctioning PRN. RN May:32-37.

Cereda, M., Villa, F., Colombo, E., Greco, G., Nacoti, M., & Pesenti, A. (2001). Closed system endotracheal suctioning maintains lung volumes during volume-controlled mechanical ventilation. Intensive Care Medicine 27:648-654.

Class, P. (1992). Nursing considerations for airway management in the PACU. Current Reviews for Post Anesthesia Care Nurses 14:1-8.

Crabtree Goodnough, S.K. (1988). Reducing tracheal injury and aspiration. Dimension of Critical Care Nursing 7:324-331.

Dailey, R.H., Simon, B., Young, G.P., & Stewart, R.D. (1992). Airway maneuvers. In The airway emergency management. St. Louis: Mosby.

Day, T., Farnell, S., & Wilson-Barnett, J. (2002), Suctioning: a review of current research recommendations. Intensive Critical Care Nursing 18:79-89.

Dean, B. (1997). Evidence-based suction management in accident and emergency vital component of airway care. Accident and Emergency Nursing 5:92-98.

Elpern, E.H. (1999). Effect of the Passy-Muir valve on pulmonary aspiration in adults with tracheostomies. Chest 116(4-S2):365S.

Fitsimones, L. (2003). Tracheostomy and ventilator speaking valves. Vital Signs April:6-8.

Frost, E.A. (1976). Tracing the tracheostomy. Annals of Otolaryngology 85:618-624.

Furtan, N.D., Dutcher, P.O., & Roberts, J.K. (1993). The safety and efficacy of bedside tracheostomy. Otolaryngology-Head and Neck Surgery 109:707-711.

Gilbert, M. (1999). Assessing the need for endotracheal suction. Paediatric Nursing 11:14-17.

Goodwell, E.W. (1934). The story of tracheostomy. British Journal of Children's Diseases 31:167-176.

Goodwell, E.W. (1934). The story of tracheostomy. British Journal of Children's Diseases 31:253-271.

Grapp, MJ. (1996). Endotracheal suctioning: ventilator vs manual delivery of hyperoxygenation breaths. American Journal of Critical Care 5:192-197.

Grossi, S.A. (1995). Closed endotracheal suction system for the prevention of hypoxemia. Rev Esc Enferm USP 29:25-33.

Jackson, C. (1909). Tracheostomy. Laryngoscope 18:285-290.

Jackson, C. (1921). High tracheostomy and other errors. The chief causes of chronic laryngeal atenosis. Surgery, Gynecology, Obstetrics 32:392-395.

Jackson, D., & Albamonte, S. (1994). Enhancing communication with the Passy-Muir valve. Pediatric Nursing 20:149-153.

Johnson, K.L., Kearney, P.A., Johnson, S.B., Niblett, J.B., MacMillan, N.L., & McClain, R.E. (1994). Closed versus open endotracheal suctioning: costs and physiologic consequences. Critical Care Medicine 22:658-666.

Kalyn, A., Blatz, S., Feuerstake, S., Paes, B., & Bautista, C. (2003). Closed suctioning of intubated neonates maintains better physiologic stability: a randomized trial. Journal of Perinatology 23:218-222.

Kirchner, J.A. (1980). Tracheostomy and its problems. Surgical Clinics of North America 60:1093-1104.

Kirimli, B., King, J.E., & Pfaeffle, H.H. (1970). Evaluation of tracheobronchial suction technique. Journal of Thoracic and Cardiovascular Surgery 59:340-344.

Lee,C,K., Ng, K.S., Tan, S.G., & Ang, R. (2001). Effect of different endotracheal suctioning systems on the cardiorespiratory parameters of ventilated patients. Annals of the Academy of Medicine Singapore 30:239-244.

Lichtman, S.W., Birnbaum, I.L., Sanfilippo, M.R., Pellicone, J.T., Damon, W.J., & King, M.L. (1995). Effect of a tracheostomy speaking valve on secretions, arterial oxygenation and olfaction: a quantitative evaluation. Journal of Speech and Hearing Research 38:549-555.

Lull, J.M., Pierson, D.J., & Tyler, M.L. (1993). Methods of airway maintenance. In Intensive respiratory care. Philadelphia: WB Saunders.

McKelvie, S. (1998). Endotracheal suctioning. Nursing in Critical Care 3:244-248.

Mocaluso, S., & Roman, M. (1994). Managing post-intubation injuries. Medsurg Nursing 3:192-202.

Montgomery, W.W. (1989). Manual of care of the Montgomery silicone tracheal T-tube. Annals of Otology, Rhinology and Laryngology 89(Suppl 73):3.

Montanari, J., & Spearing, C. (1986). Of measuring tracheal cuff pressure. Nursing 86:46-49.

Ng, K.S., Kumarasinghe, G., & Inglis, T.J. (1999). Dissemination of respiratory secretions during tracheal tube suctioning in an intensive care unit. Annals of the Academy of Medicine Singapore 28:178-182.

Noll, M.L., Hix, C.D., & Scott, G. (1990). Closed tracheal suction systems: effectiveness and nursing implications. In AACN clinical issues in critical care nursing. Philadelphia: JB Lippincott.

Panacek, E.A., Albertson, T.E., Rutherford, W.F., Fisher, C.J., & Foulke, G.E. (1989). Selections left endobronchial suctioning of the intubated patient. Chest 95:885-887.

Patton, C. (1991). The critical airway classic problems. Current Reviews for the Post Anesthesia Care Nurses 13:33-40.

Pierson, D.J., & Kacmarek, R.M. (1992). In Foundations of respiratory care. New York: Churchill Livingstone.

Pritchard, M., Flenady, W., & Woodgate, P. (2001). Preoxygenation for tracheal suctioning in intubated, ventilated newborn infants. Cochrane Database System Review 3:CD000464.

Roberts, J.T. (1994). In Clinical management of the airway. Philadelphia: WB Saunders.

Selecky, P. (1974). Tracheostomy-a review of present day indication, complications and care. Heart Lung 3:272.

St. John, R.E., & Malen, J.F. (2004). Contemporary issues in adult tracheostomy management. Critical Care Nursing Clinics North America 16:413-430.

Tracheostomy tube adult homecare guide. (1993). Irvine: Mallinckrodt Medical TPI, Inc.

Traver, G.A., Mitchell, J.T., & Flodquist-Priestly, G. (1991). Artificial airway care. In Respiratory care: a clinical approach. Gaithersberg, Md.: Aspen Publishers.

Traver, G.A., Mitchell, J.T., & Flodquist-Priestly, G. (1991). Suctioning. In Respiratory care: a clinical approach. Gaithersberg, Md.: Aspen Publishers.

Wahidi, M.M., & Ernst, A. (2003). The Montgomery T-tube tracheal stent. Clinical Chest Medicine 24:437-443.

Warnoch, C., & Porpora, K. (1994). A pediatric trache card: transforming research into practice. Pediatric Nursing 20:186-188.

Weilitz, P.B., & Dettenmeier, P.A. (1994). Back to basics test your knowledge of tracheostomy tubes. American Journal of Nursing 94:46-50.

Wood, C.J. (1998). Endotracheal suctioning: a literature review. Intensive Critical Care Nursing 14:124-136.

Wood, C.J. (1998). Can nurses safely assess the need for endotracheal suction in short-term ventilated patients, instead of using routine techniques? Intensive Care Nursing 14:170-178.

C H A P T E R 4 5

Respiratory and Cardiovascular Drug Actions

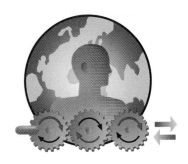

Stacy J. Laack and Arthur V. Prancan

KEY TERMS

Angiotensin-converting enzyme inhibitors
Adrenergic drugs
Alpha-adrenergic blockers
Anticholinergics
Anticholinesterase drugs
Antihistamines
Antileukotrienes
Angiotensin II receptor blockers
Beta-adrenergic blockers
Calcium-channel blockers

Cardiovascular reflex
Cholinergic drugs
Corticosteroids
Diuretics
Metered dose inhalers
Methylxanthines
Mucolytics/expectorants
Multi-dose powdered inhaler
Obstructive airway disease

The respiratory and cardiovascular systems have many built-in mechanisms for controlling their functions during health and disease. In healthy individuals, both systems act quickly and positively to maintain proper functioning under the most complicated conditions. Even during trauma or disease, these systems often overcome distress and regain normal function. Disease sometimes alters the physiology of respiration or circulation to the extent that the homeostatic mechanisms are no longer effective. In such a case, a drug with the appropriate action becomes necessary to restore normal physiological function.

Before a drug can be used effectively, the system it is to modify must be understood. How the mechanism of the drug action relates to the biological system must be clear before an effect can be predicted.

This chapter describes much of the basic respiratory and cardiovascular physiology that underlies the action of the drugs presented, with the goal of elucidating the relationship between basic physiology and the drug mechanism of action.

All pharmacological interventions for the respiratory and cardiovascular systems are not covered. Certainly no attempt has been made to describe the pharmacology of other systems or disease states. For further study, any of the texts listed in the reference section at the end of the chapter is highly recommended.

AUTONOMIC PHARMACOLOGY

This section introduces the basic aspects of drug action related to both components of the autonomic nervous system: sympathetic and parasympathetic. For both systems, synthesis, storage, and release of the chemical neurotransmitter are described to emphasize the places in the metabolic scheme where drugs can intervene. The sites of action for the adrenergic (sympathetic) and cholinergic (parasympathetic) transmitters and blockers are also described.

The autonomic nervous system controls all of the bodily functions over which the individual has no voluntary control (and which the individual might not control well given the opportunity). These functions include regulation of respiratory airway diameter, respiratory secretions, blood vessel diameter, heart rate, intestinal motility, and pupil size, among many others. It is easy to see that it might take more than the talents of a well-trained expert to keep an active person functioning day and night.

The sympathetic nervous system is the half of the autonomic system that takes a dominant role in the cardiovascular and respiratory systems when bodily activity is necessary. This includes actions such as increasing ventilation capacity, elevating blood pressure, and shunting blood flow to the skeletal muscles. Classically the sympathetic component of the autonomic nervous system has been called the fight-or-flight system. The other half of the autonomic system is called the parasympathetic nervous system. It is most important in maintaining the less exciting functions of the body like digestion, salivation, and urination. In some organs the two systems work against each other to provide very fast and very fine control. For example, the size of the pupil responds quickly to a change in light intensity. The parasympathetic system actively functions to decrease the size of the opening while the sympathetic system relaxes, thereby causing a quick decrease in pupil size. If the light is turned down, the opposite occurs just as fast. This is a good example of the antagonistic action of the two components of the autonomic nervous system.

Some organs, however, have only one innervation. Much of the arterial blood vessel network is controlled only by sympathetic nerves, whereas gastric secretion and gastric motility are primarily regulated by the parasympathetic system.

SYMPATHETIC NEUROTRANSMISSION

Sympathetic nerves transport impulses from the vasomotor center in the medulla of the brain through the spinal cord and out to the smooth muscle, heart muscle, and secretory cells. These tissues have receptor sites that will accept the norepinephrine released from the nerve ending. Norepinephrine, also called noradrenalin, is synthesized in the nerve ending only in the sympathetic neurons. It is stored in the terminal until an electric impulse reaches the terminal, then it is released into the synapse.

The norepinephrine molecule attaches to a receptor molecule on a cell surface in the immediate vicinity of its release. This drug-receptor combination causes a biological change, such as stimulation of the pacemaker cells in the heart to fire more frequently (increased heart rate). The effect is terminated when the norepinephrine is reabsorbed into the nerve terminal. About 90% of the released norepinephrine is taken back into the neuron where it is either restored into granules for future release or destroyed by the enzyme monoamine oxidase (MAO).

There are two types of sympathetic receptors: alpha and beta. The alpha-receptor is found in the arterioles, and the beta-receptor is found in the arterioles, heart, and bronchioles. Stimulation of the alpha-receptor in the arteriole causes vasoconstriction, which results in increased blood pressure. Stimulation of the beta-receptor in the arteriole causes vasodilation and lowered blood pressure. Some drugs stimulate both receptors, and in those cases the effect will be determined by the degree of alpha or beta activity of the drug. One example is norepinephrine. It has 90% alpha activity and 10% beta activity, and it always causes vasoconstriction. Epinephrine is 50% alpha and 50% beta and may cause a rise or drop in blood pressure.

Stimulation of the beta-receptor in the heart results in increased heart rate (HR) (beats per minute) and increased stroke volume (SV) (number of milliliters of blood the left ventricle pumps out into the aorta every time it contracts). Incidentally, the combination of HR and SV changes is another way to express cardiac output (CO) (milliliters of blood pumped per minute):

$$\text{beats/min (HR)} \times \text{ml/beat (SV)} = \text{ml/min (CO)}$$

This expression, cardiac output, is a common one and it constitutes half of the blood pressure regulation equation:

$$\text{CO} \times \text{TPR} = \text{BP}$$

where CO is cardiac output, TPR is total peripheral resistance, and BP is blood pressure. TPR is determined by vasoconstriction or vasodilation in the arterioles. For example, vasoconstriction increases resistance, therefore TPR and BP go up.

Stimulation of smooth muscle beta-receptors will relax these tissues wherever they are found. Respiratory airway smooth muscle will decrease tension when the beta-receptor is activated by beta-acting drugs like epinephrine or isoproterenol. The functional result will be an increase in air flow because of a larger airway diameter, otherwise referred to as bronchodilation. Likewise, blood vessels respond to beta-acting drugs by dilating as well, allowing a greater rate of flow. In this case, TPR has decreased and blood pressure will drop.

Adrenergic (Sympathomimetic) Drugs

Norepinephrine (Levarterenol, Levophed)

As mentioned previously, norepinephrine (Levarterenol, Levophed) is a mixed-activity drug (90% alpha, 10% beta). It stimulates beta-receptors in the heart, which results in an increase of heart rate and stroke volume (increased cardiac output). In the arterioles, norepinephrine causes vasoconstriction via the alpha-receptor, resulting in increased total peripheral resistance. The total effect is an increase in blood pressure. Norepinephrine has little effect on the bronchioles. This drug is given only intravenously, and it is reserved for use in hypotensive emergencies to raise blood pressure, therefore preserving blood supply to the brain and heart. The natural sympathetic compounds are known as catecholamines.

Epinephrine (Adrenalin)

Epinephrine (Adrenalin) is also a mixed-activity drug (50% alpha, 50% beta). It is naturally produced in the adrenal medulla and can be released during sympathetic nervous system activation. When this occurs, it acts as a circulating hormone, stimulating both alpha- and beta-receptors. This drug will increase heart rate and stroke volume and may slightly increase or decrease total peripheral resistance at the arterioles. In any case, cardiac output always goes up; blood pressure may go up or down slightly.

In the bronchioles, epinephrine exerts a dramatic dilating effect that is mediated by the beta-receptor. Epinephrine can be administered by inhalant aerosol to reverse a broncho-constrictive episode. It is also administered intramuscularly and subcutaneously to treat asthma, anaphylactic reactions to an allergic response, cardiac arrest, heart block, and as a mild vasoconstriction to keep local anesthetics at the injection site.

Isoproterenol (Isuprel)

Isoproterenol (Isuprel) is a synthetic compound that has 100% beta activity. This means that it can increase heart rate and stroke volume to produce a great rise in cardiac output, and it stimulates the beta-receptor on the arterioles to cause a profound vasodilation. The final result can be a high cardiac output with low blood pressure. This drug improves blood circulation in shock patients by increasing local blood flow (vasodilation) and elevating cardiac output. Isoproterenol has been useful for treating acute asthmatic conditions because of its bronchodilating action; however, it is seldom used due to the development of new, safer, beta$_2$ selective drugs.

Phenylephrine (Isophrin, Neo-Synephrine) and Metaraminol

Both phenylephrine (Isophrin, Neo-Synephrine) and metaraminol are powerful and prolonged stimulators of alpha-receptors. The action is directly on the receptor site itself. The response to the administration of either of these drugs is a rise in blood pressure because of vasoconstriction accompanied by a reflex bradycardia, which causes a decrease in cardiac output. Reflex alterations of cardiovascular function are explained later in this chapter. The primary usefulness of these drugs is in various hypotensive states. Phenylephrine is used as a nasal decongestant, mydriatic, and for the relief of paroxysmal atrial tachycardia. Phenylephrine affords relief from the tachycardia because it increases blood pressure and evokes the cardiovascular reflex that is marked by high vagal tone and bradycardia.

Ephedrine

Ephedrine has both alpha and beta activity as direct effects and it also causes release of epinephrine and norepinephrine. Its pharmacological actions are similar to epinephrine, with the main exception that duration of action of ephedrine is longer. Ephedrine increases cardiac output and vascular resistance, resulting in increased blood pressure. Ephedrine also causes bronchial muscle relaxation, which is less potent than that of epinephrine but has a longer duration. Although this drug has been useful in controlling milder cases of bronchoconstriction, it is also seldom used due to the development of new beta$_2$ selective drugs.

Amphetamine (Dextroamphetamine, Dexedrine)

Amphetamine (Dextroamphetamine, Dexedrine) drug has pharmacological properties related to the catecholamines because it causes release of norepinephrine from the nerve terminal. Amphetamine has both alpha- and beta-receptor activity, although indirectly, through its release of norepinephrine. The usual cardiovascular response is an increase in blood pressure often accompanied by a reflex bradycardia. Amphetamine also has potent central nervous system (CNS) activity. It is a stimulant of the medullary respiratory center, and it can antagonize drug-related central nervous system depression. Respiratory depression often accompanies overdoses of CNS depressant drugs and this effect may be overcome by amphetamine. This drug is usually used for its CNS effects and not for peripheral cardiovascular or respiratory effects.

Beta$_2$-Receptor Stimulants

As mentioned above, there are several drugs that act primarily at the beta$_2$ smooth muscle receptor site, causing selective actions in the bronchioles and arterioles but not in the heart. These drugs will produce a bronchodilation without increasing cardiac output. This particular lack of cardiovascular effect makes them safer than drugs like isoproterenol or ephedrine in treatment of bronchial asthma. This class of drugs is currently part of the mainstay of treatment for asthma and chronic obstructive pulmonary disease (COPD). The drugs are albuterol (Proventil, Ventolin), metaproterenol (Alupent, Metaprel), terbutaline (Brethine, Bricanyl), isoetharine (Bronkosol, Bronkometer), Pirbuterol (Maxair), Bitolterol (Tornalate), and salmeterol (Serevent).

Alpha-Adrenergic Blocking Drugs

The alpha-adrenergic blocking class of drugs should be not be used as monotherapy because of their propensity to cause fluid retention. When combined with diuretics, there is no evidence to contraindicate their use. Diuretics are drugs that act on the kidney to increase the formation of urine, therefore decreasing blood volume and fluid accumulation.

Phentolamine (Regitine)

Phentolamine (Regitine) is a competitive alpha-receptor blocker. Its action is reversible. This drug prevents the hypertensive effect of norepinephrine and reverses the blood pressure elevating effect of epinephrine (epinephrine reversal). Epinephrine reversal looks like an isoproterenol effect with high cardiac output and low blood pressure. Phentolamine may be used clinically as a vasodilator. It is useful in the emergency treatment of hypertensive patients who have pheochromocytoma, which is a tumor that grows most commonly on the adrenal glands. The tumor produces epinephrine and norepinephrine and may be responsible for one aspect of a clinical hypertension.

Phenoxybenzamine (Dibenzyline)

Phenoxybenzamine (Dibenzyline) is also an alpha-adrenergic blocking agent. It has effects similar to phentolamine in the cardiovascular system but it is less reversible. This is the drug of choice for preoperative management of pheochromocytoma. This drug is gaining some usefulness in the treatment of shock syndromes characterized by high vascular tone.

Prazosin (Minipress), Doxazosin (Cardura), and Terazosin (Hytrin)

Prazosin (Minipress), doxazosin (Cardura), and terazosin (Hytrin) are alpha$_1$ selective for arterioles and venules and are the most useful drugs in this class to deal with hypertension. They also have a dilatory effect on urethral smooth muscle and are therefore useful agents in males with enlarged prostates. Although they act by vasodilation, these drugs exert minimal reflex tachycardia because they do not potentiate the vasomotor center and the increased venous capacitance reduces venous return and cardiac output.

Beta-Adrenergic Blocking Drugs (β-Blockers)

The beta-blocker class of drugs is highly effective for the treatment of hypertension. They are commonly prescribed in conjunction with diuretics.

Propranolol (Inderal)

Propranolol (Inderal) is a beta-adrenergic blocker. This drug occupies the beta-receptor sites of the heart, the blood vessels, and the bronchioles. It prevents the beta-adrenergic effect usually seen with drugs like epinephrine, norepinephrine, and isoproterenol. In the arterioles, when epinephrine is given after propranolol, the usual mixed alpha and beta effect is eliminated, leaving only an alpha-adrenergic action. This causes profound vasoconstriction, allowing greater increase in blood pressure than is normally seen with epinephrine alone. In the heart the beta-receptors are blocked and, because there are no alpha-adrenergic receptors in this organ, all effects of catecholamine drugs on the heart are effectively eliminated, allowing the vagal influence on the heart to predominate. Propranolol decreases the heart's requirement for oxygen because it blocks the cardiac stimulant action of norepinephrine. In the respiratory system the administration of propranolol results in bronchoconstriction. This effect is increased dramatically in patients who are susceptible to asthma. The main use for propranolol is in conditions related to hypertension and tachycardia, where a decrease in cardiac output is beneficial.

Metoprolol (Lopressor) and Atenolol (Tenormin)

Metoprolol (Lopressor) and atenolol (Tenormin) are beta-adrenergic antagonists that have been designed to be cardioselective. This offers an advantage in safety when a beta-blocker must be used in patients with asthma because this disease would be aggravated if respiratory beta-receptors were blocked. The natural beta-adrenergic agonist, epinephrine, is a bronchodilator, and an important class of bronchodilating drugs acts at bronchiolar beta-adrenergic receptors.

Sympatholytic Drugs

The sympatholytic drugs are highly effective as antihypertensive agents; however, their clinical utility is limited by their side-effects profile.

Reserpine

Reserpine is an alkaloid of *Rauwolfia serpentina,* also known as the Indian snake root plant. There are many commercial preparations of this compound, but it is widely sold as the simple plant extract. This compound depletes norepinephrine from the nerve endings in the various tissues of the body that produce and store norepinephrine, including the brain. The depletion takes several days to accomplish, and it may take several weeks to restore catecholamine levels to normal after therapy is discontinued. During this time, there is a decrease in catecholamine response to sympathetic stimulation. Blood pressure in humans does not drop dramatically with therapeutic doses of reserpine, but when reserpine is used in combination with diuretics or other antihypertensive agents, a significant antihypertensive effect is obtained. Reserpine is used in this way to treat essential hypertension. One serious side effect related to reserpine use is the behavioral modification that can result in severe depression and suicide.

Guanethidine (Ismelin)

Guanethidine (Ismelin) is an adrenergic neuron-blocking agent that works by replacing norepinephrine in the nerve terminal. Norepinephrine is usually taken up by the nerve terminal after its discharge and is reused to maintain granule concentrations. Guanethidine takes the place of norepinephrine in the granules and prevents the reuptake of norepinephrine, thereby causing its metabolism outside of the neuron and its eventual depletion. The result on the cardiovascular system of this action is postural hypotension. The patient is unable to control blood pressure by sympathetic activity. This drug is no longer commonly used in the treatment of hypertension.

Methyldopa (Aldomet) and Clonidine (Catapress)

Methyldopa (Aldomet) and clonidine (Catapress) decrease the activity of the sympathetic nervous system at its control center in the brain. The consequence is a total decrease in sympathetic activity in the heart and blood vessels, which leads to a reduction in blood pressure. Methyldopa remains the drug of choice for nonemergent hypertension in pregnancy.

Clonidine comes in a patch form (transdermal administration), which is a longer acting preparation that decreases the deleterious side effect of rebound hypertension.

PARASYMPATHETIC NEUROTRANSMISSION

The center for parasympathetic control is the vagal nucleus in the medulla. The vagus nerves pass through the spinal cord and out to the heart, the smooth muscle, and exocrine glands (salivary glands and pancreas). In all of these tissues, acetylcholine (ACh) is released from the nerve terminals and combines with receptor sites to cause an effect such as bradycardia (slowing of the heart) or an increase in gastric motility. ACh is found in many parts of the central and peripheral nervous system. ACh is the only transmitter used in the parasympathetic system. It is used to transmit impulses from the nerve that comes out of the spinal cord to the nerve that finally reaches the cells in the organ being affected. This connection is called a ganglion and exists in both sympathetic and parasympathetic systems. ACh is also the neurotransmitter that makes the connection between the voluntary (somatic) nerves and the skeletal muscle.

There are two types of receptors in the central and peripheral nervous systems. ACh affects both, but some drugs affect only one and not the other. The two types of receptors are called nicotinic and muscarinic. They are named after the drugs that selectively stimulate them. Nicotine stimulates only those receptors in the ganglia and at the neuromuscular junction. The muscarinic receptor site is found everywhere a parasympathetic nerve terminal synapses at a tissue. The biological effects usually attributed to the parasympathetic nervous system, such as bradycardia, salivation, and broncho-constriction, are produced when the muscarinic receptors are stimulated. It is also possible to stimulate muscarinic receptors indirectly with a nicotinic drug by activating the parasympathetic ganglia. In a similar way, it is possible to stimulate the entire sympathetic nervous system. The neurotransmitter at the sympathetic ganglia is ACh, and it affects nicotinic receptor sites there. One of the toxic effects of ACh, and drugs that act like it, is hypertension with tachycardia, which is the result of stimulation of the sympathetic post-ganglionic fibers.

To better understand the action of ACh and related drugs, let us consider the synthesis, release, and inactivation of this transmitter. ACh is synthesized inside the nerve terminal from acetyl-CoA and choline. The ACh is then stored in granules and released out into the synapse when an action potential reaches the terminal. The ACh molecule attaches to a receptor site, muscarinic or nicotinic, or to the enzyme that breaks it apart. Combination with the receptor site results in biological action, and coupling with the enzyme ends in destruction. The enzyme, acetylcholinesterase, is found at all cholinergic synaptic sites. A nonspecific variety of the enzyme is also prevalent in many other tissues. It too will break down ACh. The final action of either enzyme is the production of acetic acid and choline. The acetic acid is washed away for further metabolism, and the choline is reabsorbed into the nerve terminal for resynthesis to ACh.

Cholinergic Drugs

Acetylcholine

ACh is the endogenous cholinergic transmitter that accounts for nicotinic and muscarinic actions within the autonomic nervous system. It is rapidly hydrolyzed by acetylcholinesterase and the nonspecific cholinesterase and therefore has a short duration of action if administered parenterally. This makes ACh a poor drug. Nicotinic effects of ACh are (1) stimulation of parasympathetic ganglia, causing occurrence of all muscarinic effects, (2) stimulation of sympathetic ganglia, causing increase in vascular resistance and cardiac output to produce hypertension, and (3) stimulation of the neuromuscular junction (NMJ) at the skeletal muscle (muscle contraction and movement). Muscarinic effects of ACh are bradycardia, salivation, pinpoint pupils, bronchial constriction, gastric and intestinal hypermotility, increased gastric acid and mucous secretion, and facilitated urination. Toxic effects of cholinergic stimulation include diarrhea, urinary incontinence, bradycardia, bronchoconstriction, excessive salivation, CNS excitement, and respiratory collapse. In all of these toxic effects, atropine, a competitive muscarinic blocker, is the antidote of choice.

Bethanecol (Urecholine)

Bethanecol (Urecholine) is a synthetic choline ester that is not destroyed as easily as ACh by cholinesterase enzymes. It is useful in treating patients with urinary retention and paralytic ileus, and it is administered orally or sub-cutaneously. The side effects and toxicities for this drug are the same as those for ACh. Because the drug is not given intravenously, however, cardiac and respiratory effects are minimized.

Carbachol (Carcholin)

Carbachol (Carcholin) is a mixed nicotinic and muscarinic drug because it releases ACh from the nerve ending, producing the expected cholinergic effects at all receptor sites. The drug is useful for treatment of glaucoma (applied topically), paralytic ileus, and urinary retention (orally and subcutaneously).

Pilocarpine (Pilocar, Salagen)

Pilocarpine (Pilocar) is a cholinomimetic that is useful in ophthalmology as an antiglaucoma agent. Cholinergic compounds decrease intraocular pressure by relieving the obstruction to the canal of Schlemm, a drainage circuit for the eye. Miosis (pinpoint pupils) is one feature of cholinergic therapy and may be beneficial to glaucoma treatment because the muscular base of the relaxed iris may contribute to the drainage block. Another use of pilocarpine (Salagen) is to promote salivary flow in patients with a ganglionic blockade.

Anticholinesterase Drugs

Before proceeding to specific anticholinesterase drugs, it is important to understand the basic mechanism of action for these compounds. Acetylcholinesterase is the enzyme responsible for destroying ACh at the various nerve junctions where it is released. The class of drugs that interfere with this function is called anticholinesterases. These drugs attach to the enzyme and thereby block the enzymatic hydrolysis of ACh, causing ACh to accumulate outside of the nerve ending. This results in a greater response than normal to any cholinergic nerve stimulation. Some of these anticholinesterases are relatively short-acting compounds and are therapeutically important, whereas others are extremely long-lasting and potent compounds that are important only as poisons. The long-acting compounds have been used as insecticides and as nerve gases in chemical warfare. The therapeutically useful anticholinesterases are beneficial in problems related to the eye, intestine, and the skeletal neuromuscular junction (NMJ). In these applications, these drugs increase the amount of ACh available for activity, an effect that is especially important in cases where the synthesis or release of ACh is lower than normal, as in myasthenia gravis.

There is great medical interest in the toxicology of the anticholinesterases, especially the extremely potent irreversible anticholinesterases. Toxicity due to these compounds is not uncommon and is often severe. When a toxic irreversible anticholinesterase, such as diisopropylfluorophosphate (DFP) or sarin, is ingested, inhaled, or absorbed across the skin, a great variety of toxic cholinergic effects are seen. The first effects seen after exposure to an anticholinesterase are often ocular and respiratory effects. In the eyes, marked miosis is produced quickly. In the respiratory system, broncho-constriction and bronchial secretions combine to produce tightness in the chest and wheezing. Gastrointestinal symptoms include nausea, vomiting, cramps, and diarrhea. Other muscarinic effects are severe salivation, involuntary defecation and urination, sweating, lacrimation, bradycardia, and hypotension.

Further effects of anticholinesterases are related to nicotinic functions of ACh. These include skeletal muscle twitching, weakness, and paralysis. CNS effects include depression of the respiratory and cardiovascular control centers, leading to respiratory collapse. At the time of death, respiratory paralysis is evident and it is because of a combination of bronchoconstriction, bronchosecretions, respiratory muscle paralysis from overstimulation, and CNS/control center depression. The treatment of this toxicity is closely related to preserving respiratory function. Administration of atropine, a muscarinic blocker, will effectively decrease bronchoconstriction and secretion. Another drug, pralidoxime (Protopam), is used to reactivate the acetylcholinesterase. It is most effective shortly after exposure to the toxic agent because it breaks down the anticholinesterase so it can be removed from the enzyme site. Additional measures are related to physiological support of the patient. Maintenance

of an airway, artificial respiration, and oxygen administration are important therapeutic applications for these patients.

Physostigmine (Eserine)

Physostigmine (Eserine) is useful in glaucoma and in selected therapeutic measures where a cholinergic effect is beneficial. It can also be used as an antidote for various anticholinergic agents. It functions as an indirect cholinomimetic by blocking the acetylcholinesterase.

Neostigmine (Prostigmine)

Neostigmine (Prostigmine) is useful in patients with non-obstructive paralytic ileus to increase tone and motility of the small and large intestines. It is also useful for stimulating skeletal NMJ. Neostigmine is used for treating myasthenia gravis because it indirectly increases ACh at the NMJ and it acts directly at the nicotinic receptor site itself. The disease is marked by subnormal response to ACh, resulting in skeletal muscle weakness. Neostigmine temporarily restores muscle strength.

Edrophonium (Tensilon)

Edrophonium (Tensilon) is a very short-acting anti-cholinesterase. It is primarily useful as a diagnostic agent in myasthenia gravis to reveal, for a few minutes, whether the dose of neostigmine is appropriate. A longer-acting drug would risk a serious cholinergic toxicity if the neostigmine dose was already at the therapeutic limit.

Donepezil (Aricept), Rivastigmine (Exelon), and Galantamine (Reminyl)

Donepezil (Aricept), rivastigmine (Exelon), and galantamine (Reminyl) increase ACh levels, which are found to be decreased in patients with Alzheimer's disease. These drugs are not only efficacious in improving cognition but are found to improve activities of daily living and other neuropsychiatric symptoms. Donepezil (Aricept) is currently most often prescribed due to the advantage of once-a-day dosing.

Cholinergic Blocking Drugs (Anticholinergics)

Cholinergic antagonists block the various receptor sites where ACh is a transmitter. There are specific blocking drugs for each type of ACh receptor. Atropine blocks all cholinergic action right at the muscarinic receptor site on smooth muscle, exocrine glands, and myocardium. The cholinergic antagonist curare works only at the neuromuscular junction to block the nicotinic effect of ACh, resulting in paralysis of skeletal muscle. Still another type of nicotinic blocker is the ganglionic blocker hexamethonium, which blocks both sympathetic and parasympathetic ganglia by occupying the ACh receptor there. These drugs are useful wherever sympathetic or parasympathetic tone needs to be decreased. It is possible to selectively inhibit cholinergic effects in the body to produce a desired effect or to eliminate an undesirable effect. Because of this selectiveness, cholinergic antagonists have widespread use in many areas of medicine.

Atropine

Atropine is an extract from the plant *Atropa belladonna,* also known as the deadly nightshade. Another plant extract, scopolamine, has action similar to atropine. Atropine works by establishing a competitive blockage at the muscarinic receptor site, which is the effector at all tissues innervated by the parasympathetic nervous system. This blockade is selective for the tissue effect of the parasympathetic system and does not counteract the nicotinic ganglionic effects or the nicotinic effects at the NMJ.

Because heart rate is controlled by both sympathetic and parasympathetic tone, atropine will eliminate the parasympathetic effect on the heart, allowing the sympathetic system to increase heart rate and stroke volume to cause an increase in cardiac output. In fact, tachycardia may occur after atropine administration. In cases where bradycardia exists because of high vagal tone, atropine can be used to reverse this depression.

In the respiratory tract, atropine is a bronchodilator. It is also possible to delay respiratory depression associated with anesthetic, tranquilizing, and anticholinesterase drugs by using atropine, either as a pretreatment agent or as an antidote during overdose.

Atropine is used widely as preanesthetic medication to prevent bronchiolar secretions and laryngeal spasm, as well as bradycardia. A more general medical use for atropine exists as an emergency tool. It is the antidote of choice for all cholinergic toxicities.

One of the most important clinical uses for atropine is in the gastrointestinal (GI) tract as an antiulcer and antispasmodic agent. This drug acts to decrease motility in the GI tract so that other antiulcer agents can remain in contact with the GI mucosa longer, and it is possible that it also decreases acid secretion. Other problems related to hypermotility of the GI tract are treated with atropine, mainly to decrease gastric muscle activity during treatment of conditions such as cramping and diarrhea.

In ophthalmology, atropine is useful for producing mydriasis, which is pupillary dilation. It is contraindicated in glaucoma patients because it may precipitate an acute attack.

Atropine itself is also capable of producing toxic effects. These are mydriasis, tachycardia, dry mouth, constipation, and urinary retention. Effects related to the CNS are also apparent and include initial sedation followed by delirium and hallucinations, which lead to a coma. In severe toxicities the patient convulses and experiences severe respiratory depression, which may be the final course. Anticholinesterase drugs, such as physostigmine and neostigmine, are effective antidotes for atropine because they increase the amount of ACh that will compete with atropine for the receptor site.

Ipratropium (Atrovent) and Tiotropium (Spiriva)

Ipratropium (Atrovent) is a synthetic analog of atropine and is more frequently used than atropine in the treatment of asthma. It has also proved useful in the treatment of chronic obstructive pulmonary disease (COPD). It is administered in aerosolized form. This route provides the advantage of maximal concentration at the bronchial target tissue with limited systemic effects. Tiotropium (Spiriva) is a long-acting anticholinergic, exhibiting bronchodilation in the lungs with indications for COPD. Like ipratropium, it exerts site-specific effects. Tiotropium is a dry powder that is inhaled.

Homatropine (Novatrin) and Cyclopentolate (Cyclogyl)

Homatropine (Novatrin) and cyclopentolate (Cyclogyl) are anticholinergic drugs related in action to atropine. They are useful in ophthalmology to produce mydriasis.

Dicyclomine (Bentyl)

Dicyclomine (Bentyl) is considered very useful in the gastrointestinal tract to decrease secretions and motility. It is sometimes called a chemical vagotomy.

Trihexyphenidyl HCL (Artane) and Benztropine Mesylate (Cogentin)

Trihexyphenidyl HCL (Artane) and benztropine mesylate (Cogentin) are primarily antiparkinson drugs that enter the CNS to reverse the imbalance between the cholinergic and dopaminergic systems in this disease. They have some of the same side effects as atropine.

Trimethaphan (Arphonad) and Mecamylamine (Inversine)

Trimethaphan (Arphonad) and mecamylamine (Inversine) are currently the only ganglionic blockers available in the United States. They block the ACh receptor site in the ganglia in both the sympathetic and parasympathetic nervous systems. Because of their blocking action at the sympathetic ganglion, these drugs will produce a postural hypotension. They will also decrease cholinergic effects at the parasympathetic effector sites because they block the ganglia for the entire parasympathetic nervous system as well. This means that a patient may experience blurred vision, dry mouth, and tachycardia, as well as other atropine-like peripheral effects. They have been surpassed by many other drugs to control hypertension. Their only remaining use is occasionally for the initial control of blood pressure in patients with an aortic dissection who have preexisting contraindications to other drugs. Another clinical use is to induce controlled hypotension during surgery to minimize blood loss.

CARDIOVASCULAR REFLEX

The cardiovascular reflex involves many of the components of the autonomic nervous system to maintain a normal blood pressure. This mechanism is important for maintaining blood pressure within certain limits during all phases of physical activity. Even the simple act of standing from a seated position requires prompt compensation by this reflex system. If in some way this reflex is interrupted, a condition known as orthostatic hypotension will exist. A common manifestation of this condition is fainting upon standing because of inadequate blood flow to the brain. This section is devoted to the functional aspects of the reflex after a change in blood pressure.

Carotid Baroreceptors

Neuronal elements, known as baroreceptors, exist in the sinus of the carotid arteries supplying the brain. These are stretch receptors that fire electrical impulses at a rate directly related to blood pressure. As the pressure in the artery increases, the vessel wall (and baroreceptor) stretches, causing an increase in the receptor firing rate. Conversely, a decrease in blood pressure results in a decrease in stretch receptor firing rate. This firing rate signal is sent directly to the brain, where the vasomotor center and vagal nucleus respond to it.

Functional Reflex

As an example to demonstrate this reflex, let us assume we have just experienced a loss of blood pressure. The carotid baroreceptors shorten and slow their firing. This message is then delivered to the brain, and the vasomotor center responds by increasing sympathetic nerve activity. This control always responds to information regarding blood pressure in the carotid artery by directly opposing the baroreceptors. If the pressure had risen, the baroreceptors would have increased their firing rate and the vasomotor center would have responded by slowing the sympathetic nerve firing rate. Because blood pressure in this example is low, the vasomotor center increases sympathetic nerve firing, resulting in increased release of norepinephrine from the nerves that reach the heart and arterioles. Norepinephrine increases the heart rate and stroke volume, thereby producing an increase in cardiac output. In the arterioles, norepinephrine stimulates the alpha-receptors, producing vasoconstriction, which results in increased resistance and ultimately raised blood pressure. A third component of the sympathetic nervous system can be involved during sympathetic activation: epinephrine released from the adrenal medulla also increases cardiac output. Meanwhile the vagal nucleus responds to the decreased baroreceptor firing by decreasing its own activity. The vagus nerve to the heart releases less ACh, allowing the sympathetic effect to predominate. The total effect becomes an increase in blood pressure, which is the response required to return the systemic pressure to normal. If the original pressure alteration had been an increase to above normal blood pressure, the opposite reflexive actions would have occurred to return pressure to a normal range. The predominant effect would have been an increase in vagal nerve tone to release high amounts of ACh at the heart, causing a dramatic slowing of heart rate accompanied by a decrease in stroke volume. This combination produces a decrease in cardiac output. The sympathetic system would have responded to the increased baroreceptor firing by decreasing firing in all sympathetic nerves, thereby decreasing norepinephrine and epinephrine release. All of these factors combine to decrease blood pressure to normal.

OTHER DRUG CLASSES USED IN THE TREATMENT OF HYPERTENSION

As mentioned in the previous sections, there are many drugs that have the potential to affect blood pressure, cardiac output, heart rate, etc. Many studies have been done to establish appropriate guidelines for patients with hypertension, which is an important risk factor for heart disease and stroke. The Antihypertensive and Lipid Lowering Treatment to Prevent Heart Attack Trial (ALLHAT) found that it takes at least two medications of different classes to treat most cases of mild hypertension, and three to four medications for those with severe hypertension (Davis, et al, 2004). The JNC 7 report (2003) recommends starting patients on a two-drug regimen in which one of the drugs is a diuretic. There are many types of diuretics, all classified according to which part of the kidney is affected and what type of action is performed. Some examples are hydrochlorothiazide (HCTZ) (HydroDIURIL), furosemide (Lasix), and spironolactone (Aldactone). In addition to the diuretics and beta-blockers discussed previously, there are angiotensin-converting enzyme (ACE) inhibitors, angiotensin II receptor blockers (ARBs), calcium-channel blockers, and many drugs that combine two of these classes. These drugs are commonly used for the treatment of hypertension but are also used in heart failure and other heart diseases.

ACE inhibitors and ARBs affect a cascade of events that ultimately leads to an increase in blood pressure. This is known as the renin-angiotensin system. The endogenous components of this system effect vascular tone and thereby affect blood pressure. Renin is an enzyme produced by the kidneys and released in response to changes in blood pressure. When renin is circulated throughout the bloodstream, it comes in contact with angiotensinogen, which is synthesized by the liver and circulates throughout the body. The angiotensinogen is then converted to angiotensin I. With the aid of ACE, angiotensin I is converted to angiotensin II, which has vasoconstricting effects. Bradykinins are inflammatory mediators that are also broken down by ACE. ACE inhibitors block the enzyme and do not allow angiotensin I to be converted or bradykinins to be broken down. Excessive bradykinins can cause many systemic effects, one of them being chronic cough. Some patients need to be taken off their ACE inhibitor for that reason. Two examples of the many ACE inhibitors commonly used are enalapril (Vasotec) and lisinopril (Prinivil). Another class of drugs known as the ARBs has helped eliminate chronic cough as well as many other side effects. ARBs work by blocking the receptor to which angiotensin II binds. Therefore, angiotensin II is not able to exert its vasoconstrictive effects on the body, and the result is a decrease in blood pressure. Some examples of ARBs are losartan (Cozaar), candesartan (Atacand), and valsartan (Diovan).

Calcium-channel blockers are another class of drugs used to treat HTN, but are unrelated to the renin-angiotensin system. There are calcium channels on the cardiac myocytes that, when activated, increase heart rate and contractility as well as vasoconstriction. Therefore, when these channels are blocked, the opposite occurs: heart rate, contractility, and vasodilation decrease. In addition to the treatment of hypertension, calcium-channel blockers can be used in heart failure and other heart diseases. Some examples of calcium-channel blockers are diltiazem (Cardizem), nifedipine (Procardia-XL), and verapamil (Calan).

The ACE inhibitors, ARBs, and calcium-channel blockers have many side effects and contraindications that are not discussed here but can be reviewed in any of the texts referenced herein. Although they all have different mechanisms of action, they all work towards reducing blood pressure and decreasing the risk of heart damage.

DRUGS USED IN OBSTRUCTIVE AIRWAY DISEASE

Patients suffering from asthma or COPD (emphysema or chronic bronchitis) may have an obstructed airway for several reasons. Acute asthmatic obstruction and some chronic airway obstruction are due to bronchial smooth muscle contraction, which results in a smaller diameter airway. Inflamed passageways, which are swollen because of edema, may also constitute an airway obstruction. A further complication seen in many respiratory diseases is the thickening and collection of secretions that cannot be eliminated from the respiratory tree and subsequently block the airway. In this section the various drugs that can reverse smooth muscle contraction, inflammatory edema, and collection of secretions are presented.

A variety of therapeutic mechanisms are useful against this collection of obstructive conditions. The single most effective mechanism for relief of smooth muscle spasm is the aerosolized beta$_2$ activity that is available in some of the adrenergic agents. Other useful mechanisms aim at potentiating the beta activity of adrenergic agents, decongesting the inflamed airway, decreasing release of histamine, and, in a broader approach, generally stabilizing cells that can release mediators of the disease, thereby lowering the severity of the disease. The following drugs will be discussed in regards to their actions in obstructive airway disease.

Adrenergic (Sympathomimetic) Drugs

Epinephrine (Adrenalin)

The muscle relaxant bronchodilator effect attributed to the beta-adrenergic sympathomimetic compounds is most commonly required for asthmatic or allergic emergencies. During a severe exacerbation of asthma when a patient is unable to coordinate aerosolized treatments, epinephrine can be given via subcutaneous routes. It is commonly used in systemic anaphylactic reactions as well. As mentioned earlier, epinephrine has 50% beta-adrenergic activity and exerts a great bronchodilating effect. Epinephrine may cause an anxiety reaction in a patient along with headache, palpitations, and respiratory difficulty. It can also cause serious cardiac reactions (dysrhythmias), which have resulted in death.

Ephedrine

Ephedrine is a sympathomimetic that acts by liberating norepinephrine and epinephrine from storage sites in addition to possibly directly effecting adrenergic receptors. Its usefulness and side effects are similar to those of epinephrine. Because of the development of more efficacious and beta$_2$-selective agonists, it is used infrequently in the treatment of asthma.

Albuterol (Proventil, Ventolin), Metaproterenol (Alupent, Metaprel), Terbutaline (Brethine, Bricanyl), Pirbuterol (Maxair), and Salmeterol (Serevent)

Albuterol (Proventil, Ventolin), metaproterenol (Alupent, Metaprel), terbutaline (Brethine, Bricanyl), pirbuterol (Maxair), and salmeterol (Serevent) are isoproterenol analogs that are specific beta$_2$-receptor agonists. They therefore exert most of their action on respiratory or vascular smooth muscle but have little effect on the heart. They are useful compounds for selectively relaxing bronchial smooth muscles in asthma and COPD. The major advantage of these drugs is that their action on the heart is minimal or absent, and their potential for inducing cardiac toxicities is correspondingly reduced. Although these beta agonists can be given orally, they are most often given by inhalation, which minimizes their systemic absorption and potential for side effects. Salmeterol (Serevent) is a long-acting beta$_2$ agonist, and is recommended to be used in combination with an inhaled steroid for the treatment of asthma.

Anticholinergics

Ipratropium (Atrovent) and Tiotropium (Spiriva)

Ipratropium (Atrovent), mentioned earlier in this chapter, is a synthetic analog of atropine used for its bronchodilatory effects. It is commonly used in conjunction with a beta$_2$ agonist to provide effective control in chronic stable asthma and in acute exacerbations of asthma. It has also proved useful in the treatment of symptomatic COPD. There is a wide variability in response to the medication from patient to patient, and this is thought to be from the difference in parasympathetic tone in individuals. Due to its aerosolized form, it provides maximal concentration at the bronchial target tissue with limited systemic effects. As mentioned before, tiotropium (Spiriva) is a new anticholinergic on the market used in COPD patients as well. It can be taken in once-a-day doses and is indicated only for maintenance treatment. It is dispensed in a powder form, from a multi-dose powder inhaler.

Methylxanthines

Methylxanthines have effects similar to the catecholamines in the respiratory and cardiovascular systems. This similarity in effect may be due to the elevation of cyclic adenosine mono-phosphate (AMP.) Both the catecholamines and methylxanthines are known to produce elevated cyclic AMP levels in the tissues they stimulate. The catecholamines activate adenylate cyclase, the enzyme that converts adenosine triphosphate (ATP) to cyclic AMP. The newly formed cyclic AMP exerts its effects on the local tissue (e.g., bronchial muscle relaxation) and is inactivated by the enzyme phosphodiesterase. The methylxanthines inhibit phosphodiesterase, conserving cyclic AMP and thereby promoting its effects. Additional actions of methylxanthines may be direct smooth muscle relaxation that could increase airway diameter, and antagonism of adenosine, which is bronchoconstricting.

Theophylline and Aminophylline

Theophylline and aminophylline are structurally very similar to caffeine. Treatment with either of these drugs is recommended only for patients with moderate or severe persistent asthma who are receiving other controller medications, such as inhaled steroids or antileukotrienes, but whose asthma is still not adequately controlled. They are given orally or intravenously and can be used in the inpatient or outpatient setting. In either situation, drug levels in the blood must be monitored due to the toxic effects and the difference in metabolism between patients. Theophylline and aminophylline are not frequently seen in use due to the advances in other asthma therapies.

Corticosteroids

The antiinflammatory steroids are related to the naturally occurring glucocorticoid cortisol (prednisone, methyl-prednisolone, and beclomethasone). Many compounds have been synthetically derived to produce a variety of anti-inflammatory potencies. The usefulness of corticosteroids in treating respiratory diseases depends on the ability of these drugs to depress the symptoms of inflamed tissue. The mechanism of action for the drugs, however, has not clearly been defined. Some specific effects of corticosteroids that relate to the antiinflammatory action are decreased capillary dilation and permeability, and stabilization of lysosomal membranes in white blood cells. In addition, these compounds decrease the synthesis of compounds that can promote broncho-obstructive disease-prostaglandins and leukotrienes. The long-term use of the corticosteroids is recommended only after other measures fail. The reason for this caution is that they produce serious side effects and permanent changes if used for two weeks or longer. After one week of cortico-steroid therapy, behavioral changes and acute peptic ulcers may be observed. When longer therapy is instituted and adrenal suppression occurs, however, the patient requires supplemental corticosteroid therapy until normal adrenal cortex function is restored. This state of insufficiency may last for as long as several months after suppression. Most patients who receive corticosteroids for long-term therapy develop a condition called Cushing's syndrome. It is characterized by wasting of muscles because of protein breakdown and by redistribution of fat from the extremities to the face and trunk. Eventually these patients develop osteoporosis and diabetes. Other serious complications are peptic ulcers, psychosis, glaucoma, intercranial hypertension, and growth retardation. The time to onset of side effects can be prolonged and the severity of effects can be minimized by applying dosing strategies that provide antiinflammatory benefit in the lung at low systemic doses. Corticosteroids can be given at low doses in alternate-day administration or by inhalation in a form that is not systemically absorbed.

Budesonide (Pulmicort), Flunisolide (Aerobid), Fluticasone (Flovent), and Triamcinolone (Azmacort)

In the treatment of persistent asthma, inhaled steroids are shown to be effective and safer treatments. They do not modify the progression of the disease; however they improve the day-to-day symptoms. Some examples of these are budesonide (Pulmicort), flunisolide (Aerobid), fluticasone (Flovent), and triamcinolone (Azmacort). Oral steroids such as methylprednisolone or prednisone are reserved for acute exacerbations of asthma. In a life-threatening situation, intra-venous methylprednisolone can be given and then switched to oral administration and tapered off over two to three weeks. If the patient is not on an inhaled steroid at this time, one is initiated. In rare cases when a patient has continued difficulty controlling asthma, the steroids can be taken every other day. This type of treatment is not routinely recommended due to the deleterious side effects of chronic steroid use. In the treatment of severe COPD with multiple exacerbations, evidence shows that inhaled steroids in combination with beta$_2$ agonists reduce the frequency and severity of the exacerbations. An example of a steroid/ beta$_2$ agonist is fluticasone/salmeterol (Advair Diskus). As in the treatment of asthma, oral steroids (methlyprednisolone, prednisone) are reserved for acute exacerbations of COPD, and usually patients are sent home on a short, tapered course.

Antihistamine

Cromolyn Sodium (Intal) and Nedocromil Sodium (Tilade)

Cromolyn sodium (Intal) and nedocromil sodium (Tilade) can prevent asthma attacks resulting from specific stimulants, such as exercise or allergen exposure. The mechanism of action is probably the stabilization of the mast cell that synthesizes, stores, and releases histamine. Because histamine can precipitate broncho-obstructive reactions, these drugs are useful by preventing its release. They are administered by inhalation and are frequently used in the pediatric population and/or when a specific stimulant is identified.

Antileukotrienes

Zileuton (Zyflo), Zafirlukast (Accolate), and Montelukast (Singulair)

Leukotrienes are eicosanoids that are prevalent in many body tissues. In the lungs they are potent bronchoconstrictors that can be up to 1000 times more potent than histamine. They also are responsible for increasing mucus production and they enhance eosinophil and basophil influx into the airways. The development of the class of drugs referred to as antileukotrienes works in two ways. They are classified as either leukotriene-synthesis inhibitors (zileuton) or they are leukotriene-receptor antagonists (zafirlukast and montelukast). They have been proven to be effective as prophylactic treatment in mild cases of asthma, but there are no clear guidelines for moderate or severe asthma treatment. They are currently used as monotherapy for mild asthma or in conjunction with inhaled steroids for more severe asthma. Most studies show that they moderately improve lung function and decrease symptoms and exacerbations. These drugs are dispensed in oral form.

Mucolytics and Expectorants

Acetylcysteine (Mucomyst)

Acetylcysteine (Mucomyst) is a mucolytic that acts by breaking the chemical bonds that hold together the large protein structure that contributes to the viscosity of mucus. Mucolytics are inhaled to liquify mucus so that it can be moved out of the bronchial tract to prevent airway obstruction. Side effects associated with these drugs are bronchospasm, nausea, and vomiting. Acetylcysteine also inactivates the penicillin antibiotics and is contraindicated in their presence. Mucolytics are used in conjunction with other medications in COPD or asthma, but they are most commonly used in patients with upper respiratory illnesses. They are usually administered by inhalation.

Guaifenesin (Mucinex)

Guaifenesin (Mucinex) is an expectorant that acts by increasing production of respiratory secretions, therefore encouraging their ejection and making coughs more productive. It can be used in chronic disease, but most commonly is used in acute respiratory illnesses. It is dispensed in oral form. The primary side effect is gastrointestinal upset.

DRUG INHALATION DEVICES

Most drugs administered by inhalation in respiratory disease are delivered by pressurized metered-dose inhalers (MDI) (Figure 45-1) or nebulizers. MDIs rely on pressurized chloroflurocarbon or hydrofluoroalkane propellants to deliver very small drug particles (less than 5-micron diameter) into the airway. Each activation of the metered valve allows an accurately determined volume (dose) of propellant and drug

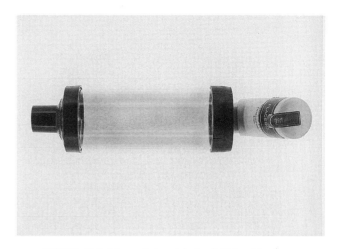

FIGURE 45-1 Metered-dose inhaler (MDI) with spacer.

mixture to be released at a high velocity. A nebulizer is a machine that delivers the drug after it has been aerosolized with room air. One important advantage of a nebulizer is that the patient does not need hand/breathing coordination, which is further discussed below. The nebulizer, however, is not portable like an MDI and is more expensive than an MDI.

The delivery of drugs to the site of action in the airway by any type of inhalation is inefficient, and therefore, correct technique in MDI use is an important concern. The MDI will allow delivery of 20% of the metered drug to the airway if the patient correctly coordinates the proper rate of inhalation with activation of the device and then adequately holds his or her breath before exhalation. It is estimated that 50% or fewer patients manage the drug delivery correctly. In response, patient education on correct MDI technique is an important part of therapy, and additional devices, called spacers, have been developed to allow success with variations in technique. The spacers come in various configurations, but they all provide a chamber between the patient and the MDI, which can be charged with the drug-propellant mixture that is then inhaled without concern for critical timing. Patients with poor MDI technique should benefit from the addition of a spacer (see Figure 45.1).

An alternative to the MDI, for patients who have difficulty with the inhalation technique, is the single-dose or multi-dose powder inhaler (Figure 45-2). This device offers a drug compounded into a fine powder that is delivered from a container on simple inhalation by the patient. Coordination of drug delivery is simple and not a problem because only inspiration by the patient drives powder delivery to the airway. The method offers the same or lower efficacy of drug delivery (6% to 20%) compared with MDI. Also, a relatively high airflow is needed to suspend the powder properly. Therefore, young children and the elderly may not benefit from this type of device. Overall, studies have shown that if the patient uses the correct technique, each of the delivery devices provides similar outcomes (Dolovich, et al, 2005).

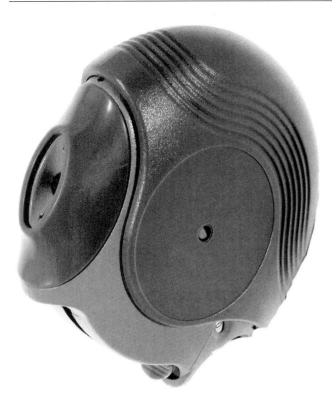

FIGURE 45-2 Multi-dose powder inhaler.

Review Questions

1. Why is it important to have an understanding of the system that a drug is to modify?
2. Describe the function of beta-blockers, diuretics, ACE inhibitors, and ARBs in the treatment of high blood pressure.
3. What is the cardiovascular reflex and why is it important to physical therapists?
4. What is the pharmacologic rationale for treatment of patients with obstructive airway disease?
5. Why is a patient's compliance with medications a concern of the physical therapist?

REFERENCES

Ciccone, C.D. (Ed). (2002). Pharmacology in Rehabilitation, ed 3. Pennsylvania: F.A. Davis Company.

Davis, B.R., Furberg, C.D., Jackson T.W. Jr., Cutler, J.A., & Whelton, P. (2004). ALLHAT: setting the record straight. Annals of Internal Medicine 141:39-46.

Dolovich, M.B., Ahrens, R.C., Hess, D.R., Anderson, P., Dhand, R., Rau, J.L., Smaldone, G.C., Guyatt, G. American College of Chest Physicians, & American College of Asthma, Allergy, and Immunology. (2005). Device selection and outcomes of aerosol therapy: evidence-based guidelines: American college of chest physicians/American college of asthma, allergy, and immunology. Chest 127:335-71.

Goldman, L., & Ausiello, D. (Eds). (2004). Cecil textbook of medicine, ed 22. Pennsylvania: Saunders.

Hardman, J., Gilman, A.G., Limbird, L., & Rall, T.W. (Eds). (2001). The pharmacological basis of therapeutics. New York: McGraw-Hill Companies.

Katzung, B.G. (Ed). (2004). Basic and clinical pharmacology, ed 9. New York: McGraw-Hill Companies.

National Heart, Lung, and Blood Institute. (2003). The seventh report of the Joint National Committee on Prevention, Detection, Evaluation, and Treatment of High Blood Pressure (NIH Publication No. 03-5233). Washington, D.C.: U.S. Government Printing Office.

Tintinalli, J.E. (Ed). (2004). Emergency medicine: a comprehensive study guide. New York: McGraw-Hill Companies.

G L O S S A R Y

Acid-base balance: A condition that exists when the net rate at which the body produces acids or bases equals the net rate at which acids or bases are excreted. The result of acid-base balance is a stable concentration of hydrogen ions in body fluids. The amount of acid or base in the arterial blood is measured by pH.

Acidosis: A process causing acidemia, which is a blood pH of less than 7.38.

Acute exacerbation of chronic airflow limitation: An increase in the severity of the signs and symptoms of chronic airflow limitation, usually triggered by infection, inflammation, or increased sputum production.

Acute lung injury: Injury to the lung characterized by a clinical spectrum of parenchymal lung dysfunction resulting from multiple etiologies and leading to alveolar capillary membrane leaking (high protein content). Mild-to-moderate injury results in noncardiogenic edema, and severe injury results in adult respiratory distress syndrome. The hallmarks of worsening lung injury include refractory hypoxemia, right-to-left shunt, and reduced lung compliance.

Adult respiratory distress syndrome (ARDS): A respiratory syndrome characterized by respiratory insufficiency and hypoxemia. Triggers include aspiration of a foreign body, cardiopulmonary bypass surgery, gram-negative sepsis, multiple blood transfusions, oxygen toxicity, trauma, pneumonia, and other respiratory infection.

Aerosol: Nebulized particles suspended in a gas or air.

Airway clearance: The removal of mucus and foreign material from the airways.

Airway-clearance deficits: Deficits in the ability to remove mucus and foreign material from the airways.

Alveolar proteinosis: A disorder marked by the accumulation of plasma proteins, lipoproteins, and other blood components in the alveoli of the lungs. The cause is unknown and clinical symptoms vary, although only the lungs are affected. Some patients are asymptomatic, whereas others show dyspnea and an unproductive cough.

Alveolar ventilation: The volume of inspired air that reaches the alveolar level and participates in gas exchange, measured by PCO_2.

Alveolitis: An allergic pulmonary reaction to the inhalation of antigenic substances characterized by acute episodes of dyspnea, cough, sweating, fever, weakness, and pain in the joints and muscles lasting from 12 to 18 hours. Recurrent episodes may lead to chronic obstructive lung disease with weight loss, increasing exertional dyspnea, and interstitial fibrosis.

Anesthesia: The absence of normal sensation, especially sensitivity to pain, as induced by an anesthetic substance or by hypnosis or as occurs with traumatic or pathophysiological damage to nerve tissue.

Angina: (often angina pectoris) A paroxysmal thoracic pain caused most often by myocardial anoxia as a result of atherosclerosis of the coronary arteries. The pain usually radiates down the inner aspect of the left arm and is frequently accompanied by a feeling of suffocation and impending death. Attacks of angina pectoris are often related to exertion, emotional stress, and exposure to intense cold.

Ankylosing spondylitis: A chronic inflammatory disease of unknown origin, first affecting the spine and adjacent structures and commonly progressing to eventual fusion (ankylosis) of the involved joints. In addition to the spine, the joints of the hip, shoulder, neck, ribs, and jaw are often involved. Physical therapy aids in keeping the spine as erect as possible to prevent flexion contractures. In advanced cases, surgery may be performed to straighten a badly deformed spine.

Arrhythmia: An abnormal heart rhythm represented by an irregularity of the timing or appearance of the ECG tracing. This term is often used synonymously with dysrhythmia.

Arterial blood gas: A test to evaluate the acid-base balance and partial pressures of oxygen and carbon dioxide in the arterial blood.

Arteriovenous-oxygen difference (a-vo$_2$ difference): The difference between the oxygen content in arterial blood versus venous blood.

Artifact: Extraneous deflection of the ECG waveform caused by movement or electrical interference. Artifact may be mistaken for a dysrhythmia.

Artificial airway: A plastic or rubber device that can be inserted into the upper or lower respiratory tract to facilitate ventilation or the removal of secretions.

Assessment: An evaluation or appraisal of a condition.

Assisted cough: Physical assistance with coughing, provided either by the patient or an assistant.

Asthma: A respiratory disorder characterized by recurring episodes of paroxysmal dyspnea, wheezing on expiration/inspiration because of constriction of the bronchi, coughing, and viscous mucoid bronchial secretions. Treatment may include elimination of the causative agent, hyposensitization, aerosol or oral bronchodilators, beta-adrenergic drugs, methylxanthines, and short-term use of corticosteroids.

Atelectasis: An abnormal condition characterized by the collapse of lung tissue, preventing the respiratory exchange of carbon dioxide and oxygen. Symptoms may include diminished breath sounds, a mediastinal shift toward the side of the collapse, fever, and increasing dyspnea.

Atherosclerosis: A common arterial disorder characterized by yellowish plaques of cholesterol, lipids, and cellular debris in the inner layers of the walls of large and medium-sized arteries. The vessel walls become thick, fibrotic, and calcified, and the lumen narrows, resulting in reduced blood flow to organs normally supplied by the artery. Antilipidemic agents do not reverse atherosclerosis, but a diet low in cholesterol, calories, and saturated fats, adequate exercise, and the avoidance of smoking and stress may help prevent the disorder.

Blood: The liquid pumped by the heart through all the arteries, veins, and capillaries. Blood is composed of a clear yellow fluid (called plasma), the formed elements, and a series of cell types with different functions. The major function of the blood is to transport oxygen and nutrients to the cells and remove carbon dioxide and other waste products from the cells for detoxification and elimination.

Body mechanics: Using one's body effectively to prevent injury.

Bradycardia: An abnormally slow heart rate.

Bradypnea: A decreased respiratory rate under 10 breaths per minute.

Bronchiectasis: An abnormal condition of the bronchial tree characterized by irreversible dilatation and destruction of the bronchial walls. Symptoms of bronchiectasis include a constant cough productive of copious purulent sputum, hemoptysis, chronic sinusitis, clubbing of fingers, and persistent moist, coarse rales. Treatment includes mobilization, frequent postural drainage, antibiotics, and, rarely, surgical resection of the affected part of the lungs.

Bronchiolitis: An acute viral infection of the lower respiratory tract that occurs primarily in infants under 18 months of age, characterized by expiratory wheezing, respiratory distress, inflammation, and obstruction at the level of the bronchioles.

Bronchitis: An acute or chronic inflammation of the mucous membranes of the tracheobronchial tree. Acute bronchitis is characterized by a productive cough, fever, hypertrophy of mucous-secreting structures, and back pain. Most common in adults, it is often a complication of cystic fibrosis in children. Treatment includes the cessation of cigarette smoking, avoidance of airway irritants, the use of expectorants, and postural drainage. Currently, prophylactic antibiotics, steroids, and desensitization therapy are not recommended.

Bronchopulmonary dysplasia: An iatrogenic condition observed in neonates that resembles chronic airflow limitation and is associated with positive pressure mechanical ventilation and oxygen therapy.

Burns: An injury to tissues of the body caused by heat, electricity, chemicals, radiation, or gases in which the extent of the injury is determined by both the amount of exposure of the cell to the agent and the nature of the agent. Treatment of burns includes pain relief, careful asepsis, prevention of infection, maintenance of the balance of body fluids and electrolytes, and good nutrition. Severe burns of any origin may cause shock, which is treated before the wound.

Cardiac output (Q): The amount of blood ejected from the heart into the aorta each minute.

Cardiac rehabilitation: A supervised program of progressive exercise, psychological support, and education or training to enable a patient who has had a myocardial infarction to resume the activities of daily living on an independent basis. Special training may be needed to adapt the patient to a new occupation and lifestyle.

Cardiopulmonary failure: Progressive insufficiency of cardiopulmonary function resulting in significant impairment of cardiac output and/or ventilation that cannot be adequately compensated without ventilatory support.

Cardiopulmonary function: Integrated function of the heart and lungs.

Cardiopulmonary unit: The heart and lungs, which function interdependently as a unit.

Catabolic: Relating to catabolism, which is the breaking down in the body of complex chemical compounds into simpler compounds, often accompanied by the liberation of energy.

Cellular respiration: The processes involved with cellular metabolism, including energy transfer, oxygen utilization, and carbon dioxide production.

Cerebral palsy: A motor function disorder caused by a permanent, nonprogressive brain defect or lesion present at birth or shortly thereafter. Early identification of the disorder facilitates the handling of infants with cerebral palsy and the initiation of an exercise and training program. Treatment is individualized and may include the use of braces, surgical correction of deformities, speech therapy, and various indicated drugs, such as muscle relaxants and anticonvulsants.

Childhood asthma: Reversible airway hyperreactivity and edema affecting children that is often triggered by dust or animals. It is hallmarked by narrowing of the airways, wheezing, shortness of breath, accessory muscle use, and impaired oxygenation.

Chronic bronchitis: Lung condition characterized by the presence of a chronic productive cough for at least 3 months in each of 2 successive years.

Chronic renal insufficiency: Impaired function of the kidneys manifested by impaired blood urea nitrogen, creatinine clearance, and reduced urinary output. Renal insufficiency may precipitate renal failure.

Chronic airflow limitation: A more precise term for chronic obstructive pulmonary disease (e.g., chronic bronchitis and emphysema).

Clinical decision making: The process of making decisions based on a thorough history, assessment, integration of the results of laboratory tests and investigations, and the patient's needs and wants.

Complications with coughing: Complications associated with an impaired cough (e.g., impaired mucociliary transport, mucous accumulation, pulmonary aspiration, and increased risk of infection).

Congestive heart failure (CHF): An abnormal condition that reflects impaired cardiac pumping, caused by myocardial infarction, ischemic heart disease, or cardiomyopathy. Failure of the ventricle to eject blood efficiently results in volume overload, chamber dilatation, and elevated intracardiac pressure. Retrograde transmission of increased hydrostatic pressure from the left heart causes pulmonary congestion; elevated right heart pressure causes systemic venous congestion and peripheral edema.

Connective tissue dysfunction: Impaired function of connective tissue observed in connective tissue and vascular collagen conditions.

Continuity of care: The provision of continuous care from one setting to another (e.g., inpatient to outpatient facilities).

Controlled breathing: Teaching a patient ventilatory strategies to exert cognitive control over ineffective breathing patterns.

Control of breathing: The central and peripheral regulation and control mechanisms of breathing.

Control of the heart: The central and peripheral regulation and control mechanisms of the heart.

Coronary artery disease: Any one of the abnormal conditions that may affect the arteries of the heart and produce various pathological effects, especially the reduced flow of oxygen and nutrients to the myocardium. Any of the coronary artery diseases, such as coronary atherosclerosis, coronary arteritis, or fibromuscular hyperplasia of the coronary arteries, may produce the common characteristic symptom of angina pectoris. Studies over the last 30 years confirm that coronary atherosclerosis occurs most frequently in populations with regular diets high in calories, total fat, saturated fat, cholesterol, and refined carbohydrates. Other risk factors include cigarette smoking, hypertension, serum cholesterol levels, coffee intake, alcohol intake, deficiencies of vitamins C and E, water hardness, hypoxia, carbon monoxide, social overcrowding, heredity, climate, and viruses.

Cough: A sudden, audible expulsion of air from the lungs. Coughing is preceded by inspiration—the glottis is partially closed, and the accessory muscles of expiration contract to expel the air forcibly from the respiratory passages. Coughing is an essential protective response that serves to clear the lungs, bronchi, or trachea of irritants and secretions or to prevent aspiration of foreign material into the lungs. It is a common symptom of diseases of the chest and larynx. Because the function of coughing is to clear the respiratory tract of secretions, it is important that the cough bring out accumulated debris. Where it does not, because of weakness or inhibition of the force of the cough caused by pain, instruction and assistance in effective coughing and deep-breathing exercises are required.

Cough pump: The integrated thoracic and abdominal mechanisms involved in cough resulting in forced expiration and evacuation and clearance of the airways.

Cough stages: The stages of cough include maximal inspiration, closure of the glottis, increased intraabdominal pressure, opening of the glottis, and forced expiration.

Cystic fibrosis: An inherited disorder of the exocrine glands that causes exocrine gland production of abnormally thick secretions of mucus, elevation of sweat electrolytes, increased organic and enzymatic constituents of saliva, and overactivity of the autonomic nervous system. The glands most affected are those in the pancreas, the respiratory system, and the sweat glands. Because there is no known cure, treatment is directed at the prevention of respiratory infections, which are the most frequent cause of death. Mucolytic agents and bronchodilators are used to help liquefy the thick, tenacious mucus. Physical therapy measures, such as exercise, postural drainage, and breathing exercises, can also dislodge secretions. Life expectancy in cystic fibrosis has improved markedly over the past several decades, and with early diagnosis and treatment, most patients can be expected to reach adulthood.

Dead space: The amount of lung in contact with ventilating gases but not in contact with pulmonary blood flow. Alveolar dead space refers to alveoli that are ventilated by the pulmonary circulation but not perfused. The condition may exist when pulmonary circulation is obstructed, as by a thromboembolus. Anatomical dead space is an area in the trachea, bronchi, and air passages containing air that does not reach the alveoli during respiration. As a general rule, the volume of air in the anatomical dead space in millimeters is approximately equal to the weight in pounds of the involved individual. Certain lung disorders, such as emphysema, increase the amount of anatomical dead space. Physiological dead space is an area in the respiratory system that includes the anatomical dead space together with the space in the alveoli occupied by air that does not contribute to the oxygen-carbon dioxide exchange.

Denervation of heart: The transplanted heart initially loses its innervation (i.e., it is denervated and relies on exogenous catecholamines for cardiac acceleration and deceleration).

Dependent patients: Patients who are unable to help themselves.

Depolarization: Changes in ionic concentrations across muscle cell membranes leading to contraction of the cell.

Diabetes: A clinical condition characterized by the excessive excretion of urine. The excess may be caused by a deficiency of antidiuretic hormone (ADH), as in diabetes insipidus, or it may be the polyuria resulting from the hyperglycemia occurring in diabetes mellitus.

Diaphragmatic breathing pattern: Involves teaching patients with COPD how to relax the accessory muscles and perform controlled diaphragmatic breathing.

Diffusion: The process in which solid, particulate matter in a fluid moves from an area of higher concentration to an area of lower concentration, resulting in an even distribution of the particles in the fluid. No energy is required.

Documentation: Written material associated with the history, the compilation of laboratory reports and investigations, and the results of clinical assessment.

Dyspnea: The sensation of difficulty in breathing.

Electrocardiographic monitoring: Electrocardiographic monitoring involving electrode placement on the chest wall and on the limbs for a 12-lead ECG. Such monitoring provides a tracing of the electrical activity of the heart.

Echocardiography: Evaluation of cardiac structure and function by using the properties of sound. Quantitative and qualitative measurements can be derived. The most common types include two-dimensional, Doppler, and transesophageal.

Ejection fraction: The amount of ventricular volume ejected with each heart beat. Expressed as a percent, ejection fraction is determined by the following equation: [(end-diastolic volume − end-systolic volume) × 100]/end-diastolic volume.

Electrocardiogram (ECG): The tracing produced by the sequential depolarization and repolarization of myocardial cells as detected by surface electrodes placed on the skin.

Electromechanical coupling: The coupling of electrical and mechanical events of the heart to effect cardiac output.

Electromyographic (EMG) power spectrum: Electromyography is the process of recording the electrical activity of muscle on a cathode-ray oscilloscope. The electromyographic (EMG) power spectrum is the full range of electrical activity of the muscle.

Emphysema: Lung condition characterized by an abnormal, permanent enlargement of the air spaces distal to the terminal bronchioles accompanied by destruction of their walls.

Endocardial cushion defect: Any cardiac defect resulting from the failure of the endocardial cushions in the embryonic heart to fuse and form the atrial septum.

Endocrine function: The function of the endocrine glands responsible for normal physiological function.

Evidence-based practice: Practice based on evidence from the physiologic and scientific literature.

Exercise: (1) The performance of any physical activity for the purpose of conditioning the body, improving health, or maintaining fitness, or as a means of therapy for correcting a deformity or restoring the organs and bodily functions to a state of health. (2) Any action, skill, or maneuver that exerts the muscles and is performed repeatedly in order to develop or strengthen the body or any of its parts. (3) To use a muscle or part of the body in a repetitive manner to maintain or develop its strength. The physical therapist constantly assesses the patient's needs and provides the proper type and amount of exercise, taking into account the patient's physical or mental limitations. Exercise has a beneficial effect on each of the body systems, although in excess it can lead to the breakdown of tissue and cause injury.

Exercise blood gases: Blood gases taken before, during, and after exercise to determine the effect of exercise on oxygen transport.

Exercise stress: Physical stress imposed by movement (i.e., mobilization and exercise.)

Expiratory reserve volume (ERV): The maximum volume of gas that can be expired from the resting expiratory level.

Extrinsic factors: Factors related to the patient's care that contribute to cardiopulmonary dysfunction and impaired gas exchange.

Fluid and electrolyte status: The status of blood volume and distribution, and the status of electrolyte balance in the body; fluid balance often has a direct effect on electrolytes.

Forced expiratory volume in one second (FEV$_1$): Amount of air expired in one second during a forced exhalation after a maximal inhalation.

Forced vital capacity (FVC): Total amount of air exhaled during a forced exhalation after a maximal inhalation.

Functional residual capacity: Volume of gas in the lungs at the end of a normal expiration. Functional residual capacity is equal to the residual volume plus the expiratory reserve volume.

Function optimization: Optimal functioning of the patient as a whole person based on optimal physiological functioning at an organ system level.

Gas exchange: The movement of oxygen and carbon dioxide between the pulmonary capillary blood and the alveolar tissue and between the systemic capillary blood and peripheral tissue cells.

Gastrointestinal dysfunction: Abnormal function of the gastrointestinal system.

Gravitational stress: Stress imposed on the human body by gravity and its physiological effects.

Gravity: The heaviness or weight of an object resulting from the universal effect of the attraction between any body of matter and any planetary body. The force of the attraction depends on the relative masses of the bodies and on the distance between them.

Head injury: Any traumatic damage to the head resulting from blunt or penetrating trauma of the skull. Blood vessels, nerves, and meninges can be torn; bleeding, edema, and ischemia may result.

Health behavior: An action taken by a person to maintain, attain, or regain good health and to prevent illness. Health behavior reflects a person's health beliefs. Some common health behaviors are exercising regularly, eating a balanced diet, and obtaining necessary inoculations.

Heart: The muscular, cone-shaped organ, about the size of a clenched fist, that pumps blood throughout the body and beats normally about 70 times per minute by coordinated nerve impulses and muscular contractions. Enclosed in pericardium, the heart rests on the diaphragm between the lower borders of the lungs, occupying the middle of the mediastinum. The sinoatrial node of the heart sets the rate. Other factors affecting the heartbeat are emotion, exercise, hormones, temperature, pain, and stress.

Heart-lung interdependence: The heart and lung are structurally and functionally interdependent and form a cardiopulmonary unit.

Hemiplegia: Paralysis of one side of the body.

Hemodynamic status: Status of the heart and its capacity to effect blood movement to perfuse the tissues of the body.

Hibernating myocardium: Contractile dysfunction of the myocardium resulting from prolonged ischemia, appearing as a regional wall motion abnormality.

Home care: A health service provided in the patient's place of residence for the purposes of promoting, maintaining, or restoring health or minimizing the effects of illness and disability.

Humidity: Pertaining to the level of moisture in the atmosphere, the amount varying with the temperature. The percentage is usually represented in terms of relative humidity, with 100% being the point of air saturation or level at which the air can absorb no additional water.

Hyaline membrane disease: Disease of the newborn, characterized by airless alveoli, inelastic lungs, more than 60 respirations a minute, nasal flaring, intercostal and subcostal retractions, grunting on expiration, and peripheral edema. The condition occurs most often in premature babies. The disease is self-limited; the infant dies in three to five days or completely recovers with no after-effects. Treatment includes measures to correct shock, acidosis, and hypoxemia and use of positive airway pressure to prevent alveolar collapse. This is also called *respiratory distress syndrome (RDS) of the newborn.*

Hypercapnia: The presence of an abnormally large amount of carbon dioxide in the circulating blood.

Hyperpnea: Rapid, shallow breathing.

Hypertension: A common, often asymptomatic disorder characterized by elevated blood pressure persistently exceeding 140/90 mm Hg. Patients with high blood pressure are advised to follow a low-sodium, low-saturated-fat diet, reduce calories to control obesity, exercise, avoid stress, and take adequate rest.

Hypoxemia: A low level of oxygen in the blood, often characterized by a PaO_2 of less than 80 mm Hg.

Immune function: Function of the immunological system and its components to effect optimal immunological protection.

Immunological dysfunction: Abnormal function of the immunological system.

Immunosuppression: Of or pertaining to a substance or procedure that lessens or prevents an immune response.

Inspiratory capacity (IC): Maximum volume of gas that can be inhaled from the resting expiratory level. Equal to the sum of the tidal volume and the inspiratory reserve volume, it is measured with a spirometer.

Inspiratory muscle training: Resistance ventilatory training designed to increase the strength and endurance of the inspiratory muscles.

Inspiratory resistance breathing: A method of respiratory muscle training that includes normal ventilation with added external threshold loading on inspiration and consists of 15 to 30 minutes of training five days per week. External loading is increased from 30% of maximal inspiratory pressure to 60% of maximal inspiratory pressure as the patient's tolerance increases.

Inspiratory reserve volume: Maximum volume of gas that can be inspired from the end-tidal inspiratory level.

Intermittent positive pressure breathing (IPPB): A form of assistive or controlled respiration produced by a ventilatory apparatus in which compressed gas is delivered under positive pressure into the patient's airways until a preset pressure is reached. Passive exhalation is allowed through a valve, and the cycle begins again as the flow of gas is triggered by inhalation. This is also called *intermittent positive pressure ventilation (IPPV).*

Interstitial pulmonary fibrosis: A classification of restrictive lung disease including conditions that result in a final common pathway of bouts of chronic lung infection and irreversible fibrosis.

Intraaortic balloon counter pulsation: Procedure for assisting left ventricular function and coronary perfusion that involves inserting a balloon into the femoral artery. The inflation and deflation of the balloon is synchronized with the ECG such that the balloon inflates during diastole and deflates during systole.

Intracardiac pressures: Pressures within the chambers of the heart. Optimal movement of blood through the heart depends on pressure gradients throughout the heart. Normal pressures within each heart chamber are within a restricted range.

Intracranial pressure monitoring: Invasive monitoring instituted to measure changes in cranial pressure usually resulting from increased volume of the brain because of injury, bleeding, fluid accumulation, or an intracranial mass.

Isocapnic hyperpnea: A method of respiratory muscle training that includes high ventilation with low external loading consisting of sustained periods of hyperpnea lasting 15 to 30 minutes daily for several weeks with the addition of carbon dioxide to maintain a normal level.

Jacobsen's progressive relaxation exercise: A technique involving contraction followed by relaxation to progressively relax muscle groups.

Kidneys: A pair of bean-shaped urinary organs in the dorsal part of the abdomen, one on each side of the vertebral column. The kidneys produce and eliminate urine through a complex filtration network and reabsorption system comprising more than 2 million nephrons. All the blood in the body passes through the kidneys about 20 times every hour but only about one fifth of the plasma is filtered by the nephrons during that period. The kidneys remove water as urine and return water that has been filtered to the blood plasma, thus helping to maintain the water balance of the body. Hormones, especially the antidiuretic hormone (ADH) produced by the pituitary gland, control the function of the kidneys in regulating the water content of the body.

Kyphoscoliosis: An abnormal condition characterized by an anteroposterior curvature and a lateral curvature of the spine. It occurs in children and adults and can be associated with cor pulmonale.

Late sequelae of poliomyelitis: Late effects of poliomyelitis that may occur in poliomyelitis survivors 30 to 35 years after onset. These effects include disproportionate fatigue, weakness, pain, reduced endurance, choking and swallowing problems, altered temperature sensitivity, and psychological problems.

Learning theory: A group of concepts and principles that attempts to explain the learning process. One concept, Guthrie's contiguous conditioning premise, postulates that each response becomes permanently linked with stimuli present at the time so that contiguity rather than reinforcement is a part of the learning process.

Liver: Largest gland of the body and one of its most complex organs. More than 500 of its functions have been identified. It is divided into four lobes, contains as many as 100,000 lobules, and is served by two distinct blood supplies. Some of the major functions performed by the liver are the production of bile by hepatic cells, the secretion of glucose, proteins, vitamins, fats, and most of the other compounds used by the body, the processing of hemoglobin for vital use of its iron content, and the conversion of poisonous ammonia to area.

Lung cancer: Pulmonary malignancy attributable to cigarette smoking in 50% of cases. Lung cancer develops most often in scarred or chronically diseased lungs and is usually far advanced when detected because metastases may precede the detection of the primary lesion in the lung. Symptoms of lung cancer include persistent cough, dyspnea, purulent or blood-streaked sputum, chest pain, and repeated attacks of bronchitis or pneumonia. Surgery is the most effective treatment, but only one half of cases are operable at the time of diagnosis and of these 50% are not resectable. Thoracotomy is contraindicated if metastases are found in contralateral or scalene lymph nodes. Irradiation is used to treat localized lesions and unresectable intrathoracic tumors and as palliative therapy for metastatic lesions. Radiotherapy may also be administered after surgery to destroy remaining tumor cells and may be combined with chemotherapy.

Lung capacities: Lung volumes that consist of two or more of the four primary nonoverlapping volumes. Functional residual capacity is the sum of residual volume and expiratory reserve volume. Inspiratory capacity is the sum of the tidal volume and inspiratory reserve volume. Vital capacity is the sum of the expiratory reserve volume, the tidal volume, and the inspiratory reserve volume. Total lung capacity, at the end of maximal inspiration, is the sum of the functional residual capacity and the inspiratory capacity.

Lung compliance: Volume change per unit of pressure change in the lungs.

Lungs: Pair of light, spongy organs in the thorax, constituting the main component of the respiratory system. The two highly elastic lungs are the main mechanisms in the body for inspiring air, from which oxygen is extracted for the arterial blood system, and for exhaling carbon dioxide, which is dispersed from the venous system.

Lung volume: Volume of the lungs that may be compartmentalized into component volumes and capacities.

Malnutrition: Any disorder of nutrition. It may result from an unbalanced, insufficient, or excessive diet or from the impaired absorption, assimilation, or use of foods.

Managed care: Health care system in which there is administrative control over primary health care services in a medical group practice. Redundant facilities and services are eliminated and costs are reduced. Health education and preventive medicine are emphasized. Patients may pay a flat fee for basic family care but may be charged additional fees for secondary care services of specialists.

Measurement: The determination, expressed numerically, of the extent or quantity of a substance, energy, or time.

Mechanical ventilation: Use of artificial mechanical means to support ventilation.

Metabolic demand: The energy and oxygen demands of the body required to support metabolism. Metabolic demand fluctuates depending on the activity level of the individual, the presence of illness and increased temperature, and the requirements of healing and repair.

Method: A technique or procedure for producing a desired effect, such as a surgical procedure, a laboratory test, or a diagnostic technique.

Minute ventilation (VE): Amount of air inspired in one minute. It is the product of tidal volume and respiratory rate.

Minute ventilation: Total expired volume of air per minute.

Mobilization: Therapeutic and prescriptive application of low-intensity exercise in the management of cardiopulmonary dysfunction, usually in acutely ill patients. The primary goal of mobilization is to exploit the acute effects of exercise to optimize oxygen transport.

Morbid obesity: Excess of body fat that threatens normal bodily functions, such as respiration.

Mucous blanket: Normal layer of mucous lining the bronchopulmonary tree. This blanket provides a medium through which foreign material and bacteria can be wafted centrally by the cilia for eventual removal by coughing or swallowing.

Multiple sclerosis (MS): A progressive disease characterized by disseminated demyelination of nerve fibers of the brain and spinal cord. It begins slowly, usually in young adulthood, and continues throughout life with periods of exacerbation and remission. As the disease progresses, the intervals between exacerbations grow shorter and disability becomes greater. There is no specific treatment for the disease; corticosteroids and other drugs are used to treat the symptoms accompanying acute episodes. Physical therapy may help to postpone or prevent specific disabilities. The patient is encouraged to live as normal and active a life as possible.

Multisystem assessment: Assessment of multiple organ systems based on clinical examination and investigative laboratory reports. Such assessment helps identify all factors that contribute to deficits in oxygen transport.

Muscle endurance: Ability to sustain repetitive contraction against a given load.

Muscle strength: Maximum force that a muscle can develop with maximal stimulation.

Muscular dystrophy (MD): A group of genetically transmitted diseases characterized by progressive atrophy of symmetrical groups of skeletal muscles without evidence of involvement or degeneration of neural tissue. In all forms of muscular dystrophy there is an insidious loss of strength with increasing disability and deformity, although each type differs in the groups of muscles affected, the age of onset, the rate of progression, and the mode of genetic inheritance. The basic cause is unknown but appears to be an inborn error of metabolism. Treatment of the muscular dystrophies consists primarily of supportive measures, such as physical therapy and orthopedic procedures to minimize deformity.

Myocardial infarction: Necrosis of a portion of cardiac muscle caused by obstruction in a coronary artery from either atherosclerosis or an embolus. Also called a heart attack.

Needs assessment: Assessment of the patient's specific physical, functional, and psychological needs.

Nocturnal ventilation: Selective use of mechanical ventilation during the night. Patients with cardiopulmonary dysfunction are at greater risk during the night when they are recumbent and the respiratory drive is depressed.

Obesity: Abnormal increase in the proportion of fat cells, mainly in the viscera and subcutaneous tissues of the body. Obesity may be exogenous or endogenous. Hyperplastic obesity is caused by an increase in the number of fat cells in the increased adipose tissue mass. Hypertrophic obesity results from an increase in the size of the fat cells in the increased adipose tissue mass.

Objective: (1) A goal. (2) Of or pertaining to a phenomenon or clinical finding that is observed; not subjective. An objective finding is often described in health care as a sign, as distinguished from a symptom, which is a subjective finding.

Obstructive lung disease: Classification of lung disease referring to airflow limitation secondary to obstruction and increased airway resistance (e.g., chronic bronchitis and emphysema).

Osteoporosis: A disorder characterized by abnormal rarefaction of bone, occurring most frequently in postmenopausal women, in sedentary or immobilized individuals, and in patients on long-term steroid therapy. The disorder may cause pain, especially in the lower back, pathological fractures, loss of stature, and various deformities.

Outpatient: A patient, not hospitalized, who is being treated in an office, clinic, or other ambulatory care facility.

Oxygen (O₂): Tasteless, odorless, colorless gas essential for human respiration.

Oxygen consumption (Vo₂): The difference between the amount of inspired oxygen and the amount of oxygen exhaled. The difference between inspired and expired oxygen is a primary measure of aerobic fitness.

Oxygen delivery (Do₂): Delivery of oxygen to the tissues of the body; an essential component of oxygen transport.

Oxygen desaturation: Desaturation of oxygen from the hemoglobin molecule in the blood in response to a reduction of tissue oxygen levels.

Oxygen transport: Process by which oxygen is absorbed in the lungs by the hemoglobin in circulating deoxygenated red cells and carried to the peripheral tissues. The process is made possible because hemoglobin has the ability to combine with oxygen present at a high concentration, such as in the lungs, and to release this oxygen when the concentration is low, such as in the peripheral tissues.

Oxygen transport pathway: Pathway for oxygen delivery to the tissues from the ambient air: through the airways and lungs, across the alveolar capillary membrane, into the pulmonary circulation through the chambers of the heart via the peripheral and regional circulation to the tissues and the mitochondria where oxygen is used in cellular respiration.

Oxygen saturation: Measurement of the amount of oxygen attached to a hemoglobin molecule.

Oxyhemoglobin dissociation: Dissociation of oxygen from the hemoglobin molecule in peripheral tissues when the concentration of oxygen is low.

Parenchyma: The tissue of an organ, as distinguished from supporting or connective tissue.

Parkinson's disease: A slowly progressive, degenerative, neurological disorder characterized by resting tremor, pill rolling of the fingers, a masklike expression, shuffling gait, forward flexion of the trunk, loss of postural reflexes, and muscle rigidity and weakness. It is usually an idiopathic disease of people over 60 years of age, although it may occur in younger people, especially after acute encephalitis or carbon monoxide or metallic poisoning, particularly by reserpine or phenothiazine drugs.

Partial pressure of gases: Pressure exerted by an individual gas, a percent of the total pressure of gases.

Patent ductus arteriosus (PDA): An abnormal opening between the pulmonary artery and the aorta caused by failure of the fetal ductus arteriosus to close after birth. The defect, which is seen primarily in premature infants, allows blood from the aorta to flow into the pulmonary artery and recirculate through the lungs, where it is reoxygenated and returned to the left atrium and left ventricle, causing an increased workload on the left side of the heart and increased pulmonary vascular congestion and resistance.

Pediatric cardiac rehabilitation: Specialized cardiac rehabilitation for children instituted in the chronic stage of heart disease or after cardiovascular surgery when the patient is through the acute phase.

Pediatric pulmonary rehabilitation: Specialized pulmonary rehabilitation for children instituted in the subacute or chronic stages of lung disease or after thoracic surgery when the patient is through the acute phase.

Perfusion: Passage of a fluid through a specific organ or an area of the body.

Perioperative complications: Complications before, during, and after surgery.

Peripheral circulation: The systemic circulation, which excludes the circulation to the heart and lungs (the central circulation).

Peripheral vascular disease: Any abnormal condition that affects the blood vessels outside the heart and the lymphatic vessels.

Pneumonia: An acute inflammation of the lungs, usually caused by inhaled pneumococci of the species *Streptococcus pneumoniae*. The alveoli and bronchioles of the lungs become plugged with a fibrous exudate. Pneumonia may be caused by other bacteria, as well as by viruses, rickettsiae, and fungi.

Positron emission scans: Tomographic scans using positron emitting radionuclides. The tracers used are often taken up in the metabolic pathways of the tissues being studied (e.g., oxygen metabolism or gluclose metabolism).

Prescription: An order for medication, therapy, or a therapeutic device given by a properly authorized person to a person properly authorized to dispense or perform the order. A prescription is usually in written form and includes the name and address of the patient, the date, the [4]+ symbol (superscription), the medication prescribed (inscription), directions to the pharmacist or other dispenser (subscription), directions to the patient that must appear on the label, the prescriber's signature, and, in some instances, an identifying number.

Prevention: Any action directed toward preventing illness and promoting health to avoid the need for secondary or tertiary health care.

Primary cardiopulmonary dysfunction: Cardiopulmonary dysfunction resulting from a primary condition of the heart, lungs, or both.

Pulmonary rehabilitation: Rehabilitation of cardiopulmonary dysfunction including the acute, subacute, and chronic phases of the disease or after thoracic surgery. The long-term management includes a comprehensive program of exercise, ventilatory support, additional airway clearance interventions as needed, nutrition, stress reduction, smoking cessation, pacing and energy conservation, vocational rehabilitation, sexual rehabilitation, and education.

Pulmonary development: Anatomical and physiological development of the cardiopulmonary system during normal growth and development.

Pulmonary circulation: Blood flow through a network of vessels between the heart and the lungs for the oxygenation of blood and removal of carbon dioxide.

Quality care: Provision of holistic care in which the needs and wants of the patient are considered.

Recumbency: The state of lying down or leaning against something.

Reflex cough: A cough stimulated reflexively.

Reliability: The extent to which a test measurement or a device produces the same results with different investigators, observers, or administration of the test over time. If repeated use of the same measurement tool on the same sample produces the same consistent results, the measurement is considered reliable.

Residual volume: Volume of air remaining in the lung after a maximal expiration.

Resources: Services, personnel, and treatment options that can be drawn on to maximize treatment delivery and effectiveness.

Respiratory muscle fatigue: Loss in the capacity of a muscle under load to develop force or velocity that is reversible by rest.

Respiratory muscles: Muscles that produce volume changes of the thorax during breathing. The inspiratory muscles include the hemidiaphragms, external intercostals, scaleni, sternomastoids, trapezius, pectoralis major, pectoralis minor, subclavius, latissimus dorsi, serratus anterior, and muscles that extend the back. The expiratory muscles are the external intercostals, abdominals, and the muscles that flex the back.

Respiratory muscle weakness: Chronic loss in the capacity of a rested muscle to generate force.

Respiratory mechanics: The physical properties of the lung, including resistance and compliance characteristics.

Respiratory failure: Inability of the cardiac and pulmonary systems to maintain an adequate exchange of oxygen and carbon dioxide in the lungs. Respiratory failure may be oxygenation or hypercapniac. Treatment of respiratory failure includes maximizing ventilation, clearing the airways by suction, bronchodilators, or tracheostomy, antibiotics for infections usually present, anticoagulants for pulmonary thromboemboli, and electrolyte replacement in fluid imbalance. Oxygen may be administered in some cases; in others it may further decrease the respiratory reflex by removing the stimulus of a decreased elevated level of oxygen.

Restrictive lung disease: Category of lung disease involving restriction of the lung parenchyma and characterized by stiffness (reduced compliance) and reduced lung volume.

Rheumatoid arthritis: A chronic, destructive, sometimes deforming collagen disease that has an autoimmune component. Rheumatoid arthritis is characterized by symmetric inflammation of the synovium and increased synovial exudate, leading to thickening of the synovium and swelling of the joint. Rheumatoid arthritis usually first appears in early middle age, between 36 and 50 years of age, and most commonly in women. The course of the disease is variable but is frequently marked by remissions and exacerbation.

Risk factors: Factors that cause a person or a group of people to be particularly vulnerable to an unwanted, unpleasant, or unhealthful event. Examples include immunosuppression, which increases the incidence and severity of infection, and cigarette smoking, which increases the risk of developing a respiratory or cardiovascular disease.

Routine body positioning: Routine use of body positioning in the management of patients to minimize the negative effects of static positioning and maximize comfort. The purposes of routine body positioning are distinct from the specific goals of prescriptive body positioning, which are related to optimizing particular components of cardiopulmonary function and gas exchange.

Scleroderma: A relatively rare autoimmune disease affecting the blood vessels and connective tissue. The disease is characterized by fibrous degeneration of the connective tissue of the skin, lungs, and internal organs, especially the esophagus, digestive tract, and kidneys. Scleroderma is most common in middle-aged women.

Secretion management: Management of airway secretions.

Sedation: An induced state of quiet, calmness, or sleep, as by means of a sedative or hypnotic medication.

Sepsis and multiorgan system failure: Overwhelming systemic infection and pathogens leading to failure within multiple organ systems.

Shock: An abnormal condition of inadequate blood flow to the body's peripheral tissues, with life-threatening cellular dysfunction, hypotension, and oliguria. The condition is usually associated with inadequate cardiac output, changes in peripheral blood flow resistance and distribution, and tissue damage. Causal factors include hemorrhage, vomiting, diarrhea, inadequate fluid intake, or excessive renal loss, resulting in hypovolemia.

Skilled nursing and rehabilitation facilities: An institution or part of an institution that meets criteria for accreditation established by the sections of the Social Security Act that determine the basis for Medicaid and Medicare reimbursement for skilled nursing care, including rehabilitation and various medical and nursing procedures.

Spinal cord injury: Disruptions of the spinal cord, often associated with extensive musculoskeletal involvement. Common spinal cord injuries are vertebral fractures and dislocations, such as those commonly experienced by individuals involved in car accidents, airplane crashes, or other violent impacts. Such trauma may cause varying degrees of paraplegia and quadriplegia. Treatment of spinal cord injuries varies considerably and involves numerous approaches, such as exercise, ambulatory techniques, and special physical and psychological therapy.

Stable angina: Anginal pain that is well-controlled, medically stable, and has a predictable activity/exercise threshold.

Status asthmaticus: An acute, severe, and prolonged asthma attack. Hypoxia, cyanosis, and unconsciousness may follow. Treatment includes bronchodilators given intravenously or by aerosol inhalation, corticosteroids, controlled positive pressure ventilation, sedation, frequent therapy, and emotional support. A bronchodilator may be given by aerosol inhalation from a ventilator.

Stroke volume (SV): The amount of blood ejected from the ventricles during systole.

Stunned myocardium: Contractile dysfunction of the myocardium as a result of an acute episode of ischemia that persists even after perfusion has returned to normal.

Subacute hospitals: Hospitals that specialize in the management of nonacute conditions.

Subjective: (1) Pertaining to the essential nature of an object as perceived in the mind rather than to a thing in itself. (2) Existing only in the mind. (3) That which arises within or is perceived by the individual, as contrasted with something that is modified by external circumstances or something that may be evaluated by objective standards.

Suctioning: Use of mechanical airway suctioning that uses a catheter and negative pressure to remove oropharyngeal or airway secretions when the patient is unable to spontaneously or voluntarily take deep breaths and cough effectively.

Supraventricular: Pertaining to a feature or event occurring superior to the ventricles of the heart.

Surgery: The branch of medicine concerned with diseases and trauma requiring operative procedures.

Syncytium: The arrangement of cells, as in the myocardium, such that stimulation of one cell causes stimulation of adjacent cells, thus causing an action potential to spread from the initial focus.

Systemic disease: Dysfunction or condition affecting one or more systems.

Systemic lupus erythematosus (SLE): A chronic inflammatory disease affecting many systems of the body. The pathophysiology of the disease includes severe vasculitis, renal involvement, and lesions of the skin and nervous system. The primary cause of the disease has not been determined; viral infection or dysfunction of the immune system has been suggested. Adverse reaction to certain drugs also may cause a lupus-like syndrome. SLE occurs four times more often in women than in men.

Tachycardia: Abnormally rapid heart rate.

Tachypnea: Increased respiratory rate over 20 breaths per minute.

Thallium-201 scan: A radionuclide scan that evaluates myocardial perfusion. The tracer is taken up in the myocardium based on perfusion of the area. This agent can be used for rest studies, exercise stress studies, and pharmacological stress studies.

Thoracic cavity: The cavity enclosed by the ribs, the thoracic portion of the vertebral column, the sternum, the diaphragm, and associated muscles.

Thoracic surgery: The branch of medicine that deals with disease and injuries of the thoracic area by manipulative and operative methods.

Throat clearing: Spontaneous elicitation of a cough-like maneuver to clear secretions or an obstruction from the oropharynx that may be threatening the upper airway.

Tidal volume (TV): Amount of air inhaled and exhaled during normal ventilation. Inspiratory reserve volume, expiratory reserve volume, and tidal volume make up vital capacity.

Total lung capacity (TLC): Volume of gas in the lungs at the end of a maximum inspiration. It equals the vital capacity plus the residual capacity.

Tracheobronchial tree (TBT): Anatomic complex that includes the trachea, the bronchi, and the bronchial tubes. It conveys air to and from the lungs.

Tracheostomy: An opening through the neck into the trachea through which an indwelling tube may be inserted.

Tracheostomy tube/cuff: A tube/cuff that is positioned directly through the trachea in the neck to provide a functioning airway that bypasses the nares and oropharynx.

Transitional care units: Settings that specialize in providing care between the acute, subacute, and long-term stages of a patient's illness.

Transitional circulation: A transition from one type of blood vessel to another on moving peripherally through the circulation.

Treatment selection and prioritization: The process of selecting treatments and then prioritizing the order in which these treatments are administered. This process is based on the relative contribution of the pathogenesis that each treatment addresses with respect to oxygen transport deficiencies.

Trunk-ventilation interaction: Interrelationship of the shape and movement of the trunk or chest wall on alveolar ventilation. Trunk and ventilation interaction depends on body positioning and movement.

Tuberculosis: A chromic granulomatous infection caused by an acid-fast bacillus, mycobacterium tuberculosis, generally transmitted by the inhalation or ingestion of infected droplets and usually affecting the lungs, although infection of multiple organ systems occurs.

Type I fibers: Type of skeletal muscle fiber that is also called slow-twitch and is suitable for sustained tonic activity (e.g., the maintenance of posture or breathing, which require resistance to fatigue).

Type IIA fibers: Type of skeletal muscle fiber that is also called fast-twitch; this type of fiber is used for short-term, fast, powerful activity in which endurance to fatigue is not required.

Validity: Extent to which a device measures what it is intended to measure.

Valvular heart disease: An acquired or congenital disorder of a cardiac valve, characterized by stenosis and obstructed blood flow or by valvular degeneration and regurgitation of blood.

Ventilation: Process by which gases are moved into and out of the lungs.

Ventilatory strategies: Teaching patients to control breathing with the use of ventilatory patterns (e.g., combining inspiration with trunk extension and exhalation with trunk flexion).

Ventilation-perfusion scan: Two scans that are used to assess patients for the presence of pulmonary emboli. Criteria (BIELLO or PIOPED) are used to determine whether matched defects present with high, intermediate, or low probability of pulmonary embolus.

Ventilation and perfusion matching: Matching of ventilation and perfusion in the lungs. Optimal ventilation and perfusion matching occurs in the mid zones of the upright lung where the ratio is 0.8 to 1.0.

Vital capacity (VC): A measurement of the amount of air that can be expelled at the normal rate of exhalation after a maximum inspiration, representing the greatest possible breathing capacity. The vital capacity equals the inspiratory reserve volume plus the tidal volume plus the expiratory reserve volume. The average normal values of 4000 to 5000 ml are affected by age, physical dimensions of the chest cage, posture, and sex. The vital capacity may be reduced by a decrease in functioning lung tissue, resulting from atelectasis, edema, fibrosis, pneumonia, pulmonary resection, or tumors; by limited chest expansion, resulting from ascites, chest deformity neuromuscular disease, pneumothorax, or pregnancy; or by airway obstruction.

Work of breathing: Total amount of effort required to expand and contract the lungs; the physiological "cost" of breathing. Generally, quiet breathing consumes 2% to 3% of the oxygen consumption and requires 10% of the vital capacity. If a greater amount is used, one would say the work of breathing is increased.

INDEX

A

Abdominal binder, 378, 378f
Abdominal muscle in paralysis, 706, 707f
Abdominal pressure, 703
Abdominal thrust assist for cough, 369, 369f
Abnormal breath sound, 219
Accessory muscle
  breathing pattern using, 706, 707f
  in facilitation of ventilation, 391-394, 391b, 393b, 394b
ACE inhibitor, 792
Acetyl CoA, 40
Acetylcholine, 789, 790
Acid-base balance, 157-158
  abnormal, 641
  in intensive care unit, 233, 233t
  ventilation and, 78
Acidosis, 233t
Acquired immunodeficiency syndrome. *See* Human
    immunodeficiency virus infection
Action potential, cardiac, 170-171, 170f
Active cycle of breathing
  equipment for, 348, 348f
  ineffective and effective huffing in, 349b
  overview of, 328
  precautions for, 334
  preparation for, 348
  selection considerations for, 359t
  treatment with, 349
Active living model, 26
Activity
  baroreceptor-mediated, 268
  dynamic, 381
  as quality of life domain, 248t
Acupressure, 492
Acupuncture, 492
  for asthma, 483
  for congestive heart failure, 480t
Acute distress disorder, 241
Acute heart failure, 105
Acute lung injury, 644-647
Acute medical condition, 507-527
  acute exacerbation as
    of asthma, 516-518
    of cystic fibrosis, 518-519
    of emphysema, 514-516
    of interstitial pulmonary fibrosis, 519-520
  cardiovascular
    angina as, 522-523
    hypertension as, 521-522
    myocardial infarction as, 523-524
  overview of, 507-508

Acute medical condition, *(cont'd)*
  pulmonary
    airflow limitation as, 514-516
    alveolar proteinosis as, 514
    alveolitis as, 514
    atelectasis as, 508-509, 508b
    bronchiolitis as, 513
    bronchitis, 512-513
    pneumonia as, 509-512
    tuberculosis as, 520-521
Acute respiratory distress syndrome, 645-647
Adaptation to mobilization stimulus, 280-281
Adductor muscle, vocal cord and, 62
Adenosine triphosphate
  in cellular energetics, 266
  in muscle contraction, 42
  in oxygen transport, 40
Adherence, patient, 502
Adrenal function, testing of, 190
Adrenal insufficiency, 123, 123b
Adrenalin, 788
Adrenergic drug, 786-788
Adult respiratory distress syndrome, 644-647
  cognitive assessment in, 241
Aerobic capacity, age affecting, 686, 687
Aerobic exercise
  in ankylosing spondylitis, 586
  in chronic bronchitis, 548
  in chronic renal insufficiency, 588
  in cystic fibrosis, 519, 553
  in emphysema, 550
  hypertension and, 522, 563
  interstitial lung disease and, 554
  in lung transplantation, 728
  in multiple sclerosis, 573
  myocardial infarction and, 558
  in osteoporosis, 583
  in Parkinson's syndrome, 572
  in post polio syndrome, 578
  resistance training and, 276
  in rheumatoid arthritis, 587
  in scleroderma, 585
  in spinal cord injury, 576
  in stroke, 570, 571
  for stroke patient, 443-444
  in systemic lupus erythematosus, 584
  in thoracic deformity, 582
Aerobic metabolism
  age and, 283-284
  bed rest and, 268b
  mobilization and exercise affecting, 275

Aerosol for positive expiratory pressure breathing, 353
Aerosol system, mechanical, 761-762, 762f
Aerosol therapy, 764-765, 765f
Affective area of learning needs assessment, 498, 498b
African American
    lifestyle effects of, 9
    risk factor modification and, 18
Afterload, 44
Age
    arterial blood gases and, 161
    asthma and, 517
    in hypertension, 562
Aging patient, 685-693
    cardiac changes in, 686-689, 688t
        in aerobic capacity, 686
        in cardiac mechanics, 686-687
        exercise training and, 687, 688
        vascular and autonomic, 688, 688f, 689t
    cardiac disease and, 101
    hypertension in, 562
    osteoporosis and, 583
    pulmonary function in, 690t
        response to exercise and, 689-691, 691f
        structural and functional changes in, 689
Agitation, postoperative, 536
Air, atmospheric, 46-47
Airflow limitation
    acute, 514-516
    chronic, 546
    in emphysema, 550
Airway
    anatomy of, 62-63, 62f, 64t
    artificial, 773-784. See also Artificial airway
    in burn injury, 634
    limitation in oxygen transport and, 251b
    outcome measurement for, 258b
    oxygen transport and, 47
    suctioning of, in infant, 669-670, 674
    in trauma, 628b
Airway clearance technique, 325-376
    active cycle of breathing as, 328
        equipment for, 348, 348f
        ineffective and effective huffing in, 349b
        preparation for, 348
        treatment with, 349
    autogenic drainage as, 329-330, 329f, 349-351
        advantages and disadvantages of, 351
        equipment for, 350
        preparation for, 350, 350f
        treatment with, 350-351, 350f, 351f
    availability of, 358
    complications of, 358, 360
    contraindications to, 332-334, 333b
    cost of, 360
    coughing techniques in, 363-376. See also Cough
    effectiveness of, 358, 360
    exercise and, 332
    exercise as, 357-358

Airway clearance technique, (cont'd)
    high-frequency chest wall oscillation as, 331
        clinical application of, 355-356, 355f
    indications for, 326
    intrapulmonary percussive ventilation as, 331-332
        advantages and disadvantages of, 357
        equipment for, 356
        treatment with, 356
    in lung cancer, 555
    manual hyperinflation as
        clinical application of, 347-348, 347f
        overview of, 328
    overview of, 325-326
    percussion as, 327, 344-346, 345f
        advantages and disadvantages of, 345-346
        equipment for, 344-345
        preparation for, 345
        treatment with, 345
    positive expiratory pressure breathing as, 351-355
        advantages and disadvantages of, 355
        equipment for, 352-353, 352f
        overview of, 330-331, 351-352
        preparation for, 353-354, 353f
        treatment with, 354, 355f
    postural drainage as, 326-327, 327f, 342-344
        advantages and disadvantages of, 344, 344f
        equipment for, 343
        preparation for, 343
        technique of, 342f-343f
        treatment with, 343-344
    selection of, 334-335, 334b, 358, 359t
    shaking as, overview of, 327-328
    support for, 360
    use of, 341-342
    vibration as, overview of, 327
Airway resistance, 76-77
Alarm, ventilator, 768
Albumin, 46, 231
Alcohol syndrome, fetal, 660t
Aldomet, 788
Alexander technique, 466, 491
    for asthma, 482
Algorithm for ECG diagnosis of myocardial ischemia, 184f
Alkaline phosphatase, 191t
Alkalosis, 233t
Allergy and asthma, 91-92, 517b
Allograft vasculopathy, cardiac, 731
Alpha-adrenergic blocking agent, 787-788
Alpha-adrenergic drug, 788
Altitude, arterial blood gases and, 161
Alveolar-capillary membrane, 77
Alveolar-capillary surface area, 689
Alveolar duct, 63
Alveolar macrophage, 63-64
Alveolar proteinosis, 97-98, 98f, 514
Alveolitis, 514
Alveolus, 158

Alzheimer's disease, 15
Ambulation
   in burn injury, 635
   in stroke, 443-444, 571
Amphetamine, 788
Amyotrophic lateral sclerosis, 625
Anaerobic metabolism, 266
Analgesia, patient-controlled, 532
Analog scale for dyspnea, 140f
Anatomy, cardiopulmonary, 53-72
   breathing process and, 59-60
   of heart, 67-69, 67f-70f
   of lower airway, 62-63, 62f, 64t
   of lungs, 65, 66f, 66t
   of lymphatic circulation, 71
   of muscles of respiration
      expiratory, 59
      inspiratory, 54-59, 55f-58f
   of pulmonary circulation, 70-71
   of ribs, 54
   of sternum, 53-54
   of systemic circulation, 69-70
   of thorax, 53, 54f
      movements of, 54, 55f
   of upper airway, 60-62, 60f, 61f
Anemia, 107-108
   cardiopulmonary complications of, 122
   exercise program for, 413-414
   oxyhemoglobin dissociation curve in, 83
   sickle cell, 108
      cardiopulmonary complications of, 122
      exercise testing and training in, 447
Anesthesia, 530-531
Aneurysm, aortic, 167f
Angina, 102, 522-523
   acute, 522-523
   angina, 555
   chronic, 555-556
   grading of, 130b
   myocardial infarction and, 524, 556
   pain of, 145
   in peripheral vascular disease, 561
Angina pectoris, 102
Angiopathy, 447
Angiotensin-converting enzyme inhibitor, 792
   cardiac rehabilitation and, 414
Angiotensin II receptor blocker, 792
Ankylosing spondylitis, 586
Anorexia nervosa
   cardiopulmonary complications of, 124, 124b
   exercise testing and training in, 448
Anrep effect, 80
Anterior chest compression assisted cough,
      369-370
Antibiotic for tuberculosis, 521
Antibody, bed rest affecting, 269
Anticholinergic drug, 790-791
Anticholinesterase drug, 790

Antiinflammatory agent, 96
Antilymphocytic drug, 730
Antimetabolite, 730
Anxiety disorder, 473
Aortic aneurysm, 167f
Aortic pressure wave, 81
Aortic valve
   anatomy of, 67
   disease of, 107
Apnea
   definition of, 381b
   obstructive sleep, 102, 667
      in chronic bronchitis, 548
      in obesity, 628
Apnea, obstructive sleep
   myocardial infarction and, 557
Apneusis, 381b
Apneustic breathing, 381b
Apneustic center, 73
Appearance, general, 214-215
ARDS, 645-647
Aricept, 790
Arphonad, 791
Arrhythmia. See Dysrhythmia
Art therapy, 491
Artane, 791
Arterial blood gases, 157-163
   acid-base balance and, 157-158
   in chronic bronchitis, 547
   factors affecting, 161-162
   in intensive care unit, 233-235
   interpretation of, 160
   partial pressure of, 158-159, 158f
   in respiratory failure, 160-161
Arterial line, radial, 237f
Arterial occlusion, management of, 560
Arterial oxygen tension, in side-lying position, 316
Arterial saturation, in intensive care patient, 233-234
Arteriole, anatomy of, 70
Arthritis, rheumatoid
   exercise testing and training in, 446
   juvenile, 660t
   lung disease and, 99
   management of, 586-588
Artificial airway, 773-784
   airway care with, 777-778
   for child, 782t
   diseases requiring, 774t
   extubation or decannulation of, 782
   indications for, 773-775
   instillation of saline and, 782
   suctioning of, 778-782, 779f, 780f
      of endotracheal tube, 781
      of nasopharyngeal airway, 781
      sterile, 781-782
   tracheostomy tube as, 775-776, 776f
Asbestos exposure, 147
Ascites, in liver disorder, 121

Aspiration
  in burn injury, 635
  left main-stem bronchus, 780
Aspiration pneumonia, 663
Assessment
  of brain activity, 240
  clinical, 211-227
    auscultation in, 217-220, 217f, 218f
    of breathing pattern, 215-216
    case studies in, 225-226, 226t
    of chest wall configuration, 215-216, 216f
    diaphragmatic excursion in, 222, 222f
    of heart sounds, 220-221, 220f, 221f
    history in, 211-212
    mediate percussion in, 221-222, 222f
    palpation in, 222-224, 223f-225f
    physical examination in, 212
    of topographic landmarks, 212, 212b, 213f, 214f
    visual inspection in, 212, 214-215, 215f, 216f
  cognitive, 240-241
  of intensive care patient, 601
  learning needs, 487b, 497-499, 498b
  multisystem, 187-191
    blood, 188-189, 188t
    common tests for, 188t
    endocrine, 189-190, 190t
    immunologic, 191, 191t
    liver, 190, 191t
    peripheral vascular, 189
    rationale for, 187-188
    renal, 189, 190t
  neuromuscular, 240
  outcomes, 135
  pain, 241
  preoperative, 533-534, 534b
  of secondary cardiopulmonary dysfunction, 442
  of systemic condition, 115-116
Assessment-421, for cardiac or pulmonary rehabilitation,
    420
Assist device, left ventricular, exercise program for, 413
Asthma, 91-93, 92b, 92f, 93f
  acute exacerbation of, 516-518
  airway clearance in, 326
  cardiac, 143
  in child, 662
    exercise and, 676-677
  complementary therapy for, 481-483, 484t
  cough in, 143
  exercise program for, 417
  management of, 550-551
  obesity and, 667
  occupational, 147-148
  radiography of, 166
  respiratory muscle training in, 458
Asymmetrical breathing, 707
Asymmetrical dysfunction, facilitation of ventilation in,
    394-395, 394b
Asymmetry, thoracic, 581

Asystole, 181, 181f
Ataxia, Friedreich's, 660t
Atelectasis, 508-509, 508b
  airway clearance in, 326
  differential diagnosis of, 226t
Atenolol, 788
Atherosclerosis, 100-101
  in diabetes, 563
  as disease of civilization, 5
  lifestyle and, 5
  metabolic syndrome and, 13
  sexual dysfunction in, 556
Atherothrombosis, atherosclerosis and, 101
Athlete, wheelchair, 444
Athletic heart syndrome, 109
Atmospheric air, 46-47
ATP-CP system, in oxygen transport, 40
ATPase, in muscle contraction, 42
Atrial depolarization, 171-172
Atrial fibrillation, 178
  on electrocardiograph, 175f
Atrial flutter, 178, 178f
  clinical features of, 236t
Atrial pressure, left, 238
Atrioventricular block, 181-182, 182f
Atrioventricular defect, 660
Atrioventricular junction, 178, 178f
Atrioventricular node, 68
  in conduction system, 172
  depolarization of, 178-179
Atrium, anatomy of, 67-68
Atrophy, bed rest causing, 270
Atropine, 791
Atrovent, 791
Auscultation, 217-220, 217f, 218f
Autogenic drainage, 329, 329f
  advantages and disadvantages of, 351
  in cystic fibrosis, 519
  equipment for, 350
  preparation for, 350, 350f
  selection considerations for, 359t
  treatment with, 350-351, 350f, 351f
Autonomic nervous system
  aging and, 688-689, 689t
  cardiopulmonary complications of, 120
  heart and, 69
  supine position affecting, 314
Autonomic neuropathy, exercise testing and training in,
    447
Azathioprine, in transplantation, 730

B
Bacteremia, 648-649
Bacterial pneumonia, 510-512
Bag, ventilation, for manual hyperinflation, 347
Bagging, for intensive care patient, 604
Balloon counter pulsation device, intraaortic, in intensive
    care unit, 239, 239f

Balloon flotation catheter, pulmonary artery, 237-238
Balloon pump, intraaortic, shock and, 648
Bandura theory of learning, 496
Barometric pressure, arterial blood gases in, 161
Baroreceptor, carotid, 792
Baroreceptor-mediated activity, bed rest affecting, 268
Barrel chest, 215, 216f
Base excess/base deficit, 159
Bed rest, 267-271
    alternatives to, 270-271
    deconditioning in, 267
    exercise prescription with, 271-272
    gender differences in, 277
    hazards of, 269-270
    indications for, 271
    physiological consequences of, 268b
Behavior modification, 497
Behavior therapy, in coronary artery disease, 477
Belief, health, 4t
Bentropaine mesylate, 791
Bentyl, 791
Beta-adrenergic blocking agent, 788
    cardiac rehabilitation and, 414
    in myocardial infarction, 103
Beta$_2$-receptor stimulant, 788
Bethanecol, 789
Bigeminy, ventricular, 179-180, 180f
Bilirubin, normal values for, 191t
Binder, abdominal, 378, 378f
Bioelectromagnetics, 466, 492
Biofeedback, 491
    for asthma, 482
    for congestive heart failure, 480t
    for hypertension, 475, 475t
Biomicroelectro-potentials, 467
Biopsy, in pulmonary fibrosis, 96
Biot respiration, definition of, 381b
Bipolar magnet, 492
Bloater, blue, 87
Blood
    expectoration of, 146
        in lung cancer, 555
    limitation in oxygen transport and, 251b
    mobilization and exercise affecting, 274, 282
    outcome measurement for, 258b
    oxygen content of, 42-43
    in oxygen transport, 45-46, 82-83
    testing of, 188-189, 188t
Blood cell, 284
Blood disorder
    anemia as, 107-108
    cardiopulmonary complications of, 122, 122b
Blood flow, 46
Blood gases, arterial, 157-163. *See also* Arterial blood
        gases
Blood pressure. *See also* Hypertension
    atherosclerosis and, 101
    exercise and, 280, 282, 298, 563

Blood pressure. (*cont'd*)
    limitation in oxygen transport and, 252b
    in mobilization monitoring, 280
Blood supply to heart, 67-68, 68f
Blood vessel, atherosclerosis in, 100-101
Blood volume
    in bed rest, 270
    oxygen transport and, 45
Blue bloater, 87
Body jacket, 379-380, 379f
Body jacket/spinal orthosis, 665f
Body mechanics
    in lifting patient, 753-754, 753f, 754
    in positioning, 307-324. *See also* Position
Body work, Rosen method, 490
Bony skeleton, 165
Bowdich effect, 80
Bowel disease, inflammatory, 121
Bradycardia
    clinical features of, 236t
    sinus, 176, 177f
Brain activity assessment, 240
Brainstem disorder, 120
Breath sound, 218, 218f, 219
Breathing
    active cycle of
        equipment for, 348, 348f
        ineffective and effective huffing in, 349b
        overview of, 328
        precautions for, 334
        preparation for, 348
        selection considerations for, 359t
        treatment with, 349
    apneustic, definition of, 381b
    assessment of, 215-216
    in cerebral palsy, 575
    compensatory patterns of, 705-708
        asymmetrical, 707, 707f
        gravity eliminated, 707
        in lack of triad ventilatory muscles, 707
        lateral, 707
        paradoxical, 706, 706f
        in paralysis, 706
        shallow, 707-708
    controlled, 73-74, 74f
        in emphysema, 550
        indications for, 383b
        in primary versus secondary dysfunction, 383-384
    controlled diaphragmatic
        facilitation of, 382-383, 382b, 383b
        scoop technique of, 386-387, 386f, 387f
    in cystic fibrosis, 519
    glossopharyngeal, 397-399, 399f
    gravity and
        chest wall development and, 696, 697f-700f, 698-699,
            701t
        planes of ventilation and, 695-696, 696f, 696t
    intermittent positive pressure, 765-766, 765f

Breathing, (cont'd)
  lateral costal, 388-390, 388f, 389f
  limitation in oxygen transport and, 251b
  mechanical factors in, 75-77, 76f, 77f
  in muscular dystrophy, 581
  in myocardial infarction, 557
  in neonate, 658
  in neurological disorder, 120
  obesity and, 628
  outcome measurement for, 258b
  planes of ventilation and, 695-696, 696f
  positive expiratory pressure
    autogenic drainage compared to, 329
    overview of, 330-331
    precautions for, 334
    selection considerations for, 359t
  postural control and, 699, 701-705, 702f, 703f
  process of, 59-60
  pursed-lip, 384
    to facilitate ventilation, 384
    relaxed, 397
  soda pop model of respiratory and postural control,
      601-705, 699, 702f, 703f
    broader application of, 601-705, 699, 702f, 703f
    clinical example of, 708-713, 708f, 709t, 710t
  surgery affecting, 531
  trauma and, 630
  treatment hierarchy for, 256b
Breathing pattern terminology, 381b
Breathlessness. See Dyspnea
Bronchial breath sound, 218
Bronchial drainage
  in cystic fibrosis, 663
  overview of, 326-327, 327f
Bronchiectasis, 93-95, 94f
  airway clearance in, 326
  physical therapy for, 551-552
Bronchiole
  anatomy of, 63
  body position and, 311, 311f
Bronchiolitis, 513
Bronchiolitis obliterans, 731
Bronchitis
  acute, 512-513
  chronic, 87
    acute exacerbation of, 512-513
    differential diagnosis of, 226t
    emphysema and, 515
    management of, 546-548
Bronchoalveolar lavage, 96
Bronchopulmonary dysplasia, 661
Bronchopulmonary segment, 65, 66t
Bronchoscopy, 207
Bronchospasm, 93
Bronchovesicular breath sound, 218
Bronchus
  anatomy of, 62-63, 62f
  aspiration of, 780

Bruise, 215
Bubble positive expiratory pressure breathing, 353, 354
Buffer, 233
Buffering system, renal, 158
Bullous emphysema, 88, 89f, 514
Bundle of His, 69, 172
Burn injury, 633-635
Butterfly position, 751, 751f
Butterfly technique, 396-397, 397f
Button, tracheostomy, 777, 777f

C
Calcification in atherosclerosis, 101
Calcium, bed rest and, 270
Calcium channel blocker, 103
Cancer
  lung, 100, 554-555
  risk factors for, 6t, 14
Cannula
  oxygen, 760, 760f
  of tracheostomy tube, 775
Capillary, pulmonary, 71
Capillary hydrostatic pressure, 81
Capillary network, 70
Capillary oncotic pressure, 81
Captopril, 414
Carbachol, 789
Carbon dioxide
  end tidal, 162
  in oxygen transport, 49
  partial pressure of, 158
  transcutaneous, 162
  transport of, 83
Carbon dioxide tension, 280
Carbon monoxide poisoning, 634
Carbonic acid, 157
Carboxyhemoglobin, 634
Carcholin, 789
Cardiac action potential, 170-171, 170f
Cardiac allograft vasculopathy, 731
Cardiac asthma, 143
Cardiac chest pain, 145. See also Angina
Cardiac circulation in exercise, 267
Cardiac cycle, 81, 82f
Cardiac development, 658
Cardiac dysfunction
  in chronic bronchitis, 547
  community and, 737
  complementary therapy for, 472-481
    after cardiac surgery, 478-479, 479t
    in congestive heart failure, 479-480, 480t
    coronary artery disease, 476-478, 478t
    in coronary care unit, 480-481
    for hypertension, 474-476, 475t
    stress reduction in, 473-474, 474t
  in muscular dystrophy, 579
Cardiac dysrhythmia. See Dysrhythmia
Cardiac magnetic resonance imaging, 206-207

Cardiac mechanics, age affecting, 686-687
Cardiac output
    blood volumn and, 45
    in exercise, 266
    exercise affecting, 272
    mobilization and exercise affecting, 273
    oxygen transport and, 44, 48
    post–myocardial infarction, 104
Cardiac physiology
    in heart transplant, 727
    of lung transplant, 728
Cardiac reflex, 79-80
Cardiac rehabilitation, 405-439. *See also* Acute medical
        condition; Chronic medical condition
    in chronic dysfunction, 408-414
        anemia, 413-414
        congenital heart disease, 413
        diabetes, 414
        heart transplantation, 412-413
        hypertension, 414
        intermittent claudication, 413
        left ventricular assist device, 413
    components of, 417-421
        purpose and goals as, 417-420
        setting and team members, 420
    drugs in, 414
    evidence base and efficacy in, 405-408
    exercise in
        long-term plan for, 428
        monitoring in, 425, 425b
        testing in, 425-426
        training in, 426-428, 427b
    future directions in, 430
    heart transplant and, 727-728
    myocardial infarction and, 557
    nutrition in, 422
    phase I of, 512b
    phases of, 422
    physical therapy in, 420-421, 421f
    preadmission work-up for, 418b
    psychosocial issues in, 422
    risk reduction in, 423, 423f, 424f
    smoking cessation in, 422
Cardiac remodeling in heart failure, 106
Cardiac risk analysis, 423f
Cardiac surgery, 539-540. *See also* Surgery
    complementary therapy after, 478-479, 479t
Cardiac valve, 67-68
Cardiogenic pulmonary edema, 644
Cardiomyocyte, 172
Cardiomyopathy, diabetic, 104
Cardiopulmonary anatomy, 53-72. *See also* Anatomy,
        cardiopulmonary
Cardiopulmonary dysfunction
    in burn injury, 634
    chronic primary, 555-565
        angina as, 555-556
        diabetes mellitus as, 563-565

Cardiopulmonary dysfunction, (*cont'd*)
        hypertension as, 562-563
        metabolic syndrome as, 563-565
        myocardial infarction as, 556-558
        peripheral vascular, 560-561
        valvular, 558-560
    intensive care for, 611-624
        in chronic obstructive pulmonary disease, 613-617,
            613f, 615f, 616f
        in myocardial infarction, 619-621, 620b, 621b
        open heart surgery and, 621-623, 622b, 623f
        pathophysiology and, 611, 613
        respiratory failure and, 612t
        in restrictive lung disease, 618-619
        in status asthmaticus, 617-618
    in multisystem impairment, 715
    musculoskeletal disease causing, 581-584
        osteoporosis, 582-584
        thoracic deformity, 581-582
    neuromuscular disease causing, 569-593
        cerebral palsy, 574-575
        multiple sclerosis, 572-574
        muscular dystrophy, 578-581
        neuromuscular, 569-581
        Parkinson's syndrome, 569-572
        poliomyelitis, 577-578
        spinal cord injury, 575-577
        stroke, 569-570
    obesity in, 667
    positioning for, 309b
    vascular/connective tissue disease causing, 584-590
Cardiopulmonary manifestations of systemic condition,
        115-126. *See also* Systemic condition
Cardiopulmonary pathophysiology, 85-114. *See also*
        Pathophysiology, cardiopulmonary
Cardiopulmonary patient education. *See* Education
Cardiopulmonary physiology, 73-84. *See also* Physiology,
        cardiopulmonary
Cardiovascular disease
    chronic, 555-565
        angina as, 555-556
        diabetes mellitus and, 563-565
        hypertension as, 562-563
        metabolic syndrome and, 563-565
        myocardial infarction as, 556-558
        peripheral vascular, 560-561
        valvular, 558-560
    cough in, 144t
    exercise benefiting, 286b
    modifiable risk factors for, 6t
    positioning for, 309b
Cardiovascular reflex, 791-792
Cardiovascular surgery, 539-540. *See also* Surgery
Cardiovascular system
    bed rest affecting, 268
    mobilization and exercise affecting, 273b
    supine position affecting, 314
Cardura, 788

Care plan, 134-135
Carotid baroreceptor, 792
Cartilage, bronchial, 63
Case study
    in clinical assessment, 225-226
    of electrocardiography, 184-185, 185f
    patient as, 24-27
Casting, 630
Catapress, 788
Catecholamine
    mobilization and exercise affecting, 275
    testing for, 190
Catheter
    flow-directed pulmonary artery, 641
    pulmonary artery balloon flotation, 237-238
    suction, 780, 780f
    Swan-Ganz, 237-238
Cavity
    nasal, 61
    pericardial, 48
    peritoneal, 47
Cell
    blood, 284
    in shock, 647
Cellular energetics, 265-267
Cellular oxidation, 40, 41f, 42
Center of gravity, 753f, 754
Central chemoreceptor, 74
Central cyanosis, 215
Central nervous system. *See also* Neurological disorder;
        Neuromuscular disorder
    bed rest affecting, 269
    mobilization and exercise affecting, 273b, 275, 282-283
Central sleep-disordered breathing, 557
Central venous pressure, 238-239
Centrilobular emphysema, 87-88, 514
Cerebral palsy
    cardiopulmonary effects of, 119, 119b
    management of, 574-575
    in pediatric patient, 664-665, 665f
Cerebrospinal fluid, 74
Cerebrovascular accident, 707f
Channel, potassium, 170
Chart review, 211-212
Chemical stimulus, 74
Chemoreceptor
    central, 74
    in hypoxemia, 159
    peripheral, 74
Chest
    flail, 628b
    imaging of, 163-168
        computed tomography, 166-167
        evaluation of, 164-166, 164f, 165f
        magnetic resonance, 168-169, 168f
        projections for, 165t
    puncture wound of, 76
    relaxation of, 385

Chest, (*cont'd*)
    topographic landmarks of, 212, 212b, 213f, 214f
Chest compression, 369-370
Chest pain, 144-146. *See also* Angina
Chest percussion in infant, 668-669, 674f
Chest physical therapy
    for child, 674-676, 675f
    high-frequency chest wall oscillation and, 331
    in hyaline membrane disease, 661
    in infant, 668-674, 669f-774f, 670b, 670t
    in muscular dystrophy, 666
Chest sound, 218
Chest tube, 232-233, 232f
Chest wall
    aging and, 689
    configuration of, 215-216, 216f
    deformity of, 581-582
    in intensive care patient, 626
    of obese patient, 627-628
    in oxygen transport, 47
    pain in, 146
    in Parkinson's syndrome, 571
Chest wall exercise
    in chronic renal insufficiency, 589
    in multiple sclerosis, 573
    in osteoporosis, 583
    in rheumatoid arthritis, 588
    in spinal cord injury, 576
Chest x-ray, normal, 700f
Cheyne-Stokes respiration, 381b
Child. *See* Pediatric patient
Chinese medicine, 466, 491-492
Chiropractic medicine, 490
Cholesterol, 100
Cholinergic blocking drug, 790-791
Cholinergic drug, 789
Chronic bronchitis, 87
    acute exacerbation of, 512-513
    differential diagnosis of, 226t
    emphysema and, 515
    management of, 546-548
Chronic cough, 143
Chronic fatigue syndrome, 447-448
Chronic heart failure, 105-106
Chronic illness, self-management of, 737-738
Chronic medical condition
    cardiopulmonary, primary, 555-565
        angina as, 555-556
        diabetes mellitus as, 563-565
        hypertension as, 562-563
        metabolic syndrome as, 563-565
        myocardial infarction as, 556-558
        peripheral vascular, 560-561
        valvular, 558-560
    musculoskeletal, 581-584
    neuromuscular, 569-581
    obstructive pulmonary. *See* Chronic obstructive
            pulmonary disease

Chronic medical condition, (*cont'd*)
  overview of, 545-546
  principles of, 546b
  restrictive pulmonary, 553-555
    interstitial lung disease as, 553-554
    lung cancer as, 554-555
  vascular/connective tissue disease, 584-590
Chronic obstructive pulmonary disease, 546-553. *See also*
    specific disease
  acute exacerbation of, 514-516
  airflow limitation with, 546
  asthma as
    management of, 550-551
    pathophysiology of, 91-93, 92b, 92f, 93f
  bronchiectasis as
    management of, 551-552
    pathophysiology of, 93-95, 94f
  bronchitis as
    acute exacerbation of, 512-513
    management of, 546-548
    pathophysiology of, 87
  chest wall configuration in, 215, 216f
  complementary therapy for, 483-485, 484t
  cultural differences and, 18
  cystic fibrosis as, 552-553
  emphysema as
    management of, 548-550
    pathophysiology of, 87-91, 88f, 89f
  evidence-planning for, 11
  exercise program for, 415-416
  incentive spirometry for, 764
  intensive care for, 612-617
    management of, 613-614, 613f
    mobilization and, 614-615, 615f, 616f, 617
    positioning in, 615
  lung transplantation and, 722-723
  oxygen with exercise and, 763
  on radiograph, 166
  respiratory muscle training in, 457-458, 457t
Chronic renal disease
  management of, 588-589
  respiratory muscle training in, 459
Cigarette smoking. *See* Smoking
Cilia, 62f
Circadian rhythm
  cardiac disease and, 101
  mobilization and exercise affecting, 284
Circuit test, 2921b
Circulation
  atherosclerosis and, 101
  exercise and, 267, 273b
  fetal, 658
  mobilization and, 273b
  neonatal, 658
  peripheral
    in oxygen transport, 48
    physiology of, 81-82
  systemic, 69-70

Cirrhosis, 446
Civilization, diseases of, 5-6, 6t
Classification of function, 248, 248f, 248t
Claudication, intermittent
  exercise program for, 413
  management of, 560
Clearance, airway, 325-376. *See also* Airway clearance
Clinical assessment, 211-227. *See also* Assessment
Clinical decision making, 247, 247b, 254, 255f, 256b
Clinical reasoning, 247
Clinical trial, 24-25
Clonidine, 788
Closed suctioning, 778
Clotting factor, 46
Cluster analysis study, 159t
Coagulation
  disseminated intravascular, 46
    in liver disorder, 121
    tests for, 188-189
  mobilization and exercise affecting, 274
Coagulopathy
  cardiopulmonary complications of, 122
  testing for, 188-189
Coal worker, 147
Coefficient, utilization, 45
Cogentin, 791
Cognitive approach to stress reduction, 473
Cognitive area of learning needs assessment, 498, 498b
Cognitive assessment, 240-241
Cognitive factor, 252b
Columnar ciliated epithelium, pseudostratified, 62f
Community, 735-746
  cardiovascular concerns in, 737
  chronic illness and, 737-738
  communication and, 741-742
  documentation in, 740
  home care and, 736-737, 740-741
    exercise and, 742-743
    monitoring in, 742
    oxygen in, 743-744, 743f, 744f
    support for, 745
    therapeutic goals for, 745
  long-term care and, 738-739
  overview of, 735-736
  oxygen therapy in, 739-740
  pulmonary concerns in, 737
Community-based rehabilitation after transplantation, 729
Compensated heart failure, 106
Complementary therapy, 465-493
  body work therapy, 470-471
  for cardiovascular dysfunction, 472-481
    cardiac surgery, 478-479, 479t
    congestive heart failure, 479-480, 480t
    coronary artery disease, 476-478, 478t
    in coronary care unit, 480-481
    hypertension, 474-476, 475t
    stress reduction in, 473-474, 474t
  for chronic obstructive pulmonary disease, 483-485, 484t

Complementary therapy, (cont'd)
  energy work techniques, 466, 471-472
  examples of, 465
  holistic, 467-468
  manual therapy, 465, 470-471
  mind/body interventions, 466-467
    t'ai chi as, 469, 470t
    yoga as, 469, 471t
  movement awareness techniques, 466
  for pulmonary dysfunction, 481-485
    asthma, 481-483, 484t
    chronic obstructive pulmonary disease, 484-485
  scientific evidence for, 468
  use of, 468-469
Compliance, lung, 75
Complications, 639-644
  acute respiratory distress syndrome as, 644-647
  medical and surgical
    acid-base abnormality as, 641
    cardiac dysrhythmia as, 641
    fluid and electrolyte abnormality as, 641
    gastrointestinal, 641-642
    metabolic, 639-640
    muscular, 642
    myocardial, 641
    neurological, 642
    pulmonary, 640-641
    renal, 642
    thromboembolism as, 641
  postoperative, 532-533, 642-644
    with artificial airway, 774-775
    deep venous thrombosis as, 643, 643b
    hypoxemia, 642
    management of, 643-644
    oxygen transport and, 643b
    pain, 642-643
    pain as, 642-643
    pulmonary embolism as, 643, 643b
  of tracheostomy, 773-774
  of transplant, 730-731, 731b
Computed tomography, 166-167, 167f
  cardiac, 205
  physics of, 205
  pulmonary, 205-206, 206f
Concentrator, oxygen, 762-763, 763f
Concha, 61
Conditioning in post polio syndrome, 445
Conduction block, 181-183, 182f, 183f
Conduction system, 170-172, 170f, 171f
Congenital heart disease, exercise program for, 413
Congestive heart failure. See Heart failure
Connective tissue disease, 118, 118b
  exercise in, 286b, 446
  heart disease in, 108
Consolidation, lung, 165
Consumption. See Oxygen consumption
Continuing education, 24, 24b
Continuous positive airway pressure breathing, 763

Contract, health care, 497, 497b
Contractility, myocardial, 44
Contraction, muscle, 42, 43f
Controlled breathing
  in cystic fibrosis, 553
  diaphragmatic
    facilitation of, 382-383, 382b, 383b
    scoop technique of, 386-387, 386f, 387f
  in emphysema, 550
  indications for, 383b
  in primary versus secondary dysfunction, 383-384
  in stroke, 571
Controlled clinical trial, randomized, 24-25
COPD. See Chronic obstructive pulmonary disease
Coronary artery
  magnetic resonance imaging of, 168f
  myocardial infarction and, 102-103
Coronary artery disease, 100-109
  anemia and, 107-108
  angina pectoris and, 102
  atherosclerosis and, 100-101
  complementary therapy for, 476-478, 478t
  heart failure and, 105-107
  hypercholesterolemia and, 100
  metabolic syndrome and, 108
  myocardial infarction and, 102-105
  obstructive sleep apnea and, 102
  pulmonary hypertension and, 107
  valvular heart disease and, 107
Coronary care unit, 480-481. See also Intensive care unit
Cortical disturbance, 118
Corticosteroid, 96
Cortisol, 190
Cost of airway clearance technique, 335, 360
Costal breathing, lateral, 388-390, 388f, 389f
Costophrenic assisted cough, 368-369, 368f
Cough, 363-376
  assisted, 368-374
  in cerebral palsy, 575
  characteristics of, 143-144, 144t
  complications of, 364-365
  in cystic fibrosis, 519, 553
  eating or drinking and, 364
  evaluation of, 365-366
  instruction about, 366-368
  in intensive care patient, 626
  manually assisted, 368-371
    anterior chest compression, 369-370
    costophrenic, 368-369, 368f
    counter-rotation, 370-371, 370f
    Heimlich-type, 369, 369f
  mechanical in-exsufflator for, 374-375
  mechanics of, 365f
  in multiple sclerosis, 573
  in muscular dystrophy, 581
  open-glottis, 5165
  in osteoporosis, 583-584
  overview of, 363-364

Cough, (*cont'd*)
  positioning for, 366
  in post polio syndrome, 578
  self-assisted, 371-374
    hands-knees, rocking, 373-374, 374f
    long-sitting, 372, 372f, 373f
    prone-on-elbows, head flexion, 371-372, 372f
    short-sitting, 372-373, 373f
    standing, 374
  in spinal cord injury, 576, 632
  stages of, 365
  in trauma, 630
  treatment hierarchy for, 256b
Cough Assist Machine, 374-375
Cough pump, 364
Cough reflex, 74
  in pneumonia, 509-510
Coughing up blood, 146, 155
Counter-rotation, 395-396
Counter-rotation assisted cough, 370-371, 370f
Coupling, electromechanical, 80-82
CPAP breathing, 763
Craniosacral therapy, 490
Creatine phosphate, 40, 42
Crohn's disease, 446
Cross training, 296-297
Cryptogenic pulmonary fibrosis, 96
Cuffed tracheostomy tube, 775-776
Cultural differences, 18
Cultural factor, 249
Curve
  oxyhemoglobin dissociation, 82-83, 82f
  relaxation pressure, 75-76, 76f
  ventricular volume, 81
Cyanosis
  assessment of, 215
  hemoglobin and, 159
Cycle
  of breathing, active, 328
    equipment for, 348, 348f
    ineffective and effective huffing in, 349b
    overview of, 328
    precautions for, 334
    preparation for, 348
    selection considerations for, 359t
    treatment with, 349
  cardiac, 81, 82f
  Krebs, 40, 41f
Cyclogyl, 791
Cyclopentolate, 791
Cyclosporine, in transplantation, 730
Cylindrical bronchiectasis, 93
Cystic fibrosis
  acute exacerbation of, 518-519
  airway clearance in, 326
  exercise program for, 417
  management of, 552-553
  in pediatric patient, 662-663

Cystic fibrosis, (*cont'd*)
  exercise and, 677
  respiratory muscle training in, 458
Cytokine, 269

D
Dalton's law, 158
Dance therapy, 491
Data sheet
  for treadmill or ergometer, 291b
  for walk or circuit test, 2921b
Death, 607-608
Decannulation, 782
Decision making, 247, 247b, 254, 255f, 256b
Decompensated heart failure, 106
Deconditioning
  bed rest and, 267-271
  in lung transplantation, 728
Deep breathing
  in muscular dystrophy, 581
  trauma and, 630
Deep venous thrombosis
  mobilization and exercise affecting, 274
  myocardial infarction with, 104
  postoperative, 643
Degenerative disk disease, 146
Dementia, 15
Demyelinating disease
  cardiopulmonary effects of, 118
  multiple sclerosis as, 572
Density on radiograph, 164, 164f
Dental health, 15
Depolarization, 170
  atrial, 171-172
  of atrioventricular node, 178-179
  ventricular, 172
Depression after myocardial infarction, 557
Desaturated blood, 49
Desquamous interstitial pulmonary fibrosis, 96
Deviation, tracheal, 224, 225f
Dexedrine, 788
Dextran, 231
Dextroamphetamine, 788
Diabetes
  atherosclerosis and, 101
  cardiomyopathy in, 104
  cardiopulmonary complications of, 120, 123
  exercise program for, 414
  exercise testing and training in, 447
  heart failure with, 106
  management of, 563-565
  modifiable risk factors for, 6t
  risk factor modification for, 13
  type 2, 108, 414
Dialysis, 642
Diaphragm
  anatomy of, 55-57, 55f, 56f
  in facilitation of ventilation, 384

Diaphragm, (cont'd)
    inhibition of, 392-394, 393f, 394f
    in multisystem impairment, 703
    in paralysis of abdominal and intercostal muscles, 706, 707f
    posture and, 384
    on radiography, 165
    stretch reflex and, 74
    in supine position, 315, 315f
Diaphragmatic breathing, controlled
    facilitation of, 382-383, 382b, 383b
    scoop technique of, 386-387, 386f, 387f
    techniques of, 384b
Diaphragmatic excursion, 222, 222f
Diastole, heart valves and, 67
Diastolic function, age affecting, 686-687
Diastolic ventricular pressure, 315
Dibenzyline, 788
Dicyclomine, 791
Diffuse esophageal spasm, 146
Diffuse interstitial pulmonary fibrosis, 95-97
Diffusion
    in cardiopulmonary physiology, 77
    of gases, 158
    oxygen transport and, 39b, 43-44, 47-48
Dilation, gastric, 641-642
Discharge from intensive care unit, 606
Disease, 5-6
Disk disease, degenerative, 146
Dislodgement of artificial airway, 775
Disposable tracheostomy tube, 775-776
Disseminated intravascular coagulation, 46
    in liver disorder, 121
    tests for, 188-189
Dissociation of oxygen from hemoglobin, 43-44
Distant healing prayer, 490
Distention, jugular venous, 215
Distress. See Respiratory distress
Diuretic hormone, 268
Documentation, 740
Donation, organ, 720. See also Transplantation
Donepezil, 790
Doppler echocardiography, 202, 204
Down syndrome
    exercise testing and training in, 445-446
    heart defects with, 660t
    in pediatric patient, 665-666, 666f
Doxazosin, 788
Drainage
    autogenic
        advantages and disadvantages of, 351
        in cystic fibrosis, 519
        equipment for, 350
        overview of, 329, 329f
        preparation for, 350, 350f
        selection considerations for, 359t
        treatment with, 350, 351f
    chest tube, 232-233, 232f
    in cystic fibrosis, 663

Drainage, (cont'd)
    postural, 342-344
        advantages and disadvantages of, 344, 344f
        in burn injury, 635
        contraindications to, 332, 333b
        in cystic fibrosis, 663
        equipment for, 343
        in infant, 668, 670t, 671f-674f
        overview of, 326-327, 327f
        precautions for, 334
        preparation for, 343
        selection considerations for, 359t
        technique of, 342f-343f
        treatment hierarchy for, 256b
        treatment with, 343-344
Dressing, 381
Drinking, 364
Dromotropic effect, 48
Drug therapy
    adrenergic, 786-788
    alpha-adrenergic blocker, 787-788
    angiotensin-converting enzyme inhibitor, 792
    angiotensin II receptor blocker, 792
    anticholinesterase, 790
    autonomic pharmacology and, 785-786
    beta-adrenergic blocking agent, 788
    for cardiac rehabilitation, 414
    cardiovascular reflex and, 791-792
    cholinergic blocking, 790-791
    for disease
        angina, 555
        asthma, 551
        bronchiectasis, 552
        chronic bronchitis, 547, 548
        chronic renal insufficiency, 588
        cystic fibrosis, 553
        diabetes, 564
        emphysema, 549
        hypertension, 563
        lung cancer, 554-555
        multiple sclerosis, 573
        myocardial infarction, 103, 558
        Parkinson's syndrome, 572
        peripheral vascular, 561
        post polio syndrome, 577
        rheumatoid arthritis, 587
        scleroderma, 585
        stroke, 570
        systemic lupus erythematosus, 584
        valvular, 559
    for intensive care patient, 602-603
    in obesity, 589
    parasympathetic neurotransmission and, 789
    surgery and, 532
    sympathetic neurotransmission and, 786
    sympatholytic, 788-789
    in transplantation, 730
Duchenne muscular dystrophy, 660t, 666-667

Duct, alveolar, 63
Ductus arteriosus, 658
Dust exposure, 147-148
Dying patient, end-of-life issues and, 607-608
Dynamic activity, facilitation of ventilation in, 381
Dysphagia, cough with, 364
Dysplasia, bronchopulmonary, 661
Dyspnea, 138-143
    acute, 139
    assessment of, 216-217
    in cardiac patient, 141-142
    classification of, 142b
    definition of, 381b
    in emphysema, 515
    on exertion, 139-141, 140t
    functional, 143
    orthopnea, 142
    overview of, 138-139
    platypnea, 142
    scales of, 141, 141f, 142f
    trepopnea, 142-143
Dysrhythmia
    clinical features of, 236t
    as complication, 641
    in intensive care patient, 235-236
    lethal, 175
    in myocardial infarction, 103
Dystrophy, muscular
    Duchenne, 660t, 666-667
    intensive care for, 625
    management of, 578-581
    in pediatric patient, 666-667

E
Eating, cough with, 364
Eccentric resistance technique, 400-401
Ecchymosis, 215
Echocardiography, 202-205
    Doppler, 202, 204
    exercise, 204
    physics of, 202, 204, 204f
    in postoperative period, 537
Ectopic focus, 177
Ectopic pacemaker, 179
Edema
    pedal, 147
    pulmonary, 116
        in acute lung injury, 644
        in burn injury, 634
    in skin assessment, 215
Edrophonium, 790
Education, 495-504
    adherence and, 502
    for cardiac or pulmonary rehabilitation, 420
    content of, 501, 501b
    continuing professional, 24, 24b
    on cough, 366-367
    definition of, 495-496

Education, (cont'd)
    disease-related
        ankylosing spondylitis, 586
        in asthma, 551
        bronchiectasis, 552
        cerebral palsy, 574-575
        chronic bronchitis, 548
        chronic renal insufficiency, 588
        cystic fibrosis, 552, 553
        in diabetes, 564
        effectiveness of, 501-502
        emphysema, 549
        interstitial lung disease, 554
        muscular dystrophy, 580
        myocardial infarction and, 558
        osteoporosis, 583
        Parkinson's syndrome, 572
        peripheral vascular, 560-561
        post polio syndrome, 578
        rheumatoid arthritis, 587
        scleroderma, 585
        stroke, 570, 571
        systemic lupus erythematosus, 584
        valvular, 559
    health care contract and, 497b
    interdisciplinary team for, 502-503
    learning needs assessment for, 497-499, 498b, 499b
    learning theory and, 496-497
    lifestyle change and, 20
    methods of, 500-501, 500t
    needs-based approach to, 497
    objectives of, 496, 496b
    in spinal cord injury, 576
    teacher-learner relationship and, 501-502
    in thoracic deformity, 582
    on transplantation, 724
Edwards' syndrome, 660t
Effusion, pleural, 116
    differential diagnosis of, 226t
    on radiograph, 165
Elastic property of lung, 75
Elastic recoil, 689
Elderly. *See* Aging patient
Electrical conduction of heart, 68-69, 69f
Electrical nerve stimulation, 240, 492, 532
Electrocardiography, 169-186
    cardiac action potential and, 170-171, 170f
    case studies of, 184-185, 185f
    conduction system in, 171-172, 171f
    dysrhythmia shown on, 176-183
        conduction blocks, 181-183, 182f, 183f
        supraventricular, 176-179, 176f-179f
        ventricular, 179-181, 179f-181f
    evaluation of strip from, 173
    in exercise testing, 280
    heart rate determination in, 173-175, 174f, 175f
    heart transplantation and, 725
    of hypertension, 562-563

Electrocardiography, (cont'd)
  in intensive care unit, 235-237, 235f, 236t
  of myocardiac ischemia or infarction, 183-184, 183f, 184f
  in myocardial infarction, 557
  overview of, 169-170
  in pulmonary embolism, 643
  recording of, 172, 173f
  rhythm evaluation in, 175-176, 176f
  terminating exercise testing and, 290b
Electrode for electrocardiography, 172-173, 173f
Electrolyte
  blood tests for, 188t
  in burn injury, 634
  in intensive care unit, 230-232, 231f, 232f
Electromagnetic field therapy, pulsed, 492
Electromechanical coupling, cardiac, 80-82
Electromyography for asthma, 482
Electron beam computed tomography, 205
Embolism, pulmonary
  differential diagnosis of, 226t
  postoperative, 643
Emotional stress, 50
Emphysema
  acute exacerbation of, 514-516
  differential diagnosis of, 226t
  management of, 548-550
  pathophysiology of, 87-91, 88f, 89f
Empyema, 166f
End diastolic ventricular pressure, 315
End-of-life issues, 607-608
End-stage disease
  cardiac, 106-107
    heart transplantation and, 722
  lung, 100
    transplantation and, 722-723
  renal, 446
End tidal carbon dioxide, 162
End tidal volume, 537
Endocardial cushion defect, 660
Endocardium, 67
Endocrine disorder
  cardiopulmonary complications of, 122-123, 123b
  exercise and, 286b, 447
  laboratory testing for, 189-190, 190t
Endocrine system, 275
Endotracheal airway, suctioning of, 781
Endotracheal intubation
  complications with, 640
  postoperative, 532, 644
Energy-based therapy, 467
Energy conservation, 256b
Energy for muscle contraction, 42, 43f
Energy transport, 40, 41f, 42
Energy work technique, 466, 471-472
  for asthma, 483
  for coronary artery disease, 478, 478t
  types of, 491-492
Environmental area of learning needs assessment, 498, 498b

Eosinophilia, 97
Eosinophilic granuloma, 97
Ephedrine, 788
Epicardium, 67
Epidemiology, 27
Epinephrine, 190, 788
Epithelium, pseudostratified columnar ciliated, 62f
Equal pressure point, 328
Equation, Henderson-Hasselbalch, 157
Equipment
  for autogenic drainage, 350
  for high-frequency chest wall oscillation, 355
  for manual hyperinflation, 347
  for percussion, 343-344
  for positive expiratory pressure breathing, 352-353, 352f
  for postural drainage, 343
  for vibration/shaking, 346
Erector spinae muscle, 59
Ergometer, data sheet for, 291b
Erythrocyte disorder, cardiopulmonary complications of, 122
Erythropoietin therapy, 447
Escherichia coli pneumonia, 511
Eserine, 790
Esophagus
  pain in, 146
  in scleroderma, 585
Ethical issues in organ transplantation, 720
Ethnic differences, 18
Eupnea, 381b
Evaluation, documentation of, 134
Evidence-based planning, 8-22
  for changing health behavior, 19-22, 20b, 21b, 22t
  cultural differences and, 18-19
  epidemiological indicators in, 8-9
  exercise and, 16, 18
  health care needs addressed in, 8
  nutrition and, 15-16, 17f
  principles of, 9
  priorities in, 9-10
  for promoting healthy living, 15
  risk factor modification in
    for cancer, 14
    for dental health, 15
    for hypertension, 11-12
    for ischemic heart disease, 10-11
    for metabolic syndrome, 13
    for musculoskeletal health, 14
    for obesity, 14
    for psychological health, 14-15
    for smoking-related conditions, 11, 12t
    for stroke, 12-13
    for type 2 diabetes, 13
  for smoking cessation, 18, 18b
Evidence-based practice, 22-23, 22b
Examination
  documentation of, 134
  physical, 212

Excess fluid, 231
Excursion, diaphragmatic, 222, 222f
Exelon, 790
Exercise, 263-306
  acute response to, 272-276, 272b-274b, 275t
  aging and, 687, 689-690
  for airway clearance, 357-358
    overview of, 332
    precautions for, 334
    selection considerations for, 359t
  in angina, 555
  in ankylosing spondylitis, 586
  in asthma, 551
  asthma and, 676-677
  in bed rest, 271-272
  in burn injury, 635
  in cardiac rehabilitation, 523
  cellular energetics in, 265-267
  changing behavior and, 20
  chest wall. See Chest wall exercise
  in chronic bronchitis, 548
  in chronic renal insufficiency, 588
  components of, 278f
  in cystic fibrosis, 553, 663
  definition of, 263
  in diabetes, 564
  dyspnea and, 216-217
  in health promotion, 16, 17f, 18
  in heart failure, 106
  heart transplantation and, 724-725, 725t, 727-728
  in hypertension, 563
  of interstitial lung disease, 554
  long-term response to, 281-284
  lung transplantation and, 725-726, 728
  in multiple sclerosis, 573
  myocardial infarction and, 558
  in osteoporosis, 583
  oxygen to improve, 763
  oxygen transport and, 50
  oxygen transport in, 267
  in Parkinson's syndrome, 572
  in post polio syndrome, 578
  prescription for, 264-265
  in rheumatoid arthritis, 587
  in scleroderma, 585
  for secondary cardiopulmonary dysfunction, 441-451
  in spinal cord injury, 576
  in stroke, 571
  in systemic lupus erythematosus, 584
  in thoracic deformity, 582
  treatment hierarchy for, 256b
  in valvular disease, 560
Exercise echocardiography, 204
  in postoperative period, 537
Exercise-induced asthma, 92
Exercise pyramid, 17f
Exercise testing and training, 284, 286-295, 551
  aging and, 687

Exercise testing and training, (cont'd)
  checklist for, 297b
  for chronic cardiac dysfunction, 408-417
    anemia, 413-414
    components of program of, 417-421, 418b, 419b
    congenital heart disease, 413
    diabetes, 414
    heart failure, 409-412
    heart transplantation, 412-413
    hypertension, 414
    left ventricular assist device, 413
    preadmission workup for, 418b
    special considerations in, 423, 425-428, 426b, 427b
  for chronic pulmonary dysfunction, 414-417
    asthma, 417
    components of program of, 417-421, 418b, 419b, 428-430
    cystic fibrosis, 417
    interstitial lung disease, 416
    lung reduction surgery, 416
    lung transplantation, 416
    obstructive, 415-416
    preadmission workup for, 419b
    pulmonary hypertension, 416
  contraindications to, 287b
  criterial for terminating, 290b
  data sheet for, 291b
  indications for, 287b
  monitoring of, 295, 298
  myocardial infarction and, 557
  in peripheral vascular disease, 561
  preexercise testing in, 289b
  preparation for, 290b
  prescription for, 295-297
  procedures for, 297-298
  protocols for, 293-295, 294f
  in pulmonary rehabilitation, 429
  readiness questionnaire for, 285f
  in secondary cardiopulmonary dysfunction, 441-451
    assessment in, 442
    connective tissue disease and, 446
    endocrine disorder and, 447
    gastrointestinal disorder and, 446
    goals of, 442
    hematological disorder and, 447
    immunhodeficiency and, 447-448
    liver disorder and, 446
    musculoskeletal disorder and, 442-443
    neurological disorder and, 443-446
    nutrition-related disorder and, 448
    renal disorder and, 446-447
    rheumatoid disorder and, 446
  subjective scales in, 288b
Exertion scale, perceived, 357f
Exhalation
  aging and, 689
  in facilitation of ventilation, 381

Expectoration of blood, 146
  in lung cancer, 555
Expiration technique, forced, 328
Expiratory muscle, 59
Expiratory muscle training, 455-456
Expiratory pressure breathing, positive
    precautions for, 334
    selection considerations for, 359t
Expiratory technique, in cystic fibrosis, 519
Expiratory volume, forced, 315-316
Expulsion, in cough, 366
External manipulation of thorax, 332-333, 333b
Extraction, tissue, 48-49
Extrapulmonary effect of chronic obstructive pulmonary
      disease, 90
Extrapulmonary sound, 219
Extubation, 782
  after surgery, 535-536

F
Family history, 148
Fatigue
  chronic, 447-448
  in muscular dystrophy, 580
  patient history of, 146-147
  in post polio syndrome, 578
  in spinal cord injury, 633
Fecal impaction, 642
Feldenkrais method, 466, 474t, 491
Fetal alcohol syndrome, 660t
Fetal circulation, 658
Fever, 161
Fiber
  muscle, 42, 43f
    of heart, 69
  Purkinje, 69
Fibrillation
  atrial, 178
  ventricular, 181, 181f
    clinical features of, 236t
Fibrinogen
  in acute respiratory distress syndrome, 645
  function of, 46
  as risk factor, 6
Fibrosis
  cystic
    acute exacerbation of, 518-519
    airway clearance in, 326
    exercise program for, 417
    respiratory muscle training in, 458
  myocardial, 107
  pulmonary
    acute exacerbation of, 519-520
    connective tissue disease and, 118
    diffuse interstitial, 95-97
    lung transplantation and, 723
Fibrous pericardium, 67
Film, x-ray, 163. *See also* Radiography

Financial issues, 335, 360
FIO_2, 320
Fitness, ischemic heart disease and, 10
Fixation
  of fracture, 630
  spinal cord injury, 632
Flail chest, 628b
Flotation catheter, pulmonary artery balloon,
      237-238
Flow-directed pulmonary artery catheter, 641
Flow meter, peak, 364
Fluid
  cerebrospinal, 74
  in lung, 116
  in pedal edema, 147
  pericardial, 67
  in peritoneal cavity, 47
  pleural, 116, 117
Fluid and electrolyte balance
  in burn injury, 634
  complications with, 641
  in intensive care unit, 230-232, 231f, 232f
Fluid balance, position affecting, 314
Fluid collection system, 232-233, 232f
Fluid retention, 641
Fluid volume
  bed rest and, 268b
  limitation in oxygen transport and, 252b
Flutter, atrial, 178, 178f
Flutter valve, 353-354, 353f, 354b
  in cystic fibrosis, 519, 553
  in positive expiratory pressure breathing, 330
Fold, vocal, 703-704
Foramen ovale, closure of, 658
Forced expiration technique, 328
Forced expiratory volume, 86
  in chronic bronchitis, 547
  side-lying position and, 315-316
Foreign body, 144t
Fowler's position, 779, 779f
Fracture
  multiple, 630-631
  radiograph of, 165
  rib, 629
FRC. *See* Functional residual capacity
Fremitus, tactile, 224, 224f
Friedreich's ataxia, 660t
Function
  classification of, 248, 248f, 248t
  structure and, 248-249
Functional dyspnea, 143
Functional reflex, 792
Functional residual capacity, 75
  anesthesia and, 531
  body position and, 310-311, 310f, 311f
  in postoperative period, 537, 643
  in side-lying position, 315
Funnel chest, 216

G

Gait after stroke, 277
Galantamine, 790
Gallop, 221
Gas, arterial blood. *See* Arterial blood gases
Gas exchange
  in acute respiratory distress syndrome, 647
  in heart failure, 106
  limitation in oxygen transport and, 251b
  position and, 308
Gastric dilation, 641-642
Gastroesophageal reflux, 715f
  airway clearance in, 334
Gastrointestinal disorder
  cardiopulmonary complications of, 120-121, 121b
  as complication, 641-642
  exercise testing and training in, 446
Gastrointestinal system, exercise affecting, 273b
Gender
  bed rest and, 277
  exercise response and, 276
  health and, 9
  mobilization and exercise and, 284
Genitourinary tract, 273b
Gland, laboratory testing of, 189-190, 190t
Globulin, 46
Glossopharyngeal breathing, 397-399, 399f
Glottis, cough and, 364, 366
Glucocorticoid in transplantation, 730
Glucose
  in diabetes, 563, 564, 565
  mobilization and exercise affecting, 283
  in oxygen transport, 40
Glucose monitoring, 447
Goal
  at end-of-life, 608
  for intensive care unit management, 598-601, 599b-
    601b
  of postoperative management, 534-536, 536b
  treatment, 253
Goblet, cell, tracheal, 62
Gradient, diffusion, 44
Graft, skin, 635
Granuloma, eosinophilic, 97
Gravitational stress
  in burn injury, 635
  in oxygen transport, 49
Gravity
  in body mechanics, 753f, 754
  chest wall development and, 696, 697f-700f, 698-699,
    701t
  physiological function and, 307-308, 308f
  planes of ventilation and, 695-696, 696f, 696t
  in postural drainage, 326
  ventilation/perfusion matching and, 78
Gravity eliminated breathing, 707
Groningen Active Living Model, 26
Guanethidine, 788

Guided imagery
  for asthma, 482
  for congestive heart failure, 480t
Guidelines
  for documentation, 133-134
    content and organization of, 133-135
    purposes of, 133
  HIPAA, 135
Guillain-Barré syndrome, 625

H

Haemophilus influenzae pneumonia, 511
Hands-knees, rocking self-assisted cough, 373-374, 374f
Head and neck anatomy, 61f
Head-down position, 316
Head injury
  management of, 631-632
  pathophysiology of, 631
Healing energy, 466
Healing environment, 607
Healing prayer, 490
Health, definitions of, 3-5
Health-belief model, 4t, 497
Health care contract, 497
Health Insurance Portability and Accountability Act, 135
Heart. *See also* Cardiac *entries*
  age affecting, 686-687
  anatomy of, 67-69, 67f-70f
  athletic heart syndrome, 109
  fetal and neonatal, 658
  magnetic resonance imaging of, 206-207
  mechanical activity of, 80-81
  mobilization and exercise affecting, 283
  in multisystem assessment, 187
  outcome measurement for, 258b
  oxygen transport and, 252b
  on radiograph, 166
  reflexes of, 79-80
  sounds of, 81
  systole and diastole and, 81
  volume and pressure changes of, 81
Heart block, 181-183, 182f, 183f
  clinical features of, 236t
Heart defect, syndromes with, 660t
Heart disease
  cardiac complications of, 116
  chest pain in, 145
  congenital, exercise program for, 413
  as disease of civilization, 5
  noncardiac conditions and, 108-109
  in stroke patient, 570
Heart failure
  congestive, 105-107
    acute, 105
    chronic, 105-106
    compensated and decompensated, 106
    complementary therapy for, 479-480, 480t
    fatigue in, 147

Heart failure, (cont'd)
    fluid and electrolyte balance and, 232
    myocardial infarction with, 104
    pedal edema in, 147
    pleural effusion and, 116
    prognosis for, 106-107
  etiology of, 130b
  exercise program for, 409-412
  fluid and electrolyte balance and, 232
  left, 116
  shock and, 648
Heart rate
  on electrocardiograph, 173-175, 174f
  exercise affecting, 266, 272
  in exercise testing, 280
  exercise training and, 298
  mobilization and, 273, 280
Heart sound, 220-221, 220f, 221f
Heart surgery, 621-623, 622b
Heart transplantation. *See also* Transplantation
  acute management of, 724-725, 725t
  for end-stage cardiac disease, 722
  exercise program for, 412-413
  recipient status for, 722b
  surgical procedure for, 724
Hearts for Life program, 27
Heated aerosol, 762, 762f
Heimlich-type assisted cough, 369, 369f
Hellerwork, 490
Hematocrit, 45
Hematological disorder
  cardiopulmonary complications of, 122, 122b
  in cardiopulmonary disease, 117
  exercise testing and training in, 447
Hematological system
  mobilization and exercise affecting, 273b
  oxygen transport and, 39b
Hemiparesis, 707f
Hemiplegia, 569-571
Hemodialysis, 446
Hemodynamics
  complications with, 641
  in diabetes, 564
  mobilization and exercise affecting, 273b, 274, 282
  monitoring of, 237-239, 237f, 238f
  muscle training and, 276
  in valvular disease, 559
Hemoglobin
  arterial blood gases and, 159
  mobilization and exercise affecting, 282
  oxygen dissociating from, 43-44
  oxygen transport by, 82-83
  red blood cells transporting, 46
Hemoptysis, 146
Hemorrhage, pulmonary, 122
Hemostasis, 188-189
Hemothorax
  on radiograph, 165, 166

Hemothorax, (cont'd)
  trauma causing, 629
Henderson-Hasselbalch equation, 157
Hepatic disorder
  cardiopulmonary complications of, 121, 121b
  exercise testing and training in, 446
  testing for, 190, 191t
Hepatopulmonary syndrome, 121
  exercise testing and training in, 446
Herbal medicine, 466, 490
Hering-Breuer reflex, 74
HFCWO. *See* High-frequency chest wall oscillation
Hierarchy, physiological, of body positions, 318b
High-flow oxygen system, 761-762, 762f
High-frequency chest wall oscillation, 331, 355-356
  advantages and disadvantages of, 356
  equipment for, 355, 355f
  precautions for, 334
  preparation for, 355-356
  selection considerations for, 359t
  treatment with, 356
High-frequency oscillating ventilator in spinal cord
    injury, 633
High-pressure positive expiratory pressure breathing
  equipment for, 353
  treatment with, 354
High-resolution computed tomography, 205-206, 206f
Highly active antiretroviral therapy, 447
HIPAA guidelines, 135
Histiocytosis X, 97
History, patient, 137-149
  of chest pain, 144-146
  in clinical assessment, 211-212
  of cough, 143-144, 144t
  of dyspnea, 138-143, 138f, 140f, 140t, 141f, 142b
  family, 148
  of fatigue and weakness, 146-147
  of hemoptysis, 146
  of hoarseness, 147
  interview for, 137-138
  occupational, 147-148
  of pedal edema, 147
  of prior treatment, 148
  questionnaires in, 138
  of smoking, 148
  of wheezing, 143
Hoarseness, 147
Holistic medicine, 467-468
Homatropine, 791
Home care
  cardiopulmonary concerns in, 740
  communication in, 741-742
  exercise in, 742-743
  goals for, 745
  monitoring of, 742
  oxygen therapy in, 743, 743f, 744f
  physical therapy in, 736-737
  support for, 745

Home care, (*cont'd*)
  for transplantation patient, 729
  working in, 740-741
Homeopathic medicine, 490
Homocysteine, 101
Human immunodeficiency virus infection
  cardiopulmonary complications of, 123
  in child, 660t
  education about, 500-501
  exercise testing and training in, 447-448
  Pneumocystis carinii pneumonia in, 662
Humidity therapy, 764
Hyaline membrane disease, 661
Hydrostatic pressure, 78, 117
  capillary, 81
  interstitial, 81
Hypercapnia, 235
Hypercholesterolemia, 100
Hyperglycemia, 564
Hyperinflation
  manual
    overview of, 328
    precautions for, 333b
    selection considerations for, 359t
  radiography and, 166
Hyperoxia, 235
Hyperpnea, 381b
Hyperpnea equipment, normocapnic, 457f
Hypersecretion in chronic bronchitis, 546
Hypertension
  as acute medical condition, 521-522
  atherosclerosis and, 101
  complementary therapy for, 474-476, 475t, 476t
  drugs for, 792
  exercise program for, 414
  exercise response and, 276
  management of, 562-563
  pulmonary, 107
    chest pain in, 145
  risk factor modification for, 11-12
  systemic, 107
Hyperthyroidism
  cardiopulmonary complications of, 123, 123b
  exercise testing and training in, 447
Hypnosis, 490
Hypocapnia, 235
Hypoglycemia, 564, 565
Hypotension, 120
Hypothyroidism
  cardiopulmonary complications of, 122-123, 123b
  exercise testing and training in, 447
Hypoventilation, 381b
Hypoxemia
  chemoreceptor response to, 159
  in chronic bronchitis, 87
  in chronic obstructive pulmonary disease, 90
  in emphysema, 515, 5165
  in intensive care patient, 234

Hypoxemia, (*cont'd*)
  in liver disease, 446
  postoperative, 536, 642
  respiratory failure and, 160-161
  signs and symptoms of, 234t
Hypoxia in premature infant, 659
Hytrin, 788

I
Idiopathic pulmonary fibrosis, 96. *See also* Pulmonary
    fibrosis
Imagery, 490
  for asthma, 482
Imaging of chest, 163-168
  computed tomography, 166-167, 167f
  evaluation of, 164-166, 164f, 165f
  magnetic resonance, 168-169, 168f
  normal, 700f
  projections for, 165t
Immigration
  global health and, 9
  health beliefs and, 4
Immune modulator, 730
Immunologic disorder, 123
Immunologic function testing, 191, 191f
Immunological system, 275
Immunosuppression
  in chronic obstructive pulmonary disease, 96
  in transplantation, 730
Impaction, fecal, 642
In-exsufflator, mechanical, 374-375
Incentive spirometry, 537, 763-764, 764f
Inderal, 788
Index, oxygen transport, 39b
Indigenous peoples, 8
Infant. *See also* Pediatric patient
  chest physical therapy for, 668-674, 669f-774f, 670b, 670t
  chest wall development of, 701, 701t
  neonate, 658-659. *See also* Neonate
  premature, 659t
Infantile scoliosis, 708-713, 708f, 709t, 710t
Infarction, myocardial. *See* Myocardial infarction
Infection
  bronchiectasis and, 93-94
  in chronic obstructive pulmonary disease, 89-90
  cough in, 144t
  human immunodeficiency virus. *See* Human
      immunodeficiency virus infection
  limitation in oxygen transport and, 252b
  pneumonia, 509-512
    bacterial, 510-512
    viral, 510
  tuberculosis, 100, 520-521
Infection control in intensive care unit, 606-607
Infiltrate, pulmonary, 97
Inflammatory disease
  asthma as, 91-92
  of bowel, 121

Inflammatory disease, (cont'd)
  bronchitis as, 87
  in obstructive lung disease, 86-87
  pulmonary fibrosis, 95-96
Inflammatory mediator, 6
Inflation of tracheostomy tube cuff, 775-776
Inhalation injury, 634
Inhaler
  in asthma, 551
  metered-dose, 764, 765
Inhibition, postural, 395
Inhibition of diaphragm, 392-394, 393f, 394f
Injury. See Trauma
Innervation, cardiac, 69
Inspection, visual, 212, 214-215, 215f, 216f
Inspiration
  cough and, 366
  in facilitation of ventilation, 380-381
Inspiratory effort in chest radiograph, 165
Inspiratory mouth pressure, 633
Inspiratory muscle training, 455, 456f
Inspired oxygen, 46-47
Instillation, 604
Instruction on cough, 366-367
Insulin
  in diabetes, 564
  laboratory test of, 190
Integumentary system, 715
Intensive care unit, 229-243, 597-610, 598f
  acid-base balance in, 233, 233t
  blood gases in, 233-235
  brain activity assessment in, 240
  chest tube drainage in, 232-233, 232f
  for chronic obstructive pulmonary disease, 612-617
    management of, 613-614, 613f
    mobilization and, 614-615, 615f, 616f, 617
    positioning in, 615
  cognitive assessment in, 240-241
  electrocardiography in, 235-237, 235f, 236t
  end-of-life issues in, 607-608
  fluid and electrolyte balance in, 230-232, 231f, 232f
  fluid collection systems in, 232-233, 232f
  general clinical aspects of, 601-603
  goals of, 598-601, 599b-601b
  hemodynamic monitoring in, 237-239, 237f, 238f
  intraaortic balloon pump in, 239, 239f
  intracranial pressure measurement in, 239-240
  intravenous lines in, 230
  monitoring in, 602b
  for myocardial infarction, 619-621, 620b, 621b
  neuromuscular assessment in, 240
  nonclinical aspects of, 606-607, 606f
  for open heart surgery patient, 621-623, 622b
  overview of, 229-230, 230f
  pain assessment in, 241
  prescriptions in, 603-606, 605b
  for restrictive lung disease, 618-619
  specialized expertise for, 597-598, 598b

Intensive care unit, (cont'd)
  for status asthmaticus, 615-618
Intercostal muscle
  anatomy of, 57
  in multisystem impairment, 703
  in paralysis, 706, 707f
  stretch reflex and, 74
Interdisciplinary team, 502-503
Intermittent claudication
  exercise program for, 413
  management of, 560
Intermittent positive pressure breathing, 765-766, 765f
Internal organ, 704-705
International classification of function, 4-5, 248, 248f, 248t
Interstitial hydrostatic pressure, 81
Interstitial lung disease
  exercise program for, 416
  management of, 553-554
Interstitial pneumonia, 97
Interstitial pulmonary fibrosis
  acute exacerbation of, 519-520
  diffuse, 95-97
Interval measurement, 130-131
Intervention, 247-261
  classification of function and, 248-250, 248f, 248t
  clinical decision making in, 254, 255f, 256b, 257b
  course of treatment in, 257-259, 258b
  documentation of, 135
  overview of, 247-248
  patterns of, 254, 254b
  plan of, 254
  prescription for, 254
  problem identification for, 250-254, 250b-253b
Interview, patient, 211-212
Intima, 100-101
Intraabdominal pressure, 366
Intraaortic balloon counter pulsation device, 239, 239f
Intraaortic balloon pump, 648
Intraarterial line, 237, 237f
Intracranial pressure
  in head injury, 631-632
  in intensive care unit patient, 239-240
Intrapleural pressure
  differences in, 311
  in supine position, 314
Intrapulmonary percussive ventilation
  advantages and disadvantages of, 357
  equipment for, 356
  overview of, 331-332
  precautions for, 334
  selection considerations for, 359t
  treatment with, 356
Intrathoracic pressure
  in bronchiectasis, 551
  in chronic bronchitis, 547
  cough and, 366
  in emphysema, 550

Intravascular coagulation, disseminated, 46
  in liver disorder, 121
  tests for, 188-189
Intravenous line, 230
Intubation
  endotracheal, 532, 644
  of pediatric patient, 663-664
Inversine, 791
Ion in plasma, 46
Ipratropium, 791
Irritable bowel syndrome, 446
Ischemia, myocardial
  on electrocardiograph, 183-184, 183f, 184f
  pain of, 145
  stress reduction for, 477
Ischemic heart disease
  as disease of civilization, 5
  lifestyle and, 5-6
  risk factor modification for, 10-11
  risk factors for, 10-11
Ismelin, 788
Isometric exercise, in bed rest, 271-272
Isophrin, 788
Isoproterenol, 788
Isuprel, 788

J
Jacket, body, 379-380, 379f, 665f
Joint receptor, 74-75
Jugular venous distention, 215
Junctional rhythm, 179, 179f
Juvenile rheumatoid arthritis, 660t

K
Kidney, 189. *See also* Renal *entries*
Kinetic bed, 270-271
Kinetics
  glucose, 283
  oxygen, 234
Knee joint replacement, 164f
Krebs cycle, 40, 41f
Kyphoscoliosis, 165f, 581

L
L-dopa, 572
Labile hypertension, 522
Laboratory test, 187-191. *See also* Test
Lactic dehydrogenase, bed rest and, 271-272
Laminar airflow, 76
Landmark, topographic, 212, 212b, 213f, 214f
Laryngopharynx, anatomy of, 61
Larynx, 61-62, 62f
Laser therapy, 492
Lateral breathing, 707
Lateral costal breathing, 388-390, 388f, 389f
Latina population, 9
Lavage, bronchoalveolar
  for alveolar proteinosis, 96

Lavage, bronchoalveolar, (*cont'd*)
  in pulmonary fibrosis, 96
Law, Dalton's, 158
Lead, electrocardiographic, 172-173, 173f
Learning needs assessment, 487b, 497-499, 498b
Learning theory, 496-497
Left atrial pressure, 238
Left heart failure, 116
Left main-stem bronchus aspiration, 780
Left ventricular assist device, 413
Left ventricular pressure, 238
Lethal dysrhythmia, 175
Levarterenol, 786-788
Levophed, 786-788
Life cycle, disease and, 5-6
Lifestyle
  disease and, 5
  effecting change in, 7-8
  myocardial infarction and, 524
Lifestyle change
  physical therapist's role in, 15-22
    exercise and, 16, 17f, 18
    nutrition and, 15-16, 17f
    in smoking cessation, 18, 18f
  stages of readiness for, 20b
Lifestyle factors
  in diabetes, 564
  in hypertension, 562
Lifting patient, 753-754, 753f, 754
Lipoprotein, 101
Liver disease
  cardiopulmonary complications of, 121, 121b
  exercise testing and training in, 446
  testing for, 190, 191t
Long-sitting, body jacket for, 379-380, 379f
Long-sitting self-assisted cough, 372, 372f, 373f
Long-term care facility, 738-739
  monitoring in, 739
  physical therapy in, 736-737
Lopressor, 788
Low-density lipoprotein, 101
Low-flow oxygen system, 760-761, 760f, 760t
Lower airway, anatomy of, 62-63, 62f, 64t
Lower body negative pressure, 314
Lung
  aging and, 689
  anatomy of, 65, 66f, 66t
  anesthesia and, 531
  body position and, 311, 311f
  compliance of, 75
  in exercise, 266
  fluid and electrolyte balance and, 232
  limitation in oxygen transport and, 251b
  magnetic resonance imaging of, 207
  in multisystem assessment, 187
  outcome measurement for, 258b
  in oxygen transport, 47
  radiograph of, 165

Lung, (*cont'd*)
  shrinking, 118
  surface markings of, 65, 66f, 67f
  in tuberculosis, 521
Lung cancer, 100
  management of, 554-555
Lung disease
  airway clearance in, 334-335
  cardiac complications of, 117
  interstitial
    exercise program for, 416
    management of, 553-554
  modifiable risk factors for, 6t
  obstructive, 87-95
    asthma as, 91-93, 92b, 92f, 93f
    bronchiectasis as, 93-95, 94f
    chronic bronchitis as, 87
    cultural differences and, 18
    emphysema as, 87-91, 88f, 89f
    evidence-planning for, 11
  restrictive
    diffuse interstitial pulmonary fibrosis, 95-97
    end-stage, 100
    intensive care unit for, 618-619
    lung cancer, 100
    progressive systemic sclerosis, 100
    pulmonary alveolar proteinosis, 97-98, 98f
    pulmonary infiltrates with eosinophilia, 97
    rheumatoid arthritis, 99
    sarcoidosis, 99, 99f
    systemic lupus erythematosus, 99-100
    tuberculosis, 100
Lung field in radiograph, 164f, 165
Lung injury, acute, 644-647
Lung transplantation. *See also* Transplantation
  acute management of, 725-726, 726t
  cardiac and respiratory physiology in, 728
  end-stage disease and, 722-723
  exercise and, 416, 728-729
  rehabilitation guidelines for, 728b
Lung volume in cystic fibrosis, 519
Lung volume reduction surgery, 416
Lupus erythematosus
  lung disease in, 100
  management of, 584
  systemic, 118
Lymphatic disorder, 309b
Lymphatic system, 71, 273b
Lymphatic vessel
  hydrostatic pressure and, 117
  in oxygen transport, 47

M
Macrophage, alveolar, 63-64
Magnet therapy, 492
Magnetic resonance imaging, 168-169, 168f
  cardiac, 206-207
  physics of, 206

Magnetic resonance imaging, (*cont'd*)
  pulmonary, 207
Main stem bronchus
  anatomy of, 62-63, 62f
Main-stem bronchus
  aspiration of, 780
Malalignment, postural, 445
Malignancy
  exercise benefiting, 286b
  lung cancer, 100, 554-555
  risk factors for, 6t, 14
Malnutrition, 448
Manipulation of thorax, 332-333, 333b
Manometer for positive expiratory pressure breathing, 353
Manual airway clearance, in lung cancer, 555
Manual hyperinflation, 347f
  advantages and disadvantages of, 348
  equipment for, 347
  overview of, 328
  precautions for, 333b
  preparation for, 347
  selection considerations for, 359t
  treatment with, 347
Manual technique for vocalization, 400
Manual therapy, 465, 470-471, 489-490
Manually assisted cough, 368-371
  anterior chest compression, 369-370
  costophrenic, 368-369, 368f
  counter-rotation, 370-371, 370f
  Heimlich-type, 369, 369f
Marfan syndrome, 660t
Marketing research model, 27
Marking of lung, 65, 66f
Marrow, bone, 46
Mask
  oxygen, 761, 761f
  for positive expiratory pressure breathing, 353
Massage, 490
  for stress reduction, 474t
McEwen model of health motivation, 20
McKenzie exercise, 276
Measurement, 129-133
  to assess treatment, 257-259, 257b
  documentation of, 133, 133
  from echocardiography, 204
  interpretation of, 133
  intracranial pressure, 239-240
  objective and subjective, 132, 132f
  performance of, 132-133
  reliability of, 131
  selection of, 132
  types of, 129-131, 130b
  validity of, 131-132
Mecamylamine, 791
Mechanical aerosol system, 761-762, 762f
Mechanical body positioning, 319
Mechanical in-exsufflator, 374-375
Mechanical stimulus for cough reflex, 74

Mechanical ventilation
  in acute respiratory distress syndrome, 646
  airway clearance in, 326
  alarm management in, 768
  atelectasis and, 509
  complications with, 640
  for emphysema, 549
  invasive versus noninvasive, 766-767
  modes of, 767-768
  in muscular dystrophy, 581
  postoperative, 532
  precautions for, 768, 768f
  in spinal cord injury, 633
  weaning from, 768-769
    in intensive care unit, 604-605, 605b
    respiratory muscle training for, 459-460
Mechanics, body
  in lifting patient, 753-754, 753f, 754
  position and, 307-324. *See also* Position; Positioning
Mechanoreceptor, 75
Meconium aspiration syndrome, 661-662
Mediastinum, 164f, 166
Mediate percussion, 221-222, 222f
Medical condition, 507-544. *See also* Acute medical
    condition; Chronic medical condition; Systemic
    condition
Meditation, 490
  for congestive heart failure, 480t
  transcendental, 473, 475
Medullary respiratory center, 73
Membrane
  alveolar-capillary, 77
  mucous, tracheal, 62
Mental health, 14-15
Metabolic acidosis, 233t
Metabolic alkalosis, 233t
Metabolic demand, 265, 265b
Metabolic disorder
  in acute respiratory distress syndrome, 645-646
  cardiopulmonary complications of, 122-123,
    123b
  as complication, 639-640
Metabolic syndrome, 108
  management of, 563-565
Metabolism
  aerobic, age and, 283-284
  anaerobic, 266
  in diabetes, 563
  Krebs' cycle and, 40, 41f, 42
  mobilization and exercise affecting, 275
Metal tracheostomy tube, 775
Metaraminol, 788
Meter, peak flow, 364
Metered-dose inhaler, 764, 765
Methyldopa, 788
Metoprolol, 788
Microatelectasis, 508
Microcirculation, 48

Mind/body intervention, 466-467
  for coronary artery disease, 477
  for hypertension, 475
  other, 470
  t'ai chi as, 469, 470t
  types of, 490
  yoga as, 469, 471t
Minipress, 788
Mitochondria, shock and, 648
Mitochondrial enzyme in oxygen transport, 49
Mitral valve
  anatomy of, 67
  prolapse of, 107
Mobility
  in intensive care unit, 599, 627
  limitation in oxygen transport and, 253
  obesity and, 14
  poor, 5
  surgical outcome and, 533
Mobilization, 263-306
  in acute respiratory distress syndrome, 646
  acute response to, 272-276, 272b-274b, 275t
  adaptation to, 280-281
  aids for, 276b
  in cardiac rehabilitation, 523
  cellular energetics in, 265-267
  in cerebral palsy, 575
  definition of, 263
  long-term response to, 281-284
  in lung cancer, 555
  monitoring of, 277
  in muscular dystrophy, 580
  of obese patient, 627
  oxygen transport and, 265, 265b, 267
  physiological effects of, 272-276, 273b
  in polyneuropathy, 650f
  in postoperative period, 537-538
  prescription for, 277-278
  progression of, 278f
  soft tissue, Rolf method of, 470
  in spinal cord injury, 632
  stimuli for, 276b
  testing of, 276-277
  of thorax, 390-391, 390b
  training for, 278-279
  of trauma patient, 630
  treatment hierarchy for, 256b
Mobitz block, 182-183, 182f, 183f
Model
  of aging, 685
  Groningen active living, 26
  health belief, 4t, 497
  of health motivation, 20
  marketing research, 27
  motivational, 5
  psychobiological adaptation, 4
  soda pop, 601-705, 699, 702f, 703f
    broader application of, 713-715, 714f, 715f

Model, (*cont'd*)
    clinical example of, 708-713, 708f, 709t, 710t
    transtheoretical, 20
Modernization, global health and, 9
Monitoring
    in acute respiratory distress syndrome, 646
    in ankylosing spondylitis, 586
    in asthma, 551
    blood gas, 161-162
    of body position, 320-321
    in bronchiectasis, 552
    in cardiac rehabilitation, 425
    in cerebral palsy, 574
    in chronic bronchitis, 548
    in chronic renal insufficiency, 588
    in cystic fibrosis, 552
    in diabetes, 564
    in emphysema, 549
    glucose, 447
    hemodynamic, 237-239, 237f, 238f
    of hypertension, 562, 563
    in intensive care unit, 229-243, 602, 602b
        of acid-base balance, 233, 233t
        blood gas, 233-235
        of brain activity, 240
        of chest tube drainage, 232-233, 232f
        cognitive, 240-241
        electrocardiographic, 235-237, 235f, 236t
        of fluid and electrolyte balance, 230-232, 231f,
            232f
        of fluid collection system, 232-233, 232f
        hemodynamic, 237-239, 237f, 238f
        of intraaortic balloon pump, 239, 239f
        intracranial pressure, 239-240
        of intravenous lines, 230
        neuromuscular, 240
        overview of, 229-230, 230f
        of pain, 241
    of interstitial lung disease, 554
    in long-term care facility, 739
    in lung cancer, 554
    of mobilization, 277
    in multiple sclerosis, 573
    in muscular dystrophy, 580
    in myocardial infarction, 557, 558
    in obesity, 589
    in osteoporosis, 583
    in Parkinson's syndrome, 572
    in peripheral vascular disease, 561
    in post polio syndrome, 577
    of prone position, 317
    in pulmonary rehabilitation, 429
    in rheumatoid arthritis, 587
    in scleroderma, 585
    in spinal cord injury, 576
    of stroke patient, 570
    in systemic lupus erythematosus, 584
    in thoracic deformity, 582

Monopolar magnet, 492
Montgomery T tube, 777, 778f
Motivational model, 5
Motor area of learning needs assessment, 498, 498b
Motor impairment, 695-715
    categories of, 695, 696b
    gravity and, 695-696, 697f-699f, 698-699
    planes of ventilation and, 695-696, 696f
    respiration and postural control in, 699-715
Motor recovery plateau in stroke, 570
Motor therapy for child, 677-678, 678f
Mouth pressure, inspiratory, 633
Movement
    of cilia, 62f
    in head injury, 632
    of thorax, 54, 55f
    ventilation and perfusion and, 308
Movement awareness technique, 466, 491
Movement economy in spinal cord injury, 444
Moving patient, 755-756, 756f
Mucociliary transport
    in atelectasis, 509
    obesity and, 628
    in postoperative period, 644
    in sepsis, 650
Mucous membrane, tracheal, 62
Mucus
    in chronic bronchitis, 546
    high-frequency chest wall oscillation and, 331
Mucus plug in asthma, 93
Multidetector computed tomography, 205
Multifocal atrial tachycardia, 178
Multifocal premature ventricular complex, 180, 180f
Multiorgan system failure, 648-650, 649t, 650f
Multiple sclerosis
    intensive care for, 625
    management of, 572-574
Multisystem assessment, 187-191. *See also* Assessment,
        multisystem
Multisystem impairment
    gravity and, 695-696, 697f-699f, 698-699
    planes of ventilation and, 695-696, 696f
    respiration and postural control in, 699-715
Murmur, heart, 221
Muscle
    accessory, 391-394, 391b, 393b, 394b
    adductor, vocal cord and, 62
    bed rest and, 268b
    intercostal
        in multisystem impairment, 703
        stretch reflex and, 74
    mobilization and exercise affecting, 275
    obesity and, 667
    pelvic floor, 704
    respiratory
        in cystic fibrosis, 663
        in muscular dystrophy, 580
        in thoracic deformity, 582

Muscle atrophy, 270
Muscle contraction, 42, 43f
Muscle deconditioning in lung transplantation, 728
Muscle fiber, 42, 43f
  of heart, 69
Muscle receptor, 74-75
Muscle relaxation, progressive, 475
Muscle resistance training. *See* Resistance training
Muscle weakness
  airway clearance in, 326
  in cerebral palsy, 575
  in muscular dystrophy, 579, 581
  in post polio syndrome, 445, 578
  in spinal cord injury, 633
  in stroke, 571
Muscular dystrophy
  Duchenne, 660t, 666-667
  intensive care for, 625
  management of, 578-581
  in pediatric patient, 666-667
Musculoskeletal disorder, 117-118, 117b
  as complication, 642
  exercise testing and training in, 442
  secondary cardiopulmonary dysfunction from, 581-584
    osteoporosis, 582-584
    thoracic deformity, 581-582
  trauma causing, 628-631, 628b
    hemothorax with, 629
    management of, 629
    pathophysiology of, 628-629
    pneumothorax with, 629
    rib fracture, 629
Musculoskeletal system
  bed rest affecting, 269
  risk factor modification for, 14
Music therapy, 491
  after cardiac surgery, 479t
Myasthenia gravis, 625
Mycobacterium tuberculosis infection, 100, 520-521
Mycophenolate mofetil, in transplantation, 730
Myelomeningocele, 665
Myocardial contractility in oxygen transport, 44
Myocardial contrast echocardiography, 205
Myocardial dysfunction, 641
Myocardial fibrosis, 107
Myocardial function in oxygen transport, 48
Myocardial infarction, 102-105
  acute, 523-524
  complementary therapy after, 476
  on electrocardiograph, 183-184, 183f, 184f
  intensive care for, 619-621, 620b, 621b
  management of, 556-558
  pathophysiology of, 102-105
  respiratory failure and, 641
Myocardial ischemia
  on electrocardiograph, 183-184, 183f, 184f
  pain of, 145
  stress reduction for, 477

Myocardial perfusion
  limitation in oxygen transport and, 251b
  magnetic resonance imaging of, 207
Myocardium
  anatomy of, 67
  magnetic resonance imaging of, 207
Myofascial release, 489-490
Myofilament, 42
Myoglobin, 49
Myopathology in lung disease, 86
Myopathy, 442, 447

N
Narcotic for intensive care patient, 602-603
Nasopharynx, 61
Nasotracheal airway, 781
Naturopathy, 490
Nebulizer, 762, 762f
Neck, 215
Needs assessment, learning, 487b, 497-499, 498b
Negative pressure, lower body, 314
Neo-Synephrine, 788
Neonatal pneumonia, 663
Neonatal respiratory distress, 659
Neonate. *See also* Pediatric patient
  arterial blood gases in, 161
  chest physical therapy for, 668-674, 669f-774f, 670b, 670t
  circulation of, 658
  normal chest x-ray of, 700f
  positioning contraindications in, 333b
  premature, 659, 659t
  respiration in, 658-659
  respiratory distress syndrome in, 326
Neostigmine, 790
Nerve electrical stimulation
  peripheral, 240
  transcutaneous, 492, 532
Nervous system
  autonomic, heart and, 69
  mobilization and exercise affecting, 275
Neurolinguistic psychology, 491
Neurological disorder
  cardiopulmonary effects of, 118-120, 119b
  as complication, 642
  exercise benefiting, 286b
  respiratory muscle training in, 458-459
Neurological system, exercise affecting, 273b
Neuromuscular assessment, 240
Neuromuscular blockade, 648
Neuromuscular disorder, 569-593
  cerebral palsy, 574-575
  intensive care for, 625-627
  multiple sclerosis, 572-574
  in multisystem impairment, 706, 715
  muscular dystrophy, 578-581
  Parkinson's syndrome, 571-572
  poisoning, 625
  poliomyelitis, 577-578

Neuromuscular disorder, (*cont'd*)
  respiratory muscle training in, 458-459
  soda-pop model in, 713
  spinal cord injury, 575-577
  stroke, 569-570
Neuromuscular therapy, 490
Neuropathy
  cardiopulmonary complications of, 120
  critical illness, 642
  exercise testing and training in, 447
Neurotransmission
  parasympathetic, 789
  sympathetic, 786
Neurotransmitter, testing for, 190
Node
  atrioventricular, 68-69
    in conduction system, 172
    depolarization of, 178-179
  sinoatrial, 68-69, 171
Nominal measurement, 130
Nonbreathing mask, 761, 761f
Noncardiogenic pulmonary edema, 644
Noninvasive blood gas monitoring, 161
Noninvasive cardiac rehabilitation, 406. *See also* Cardiac
    rehabilitation
Noninvasive mechanical ventilation, 581
Noninvasive positive pressure mechanical ventilation, 549
Noninvasive pulmonary rehabilitation. *See* Pulmonary
    rehabilitation
Noninvasive therapy, 4, 7
  for intensive care unit patient, 609-610
Nonpharmacological treatment, efficacy of, 7
Noonan's syndrome, 660t
Norepinephrine, 786-788
  testing for, 190
Normocapnic hyperpnea equipment, 457f
Nose, 60
Note, content and organization of, 133-134
Novatrin, 791
Nursing home, 738-739
Nutrition
  in cardiac rehabilitation, 422
  in chronic obstructive pulmonary disease, 91
  in health promotion, 15-16, 17f
  in intensive care unit, 606
  ischemic heart disease and, 10
  in pulmonary rehabilitation, 428
Nutrition pyramid, 17f
Nutritional disorder
  cardiopulmonary complications of, 124, 124b
  exercise and, 286b, 448

O

Obesity
  cardiopulmonary complications of, 124, 124b
  childhood, 667
  exercise testing and training in, 448
  heart disease and, 109

Obesity, (*cont'd*)
  hypertension and, 107
  in intensive care patient, 627-628
  management of, 589-590
  risk factor modification for, 14
Obstruction
  in bronchiectasis, 94
  upper airway, in obesity, 628
Obstructive dysfunction in Parkinson's syndrome, 571
Obstructive lung disease, chronic, 87-95
  asthma as, 91-93, 92b, 92f, 93f
  bronchiectasis as, 93-95, 94f
  chronic bronchitis as, 87
  cultural differences and, 18
  emphysema as, 87-91, 88f, 89f
  evidence-planning for, 11
  modifiable risk factors for, 6t
Obstructive sleep apnea, 102
  in chronic bronchitis, 548
  obesity and, 628, 667
Occlusion, arterial, 560
Occupational history, 147-148
Olympic tracheostomy button, 777, 777f
Oncotic pressure, capillary, 81
Open-face mask, 761, 761f
Open-glottis cough, 5165
Open heart surgery, 621-623, 622b
Open suctioning, 778
Ordinal measurement, 130
Organ, internal, 704-705
Organ Procurement and Transplantation Network,
    719, 720
Organ transplantation, 635
Oropharynx, 61
Orthopnea, 142
Orthosis, spinal, 665f
Oscillating ventilator, 633
Oscillatory positive expiratory pressure breathing, 352-353
Osteopathic medicine, 490
Osteopenia, 442-443
Osteoporosis
  cardiopulmonary dysfunction with, 582-584
  modifiable risk factors for, 6t
  risk factor modification for, 14
  transplantation and, 730-731
Outcomes assessment, 135
Outpatient rehabilitation, posttransplant, 726-729
Overuse in post polio syndrome, 445
Oxidation, cellular, 40, 41f, 42
Oxygen
  anesthesia and, 530-531
  in blood, 42-43
  partial pressure of, 158
  shock and, 648
  to tissues, 43-44
  toxicity of, 640-641
  transcutaneous, 162
    in exercise testing, 280

Oxygen consumption, 38
  age affecting, 686
  complications with, 640
  definition of, 263-264
  factors increasing, 265, 265b
  supply-dependent, 45
Oxygen debt, 44-45
Oxygen delivery, 264, 265-266
Oxygen demand, 38
Oxygen extraction, 39b
Oxygen extraction ratio, 38, 45
Oxygen kinetics, 234
Oxygen saturation, 159
Oxygen tension, arterial, 316
Oxygen therapy
  arterial blood gases and, 161
  in burn injury, 634
  cannula for, 760, 760f
  in chronic bronchitis, 548
  in chronic obstructive pulmonary disease, 96-97
  continuous positive airway pressure breathing, 763
  in exercise, 763
  high-flow system for, 761-762, 762f
  in long-term care facility, 739-740
  low-flow system for, 760-761, 760t
  in muscular dystrophy, 580
  overview of, 759-760
  portable, 762-763, 763f
Oxygen transport, 37-51
  afterload in, 44
  in ankylosing spondylitis, 586
  atelectasis and, 509
  in bed rest, 268
  blood in, 42-43, 82-83
  blood volume and, 45-46
  in bronchiectasis, 552
  in burn injury, 635
  cardiac output in, 44
  in chronic bronchitis, 548
  in chronic renal insufficiency, 588
  complications with, 640
  in cystic fibrosis, 553
  in emphysema, 549-550
  energy transport and cellular metabolism in, 40, 41f, 42
  in exercise, 267
  factors affecting, 49-50
  formulas for determining, 38f
  hemoglobin and, 159
  of interstitial lung disease, 554
  limitations related to, 249-251, 250b, 251b, 252b, 253
  in lung cancer, 555
  measures and indexes of, 38, 39b
  metabolic demand and, 265, 265b
  in multiple sclerosis, 573
  muscle contraction and, 42, 43f
  in muscular dystrophy, 580
  myocardial contractility in, 44
  myocardial infarction and, 558

Oxygen transport, (cont'd)
  organ transplantation and, 721
  in osteoporosis, 583
  oxygen debt and, 44-45
  oxygen extraction ratio and, 45
  oxyhemoglobin dissociation and, 46
  pathway for, 45
  in peripheral vascular disease, 561
  position and, 308, 309b
  in postoperative period, 535-536, 536b, 537, 643b
  preload in, 44
  principles of, 42
  in rheumatoid arthritis, 587
  in scleroderma, 585
  in spinal cord injury, 576
  steps in, 46-49
  stroke and, 571
  systemic condition affecting, 116
  in thoracic deformity, 582
  to tissues, 43-44
  in valvular disease, 559-560
Oxygenation
  in acute respiratory distress syndrome, 646
  placental, 658
Oxyhemoglobin dissociation, 46, 82-83, 82f

P
P-R interval, 182
P wave, 69, 178
  in conduction block, 182
Pacemaker, sinoatrial node as, 171
Pain
  anginal, 102, 522-523, 555
  assessment of, 241
  postoperative, 642-643, 644
  types of, 144-146
Palpation, 222-224, 223f-225f
Pancreas, 190
Pancreatitis, 121
Panlobular emphysema, 88, 88f, 514
Paradoxical breathing, 706, 706f
Paralysis, 706, 707f
Parasympathetic neurotransmission, 789
Parkinson's syndrome
  cardiopulmonary manifestations of, 119-120, 119b
  management of, 569-572
Paroxysmal atrial tachycardia, 178, 236t
Partial pressure of carbon dioxide, peripheral
    chemoreceptors and, 74
Partial pressure of gases, 158-159
Partial rebreathing mask, 761, 761f
Passy-Muir valve, 777, 778f
Patau's syndrome, 660t
Patent ductus arteriosus, 660
Pathophysiology, cardiopulmonary, 85-114
  chronic obstructive pulmonary disease as, 86-95.
      See also Chronic obstructive pulmonary disease
  overview of, 85-86

Pathophysiology, cardiopulmonary, (*cont'd*)
  restrictive lung disease as, 95-100
    diffuse interstitial pulmonary fibrosis, 95-97
    end-stage, 100
    lung cancer, 100
    progressive systemic sclerosis, 100
    pulmonary alveolar proteinosis, 97-98, 98f
    pulmonary infiltrates with eosinophilia, 97
    rheumatoid arthritis, 99
    sarcoidosis, 99, 99f
    systemic lupus erythematosus, 99-100
    tuberculosis, 100
Pathway, oxygen transport, 45
Patient adherence, 502
Patient-controlled analgesia, 532
Patient education, 495-504. *See also* Education
Patient history, 137-149. *See also* History
Pattern, breathing, 215-216
Pattern, practice, 254, 255b
Peak exercise test
  in myocardial infarction, 558
  in peripheral vascular disease, 561
Peak flow meter, cough and, 364
Pectoralis muscle
  anatomy of, 58
  facilitation of, 391-392, 392f
Pectus carinatum, 216
Pectus excavatum, 216, 707f
Pedal edema, 147
Pediatric patient, 657-683
  airway suctioning in, in infant, 669-670, 674
  cardiac disorder in, 660-661
    atrioventricular defect, 660
    endocardial cushion defect, 660
    patent ductus arteriosus, 660
    tetralogy of Fallot, 660-661
  cardiopulmonary development in, 658-659, 659t
  chest physical therapy for
    for child, 674-676, 675f
    for neonate and infant, 668-674, 669f-774f, 670b, 670t
  diseases of civilization in, 6
  obesity and, 667
  overview of, 657
  positional rotation
    in child, 674-675
    in infant, 668, 669f, 670b, 670f
  postoperative cardiac rehabilitation in, 667-668
  postoperative care of, 676
  postural drainage in, 668, 670t, 671f-674f
  preoperative care of, 675-676
  pulmonary disorder in, 660-664
    asthma, 662
    bronchopulmonary dysplasia, 661
    in cerebral palsy, 664-665, 665f
    cystic fibrosis, 662-663
    in Down syndrome, 665-666, 666f
    hyaline membrane disease, 661
    intubation and, 663-664

Pediatric patient, (*cont'd*)
    meconium aspiration syndrome, 661-662
    in miscellaneous conditions, 667
    in muscular dystrophy, 666-667
    in myelomeningocele, 665
    pneumonia, 662
    tracheostomy and, 663-664
    transient tachypnea of newborn, 661
  tracheostomy tube for, 782t
Pelvic floor, 704-705
Pelvic position, 384-385
Perceived exertion scale, 357f
Perceptual area of learning needs assessment, 498, 498b
Percussion, 344-346, 345f
  advantages and disadvantages of, 345-346
  contraindications to, 333
  equipment for, 344-345
  in infant, 668-669, 674f
  mediate, 221-222, 222f
  overview of, 327
  preparation for, 345
  selection considerations for, 359t
  treatment with, 345
Percussionaire Impulsator, 356
Percussive ventilation, intrapulmonary, 331-332
Perfusion
  cardiopulmonary physiology and, 78
  in left heart failure, 116
  myocardial
    limitation in oxygen transport and, 251b
    magnetic resonance imaging of, 207
  in oxygen transport, 48
  in upright lung, 312
  ventilation, 78-79, 79f
Pericardial cavity, 48
Pericardial pain, 145-146
Pericardium, anatomy of, 67
Periodontitis, 15
Perioperative care, 530-542. *See also* Surgery
Peripheral chemoreceptor, 74
Peripheral circulation
  in exercise, 267
  mobilization and exercise affecting, 273b
  outcome measurement for, 258b
  in oxygen transport, 48
  physiology of, 81-82
Peripheral cyanosis, 215
Peripheral muscle deconditioning in lung transplantation, 728
Peripheral nerve electrical stimulation, 240
Peripheral nervous system, 120
Peripheral vascular disease
  in diabetes, 563
  management of, 560-561
Peripheral vascular function, 189, 189t
Peritoneal cavity, 47
Perkinje fiber, 69
Personal transmission of healing energy, 466

pH, 158
Pharynx, 61
Phenoxybenzamine, 788
Phentolamine, 788-789
Phenylephrine, 788
Physical examination, 212
Physical therapist as change agent, 15-22, 23-24, 24b
Physical therapy
    for child, 674-676, 675f
    "do no harm" and, 7-8
    high-frequency chest wall oscillation and, 331
    in hyaline membrane disease, 661
    in infant, 668-674, 669f-774f, 670b, 670t
    in muscular dystrophy, 666
    roles of, 26-27
Physiological complications of artificial airway, 774-775
Physiology, cardiopulmonary, 73-84
    cardiac events and, 80-82, 81f
    cardiac reflexes and, 79-80
    control of breathing and, 73-74, 74f
    diffusion in, 77, 78f
    in heart transplant, 727
    of lung transplant, 728
    mechanical factors in, 75-77, 76f, 77f
    oxygen transport and, 82-83, 82f
    perfusion in, 78-79, 78f-80f
    reflexes in, 74-75
    ventilation and, 77
Physostigmine, 790
Pigeon chest, 216
Pilates, 491
Pilocar, 789
Pilocarpine, 789
Pink puffer, 89, 515
Placental oxygenation, 658
Plan, treatment, 254
    documentation of, 134-135
Plane of ventilation, 695-696
Planning, evidence-based, 8-22. See also Evidence-based
        planning
Plasma
    ions in, 46
    mobilization and exercise affecting, 274
Plasma protein disorder, 122
Plastic tracheostomy tube, 775-776
Platelet, 274, 282
Platypnea, 142
Pleura
    in oxygen transport, 47
    in pneumonia, 511
Pleural effusion, 116
    differential diagnosis of, 226t
    in liver disorder, 121
    on radiograph, 165
Pleuritic pain, 145
Plug, mucus, in asthma, 93
Pneumobelt, 577
Pneumococcal pneumonia, 511

Pneumocystis carinii pneumonia, 662
Pneumonia
    acute, 509-512
    interstitial, 97
    in pediatric patient, 662
Pneumotaxic center, 73
Pneumothorax
    differential diagnosis of, 226t
    on radiograph, 165, 166
    trauma causing, 629
Poisoning
    carbon monoxide, 634
    neuromuscular, 625
Poliomyelitis
    cardiopulmonary effects of, 120
    exercise testing and training in, 445
    intensive care for, 625
    management of, 577-578
Polycythemia in bronchitis, 87
Polyneuropathy, 650f
Polypnea, 381b
Polyvinyl chloride tracheostomy tube, 775-776
Pontine respiratory center, 73
Portable oxygen, 762-763, 763f
Position. See also Positioning
    butterfly, 751, 751f
    head-down, 316
    neutral alignment in, 752-753
    physiological effects of, 309-317, 309f
    physiological hierarchy of, 318b
    prone, 316-317, 751
    side-lying, 315-316, 315f, 751
    supine, 313-315, 314f, 315f, 749-751, 750f, 751f
    upright, 752, 752f
        physiological effects of, 310-313, 311f, 312f
Positional rotation of infant, 668, 669f, 670b, 670f
Positioning, 307-324
    in acute respiratory distress syndrome, 646, 647
    in angina, 523, 555
    in burn injury, 635
    in cerebral palsy, 575
    considerations in, 320
    contraindications to, 333b
    in emphysema, 5165
    in facilitating ventilation, 377-380, 378f-380f, 384-385
    gravity and, 307-308
    indications for, 309b, 310b
    of intensive care patient, 626
    lung and, 308f
    mechanical, 319
    monitoring response to, 320-321
    in myocardial infarction, 558
    of obese patient, 627
    for optimal ventilation, 749
    to optimize oxygen transport, 309b
    in peripheral vascular disease, 561
    physiological effects of, 309-317, 309f
        of changes in, 317-318, 318f

Positioning, (cont'd)
   head-down, 316
   prone, 316-317
   side-lying, 315-316, 315f
   supine, 313-315, 314f, 315f
   upright, 310-313, 311f, 312f
  in postoperative period, 537
  for postural drainage, 326-327, 327f, 343f
  prescription for, 318-319, 318f, 319f
  prescriptive versus routine, 308-309
  in spinal cord injury, 633
  in stroke, 571
  symmetrical, 394
  treatment hierarchy for, 256b
  in valvular disease, 560
  for vocalization, 400
  in wheelchair, 380, 380f
Positive end-expiratory pressure, 317
Positive expiratory pressure breathing
  advantages and disadvantages of, 355
  autogenic drainage compared to, 329
  in cystic fibrosis, 519, 553
  equipment for, 352-353, 352f
  overview of, 330-331, 351-352
  precautions for, 334
  preparation for, 353-354, 353f
  selection considerations for, 359t
  treatment with, 354, 355f
Positive pressure breathing, intermittent, 765-766, 765f
Positive pressure mechanical ventilation for emphysema, 549
Positive pressure support, 701-702
Post polio syndrome
  exercise testing and training in, 445
  management of, 577
Postoperative complications, 642-644
  deep venous thrombosis as, 643
  hypoxemia as, 642
  management of, 643-644
  oxygen transport and, 643b
  pain as, 642-643
  pulmonary embolism as, 643
Postoperative management, 534-536, 535b
Postoperative period, 531
Posttransplant outpatient rehabilitation, 726-729
Postural control
  respiration and, soda-pop model of, 699, 701-705, 702f, 703f
  soda pop model of, 701-705, 699, 702f, 703f
   broader application of, 713-715, 714f, 715f
   clinical example of, 708-713, 708f, 709t, 710t
Postural drainage. See Drainage, postural
Postural hypotension, 120
Postural inhibition, 395
Postural malalignment in post polio syndrome, 445
Posture in postoperative period, 537-538
Potassium, 170
Potential, cardiac action, 170-171, 170f

Practice pattern, 254, 255b
Prayer
  distant healing, 490
  for self, 490
Prazosin, 788
Preadmission workup
  for cardiac rehabilitation, 418b
  for pulmonary rehabilitation, 418b
Prednisone in transplantation, 730
Preload, 44
Premature atrial complex, 177, 177f
Premature infant, 659, 659t
Premature ventricular complex, 179-180, 180f
Preoperative assessment, 533-534, 534b
Prescription
  for body positioning, 308-309
   in postoperative period, 538-539
  for exercise, 264-265, 281-284
   acute response to, 272-276, 272b-274b, 275t
   preventive effects of, 267-271
  for intensive care patient, 603-606
   for breathing and coughing maneuvers, 603
   for secretion clearance, 603-604
   for supplemental oxygen, 603
  for mobilization, 277-278, 281-284
  for oxygen, 759-760
  of positioning, 318-319, 319f
  treatment, 254, 257
Pressure
  abdominal, 703
  aortic, 81
  barometric, 161
  bed rest and, 268b
  capillary hydrostatic, 81
  capillary oncotic, 81
  central venous, 238-239
  end diastolic ventricular, in side-lying position, 315
  hydrostatic, 78, 117
  inspiratory mouth, in spinal cord injury, 633
  interstitial hydrostatic, 81
  intraabdominal, cough and, 366
  intracranial
   in head injury, 631-632
   in intensive care unit patient, 239-240
  intrapleural
   differences in, 311
   in supine position, 314
  intrathoracic
   in bronchiectasis, 551
   in chronic bronchitis, 547
   cough and, 366
   in emphysema, 550
  left atrial, 238
  left ventricular, 238
  lower body negative, 314
  partial, 158-159
  positive, 701, 703
  pulmonary artery, 237-238

Pressure, (cont'd)
  transmural, 77
Pressure curve, relaxation, 75-76, 76f
Pressure-volume relationship, 75-76
Preterm infant, 659, 659t
Pretransplantation rehabilitation, 722-724, 723t
Prevention
  exercise and mobilization for, 272
  goals for, 253-254
  for intensive care patient, 600-601
  of secondary cardiopulmonary dysfunction, 442
  stroke, 12-13
Prioritizing, patient's learning needs, 499
Professional education, continuing, 24, 24b
Prognosis, documentation of, 134-135
Progressive muscle relaxation, for hypertension, 475
Projection, radiographic, 165t
Prolapse, mitral valve, 107
Prolonged pulmonary eosinophilia, 97
Prone-on-elbows, head flexion assisted cough, 371-372,
      372f
Prone position
  in obesity, 628
  physiological effects of, 316-317
Prophylaxis
  for intensive care patient, 600-601
  in multiple sclerosis, 574
  in spinal cord injury, 577
Propranolol, 788
Prostigmin, 790
Protein, blood tests for, 188t
Protein disorder, plasma, 122
Proteinosis
  alveolar, 514
  pulmonary alveolar, 97-98, 98f
Pseudomonas aeruginosa pneumonia, 511
Pseudostratified columnar ciliated epithelium, 62f
Psychobiological adaptation model, 4
Psychoeducational intervention
  for asthma, 481
  for chronic obstructive pulmonary disease, 484-485,
      484t
Psychological factors
  complementary therapy and, 473
  risk factor modification and, 14-15
Psychosocial factors, 249
  in cardiac rehabilitation, 422
  in coronary artery disease, 477
  at end-of-life, 608
  in ischemic heart disease, 10-11
  limitation in oxygen transport and, 252b
  in organ transplantation, 720-721
  in pulmonary rehabilitation, 428
Psychotherapy, 490
Pt CO$_2$, 162
Puffer, pink, 89
Pulmonary alveolar proteinosis, 97-98, 98f
Pulmonary artery balloon flotation catheter, 237-238

Pulmonary artery catheter, flow-directed, 641
Pulmonary artery pressure, 237-238
  in burn injury, 634
Pulmonary artery wedge pressure, 237-238
Pulmonary blood vessel, 78
Pulmonary circulation
  anatomy of, 70-71
  outcome measurement for, 258b
Pulmonary development, 658-659
Pulmonary disease. See also Lung disease; Respiratory
      entries
  chronic obstructive, 87-95. See also Chronic obstructive
      pulmonary disease
  community and, 737
  complementary therapy for, 481-485
    asthma, 481-483, 484t
  as complication, 640-641
  restrictive, 95-100
Pulmonary edema, 116
  in acute lung injury, 644
  in burn injury, 634
Pulmonary embolism
  differential diagnosis of, 226t
  postoperative, 643
Pulmonary fibrosis, 118
  acute exacerbation of, 519-520
  connective tissue disease and, 118
  diffuse interstitial, 95-97
  lung transplantation and, 723
Pulmonary fluid, 116
Pulmonary function
  aging and, 689-691, 690t, 691f
  positioning and, 310-311
  in pulmonary fibrosis, 96
Pulmonary hemorrhage, cardiopulmonary complications
      of, 122
Pulmonary hypertension, 107
  chest pain in, 145
  exercise program for, 416
  primary, 562
Pulmonary infiltrate, 97
Pulmonary magnetic resonance imaging, 207
Pulmonary rehabilitation, 428-430
  of child, 676
  in chronic dysfunction
    asthma, 417
    chronic obstructive pulmonary disease, 415-416
    cystic fibrosis, 417
    interstitial lung disease, 416
    lung transplantation, 416
    pulmonary hypertension, 416
    reduced lung volume, 416
  components of, 417-421
    purpose and goals as, 417-420
    setting and team members, 420
  drugs in, 414
  evidence base and efficacy in, 405-408
  exercise in, 429-430

Pulmonary rehabilitation, (*cont'd*)
  future directions in, 430
  nutrition in, 428
  phase I of, 512b
  phases of, 428
  physical therapy in, 420-421, 421f
  preadmission work-up for, 419b
  psychosocial issues in, 428
  risk reduction in, 428-429
  smoking cessation in, 428
Pulmonary system, mobilization and exercise affecting, 273, 273b
Pulmonary variables in oxygen transport, 39b
Pulmonic valve, anatomy of, 67
Pulsation device, intraaortic balloon counter, in intensive care unit, 239, 239f
Pulse oximetry, 161-162
Pulsed electromagnetic field therapy, 492
Pump
  cough, 364
  intraaortic balloon, shock and, 648
Puncture wound, of chest, 76
Pursed-lip breathing, 384
  to facilitate ventilation, 384
  relaxed, 397
Push-up, serratus, 394
PVC, 179-180, 180f
Pyramid
  exercise, 17f
  nutrition, 17f

Q
Q wave, 184, 184f
Qi gong
  for asthma, 483
  for congestive heart failure, 480t
  description of, 492
  for hypertension, 475t, 476t
QRS complex, 69, 172, 176
  in conduction block, 182
  in ventricular dysrhythmia, 179
Quadriplegia, respiratory muscle training in, 58
Quake, 354
Quality of life
  in diabetes, 564
  domains of, 248t
  in myocardial infarction, 557
  in peripheral vascular disease, 560
  scoliosis and, 713
  transplantation and, 731
Quiz to assess readiness to change, 21b

R
Radial arterial line, 237f
Radiography, 163-168
  computed tomography, 166-167, 167f
  evaluation of, 164-166, 164f, 165f
  magnetic resonance, 168-169, 168f

Radiography, (*cont'd*)
  of normal chest, 700f
  projections for, 165t
Randomized controlled clinical trial, 24-25
Range of motion, in spinal cord injury, 576
Range of motion exercise, treatment hierarchy for, 256b
Ratio
  oxygen extraction, 38, 45
  risk-benefit, 132
  ventilation-perfusion, 78-79
    body position and, 308, 312
Ratio measurement, 130
Readiness to change, 20b, 21b
Reasoning, clinical, 247
Rebreathing mask, 761, 761f
Receptor
  cough-irritant, 143
  joint, 74-75
  muscle, 74-75
Recoil, elastic, of lung, 75
Recumbency, 267-268. *See also* Bed rest
Red blood cell
  anemia and, 107-108
  oxygen transport and, 46
  testing of, 188
Red blood cell disorder, cardiopulmonary complications of, 122
Reflex
  cardiac, 79-80
  cardiovascular, 791-792
  cough, 74
    in pneumonia, 509-510
  functional, 792
  Hering-Breuer, 74
  Starling, 80
  stretch, 74
Reflexology, 492
Refractory period, 170
Regitine, 788-789
Rehabilitation
  cardiac. *See* Cardiac rehabilitation
  pulmonary. *See* Pulmonary rehabilitation
  for transplant patient
    after heart procedure, 724-728, 725t, 727b, 727t
    after lung procedure, 725-726, 726t, 728-729, 728b
    community or home-based, 729
    preoperative, 722-724, 723t
    surgical procedures affecting, 724
Reiki, 492
Rejection of transplant, 729-730
  heart, 726, 727
  lung, 728
Relationship, teacher-learner, 501-502
Relaxation pressure curve, 75-76, 76f
Relaxation therapy
  for asthma, 481
  complementary, 473-474, 474t
  in facilitation of ventilation, 385

Relaxation therapy, (*cont'd*)
  for hypertension, 475, 522
  for myocardial infarction, 524
  in trauma, 630
  treatment hierarchy for, 256b
Relaxed pursed-lip breathing, 397
Religion
  cardiac surgery and, 479t
  coronary care unit patient and, 480-481
Reminyl, 790
Remodeling, cardiac, 106
Renal disease
  cardiopulmonary complications of, 121-122, 122b
  heart failure with, 109
Renal disorder
  as complication, 642
  exercise testing and training in, 446-447
Renal failure
  erythropoietin therapy in, 447
  respiratory muscle training in, 459
Renal function, 189
Renal insufficiency, chronic, 588-589
Renal system
  as buffering mechanism, 158
Renal systemfunction testing of, 189
Repatterning technique, 385-386
Repiratory rate, 298
Repressive coping style, 481
Research, 24-26
Reserpine, 788
Residual capacity, functional, 315
Resistance, airway, 76-77
Resistance technique, eccentric, 400-401
Resistance training
  aerobic exercise and, 276
  after stroke, 444
  in bed rest, 271-272
  heart transplant and, 727-728
  long-term effects of, 283
Resistive breathing device, 455, 456f
Respiration
  Biot, definition of, 381b
  Cheyne-Stokes, definition of, 381b
  neonatal, 658-659
  postural control and
    broader application of, 713-715, 714f, 715f
    clinical example of, 708-713, 708f, 709t, 710t
    soda-pop model of, 699, 701-705, 702f, 703f
  trunk control and, 664t
Respiratory acidosis, 233t
Respiratory alkalosis, 233t
Respiratory care practice review
  aerosol therapy, 764-765, 765f
  humidity therapy, 764
  intermittent positive pressure breathing, 765-766, 765f
  mechanical ventilation, 766-769. *See also* Mechanical ventilation
  oxygen therapy, 759-763, 760f-763f

Respiratory care practice review, (*cont'd*)
  respiratory modalities, 763-764, 764f
  role of physical therapist, 769
Respiratory center, 73
Respiratory control, soda pop model of, 601-705, 699, 702f, 703f
  broader application of, 713-715, 714f, 715f
  clinical example of, 708-713, 708f, 709t, 710t
Respiratory disease. *See* Lung disease
Respiratory distress, 92, 92f, 644-647
  cognitive assessment in, 241
  neonatal, 326
  in premature infant, 659
Respiratory failure
  arterial blood gases in, 160-161
  cardiac dysrhythmia with, 641
  complications with, 639-640
  prone position in, 317
Respiratory infection in multiple sclerosis, 574
Respiratory modality, 763-766
  aerosol therapy, 764-765, 765f
  humidity therapy, 764
  incentive spirometry, 763-764, 764f
  intermittent positive pressure breathing, 765-766, 765f
Respiratory muscle, 56f, 58f
  aging and, 689, 689f
  in chronic obstructive pulmonary disease, 91
  cough and, 364
  diaphragm, 55-57, 55f, 56f
  expiratory, 59
  inspiratory, 54-59, 55f-58f
    erector spinae, 59
    intercostals, 57
    pectoralis, 58
    scalenes, 58
    serratus anterior, 58
    sternocleidomastoid, 57-58
    trapezius, 58
  limitation in oxygen transport and, 251b
  mobilization and exercise affecting, 283
  in muscular dystrophy, 579, 580
  in Parkinson's syndrome, 571
  in spinal cord injury, 576, 633
  in thoracic deformity, 582
Respiratory muscle training, 453-464
  assessment of
    endurance testing in, 454-456, 455t, 456f
    strength testing in, 453-454
  in asthma, 458
  in chronic obstructive pulmonary disease, 457-458, 457t
  in chronic renal failure, 459
  in cystic fibrosis, 458
  in health, 456-457
  in neurological disorder, 458-459
  in neuromuscular disorder, 458-459
  in quadriplegia, 458
  in weaning failure, 459-460

Respiratory muscle weakness, 326
Respiratory physiology of lung transplant, 728
Respiratory rate
  in exercise testing, 280
  mobilization and exercise affecting, 273
  in mobilization monitoring, 280
  reduction of, 395-397, 395b, 397f
Rest in postoperative period, 531, 644. *See also* Bed rest
Restlessness, postoperative, 536
Restrictive lung disease, 95-100. *See also* Lung disease, restrictive
  intensive care for, 626
  intensive care unit for, 618-619
Restrictive pulmonary chronic medical condition
  interstitial lung disease as, 553-554
  lung cancer as, 554-555
Retention, fluid, 641
Review of systems, 212
Rheumatoid arthritis
  exercise testing and training in, 446
  juvenile, 660t
  lung disease and, 99
  management of, 586-588
Rib
  anatomy of, 54
  fracture of, 166f, 629
Rigidity in Parkinson's syndrome, 571, 572
Risk analysis, cardiac, 423f, 424f
Risk-benefit ratio, 132
Risk factor
  for cardiopulmonary pathophysiology, 85
  in obesity, 589
  structure and function and, 248-249
Risk factor modification, 6t
  for cancer, 14
  for dental health, 15
  for ischemic heart disease, 10-11
  for musculoskeletal health, 14
  for myocardial infarction, 557
  for obesity, 14
  for psychological health, 14-15
  for smoking-related conditions, 11, 12t
  for stroke, 12-13
  for type 2 diabetes, 13
Risk reduction
  in cardiac rehabilitation, 423, 423f, 424f
  in pulmonary rehabilitation, 428-429
Risk stratification, 425b
Rivastigmine, 790
Rolf method of soft tissue mobilization, 470
Rolfing, 490
Rolling, facilitation of ventilation in, 381
Rosen method body work, 490
Rotating bed, 270-271
Rotation
  counter, 395-396
  positional, of infant, 668, 669f, 670b, 670f

S
S-T segment, in myocardial ischemia, 183-184
S-T segment depression, 183
Sac, alveolar, 63
Saccular bronchiectasis, 93, 94f
Salagen, 789
Sarcoidosis, pulmonary, 99, 99f
Scale, perceived exertion, 357f
Scalene muscle
  anatomy of, 58
  facilitation of, 392
Scar, 215
Scientific evidence for complementary therapy, 468
Scleroderma
  cardiopulmonary manifestations of, 118
  of lung, 100
  management of, 585-586
Scoliosis
  clinical example of, 708-715, 708f, 709t, 710t, 714f
  exercise testing and training in, 443
Scoop technique of controlled diaphragmatic breathing, 386-387, 386f, 387f
Secondary cardiopulmonary dysfunction
  in intensive care patient, 625-637
    burn injury causing, 633-635
    head injury causing, 631-632, 631f, 632b
    musculoskeletal trauma causing, 628-631, 628b
    neuromuscular disease causing, 625-627
    obesity causing, 627-628
    organ transplantation and, 635
    spinal cord injury causing, 632-633
  musculoskeletal causes of, 581-584
    in intensive care patient, 628-631, 628b
    osteoporosis, 582-584
    thoracic deformity, 581-582
  neuromuscular causes of, 569-593
    cerebral palsy, 574-575
    in intensive care patient, 625-627
    multiple sclerosis, 572-574
    muscular dystrophy, 578-581
    Parkinson's syndrome, 571-572
    poliomyelitis, 577-578
    respiratory muscle training in, 458-459
    spinal cord injury, 575-577
    stroke, 569-570
Secretion. *See also* Airway clearance technique
  in atelectasis, 509
  in bronchiectasis, 551
  in burn injury, 635
  in cerebral palsy, 575
  in chronic bronchitis, 546
  in cystic fibrosis, 519
  in emphysema, 5165
Sedation, postoperative, 532
Segment, bronchopulmonary, 65, 66t
Self-assisted cough, 371-374
  hands-knees, rocking, 373-374, 374f
  long-sitting, 372, 372f, 373f

Self-assisted cough, (cont'd)
   prone-on-elbows, head flexion, 371-372, 372f
   short-sitting, 372-373, 373f
   standing, 374
Self-efficacy, 496
Self-management of chronic illness, 737-738
Semi-Fowler's position, for suctioning, 779, 779f
Sepsis, 648-650
Septum, cardiac, 67-68
Serratus anterior muscle, 58
Serratus push-up, 394
Seventh-day Adventist lifestyle, 9
Sexual dysfunction in atherosclerosis, 556
Shaking, 346-347
   advantages and disadvantages of, 347
   equipment for, 346
   overview of, 327-328
   preparation for, 346
   selection considerations for, 359t
   treatment with, 346-347
Shallow breathing, 707-708
Shock, 647-648
   management of, 648
   pathophysiology of, 647-648
Short-sitting self-assisted cough, 372-373, 373f
Shortness of breath, 89. See also Dyspnea
Shoulder, relaxation of, 385
Shrinking lung syndrome, 118
Sickle cell anemia, 108
   cardiopulmonary complications of, 122
   exercise testing and training in, 447
Side-lying position, 315-316, 315f
Silica exposure, 147
Simple pulmonary eosinophilia, 97
Sinoatrial node, 68-69, 171
Sinus bradycardia, 176, 177f
   clinical features of, 236t
Sinus rhythm, normal, 175-176, 176f
Sinus tachycardia, 176-177, 177f
   clinical features of, 236t
Sitting position, 381
Skeleton in chest radiograph, 165
Skin
   assessment of, 215
   in multisystem impairment, 715
   turgor of, 231
Skin graft, 635
Sleep
   arterial blood gases in, 161
   emphysema and, 549
   myocardial infarction and, 524
   in postoperative period, 531
Sleep apnea, 102
   in chronic bronchitis, 548
   myocardial infarction and, 557
   in obesity, 628, 667
Sleep disorder in myocardial infarction, 557
Small-volume nebulizer, 764, 765

Smoking
   atherosclerosis and, 101
   chronic bronchitis and, 87, 546-547
   chronic obstructive pulmonary disease and, 85
   consequences of, 12b
   disease related to, 5
   emphysema and, 548
   history of, 148
   in peripheral vascular disease, 561
   risk factor modification for, 11, 12t
Smoking cessation
   in cardiac rehabilitation, 422
   physical therapist's role in, 18, 18f
   in pulmonary rehabilitation, 428
Sniffing, 385-386
Social-cognitive theory, 496
Social support
   after cardiac surgery, 479t
   in stroke, 571
Soda pop model of respiratory and postural control,
      601-705, 699, 702f, 703f
   broader application of, 713-715, 714f, 715f
   clinical example of, 708-713, 708f, 709t, 710t
Soft tissue mobilization, Rolf method of, 470
Soma, 490
Sound
   breath, 218, 218f
   extrapulmonary, 219
   heart, 220, 220f, 221f
   lung, 232
   voice, 219-220
Spasm, diffuse esophageal, 146
Speed, gait, after stroke, 277
Spina bifida, 665
Spinal cord injury
   cardiopulmonary effects of, 120
   exercise testing and training after, 444
   management of, 575-577
      in intensive care unit, 632-633
   pathophysiology of, 632
Spinal disorder, pain of, 146
Spinal orthosis, 665f
Spine in osteoporosis, 583
Spiriva, 791
Spirometry
   incentive, 763-764, 764f
   in postoperative period, 537
Spondylitis, ankylosing, 586
Sputum
   in bronchiectasis, 95
   in bronchitis, 87, 512, 546
   high-frequency chest wall oscillation and, 331
Stable angina, 102
Standing
   controlled breathing and, 387, 387f
   facilitation of ventilation in, 382
Staphylococcal pneumonia, 511
Starling reflex, 80

Starvation, 124, 124b
Status asthmaticus, 93, 615-618
Sterile suctioning, 781-782
Sternocleidomastoid muscle
    anatomy of, 57-58
    facilitation of, 392
Sternum, 53-54
Stethoscope, 217-219, 217f, 218f
Stiffening of chest wall, 689
Stimulation
    peripheral nerve electrical, 240
    transcutaneous electrical nerve, 492
        postoperative, 532
Stimulus
    exercise, in bed rest, 271-272
    mobilization, 276b
        adaptation to, 280-281
Strength training in osteoporosis, 583
Strengthening exercise, in emphysema, 550
Streptococcus pyrogenes pneumonia, 511
Stress
    in cystic fibrosis, 519
    exercise, 264-265
    gravitational, in burn injury, 635
    immigration and, 4
    myocardial infarction and, 557
    in oxygen transport, 49-50
Stress reduction
    complementary therapy for, 473-474, 474t
        in coronary artery disease, 476
        for hypertension, 475
    in myocardial ischemia, 477
Stress ulcer, 641
Stretch reflex, 74
Stroke
    cardiopulmonary effects of, 118-119, 119b
    exercise testing and training after, 443-444
    intensive care for, 625
    modifiable risk factors for, 6t
    restricted mobility in, 276
    risk factor modification for, 12-13
Stroke volume in exercise, 266, 272, 273
Structure and function, 248-249
Subjunctional tachycardia, 236t, 237
Subsegmental bronchus, 63
Suctioning
    of articial airway, 778-782, 779f, 780f
    of infant, 669-670, 674
    in postoperative period, 644
    treatment hierarchy for, 256b
Supine position, 313-315, 314f, 315f, 779, 779f
Supplemental oxygen. See also Oxygen therapy
    anesthesia and, 530-531
    in chronic bronchitis, 548
    in muscular dystrophy, 580
Supply-dependent oxygen consumption, 45
Support group, 490

Supraventricular dysrhythmia, 176-179, 176f-179f
    tachycardia, 177-178, 178f, 236t
Surface marking of lung, 65, 66f, 67f
Surgery, 529-542
    anesthesia and, 530-531
    cardiopulmonary consequences of, 530
    cardiovascular, 539-540
    complications prevention in, 532-533
    drug therapy with, 532
    learning needs assessment, 499, 499b
    lung volume reduction, 416
    mobilization after, 536b
    outcome of, 533
    oxygen transport and, 535b
    postoperative management after, 534-536
        prescription for, 537-539
        rationale for, 537
    postoperative period and, 531
    preoperative assessment for, 533-534
    thoracic, 539
    transplantation, 721-722. See also
        Transplantation
    for tuberculosis, 521
SV. See Stroke volume
Swallowing, cough and, 364
Swan-Ganz catheter, 237-238
Symmetrical positioning, 394
Sympathetic nervous system, 275
Sympathetic neurotransmission, 786
Sympatholytic drug, 788-789
Sympathomimetic drug, 786-788
Syncope, heart disease in, 108
Syncopy, tussive, 364-365
System review, 212
Systemic blood pressure. See Blood pressure
Systemic condition. See also Acute medical condition;
        Chronic medical condition
    cardiac, 116
    of connective tissue, 118, 118b
    diagnosis of, 115-116
    endocrine, 122-123, 123b
    gastrointestinal, 120-121, 121b
    hematological, 122, 122b
    hepatic, 121, 121b
    immunological, 123
    musculoskeletal, 117-118, 117b
    neurological, 118-120, 119b
    nutritional, 124, 124b
    oxygen transport and, 116t
    pulmonary, 117
    renal, 121-122, 122b
Systemic lupus erythematosus, 118
    of lung, 99-100
    management of, 584
Systole
    age affecting, 686-687
    heart valves and, 67

T

T cell in transplantation, 730
T wave, 184
Table, tilt, 271
Tachycardia, 176-177
    atrial, 178
    clinical features of, 236t
    sinus, 176-177, 177f
    supraventricular, 177-178, 178f
    surgery and, 531
Tachypnea
    definition of, 381b
    surgery and, 531
    transient, of newborn, 661
Tactile fremitus, 224, 224f
T'ai chi, 469, 470t
    after cardiac surgery, 479t
    for coronary artery disease, 477-478
    description of, 491
    for stress reduction, 474t
Teacher-learner relationship, 501-502
Teaching. *See also* Education
    about cardiac or pulmonary rehabilitation, 420
    of controlled breathing, 383b
Team
    for cardiac or pulmonary rehabilitation, 420
    in intensive care unit, 606
    interdisciplinary, 502-503
Temperature, 161
Tenormin, 788
TENS units, 492
Tensilon, 790
Tension, arterial oxygen, 316
Tension pneumothorax, 628b
Terazosin, 788
Terminal bronchiole, 63
Terminology, breathing pattern, 381b
Test, 193-209
    angiographic, 199, 202
    bronchoscopic, 207
    computed tomography, 205-206, 206f
    echocardiographic, 202-205
        Doppler, 202, 204
        exercise, 204
        measurements derived from, 204
        myocardial contrast, 205
        physics of, 202, 204, 204f
        transesophageal, 204-205
    interpretation of, 133
    laboratory, 187-191
        of blood, 188-189, 188t
        common tests for, 188t
        endocrine, 189-190, 190t
        immunologic, 191, 191t
        of liver, 190, 191t
        peripheral vascular, 189
        rationale for, 187-188
        renal, 189, 190t

Test, (*cont'd*)
    nuclear
        of cardiovascular system, 195-199, 197t, 198f
        of pulmonary function, 199, 200f-201f
    nuclear imaging, 194-195, 194f
    overview of, 193-194
Testing
    exercise, 284, 286-295, 286b, 287, 288t, 289b-292b
    mobilization, 276-277
Tetralogy of Fallot, 660-661
Tetraplegia, 379f
ThAIRapy Vest, 331
Therapeutic massage, 474t
Therapeutic touch, 492
Thoracic aortic aneurysm, 167f
Thoracic deformity, 581-582
Thoracic surgery, 539. *See also* Surgery
Thoracic trauma, 120
Thorax
    anatomy of, 53, 54f
    anterior view of, 213f
    external manipulation of, 332-333, 333b
    lung compliance and, 75
    mobilization of, 390-391, 390b
Threshold loading device, 455, 456f
Thromboembolism
    in chronic obstructive pulmonary disease, 91
    as complication, 641
Thrombosis
    atherosclerosis and, 101
    deep venous
        mobilization and exercise affecting, 274
        postoperative, 643
    myocardial infarction with, 104
Thyroid disorder
    atherosclerosis and, 101
    cardiopulmonary complications of, 122-123, 123b
    exercise testing and training in, 447
    hypertension and, 107
    testing for, 190, 190t
Thyroxine, 190, 190t
Tilt table, 271
Timing in lateral costal breathing, 389-390
Tiotropium, 791
Tissue
    outcome measurement for, 258b
    oxygen use by, 48-49
Tissue oxygenation, 252b
Tissue perfusion, 252b
Tools for learning needs assessment, 497-498
Topograpjhic landmark, 212, 212b, 213f, 214f
Total joint replacement, 164f
Touch, therapeutic, 492
Toxicity, oxygen, 640-641
Trachea
    anatomy of, 62, 62f
    goblet cell of, 62
Tracheal deviation, 224, 225f

Tracheostomy
    complications of, 773-774
    in pediatric patient, 663-664
    suctioning of, 781
Tracheostomy button, 777, 777f
Tracheostomy tube
    metal, 775
    polyvinyl chloride, 775-776
Traction, 630
Traditional Chinese medicine, 466, 491-492
Trager approach, 466, 491
Training
    mobilization, 278-279
    resistance
        aerobic exercise and, 276
        in bed rest, 271-272
        long-term effects of, 283
    strength, 583
Transcendental meditation, 473
    for hypertension, 475
Transcutaneous carbon dioxide, 162
Transcutaneous electrical nerve stimulation, 492
    postoperative, 532
Transcutaneous oxygen, 280
Transcutaneous oxygenation, 162
Transesophageal echocardiography, 204-205
Transient tachypnea of newborn, 661
Transmural pressure, 77
Transplantation, 719-733
    background of, 719-720
    complications of, 730-731, 731b
    drug therapy for, 729-730, 730t
    ethical considerations in, 720
    heart, exercise program for, 412-413
    lung, exercise program for, 416
    national data on, 720t
    organ donation for, 720
    oxygen transport and, 721
    psychosocial considerations in, 720-721
    recipient status for, 722t
    rehabilitation and
        after heart procedure, 724-728, 725t, 727b, 727t
        after lung procedure, 725-726, 726t, 728-729, 728b
        community or home-based, 729
        preoperative, 722-724, 723t
        surgical procedures affecting, 724
    secondary cardiopulmonary dysfunction in, 635
    surgical and medical considerations in, 721-722
    waiting list criteria for, 720b
Transport
    of carbon dioxide, 83
    mucociliary, 644
    oxygen, 37-51. See also Oxygen transport
Transtheoretical model, 20
Trapezius muscle
    anatomy of, 58
    facilitation of, 392

Trauma
    in atherosclerosis, 100-101
    burn, 633-635
    head
        management of, 631-632
        pathophysiology of, 631
    lung injury, 644-647
    musculoskeletal, 627-629, 627b
        multiple, 630-631
        multiple fracture, 630-631
        pneumothorax/hemothorax, 628b, 629
        rib fracture, 629
    spinal cord, 575-577
        cardiopulmonary effects of, 120
        exercise testing and training after, 444
        management of, 575-577, 632-633
        pathophysiology of, 632
    thoracic, cardiopulmonary effects of, 120
Treadmill
    data sheet for, 291b
    for stroke patient, 443
Treatment
    course of, 257-259
    goal of, 253-254, 256b
    plan of, 254
    prescription for, 254, 257
Tree, tracheobronchial, 62, 62f
Trendelenburg position, contraindications to, 333b
Trepopnea, 142-143
Trial, randomized controlled clinical, 24-25
Tricuspid valve, anatomy of, 67
Trigger, asthma, 550, 551
Trihexyphenidyl, 791
Triiodothyronine, testing for, 190, 190t
Trimethaphan, 791
Trisomy 13, 660t
Trisomy 18, 660t
Trisomy 21, 660t
Trunk control and respiration, 664t
Tube
    chest, 232-233, 232f
    tracheostomy, 775-776
Tuberculosis, 100
Tubular breath sound, 219
Tumor, cough in, 144t
Turbulent airflow, 76
Turgor, skin, 231
Turner's syndrome, 660t
Tussive syncopy, 364-365
Type 2 diabetes mellitus, 108

U
Ulcer, stress, 641
Unstable angina, 102
Upper accessory muscle, 706, 707f
Upper airway
    anatomy of, 60-62, 60f, 61f
    in obesity, 628

Upper chest inhibition, 388-389
Upright position
    physiological effects of, 310-313, 311f, 312f
    in postoperative period, 537-538
Urbanization, global health and, 9
Utilization coefficient, 45

V
Validity of measurement, 131-132
Valve
    flutter, 353-354, 353f, 354b
        in cystic fibrosis, 519, 553
    heart, 67-68
        disease of, 107, 558-560
    Passy-Muir, 777, 778f
V$_A$Q. *See* Ventilation-perfusion ratio
Variability of measurement, 131
Variant angina, 102
Varicose bronchiectasis, 93, 94f
Vascular/connective tissue disease
    ankylosing spondylitis as, 586
    chronic renal insufficiency, 588-589
    rheumatoid arthritis as, management of, 586-588
    scleroderma as, 585-586
    systemic lupus erythematosus as, 584
Vascular disease
    atherosclerosis and, 101
    lifestyle and, 5-6
    peripheral, 560-561
Vascular system
    aging and, 688-689, 688f, 689t
    anatomy of
        pulmonary, 70-71
        systemic, 69-70
    tests of, 189, 189t
Vasculopathy, cardiac allograft, 731
Vena cava, 70-71
Venous distention, jugular, 215
Venous insufficiency, 560
Venous pressure, central, 238-239
Venous stasis, 561
Venous thrombosis
    bed rest causing, 270
    in chronic obstructive pulmonary disease, 91
    deep
        mobilization and exercise affecting, 274
        postoperative, 643
    myocardial infarction with, 104
Ventilation, 77
    alveolar, 158
    intrapulmonary percussive, 331-332
    in left heart failure, 116
    mechanical. *See* Mechanical ventilation
    motor therapy for child and, 677-678, 678f
    oxygen transport and, 39b, 47
    perfusion and, 78-79, 79f
    in post polio syndrome, 578
    postoperative pain and, 643

Ventilation, (*cont'd*)
    regional differences in, 311f, 312f
    in spinal cord injury, 633
    in thoracic deformity, 582
    in trauma, 628b
Ventilation bag, 347
Ventilation pattern, facilitation of
    of accessory muscles, 391-394, 391b, 393b, 394b
    in asymmetrical dysfunction, 394-395, 394b
    controlled diaphragmatic breathing, 382-383, 382b, 383b, 384
        scoop technique of, 386-387, 386f, 387f
    diaphragm and posture in, 384
    glossopharyngeal breathing, 397-399, 399f
    lateral costal breathing, 388-390, 388f, 390f
    mobilization of thorax in, 390-391, 390b
    positioning in, 377-380, 378f-380f, 384-385
    in primary versus secondary dysfunction, 383-384
    pursed-lip breathing, 384
    reducing respiratory rate in, 395-397, 395b, 397f
    relaxation in, 385
    repatterning technique in, 385-386
    in simple therapy tasks, 380-382
    vocalization skills in, 399-401, 400b
Ventilation-perfusion ratio, 78-79
    body position and, 308, 312
    side-lying position and, 315-316
Ventilatory device in cystic fibrosis, 553
Ventilatory muscle training
    in cystic fibrosis, 663
    in spinal cord injury, 576
Ventricle, 172
Ventricular assist device
    exercise and, 413
    shock and, 648
Ventricular bigeminy, 179-180, 180f
Ventricular couplet, 180, 180f
Ventricular depolarization, 172
Ventricular dysrhythmia, 179-181, 179f-181f
Ventricular fibrillation, 181, 181f
    clinical features of, 236t, 237
Ventricular pressure
    end diastolic, 315
    left, 238
Ventricular tachycardia, 236t, 237
Ventricular volume curve, 81
Venturi mask, 761, 762f
Venule, 70
Verbal technique, 401
Vertebra in osteoporosis, 583
Vesicular breath sound, 218
Vessel, lymphatic
    hydrostatic pressure and, 117
    in oxygen transport, 47
Vest for high-frequency chest wall oscillation, 331, 355
Vestibule, nasal, 61
Vibration, 346f
    advantages and disadvantages of, 347

Vibration, (cont'd)
  equipment for, 346
  in infant, 668-669, 674f
  overview of, 327
  preparation for, 346
  selection considerations for, 359t
  treatment with, 346-347
Viral pneumonia, 510
Virus infection, human immunodeficiency. *See* Human
    immunodeficiency virus infection
Viscosity of blood, 45
Visual analog scale for dyspnea, 140f
Visual inspection, 212, 214-215, 215f, 216f
VO$_2$, 266
Vocal cord, 62
Vocal fold, 703-704
Vocalization skills, 399-401, 400b
Voice sound, 219-220
Volume
  blood, 45
  fluid, 252b
  forced expiratory, 315-316
  lung, 519
  stroke
    exercise affecting, 272
    mobilization and exercise affecting, 273
Volume curve, ventricular, 81
Volume reduction surgery of lung, 416
VO$_2$max, 264
VO$_2$peak, 264

W
Walk test, data sheet for, 2921b
Walking
  after stroke, 443
  controlled breathing and, 387, 387f
Wall
  chest
    configuration of, 215-216, 216f
    in oxygen transport, 47
    pain in, 146
  myocardial, 104

Wave, aortic pressure, 81
Weakness
  in cerebral palsy, 575
  gravity eliminated breathing in, 707
  history of, 146-147
  in muscular dystrophy, 579, 580, 581
  in post polio syndrome, 445, 578
  respiratory muscle, 326
  in spinal cord injury, 633
  in stroke, 571
Weaning from mechanical ventilation
  failure of, 459-460
  in intensive care unit, 604-605, 605b
Weight. *See also* Obesity
  bed rest and, 268b
  in cardiac rehabilitation, 422
  fluid and electrolyte balance and, 231-232
  in pulmonary rehabilitation, 428
Weight loss, 589
Wenckebach block, 182
Wheelchair
  positioning in, 380, 380f
  in stroke, 571
Wheelchair athlete, 444
Wheezing, 143
White blood cell, 284
Whole-lung lavage, 96
Williams syndrome, 660t
World Health Organization
  classification of function of, 248, 248f
  health defined by, 3-4
Wound, puncture, of chest, 76

Y
Yoga, 469, 471t, 491
  for asthma, 482, 483t
  for chronic obstructive pulmonary disease, 485
  for congestive heart failure, 480t
  for hypertension, 475, 475t
  for stress reduction, 474t